Place-of-Service Codes for Professional Claims

Listed below are place-of-service codes and descriptions. These codes should be used on professional claims to specify the entity where service(s) were rendered. Check with individual payers (eg, Medicare, Medicaid, other private insurance) for reimbursement policies regarding these codes. If you would like to comment on a code(s) or description(s), please send your request to posinfo@cms.hhs.gov.

Place of Service Code(s)	Place of Service Name	Place of Service Description
01	Pharmacy	A facility or location where drugs and other medically related items and services are sold, dispensed, or otherwise provided directly to patients. (effective 10/1/05)
02	Unassigned	N/A
03	School	A facility whose primary purpose is education.
04	Homeless shelter	A facility or location whose primary purpose is to provide temporary housing to homeless individuals (eg, emergency shelters, individual or family shelters).
05	Indian Health Service freestanding facility	A facility or location, owned and operated by the Indian Health Service, which provides diagnostic, therapeutic (surgical and nonsurgical), and rehabilitation services to American Indians and Alaska Natives who do not require hospitalization.
06	Indian Health Service provider-based facility	A facility or location, owned and operated by the Indian Health Service, which provides diagnostic, therapeutic (surgical and nonsurgical), and rehabilitation services rendered by, or under the supervision of, physicians to American Indians and Alaska Natives admitted as inpatients or outpatients.
07	Tribal 638 freestanding facility	A facility or location owned and operated by a federally recognized American Indian or Alaska Native tribe or tribal organization under a 638 agreement which provides diagnostic, therapeutic (surgical and nonsurgical), and rehabilitation services to tribal members who do not require hospitalization.
08	Tribal 638 provider-based facility	A facility or location owned and operated by a federally recognized American Indian or Alaska Native tribe or tribal organization under a 638 agreement which provides diagnostic, therapeutic (surgical and nonsurgical), and rehabilitation services to tribal members admitted as inpatients or outpatients.
09	Prison-Correctional facility	A prison, jail, reformatory, work farm, detention center, or any other similar facility maintained by either Federal, State, or local authorities for the purpose of confinement or rehabilitation of adult or juvenile criminal offenders.
10	Unassigned	N/A
11	Office	Location, other than a hospital, skilled nursing facility (SNF), military treatment facility, community health center, State or local public health clinic, or intermediate care facility (ICF), where the health professional routinely provides health examinations, diagnosis, and treatment of illness or injury on an ambulatory basis.
12	Home	Location, other than a hospital or other facility, where the patient receives care in a private residence.
13	Assisted living facility	Congregate residential facility with self-contained living units providing assessment of each resident's needs and on-site support 24 hours a day, seven days a week, with the capacity to deliver or arrange for services including some health care and other services.
14	Group home	A residence, with shared living areas, where clients receive supervision and other services such as social and/or behavioral services, custodial service, and minimal services (eg, medication administration). (effective 4/1/04)
15	Mobile unit	A facility or unit that moves from place to place and is equipped to provide preventive, screening, diagnostic, and/or treatment services.
16	Temporary lodging	A short term accommodation such as a hotel, camp ground, hostel, cruise ship, or resort where the patient receives care, and which is not identified by any other POS code.
17	Walk-in retail health clinic	A walk-in health clinic, other than an office, urgent care facility, pharmacy, or independent clinic, which is not described by any other Place of Service code, that is located within a retail operation and provides on an ambulatory basis, preventive and primary care services. (This code is available for use immediately with a final effective date of May 1, 2010.)
18-19	Unassigned	N/A
20	Urgent care facility	Location, distinct from a hospital emergency department, an office, or a clinic, whose purpose is to diagnose and treat illness or injury for unscheduled, ambulatory patients seeking immediate medical attention.
21	Inpatient hospital	A facility, other than psychiatric, which primarily provides diagnostic, therapeutic (both surgical and nonsurgical), and rehabilitation services by, or under, the supervision of physicians to patients admitted for a variety of medical conditions.
22	Outpatient hospital	A portion of a hospital that provides diagnostic, therapeutic (both surgical and nonsurgical), and rehabilitation services to sick or injured persons who do not require hospitalization or institutionalization.
23	Emergency Room—hospital	A portion of a hospital where emergency diagnosis and treatment of illness or injury is provided.
24	Ambulatory surgical center	A freestanding facility, other than a physician's office, where surgical and diagnostic services are provided on an ambulatory basis.
25	Birthing center	A facility, other than a hospital's maternity facilities or a physician's office, which provides a setting for labor, delivery, and immediate postpartum care as well as immediate care of newborn infants.
26	Military treatment facility	A medical facility operated by one or more of the Uniformed Services. Military treatment facility (MTF) also refers to certain former US Public Health Service (USPHS) facilities now designated as Uniformed Service Treatment Facilities (USTF).
27-30	Unassigned	N/A

31	Skilled nursing facility	A facility that primarily provides inpatient skilled nursing care and related services to patients who require medical, nursing, or rehabilitative services but does not provide the level of care or treatment available in a hospital.
32	Nursing facility	A facility that primarily provides to residents skilled nursing care and related services for the rehabilitation of injured, disabled, or sick persons, or, on a regular basis, health-related care services above the level of custodial care to other than mentally retarded individuals.
33	Custodial care facility	A facility that provides room, board, and other personal assistance services, generally on a long-term basis, and does not include a medical component.
34	Hospice	A facility, other than a patient's home, in which palliative and supportive care are provided for terminally ill patients and their families.
35-40	Unassigned	N/A
41	Ambulance—land	A land vehicle specifically designed, equipped, and staffed for lifesaving and transporting the sick or injured.
42	Ambulance—air or water	An air or water vehicle specifically designed, equipped, and staffed for lifesaving and transporting the sick or injured.
43-48	Unassigned	N/A
49	Independent clinic	A location, not part of a hospital and not described by any other Place of Service code, that is organized and operated to provide preventive, diagnostic, therapeutic, rehabilitative, or palliative services to outpatients only. (effective 10/1/03)
50	Federally qualified health center	A facility located in a medically underserved area that provides Medicare beneficiaries preventive primary medical care under the general direction of a physician.
51	Inpatient psychiatric facility	A facility that provides inpatient psychiatric services for the diagnosis and treatment of mental illness on a 24-hour basis, by or under the supervision of a physician.
52	Psychiatric facility— partial hospitalization	A facility for the diagnosis and treatment of mental illness that provides a planned therapeutic program for patients who do not require full-time hospitalization but who need broader programs than are possible from outpatient visits to a hospital-based or hospital-affiliated facility.
53	Community mental health center	A facility that provides the following services: outpatient services, including specialized outpatient services for children, the elderly, individuals who are chronically ill, and residents of the CMHC's community mental health area who have been discharged from inpatient treatment at a mental health facility; 24-hour a day emergency care services; day treatment, other partial hospitalization services, or psychosocial rehabilitation services; screening for patients being considered for admission to State mental health facilities to determine the appropriateness of such admission; and consultation and education services.
54	Intermediate care facility/mentally retarded	A facility that primarily provides health-related care and services above the level of custodial care to mentally retarded individuals but does not provide the level of care or treatment available in a hospital or SNF.
55	Residential substance abuse treatment facility	A facility which provides treatment for substance (alcohol and drug) abuse to live-in residents who do not require acute medical care. Services include individual and group therapy and counseling, family counseling, laboratory tests, drugs and supplies, psychological testing, and room and board.
56	Psychiatric residential treatment center	A facility or distinct part of a facility for psychiatric care which provides a total 24-hour therapeutically planned and professionally staffed group living and learning environment.
57	Nonresidential substance abuse treatment facility	A location that provides treatment for substance (alcohol and drug) abuse on an ambulatory basis. Services include individual and group therapy and counseling, family counseling, laboratory tests, drugs and supplies, and psychological testing.
58-59	Unassigned	N/A
60	Mass immunization center	A location where providers administer pneumococcal pneumonia and influenza virus vaccinations and submit these services as electronic media claims or paper claims or by using the roster billing method. This generally takes place in a mass immunization setting, such as a public health center, pharmacy, or mall but may include a physician office setting.
61	Comprehensive inpatient rehabilitation facility	A facility that provides comprehensive rehabilitation services under the supervision of a physician to inpatients with physical disabilities. Services include physical therapy, occupational therapy, speech pathology, social or psychological services, and orthotics and prosthetics services.
62	Comprehensive outpatient rehabilitation facility	A facility that provides comprehensive rehabilitation services under the supervision of a physician to outpatients with physical disabilities. Services include physical therapy, occupational therapy, and speech pathology services.
63-64	Unassigned	N/A
65	End-stage renal disease treatment facility	A facility, other than a hospital, that provides dialysis treatment, maintenance, and/or training to patients or caregivers on an ambulatory or home-care basis.
66-70	Unassigned	N/A
71	Public health clinic	A facility maintained by either State or local health departments that provides ambulatory primary medical care under the general direction of a physician.
72	Rural health clinic	A certified facility located in a rural, medically underserved area that provides ambulatory primary medical care under the general direction of a physician.
73-80	Unassigned	N/A
81	Independent laboratory	A laboratory certified to perform diagnostic and/or clinical tests independent of an institution or a physician's office.
82-98	Unassigned	N/A
99	Other place of service	Other place of service not identified above.

Use these tabs to mark important pages in your CPT® 2013 Professional Edition codebook for quick reference and review.

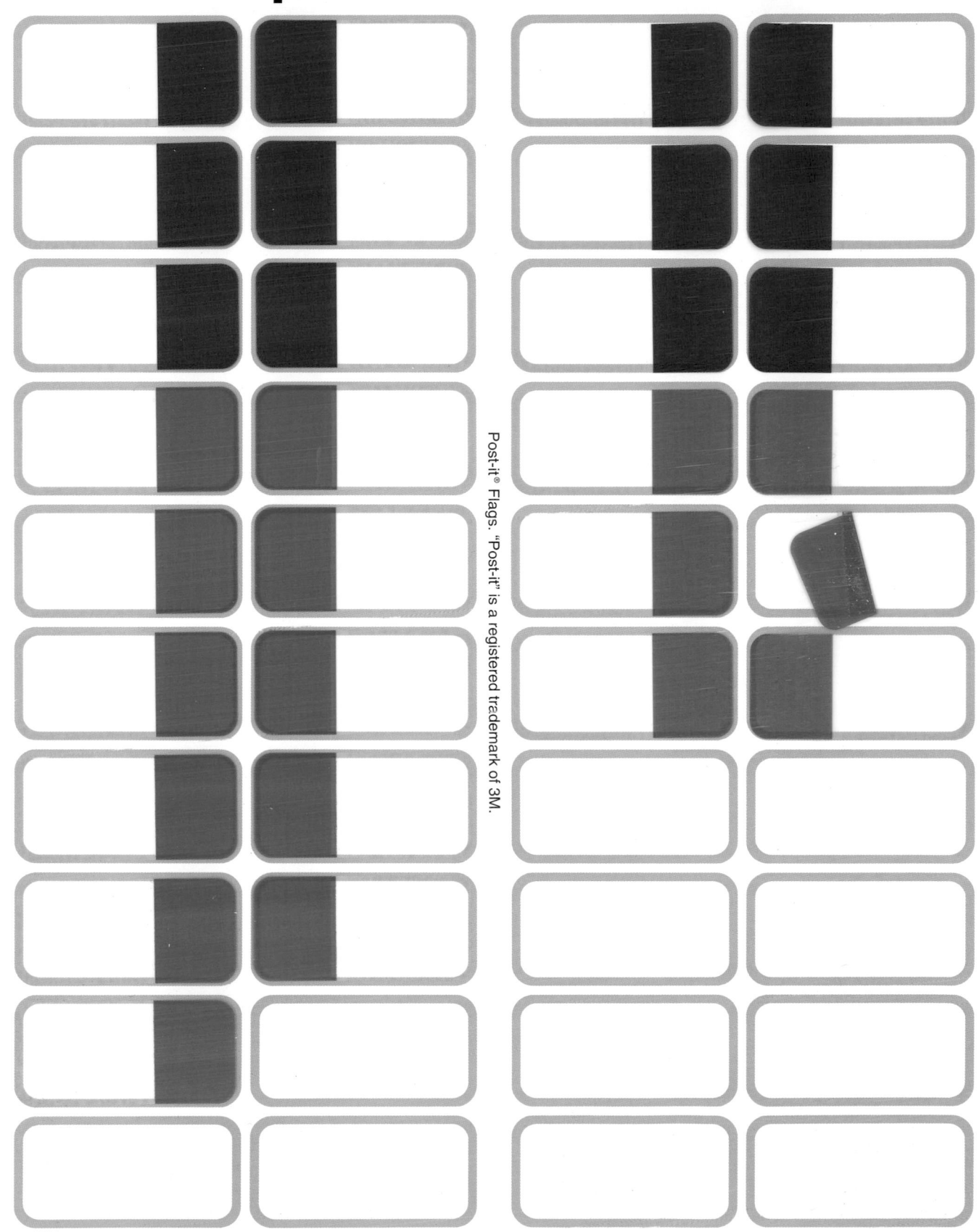

Customize your CPT® 2013 Professional codebook and make it work for you.

These removable and reusable tabs can be used to flag the code sections and codes that you refer to regularly.

- Use the **red** tabs to flag the Evaluation and Management, Radiology, Category II, and Category III sections.

- Use the **blue** tabs to flag Anesthesia, Pathology and Laboratory, and the Appendices.

- Use the **green** tabs to flag the Surgery and Medicine sections.

- Use the **yellow** tabs to flag codes that you commonly use in your practice, codes that you need to research further, or personal notes that you've written into your codebook.

AMA Coding Workshops

Learn about the latest changes to *CPT 2013 Professional* by attending our popular CPT Changes workshop. Mark your calendar now for these December 2012 dates and locations:

December 3 — Baltimore
December 3 — New Brunswick, NJ
December 5 — Irving, TX
December 10 — Las Vegas
December 13 — Atlanta

Visit **ama-assn.org/go/cptchangesworkshops** for more information, access to online registration, and early-bird savings.

Still need to prepare for ICD-10? Need to know more about ICD-10-CM coding? Pair an ICD-10-CM workshop with your CPT Changes workshop.

For more information, visit **ama-assn.org/go/icd10workshops.**

current procedural terminology

cpt®
2013
Professional Edition

Michelle Abraham, MHA, CCS-P
Jay T. Ahlman
Angela J. Boudreau
Judy Connelly
Lia Levreau-Davis, CCP
Desiree D. Evans, AAS

Rejina L. Glenn
DeHandro Hayden, BS
Grace M. Kotowicz, RN, BS
Janette Meggs, RHIA
Marie L. Mindeman, BA, RHIT
Karen E. O'Hara, BS, CCS-P

Mary R. O'Heron, RHIA
Danielle Pavloski, BS, RHIT, CCS-P
Desiree Rozell, MPA
Lianne Stancik, RHIT
Ada Walker, CCA
Arletrice Watkins, MHA, RHIA

AMERICAN MEDICAL
ASSOCIATION

Executive Vice President, Chief Executive Officer: James L. Madara, MD
Chief Operating Officer: Bernard L. Hengesbaugh
Senior Vice President, Publishing and Business Services: Robert A. Musacchio, PhD
Vice President, Business Operations: Vanessa Hayden
Vice President, CPT and Physician Practice Solutions: Jay Ahlman
Director, CPT Coding and Regulatory Services: Marie Mindeman
Manager, Book and Product Development and Production: Nancy Baker
Senior Developmental Editor: Lisa Chin-Johnson
Production Specialist: Mary Ann Albanese
Director, Sales, Marketing and Strategic Relationships: Joann Skiba
Director, Sales and Business Products: Mark Daniels
Director, Marketing: Erin Kalitowski
Marketing Manager: Carol Brockman

Professional ISBN: 978-1-60359-684-8
ISSN: 0276-8283

1st Edition printed 1966
2nd Edition printed 1970
3rd Edition printed 1973
4th Edition printed 1977
Revised: 1978, 1979, 1980, 1981, 1982, 1984, 1985, 1986, 1987, 1988,
1989, 1990, 1991, 1992, 1993, 1994, 1995, 1996, 1997, 1998, 1999,
2000, 2001, 2002, 2003, 2004, 2005, 2006, 2007, 2008, 2009, 2010, 2011, 2012

To purchase additional CPT products, contact the American Medical Association Customer Service
at 800 621-8335.

To request a license for distribution of products containing or reprinting CPT codes and/or guidelines,
please see our Web site at www.ama-assn.org/go/cpt or contact the American Medical Association CPT
Intellectual Property Services, 515 N. State Street, Chicago, Illinois 60654, 312 464-5022.

AC36:EP054113:12-P-001:9/12
AC36:EP888813:12-P-001:9/12

Foreword

Current Procedural Terminology (CPT®), Fourth Edition, is a listing of descriptive terms and identifying codes for reporting medical services and procedures performed by physicians. The purpose of the terminology is to provide a uniform language that will accurately describe medical, surgical, and diagnostic services, and will thereby provide an effective means for reliable nationwide communication among physicians, patients, and third parties. *CPT 2013* is the most recent revision of a work that first appeared in 1966.

CPT descriptive terms and identifying codes currently serve a wide variety of important functions in the field of medical nomenclature. The CPT code set is useful for administrative management purposes such as claims processing and for the development of guidelines for medical care review. The uniform language is also applicable to medical education and outcomes, health services, and quality research by providing a useful basis for local, regional, and national utilization comparisons. The CPT code set is the most widely accepted nomenclature for the reporting of physician procedures and services under government and private health insurance programs. In 2000, the CPT code set was designated by the Department of Health and Human Services as the national coding standard for physician and other health care professional services and procedures under the Health Insurance Portability and Accountability Act (HIPAA). This means that for all financial and administrative health care transactions sent electronically, the CPT code set will need to be used.

The changes that appear in this revision have been prepared by the CPT Editorial Panel with the assistance of physicians representing all specialties of medicine, and with important contributions from many third-party payers and governmental agencies.

The American Medical Association trusts that this revision will continue the usefulness of its predecessors in identifying, describing, and coding medical, surgical, and diagnostic services.

Acknowledgments

Publication of the annual CPT codebook represents many challenges and opportunities. From reconciling the many differences of opinion about the best way to describe a procedure, to the last details on placement of a semicolon, many individuals and organizations devote their energies and expertise to the preparation of this revision.

The editorial staff wishes to express sincere thanks to the many national medical specialty societies, health insurance organizations and agencies, and individual physicians and other health professionals who have made contributions.

Thanks are due to Robert A. Musacchio, PhD, Sr VP, American Medical Association; Claudia Bonnell, Blue Cross and Blue Shield Association; Nelly Leon-Chisen, American Hospital Association; Sue Bowman, RHIA, American Health Information Management Association; and Raemarie Jiminez, CPC, American Academy of Professional Coders for their invaluable assistance in enhancing the CPT code set.

For their assistance in development of the CPT Category II codes:

Ronald A. Gabel, MD
Darryl T. Gray, MD, ScD
Sam J. W. Romeo, MD, MBA

We recognize the following people for efforts in working with the Physician Consortium for Performance Improvement® (PCPI™) and other quality measurement organizations:

Mark Antman, DDS, MBA
Katherine Ast, MSW, LCSW
Kendra Hanley, MS
Diedra D. Joseph, MPH
Karen S. Kmetik, PhD
Marjorie C. Rallins, DPM
Kimberly Smuk, BS, RHIA
Beth Tapper, MA
Samantha Tierney, MPH
Jennifer Trajkovski, MJ, RHIT

AMA CPT Editorial Panel

Chair
Peter A. Hollmann, MD*
Vice-Chair
Kenneth P. Brin, MD, PhD, FACC*

Albert E. Bothe, Jr, MD, FACS
Boyd R. Buser, DO, FACOFP
Patrick J. Cafferty, MPAS, PA-C*
Leslie F. Davidson, PhD, OTR/L†
Frank J. Dubeck, Jr, MD, FACP*
Richard Duszak, Jr, MD, FACR*
David A. Ellington, MD
Ronald A. Gabel, MD
Edith Hambrick, MD, JD†
M. Bradford Henley, MD, MBA
Christopher L. Jagmin, MD†
Katharine Krol, MD†
Victor L. Lewis, MD
Julia M. Pillsbury, DO, FAAO, FACOP†
Antonio E. Puente, PhD
Kenneth B. Simon, MD, MBA*
Mark S. Synovec, MD*

Secretary
Marie L. Mindeman, BA, RHIT

*Member of the CPT Executive Committee
†New Panel Member April 2011, 2012
‡New Advisors

AMA CPT Advisory Committee

Academy of Pharmaceutical Physicians and Investigators
Grant P. Bagley, MD
American Academy of Allergy, Asthma and Immunology
Donald W. Aaronson, MD, JD, MPH
American Academy of Child & Adolescent Psychiatry
David I. Berland, MD
Benjamin N. Shain, MD, PhD‡
American Academy of Dermatology
Alexander Miller, MD
American Academy of Disability Evaluating Physicians
Douglas W. Martin, MD, FAADEP, FACOEM
American Academy of Family Physicians
Robert J. Carr, Jr, MD
Gretchen M. Dickson, MD, MBA
American Academy of Neurology
Marc R. Nuwer, MD, PhD
Bruce H. Cohen, MD, FAAN
American Academy of Ophthalmology
Michael X. Repka, MD
American Academy of Orthopaedic Surgeons
Richard J. Friedman, MD, FACSC
American Academy of Otolaryngic Allergy
Paul T. Fass, MD, FACS
Bryan D. Leatherman, MD
American Academy of Otolaryngology Head and Neck Surgery
Bradley F. Marple, MD, FAAOA
Brendan C. Stack, Jr, MD, FACS, FACE
American Academy of Pain Medicine
Eduardo M. Fraifeld, MD
Lee T. Snook, Jr, MD, FACP, DABPM
American Academy of Pediatrics
Richard A. Molteni, MD
Sanjeev Y. Tuli, MD, MEME, FAAP‡

American Academy of Physical Medicine and Rehabilitation
Francis P. Lagattuta, MD
Jeffrey S. Brault, DO‡
American Academy of Sleep Medicine
Amy J. Aronsky, DO, FAAP, FACOP‡
William C. Sherrill, Jr, MD‡
American Association for Clinical Chemistry
Robert L. Murray, JD, PhD
American Association for Thoracic Surgery
Kirk R. Kanter, MD
Stephen J. Lahey, MD
American Association of Clinical Endocrinologists
Eric A. Orzeck, MD, FACP, FACE
American Association of Neurological Surgeons
R. Patrick Jacob, MD
American Association of Neuromuscular and Electrodiagnostic Medicine
Andrea J. Boon, MD
American Association of Public Health Physicians
Arvind K. Goyal, MD, MPH, FAAFP, FACPM
American Clinical Neurophysiology Society
Marc R. Nuwer, MD, PhD
American College of Allergy, Asthma and Immunology
Gary N. Gross, MD
American College of Cardiology
Robert N. Piana, MD, FACC
Patricio A. Frais, MD, FACC
American College of Chest Physicians
Steve G. Peters, MD
Michael E. Nelson, MD, FCCP
American College of Emergency Physicians
Kenneth L. DeHart, MD, FACEP
American College of Gastroenterology
Daniel C. DeMarco, MD, FACG
American College of Medical Genetics
David B. Flannery, MD
American College of Medical Quality
Joel Grossman, MD
American College of Mohs Surgery
David B. Pharis, MD, PC
American College of Nuclear Medicine
Scott C. Bartley, MD
American College of Occupational and Environmental Medicine
Lee S. Glass, MD, JD
American College of Physicians
R. Scott Hanson, MD, MPH
Jeannine Z. Engel, MD, FACP
American College of Preventive Medicine
Ryung Suh, MD, MPP, MBA, MPH
American College of Radiation Oncology
Andy W. Su, MD
Paul E. Wallner, DO, FACR, FAOCR, FASTRO, FACRO
American College of Radiology
Daniel Picus, MD, FACR, RCC
American College of Rheumatology
Gerald M. Eisenberg, MD, FACP, FACR
Robert J. Lloyd, MD, FACR
American College of Surgeons
Linda M. Barney, MD, FACS
Mark T. Savarise, MD, FACS
American Congress of Obstetricians and Gynecologists
Jordan G. Pritzker, MD, MBA, FACOG
Jon K. Hathaway, MD, PhD
American Gastroenterological Association
Joel V. Brill, MD, AGAF, FASGE, FACG, CHCQM

American Geriatric Society
Robert A. Zorowitz, MD, MBA, FACP, AGSF, CMD
American Institute of Ultrasound in Medicine
Harvey L. Nisenbaum, MD
American Medical Directors Association
Dennis L. Stone, MD, MBA
American Orthopaedic Association
Blair C. Filler, MD
American Orthopaedic Foot and Ankle Society
Walter J. Pedowitz, MD
David I. Pedowitz, MD
American Osteopathic Association
Judith A. O'Connell, DO, FAAO
Robert B. Goldberg, DO‡
American Psychiatric Association
David K. Nace, MD
Jeremy S. Musher, MD, DFAPA‡
American Roentgen Ray Society
Mark D. Alson, MD
American Society for Aesthetic Plastic Surgery, Inc.
Paul R. Weiss, MD
American Society for Clinical Pathology
Lee H. Hilborne, MD, MPH, FASCP
American Society for Dermatologic Surgery
Murad Alam, MD
Jeremy S. Bordeaux, MD, MPH
American Society for Gastrointestinal Endoscopy
Glenn D. Littenberg, MD, FACP
Christopher Y. Kim, MD, MBA, FACG, FASGE, AGAF, FACP
American Society for Radiation Oncology
David C. Beyer, MD, FACR, FACRO, FASTRO
American Society for Reproductive Medicine
John T. Queenan, Jr, MD, FACOG
American Society for Surgery of the Hand
Daniel J. Nagle, MD
American Society of Abdominal Surgeons
Louis F. Alfano, Jr, MD
American Society of Anesthesiologists
Peter A. Goldzweig, DO
American Society of Cataract and Refractive Surgery
Stephen S. Lane, MD
American Society of Clinical Oncology
William C. Penley, MD
American Society of Colon and Rectal Surgeons
James I. Merlino, MD
American Society of Cytopathology
Carol A. Filomena, MD
American Society of General Surgeons
Charles Drueck, III, MD, FACS
American Society of Hematology
Samuel M. Silver, MD, PhD, FACP, FAHA
American Society of Interventional Pain Physicians
Frank J. E. Falco, MD
American Society of Neuroradiology
Jacqueline A. Bello, MD, FACR
Raymond K. Tu, MD‡
American Society of Ophthalmic Plastic and Reconstructive Surgery
L. Neal Freeman, MD, MBA, CCS-P, FACS
American Society of Oral Maxillofacial Surgeons
Anthony M. Spina, DDS, MD
Joseph F. Piecuch, DMD, MD
American Society of Plastic Surgeons
Raymond V. Janevicius, MD
Deborah S. Bash, MD‡

American Thoracic Society
Stephen P. Hoffmann, MD
Kathrin Nicolacakis, MD
American Urological Association
Jeffrey A. Dann, MD, MBA
Ronald P. Kaufman, Jr, MD, FACS
Association of University Radiologists
Robert K. Zeman, MD, FACR
College of American Pathologists
Michael D. McEachin, MD
Congress of Neurological Surgeons
Joseph S. Cheng, MD
Heart Rhythm Society
Amit J. Shanker, MD
Infectious Disease Society of America
Steven K. Schmitt, MD
International Spinal Intervention Society
Scott I. Horn, DO
Claire Tibiletti, MD
National Association of Medical Examiners
Paul A. Raslavicus, MD, MHA, CPE
North American Spine Society
William Mitchell, MD
David R. O'Brien, Jr, MD
Radiological Society of North America
Timothy A. Crummy, MD
Renal Physicians Association
Chester A. Amedia, Jr, MD, FACP
Richard J. Hamburger, MD
Society for Investigative Dermatology
Stephen P. Stone, MD
Society for Vascular Surgery
Sean P. Roddy, MD, FACS
Society of American Gastrointestinal Endoscopic Surgeons
Michael B. Edye, MD
Society of Critical Care Medicine
George A. Sample, MD, FCCP
Society of Interventional Radiology
Donald F. Denny, Jr, MD
Timothy L. Swan, MD‡
Society of Nuclear Medicine
Gary L. Dillehay, MD, FACNP, FACR‡
Society of Thoracic Surgeons
Francis C. Nichols, III, MD
Jeffrey P. Jacobs, MD, FACS, FACC, FCCP
The Endocrine Society
Richard A. Guthrie, MD
The Triological Society
Richard W. Waguespack, MD, FACS
United States and Canadian Academy of Pathology
David S. Wilkinson, MD, PhD

AMA Health Care Professionals Advisory Committee (HCPAC)

Peter A. Hollmann, MD*, Co-Chair
AMA CPT Editorial Panel
Patrick J. Cafferty, MPAS, PA-C, Co-Chair
Antonio E. Puente, PhD, Co-Chair
AMA CPT Editorial Panel
American Academy of Audiology
Brad A. Stach, PhD‡
Paul M. Pessis, AuD‡
Academy of Nutrition and Dietetics
Keith-Thomas Ayoob, EdD, RN, FADA
American Academy of Physician Assistants
Terry E. Carlisle, PA-C, MPAS
American Association of Naturopathic Physicians
Wendell B. Milliman, ND
Eva Miller, ND
American Association for Respiratory Care
Susan Rinaldo-Gallo, Med, RRT
American Chiropractic Association
Craig S. Little, DC, FACO
American Massage Therapy Association
Susan B. Rosen, LPM
American Nurses Association
Julie E. Chicoine, JD, RN, CPC
American Occupational Therapy Association
Leslie F. Davidson, PhD, OTR/L
Mary Jo McGuire, MS, OTR/L, FAOTA‡
American Optometric Association
Douglas C. Morrow, OD
Rebecca H. Warton, OD
American Physical Therapy Association
Helene M. Fearon, PT
American Podiatric Medical Association
Phillip E. Ward, DPM
Ira H. Krause, DPM
American Psychological Association
Neil H. Pliskin, PhD
American Speech Hearing Association
R. Wayne Holland, EdD, CCC-SLP
Stuart G. Trembath, MA, CCC-A
National Athletic Trainers' Association
William T. Griffin, MA, LAT, ATC
Karen D. Fennell, MS, ATC, LAT
National Association of Social Workers
Mirean F. Coleman, LICSW
National Society of Genetic Counselors
Leslie H. Cohen, MS, CGC
Pharmacist Services Technical Advisory Coalition
Daniel E. Buffington, PharmD, MBA

Contents

Introduction

Current Procedural Terminology (CPT®), Fourth Edition, is a set of codes, descriptions, and guidelines intended to describe procedures and services performed by physicians and other health care professionals. The CPT code set is also used by other entities to report outpatient services. Each procedure or service is identified with a five-digit code. The use of CPT codes simplifies the reporting of services.

Inclusion of a descriptor and its associated five-digit code number in the CPT codebook is based on whether the procedure is consistent with contemporary medical practice and is performed by many individuals in clinical practice in multiple locations. Inclusion in the CPT codebook does not represent endorsement by the American Medical Association (AMA) of any particular diagnostic or therapeutic procedure. Inclusion or exclusion of a procedure does not imply any health insurance coverage or reimbursement policy.

The CPT code set is published annually in the late summer or early fall as both electronic data files and books. The release of CPT data files on the Internet typically precedes the book by several weeks. In any case, January 1 is the effective date for use of the update of the CPT code set. The interval between the release of the update and the effective date is considered the implementation period and is intended to allow physicians and other providers, payers, and vendors to incorporate CPT changes into their systems. The exceptions to this schedule of release and effective dates are CPT Category III and vaccine product codes, which are released twice a year on January 1 or July 1 with effective dates for use six months later, and CPT Category II codes. Changes to the CPT code set are meant to be applied prospectively from the effective date.

The main body of the Category I section is listed in six sections. Each section is divided into subsections with anatomic, procedural, condition, or descriptor subheadings. The procedures and services with their identifying codes are presented in numeric order with one exception—the entire **Evaluation and Management** section (99201-99499) appears at the beginning of the listed procedures. These items are used by most physicians in reporting a significant portion of their services.

Section Numbers and Their Sequences

Evaluation and Management	99201-99499
Anesthesiology	00100-01999, 99100-99140
Surgery	10021-69990
Radiology (Including Nuclear Medicine and Diagnostic Ultrasound)	70010-79999
Pathology and Laboratory	80047-89398
Medicine (except Anesthesiology)	90281-99199, 99500-99607

The first and last code numbers and the subsection name of the items appear at the top margin of most pages (eg, "11010-11306 Surgery/Integumentary System"). The continuous pagination of the CPT codebook is found on the lower margin of each page along with explanation of any code symbols that are found on that page.

Instructions for Use of the CPT Codebook

Select the name of the procedure or service that accurately identifies the service performed. Do not select a CPT code that merely approximates the service provided. If no such specific code exists, then report the service using the appropriate unlisted procedure or service code. In surgery, it may be an operation; in medicine, a diagnostic or therapeutic procedure; in radiology, a radiograph. Other additional procedures performed or pertinent special services are also listed. When necessary, any modifying or extenuating circumstances are added. Any service or procedure should be adequately documented in the medical record.

It is important to recognize that the listing of a service or procedure and its code number in a specific section of this book does not restrict its use to a specific specialty group. Any procedure or service in any section of this book may be used to designate the services rendered by any qualified physician or other qualified health care professional or entity (eg, hospital, clinical laboratory, home health agency).

A "physician or other qualified health care professional" is an individual who is qualified by education, training, licensure/regulation (when applicable), and facility privileging (when applicable) who performs a professional service within his/her scope of practice and independently reports that professional service. These professionals are distinct from "clinical staff." A clinical staff member is a person who works under the supervision of a physician or other qualified health care professional and who is allowed by law, regulation, and facility policy to perform or assist in the performance of a specified professional service, but who does not individually report that professional service. Other policies may also affect who may report specific services.

►Throughout the CPT code set the use of terms such as "physician," "qualified health care professional," or "individual" is not intended to indicate that other entities may not report the service. In selected instances, specific instructions may define a service as limited to professionals or limited to other entities (eg, hospital or home health agency).◄

Instructions, typically included as parenthetical notes with selected codes, indicate that a code should not be reported with another code or codes. These instructions are intended to prevent errors of significant probability and are not all inclusive. For example, the code with such instructions may be a component of another code and therefore it would be incorrect to report both codes even when the component service is performed. These instructions are not intended as a listing of all possible code combinations that should not be reported, nor do they indicate all possible code combinations that are appropriately reported. When reporting codes for services provided, it is important to assure the accuracy and quality of coding through verification of the intent of the code by use of the related guidelines, parenthetical instructions, and coding resources, including *CPT Assistant* and other publications resulting from collaborative efforts of the American Medical Association with the medical specialty societies (ie, *Clinical Examples in Radiology*).

Format of the Terminology

The CPT code set has been developed as stand-alone descriptions of medical procedures. However, some of the procedures in the CPT codebook are not printed in their entirety but refer back to a common portion of the procedure listed in a preceding entry. This is evident when an entry is followed by one or more indentations. This is done in an effort to conserve space.

Example

25100   Arthrotomy, wrist joint; with biopsy

25105   with synovectomy

Note that the common part of code 25100 (the part before the semicolon) should also be considered part of code 25105. Therefore, the full procedure represented by code 25105 should read:

25105   Arthrotomy, wrist joint; with synovectomy

Requests to Update the CPT Nomenclature

The effectiveness of the CPT nomenclature depends on constant updating to reflect changes in medical practice. This can only be accomplished through the interest and timely suggestions of practicing physicians, medical specialty societies, state medical associations, and other organizations and agencies. Accordingly, the AMA welcomes correspondence, inquiries, and suggestions concerning old and new procedures, as well as other matters such as codes and indices.

To submit a suggestion to add, delete, or revise codes contained in the CPT codebook, please contact:

CPT Editorial Research & Development
American Medical Association
515 North State Street
Chicago, Illinois 60654

Coding change request forms are available at the AMA's CPT Web site: www.ama-assn.org/ama/pub/category/3866.html.

All proposed changes of the CPT codebook will be considered by the CPT Editorial Panel with consultation of appropriate medical specialty societies.

Guidelines

Specific guidelines are presented at the beginning of each of the sections. These guidelines define items that are necessary to appropriately interpret and report the procedures and services contained in that section. For example, in the **Medicine** section, specific instructions are provided for handling unlisted services or procedures, special reports, and supplies and materials provided. Guidelines also provide explanations regarding terms that apply only to a particular section. For instance, **Radiology Guidelines** provide a definition of the unique

term, "radiological supervision and interpretation." While in **Anesthesia,** a discussion of reporting time is included.

Add-on Codes

Some of the listed procedures are commonly carried out in addition to the primary procedure performed. These additional or supplemental procedures are designated as add-on codes with the ✚ symbol and they are listed in **Appendix D** of the CPT codebook. Add-on codes in *CPT 2013* can be readily identified by specific descriptor nomenclature that includes phrases such as "each additional" or "(List separately in addition to primary procedure)."

The add-on code concept in *CPT 2013* applies only to add-on procedures or services performed by the same physician. Add-on codes describe additional intra-service work associated with the primary procedure, eg, additional digit(s), lesion(s), neurorrhaphy(s), vertebral segment(s), tendon(s), joint(s).

Add-on codes are always performed in addition to the primary service or procedure and must never be reported as a stand-alone code. All add-on codes found in the CPT codebook are exempt from the multiple procedure concept (see the modifier 51 definition in **Appendix A**).

Modifiers

A modifier provides the means to report or indicate that a service or procedure that has been performed has been altered by some specific circumstance but not changed in its definition or code. Modifiers also enable health care professionals to effectively respond to payment policy requirements established by other entities. The judicious application of modifiers obviates the necessity for separate procedure listings that may describe the modifying circumstance. Modifiers may be used to indicate to the recipient of a report that:

- A service or procedure had both a professional and technical component.

- A service or procedure was performed by more than one physician and/or in more than one location.

- A service or procedure was increased or reduced.

- Only part of a service was performed.

- An adjunctive service was performed.

- A bilateral procedure was performed.

- A service or procedure was provided more than once.

- Unusual events occurred.

Example

A physician providing diagnostic or therapeutic radiology services, ultrasound, or nuclear medicine services in a hospital would add modifier 26 to report the professional component.

73090 with modifier 26 = Professional component only for an X-ray of the forearm

Example

Two surgeons may be required to manage a specific surgical problem. When two surgeons work together as primary surgeons performing distinct part(s) of a procedure, each surgeon should report his/her distinct operative work by adding modifier 62 to the procedure code and any associated code(s) for that procedure as long as both surgeons continue to work together as primary surgeons. Each surgeon should report the co-surgery once using the same procedure code. Modifier 62 would be applicable. For instance, a neurological surgeon and an otolaryngologist are working as co-surgeons in performing transphenoidal excision of a pituitary neoplasm.

The first surgeon would report:

61548 62 = Hypophysectomy or excision of pituitary tumor, transnasal or transseptal approach, nonstereotactic + two surgeons modifier

AND the second surgeon would report:

61548 62 = Hypophysectomy or excision of pituitary tumor, transnasal or transseptal approach, nonstereotactic + two surgeons modifier

If additional procedure(s) (including add-on procedure[s]) are performed during the same surgical session, separate code(s) may also be reported with modifier 62 added. It should be noted that if a co-surgeon acts as an assistant in the performance of additional procedure(s) during the same surgical session, those services may be reported using separate procedure code(s) with modifier 80 or modifier 82 added, as appropriate. A complete listing of modifiers is found in **Appendix A.**

Place of Service and Facility Reporting

►Some codes have specified places of service (eg, evaluation and management codes are specific to a setting). Other services and procedures may have instructions specific to the place of service (eg, therapeutic, prophylactic, and diagnostic injections and infusions). The CPT code set is designated for reporting physician and qualified health care professional services. It is also the designated code set for reporting services provided by organizations or facilities (eg, hospitals) in specific circumstances. Throughout the CPT code set, the use of terms such as "physician," "qualified health care professional," or "individual" is not intended to indicate that other entities may not report the service. In selected instances, specific instructions may define a service as limited to professionals or limited to other entities (eg, hospital or home health agency). The CPT code set uses the term *facility* to describe such providers and the term *nonfacility* to describe services settings or circumstances in which no facility reporting may occur. Services provided in the home by an agency are facility services. Services provided in the home by a physician or qualified health care professional who is not a representative of the agency are nonfacility services.◄

Unlisted Procedure or Service

It is recognized that there may be services or procedures performed by physicians or other qualified health care professionals that are not found in the CPT code set. Therefore, a number of specific code numbers have been designated for reporting unlisted procedures. When an unlisted procedure number is used, the service or procedure should be described (see specific section guidelines). Each of these unlisted procedural code numbers (with the appropriate accompanying topical entry) relates to a specific section of the book and is presented in the guidelines of that section.

In some cases alternative coding and procedural nomenclature as contained in other code sets may allow appropriate reporting of a more specific code. CPT references to use an unlisted procedure code do not preclude the reporting of an appropriate code that may be found in other code sets.

Results, Testing, Interpretation, and Report

Results are the technical component of a service. Testing leads to results; results lead to interpretation. Reports are the work product of the interpretation of test results. Certain procedures or services described in CPT involve a technical component (eg, tests) which produce "results" (eg, data, images, slides). For clinical use, some of these results require interpretation. Some CPT descriptors specifically require interpretation and reporting to report that code.

Special Report

A service that is rarely provided, unusual, variable, or new may require a special report. Pertinent information should include an adequate definition or description of the nature, extent, and need for the procedure and the time, effort, and equipment necessary to provide the service.

Time

►The CPT code set contains many codes with a time basis for code selection. The following standards shall apply to time measurement, unless there are code or code-range–specific instructions in guidelines, parenthetical instructions, or code descriptors to the contrary. Time is the face-to-face time with the patient. Phrases such as "interpretation and report" in the code descriptor are not intended to indicate in all cases that report writing is part of the reported time. A unit of time is attained when the mid-point is passed. For example, an hour is attained when 31 minutes have elapsed (more than midway between zero and sixty minutes). A second hour is attained when a total of 91 minutes have elapsed. When codes are ranked in sequential typical times and the actual time is between two typical times, the code with the typical time closest to the actual time is used. See also the Evaluation and Management (E/M) Services Guidelines. When another service is performed concurrently with a time-based service, the time associated with the concurrent service should not be included in the time used for reporting the time-based service. Some services measured in units other than days extend across calendar dates. When this occurs a continuous service does not reset and create a first hour. However, any disruption in the service does create a new initial service. For example, if intravenous hydration (96360, 96361) is given from 11 PM to 2 AM, 96360 would be reported once and 96361 twice. For facility reporting on a single date of service or for continuous services that last beyond midnight (ie, over a range of dates), report the total units of time provided continuously. However, if instead of a continuous infusion, a medication was given by intravenous push at 10 PM and 2 AM, as the service was not continuous, both administrations would be reported as initial (96374) and sequential (96376), as: (1) no other infusion services were performed; and (2) the push of the same drug was performed more than 30 minutes beyond the initial administration. For facility reporting per single calendar date, both administrations would be reported as initial (96374). For continuous services that last beyond midnight, use the date in which the service began and report the total units of time provided continuously.◄

Code Symbols

A summary listing of additions, deletions, and revisions applicable to the CPT codebook is found in **Appendix B.** New procedure numbers added to the CPT codebook are identified throughout the text with the symbol ● placed before the code number. In instances where a code revision has resulted in a substantially altered procedure descriptor, the symbol ▲ is placed before the code number. The symbols ► ◄ are used to indicate new and revised text other than the procedure descriptors. These symbols indicate CPT Editorial Panel actions. The symbol ○ is used to indicate reinstated/recycled code. The AMA reserves the right to correct typographical errors and make stylistic improvements.

CPT add-on codes are annotated by the symbol ✚ and are listed in **Appendix D.** The symbol ⊘ is used to identify codes that are exempt from the use of modifier 51 but have not been designated as CPT add-on procedures or services. A list of codes exempt from modifier 51 usage is included in **Appendix E.** The symbol ⊙ is used to identify codes that include moderate sedation (see **Appendix G**). The symbol ✗ is used to identify codes for vaccines that are pending FDA approval (see **Appendix K**). The symbol # is used to identify codes that are listed out of numerical sequence (see **Appendix N**).

Resequenced codes that are not placed numerically are identified with the # symbol, and a reference placed numerically (eg, Code is out of numerical sequence. See...) as a navigational alert to direct the user to the location of the out-of-sequence code (see **Appendix N**). Resequencing is utilized to allow placement of related concepts in appropriate locations within the families of codes regardless of the availability of numbers for sequential numerical placement.

Alphabetical Reference Index

This codebook features an expanded alphabetical index that includes listings by procedure and anatomic site. Procedures and services commonly known by their eponyms or other designations are also included.

CPT 2013 in Electronic Formats

CPT 2013 procedure codes and descriptions are available on CD-ROM as data files and electronic software. Data files are available in ASCII and EBCDIC formats and can be imported into any billing and claims reporting software that accepts a text (.TXT) file format. *CPT 2013 Electronic Professional* software, with *Netter's Atlas of Human Anatomy for CPT Coding,* provides access to the entire *CPT 2013 Professional Edition* codebook on your desktop. Easy-to-use and fully searchable, this invaluable software contains all of the favorite *CPT Professional* features plus CPT codes and quick linking access between CPT codes, guidelines, modifiers, appendices, index, and more. For more information call (800) 621-8335 or visit *www.amabookstore.com.*

References to AMA Resources

The symbols ➔ and ➔ appear after many codes throughout this codebook and indicate that the AMA has published reference material regarding that particular code.

The symbol ➔ refers to the *CPT Assistant* monthly newsletter and *CPT Changes: An Insider's View,* an annual book with all of the coding changes for the current year. The symbol ➔ refers to the quarterly newsletter *Clinical Examples in Radiology.*

Example

36598 Contrast injection(s) for radiologic evaluation of existing central venous access device, including fluoroscopy, image documentation and report

➔ *CPT Changes: An Insider's View* 2006

➔ *Clinical Examples in Radiology* Winter 2006:15

(For placement of centrally inserted non-tunneled central venous catheter, without subcutaneous port or pump, age 5 years or older, use 36556)

In this example, the green reference symbol indicates that in the 2006 edition of *CPT Changes: An Insider's View* material is available that may assist in understanding the application of the code. The red reference symbol indicates that the 2006 Winter issue of *Clinical Examples in Radiology* (page 15) should be consulted.

Subscriptions to *CPT Assistant* and *Clinical Examples in Radiology* can be purchased by calling the AMA's Unified Service Center at (800) 621-8335. Individual back issues are available for purchase and immediate download at *www.amabookstore.com.*

An archive software product with every issue of *CPT Assistant* is also available. *CPT Assistant Archives 1990-2012* provides convenient access 20 years of *CPT Assistant* newsletter articles on your de... Search past issues of the AMA's authoritative coding new... by keyword, phrase, CPT code number, newsletter issue, article index, or codebook table of contents. This product offers simple search capabilities and a complete historical CPT code list from 1990-2012 that references when a code was added, deleted, and/or revised. Call (800) 621-8335 or visit *www.amabookstore.com* for more information.

Current and past editions of *CPT Changes: An Insider's View* can be purchased by calling the AMA's Unified Service Center at (800) 621-8335 or visiting *www.amabookstore.com.*

In addition, an archives software product with all content from past and present editions of *CPT Changes: An Insider's View* is available. *CPT Changes Archives 2000-2012* provides access to current and historical CPT code and guideline changes on your computer desktop. Search by keyword, phrase, CPT code number, edition, and CPT codebook table of contents. For more information, call (800) 621-8335 or visit *www.amabookstore.com.*

Illustrated Anatomical and Procedural Review

It is essential that coders have a thorough understanding of medical terminology and anatomy to code accurately. The following section reviewing the basics of vocabulary and anatomy can be used as a quick reference to help you with your coding. It is not intended as a replacement for up-to-date medical dictionaries and anatomy texts, which are essential tools for accurate coding.

Prefixes, Suffixes, and Roots

Although medical terminology may seem complex, many medical terms can be broken into component parts, which makes them easier to understand. Many of these terms are derived from Latin or Greek words, but some include the names of physicians.

Prefixes are word parts that appear at the beginning of a word and modify its meaning; suffixes are found at the end of words. By learning what various prefixes and suffixes mean, it is possible to decipher the meaning of a word quickly. The following lists are a quick reference for some common prefixes and suffixes.

Numbers

Prefix	Meaning	Example
mono-, uni-	one	monocyte, unilateral
bi-	two	bilateral
tri-	three	triad
quadr-	four	quadriplegia
hex-, sex-	six	hexose
diplo-	double	diplopia

Surgical Procedures

Suffix	Meaning	Example
-centesis	puncture a cavity to remove fluid	amniocentesis
-ectomy	surgical removal (excision)	appendectomy
-ostomy	a new permanent opening	colostomy
-otomy	cutting into (incision)	tracheotomy
-orrhaphy	surgical repair/suture	herniorrhaphy
-opexy	surgical fixation	nephropexy
-oplasty	surgical repair	rhinoplasty
-otripsy	crushing, destroying	lithotripsy

Conditions

Prefix	Meaning	Example
ambi-	both	ambidextrous
aniso-	unequal	anisocoria
dys-	bad, painful, difficult	dysphoria
eu-	good, normal	euthanasia
hetero-	different	heterogeneous
homo-	same	homogeneous
hyper-	excessive, above	hypergastric
hypo-	deficient, below	hypogastric
iso-	equal, same	isotonic
mal-	bad, poor	malaise
megalo-	large	megalocardia

Suffix	Meaning	Example
-algia	pain	neuralgia
-asthenia	weakness	myasthenia
-emia	blood	anemia
-iasis	condition of	amebiasis
-itis	inflammation	appendicitis
-lysis	destruction, break down	hemolysis
-lytic	destroy, break down	hemolytic
-oid	like	lipoid
-oma	tumor	carcinoma
-opathy	disease of	arthropathy
-orrhagia	hemorrhage	menorrhagia
-orrhea	flow or discharge	amenorrhea
-osis	abnormal condition of	tuberculosis
-paresis	weakness	hemiparesis
-plasia	growth	hyperplasia
-plegia	paralysis	paraplegia
-pnea	breathing	apnea

Directions and Positions

Prefix	Meaning	Example
ab-	away from	abduction
ad-	toward	adduction
ecto, exo-	outside	ectopic, exocrine
endo-	within	endoscope
epi-	upon	epigastric
infra-	below, under	infrastructure
ipsi-	same	ipsilateral
meso-	middle	mesopexy
meta-	after, beyond, transformation	metastasis
peri-	surrounding	pericardium
retro-	behind, back	retroversion
trans-	across, through	transvaginal

Word	Meaning
anterior or ventral	at or near the front surface of the body
posterior or dorsal	at or near the back surface of the body
superior	above
inferior	below
lateral	side
distal	farthest from center
proximal	nearest to center
medial	middle
supine	face up or palm up
prone	face down or palm down
sagittal	vertical body plane, divides the body into equal right and left sides
transverse	horizontal body plane, divides the body into top and bottom sections
coronal	vertical body plane, divides the body into front and back sections

Additional References

For best coding results, you will need to use other reference materials in addition to your coding books. These references include a medical dictionary and one or more anatomy books that can be purchased from the American Medical Association by calling (800) 621-8335.

Medical Dictionaries

Stedman's CPT® Dictionary, 2nd ed.
Chicago, IL: American Medical Association, 2009.
OP300609

Merriam-Webster's Medical Desk Dictionary.
Springfield, Mass: Merriam Webster.
OP941493

Stedman's Medical Dictionary. 27th ed.
Baltimore, Md: Williams & Wilkins; 2000.
OP982900

Anatomy References

Kirschner, CG. *Netter's Atlas of Human Anatomy for CPT® Coding, 2nd ed.*
Chicago, Ill: American Medical Association; 2005.
OP490609

Kirschner, CG. *Netter's Atlas of Human Anatomy for CPT® and ICD-9-CM Coding Series: Musculoskeletal.*
Chicago, Ill: American Medical Association
OP492206

Netter, FH. *Atlas of Human Anatomy.* 3rd ed.
East Hanover, NJ: Novartis; 2003.
OP936798

Lists of Illustrations

To further aid coders in properly assigning CPT codes, the codebook contains a number of anatomical and procedural illustrations.

Anatomical Illustrations

Thirty-one anatomical illustrations are located on the following pages:

Procedural Illustrations

Procedural illustrations are placed throughout the codebook and are associated with the following specific CPT codes.

CPT Code(s)	Illustration Title
11005	Debridement of Abdominal Wall
11200, 11201	Removal of Skin Tags
11423, 11600, 11606, 11642	Measuring and Coding the Removal of a Lesion
11719-11765	Lateral Nail View
11719-11765	Dorsal Nail View
14000-14061	Adjacent Tissue Repairs
15731	Axial Pattern Forehead Flap
16000	Calculation of Total Body Surface Area (TBSA) Burn
17004	Destruction, Benign or Premalignant Lesions
20552, 20553	Trigger Point Injection
20610	Arthrocentesis, Aspiration, or Injection of Major Joint or Bursa
20664	Halo Application for Thin Skull Osteology
20690	Uniplane External Fixation System
20692	Multiplane External Fixation System
21196	Reconstruction of Mandibular Rami
22520	Percutaneous Vertebroplasty
22548	Arthrodesis (Anterior Transoral Technique)
22554	Anterior Approach for Cervical Fusion
22558	Anterior Approach for Lumbar Fusion (Anterior Retroperitoneal Exposure)
22840	Non-Segmental Spinal Instrumentation
22842-22844	Segmental Spinal Instrumentation
22851	Spinal Prosthetic Devices
27125	Partial Hip Replacement With or Without Bipolar Prosthesis
27130	Total Hip Replacement
27235	Percutaneous Treatment of Femoral Fracture
27236	Open Treatment of Femoral Fracture
28290	Hallux Valgus Correction
28292	Keller-Type Procedure
28293	Keller-Mayo Procedure With Implant
28294	Joplin Procedure
28296	Mitchell Procedure
28297	Lapidus-Type Procedure
28298	Phalanx Osteotomy
28299	Double Osteotomy
29824	Arthroscopy, Shoulder, Distal Claviculectomy (Mumford Procedure)
29870-29887	Arthroscopy of the Knee
29894-29899	Arthroscopy of the Ankle
30465	Surgical Repair of Vestibular Stenosis
31070	Sinusotomy, Frontal
31231-31294	Sinus Endoscopy
31622-31656	Bronchoscopy

CPT Code(s)	Illustration Title
32554, 32555	Thoracentesis
32601-32665	Thoracoscopy
33210	Temporary Pacemaker
33212, 33214A	Implanted Pacemaker—Single Chamber
33212, 33214B	Implanted Pacemaker—Two Chambers
33224-33226	Biventricular Pacing
33510-33516A	Coronary Artery Bypass—Venous Grafting Only—Single Graft
33510-33516B	Coronary Artery Bypass—Venous Grafting Only—Three Coronary Grafts
33517-33530	Coronary Artery Bypass—Combined Arterial-Venous Grafting
33517-33530	Coronary Artery Bypass—Sequential Combined Arterial-Venous Grafting
33621	Initial Hybrid Palliation
33622	Hybrid Reconstruction
33820	Patent Ductus Arteriosus
33864	Aortic Root Remodeling: Coronary Arteries Replanted
33979	Insertion of Implantable Single Ventricle Assist Device
34802	Endovascular Repair of Abdominal Aortic Aneurysm
35371-35372	Thromboendarterectomy
35571	Bypass Graft, Vein
35600	Harvest of Upper Extremity Artery
36002	Injection Procedure (eg, Thrombin) for Percutaneous Treatment of Extremity Pseudoaneurysm
36222-36228	Angiography, Carotid Artery
36555-36556	Insertion of Non-Tunneled Centrally Inserted Central Venous Catheter
36557-36558	Insertion of Tunneled Central Venous Catheter
36570-36571, 36576, 36578	Implantable Venous Access Port
36821	Arteriovenous Anastomosis, Direct
36822	Insertion of Cannulas for Prolonged Extracorporeal Circulation Membrane Oxygenation (ECMO)
36825-36830	Arteriovenous Fistula
37191	Vena Cava Filter
37220, 37222	Transluminal Ballon Angioplasty
37220-37235	Iliac and Lower Extremity Arterial Anatomy Territory
37700	Ligation and Division of Long Saphenous Vein
38230	Bone Marrow Harvesting for Transplantation
43235	Upper Gastrointestinal Endoscopy
43260	Endoscopic Retrograde Cholangiopancreatography (ERCP)
43280	Laparoscopic Fundoplasty
43227, 43328	Nissen Fundoplasty
43753	Gastric Intubation
43846	Gastric Bypass for Morbid Obesity
44127	Enterectomy, Resection for Congenital Atresia

Figure 1A
Body Planes — 3/4 View

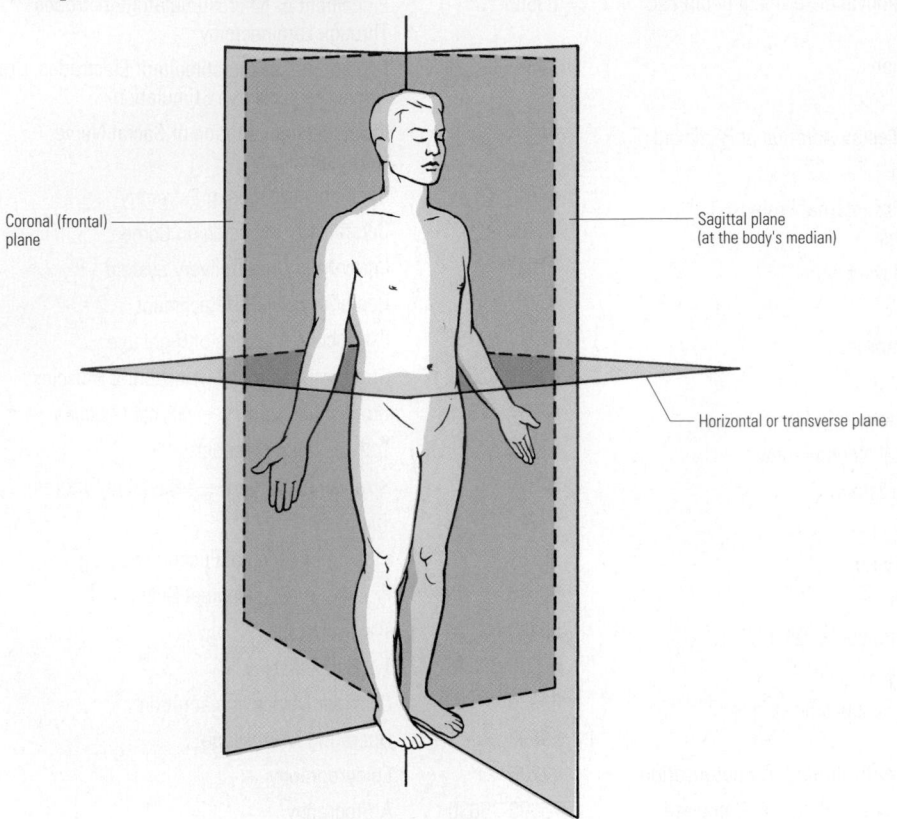

Coronal (frontal) plane

Sagittal plane (at the body's median)

Horizontal or transverse plane

Figure 1B
Body Aspects — Side View

Superior (cranial) aspect

Posterior aspect

Anterior aspect

Dorsal surface of hand

Palmar surface of hand

Dorsal surface of foot

Plantar surface of foot

Inferior aspect

Figure 1C
Body Planes — Front View

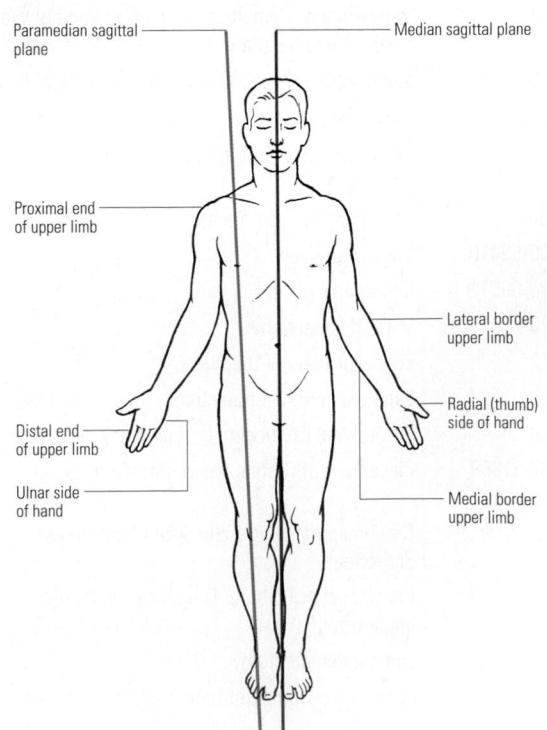

Paramedian sagittal plane

Median sagittal plane

Proximal end of upper limb

Lateral border upper limb

Radial (thumb) side of hand

Distal end of upper limb

Ulnar side of hand

Medial border upper limb

Molecular Pathology

The 2013 edition of the CPT code set contains 116 Molecular Pathology codes. These codes represent one of the largest single expansions to the CPT code set. Because the field of molecular pathology (or "molecular diagnostics") is rapidly evolving,—due in part to significant efforts to understand the molecular basis of disease, including the Human Genome Project—medicine's knowledge about the very basic elements of human medical affliction is highlighted and elucidated more than ever. Consequently, the number of new molecular pathology procedures and new diagnostic approaches, mainly in the area of genetic and molecular medicine, has increased dramatically in just the last decade.

Molecular and genetic medicine offers an incredible opportunity to understand who is at risk for particular conditions, to sort out specific clinical diagnoses for patients who present with constellations of signs and symptoms that are nonspecific, and to guide therapy by identifying optimal interventions based on the results of genetic testing for the patient's condition.

During the last decade, the CPT Editorial Panel, with guidance from pathologists and other laboratory and clinical experts, developed an initial set of codes to describe molecular pathology services. When initially created, only a few molecular pathology procedures were available, but the experts realized that whatever system was created would only be a "stopgap" solution to a much bigger diagnostic environment that was emerging. For the most part, the initial effort created a set of methodological codes that described the various techniques available to arrive at a diagnosis. Because most molecular tests employ a number of techniques (eg, extraction, amplification, in situ hybridization), these tests (excluding those describing most infectious agents) were coded using a "stack" of molecular pathology methodologic codes (CPT codes 83890-83914) that were placed in the Chemistry subsection of the Pathology and Laboratory section of the CPT code set. The stacked codes allowed tests to be reported by selecting from the menu of tests the methodologies used to reach the final result.

However, these methodological codes presented several challenges. First, these represented individual methodologies that required reporting a few to many stacked methodological molecular pathology procedures to arrive at a single result, and often required reporting multiple units of service, to describe that result. Second, although it is common for several molecular pathology procedures to be ordered and performed simultaneously, depending on the clinical indication and differential diagnosis, all of these services must be described by the same set of methodological CPT codes. Lastly, the lack of analyte-specificity in the methodological codes prevented providers and payers from communicating efficiently about the specific services provided and the relevant diagnostic information obtained.

In response to the need to identify more specific information about molecular pathology tests performed, the CPT code set also included a listing of genetic testing modifiers (previous Appendix I) to append to the stacking codes and identify the specific genetically linked conditions and diseases related to the test. However, the genetic testing modifiers were problematic for some providers and payers who lacked the ability to easily accept claims that included molecular pathology codes with former Appendix I modifiers.

When the stacking molecular pathology codes and the former Appendix I were originally established, the CPT Editorial Panel recognized that the rapid development of molecular pathology would soon exceed the capacity of the modifier system to accommodate new codes. These reporting mechanisms were created as an initial step, with the understanding that development of a more robust solution would be needed in the future when the test methodologies began to exhibit more established and standardized protocols.

Given the lack of specificity associated with the methodological molecular pathology codes, payers and others were unable to associate a specific test with a clear indication using the genetic testing modifiers. With the explosion of new molecular pathology procedures across the field of diagnostic medicine, the impetus for creating a long-term solution for coding molecular pathology procedures became even more urgent. In December 2009, the CPT Editorial Panel created the Molecular Pathology Workgroup and charged the group with creating a code structure to respond to the needs of all stakeholders, providing the flexibility and specificity to accommodate both current molecular pathology procedures and future expansion. The Molecular Pathology Workgroup (Workgroup) began the most intensive and complex workgroup efforts in the history of the CPT Editorial Panel. To assure relevance in the Workgroup's outcome, participation was solicited from all sectors, including pathologists, other laboratorians and clinicians, representatives of academic and national reference laboratories, government and government contractors, private payers, and industry.

As a result of the Workgroup's efforts, the Editorial Panel approved a two-tier system structure created for the Molecular Pathology section of the CPT code set, to allow categorization of the most commonly performed molecular pathology tests with unique and analyte-specific Tier 1 codes. The lower volume, but medically useful and commonly performed tests were then grouped into the appropriate Tier 2 category.

Typical patient and service descriptions that describe the clinical indication and services provided for each test are available. Tier 1 and Tier 2 codes capture 90 to 95% of current molecular pathology procedures, and therefore, account for the vast majority of procedures performed. With the completion of the initial code set for molecular pathology, the stacking codes (83890-83914) and Appendix I have been deleted and will not be available for reporting after December 31, 2012.

It is important to be aware that different Medicare contractors may have different policies regarding claims submission for reporting molecular pathology services. Some payers have determined that when a specific procedure is described by either a Tier 1 or Tier 2 code, the new Tier 1 or Tier 2 code should be used to describe that service. For these payers, only when a new Tier 1 or Tier 2 code does not exist, should the unlisted molecular pathology code 81479 be reported. Coders and providers must ensure that they are aware of payer-specific requirements for submitting claims for molecular pathology services in 2013.

When information is available, updates to the molecular pathology codes will be found on the CPT Web site at www.ama-assn.org/ama/pub/physician-resources/solutions-managing-your-practice/coding-billing-insurance/cpt/about-cpt/mopath-codes.page and in future *CPT Assistant* articles to insure that readers are informed of anticipated changes to and education on the use of the code set.

The Tier 1 section contains 105 codes (81200-81383) and describes specific gene and genomic procedures. Placement of a test in the Tier 1 grouping is based on statistical genetic test frequency data provided by Workgroup members representing the laboratories. Further statistical data from the national genetic test repositories (eg, GeneTests, available at www.ncbi.nlm.nih.gov/sites/GeneTests) provided additional information to support the determinations of placement of tests within the new molecular pathology structure.

Tier 2 contains nine codes (81400-81408) that are used to report molecular pathology procedures that are not specifically described in the Tier 1 molecular pathology codes (81200-81383).

The Tier 2 codes categorize molecular pathology services based on the complexity of the methodologies to perform these tests and the relative resources required to perform those tests. Since the prospect of creating a unique code for each gene was not possible, the two-tier system provides greater efficiency in the potential future development of thousands of molecular pathology tests. For new Tier 1 tests or tests that are ready to migrate from Tier 2 categorization to a Tier 1 specific code, a process and code change application have been developed to accommodate introduction of these new codes.

Tier 2 codes are not to be self-assigned, which means that a Tier 2 code cannot be used for an analysis unless it is listed under that code in the CPT codebook.

Features of the Molecular Diagnostics Code Set

An important part of the Molecular Pathology code subsection includes the guidelines and definitions to give users immediate access to the nomenclature and definitions of this technology to better understand and more accurately report these codes. Those unfamiliar with molecular pathology will find this section of the CPT 2013 code set to be educational.

Detailed guidelines, beginning on page 421 of *CPT 2013 Professional Edition,* and parenthetical notes added throughout the Molecular Pathology section provide instructions to guide appropriate reporting of the molecular pathology codes. Before reporting molecular pathology services, it is important to become familiar with the terms and their definitions in order to appropriately report the codes within the Molecular Pathology subsection.

Frequently Asked Questions

Question: I recently attended a teleconference regarding the new molecular pathology CPT codes. Presenters said that a laboratory can crosswalk within Tier 2 if your "gene" (analyte) was not listed under Tier 2. Is this true?

Answer: No. Do not self-assign a Tier 2 molecular pathology code for an analysis that is not listed in the CPT codebook. Please note the following statement in the introduction of the Tier 2 code set that applies to molecular pathology coding in the CPT 2013 code set:

> Use the appropriate molecular pathology procedure level code that includes the specific analyte found listed after the code descriptor. If the analyte tested is not listed below one of the Tier 2 codes or is not represented by a Tier 1 code, use the unlisted molecular pathology procedure code 81479.

Question: My lab does screening for cystic fibrosis variants. However, we test for more variants than are named in the American College of Medical Genetics/American College of Obstetricians and Gynecologists' (ACMG/ACOG) guidelines. Do we report only code 81220 or is there an additional code or codes that should be reported for the other variants?

Answer: The code choices for cystic fibrosis (CFTR) gene analysis are:

81220	*CFTR (cystic fibrosis transmembrane conductance regulator)* (eg, cystic fibrosis) gene analysis; common variants (eg, ACMG/ACOG guidelines)
81221	known familial variants
81222	duplication/deletion variants
81223	full gene sequence
81224	intron 8 poly-T analysis (eg, male infertility)

If your laboratory is evaluating a specimen for duplication/deletion variants (81222) or performing full gene sequencing (81223), these codes should be used to report those services. Consistent with CPT convention, the "eg" that precedes "ACMG/ACOG guidelines" indicates that this is an example of common variants and not a restrictive code. Other common variant services can and should be reported using code 81220. Hence, if your laboratory is testing for other variants in addition to those within the ACMG/ACOG guidelines, they are not separately reported.

Question: How do you know what CPT codes to use for the various cystic fibrosis tests?

What code is used for cystic fibrosis screening?

Answer: Cystic fibrosis transmembrane conductance regulator (CFTR) testing is reported with codes 81220-81224. For code descriptors of these codes, please see previous question's answer. If your laboratory is evaluating a patient for common variants such as a cystic fibrosis screening exam, report code 81220. If, based on patient history or other indications, testing is indicated for duplication/deletion variants or there is a need to perform full gene sequencing, code 81222 or code 81223 should be used, respectively.

Question: How is 5T coded when it is performed by itself?

Answer: Report code 81224, *CFTR (cystic fibrosis transmembrane conductance regulator)* (eg, cystic fibrosis) gene analysis; intron 8 poly-T analysis (eg, male infertility), for 5T analysis.

Question: When a code descriptor lists two genes and only one of those two genes is tested, how should this be coded? For example, code 81331, *SNRPN/UBE3A (small nuclear ribonucleoprotein polypeptide N and ubiquitin protein ligase E3A) (eg, Prader-Willi syndrome and/or Angelman syndrome)*, methylation analysis?

Answer: As a part of the consideration for inclusion of codes in the molecular pathology code set, potential analytes were identified, with further consideration given to the clinical utility of the analyses. In some cases, due to clinical or molecular concerns, two genes were combined into a single code, and, in some cases, specific analyses were required. In the case of code 81331, both SNRPN and UBE3A must be evaluated by methylation analysis in order to use that code. If only SNRPN or UBE3A is tested, or SNRPN and UBE3A are both tested using techniques other than methylation analyses, this code cannot be used. If only one gene is reported because that procedure is not described by code 81331, it will be necessary to report the unlisted molecular pathology code 81479 to describe that service.

Question: What are the Factor V Leiden variants that are covered in the Factor V code, 81241, *F5 (coagulation Factor V) (eg, hereditary hypercoagulability) gene analysis, Leiden variant?* The code states "variant," implying the test is for only one variant. Should more than one unit of service be used when multiple variants are examined?

Answer: No. Code 81241 is specific for the Leiden variant of coagulation Factor V (R506Q). If one analyzes for the other clinically performed HR2 variant (H1327R), one would use code 81400, *Molecular pathology procedure, Level 1 (eg, identification of single germline variant [eg, SNP] by techniques such as restriction enzyme digestion or melt curve analysis)*, because this code includes the HR2 variant. Two units of code 81241 would not be appropriate.

Question: Please explain the use of *ie* and *eg* in the descriptors of the molecular pathology codes.

Answer: The use of ie, and eg, is very specific in CPT nomenclature, although often misused in English. These are abbreviations for Latin phrases, whose meanings are as follows: ie means "that is" or "in other words;" and eg means "for example."

When a code descriptor in the CPT codebook has a parenthetical note that begins with *ie*, this means that the term that follows clarifies the intent of the word or phrase preceding the parenthetical statement. If the content of the parenthetical is not met, then the code should not be used. For example, code 81245, *FLT3 (fms-related tyrosine kinase 3) (eg, acute myeloid leukemia), gene analysis, internal tandem duplication (ITD) variants (ie, exons 14, 15)*, requires analysis for internal tandem duplication variants in exons 14 and 15.

In contrast, when a code descriptor in the CPT codebook has a parenthetical note that begins with *eg*, it means that the following language represents an example or examples of the intent of the word or phrase preceding the parenthetical statement. For example, code 81205, *BCKDHB (branched-chain keto acid dehydrogenase E1, beta polypeptide) (eg, Maple syrup urine disease) gene analysis, common variants (eg, R183P, G278S, E422X)*, which may include testing for R183P, G278S, E422X, or other common variants in BCKDHB. However, as the code specifically indicates variants, more than one variant must be tested in order to use this code.

Question: Why are the qualitative and quantitative codes listed together with the qualified phrase, "if performed"?

Answer: The use of "if performed" in CPT nomenclature is used to clarify, and more precisely specify the use of a code versus the more traditional "with or without" or "and/or" terminology. It allows for the use of a single code for the majority of instances when the first service is performed alone, as well as the minority of cases when the second service is also performed. For example, code 81301, *Microsatellite instability analysis (eg, hereditary nonpolyposis colorectal cancer, Lynch syndrome) of markers for mismatch repair deficiency (eg, BAT25, BAT26), includes comparison of neoplastic and normal tissue, if performed.*

Regarding the use of code 81301 for microsatellite instability analysis, if the laboratory performs the analysis on either neoplastic tissue or on both neoplastic and normal tissue (for comparison), one unit of code 81301 should be reported.

Question: If both BRCA1 and BRCA2 are performed, would two codes be used?

Answer: When the Tier 1 and Tier 2 code sets were added, different analyses were not packaged into analyte panels. This principle holds true for BRCA1 and BRCA2 testing. If both are performed, the appropriate code for BRCA1 (81214 or 81215) and the appropriate code for BRCA2 (81216 or 81217) should be used.

Question: It is understood that the intent of adding the Molecular Pathology coding section was to provide individual CPT codes for molecular pathology tests. Is this always the case?

Answer: When a single analyte is tested, it is generally reported using a single code when the analyte is identified in the Tier 1 or Tier 2 list. Please note the guidelines for molecular pathology in the Pathology and Laboratory section of the CPT codebook on page 421:

> The molecular pathology codes include all analytical services performed in the test (eg, cell lysis, nucleic acid stabilization, extraction, digestion, amplification, and detection). Any procedures required prior to cell lysis (eg, microdissection, codes 88380 and 88381) should be reported separately.

Question: The CPT 2012 Tier 2 guidelines instructed that "if the analyte tested is not listed under one of the Tier 2 codes or is not represented by a Tier 1 code, use the appropriate methodology codes in the 83890-83914 and 88384-88386 series." How has this changed for 2013?

Answer: The stacking codes 83890-83914 and 88384-88386 were deleted for 2013 and unlisted molecular pathology code, 81479, replaces these codes. In addition, the list of specifically identified molecular pathology codes was expanded this year particularly with the addition of many new analytes to the Tier 2 codes.

Question: How do I code intermediate resolution in human leukocyte antigen (HLA) system testing?

Answer: Note the comment in the HLA Molecular Pathology introduction of the CPT code set: "Both low and intermediate resolution are considered low resolution for code assignment." Therefore, select from the low-resolution code series (81370-81377).

Question: What are the alleles or allele-group specific HLA codes?

Answer: The molecular pathology HLA code set (81370-81383) contains four codes to be used to code for individual alleles, allele groups, or antigen equivalents. Each is followed by an important parenthetical note that provides instruction regarding the use of these codes. These codes should be used when HLA testing is done by molecular techniques.

81374   HLA Class I typing, low resolution (eg, antigen equivalents); one antigen equivalent (eg, *B*27*), each

(When testing for presence or absence of more than 2 antigen equivalents at a locus, use 81373 for each locus tested)

81377   HLA Class II typing, low resolution (eg, antigen equivalents); one antigen equivalent, each

(When testing for presence or absence of more than 2 antigen equivalents at a locus, use 81376 for each locus)

81381   HLA Class I typing, high resolution (ie, alleles or allele groups); one allele or allele group (eg, *B*57:01P*), each

(When testing for the presence or absence of more than 2 alleles or allele groups at a locus, use 81380 for each locus)

81383   HLA Class II typing, high resolution (ie, alleles or allele groups); one allele or allele group (eg, *HLA-DQB1*06:02P*), each

(When testing for the presence or absence of more than 2 alleles or allele groups at a locus, use 81382 for each locus)

When performing analysis for a specific allele, allele group or antigen equivalent, the appropriate code(s) from the above group should be reported for low resolution or high resolution and HLA Class I or II. However, if more than two alleles or allele groups are being tested, the corresponding locus code (81373, 81376, 81380, or 81382) should be reported using the direction contained in the appropriate parenthetical.

Question: What are the locus-specific HLA codes?

Answer: The molecular pathology HLA code set (81370-81388) contains four codes that are used to code for individual HLA loci. Each is followed by an important parenthetical that provides instruction regarding the use of these codes. These codes should be used when HLA testing is done by molecular techniques.

81373   HLA Class I typing, low resolution (eg, antigen equivalents); one locus (eg, *HLA-A, -B, or -C*), each

(When performing a complete Class I *[HLA-A, -B, and -C]* low resolution HLA typing, use 81372)

(When the presence or absence of a single antigen equivalent is reported using low resolution testing, use 81374)

81376   HLA Class II typing, low resolution (eg, antigen equivalents); one locus (eg, *HLA-DRB1/3/4/5, -DQB1, -DQA1, -DPB1, or -DPA1*), each

(When low resolution typing is performed for *HLA-DRB1/3/4/5* and -DQB1, use 81375)

(For low resolution typing, *HLA-DRB1/3/4/5* should be treated as a single locus)

81380   HLA Class I typing, high resolution (ie, alleles or allele groups); one locus (eg, *HLA-A, -B, or -C*), each

(When a complete Class I high resolution typing for *HLA-A, -B, and -C* is performed, use 81379)

(When the presence or absence of a single allele or allele group is reported using high resolution testing, use 81381)

81382   HLA Class II typing, high resolution (ie, alleles or allele groups); one locus (eg, *HLA-DRB1, -DRB3, -DRB4, -DRB5, -DQB1, -DQA1, -DPB1, or -DPA1*), each

(When only the presence or absence of a single allele or allele group is reported using high resolution testing, use 81383)

When performing an analysis for a single HLA locus, for low resolution or high resolution, for either HLA class I or II, the appropriate code(s) from this group should be used. When testing for one or two individual alleles (ie, antigen equivalents), use the corresponding individual single allele CPT code (81374, 81377, 81381, or 81383). CPT codes 81373, 81376, 81380, and 81382 should not be used for complete HLA typing. Rather, as indicated in the parenthetical note, the complete HLA typing codes should be used.

Question: When would tissue typing codes 83812-86813 be used instead of the molecular pathology HLA codes?

Answer: Use the traditional HLA codes 86812-86817 only for serologic testing. When using molecular pathology techniques, use codes 81370-81383.

Question: Code 81265 for maternal cell testing is for the patient and comparative specimen. When would code 81266 be used and would it ever have more than one unit of service?

Answer: Code 81266 is an add-on code that would be used, as noted in the parenthetical note that follows the code, in addition to code 81265 in situations in which additional specimens are required for Short Tandem Repeat (STR) comparative analyses. Such examples are included in the parenthetical note of the code, as stated in the CPT code set: "(eg, additional cord blood donor, additional fetal samples from different cultures, or additional zygosity in multiple birth pregnancies)." Because code 81266 is reported once for each additional specimen, it would be appropriate for more than one unit of service of the code to be reported when more than one additional specimen is analyzed.

81265   Comparative analysis using Short Tandem Repeat (STR) markers; patient and comparative specimen (eg, pretransplant recipient and donor germline testing, posttransplant non-hematopoietic recipient germline [eg, buccal swab or other germline tissue sample] and donor testing, twin zygosity testing, or maternal cell contamination of fetal cells)

+81266   each additional specimen (eg, additional cord blood donor, additional fetal samples from different cultures, or additional zygosity in multiple birth pregnancies) (List separately in addition to code for primary procedure)

Question: There is a gene test with one CPT code. However, microdissection is used in preparation for the test to be performed. Is it appropriate to report codes for both the test and the microdissection?

Answer: Yes. Please note the guidelines for molecular pathology in the Pathology and Laboratory section of the CPT codebook on page 412:

The molecular pathology codes include all analytical services performed in the test (eg, cell lysis, nucleic acid stabilization, extraction, digestion, amplification, and detection). Any procedures required prior to cell lysis (eg, microdissection, codes 88380 and 88381) should be reported separately.

Question: How do you know which Fragile X code to use for what procedure? Additional clarity is needed to define the difference between "evaluation" and "characterization" of alleles.

Answer: According to the molecular pathology codes and instructions, report code 81243 for Fragile X testing when detecting an expansion of CGG repeats, and report code 81244 for the determination of methylation status of the promoter.

Question: It seems that code 81244 is to only be used with Southern blotting analysis. Is that true? Would it also be used if methylation status is determined by a method other than Southern blotting?

Answer: While Southern analysis is the most common method currently performed to characterize expanded alleles for methylation, code 81244, *FMR1 (Fragile X mental retardation 1) (eg, fragile X mental retardation) gene analysis; characterization of alleles (eg, expanded size and methylation status)*, does not specify methodology. If a laboratory characterizes alleles using other methodologies, this code may also be reported.

Question: In reviewing the molecular pathology CPT codes, three codes are listed for BCR-ABL:

81206   *BCR/ABL1 (t(9;22))* (eg, chronic myelogenous leukemia) translocation analysis; major breakpoint, qualitative or quantitative

81207   minor breakpoint, qualitative or quantitative

81208   other breakpoint, qualitative or quantitative

Does major breakpoint refer to the p210 breakpoints (e13/314:a2) and minor breakpoint to the p190 (e1:a2) breakpoint? Alternatively, are p210 and p190 considered major breakpoints with the less common breakpoints relegated to minor and other?

Answer: Major breakpoint encompasses those exons leading to p210 and minor breakpoint encompasses p190, as postulated. The major breakpoint (code 81206) in BCR/ABL1 is p210 (ie, e13a2, e14a2; b2a2). The minor breakpoint (code 81207) is p190 (ie, e1a2). Other breakpoints (code 81208) could include p230.

Question: Is it appropriate to report code 81229 for array-based comparative genomic hybridization (aCGH) for oncologic indications, as it is the same technology?

Answer: No. Cytogenomic constitutional (genome-wide) microarray analysis (codes 81228 and 81229) should not be used for oncologic indications. Report Tier 2 Molecular Pathology procedure, Level 7 (code 81406) because it includes this specific analysis:

▲ **81406**   Molecular pathology procedure, Level 7 (eg, analysis of 11-25 exons by DNA sequence analysis, mutation scanning or duplication/deletion variants of 26-50 exons, cytogenomic array analysis for neoplasia)

Cytogenomic microarray analysis, neoplasia (eg, interrogation of copy number, and loss-of-heterozygosity via single nucleotide polymorphism [SNP]-based comparative genomic hybridization [CGH] microarray analysis)

Question: Our laboratory tests for JAK2 sequencing on exon 12 and exon 13. Is it appropriate to report code 81403 twice?

Answer: No. Code 81403 is used to report JAK2 testing and indicates "exon 12 sequence and exon 13 sequence, if performed." This phrase indicates that one unit of code 81430 is reported when either exon 12 alone or both exon 12 and 13 are sequenced.

▲ **81403**   Molecular pathology procedure, Level 4 (eg, analysis of single exon by DNA sequence analysis, analysis of >10 amplicons using multiplex PCR in 2 or more independent reactions, mutation scanning or duplication/deletion variants of 2-5 exons) JAK2 (Janus kinase 2) (eg, myeloproliferative disorder), exon 12 sequence and exon 13 sequence, if performed

EVALUATION AND MANAGEMENT TABLES

Office or Other Outpatient Services

Patient: New
Required Components: 3/3

Code	99201	99202	99203	99204	99205
Required Key Components					
History and Exam (#1 and #2)					
Problem-Focused	X				
Expanded Problem-Focused		X			
Detailed			X		
Comprehensive				X	X
Medical Decision Making (Complexity) (#3)					
Straightforward	X	X			
Low			X		
Moderate				X	
High					X
Contributory Factors					
Presenting Problem (Severity) (#1)					
Self-limited or Minor	X				
Low to Moderate		X			
Moderate			X		
Moderate to High				X	X
Counseling (#2) See E/M Guidelines					
Coordination of Care (#3) See E/M Guidelines					
Typical Face-to-Face Time (#4)					
Minutes	10	20	30	45	60

Initial Observation Care

Patient: New or Established
Required Components: 3/3

Code	99218	99219	99220
Required Key Components			
History and Exam (#1 and #2)			
Detailed or Comprehensive	X		
Comprehensive		X	X
Medical Decision Making (Complexity) (#3)			
Straightforward or Low	X		
Moderate		X	
High			X
Contributory Factors			
Presenting Problem (Severity) (#1)			
Low	X		
Moderate		X	
High			X
Counseling (#2) See E/M Guidelines			
Coordination of Care (#3) See E/M Guidelines			
Bedside/Unit/Floor Time (#4)			
Minutes	30	50	70

Subsequent Observation Care

Patient: New or Established
Required Components: 2/3

Code	99224	99225	99226
Required Key Components			
Interval History and Exam (#1 and #2)			
Problem-Focused	X		
Expanded Problem-Focused		X	
Detailed			X
Medical Decision Making (Complexity) (#3)			
Straightforward or Low	X		
Moderate		X	
High			X
Contributory Factors			
Presenting Problem (Severity) (#1)			
Stable/Recovering/Improving	X		
Inadequate Response to Therapy/ Minor Complication Development		X	
Unstable/Significant Complication/Significant New Problem			X
Counseling (#2) See E/M Guidelines			
Coordination of Care (#3), See E/M Guidelines			
Bedside/Unit/Floor Time (#4)			
Minutes	15	25	35

Office or Other Outpatient Services

Patient: Established
Required Components: 2/3

Code	99211	99212	99213	99214	99215
Required Key Components					
History and Exam (#1 and #2)					
Problem-Focused	N/A	X			
Expanded Problem-Focused			X		
Detailed				X	
Comprehensive					X
Medical Decision Making (Complexity) (#3)					
Straightforward	N/A	X			
Low			X		
Moderate				X	
High					X
Contributory Factors					
Presenting Problem (Severity) (#1)					
Minimal	X				
Self-Limited or Minor		X			
Low to Moderate			X		
Moderate to High				X	X
Counseling (#2) See E/M Guidelines					
Coordination of Care (#3) See E/M Guidelines					
Typical Face-to-Face Time (#4)					
Minutes	5	10	15	25	40

Initial Hospital Care

Patient: New or Established
Required Components: 3/3

Code	99221	99222	99223
Required Key Components			
History and Exam (#1 and #2)			
Detailed or Comprehensive	X		
Comprehensive		X	X
Medical Decision Making (Complexity) (#3)			
Straightforward or Low	X		
Moderate		X	
High			X
Contributory Factors			
Presenting Problem (Severity) (#1)			
Low	X		
Moderate		X	
High			X
Counseling (#2) See E/M Guidelines			
Coordination of Care (#3) See E/M Guidelines			
Bedside/Unit/Floor Time (#4)			
Minutes	30	50	70

Subsequent Hospital Care

Patient: New or Established
Required Components: 2/3

Code	99231	99232	99233
Required Key Components			
Interval History and Exam (#1 and #2)			
Problem-Focused	X		
Expanded Problem-Focused		X	
Detailed			X
Medical Decision Making (Complexity) (#3)			
Straightforward or Low	X		
Moderate		X	
High			X
Contributory Factors			
Presenting Problem (Severity) (#1)			
Stable/Recovering/Improving	X		
Responding Inadequately/ Minor Complication		X	
Unstable/Significant Complication/New Problem			X
Counseling (#2) See E/M Guidelines			
Coordination of Care (#3) See E/M Guidelines			
Bedside/Unit/Floor Time (#4)			
Minutes	15	25	35

Office or Other Outpatient Consultations

Patient: New or Established
Required Components: 3/3

Code	99241	99242	99243	99244	99245
Required Key Components					
History and Exam (#1 and #2)					
Problem-Focused	X				
Expanded Problem-Focused		X			
Detailed			X		
Comprehensive				X	X
Medical Decision Making (Complexity) (#3)					
Straightforward	X	X			
Low			X		
Moderate				X	
High					X
Contributory Factors					
Presenting Problem (Severity) (#1)					
Self-limited or Minor	X				
Low to Moderate		X			
Moderate			X		
Moderate to High				X	X
Counseling (#2) See E/M Guidelines					
Coordination of Care (#3) See E/M Guidelines					
Typical Face-to-Face Time (#4)					
Minutes	15	30	40	60	80

Inpatient Consultations

Patient: New or Established
Required Components: 3/3

Code	99251	99252	99253	99254	99255
Required Key Components					
History and Exam (#1 and #2)					
Problem-Focused	X				
Expanded Problem-Focused		X			
Detailed			X		
Comprehensive				X	X
Medical Decision Making (Complexity) (#3)					
Straightforward	X	X			
Low			X		
Moderate				X	
High					X
Contributory Factors					
Presenting Problem (Severity) (#1)					
Self-limited or Minor	X				
Low to Moderate		X			
Moderate			X		
Moderate to High				X	X
Counseling (#2) See E/M Guidelines					
Coordination of Care (#3) See E/M Guidelines					
Bedside/Unit/Floor Time (#4)					
Minutes	20	40	55	80	110

Subsequent Nursing Facility Care

Patient: New or Established
Required Components: 2/3

Code	99307	99308	99309	99310
Required Key Components				
History and Exam (#1 and #2)				
Problem-Focused	X			
Expanded Problem-Focused		X		
Detailed			X	
Comprehensive				X
Medical Decision Making (Complexity) (#3)				
Straightforward	X			
Low		X		
Moderate			X	
High				X
Contributory Factors				
Presenting Problem (Severity) (#1)				
Stable/Recovering/Improving	X			
Responding Inadequately to Therapy/ Minor Complication		X		
Significant Complication/ Significant New Problem			X	
Unstable/Significant New Problem Requiring Immediate Physician Attention				X
Counseling and Coordination of Care (#2 and #3) Counseling and/or coordination of care with other providers or agencies are provided consistant with the nature of the problem(s) and the patient's and/or family's needs.				
Bedside/Unit/Floor Time (#4)				
Minutes	10	15	25	35

Observation or Inpatient Care Services (Including Admission and Discharge Services)

Patient: New or Established
Required Components: 3/3

Code	99234	99235	99236
Required Key Components			
History and Exam (#1 and #2)			
Detailed or Comprehensive	X		
Comprehensive		X	X
Medical Decision Making (Complexity) (#3)			
Straightforward or Low	X		
Moderate		X	
High			X
Contributory Factors			
Presenting Problem (Severity) (#1)			
Low	X		
Moderate		X	
High			X
Counseling (#2) See E/M Guidelines			
Coordination of Care (#3) See E/M Guidelines			
Typical Time (#4)			
N/A			

Initial Nursing Facility Care

Patient: New or Established
Required Components: 3/3

Code	99304	99305	99306
Required Key Components			
History and Exam (#1 and #2)			
Detailed or Comprehensive	X		
Comprehensive		X	X
Medical Decision Making (Complexity) (#3)			
Straightforward or Low	X		
Moderate		X	
High			X
Contributory Factors			
Presenting Problem (Severity) (#1)			
Low	X		
Moderate		X	
High			X
Counseling and Coordination of Care (#2 and #3) Counseling and/or coordination of care with other providers or agencies are provided consistant with the nature of the problem(s) and the patient's and/or family's needs.			
Bedside/Unit/Floor Time (#4)			
Minutes	25	35	45

Emergency Department Services

Patient: New or Established
Required Components: 3/3

Code	99281	99282	99283	99284	99285
Required Key Components					
History and Exam (#1 and #2)					
Problem-Focused	X				
Expanded Problem-Focused		X	X		
Detailed				X	
Comprehensive					X
Medical Decision Making (Complexity) (#3)					
Straightforward	X				
Low		X			
Moderate			X	X	
High					X
Contributory Factors					
Presenting Problem (Severity) (#1)					
Self-limited or Minor	X				
Low to Moderate		X			
Moderate			X		
High				X	
High Severity/ Immediate Significant Threat to Life or Physiological Function					X
Counseling and Coordination of Care (#2 and #3) Counseling and/or coordination of care with other providers or agencies are provided consistant with the nature of the problem(s) and the patient's and/or family's needs.					
Typical Time (#4)					
N/A					

Domiciliary, Rest Home (eg, Boarding Home), or Custodial Care Services

Patient: New
Required Components: 3/3

Code	99324	99325	99326	99327	99328
Required Key Components					
History and Exam (#1 and #2)					
Problem-Focused	X				
Expanded Problem-Focused		X			
Detailed			X		
Comprehensive				X	X
Medical Decision Making (Complexity) (#3)					
Straightforward	X				
Low		X			
Moderate			X	X	
High					X
Contributory Factors					
Presenting Problem (Severity) (#1)					
Low	X				
Moderate		X			
Moderate to High			X		
High				X	
Unstable/Significant New Problem Requiring Immediate Physician Attention					X
Counseling (#2) See E/M Guidelines					
Coordination of Care (#3) See E/M Guidelines					
Typical Time (#4)					
Minutes	20	30	45	60	75

Domiciliary, Rest Home (eg, Boarding Home), or Custodial Care Services

Patient: Established
Required Components: 2/3

Code	99334	99335	99336	99337
Required Key Components				
History and Exam (#1 and #2)				
Problem-Focused	X			
Expanded Problem-Focused		X		
Detailed			X	
Comprehensive				X
Medical Decision Making (Complexity) (#3)				
Straightforward	X			
Low		X		
Moderate			X	
Moderate to High				X
Contributory Factors				
Presenting Problem (Severity) (#1)				
Self-limited or Minor	X			
Low to Moderate		X		
Moderate to High			X	
Moderate to High/ Unstable/ Significant Complication/New Problem				X
Counseling (#2) See E/M Guidelines				
Coordination of Care (#3) See E/M Guidelines				
Typical Time (#4)				
Minutes	15	25	40	60

Home Services

Patient: New
Required Components: 3/3

Code	99341	99342	99343	99344	99345
Required Key Components					
History and Exam (#1 and #2)					
Problem-Focused	X				
Expanded Problem-Focused		X			
Detailed			X		
Comprehensive				X	X
Medical Decision Making (Complexity) (#3)					
Straightforward	X				
Low		X			
Moderate			X	X	
High					X
Contributory Factors					
Presenting Problem (Severity) (#1)					
Low	X				
Moderate		X			
Moderate to High			X		
High				X	
Unstable/Significant New Problem					X
Counseling (#2) See E/M Guidelines					
Coordination of Care (#3) See E/M Guidelines					
Typical Face-to-Face Time (#4)					
Minutes	20	30	45	60	75

Home Services

Patient: Established
Required Components: 2/3

Code	99347	99348	99349	99350
Required Key Components				
History and Exam (#1 and #2)				
Problem-Focused	X			
Expanded Problem-Focused		X		
Detailed			X	
Comprehensive				X
Medical Decision Making (Complexity) (#3)				
Straightforward	X			
Low		X		
Moderate			X	
Moderate to High				X
Contributory Factors				
Presenting Problem (Severity) (#1)				
Self-limited or Minor	X			
Low to Moderate		X		
Moderate to High			X	
Moderate to High/Unstable/Significant New Problem				X
Counseling (#2) See E/M Guidelines				
Coordination of Care (#3) See E/M Guidelines				
Typical Time (#4)				
Minutes	15	25	40	60

Initial Inpatient Neonatal and Pediatric Critical Care

Code	99468	99471	99475	99291-99292
Age	28 days or less	29 days to 24 mos	2-5 yrs	6 yrs +

Subsequent Inpatient Neonatal and Pediatric Critical Care

Code	99469	99472	99476	99291-99292
Age	28 days or less	29 days to 24 mos	2-5 yrs	6 yrs +

Initial Neonatal Intensive Care

Code	99477
Age	28 days of age or younger
Weight	1500-5000 gms +
Presenting Problem	Requires Intensive Observation, Frequent Interventions/Other Intensive Care Services

Continuing Neonatal and Infant Inpatient Low Birth-Weight Intensive Care

Code	99478	99479	99480	See 99231-99233
Age	28 days of age or less			
Weight	1500 gms or less	1500-2500 gms	2501-5000 gms	+5000 gms
Presenting Problem	Recovering			

Critical Care Time Reporting

Total Duration of Critical Care	CPT Codes
Less than 30 minutes	Appropriate E/M codes
30-74 minutes (1/2 hour - 1 hour 14 minutes)	99291 X 1
75-104 minutes (1 hour 15 minutes - 1 hour 44 minutes)	99291 X 1 and 99292 X 1
105-134 minutes (1 hour 45 minutes - 2 hours 14 minutes)	99291 X 1 and 99292 X 2
135-164 minutes (2 hours 15 minutes - 2 hours 44 minutes)	99291 X 1 and 99292 X 3
165-194 minutes (2 hours 45 minutes - 3 hours 14 minutes)	99291 X 1 and 99292 X 4
195 minutes or more (3 hours 15 minutes or more)	99291 and 99292 as appropriate

Evaluation and Management (E/M) Services Guidelines

The following is a listing of headings and subheadings that appear within the Integumentary System section of the CPT codebook. The subheadings or subsections denoted with asterisks (*) below have special instructions unique to that section. Where these are indicated, special "notes" or guidelines will be presented preceding those procedural terminology listings, referring to that subsection specifically.

Evaluation and Management

Evaluation and Management (E/M) Services Guidelines

In addition to the information presented in the Introduction, several other items unique to this section are defined or identified here.

Classification of Evaluation and Management (E/M) Services

▶The E/M section is divided into broad categories such as office visits, hospital visits, and consultations. Most of the categories are further divided into two or more subcategories of E/M services. For example, there are two subcategories of office visits (new patient and established patient) and there are two subcategories of hospital visits (initial and subsequent). The subcategories of E/M services are further classified into levels of E/M services that are identified by specific codes. This classification is important because the nature of work varies by type of service, place of service, and the patient's status.◀

The basic format of the levels of E/M services is the same for most categories. First, a unique code number is listed. Second, the place and/or type of service is specified, eg, office consultation. Third, the content of the service is defined, eg, comprehensive history and comprehensive examination. (See "Levels of E/M Services," page 6, for details on the content of E/M services.) Fourth, the nature of the presenting problem(s) usually associated with a given level is described. Fifth, the time typically required to provide the service is specified. (A detailed discussion of time is provided on page 7.)

Definitions of Commonly Used Terms

Certain key words and phrases are used throughout the E/M section. The following definitions are intended to reduce the potential for differing interpretations and to increase the consistency of reporting by physicians in differing specialties. E/M services may also be reported by other qualified health care professionals who are authorized to perform such services within the scope of their practice.

New and Established Patient

▶Solely for the purposes of distinguishing between new and established patients, **professional services** are those face-to-face services rendered by physicians and other qualified health care professionals who may report evaluation and management services reported by a specific CPT code(s). A new patient is one who has not received any professional services from the physician/ qualified health care professional or another physician/ qualified health care professional of the **exact** same specialty **and subspecialty** who belongs to the same group practice, within the past three years.

An established patient is one who has received professional services from the physician/qualified health care professional or another physician/qualified health care professional of the **exact** same specialty **and subspecialty** who belongs to the same group practice, within the past three years. See Decision Tree.

In the instance where a physician/qualified health care professional is on call for or covering for another physician/qualified health care professional, the patient's encounter will be classified as it would have been by the physician/qualified health care professional who is not available. When advanced practice nurses and physician assistants are working with physicians, they are considered as working in the exact same specialty and exact same subspecialties as the physician.◀

No distinction is made between new and established patients in the emergency department. E/M services in the emergency department category may be reported for any new or established patient who presents for treatment in the emergency department.

The decision tree on page 5 is provided to aid in determining whether to report the E/M service provided as a new or an established patient encounter.

─── *Coding Tip* ───

Instructions for Use of the CPT Codebook

When advanced practice nurses and physician assistants are working with physicians they are considered as working in the exact same specialty and exact same subspecialties as the physician. A "physician or other qualified health care professional" is an individual who is qualified by education, training, licensure/regulation (when applicable), and facility privileging (when applicable) who performs a professional service within his or her scope of practice and independently reports that professional services. These professionals are distinct from "clinical staff." A clinical staff member is a person who works under the supervision of a physician or other qualified health care professional, and who is allowed by law, regulation and facility policy to perform or assist in the performance of a specific professional service, but does not individually report that professional service. Other policies may also affect who may report specific services.

CPT Coding Guidelines, Introduction, Instructions for Use of the CPT Codebook

Chief Complaint

A chief complaint is a concise statement describing the symptom, problem, condition, diagnosis, or other factor that is the reason for the encounter, usually stated in the patient's words.

Concurrent Care and Transfer of Care

►Concurrent care is the provision of similar services (eg, hospital visits) to the same patient by more than one physician or other qualified health care professional on the same day. When concurrent care is provided, no special reporting is required. Transfer of care is the process whereby a physician or other qualified health care professional who is providing management for some or all of a patient's problems relinquishes this responsibility to another physician or other qualified health care professional who explicitly agrees to accept this responsibility and who, from the initial encounter, is not providing consultative services. The physician or other qualified health care professional transferring care is then no longer providing care for these problems though he or she may continue providing care for other conditions when appropriate. Consultation codes should not be reported by the physician or other qualified health care professional who has agreed to accept transfer of care before an initial evaluation but are appropriate to report if the decision to accept transfer of care cannot be made until after the initial consultation evaluation, regardless of site of service.◄

Decision Tree for New vs Established Patients

Decision Tree for New vs Established Patients

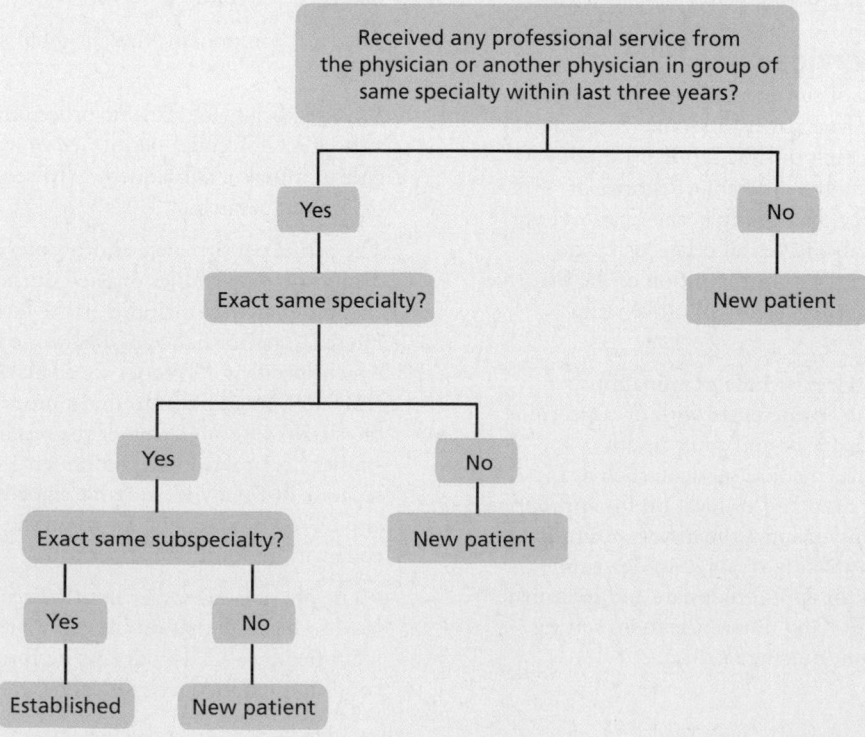

Evaluation/Management

Counseling

Counseling is a discussion with a patient and/or family concerning one or more of the following areas:

- Diagnostic results, impressions, and/or recommended diagnostic studies
- Prognosis
- Risks and benefits of management (treatment) options
- Instructions for management (treatment) and/or follow-up
- Importance of compliance with chosen management (treatment) options
- Risk factor reduction
- Patient and family education

Family History

A review of medical events in the patient's family that includes significant information about:

- The health status or cause of death of parents, siblings, and children
- Specific diseases related to problems identified in the Chief Complaint or History of the Present Illness, and/or System Review
- Diseases of family members that may be hereditary or place the patient at risk

History of Present Illness

A chronological description of the development of the patient's present illness from the first sign and/or symptom to the present. This includes a description of location, quality, severity, timing, context, modifying factors, and associated signs and symptoms significantly related to the presenting problem(s).

Levels of E/M Services

Within each category or subcategory of E/M service, there are three to five levels of E/M services available for reporting purposes. Levels of E/M services are **not** interchangeable among the different categories or subcategories of service. For example, the first level of E/M services in the subcategory of office visit, new patient, does not have the same definition as the first level of E/M services in the subcategory of office visit, established patient.

The levels of E/M services include examinations, evaluations, treatments, conferences with or concerning patients, preventive pediatric and adult health supervision, and similar medical services, such as the determination of the need and/or location for appropriate care. Medical screening includes the history, examination, and medical decision-making required to determine the need and/or location for appropriate care and treatment of the patient (eg, office and other outpatient setting, emergency department, nursing facility).

▶The levels of E/M services encompass the wide variations in skill, effort, time, responsibility, and medical knowledge required for the prevention or diagnosis and treatment of illness or injury and the promotion of optimal health. Each level of E/M services may be used by all physicians or other qualified health care professionals.◀

The descriptors for the levels of E/M services recognize seven components, six of which are used in defining the levels of E/M services. These components are:

- History
- Examination
- Medical decision making
- Counseling
- Coordination of care
- Nature of presenting problem
- Time

The first three of these components (history, examination, and medical decision making) are considered the **key** components in selecting a level of E/M services. (See "Determine the Extent of History Obtained," page 9.)

The next three components (counseling, coordination of care, and the nature of the presenting problem) are considered **contributory** factors in the majority of encounters. Although the first two of these contributory factors are important E/M services, it is not required that these services be provided at every patient encounter.

▶Coordination of care with other physicians, other health care professionals, or agencies without a patient encounter on that day is reported using the case management codes.◀

The final component, time, is discussed in detail on page 7.

Any specifically identifiable procedure (ie, identified with a specific CPT code) performed on or subsequent to the date of initial or subsequent E/M services should be reported separately.

The actual performance and/or interpretation of diagnostic tests/studies ordered during a patient encounter are not included in the levels of E/M services. Physician performance of diagnostic tests/studies for which specific CPT codes are available may be reported separately, in addition to the appropriate E/M code. The physician's interpretation of the results of diagnostic tests/studies (ie, professional component) with preparation of a separate distinctly identifiable signed written report may also be reported separately, using the appropriate CPT code with modifier 26 appended.

▶The physician or other health care professional may need to indicate that on the day a procedure or service identified by a CPT code was performed, the patient's condition required a significant separately identifiable

E/M service above and beyond other services provided or beyond the usual preservice and postservice care associated with the procedure that was performed. The E/M service may be caused or prompted by the symptoms or condition for which the procedure and/or service was provided. This circumstance may be reported by adding modifier 25 to the appropriate level of E/M service. As such, different diagnoses are not required for reporting of the procedure and the E/M services on the same date.◄

Nature of Presenting Problem

A presenting problem is a disease, condition, illness, injury, symptom, sign, finding, complaint, or other reason for encounter, with or without a diagnosis being established at the time of the encounter. The E/M codes recognize five types of presenting problems that are defined as follows:

►*Minimal:* A problem that may not require the presence of the physician or other qualified health care professional, but service is provided under the physician's or other qualified health care professional's supervision.◄

Self-limited or minor: A problem that runs a definite and prescribed course, is transient in nature, and is not likely to permanently alter health status OR has a good prognosis with management/compliance.

Low severity: A problem where the risk of morbidity without treatment is low; there is little to no risk of mortality without treatment; full recovery without functional impairment is expected.

Moderate severity: A problem where the risk of morbidity without treatment is moderate; there is moderate risk of mortality without treatment; uncertain prognosis OR increased probability of prolonged functional impairment.

High severity: A problem where the risk of morbidity without treatment is high to extreme; there is a moderate to high risk of mortality without treatment OR high probability of severe, prolonged functional impairment.

Past History

A review of the patient's past experiences with illnesses, injuries, and treatments that includes significant information about:

- Prior major illnesses and injuries
- Prior operations
- Prior hospitalizations
- Current medications
- Allergies (eg, drug, food)
- Age appropriate immunization status
- Age appropriate feeding/dietary status

Social History

An age appropriate review of past and current activities that includes significant information about:

- Marital status and/or living arrangements
- Current employment
- Occupational history
- Use of drugs, alcohol, and tobacco
- Level of education
- Sexual history
- Other relevant social factors

System Review (Review of Systems)

An inventory of body systems obtained through a series of questions seeking to identify signs and/or symptoms that the patient may be experiencing or has experienced. For the purposes of the CPT codebook the following elements of a system review have been identified:

- Constitutional symptoms (fever, weight loss, etc)
- Eyes
- Ears, nose, mouth, throat
- Cardiovascular
- Respiratory
- Gastrointestinal
- Genitourinary
- Musculoskeletal
- Integumentary (skin and/or breast)
- Neurological
- Psychiatric
- Endocrine
- Hematologic/lymphatic
- Allergic/immunologic

The review of systems helps define the problem, clarify the differential diagnosis, identify needed testing, or serves as baseline data on other systems that might be affected by any possible management options.

Time

►The inclusion of time in the definitions of levels of E/M services has been implicit in prior editions of the CPT codebook. The inclusion of time as an explicit factor beginning in *CPT 1992* is done to assist in selecting the most appropriate level of E/M services. It should be recognized that the specific times expressed in the visit code descriptors are averages and, therefore, represent a range of times that may be higher or lower depending on actual clinical circumstances.

Time is **not** a descriptive component for the emergency department levels of E/M services because emergency department services are typically provided on a variable intensity basis, often involving multiple encounters with several patients over an extended period of time.

Therefore, it is often difficult to provide accurate estimates of the time spent face-to-face with the patient.

Studies to establish levels of E/M services employed surveys of practicing physicians to obtain data on the amount of time and work associated with typical E/M services. Since "work" is not easily quantifiable, the codes must rely on other objective, verifiable measures that correlate with physicians' estimates of their "work." It has been demonstrated that estimations of **intraservice** time (as explained on the next page), both within and across specialties, is a variable that is predictive of the "work" of E/M services. This same research has shown there is a strong relationship between intraservice time and total time for E/M services. Intraservice time, rather than total time, was chosen for inclusion with the codes because of its relative ease of measurement and because of its direct correlation with measurements of the total amount of time and work associated with typical E/M services.◄

Intraservice times are defined as **face-to-face** time for office and other outpatient visits and as **unit/floor** time for hospital and other inpatient visits. This distinction is necessary because most of the work of typical office visits takes place during the face-to-face time with the patient, while most of the work of typical hospital visits takes place during the time spent on the patient's floor or unit. When prolonged time occurs in either the office or the inpatient areas, the appropriate add-on code should be reported.

►*Face-to-face time (office and other outpatient visits and office consultations):* For coding purposes, face-to-face time for these services is defined as only that time spent face-to-face with the patient and/or family. This includes the time spent performing such tasks as obtaining a history, performing an examination, and counseling the patient.

Time is also spent doing work before or after the face-to-face time with the patient, performing such tasks as reviewing records and tests, arranging for further services, and communicating further with other professionals and the patient through written reports and telephone contact.◄

This **non-face-to-face** time for office services—also called pre- and postencounter time—is not included in the time component described in the E/M codes. However, the pre- and post-non-face-to-face work associated with an encounter was included in calculating the total work of typical services in physician surveys.

Thus, the face-to-face time associated with the services described by any E/M code is a valid proxy for the total work done before, during, and after the visit.

►*Unit/floor time (hospital observation services, inpatient hospital care, initial inpatient hospital consultations, nursing facility):* For reporting purposes, intraservice time for these services is defined as unit/floor time, which includes the time present on the patient's hospital unit and at the bedside rendering services for that patient. This includes the time to establish and/or

review the patient's chart, examine the patient, write notes, and communicate with other professionals and the patient's family.◄

In the hospital, pre- and post-time includes time spent off the patient's floor performing such tasks as reviewing pathology and radiology findings in another part of the hospital.

This pre- and postvisit time is not included in the time component described in these codes. However, the pre- and postwork performed during the time spent off the floor or unit was included in calculating the total work of typical services in physician surveys.

Thus, the unit/floor time associated with the services described by any code is a valid proxy for the total work done before, during, and after the visit.

Unlisted Service

An E/M service may be provided that is not listed in this section of the CPT codebook. When reporting such a service, the appropriate unlisted code may be used to indicate the service, identifying it by "Special Report," as discussed in the following paragraph. The "Unlisted Services" and accompanying codes for the E/M section are as follows:

99429 **Unlisted preventive** medicine service

99499 **Unlisted evaluation and management** service

Special Report

An unlisted service or one that is unusual, variable, or new may require a special report demonstrating the medical appropriateness of the service. Pertinent information should include an adequate definition or description of the nature, extent, and need for the procedure and the time, effort, and equipment necessary to provide the service. Additional items that may be included are complexity of symptoms, final diagnosis, pertinent physical findings, diagnostic and therapeutic procedures, concurrent problems, and follow-up care.

Clinical Examples

►Clinical examples of the codes for E/M services are provided to assist in understanding the meaning of the descriptors and selecting the correct code. The clinical examples are listed in Appendix C. Each example was developed by the specialties shown.

The same problem, when seen by different specialties, may involve different amounts of work. Therefore, the appropriate level of encounter should be reported using the descriptors rather than the examples.

The examples have been tested for validity and approved by the CPT Editorial Panel. Specialties were given the examples and asked to assign a code or assess the amount of time and work involved. Only examples that were rated consistently have been included in Appendix C.◄

Instructions for Selecting a Level of E/M Service

Review the Reporting Instructions for the Selected Category or Subcategory

Most of the categories and many of the subcategories of service have special guidelines or instructions unique to that category or subcategory. Where these are indicated, eg, "Inpatient Hospital Care," special instructions will be presented preceding the levels of E/M services.

Review the Level of E/M Service Descriptors and Examples in the Selected Category or Subcategory

The descriptors for the levels of E/M services recognize seven components, six of which are used in defining the levels of E/M services. These components are:

- History
- Examination
- Medical decision making
- Counseling
- Coordination of care
- Nature of presenting problem
- Time

The first three of these components (ie, history, examination, and medical decision making) should be considered the **key** components in selecting the level of E/M services. An exception to this rule is in the case of visits that consist predominantly of counseling or coordination of care (see numbered paragraph 3, page 10).

The nature of the presenting problem and time are provided in some levels to assist the physician in determining the appropriate level of E/M service.

Determine the Extent of History Obtained

The extent of the history is dependent upon clinical judgment and on the nature of the presenting problem(s). The levels of E/M services recognize four types of history that are defined as follows:

Problem focused: Chief complaint; brief history of present illness or problem.

Expanded problem focused: Chief complaint; brief history of present illness; problem pertinent system review.

Detailed: Chief complaint; extended history of present illness; problem pertinent system review extended to include a review of a limited number of additional systems; **pertinent** past, family, and/or social history **directly related to the patient's problems.**

Comprehensive: Chief complaint; extended history of present illness; review of systems that is directly related to the problem(s) identified in the history of the present illness plus a review of all additional body systems; **complete** past, family, and social history.

The comprehensive history obtained as part of the preventive medicine E/M service is not problem-oriented and does not involve a chief complaint or present illness. It does, however, include a comprehensive system review and comprehensive or interval past, family, and social history as well as a comprehensive assessment/history of pertinent risk factors.

Determine the Extent of Examination Performed

The extent of the examination performed is dependent on clinical judgment and on the nature of the presenting problem(s). The levels of E/M services recognize four types of examination that are defined as follows:

Problem focused: A limited examination of the affected body area or organ system.

Expanded problem focused: A limited examination of the affected body area or organ system and other symptomatic or related organ system(s).

Detailed: An extended examination of the affected body area(s) and other symptomatic or related organ system(s).

Comprehensive: A general multisystem examination or a complete examination of a single organ system. **Note:** The comprehensive examination performed as part of the preventive medicine E/M service is multisystem, but its extent is based on age and risk factors identified.

For the purposes of these CPT definitions, the following body areas are recognized:

- Head, including the face
- Neck
- Chest, including breasts and axilla
- Abdomen
- Genitalia, groin, buttocks
- Back
- Each extremity

For the purposes of these CPT definitions, the following organ systems are recognized:

- Eyes
- Ears, nose, mouth, and throat
- Cardiovascular
- Respiratory
- Gastrointestinal
- Genitourinary
- Musculoskeletal
- Skin
- Neurologic
- Psychiatric
- Hematologic/lymphatic/immunologic

Determine the Complexity of Medical Decision Making

Medical decision making refers to the complexity of establishing a diagnosis and/or selecting a management option as measured by:

- The number of possible diagnoses and/or the number of management options that must be considered
- The amount and/or complexity of medical records, diagnostic tests, and/or other information that must be obtained, reviewed, and analyzed
- The risk of significant complications, morbidity, and/or mortality, as well as comorbidities, associated with the patient's presenting problem(s), the diagnostic procedure(s), and/or the possible management options

Four types of medical decision making are recognized: straightforward, low complexity, moderate complexity, and high complexity. To qualify for a given type of decision making, two of the three elements in Table 1 must be met or exceeded.

Comorbidities/underlying diseases, in and of themselves, are not considered in selecting a level of E/M services *unless* their presence significantly increases the complexity of the medical decision making.

Select the Appropriate Level of E/M Services Based on the Following

1. For the following categories/subcategories, **all of the key components,** ie, history, examination, and medical decision making, must meet or exceed the stated requirements to qualify for a particular level of E/M service: office, new patient; hospital observation services; initial hospital care; office consultations; initial inpatient consultations; emergency department services; initial nursing facility care; domiciliary care, new patient; and home, new patient.

2. For the following categories/subcategories, **two of the three key components** (ie, history, examination, and medical decision making) must meet or exceed the stated requirements to qualify for a particular level of E/M services: office, established patient; subsequent hospital care; subsequent nursing facility care; domiciliary care, established patient; and home, established patient.

►3. When counseling and/or coordination of care dominates (more than 50%) the encounter with the patient and/or family (face-to-face time in the office or other outpatient setting or floor/unit time in the hospital or nursing facility), then **time** shall be considered the key or controlling factor to qualify for a particular level of E/M services. This includes time spent with parties who have assumed responsibility for the care of the patient or decision making whether or not they are family members (eg, foster parents, person acting in loco parentis, legal guardian). The extent of counseling and/or coordination of care must be documented in the medical record.◄

Table 1
Complexity of Medical Decision Making

Number of Diagnoses or Management Options	Amount and/or Complexity of Data to be Reviewed	Risk of Complications and/or Morbidity or Mortality	Type of Decision Making
minimal	minimal or none	minimal	**straightforward**
limited	limited	low	**low complexity**
multiple	moderate	moderate	**moderate complexity**
extensive	extensive	high	**high complexity**

Evaluation and Management

Office or Other Outpatient Services

▶The following codes are used to report evaluation and management services provided in the office or in an outpatient or other ambulatory facility. A patient is considered an outpatient until inpatient admission to a health care facility occurs.◀

To report services provided to a patient who is admitted to a hospital or nursing facility in the course of an encounter in the office or other ambulatory facility, see the notes for initial hospital inpatient care (page 15) or initial nursing facility care (page 25).

▶For services provided in the emergency department, see 99281-99285.◀

For observation care, see 99217-99226.

For observation or inpatient care services (including admission and discharge services), see 99234-99236.

—— *Coding Tip* ——

Determination of Patient Status as New or Established Patient

Solely for the purposes of distinguishing between new and established patients, **professional services** are those face-to-face services rendered by physicians and other qualified health care professionals who may report evaluation and management services reported by a specific CPT code(s). A new patient is one who has not received any professional services from the physician/qualified health care professional or another physician/qualified health care professional of the **exact** same specialty and subspecialty who belongs to the same group practice, within the past three years.

An established patient is one who has received professional services from the physician/qualified health care professional or another physician/qualified health care professional of the **exact** same specialty and **subspecialty** who belongs to the same group practice, within the past three years.

In the instance where a physician/qualified health care professional is on call for or covering for another physician/qualified health care professional, the patient's encounter will be classified as it would have been by the physician/qualified health care professional who is not available. When advanced practice nurses and physician assistants are working with physicians they are considered as working in the exact same specialty and exact same subspecialties as the physician.

CPT Coding Guidelines, Evaluation and Management, Definitions of Commonly Used Terms, New and Established Patient

New Patient

▲ **99201**   **Office or other outpatient visit** for the evaluation and management of a new patient, which requires these 3 key components:

■ **A problem focused history;**
■ **A problem focused examination;**
■ **Straightforward medical decision making.**

Counseling and/or coordination of care with other physicians, other qualified health care professionals, or agencies are provided consistent with the nature of the problem(s) and the patient's and/or family's needs.

Usually, the presenting problem(s) are self limited or minor. Typically, 10 minutes are spent face-to-face with the patient and/or family.

➔ *CPT Assistant* Winter 91:11, Spring 92:13, 24, Summer 92:1, 24, Spring 93:34, Summer 93:2, Fall 93:9, Spring 95:1, Summer 95:4, Fall 95:9, Jul 98:9, Sep 98:5, Jun 99:8, Feb 00:3, 9, 11, Aug 01:2, Oct 04:11, Mar 05:11, Apr 05:1, May 05:1, Jun 05:11, Dec 05:10, Feb 06:14, May 06:1, Jun 06:1, Aug 06:12, Oct 06:15, Apr 07:11, Sep 07:1, Nov 08:10, Mar 09:3, Aug 09:5, Dec 09:9, Jul 10:10, Jan 11:3, Jan 12:5, Mar 12:4, 8, Apr 12:10; *CPT Changes: An Insider's View* 2011, 2013

➔ *Clinical Examples in Radiology* Winter 12:9

▲ **99202**   **Office or other outpatient visit** for the evaluation and management of a new patient, which requires these 3 key components:

■ **An expanded problem focused history;**
■ **An expanded problem focused examination;**
■ **Straightforward medical decision making.**

Counseling and/or coordination of care with other physicians, other qualified health care professionals, or agencies are provided consistent with the nature of the problem(s) and the patient's and/or family's needs.

Usually, the presenting problem(s) are of low to moderate severity. Typically, 20 minutes are spent face-to-face with the patient and/or family.

➔ *CPT Assistant* Winter 91:11, Spring 92:13, 24, Summer 92:1, 24, Spring 93:34, Summer 93:2, Fall 93:9, Spring 95:1, Summer 95:4, Fall 95:9, Jul 98:9, Sep 98:5, Feb 00:11, Aug 01:2, Apr 02:14, Oct 04:10, Apr 05:1, 3, Jun 05:11, Dec 05:10, May 06:1, Jun 06:1, Oct 06:15, Apr 07:11, Sep 07:1, Mar 09:3, Aug 09:5, Dec 09:9, Jan 11:3, Mar 12:4, 8; *CPT Changes: An Insider's View* 2013

➔ *Clinical Examples in Radiology* Winter 12:9

▲ **99203**   **Office or other outpatient visit** for the evaluation and management of a new patient, which requires these 3 key components:

■ **A detailed history;**
■ **A detailed examination;**
■ **Medical decision making of low complexity.**

Counseling and/or coordination of care with other physicians, other qualified health care professionals, or agencies are provided consistent with the nature of the problem(s) and the patient's and/or family's needs.

Usually, the presenting problem(s) are of moderate severity. Typically, 30 minutes are spent face-to-face with the patient and/or family.

➔ *CPT Assistant* Winter 91:11, Spring 92:14, 24, Summer 92:1, 24, Spring 93:34, Summer 93:2, Fall 93:9, Spring 95:1, Summer 95:4, Fall 95:9, Jul 98:9, Sep 98:5, Feb 00:11, Aug 01:2, Apr 02:14, Oct 04:10, Feb 05:9, Apr 05:1, 3, Jun 05:11, Dec 05:10, May 06:1, Jun 06:1, Oct 06:15, Apr 07:11, Sep 07:1, Mar 09:3, Aug 09:5, Dec 09:9, Jan 11:3, Mar 12:4, 8; *CPT Changes: An Insider's View* 2013

➔ *Clinical Examples in Radiology* Winter 12:9

▲ **99204** **Office or other outpatient visit** for the evaluation and management of a new patient, which requires these 3 key components:

- **A comprehensive history;**
- **A comprehensive examination;**
- **Medical decision making of moderate complexity.**

Counseling and/or coordination of care with other physicians, other qualified health care professionals, or agencies are provided consistent with the nature of the problem(s) and the patient's and/or family's needs.

Usually, the presenting problem(s) are of moderate to high severity. Typically, 45 minutes are spent face-to-face with the patient and/or family.

➔ *CPT Assistant* Winter 91:11, Spring 92:14, 24, Summer 92:1, 24, Spring 93:34, Summer 93:2, Fall 93:9, Spring 95:1, Summer 95:4, Fall 95:9, Jul 98:9, Sep 98:5, Feb 00:11, Aug 01:2, Apr 02:14, May 02:1, Oct 04:10, Apr 05:1, 3, Jun 05:11, Dec 05:10, May 06:1, Jun 06:1, Oct 06:15, Apr 07:11, Sep 07:1, Mar 09:3, Aug 09:5, Dec 09:9, Jan 11:3, Mar 12:4, 8; *CPT Changes: An Insider's View* 2013

➔ *Clinical Examples in Radiology* Winter 12:9

▲ **99205** **Office or other outpatient visit** for the evaluation and management of a new patient, which requires these 3 key components:

- **A comprehensive history;**
- **A comprehensive examination;**
- **Medical decision making of high complexity.**

Counseling and/or coordination of care with other physicians, other qualified health care professionals, or agencies are provided consistent with the nature of the problem(s) and the patient's and/or family's needs.

Usually, the presenting problem(s) are of moderate to high severity. Typically, 60 minutes are spent face-to-face with the patient and/or family.

➔ *CPT Assistant* Winter 91:11, Spring 92:14, 24, Summer 92:1, 24, Spring 93:34, Summer 93:2, Fall 93:9, Spring 95:1, Summer 95:4, Fall 95:9, Jul 98:9, Sep 98:5, Feb 00:11, Aug 01:2, Apr 02:2, May 02:1, Oct 04:10, Apr 05:1, 3, Jun 05:11, Dec 05:10, May 06:1, Jun 06:1, Oct 06:15, Apr 07:11, Sep 07:1, Mar 09:3, Aug 09:5, Dec 09:9, Jul 10:4, Jan 11:3, Jan 12:3, Mar 12:4, 8; *CPT Changes: An Insider's View* 2013

➔ *Clinical Examples in Radiology* Winter 12:9

Established Patient

▲ **99211** **Office or other outpatient visit** for the evaluation and management of an established patient, that may not require the presence of a physician or other qualified health care professional. Usually, the presenting problem(s) are minimal. Typically, 5 minutes are spent performing or supervising these services.

➔ *CPT Assistant* Winter 91:11, Spring 92:14, 24, Summer 92:1, 24, Spring 93:34, Summer 93:2, Fall 93:9, Spring 95:1, Summer 95:4, Fall 95:9, Oct 96:10, Feb 97:9, May 97:4, Jul 98:9, Sep 98:5, Oct 99:9, Feb 00:11, Aug 01:2, Jan 02:2, Oct 04:10, Feb 05:15, Mar 05:11, Apr 05:1, 3, May 05:1, Jun 05:11, Nov 05:1, Dec 05:10, Feb 06:14, May 06:1, Jun 06:1, Jul 06:19, Oct 06:15, Nov 06:21, Apr 07:11, Jul 07:1, Sep 07:1, Dec 07:9, Mar 08:3, Aug 08:13, Mar 09:3, Aug 09:5, Apr 10:10, Jan 11:3, Jan 12:3, Mar 12:4, 8, Apr 12:10; *CPT Changes: An Insider's View* 2013

▲ **99212** **Office or other outpatient visit** for the evaluation and management of an established patient, which requires at least 2 of these 3 key components:

- **A problem focused history;**
- **A problem focused examination;**
- **Straightforward medical decision making.**

Counseling and/or coordination of care with other physicians, other qualified health care professionals, or agencies are provided consistent with the nature of the problem(s) and the patient's and/or family's needs.

Usually, the presenting problem(s) are self limited or minor. Typically, 10 minutes are spent face-to-face with the patient and/or family.

➔ *CPT Assistant* Winter 91:11, Spring 92:14, 24, Summer 92:1, 24, Spring 93:34, Summer 93:2, Fall 93:9, Spring 95:1, Summer 95:4, Fall 95:9, Jul 98:9, Sep 98:5, Feb 00:11, Jun 00:11, Aug 01:2, Jan 02:2, May 02:3, Apr 04:14, Oct 04:10, Apr 05:1, 3, Jun 05:11, Dec 05:10, May 06:1, Jun 06:1, 11, Sep 06:8, Oct 06:15, Apr 07:11, Jul 07:1, Sep 07:1, Mar 08:3, Mar 09:3, Aug 09:5, Feb 10:13, Jul 10:4, Sep 10:4, Jan 11:3, Jun 11:3, Mar 12:4, 8, Apr 12:17; *CPT Changes: An Insider's View* 2013

▲ **99213** **Office or other outpatient visit** for the evaluation and management of an established patient, which requires at least 2 of these 3 key components:

- **An expanded problem focused history;**
- **An expanded problem focused examination;**
- **Medical decision making of low complexity.**

Counseling and coordination of care with other physicians, other qualified health care professionals, or agencies are provided consistent with the nature of the problem(s) and the patient's and/or family's needs.

Usually, the presenting problem(s) are of low to moderate severity. Typically, 15 minutes are spent face-to-face with the patient and/or family.

➔ *CPT Assistant* Winter 91:11, Spring 92:14, 24, Summer 92:1, 24, Spring 93:34, Summer 93:2, Fall 93:9, Spring 95:1, Summer 95:4, Fall 95:9, Jan 97:10, Jul 98:9, Sep 98:5, Aug 01:2, May 02:3, Oct 03:5, Apr 04:14, Oct 04:10, Mar 05:11, Apr 05:1, 3, Jun 05:11, Dec 05:10, May 06:1, Jun 06:1, 11, Sep 06:8, Oct 06:15, Apr 07:11, Jul 07:1, Sep 07:1, Mar 08:3, Mar 09:3, Aug 09:5, Sep 10:4, Jan 11:3, Jun 11:3, Mar 12:4, 8; *CPT Changes: An Insider's View* 2013

▲ **99214**   **Office or other outpatient visit** for the evaluation and management of an established patient, which requires at least 2 of these 3 key components:

- **A detailed history;**
- **A detailed examination;**
- **Medical decision making of moderate complexity.**

Counseling and/or coordination of care with other physicians, other qualified health care professionals, or agencies are provided consistent with the nature of the problem(s) and the patient's and/or family's needs.

Usually, the presenting problem(s) are of moderate to high severity. Typically, 25 minutes are spent face-to-face with the patient and/or family.

➔ *CPT Assistant* Winter 91:11, Spring 92:15, 24, Summer 92:1, 24, Spring 93:34, Summer 93:2, Fall 93:9, Spring 95:1, Summer 95:4, Fall 95:9, May 97:4, Jul 98:9, Sep 98:5, Aug 01:2, Jan 02:2, May 02:1-2, Oct 03:5, Apr 04:14, Oct 04:10, Apr 05:1, 3, Jun 05:11, Dec 05:10, May 06:1, Jun 06:1, 11, Sep 06:8, Oct 06:15, Apr 07:11, Jul 07:1, Sep 07:1, Mar 08:3, Mar 09:3, Aug 09:5, Sep 10:4, Jan 11:3, Jun 11:3, Mar 12:4, 8; *CPT Changes: An Insider's View* 2013

▲ **99215**   **Office or other outpatient visit** for the evaluation and management of an established patient, which requires at least 2 of these 3 key components:

- **A comprehensive history;**
- **A comprehensive examination;**
- **Medical decision making of high complexity.**

Counseling and/or coordination of care with other physicians, other qualified health care professionals, or agencies are provided consistent with the nature of the problem(s) and the patient's and/or family's needs.

Usually, the presenting problem(s) are of moderate to high severity. Typically, 40 minutes are spent face-to-face with the patient and/or family.

➔ *CPT Assistant* Winter 91:11, Spring 92:15, 24, Summer 92:1, 24, Spring 93:34, Summer 93:2, Fall 93:9, Spring 95:1, Summer 95:4, Fall 95:9, Jan 97:10, Jul 98:9, Sep 98:5, Aug 01:2, Jan 02:2, May 02:1, 3, Apr 04:14, Oct 04:10, Mar 05:11, Apr 05:1, 3, Jun 05:11, Dec 05:10, May 06:1, Jun 06:1, 11, Sep 06:8, Oct 06:15, Apr 07:11, Jul 07:1, Sep 07:1, Mar 08:3, Mar 09:3, Aug 09:5, Jul 10:4, Sep 10:4, Jan 11:3, Jun 11:3, Jan 12:3, Mar 12:4, 8, Apr 12:10; *CPT Changes: An Insider's View* 2013

Hospital Observation Services

The following codes are used to report evaluation and management services provided to patients designated/admitted as "observation status" in a hospital. It is not necessary that the patient be located in an observation area designated by the hospital.

If such an area does exist in a hospital (as a separate unit in the hospital, in the emergency department, etc.), these codes are to be utilized if the patient is placed in such an area.

For definitions of key components and commonly used terms, please see **Evaluation and Management Services Guidelines.**

—— *Coding Tip* ——

The Significance of Time as a Factor in Selection of an Evaluation and Management Code

The inclusion of time as an explicit factor beginning in CPT 1992 is done to assist in selecting the most appropriate level of E/M services. It should be recognized that the specific times expressed in the visit code descriptors are averages and, therefore, represent a range of times that may be higher or lower depending on actual clinical circumstances.

Intraservice times are defined as **face-to-face** time for office and other outpatient visits and as **unit/floor** time for hospital and other inpatient visits. This distinction is necessary because most of the work of typical office visits takes place during the face-to-face time with the patient, while most of the work of typical hospital visits takes place during the time spent on the patient's floor or unit.

Unit/floor time (hospital observation services, inpatient hospital care, initial inpatient hospital consultations, nursing facility):

For reporting purposes, intraservice time for these services is defined as unit/floor time, which includes the time present on the patient's hospital unit and at the bedside rendering services for that patient. This includes the time to establish and/or review the patient's chart, examine the patient, write notes, and communicate with other professionals and the patient's family.

In the hospital, pre- and post-time includes time spent off the patient's floor performing such tasks as reviewing pathology and radiology findings in another part of the hospital.

This pre- and postvisit time is not included in the time component described in these codes. However, the pre- and post-work performed during the time spent off the floor or unit was included in calculating the total work of typical services in physician surveys.

Thus, the unit/floor time associated with the services described by any code is a valid proxy for the total work done before, during, and after the visit.

CPT Coding Guidelines, Evaluation and Management, Definitions of Commonly Used Term, Time

Observation Care Discharge Services

Observation care discharge of a patient from "observation status" includes final examination of the patient, discussion of the hospital stay, instructions for continuing care, and preparation of discharge records. For observation or inpatient hospital care including the admission and discharge of the patient on the same date, see codes 99234-99236 as appropriate.

▲ **99217** **Observation care discharge** day management (This code is to be utilized to report all services provided to a patient on discharge from "observation status" if the discharge is on other than the initial date of "observation status." To report services to a patient designated as "observation status" or "inpatient status" and discharged on the same date, use the codes for Observation or Inpatient Care Services [including Admission and Discharge Services, 99234-99236 as appropriate.])

→ *CPT Assistant* Nov 97:2, Mar 98:1, May 98:3, Sep 98:5, Sep 00:3, May 05:1, Nov 05:10, Sep 06:8, Dec 06:14, Sep 10:4, Jun 11:3, Jul 12:10, 11, 14; *CPT Changes: An Insider's View* 2013

Initial Observation Care

New or Established Patient

▶The following codes are used to report the encounter(s) by the supervising physician or other qualified health care professional with the patient when designated as "observation status." This refers to the initiation of observation status, supervision of the care plan for observation and performance of periodic reassessments. For observation encounters by other physicians, see office or other outpatient consultation codes (99241-99245) or subsequent observation care codes (99224-99226) as appropriate.

To report services provided to a patient who is admitted to the hospital after receiving hospital observation care services on the same date, see the notes for initial hospital inpatient care (page 15). For observation care services on other than the initial or discharge date, see subsequent observation services codes (99224-99226). For a patient admitted to the hospital on a date subsequent to the date of observation status, the hospital admission would be reported with the appropriate initial hospital care code (99221-99223). For a patient admitted and discharged from observation or inpatient status on the same date, the services should be reported with codes 99234-99236 as appropriate. Do not report observation discharge (99217) in conjunction with a hospital admission (99221-99223).

When "observation status" is initiated in the course of an encounter in another site of service (eg, hospital emergency department, office, nursing facility) all evaluation and management services provided by the supervising physician or other qualified health care professional in conjunction with initiating "observation status" are considered part of the initial observation care when performed on the same date. The observation care level of service reported by the supervising physician or other qualified health care professional should include the services related to initiating "observation status" provided in the other sites of service as well as in the observation setting.

Evaluation and management services including new or established patient office or other outpatient services including (99201-99215), emergency department services (99281-99285), nursing facility services (99304-99318), domiciliary, rest home, or custodial care services (99324-99337), home services (99341-99350), and preventive medicine services (99381-99429) on the same date related to the admission to "observation status" should not be reported separately.◀

These codes may not be utilized for post-operative recovery if the procedure is considered part of the surgical "package." These codes apply to all evaluation and management services that are provided on the same date of initiating "observation status."

▲ **99218** **Initial observation care,** per day, for the evaluation and management of a patient which requires these 3 key components:

■ **A detailed or comprehensive history;**

■ **A detailed or comprehensive examination; and**

■ **Medical decision making that is straightforward or of low complexity.**

Counseling and/or coordination of care with other physicians, other qualified health care professionals, or agencies are provided consistent with the nature of the problem(s) and the patient's and/or family's needs.

Usually, the problem(s) requiring admission to "observation status" are of low severity. Typically, 30 minutes are spent at the bedside and on the patient's hospital floor or unit.

→ *CPT Assistant* Spring 93:34, Fall 95:9, Nov 97:2, Mar 98:1, Sep 98:5, Sep 00:3, Jan 03:10, Aug 04:11, May 05:1, Nov 05:10, Sep 06:8, Dec 06:14, Sep 10:4, Oct 10:6, Jun 11:3, Jul 12:11, 14; *CPT Changes: An Insider's View* 2012, 2013

▲ **99219** **Initial observation care,** per day, for the evaluation and management of a patient, which requires these 3 key components:

■ **A comprehensive history;**

■ **A comprehensive examination; and**

■ **Medical decision making of moderate complexity.**

Counseling and/or coordination of care with other physicians, other qualified health care professionals, or agencies are provided consistent with the nature of the problem(s) and the patient's and/or family's needs.

Usually, the problem(s) requiring admission to "observation status" are of moderate severity. Typically, 50 minutes are spent at the bedside and on the patient's hospital floor or unit.

→ *CPT Assistant* Spring 93:34, Fall 95:16, Nov 97:2, Mar 98:1, Sep 98:5, Sep 00:3, Jan 03:10, Aug 04:11, Nov 05:10, Sep 06:8, Dec 06:14, Sep 10:4, Oct 10:6, Jun 11:3, Jul 12:11, 14; *CPT Changes: An Insider's View* 2012, 2013

▲ **99220** **Initial observation care,** per day, for the evaluation and management of a patient, which requires these 3 key components:

■ **A comprehensive history;**

■ **A comprehensive examination; and**

■ **Medical decision making of high complexity.**

Counseling and/or coordination of care with other physicians, other qualified health care professionals, or agencies are provided consistent with the nature of the problem(s) and the patient's and/or family's needs.

Usually, the problem(s) requiring admission to "observation status" are of high severity. Typically, 70 minutes are spent at the bedside and on the patient's hospital floor or unit.

➔ *CPT Assistant* Spring 93:34, Fall 95:16, Nov 97:2, Mar 98:1, Sep 98:5, Sep 00:3, Jan 03:10, Aug 04:11, Nov 05:10, Sep 06:8, Dec 06:14, Sep 10:4, Oct 10:6, Jun 11:3, Jul 12:11; *CPT Changes: An Insider's View* 2012, 2013

Subsequent Observation Care

►All levels of subsequent observation care include reviewing the medical record and reviewing the results of diagnostic studies and changes in the patient's status (ie, changes in history, physical condition, and response to management) since the last assessment.◄

#▲ 99224   **Subsequent observation care,** per day, for the evaluation and management of a patient, which requires at least 2 of these 3 key components:

- **Problem focused interval history;**
- **Problem focused examination;**
- **Medical decision making that is straightforward or of low complexity.**

Counseling and/or coordination of care with other physicians, other qualified health care professionals, or agencies are provided consistent with the nature of the problem(s) and the patient's and/or family's needs.

Usually, the patient is stable, recovering, or improving. Typically, 15 minutes are spent at the bedside and on the patient's hospital floor or unit.

➔ *CPT Assistant* Jun 11:3, Aug 11:11, Jul 12:10, 11; *CPT Changes: An Insider's View* 2011, 2013

#▲ 99225   **Subsequent observation care,** per day, for the evaluation and management of a patient, which requires at least 2 of these 3 key components:

- **An expanded problem focused interval history;**
- **An expanded problem focused examination;**
- **Medical decision making of moderate complexity.**

Counseling and/or coordination of care with other physicians, other qualified health care professionals, or agencies are provided consistent with the nature of the problem(s) and the patient's and/or family's needs.

Usually, the patient is responding inadequately to therapy or has developed a minor complication. Typically, 25 minutes are spent at the bedside and on the patient's hospital floor or unit.

➔ *CPT Assistant* Jun 11:3, Aug 11:11, Jul 12:10, 11; *CPT Changes: An Insider's View* 2011, 2013

#▲ 99226   **Subsequent observation care,** per day, for the evaluation and management of a patient, which requires at least 2 of these 3 key components:

- **A detailed interval history;**
- **A detailed examination;**
- **Medical decision making of high complexity.**

Counseling and/or coordination of care with other physicians, other qualified health care professionals, or agencies are provided consistent with the nature of the problem(s) and the patient's and/or family's needs.

Usually, the patient is unstable or has developed a significant complication or a significant new problem. Typically, 35 minutes are spent at the bedside and on the patient's hospital floor or unit.

➔ *CPT Assistant* Jun 11:3, Aug 11:11, Jul 12:10, 11; *CPT Changes: An Insider's View* 2011, 2013

Hospital Inpatient Services

►The following codes are used to report evaluation and management services provided to hospital inpatients. Hospital inpatient services include those services provided to patients in a "partial hospital" setting. These codes are to be used to report these partial hospitalization services. See also psychiatry notes in the full text of the CPT code set.◄

For definitions of key components and commonly used terms, please see **Evaluation and Management Services Guidelines.** For Hospital Observation Services, see 99218-99220, 99224-99226. For a patient admitted and discharged from observation or inpatient status on the same date, the services should be reported with codes 99234-99236 as appropriate.

—— *Coding Tip* ——

The Significance of Time as a Factor in Selection of an Evaluation and Management Code

The inclusion of time as an explicit factor beginning in CPT 1992 is done to assist in selecting the most appropriate level of E/M services. It should be recognized that the specific times expressed in the visit code descriptors are averages and, therefore, represent a range of times that may be higher or lower depending on actual clinical circumstances.

Intraservice times are defined as **face-to-face** time for office and other outpatient visits and as **unit/floor** time for hospital and other inpatient visits. This distinction is necessary because most of the work of typical office visits takes place during the face-to-face time with the patient, while most of the work of typical hospital visits takes place during the time spent on the patient's floor or unit.

Unit/floor time (hospital observation services, inpatient hospital care, initial inpatient hospital consultations, nursing facility):

For reporting purposes, intraservice time for these services is defined as unit/floor time, which includes the time present on the patient's hospital unit and at the bedside rendering services for that patient. This includes the time to establish and/or review the patient's chart, examine the patient, write notes, and communicate with other professionals and the patient's family.

In the hospital, pre- and post-time includes time spent off the patient's floor performing such tasks as reviewing pathology and radiology findings in another part of the hospital.

This pre- and postvisit time is not included in the time component described in these codes. However, the pre- and post-work performed during the time spent off the floor or unit was included in calculating the total work of typical services in physician surveys.

Thus, the unit/floor time associated with the services described by any code is a valid proxy for the total work done before, during, and after the visit.

CPT Coding Guidelines, Evaluation and Management, Definitions of Commonly Used Terms, Time

Initial Hospital Care

New or Established Patient

The following codes are used to report the first hospital inpatient encounter with the patient by the admitting physician.

For initial inpatient encounters by physicians other than the admitting physician, see initial inpatient consultation codes (99251-99255) or subsequent hospital care codes (99231-99233) as appropriate.

For admission services for the neonate (28 days of age or younger) requiring intensive observation, frequent interventions, and other intensive care services, see 99477.

►When the patient is admitted to the hospital as an inpatient in the course of an encounter in another site of service (eg, hospital emergency department, observation status in a hospital, office, nursing facility) all evaluation and management services provided by that physician in conjunction with that admission are considered part of the initial hospital care when performed on the same date as the admission. The inpatient care level of service reported by the admitting physician should include the services related to the admission he/she provided in the other sites of service as well as in the inpatient setting.

Evaluation and management services including new or established patient office or other outpatient services (99201-99215), emergency department services (99281-99285), nursing facility services (99304-99318), domiciliary, rest home, or custodial care services (99324-99337), home services (99341-99350), and preventive medicine services (99381-99397) on the same date

related to the admission to "observation status" should **not** be reported separately. For a patient admitted and discharged from observation or inpatient status on the same date, the services should be reported with codes 99234-99236 as appropriate.◄

▲ **99221**   **Initial hospital care,** per day, for the evaluation and management of a patient, which requires these 3 key components:

- **A detailed or comprehensive history;**
- **A detailed or comprehensive examination; and**
- **Medical decision making that is straightforward or of low complexity.**

Counseling and/or coordination of care with other physicians, other qualified health care professionals, or agencies are provided consistent with the nature of the problem(s) and the patient's and/or family's needs.

Usually, the problem(s) requiring admission are of low severity. Typically, 30 minutes are spent at the bedside and on the patient's hospital floor or unit.

➔ *CPT Assistant* Winter 91:11, Spring 92:14, 24, Summer 92:10, 24, Fall 92:1, Spring 93:34, Spring 95:1, Fall 95:9, Jul 96:11, Sep 96:10, Nov 97:2, Mar 98:1, Sep 98:5, Jan 02:2-3, Apr 03:26, Apr 04:14, Aug 04:11, May 05:1, Sep 06:8, Jul 07:12, Jul 12:12; *CPT Changes: An Insider's View* 2013

▲ **99222**   **Initial hospital care,** per day, for the evaluation and management of a patient, which requires these 3 key components:

- **A comprehensive history;**
- **A comprehensive examination; and**
- **Medical decision making of moderate complexity.**

Counseling and/or coordination of care with other physicians, other qualified health care professionals, or agencies are provided consistent with the nature of the problem(s) and the patient's and/or family's needs.

Usually, the problem(s) requiring admission are of moderate severity. Typically, 50 minutes are spent at the bedside and on the patient's hospital floor or unit.

➔ *CPT Assistant* Winter 91:11, Spring 92:14, 24, Summer 92:10, 24, Fall 92:1, Spring 93:34, Spring 95:1, Fall 95:9, Jul 96:11, Sep 96:10, Nov 97:2, Mar 98:1, Sep 98:5, Jan 02:2-3, Apr 03:26, Apr 04:14, Aug 04:11, Sep 06:8, Jul 07:12, Jul 12:12; *CPT Changes: An Insider's View* 2013

▲ **99223**   **Initial hospital care,** per day, for the evaluation and management of a patient, which requires these 3 key components:

- **A comprehensive history;**
- **A comprehensive examination; and**
- **Medical decision making of high complexity.**

Counseling and/or coordination of care with other physicians, other qualified health care professionals, or agencies are provided consistent with the nature of the problem(s) and the patient's and/or family's needs.

Usually, the problem(s) requiring admission are of high severity. Typically, 70 minutes are spent at the bedside and on the patient's hospital floor or unit.

➡ *CPT Assistant* Winter 91:11, Spring 92:14, 24, Summer 92:10, 24, Fall 92:1, Spring 93:34, Spring 95:1, Fall 95:9, Jul 96:11, Sep 96:10, Nov 97:2, Mar 98:1, Sep 98:5, Jan 02:2-3, Apr 03:26, Apr 04:14, Aug 04:11, Sep 06:8, Jul 07:12, Jul 12:12; *CPT Changes: An Insider's View* 2013

99224   Code is out of numerical sequence. See 99224-99226

99225   Code is out of numerical sequence. See 99224-99226

99226   Code is out of numerical sequence. See 99224-99226

Subsequent Hospital Care

▶All levels of subsequent hospital care include reviewing the medical record and reviewing the results of diagnostic studies and changes in the patient's status (ie, changes in history, physical condition and response to management) since the last assessment.◀

▲ **99231**   **Subsequent hospital care,** per day, for the evaluation and management of a patient, which requires at least 2 of these 3 key components:

- **A problem focused interval history;**
- **A problem focused examination;**
- **Medical decision making that is straightforward or of low complexity.**

Counseling and/or coordination of care with other physicians, other qualified health care professionals, or agencies are provided consistent with the nature of the problem(s) and the patient's and/or family's needs.

Usually, the patient is stable, recovering or improving. Typically, 15 minutes are spent at the bedside and on the patient's hospital floor or unit.

➡ *CPT Assistant* Winter 91:11, Spring 92:14, 24, Summer 92:10, 24, Fall 92:1, Spring 93:34, Spring 95:1, Fall 95:16, Nov 97:2, Sep 98:5, Jan 99:10, Nov 99:5, Aug 01:2, Jan 02:2-3, Apr 04:14, Aug 04:11, Mar 05:11, May 05:1, May 06:1, 16, Jul 06:4, Mar 07:9, Jul 07:1, Mar 09:3, Dec 09:9, Jun 11:3, Jul 12:12; *CPT Changes: An Insider's View* 2013

▲ **99232**   **Subsequent hospital care,** per day, for the evaluation and management of a patient, which requires at least 2 of these 3 key components:

- **An expanded problem focused interval history;**
- **An expanded problem focused examination;**
- **Medical decision making of moderate complexity.**

Counseling and/or coordination of care with other physicians, other qualified health care professionals, or agencies are provided consistent with the nature of the problem(s) and the patient's and/or family's needs.

Usually, the patient is responding inadequately to therapy or has developed a minor complication. Typically, 25 minutes are spent at the bedside and on the patient's hospital floor or unit.

➡ *CPT Assistant* Winter 91:11, Spring 92:14, 24, Summer 92:10, 24, Fall 92:1, Spring 93:34, Spring 95:1, Fall 95:16, Nov 97:2, Sep 98:5, Jan 99:10, Nov 99:5, Jan 00:11, Aug 01:2, Apr 04:14, Aug 04:11, May 06:1, 16, Jul 06:4, Mar 07:9, Jul 07:1, Mar 09:3, Dec 09:9, Jun 11:3, Jul 12:12; *CPT Changes: An Insider's View* 2013

▲ **99233**   **Subsequent hospital care,** per day, for the evaluation and management of a patient, which requires at least 2 of these 3 key components:

- **A detailed interval history;**
- **A detailed examination;**
- **Medical decision making of high complexity.**

Counseling and/or coordination of care with other physicians, other qualified health care professionals, or agencies are provided consistent with the nature of the problem(s) and the patient's and/or family's needs.

Usually, the patient is unstable or has developed a significant complication or a significant new problem. Typically, 35 minutes are spent at the bedside and on the patient's hospital floor or unit.

➡ *CPT Assistant* Winter 91:11, Spring 92:14, 24, Summer 92:10, 24, Fall 92:1, Spring 93:34, Spring 95:1, Fall 95:16, Nov 97:2, Sep 98:5, Jan 99:10, Nov 99:5, Aug 01:2, Apr 04:14, Aug 04:11, May 06:1, 16, Jul 06:4, Mar 07:9, Jul 07:1, Mar 09:3, Dec 09:9, Jun 11:3, Jul 12:12; *CPT Changes: An Insider's View* 2013

Observation or Inpatient Care Services (Including Admission and Discharge Services)

▶The following codes are used to report observation or inpatient hospital care services provided to patients admitted and discharged on the same date of service. When a patient is admitted to the hospital from observation status on the same date, only the initial hospital care code should be reported. The initial hospital care code reported by the admitting physician or other qualified health care professional should include the services related to the observation status services he/she provided on the same date of inpatient admission.

When "observation status" is initiated in the course of an encounter in another site of service (eg, hospital emergency department, office, nursing facility) all evaluation and management services provided by the supervising physician or other qualified health care professional in conjunction with initiating "observation status" are considered part of the initial observation care when performed on the same date. The observation care level of service should include the services related to initiating "observation status" provided in the other sites of service as well as in the observation setting when provided by the same individual.◀

Evaluation/Management

For patients admitted to observation or inpatient care and discharged on a different date, see codes 99218-99220, 99224-99226, 99217, or 99221-99223, 99238 and 99239.

▲ **99234**   **Observation or inpatient hospital care,** for the evaluation and management of a patient including admission and discharge on the same date, which requires these 3 key components:

- **A detailed or comprehensive history;**
- **A detailed or comprehensive examination; and**
- **Medical decision making that is straightforward or of low complexity.**

Counseling and/or coordination of care with other physicians, other qualified health care professionals, or agencies are provided consistent with the nature of the problem(s) and the patient's and/or family's needs.

Usually the presenting problem(s) requiring admission are of low severity. Typically, 40 minutes are spent at the bedside and on the patient's hospital floor or unit.

➥ *CPT Assistant* Nov 97:2, Mar 98:2, May 98:1, Sep 98:5, Jan 00:11, Sep 00:3, Jan 02:2, Jun 02:10, Jan 03:10, May 05:1, Nov 05:10, Sep 06:8, Dec 06:14, Sep 10:4, Jun 11:3, Jul 12:14; *CPT Changes: An Insider's View* 2013

▲ **99235**   **Observation or inpatient hospital care,** for the evaluation and management of a patient including admission and discharge on the same date, which requires these 3 key components:

- **A comprehensive history;**
- **A comprehensive examination; and**
- **Medical decision making of moderate complexity.**

Counseling and/or coordination of care with other physicians, other qualified health care professionals, or agencies are provided consistent with the nature of the problem(s) and the patient's and/or family's needs.

Usually the presenting problem(s) requiring admission are of moderate severity. Typically, 50 minutes are spent at the bedside and on the patient's hospital floor or unit.

➥ *CPT Assistant* Nov 97:2, Mar 98:2, May 98:1, Sep 98:5, Jan 00:11, Sep 00:3, Jan 02:2, Jun 02:10, Jan 03:10, Nov 05:10, Sep 06:8, Dec 06:14, Sep 10:4, Jun 11:3, Jul 12:14; *CPT Changes: An Insider's View* 2013

▲ **99236**   **Observation or inpatient hospital care,** for the evaluation and management of a patient including admission and discharge on the same date, which requires these 3 key components:

- **A comprehensive history;**
- **A comprehensive examination; and**
- **Medical decision making of high complexity.**

Counseling and/or coordination of care with other physicians, other qualified health care professionals, or agencies are provided consistent with the nature of the problem(s) and the patient's and/or family's needs.

Usually the presenting problem(s) requiring admission are of high severity. Typically, 55 minutes are spent at the bedside and on the patient's hospital floor or unit.

➥ *CPT Assistant* Nov 97:2, Mar 98:2, May 98:1, Sep 98:5, Jan 00:11, Sep 00:3, Jan 02:2, Jun 02:10, Jan 03:10, Nov 05:10, Sep 06:8, Dec 06:14, Sep 10:4, Jun 11:3, Jul 12:14; *CPT Changes: An Insider's View* 2013

Hospital Discharge Services

The hospital discharge day management codes are to be used to report the total duration of time spent by a physician for final hospital discharge of a patient. The codes include, as appropriate, final examination of the patient, discussion of the hospital stay, even if the time spent by the physician on that date is not continuous, instructions for continuing care to all relevant caregivers, and preparation of discharge records, prescriptions and referral forms. For a patient admitted and discharged from observation or inpatient status on the same date, the services should be reported with codes 99234-99236 as appropriate.

99238   **Hospital discharge day management**; 30 minutes or less

➥ *CPT Assistant* Fall 92:1, Spring 93:4, Nov 97:4, Mar 98:3, 11, May 98:2, Jan 99:10, Jan 02:2, Aug 04:11, May 05:1, Sep 06:8, Nov 09:10, Dec 09:9, Jul 11:16, Jul 12:10, 12

99239   more than 30 minutes

➥ *CPT Assistant* Nov 97:4, Mar 98:3, 11, May 98:2, Jan 99:10, Jan 02:2, Aug 04:11, Sep 06:8, Nov 09:10, Dec 09:9, Jul 11:16, Jul 12:12

▶(These codes are to be utilized by the physician to report all services provided to a patient on the date of discharge, if other than the initial date of inpatient status. To report services to a patient who is admitted as an inpatient and discharged on the same date, see codes 99234-99236 for observation or inpatient hospital care including the admission and discharge of the patient on the same date. To report concurrent care services provided by a physician[s] other than the ordering physician or another qualified health care professional, use subsequent hospital care codes [99231-99233] on the day of discharge.)◀

(For Observation Care Discharge, use 99217)

(For observation or inpatient hospital care including the admission and discharge of the patient on the same date, see 99234-99236)

(For Nursing Facility Care Discharge, see 99315, 99316)

(For discharge services provided to newborns admitted and discharged on the same date, use 99463)

Consultations

▶A consultation is a type of evaluation and management service provided at the request of another physician or appropriate source to either recommend care for a specific condition or problem or to determine whether to accept responsibility for ongoing management of the patient's entire care or for the care of a specific condition or problem.◄

A physician consultant may initiate diagnostic and/or therapeutic services at the same or subsequent visit.

A "consultation" initiated by a patient and/or family, and not requested by a physician or other appropriate source (eg, physician assistant, nurse practitioner, doctor of chiropractic, physical therapist, occupational therapist, speech-language pathologist, psychologist, social worker, lawyer, or insurance company), is not reported using the consultation codes but may be reported using the office visit, home service, or domiciliary/rest home care codes as appropriate.

The written or verbal request for consult may be made by a physician or other appropriate source and documented in the patient's medical record by either the consulting or requesting physician or appropriate source. The consultant's opinion and any services that were ordered or performed must also be documented in the patient's medical record and communicated by written report to the requesting physician or other appropriate source.

If a consultation is mandated (eg, by a third-party payer) modifier 32 should also be reported.

Any specifically identifiable procedure (ie, identified with a specific CPT code) performed on or subsequent to the date of the initial consultation should be reported separately.

►If subsequent to the completion of a consultation the consultant assumes responsibility for management of a portion or all of the patient's condition(s), the appropriate **Evaluation and Management** services code for the site of service should be reported. In the hospital or nursing facility setting, the consultant should use the appropriate inpatient consultation code for the initial encounter and then subsequent hospital or nursing facility care codes. In the office setting, the consultant should use the appropriate office or other outpatient consultation codes and then the established patient office or other outpatient services codes.◄

To report services provided to a patient who is admitted to a hospital or nursing facility in the course of an encounter in the office or other ambulatory facility, see the notes for Initial Hospital Inpatient Care (page 15) or Initial Nursing Facility Care (page 25).

For definitions of key components and commonly used terms, please see **Evaluation and Management Services Guidelines.**

Office or Other Outpatient Consultations

New or Established Patient

►The following codes are used to report consultations provided in the office or in an outpatient or other ambulatory facility, including hospital observation services, home services, domiciliary, rest home, or emergency department (see the preceding consultation definition above). Follow-up visits in the consultant's office or other outpatient facility that are initiated by the consultant or patient are reported using the appropriate codes for established patients, office visits (99211-99215), domiciliary, rest home (99334-99337), or home (99347-99350). If an additional request for an opinion or advice regarding the same or a new problem is received from another physician or other appropriate source and documented in the medical record, the office consultation codes may be used again. Services that constitute transfer of care (ie, are provided for the management of the patient's entire care or for the care of a specific condition or problem) are reported with the appropriate new or established patient codes for office or other outpatient visits, domiciliary, rest home services, or home services.◄

─── *Coding Tip* ───

Definition of Transfer of Care

Transfer of care is the process whereby a physician or other qualified health care professional who is providing management for some or all of a patient's problems relinquishes this responsibility to another physician or other qualified health care professional who explicitly agrees to accept this responsibility and who, from the initial encounter, is not providing consultative services. The physician or other qualified health care professional transferring care is then no longer providing care for these problems though he or she may continue providing care for other conditions when appropriate. Consultation codes should not be reported by the physician or other qualified health care professional who has agreed to accept transfer of care before an initial evaluation but are appropriate to report if the decision to accept transfer of care cannot be made until after the initial consultation evaluation, regardless of site of service.

CPT Coding Guidelines, Evaluation and Management, Definitions of Commonly Used Terms, Concurrent Care and Transfer of Care

▲ **99241**   **Office consultation** for a new or established patient, which requires these 3 key components:

   ▪ **A problem focused history;**
   ▪ **A problem focused examination; and**
   ▪ **Straightforward medical decision making.**

   Counseling and/or coordination of care with other physicians, other qualified health care professionals, or agencies are provided consistent with the nature of the problem(s) and the patient's and/or family's needs.

Usually, the presenting problem(s) are self limited or minor. Typically, 15 minutes are spent face-to-face with the patient and/or family.

→ *CPT Assistant* Winter 91:11, Spring 92:4, 23-24, Summer 92:12, Spring 93:4, Spring 95:1, Oct 97:1, Sep 98:5, Jun 99:10, Apr 00:10, Aug 01:3, Jan 02:2, Jul 02:2, Sep 02:11, May 05:1, Dec 05:10, Jan 06:46, May 06:1, 16, Jun 06:1, Sep 06:8, Jan 07:28, Apr 07:11, Jul 07:1, May 08:13, Nov 08:10, Aug 09:9, Jan 10:3, Jul 10:4, Jun 11:3, Apr 12:10; *CPT Changes: An Insider's View* 2013

→ *Clinical Examples in Radiology* Summer 09:3

▲ **99242** **Office consultation** for a new or established patient, which requires these 3 key components:

- **An expanded problem focused history;**
- **An expanded problem focused examination; and**
- **Straightforward medical decision making.**

Counseling and/or coordination of care with other physicians, other qualified health care professionals, or agencies are provided consistent with the nature of the problem(s) and the patient's and/or family's needs.

Usually, the presenting problem(s) are of low severity. Typically, 30 minutes are spent face-to-face with the patient and/or family.

→ *CPT Assistant* Winter 91:11, Spring 92:4, 23-24, Summer 92:12, Spring 93:2, 34, Spring 95:1, Oct 97:1, Sep 98:5, Aug 01:3, Jan 02:2, Jul 02:2, Sep 02:11, Dec 05:10, May 06:1, 16, Jun 06:1, Sep 06:8, Apr 07:11, Jul 07:1, Jan 10:3, Jun 11:3; *CPT Changes: An Insider's View* 2000, 2013

→ *Clinical Examples in Radiology* Summer 09:3

▲ **99243** **Office consultation** for a new or established patient, which requires these 3 key components:

- **A detailed history;**
- **A detailed examination; and**
- **Medical decision making of low complexity.**

Counseling and/or coordination of care with other physicians, other qualified health care professionals, or agencies are provided consistent with the nature of the problem(s) and the patient's and/or family's needs.

Usually, the presenting problem(s) are of moderate severity. Typically, 40 minutes are spent face-to-face with the patient and/or family.

→ *CPT Assistant* Winter 91:11, Spring 92:4, 23-24, Summer 92:12, Spring 93:2, 34, Spring 95:1, Oct 97:1, Sep 98:5, Aug 01:3, Jan 02:2, Jul 02:2, Sep 02:11, Oct 03:5, Dec 05:10, May 06:1, 16, Jun 06:1, Sep 06:8, Apr 07:11, Jul 07:1, Jan 10:3, Jun 11:3; *CPT Changes: An Insider's View* 2013

→ *Clinical Examples in Radiology* Summer 09:3

▲ **99244** **Office consultation** for a new or established patient, which requires these 3 key components:

- **A comprehensive history;**
- **A comprehensive examination; and**
- **Medical decision making of moderate complexity.**

Counseling and/or coordination of care with other physicians, other qualified health care professionals, or agencies are provided consistent with the nature of the problem(s) and the patient's and/or family's needs.

Usually, the presenting problem(s) are of moderate to high severity. Typically, 60 minutes are spent face-to-face with the patient and/or family.

→ *CPT Assistant* Winter 91:11, Spring 92:3, 23-24, Summer 92:12, Spring 93:2, 34, Spring 95:1, Oct 97:1, Sep 98:5, Aug 01:3, Jan 02:2, Jul 02:2, Sep 02:11, Oct 03:5, Dec 05:10, May 06:1, 16, Jun 06:1, Sep 06:8, Apr 07:11, Jul 07:1, Jan 10:3, Jun 11:3; *CPT Changes: An Insider's View* 2013

→ *Clinical Examples in Radiology* Summer 09:2, 3

▲ **99245** **Office consultation** for a new or established patient, which requires these 3 key components:

- **A comprehensive history;**
- **A comprehensive examination; and**
- **Medical decision making of high complexity.**

Counseling and/or coordination of care with other physicians, other qualified health care professionals, or agencies are provided consistent with the nature of the problem(s) and the patient's and/or family's needs.

Usually, the presenting problem(s) are of moderate to high severity. Typically, 80 minutes are spent face-to-face with the patient and/or family.

→ *CPT Assistant* Winter 91:11, Spring 92:4, 23-24, Summer 92:12, Spring 93:2, 34, Spring 95:1, Oct 97:1, Sep 98:5, Aug 01:2, Jan 02:2, Jul 02:2, Sep 02:11, Dec 05:10, May 06:1, 16, Jun 06:1, Sep 06:8, Apr 07:11, Jul 07:1, Jan 10:3, Jul 10:4, Jun 11:3, Apr 12:10; *CPT Changes: An Insider's View* 2013

→ *Clinical Examples in Radiology* Summer 09:3

Inpatient Consultations

New or Established Patient

▶The following codes are used to report physician or other qualified health care professional consultations provided to hospital inpatients, residents of nursing facilities, or patients in a partial hospital setting. Only one consultation should be reported by a consultant per admission. Subsequent services during the same admission are reported using subsequent hospital care codes (99231-99233) or subsequent nursing facility care codes (99307-99310), including services to complete the initial consultation, monitor progress, revise recommendations, or address a new problem. Use subsequent hospital care codes (99231-99233) or subsequent nursing facility care codes (99307-99310) to report transfer of care services (see page 4, Concurrent Care and Transfer of Care definitions).

When an inpatient consultation is performed on a date that a patient is admitted to a hospital or nursing facility, all evaluation and management services provided by the consultant related to the admission are reported with the inpatient consultation service code (99251-99255). If a patient is admitted after an outpatient consultation (office, emergency department, etc), and the patient is not seen on the unit on the date of admission, only report the outpatient consultation code (99241-99245). If the patient is seen by the consultant on the unit on the date of admission, report all evaluation and management services provided by the consultant related to the admission with either the inpatient consultation code (99251-99255) or with the initial inpatient admission service code (99221-99223). Do not report both an outpatient consultation (99241-99245) and inpatient consultation (99251-99255) for services related to the same inpatient stay. When transfer of care services are provided on a date subsequent to the outpatient consultation, use the subsequent hospital care codes (99231-99233) or subsequent nursing facility care codes (99307-99310).◄

▲ **99251**   **Inpatient consultation** for a new or established patient, which requires these 3 key components:

- **A problem focused history;**
- **A problem focused examination; and**
- **Straightforward medical decision making.**

Counseling and/or coordination of care with other physicians, other qualified health care professionals, or agencies are provided consistent with the nature of the problem(s) and the patient's and/or family's needs.

Usually, the presenting problem(s) are self limited or minor. Typically, 20 minutes are spent at the bedside and on the patient's hospital floor or unit.

➔ *CPT Assistant* Winter 91:11, Spring 92:16, 23-24, Summer 92:12, Spring 93:34, Spring 95:1, Oct 97:1, Sep 98:5, Aug 01:3, Sep 02:11, May 05:1, May 06:1, 16, Jun 06:1, Jul 06:19, Jul 07:1, Jan 10:3; *CPT Changes: An Insider's View* 2007, 2013

➔ *Clinical Examples in Radiology* Summer 09:3

▲ **99252**   **Inpatient consultation** for a new or established patient, which requires these 3 key components:

- **An expanded problem focused history;**
- **An expanded problem focused examination; and**
- **Straightforward medical decision making.**

Counseling and/or coordination of care with other physicians, other qualified health care professionals, or agencies are provided consistent with the nature of the problem(s) and the patient's and/or family's needs.

Usually, the presenting problem(s) are of low severity. Typically, 40 minutes are spent at the bedside and on the patient's hospital floor or unit.

➔ *CPT Assistant* Winter 91:11, Spring 92:16, 23-24, Summer 92:12, Summer 93:34, Spring 95:1, Oct 97:1, Sep 98:5, Aug 01:4, Sep 02:11, May 06:1, 16, Jun 06:1, Jul 06:19, Jul 07:1, Jan 10:3; *CPT Changes: An Insider's View* 2007, 2013

➔ *Clinical Examples in Radiology* Summer 09:3

▲ **99253**   **Inpatient consultation** for a new or established patient, which requires these 3 key components:

- **A detailed history;**
- **A detailed examination; and**
- **Medical decision making of low complexity.**

Counseling and/or coordination of care with other physicians, other qualified health care professionals, or agencies are provided consistent with the nature of the problem(s) and the patient's and/or family's needs.

Usually, the presenting problem(s) are of moderate severity. Typically, 55 minutes are spent at the bedside and on the patient's hospital floor or unit.

➔ *CPT Assistant* Winter 91:11, Spring 92:16, 23-24, Summer 92:12, Summer 93:34, Spring 95:1, Oct 97:1, Sep 98:5, Aug 01:4, Sep 02:11, May 06:1, 16, Jun 06:1, Jul 06:19, Jul 07:1, Jan 10:3; *CPT Changes: An Insider's View* 2007, 2013

➔ *Clinical Examples in Radiology* Summer 09:3

▲ **99254**   **Inpatient consultation** for a new or established patient, which requires these 3 key components:

- **A comprehensive history;**
- **A comprehensive examination; and**
- **Medical decision making of moderate complexity.**

Counseling and/or coordination of care with other physicians, other qualified health care professionals, or agencies are provided consistent with the nature of the problem(s) and the patient's and/or family's needs.

Usually, the presenting problem(s) are of moderate to high severity. Typically, 80 minutes are spent at the bedside and on the patient's hospital floor or unit.

➔ *CPT Assistant* Winter 91:11, Spring 92:16, 23-24, Summer 92:12, Summer 93:34, Spring 95:1, Oct 97:1, Sep 98:5, Aug 01:4, Sep 02:11, May 06:1, 16, Jun 06:1, Jul 06:19, Jul 07:1, Jan 10:3; *CPT Changes: An Insider's View* 2007, 2013

➔ *Clinical Examples in Radiology* Summer 09:3

▲ **99255**   **Inpatient consultation** for a new or established patient, which requires these 3 key components:

- **A comprehensive history;**
- **A comprehensive examination; and**
- **Medical decision making of high complexity.**

Counseling and/or coordination of care with other physicians, other qualified health care professionals, or agencies are provided consistent with the nature of the problem(s) and the patient's and/or family's needs.

Usually, the presenting problem(s) are of moderate to high severity. Typically, 110 minutes are spent at the bedside and on the patient's hospital floor or unit.

➔ *CPT Assistant* Winter 91:11, Spring 92:16, 23-24, Summer 92:12, Summer 93:34, Spring 95:1, Oct 97:1, Sep 98:5, Aug 01:4, Sep 02:11, May 06:1, 16, Jun 06:1, Jul 06:19, Jul 07:1, Jan 10:3; *CPT Changes: An Insider's View* 2007, 2013

➔ *Clinical Examples in Radiology* Summer 09:3

Emergency Department Services

New or Established Patient

The following codes are used to report evaluation and management services provided in the emergency department. No distinction is made between new and established patients in the emergency department.

An emergency department is defined as an organized hospital-based facility for the provision of unscheduled episodic services to patients who present for immediate medical attention. The facility must be available 24 hours a day.

For critical care services provided in the emergency department, see Critical Care notes and 99291, 99292.

For evaluation and management services provided to a patient in an observation area of a hospital, see 99217-99220.

For observation or inpatient care services (including admission and discharge services), see 99234-99236.

— *Coding Tip* —

Time as a Factor in the Emergency Department Setting

Time is **not** a descriptive component for the emergency department levels of E/M services because emergency department services are typically provided on a variable intensity basis, often involving multiple encounters with several patients over an extended period of time. Therefore, it is often difficult for physicians to provide accurate estimates of the time spent face-to-face with the patient.

CPT Coding Guidelines, Evaluation and Management, Definitions of Commonly Used Terms, Time

▲ **99281** **Emergency department visit** for the evaluation and management of a patient, which requires these 3 key components:

- **A problem focused history;**
- **A problem focused examination; and**
- **Straightforward medical decision making.**

Counseling and/or coordination of care with other physicians, other qualified health care professionals, or agencies are provided consistent with the nature of the problem(s) and the patient's and/or family's needs.

Usually, the presenting problem(s) are self limited or minor.

➲ *CPT Assistant* Winter 91:11, Spring 92:24, Summer 92:18, Spring 93:34, Spring 95:1, Feb 96:3, Sep 98:5, Jan 00:11, Feb 00:11, Sep 00:3, Apr 02:14, Jul 02:2, Nov 05:10, Feb 06:14, Dec 06:14, Dec 07:13; *CPT Changes: An Insider's View* 2013

▲ **99282** **Emergency department visit** for the evaluation and management of a patient, which requires these 3 key components:

- **An expanded problem focused history;**
- **An expanded problem focused examination; and**
- **Medical decision making of low complexity.**

Counseling and/or coordination of care with other physicians, other qualified health care professionals, or agencies are provided consistent with the nature of the problem(s) and the patient's and/or family's needs.

Usually, the presenting problem(s) are of low to moderate severity.

➲ *CPT Assistant* Winter 91:11, Spring 92:24, Summer 92:18, Spring 93:34, Spring 95:1, Summer 95:1, Feb 96:3, Sep 98:5, Jan 00:11, Feb 00:11, Sep 00:3, Apr 02:14, Jul 02:2, Nov 05:10, Feb 06:14, Dec 06:14, Dec 07:13; *CPT Changes: An Insider's View* 2013

▲ **99283** **Emergency department visit** for the evaluation and management of a patient, which requires these 3 key components:

- **An expanded problem focused history;**
- **An expanded problem focused examination; and**
- **Medical decision making of moderate complexity.**

Counseling and/or coordination of care with other physicians, other qualified health care professionals, or agencies are provided consistent with the nature of the problem(s) and the patient's and/or family's needs.

Usually, the presenting problem(s) are of moderate severity.

➲ *CPT Assistant* Winter 91:11, Spring 92:24, Summer 92:18, Spring 93:34, Spring 95:1, Feb 96:3, Sep 98:5, Jan 00:11, Feb 00:11, Sep 00:3, Apr 02:14, Jul 02:2, Nov 05:10, Feb 06:14, Dec 06:14, Dec 07:13; *CPT Changes: An Insider's View* 2013

▲ **99284** **Emergency department visit** for the evaluation and management of a patient, which requires these 3 key components:

- **A detailed history;**
- **A detailed examination; and**
- **Medical decision making of moderate complexity.**

Counseling and/or coordination of care with other physicians, other qualified health care professionals, or agencies are provided consistent with the nature of the problem(s) and the patient's and/or family's needs.

Usually, the presenting problem(s) are of high severity, and require urgent evaluation by the physician or other qualified health care professionals but do not pose an immediate significant threat to life or physiologic function.

➲ *CPT Assistant* Winter 91:11, Spring 92:24, Summer 92:18, Spring 93:34, Spring 95:1, Summer 95:1, Feb 96:3, Sep 98:5, Jan 00:11, Feb 00:11, Sep 00:3, Apr 02:14, Jul 02:2, Nov 05:10, Feb 06:14, Dec 06:14, Dec 07:13; *CPT Changes: An Insider's View* 2013

▲ **99285** **Emergency department visit** for the evaluation and management of a patient, which requires these 3 key components within the constraints imposed by the urgency of the patient's clinical condition and/or mental status:

- **A comprehensive history;**
- **A comprehensive examination; and**
- **Medical decision making of high complexity.**

Counseling and/or coordination of care with other physicians, other qualified health care professionals, or agencies are provided consistent with the nature of the problem(s) and the patient's and/or family's needs.

Usually, the presenting problem(s) are of high severity and pose an immediate significant threat to life or physiologic function.

➔ *CPT Assistant* Winter 91:11, Spring 92:24, Summer 92:18, Spring 93:34, Spring 95:1, Summer 95:1, Feb 96:3, Aug 98:8, Sep 98:5, Nov 99:23, Jan 00:11, Feb 00:11, Sep 00:3, Apr 02:14, Jul 02:2, Sep 02:11, Mar 05:11, Nov 05:10, Feb 06:14, Dec 06:14, Dec 07:13; *CPT Changes: An Insider's View* 2000, 2013

Coding Tip

Emergency Department Classification of New vs Established Patient

No distinction is made between new and established patients in the emergency department. E/M services in the emergency department category may be reported for any new or established patient who presents for treatment in the emergency department.

CPT Coding Guidelines, Evaluation and Management, Definitions of Commonly Used Terms, New and Established Patient

---

Other Emergency Services

▶In directed emergency care, advanced life support, the physician or other qualified health care professional is located in a hospital emergency or critical care department, and is in two-way voice communication with ambulance or rescue personnel outside the hospital. Direction of the performance of necessary medical procedures includes but is not limited to: telemetry of cardiac rhythm; cardiac and/or pulmonary resuscitation; endotracheal or esophageal obturator airway intubation; administration of intravenous fluids and/or administration of intramuscular, intratracheal or subcutaneous drugs; and/or electrical conversion of arrhythmia.◀

▲ **99288**   **Physician or other qualified health care professional direction of** emergency medical systems (EMS) emergency care, advanced life support

➔ *CPT Assistant* Summer 92:18, May 05:1, Nov 07:5; *CPT Changes: An Insider's View* 2013

(99289 has been deleted. To report, use 99466)

(99290 has been deleted. To report, use 99467)

Critical Care Services

▶Critical care is the direct delivery by a physician(s) or other qualified health care professional of medical care for a critically ill or critically injured patient. A critical illness or injury acutely impairs one or more vital organ systems such that there is a high probability of imminent or life threatening deterioration in the patient's condition. Critical care involves high complexity decision making to assess, manipulate, and support vital system function(s) to treat single or multiple vital organ system failure and/or to prevent further life threatening deterioration of the patient's condition. Examples of vital organ system failure include, but are not limited to: central nervous system failure, circulatory failure, shock, renal, hepatic, metabolic, and/or respiratory failure. Although critical care typically requires interpretation of multiple physiologic parameters and/or application of advanced technology(s), critical care may be provided in life threatening situations when these elements are not present. Critical care may be provided on multiple days, even if no changes are made in the treatment rendered to the patient, provided that the patient's condition continues to require the level of attention described above.◀

Providing medical care to a critically ill, injured, or post-operative patient qualifies as a critical care service only if both the illness or injury and the treatment being provided meet the above requirements. Critical care is usually, but not always, given in a critical care area, such as the coronary care unit, intensive care unit, pediatric intensive care unit, respiratory care unit, or the emergency care facility.

▶Inpatient critical care services provided to infants 29 days through 71 months of age are reported with pediatric critical care codes 99471-99476. The pediatric critical care codes are reported as long as the infant/young child qualifies for critical care services during the hospital stay through 71 months of age. Inpatient critical care services provided to neonates (28 days of age or younger) are reported with the neonatal critical care codes 99468 and 99469. The neonatal critical care codes are reported as long as the neonate qualifies for critical care services during the hospital stay through the 28th postnatal day. The reporting of the pediatric and neonatal critical care services is not based on time or the type of unit (eg, pediatric or neonatal critical care unit) and it is not dependent upon the type of physician or other qualified health care professional delivering the care. To report critical care services provided in the outpatient setting (eg, emergency department or office), for neonates and pediatric patients up through 71 months of age, see the critical care codes 99291, 99292. If the same individual provides critical care services for a neonatal or pediatric patient in both the outpatient and inpatient settings on the same day, report only the appropriate neonatal or pediatric critical care code 99468-99472 for all critical care services provided on that day. Also report 99291-99292 for neonatal or pediatric critical care services provided by the individual providing critical care at one facility but transferring the patient to another facility. Critical care services provided by a second individual of a different specialty not reporting a per day neonatal or pediatric critical care code can be reported with codes 99291, 99292. For additional instructions on reporting

---

these services, see the Neonatal and Pediatric Critical Care section and codes 99468-99476.◄

Services for a patient who is not critically ill but happens to be in a critical care unit are reported using other appropriate E/M codes.

►Critical care and other E/M services may be provided to the same patient on the same date by the same individual.◄

For reporting by professionals, the following services are included in critical care when performed during the critical period by the physician(s) providing critical care: the interpretation of cardiac output measurements (93561, 93562), chest X-rays (71010, 71015, 71020), pulse oximetry (94760, 94761, 94762), blood gases, and information data stored in computers (eg, ECGs, blood pressures, hematologic data [99090]); gastric intubation (43752, 43753); temporary transcutaneous pacing (92953); ventilatory management (94002-94004, 94660, 94662); and vascular access procedures (36000, 36410, 36415, 36591, 36600). Any services performed that are not included in this listing should be reported separately. Facilities may report the above services separately.

►Codes 99291, 99292 should be reported for the attendance during the transport of critically ill or critically injured patients older than 24 months of age to or from a facility or hospital. For transport services of critically ill or critically injured pediatric patients 24 months of age or younger, see 99466, 99467.

Codes 99291, 99292 are used to report the total duration of time spent in provision of critical care services to a critically ill or critically injured patient, even if the time spent providing care on that date is not continuous. For any given period of time spent providing critical care services, the individual must devote his or her full attention to the patient and, therefore, cannot provide services to any other patient during the same period of time.◄

Time spent with the individual patient should be recorded in the patient's record. The time that can be reported as critical care is the time spent engaged in work directly related to the individual patient's care whether that time was spent at the immediate bedside or elsewhere on the floor or unit. For example, time spent on the unit or at the nursing station on the floor reviewing test results or imaging studies, discussing the critically ill patient's care with other medical staff or documenting critical care services in the medical record would be reported as critical care, even though it does not occur at the bedside. Also, when the patient is unable or lacks capacity to participate in discussions, time spent on the floor or unit with family members or surrogate decision makers obtaining a medical history, reviewing the patient's condition or prognosis, or discussing treatment or limitation(s) of treatment may be reported as critical care, provided that the conversation bears directly on the management of the patient.

►Time spent in activities that occur outside of the unit or off the floor (eg, telephone calls whether taken at home, in the office, or elsewhere in the hospital) may not be reported as critical care since the individual is not immediately available to the patient. Time spent in activities that do not directly contribute to the treatment of the patient may not be reported as critical care, even if they are performed in the critical care unit (eg, participation in administrative meetings or telephone calls to discuss other patients). Time spent performing separately reportable procedures or services should not be included in the time reported as critical care time. No individual may report remote real-time interactive video-conferenced critical care services (0188T, 0189T) for the period in which any other physician or qualified health care professional reports codes 99291, 99292.

Code 99291 is used to report the first 30-74 minutes of critical care on a given date. It should be used only once per date even if the time spent by the individual is not continuous on that date. Critical care of less than 30 minutes total duration on a given date should be reported with the appropriate E/M code.◄

Code 99292 is used to report additional block(s) of time, of up to 30 minutes each beyond the first 74 minutes. (See the following table.)

The following examples illustrate the correct reporting of critical care services:

Total Duration of Critical Care Codes

Total Duration of Critical Care	Codes
less than 30 minutes	appropriate E/M codes
30-74 minutes (30 minutes - 1 hr. 14 min.)	99291 X 1
75-104 minutes (1 hr. 15 min. - 1 hr. 44 min.)	99291 X 1 AND 99292 X 1
105-134 minutes (1 hr. 45 min. - 2 hr. 14 min.)	99291 X 1 AND 99292 X 2
135-164 minutes (2 hr. 15 min. - 2 hr. 44 min.)	99291 X 1 AND 99292 X 3
165-194 minutes (2 hr. 45 min. - 3 hr. 14 min.)	99291 X 1 AND 99292 X 4
195 minutes or longer (3 hr. 15 min. - etc.)	99291 and 99292 as appropriate (see illustrated reporting examples above)

99291 **Critical care, evaluation and management** of the critically ill or critically injured patient; first 30-74 minutes

➜ *CPT Assistant* Summer 92:18, Summer 93:1, Summer 95:1, Jan 96:7, Apr 97:3, Dec 98:6, Nov 99:3, Apr 00:6, Sep 00:1, Dec 00:15, Jul 02:2, Feb 03:15, Oct 03:2, Aug 04:7, 10, Oct 04:14, May 05:1, Jul 05:15, Nov 05:10, Jul 06:4, Dec 06:13, Nov 07:5, Jan 09:5, Mar 09:3, Jul 09:10, Aug 11:10, Sep 11:3, Jul 12:13

+ 99292   each additional 30 minutes (List separately in
               addition to code for primary service)

➔ *CPT Assistant* Summer 92:18, Summer 93:1, Summer 95:1,
   Jan 96:7, Apr 97:3, Dec 98:6, Nov 99:3, Apr 00:6, Sep 00:1,
   Dec 00:15, Feb 03:15, Oct 03:2, Aug 04:10, Oct 04:14,
   Jul 05:15, Nov 05:10, Jul 06:4, Dec 06:13, Nov 07:5,
   Jan 09:5, Mar 09:3, Aug 11:10, Sep 11:3

(Use 99292 in conjunction with 99291)

───── *Coding Tip* ─────

Services Included in Critical Care Services

For reporting by professionals, the following services are
included in critical care when performed during the critical
period by the physician(s) providing critical care: the
interpretation of cardiac output measurements (93561,
93562), chest X-rays (71010, 71015, 71020), pulse oximetry
(94760, 94761, 94762), blood gases, and information data
stored in computers (eg, ECGs, blood pressures, hematologic
data [99090]; gastric intubation (43752, 43753); temporary
transcutaneous pacing (92953); ventilatory management
(94002-94004, 94660, 94662); and vascular access
procedures (36000, 36410, 36415, 36591, 36600). Any
services performed that are not listed above should be
reported separately. Facilities may report the above services
separately.

CPT Coding Guideline, Critical Care

(99293 has been deleted. To report, use 99471)

(99294 has been deleted. To report, use 99472)

(99295 has been deleted. To report, use 99468)

(99296 has been deleted. To report, use 99469)

(99298 has been deleted. To report, use 99478)

(99299 has been deleted. To report, use 99479)

(99300 has been deleted. To report, use 99480)

Nursing Facility Services

The following codes are used to report evaluation and
management services to patients in nursing facilities
(formerly called skilled nursing facilities [SNFs],
intermediate care facilities [ICFs], or long-term care
facilities [LTCFs]).

These codes should also be used to report evaluation and
management services provided to a patient in a
psychiatric residential treatment center (a facility or a
distinct part of a facility for psychiatric care, which
provides a 24-hour therapeutically planned and
professionally staffed group living and learning
environment). If procedures such as medical
psychotherapy are provided in addition to evaluation and
management services, these should be reported in
addition to the evaluation and management services
provided.

Nursing facilities that provide convalescent, rehabilitative,
or long term care are required to conduct comprehensive,
accurate, standardized, and reproducible assessments of
each resident's functional capacity using a Resident
Assessment Instrument (RAI). All RAIs include the
Minimum Data Set (MDS), Resident Assessment
Protocols (RAPs), and utilization guidelines. The MDS is
the primary screening and assessment tool; the RAPs
trigger the identification of potential problems and
provide guidelines for follow-up assessments.

►Physicians and other qualified health care professionals
have a central role in assuring that all residents receive
thorough assessments and that medical plans of care are
instituted or revised to enhance or maintain the residents'
physical and psychosocial functioning. This role includes
providing input in the development of the MDS and a
multi-disciplinary plan of care, as required by regulations
pertaining to the care of nursing facility residents.◄

Two major subcategories of nursing facility services are
recognized: Initial Nursing Facility Care and Subsequent
Nursing Facility Care. Both subcategories apply to new or
established patients.

For definitions of key components and commonly used
terms, please see **Evaluation and Management Services
Guidelines.**

(For care plan oversight services provided to nursing
facility residents, see 99379-99380)

Initial Nursing Facility Care

New or Established Patient

►When the patient is admitted to the nursing facility in
the course of an encounter in another site of service (eg,
hospital emergency department, office), all evaluation
and management services provided by that physician in
conjunction with that admission are considered part of
the initial nursing facility care when performed on the
same date as the admission or readmission. The nursing
facility care level of service reported by the admitting
physician should include the services related to the
admission he/she provided in the other sites of service as
well as in the nursing facility setting.◄

Hospital discharge or observation discharge services
performed on the same date of nursing facility admission
or readmission may be reported separately. For a patient
discharged from inpatient status on the same date of
nursing facility admission or readmission, the hospital
discharge services should be reported with codes 99238,
99239 as appropriate. For a patient discharged from
observation status on the same date of nursing facility
admission or readmission, the observation care discharge
services should be reported with code 99217. For a
patient admitted and discharged from observation or
inpatient status on the same date, see codes 99234-
99236.

(For nursing facility care discharge, see 99315, 99316)

─── *Coding Tip* ───

The Significance of Time as a Factor in Selection of an Evaluation and Management Code

The inclusion of time as an explicit factor beginning in CPT 1992 is done to assist in selecting the most appropriate level of E/M services. It should be recognized that the specific times expressed in the visit code descriptors are averages and, therefore, represent a range of times that may be higher or lower depending on actual clinical circumstances.

Intraservice times are defined as **face-to-face** time for office and other outpatient visits and as **unit/floor** time for hospital and other inpatient visits. This distinction is necessary because most of the work of typical office visits takes place during the face-to-face time with the patient, while most of the work of typical hospital visits takes place during the time spent on the patient's floor or unit.

Unit/floor time (hospital observation services, inpatient hospital care, initial inpatient hospital consultations, nursing facility):

For reporting purposes, intraservice time for these services is defined as unit/floor time, which includes the time present on the patient's hospital unit and at the bedside rendering services for that patient. This includes the time to establish and/or review the patient's chart, examine the patient, write notes, and communicate with other professionals and the patient's family.

In the hospital, pre- and post-time includes time spent off the patient's floor performing such tasks as reviewing pathology and radiology findings in another part of the hospital.

This pre- and postvisit time is not included in the time component described in these codes. However, the pre- and post-work performed during the time spent off the floor or unit was included in calculating the total work of typical services in physician surveys.

Thus, the unit/floor time associated with the services described by any code is a valid proxy for the total work done before, during, and after the visit.

CPT Coding Guidelines, Evaluation and Management, Definitions of Commonly Used Terms Time

▲ 99304 Initial nursing facility care, per day, for the evaluation and management of a patient, which requires these 3 key components:

■ **A detailed or comprehensive history;**

■ **A detailed or comprehensive examination; and**

■ **Medical decision making that is straightforward or of low complexity.**

Counseling and/or coordination of care with other physicians, other qualified health care professionals, or agencies are provided consistent with the nature of the problem(s) and the patient's and/or family's needs.

Usually, the problem(s) requiring admission are of low severity. Typically, 25 minutes are spent at the bedside and on the patient's facility floor or unit.

➔ *CPT Assistant* Jul 10:4, Jan 11:3, Jun 11:3, Jan 12:3, Jul 12:12; *CPT Changes: An Insider's View* 2006, 2008, 2010, 2013

▲ 99305 Initial nursing facility care, per day, for the evaluation and management of a patient, which requires these 3 key components:

■ **A comprehensive history;**

■ **A comprehensive examination; and**

■ **Medical decision making of moderate complexity.**

Counseling and/or coordination of care with other physicians, other qualified health care professionals, or agencies are provided consistent with the nature of the problem(s) and the patient's and/or family's needs.

Usually, the problem(s) requiring admission are of moderate severity. Typically, 35 minutes are spent at the bedside and on the patient's facility floor or unit.

➔ *CPT Assistant* Jan 11:3, Jun 11:3, Jul 12:12; *CPT Changes: An Insider's View* 2006, 2008, 2010, 2013

▲ 99306 Initial nursing facility care, per day, for the evaluation and management of a patient, which requires these 3 key components:

■ **A comprehensive history;**

■ **A comprehensive examination; and**

■ **Medical decision making of high complexity.**

Counseling and/or coordination of care with other physicians, other qualified health care professionals, or agencies are provided consistent with the nature of the problem(s) and the patient's and/or family's needs.

Usually, the problem(s) requiring admission are of high severity. Typically, 45 minutes are spent at the bedside and on the patient's facility floor or unit.

➔ *CPT Assistant* Jan 11:3, Jun 11:3, Jan 12:3, Jul 12:12; *CPT Changes: An Insider's View* 2006, 2008, 2010, 2013

Subsequent Nursing Facility Care

►All levels of subsequent nursing facility care include reviewing the medical record and reviewing the results of diagnostic studies and changes in the patient's status (ie, changes in history, physical condition, and response to management) since the last assessment by the physician or other qualified health care professional.◄

▲ 99307 Subsequent nursing facility care, per day, for the evaluation and management of a patient, which requires at least 2 of these 3 key components:

■ **A problem focused interval history;**

■ **A problem focused examination;**

■ **Straightforward medical decision making.**

Counseling and/or coordination of care with other physicians, other qualified health care professionals, or agencies are provided consistent with the nature of the problem(s) and the patient's and/or family's needs.

Usually, the patient is stable, recovering, or improving. Typically, 10 minutes are spent at the bedside and on the patient's facility floor or unit.

➔ *CPT Assistant* May 06:1, 16, Jun 06:1, 19, Mar 07:9, Jul 07:1, Jul 09:3, 8, Jan 11:3, Jan 12:3, Jul 12:12; *CPT Changes: An Insider's View* 2006, 2008, 2010, 2013

▲ **99308** Subsequent nursing facility care, per day, for the evaluation and management of a patient, which requires at least 2 of these 3 key components:

- **An expanded problem focused interval history;**
- **An expanded problem focused examination;**
- **Medical decision making of low complexity.**

Counseling and/or coordination of care with other physicians, other qualified health care professionals, or agencies are provided consistent with the nature of the problem(s) and the patient's and/or family's needs.

Usually, the patient is responding inadequately to therapy or has developed a minor complication. Typically, 15 minutes are spent at the bedside and on the patient's facility floor or unit.

➔ *CPT Assistant* May 06:1, 16, Jun 06:1, 19, Mar 07:9, Jul 07:1, Jul 09:3, 8, Jan 11:3, Jul 12:12; *CPT Changes: An Insider's View* 2006, 2008, 2010, 2013

▲ **99309** Subsequent nursing facility care, per day, for the evaluation and management of a patient, which requires at least 2 of these 3 key components:

- **A detailed interval history;**
- **A detailed examination;**
- **Medical decision making of moderate complexity.**

Counseling and/or coordination of care with other physicians, other qualified health care professionals, or agencies are provided consistent with the nature of the problem(s) and the patient's and/or family's needs.

Usually, the patient has developed a significant complication or a significant new problem. Typically, 25 minutes are spent at the bedside and on the patient's facility floor or unit.

➔ *CPT Assistant* May 06:1, 16, Jun 06:1, 19, Mar 07:9, Jul 07:1, Jul 09:3, 8, Jan 11:3, Jul 12:12; *CPT Changes: An Insider's View* 2006, 2008, 2010, 2013

▲ **99310** Subsequent nursing facility care, per day, for the evaluation and management of a patient, which requires at least 2 of these 3 key components:

- **A comprehensive interval history;**
- **A comprehensive examination;**
- **Medical decision making of high complexity.**

Counseling and/or coordination of care with other physicians, other qualified health care professionals, or agencies are provided consistent with the nature of the problem(s) and the patient's and/or family's needs.

The patient may be unstable or may have developed a significant new problem requiring immediate physician attention. Typically, 35 minutes are spent at the bedside and on the patient's facility floor or unit.

➔ *CPT Assistant* May 06:1, 16, Jun 06:1, 19, Mar 07:9, Jul 07:1, Jul 09:3, 8, Jul 10:4, Jan 11:3, Jan 12:3, Jul 12:12; *CPT Changes: An Insider's View* 2006, 2008, 2010, 2013

Nursing Facility Discharge Services

▶The nursing facility discharge day management codes are to be used to report the total duration of time spent by a physician or other qualified health care professional for the final nursing facility discharge of a patient. The codes include, as appropriate, final examination of the patient, discussion of the nursing facility stay, even if the time spent on that date is not continuous. Instructions are given for continuing care to all relevant caregivers, and preparation of discharge records, prescriptions and referral forms.◀

99315 Nursing facility discharge day management; 30 minutes or less

➔ *CPT Assistant* Nov 97:5-6, Sep 98:5, May 02:19, Nov 02:11, May 05:1, Jul 09:3, Jan 11:3, Jan 12:3, Jul 12:12

99316 more than 30 minutes

➔ *CPT Assistant* Nov 97:5-6, Sep 98:5, May 02:19, Nov 02:11, Jul 09:3, Jan 11:3, Jul 12:12

Other Nursing Facility Services

▲ **99318** Evaluation and management of a patient involving an annual nursing facility assessment, which requires these 3 key components:

- **A detailed interval history;**
- **A comprehensive examination; and**
- **Medical decision making that is of low to moderate complexity.**

Counseling and/or coordination of care with other physicians, other qualified health care professionals, or agencies are provided consistent with the nature of the problem(s) and the patient's and/or family's needs.

Usually, the patient is stable, recovering, or improving. Typically, 30 minutes are spent at the bedside and on the patient's facility floor or unit.

➔ *CPT Assistant* Jan 11:3, Jan 12:3; *CPT Changes: An Insider's View* 2006, 2008, 2010, 2013

(Do not report 99318 on the same date of service as nursing facility services codes 99304-99316)

Domiciliary, Rest Home (eg, Boarding Home), or Custodial Care Services

The following codes are used to report evaluation and management services in a facility which provides room, board and other personal assistance services, generally on a long-term basis. They also are used to report evaluation and management services in an assisted living facility.

The facility's services do not include a medical component.

For definitions of key components and commonly used terms, please see **Evaluation and Management Services Guidelines**.

▶(For care plan oversight services provided to a patient in a domiciliary facility under the care of a home health agency, see 99374, 99375, and for hospice agency, see 99377, 99378. For care plan oversight provided to a patient under hospice or home health agency care, see 99339, 99340)◀

New Patient

▲ **99324** Domiciliary or rest home visit for the evaluation and management of a new patient, which requires these 3 key components:

- **A problem focused history;**
- **A problem focused examination; and**
- **Straightforward medical decision making.**

Counseling and/or coordination of care with other physicians, other qualified health care professionals, or agencies are provided consistent with the nature of the problem(s) and the patient's and/or family's needs.

Usually, the presenting problem(s) are of low severity. Typically, 20 minutes are spent with the patient and/or family or caregiver.

➜ *CPT Assistant* Jan 06:1, Jun 06:1, Jul 09:8, Aug 09:5, Jan 11:3, Jan 12:3, Apr 12:10; *CPT Changes: An Insider's View* 2006, 2013

▲ **99325** Domiciliary or rest home visit for the evaluation and management of a new patient, which requires these 3 key components:

- **An expanded problem focused history;**
- **An expanded problem focused examination; and**
- **Medical decision making of low complexity.**

Counseling and/or coordination of care with other physicians, other qualified health care professionals, or agencies are provided consistent with the nature of the problem(s) and the patient's and/or family's needs.

Usually, the presenting problem(s) are of moderate severity. Typically, 30 minutes are spent with the patient and/or family or caregiver.

➜ *CPT Assistant* Jan 06:1, Jun 06:1, Jul 09:8, Aug 09:5, Jan 11:3; *CPT Changes: An Insider's View* 2006, 2013

▲ **99326** Domiciliary or rest home visit for the evaluation and management of a new patient, which requires these 3 key components:

- **A detailed history;**
- **A detailed examination; and**
- **Medical decision making of moderate complexity.**

Counseling and/or coordination of care with other physicians, other qualified health care professionals, or agencies are provided consistent with the nature of the problem(s) and the patient's and/or family's needs.

Usually, the presenting problem(s) are of moderate to high severity. Typically, 45 minutes are spent with the patient and/or family or caregiver.

➜ *CPT Assistant* Jan 06:1, Jun 06:1, Jul 09:8, Aug 09:5, Jan 11:3; *CPT Changes: An Insider's View* 2006, 2013

▲ **99327** Domiciliary or rest home visit for the evaluation and management of a new patient, which requires these 3 key components:

- **A comprehensive history;**
- **A comprehensive examination; and**
- **Medical decision making of moderate complexity.**

Counseling and/or coordination of care with other physicians, other qualified health care professionals, or agencies are provided consistent with the nature of the problem(s) and the patient's and/or family's needs.

Usually, the presenting problem(s) are of high severity. Typically, 60 minutes are spent with the patient and/or family or caregiver.

➜ *CPT Assistant* Jan 06:1, Jun 06:1, Jul 09:8, Aug 09:5, Jan 11:3; *CPT Changes: An Insider's View* 2006, 2013

▲ **99328** Domiciliary or rest home visit for the evaluation and management of a new patient, which requires these 3 key components:

- **A comprehensive history;**
- **A comprehensive examination; and**
- **Medical decision making of high complexity.**

Counseling and/or coordination of care with other physicians, other qualified health care professionals, or agencies are provided consistent with the nature of the problem(s) and the patient's and/or family's needs.

Usually, the patient is unstable or has developed a significant new problem requiring immediate physician attention. Typically, 75 minutes are spent with the patient and/or family or caregiver.

➜ *CPT Assistant* Jan 06:1, Jun 06:1, Jul 09:8, Aug 09:5, Jan 11:3, Jan 12:3; *CPT Changes: An Insider's View* 2006, 2013

Established Patient

▲ **99334** Domiciliary or rest home visit for the evaluation and management of an established patient, which requires at least 2 of these 3 key components:

- **A problem focused interval history;**
- **A problem focused examination;**
- **Straightforward medical decision making.**

Counseling and/or coordination of care with other physicians, other qualified health care professionals, or agencies are provided consistent with the nature of the problem(s) and the patient's and/or family's needs.

Usually, the presenting problem(s) are self-limited or minor. Typically, 15 minutes are spent with the patient and/or family or caregiver.

➔ *CPT Assistant* Jan 06:1, Jun 06:1, Jul 07:1, Jul 09:8, Aug 09:5, Jan 11.3, Jan 12:3; *CPT Changes: An Insider's View* 2006, 2013

▲ **99335** Domiciliary or rest home visit for the evaluation and management of an established patient, which requires at least 2 of these 3 key components:

- **An expanded problem focused interval history;**
- **An expanded problem focused examination;**
- **Medical decision making of low complexity.**

Counseling and/or coordination of care with other physicians, other qualified health care professionals, or agencies are provided consistent with the nature of the problem(s) and the patient's and/or family's needs.

Usually, the presenting problem(s) are of low to moderate severity. Typically, 25 minutes are spent with the patient and/or family or caregiver.

➔ *CPT Assistant* Jan 06:1, Jun 06:1, Jul 07:1, Jul 09:8, Aug 09:5, Jan 11.3; *CPT Changes: An Insider's View* 2006, 2013

▲ **99336** Domiciliary or rest home visit for the evaluation and management of an established patient, which requires at least 2 of these 3 key components:

- **A detailed interval history;**
- **A detailed examination;**
- **Medical decision making of moderate complexity.**

Counseling and/or coordination of care with other physicians, other qualified health care professionals, or agencies are provided consistent with the nature of the problem(s) and the patient's and/or family's needs.

Usually, the presenting problem(s) are of moderate to high severity. Typically, 40 minutes are spent with the patient and/or family or caregiver.

➔ *CPT Assistant* Jan 06:1, Jun 06:1, Jul 07:1, Jul 09:8, Aug 09:5, Jan 11.3; *CPT Changes: An Insider's View* 2006, 2013

▲ **99337** Domiciliary or rest home visit for the evaluation and management of an established patient, which requires at least 2 of these 3 key components:

- **A comprehensive interval history;**
- **A comprehensive examination;**
- **Medical decision making of moderate to high complexity.**

Counseling and/or coordination of care with other physicians, other qualified health care professionals, or agencies are provided consistent with the nature of the problem(s) and the patient's and/or family's needs.

Usually, the presenting problem(s) are of moderate to high severity. The patient may be unstable or may have developed a significant new problem requiring immediate physician attention. Typically, 60 minutes are spent with the patient and/or family or caregiver.

➔ *CPT Assistant* Jan 06:1, Jun 06:1, Jul 07:1, Jul 09:8, Aug 09:5, Jan 11:3, Jan 12:3, Apr 12:10; *CPT Changes: An Insider's View* 2006, 2013

Domiciliary, Rest Home (eg, Assisted Living Facility), or Home Care Plan Oversight Services

(For instructions on the use of 99339, 99340, see introductory notes for 99374-99380)

(For care plan oversight services for patients under the care of a home health agency, hospice, or nursing facility, see 99374-99380)

(Do not report 99339, 99340 for time reported with 98966-98969, 99441-99444)

99339 Individual physician supervision of a patient (patient not present) in home, domiciliary or rest home (eg, assisted living facility) requiring complex and multidisciplinary care modalities involving regular physician development and/or revision of care plans, review of subsequent reports of patient status, review of related laboratory and other studies, communication (including telephone calls) for purposes of assessment or care decisions with health care professional(s), family member(s), surrogate decision maker(s) (eg, legal guardian) and/or key caregiver(s) involved in patient's care, integration of new information into the medical treatment plan and/or adjustment of medical therapy, within a calendar month; 15-29 minutes

➔ *CPT Assistant* Jan 06:1, Dec 06:4, Mar 07:11, Sep 08:3, Jul 09:5, 10, Jan 12:3; *CPT Changes: An Insider's View* 2006

99340 30 minutes or more

➔ *CPT Assistant* Jan 06:1, Dec 06:4, Mar 07:11, Sep 08:3, Jul 09:5, 10, Jan 12:3; *CPT Changes: An Insider's View* 2006

(Do not report 99339, 99340 for patients under the care of a home health agency, enrolled in a hospice program, or for nursing facility residents)

►(Do not report 99339, 99340 during the same month with 99487-99489)◄

►(Do not report 99339, 99340 when performed during the service time of codes 99495 or 99496)◄

Home Services

The following codes are used to report evaluation and management services provided in a private residence.

For definitions of key components and commonly used terms, please see **Evaluation and Management Services Guidelines.**

►(For care plan oversight services provided to a patient in the home under the care of a home health agency, see 99374, 99375, and for hospice agency, see 99377, 99378. For care plan oversight provided to a patient under hospice or home health agency care, see 99339, 99340)◄

New Patient

▲ **99341** **Home visit** for the evaluation and management of a new patient, which requires these 3 key components:

- **A problem focused history;**
- **A problem focused examination; and**
- **Straightforward medical decision making.**

Counseling and/or coordination of care with other physicians, other qualified health care professionals, or agencies are provided consistent with the nature of the problem(s) and the patient's and/or family's needs.

Usually, the presenting problem(s) are of low severity. Typically, 20 minutes are spent face-to-face with the patient and/or family.

➲ *CPT Assistant* Winter 91:11, Spring 92:24, Summer 92:12, Spring 93:34, Spring 95:1, Jun 97:6, Nov 97:6-8, Oct 98:6, Oct 03:7, May 05:1, Jan 06:1, Jul 09:8, Aug 09:5, Jan 11:3, Jan 12:3, Apr 12:10; *CPT Changes: An Insider's View* 2013

▲ **99342** **Home visit** for the evaluation and management of a new patient, which requires these 3 key components:

- **An expanded problem focused history;**
- **An expanded problem focused examination; and**
- **Medical decision making of low complexity.**

Counseling and/or coordination of care with other physicians, other qualified health care professionals, or agencies are provided consistent with the nature of the problem(s) and the patient's and/or family's needs.

Usually, the presenting problem(s) are of moderate severity. Typically, 30 minutes are spent face-to-face with the patient and/or family.

➲ *CPT Assistant* Winter 91:11, Spring 92:24, Summer 92:12, Spring 93:34, Spring 95:1, Jun 97:6, Nov 97:6-8, Oct 98:6, Jan 06:1, Jul 09:8, Aug 09:5, Jan 11:3; *CPT Changes: An Insider's View* 2013

▲ **99343** **Home visit** for the evaluation and management of a new patient, which requires these 3 key components:

- **A detailed history;**
- **A detailed examination; and**
- **Medical decision making of moderate complexity.**

Counseling and/or coordination of care with other physicians, other qualified health care professionals, or agencies are provided consistent with the nature of the problem(s) and the patient's and/or family's needs.

Usually, the presenting problem(s) are of moderate to high severity. Typically, 45 minutes are spent face-to-face with the patient and/or family.

➲ *CPT Assistant* Winter 91:11, Spring 92:24, Summer 92:12, Spring 93:34, Spring 95:1, Jun 97:6, Nov 97:6-8, Oct 98:6, Jan 06:1, Jul 09:8, Aug 09:5, Jan 11:3; *CPT Changes: An Insider's View* 2013

▲ **99344** **Home visit** for the evaluation and management of a new patient, which requires these 3 key components:

- **A comprehensive history;**
- **A comprehensive examination; and**
- **Medical decision making of moderate complexity.**

Counseling and/or coordination of care with other physicians, other qualified health care professionals, or agencies are provided consistent with the nature of the problem(s) and the patient's and/or family's needs.

Usually, the presenting problem(s) are of high severity. Typically, 60 minutes are spent face-to-face with the patient and/or family.

➲ *CPT Assistant* Nov 97:6-8, Oct 98:6, Jan 06:1, Jul 09:8, Aug 09:5, Jan 11:3; *CPT Changes: An Insider's View* 2013

▲ **99345** **Home visit** for the evaluation and management of a new patient, which requires these 3 key components:

- **A comprehensive history;**
- **A comprehensive examination; and**
- **Medical decision making of high complexity.**

Counseling and/or coordination of care with other physicians, other qualified health care professionals, or agencies are provided consistent with the nature of the problem(s) and the patient's and/or family's needs.

Usually, the patient is unstable or has developed a significant new problem requiring immediate physician attention. Typically, 75 minutes are spent face-to-face with the patient and/or family.

➲ *CPT Assistant* Nov 97:6-8, Oct 98:6, Jan 06:1, Jul 09:8, Aug 09:5, Jan 11:3, Jan 12:3; *CPT Changes: An Insider's View* 2013

Established Patient

▲ **99347** **Home visit** for the evaluation and management of an established patient, which requires at least 2 of these 3 key components:

- **A problem focused interval history;**
- **A problem focused examination;**
- **Straightforward medical decision making.**

Counseling and/or coordination of care with other physicians, other qualified health care professionals, or agencies are provided consistent with the nature of the problem(s) and the patient's and/or family's needs.

Usually, the presenting problem(s) are self limited or minor. Typically, 15 minutes are spent face-to-face with the patient and/or family.

➲ *CPT Assistant* Nov 97:6-8, Oct 98:6, May 05:1, Jan 06:1, Jul 07:1, Jul 09:8, Aug 09:5, Jan 11:3, Jan 12:3; *CPT Changes: An Insider's View* 2013

▲ **99348** **Home visit** for the evaluation and management of an established patient, which requires at least 2 of these 3 key components:

- **An expanded problem focused interval history;**
- **An expanded problem focused examination;**
- **Medical decision making of low complexity.**

Counseling and/or coordination of care with other physicians, other qualified health care professionals, or agencies are provided consistent with the nature of the problem(s) and the patient's and/or family's needs.

Usually, the presenting problem(s) are of low to moderate severity. Typically, 25 minutes are spent face-to-face with the patient and/or family.

➔ *CPT Assistant* Nov 97:6-8, Oct 98:6, Jan 06:1, Jul 07:1, Jul 09:8, Aug 09:5, Jan 11:3; *CPT Changes: An Insider's View* 2013

▲ **99349**   **Home visit** for the evaluation and management of an established patient, which requires at least 2 of these 3 key components:

- **A detailed interval history;**
- **A detailed examination;**
- **Medical decision making of moderate complexity.**

Counseling and/or coordination of care with other physicians, other qualified health care professionals, or agencies are provided consistent with the nature of the problem(s) and the patient's and/or family's needs.

Usually, the presenting problem(s) are moderate to high severity. Typically, 40 minutes are spent face-to-face with the patient and/or family.

➔ *CPT Assistant* Nov 97:6-8, Oct 98:6, Jan 06:1, Jul 07:1, Jul 09:8, Aug 09:5; *CPT Changes: An Insider's View* 2013

▲ **99350**   **Home visit** for the evaluation and management of an established patient, which requires at least 2 of these 3 key components:

- **A comprehensive interval history;**
- **A comprehensive examination;**
- **Medical decision making of moderate to high complexity.**

Counseling and/or coordination of care with other physicians, other qualified health care professionals, or agencies are provided consistent with the nature of the problem(s) and the patient's and/or family's needs.

Usually, the presenting problem(s) are of moderate to high severity. The patient may be unstable or may have developed a significant new problem requiring immediate physician attention. Typically, 60 minutes are spent face-to-face with the patient and/or family.

➔ *CPT Assistant* Nov 97:6-8, Oct 98:6, Oct 03:7, Jan 06:1, Jul 07:1, Jul 09:8, Aug 09:5, Jan 12:3, Apr 12:10; *CPT Changes: An Insider's View* 2013

Prolonged Services

Prolonged Service With Direct Patient Contact

Codes 99354-99357 are used when a physician or other qualified health care professional provides prolonged service involving direct patient contact that is provided beyond the usual service in either the inpatient or outpatient setting. Direct patient contact is face-to-face and includes additional non-face-to-face services on the patient's floor or unit in the hospital or nursing facility during the same session. This service is reported in addition to the designated evaluation and management

services at any level and any other services provided at the same session as evaluation and management services. Appropriate codes should be selected for supplies provided or procedures performed in the care of the patient during this period.

Codes 99354-99355 are used to report the total duration of face-to-face time spent by a physician or other qualified health care professional on a given date providing prolonged service in the office or other outpatient setting, even if the time spent by the physician or other qualified health care professional on that date is not continuous. Codes 99356-99357 are used to report the total duration of time spent by a physician or other qualified health care professional at the bedside and on the patient's floor or unit in the hospital or nursing facility on a given date providing prolonged service to a patient, even if the time spent by the physician or other qualified health care professional on that date is not continuous.

Code 99354 or 99356 is used to report the first hour of prolonged service on a given date, depending on the place of service.

Either code should be used only once per date, even if the time spent by the physician or other qualified health care professional is not continuous on that date. Prolonged service of less than 30 minutes total duration on a given date is not separately reported because the work involved is included in the total work of the evaluation and management codes.

Code 99355 or 99357 is used to report each additional 30 minutes beyond the first hour, depending on the place of service. Either code may also be used to report the final 15-30 minutes of prolonged service on a given date. Prolonged service of less than 15 minutes beyond the first hour or less than 15 minutes beyond the final 30 minutes is not reported separately.

The use of the time based add-on codes requires that the primary evaluation and management service have a typical or specified time published in the CPT codebook.

The following examples illustrate the correct reporting of prolonged physician or other qualified health care professional service with direct patient contact in the office setting:

Total Duration of Prolonged Services	Code(s)
less than 30 minutes	Not reported separately
30-74 minutes (30 minutes - 1 hr. 14 min.)	99354 X 1
75-104 minutes (1 hr. 15 min. - 1 hr. 44 min.)	99354 X 1 AND 99355 X 1
105 or more (1 hr. 45 min. or more)	99354 X 1 AND 99355 X 2 or more for each additional 30 minutes.

Evaluation/Management

Evaluation/Management

--- *Coding Tip* ---

Reporting Service of Less than 30 Minutes

Prolonged service of less than 30 minutes total duration on a given date is not separately reported because the work involved is included in the total work of the evaluation and management codes.

CPT Coding Guidelines, Evaluation and Management, Prolonged Physician Service with Direct (Face-to-Face) Patient Contact

+ 99354 Prolonged service in the office or other outpatient setting requiring direct patient contact beyond the usual service; first hour (List separately in addition to code for office or other outpatient **Evaluation and Management** service)
→ CPT Assistant Spring 94:30, 32, May 97:3, Sep 98:5, Sep 00:2, Jul 01:2, May 05:1, Nov 05:10, Jun 08:12, Sep 08:3, Jul 09:8, Apr 12:10; CPT Changes: An Insider's View 2009, 2012

►(Use 99354 in conjunction with 99201-99215, 99241-99245, 99324-99337, 99341-99350)◄

+ 99355 each additional 30 minutes (List separately in addition to code for prolonged service)
→ CPT Assistant Spring 94:30, 32, May 97:3, Sep 98:5, Sep 00:2, Jul 01:2, Nov 05:10, Jun 08:12, Sep 08:3, Jul 09:8, Apr 12:10; CPT Changes: An Insider's View 2009, 2012

(Use 99355 in conjunction with 99354)

+ 99356 Prolonged service in the inpatient or observation setting, requiring unit/floor time beyond the usual service; first hour (List separately in addition to code for inpatient **Evaluation and Management** service)
→ CPT Assistant Spring 94:30, 32, Apr 97:3, May 97:3, Sep 98:5, Sep 00:2, Jul 01:2, Nov 05:10, Jun 08:12, Sep 08:3, Jul 09:8, Jun 11:3, Aug 11:11, Jul 12:11; CPT Changes: An Insider's View 2009, 2012

►(Use 99356 in conjunction with 99218-99220, 99221-99223, 99224-99226, 99231-99233, 99234-99236, 99251-99255, 99304-99310)◄

+ 99357 each additional 30 minutes (List separately in addition to code for prolonged service)
→ CPT Assistant Spring 94:34, Apr 97:3, May 97:3, Sep 98:5, Sep 00:2, Jul 01:2, Nov 05:10, Jun 08:12, Sep 08:3, Jul 09:8, Jun 11:3, Aug 11:11, Jul 12:11; CPT Changes: An Insider's View 2009, 2012

(Use 99357 in conjunction with 99356)

Prolonged Service Without Direct Patient Contact

Codes 99358 and 99359 are used when a prolonged service is provided that is neither face-to face time in the office or outpatient setting, nor additional unit/floor time in the hospital or nursing facility setting during the same session of an evaluation and management service and is beyond the usual physician or other qualified health care professional service time.

This service is to be reported in relation to other physician or other qualified health care professional services, including evaluation and management services at

any level. This prolonged service may be reported on a different date than the primary service to which it is related. For example, extensive record review may relate to a previous evaluation and management service performed earlier and commences upon receipt of past records. However, it must relate to a service or patient where (face-to-face) patient care has occurred or will occur and relate to ongoing patient management. A typical time for the primary service need not be established within the CPT code set.

Codes 99358 and 99359 are used to report the total duration of non-face-to-face time spent by a physician or other qualified health care professional on a given date providing prolonged service, even if the time spent by the physician or other qualified health care professional on that date is not continuous. Code 99358 is used to report the first hour of prolonged service on a given date regardless of the place of service. It should be used only once per date.

Prolonged service of less than 30 minutes total duration on a given date is not separately reported.

Code 99359 is used to report each additional 30 minutes beyond the first hour regardless of the place of service. It may also be used to report the final 15 to 30 minutes of prolonged service on a given date.

Prolonged service of less than 15 minutes beyond the first hour or less than 15 minutes beyond the final 30 minutes is not reported separately.

►Do not report 99358, 99359 for time spent in care plan oversight services (99339, 99340, 99374-99380), anticoagulant management (99363, 99364), medical team conferences (99366-99368), on-line medical evaluations (99444), or other non-face-to-face services that have more specific codes and no upper time limit in the CPT code set. Codes 99358, 99359 may be reported when related to other non-face-to-face services codes that have a published maximum time (eg, telephone services).◄

99358 **Prolonged evaluation and management service** before and/or after direct patient care; first hour
→ CPT Assistant Spring 94:34, Nov 98:3, Sep 00:3, Nov 05:10, Jun 08:12, Sep 08:3; CPT Changes: An Insider's View 2010, 2012

+ 99359 each additional 30 minutes (List separately in addition to code for prolonged service)
→ CPT Assistant Spring 94:34, Sep 00:3, Nov 05:10, Jun 08:12, Sep 08:3; CPT Changes: An Insider's View 2010, 2012

(Use 99359 in conjunction with 99358)

►(Do not report 99358, 99359 during the same month with 99487-99489)◄

►(Do not report 99358, 99359 when performed during the service time of codes 99495 or 99496)◄

►Standby Services◄

►Code 99360 is used to report physician or other qualified health care professional standby services that are requested by another individual and that involve prolonged attendance without direct (face-to-face) patient contact. Care or services may not be provided to other patients during this period. This code is not used to report time spent proctoring another individual. It is also not used if the period of standby ends with the performance of a procedure, subject to a surgical package by the individual who was on standby.

Code 99360 is used to report the total duration of time spent on a given date on standby. Standby service of less than 30 minutes total duration on a given date is not reported separately.◀

Second and subsequent periods of standby beyond the first 30 minutes may be reported only if a full 30 minutes of standby was provided for each unit of service reported.

▲ **99360**   **Standby service,** requiring prolonged attendance, each 30 minutes (eg, operative standby, standby for frozen section, for cesarean/high risk delivery, for monitoring EEG)

➔ *CPT Assistant* Spring 94:32, Apr 97:10, Aug 97:18, Nov 97:8, Nov 99:5-6, Aug 00:3, Sep 00:3, May 05:1, Nov 05:10, Nov 06:23, Mar 08:14, Feb 11:3; *CPT Changes: An Insider's View* 2013

(For hospital mandated on call services, see 99026, 99027)

(99360 may be reported in addition to 99460, 99465 as appropriate)

(Do not report 99360 in conjunction with 99464)

Case Management Services

Case management is a process in which a physician or another qualified health care professional is responsible for direct care of a patient and, additionally, for coordinating, managing access to, initiating, and/or supervising other health care services needed by the patient.

Anticoagulant Management

Anticoagulant services are intended to describe the outpatient management of warfarin therapy, including ordering, review, and interpretation of International Normalized Ratio (INR) testing, communication with patient, and dosage adjustments as appropriate.

When reporting these services, the work of anticoagulant management may not be used as a basis for reporting an evaluation and management (E/M) service or care plan oversight time during the reporting period. Do not report these services with 98966-98969, 99441-99444 when telephone or on-line services address anticoagulation with warfarin management. If a significant, separately identifiable E/M service is performed, report the appropriate E/M service code using modifier 25.

These services are outpatient services only. When anticoagulation therapy is initiated or continued in the inpatient or observation setting, a new period begins after

discharge and is reported with 99364. Do not report 99363-99364 with 99217-99239, 99291-99292, 99304-99318, 99471-99480 or other code(s) for physician review, interpretation, and patient management of home INR testing for a patient with mechanical heart valve(s).

Any period less than 60 continuous outpatient days is not reported. If less than the specified minimum number of services per period are performed, do not report the anticoagulant management services (99363-99364).

99363   Anticoagulant management for an outpatient taking warfarin, physician review and interpretation of International Normalized Ratio (INR) testing, patient instructions, dosage adjustment (as needed), and ordering of additional tests; initial 90 days of therapy (must include a minimum of 8 INR measurements)

➔ *CPT Assistant* Sep 07:1, Jul 09:5; *CPT Changes: An Insider's View* 2007

99364   each subsequent 90 days of therapy (must include a minimum of 3 INR measurements)

➔ *CPT Assistant* Sep 07:1, Jul 09:5; *CPT Changes: An Insider's View* 2007

▶(Do not report 99363, 99364 during the same month with 99487-99489)◀

▶(Do not report 99363, 99364 when performed during the service time of codes 99495 or 99496)◀

Medical Team Conferences

Medical team conferences include face-to-face participation by a minimum of three qualified health care professionals from different specialties or disciplines (each of whom provide direct care to the patient), with or without the presence of the patient, family member(s), community agencies, surrogate decision maker(s) (eg, legal guardian), and/or caregiver(s). The participants are actively involved in the development, revision, coordination, and implementation of health care services needed by the patient. Reporting participants shall have performed face-to-face evaluations or treatments of the patient, independent of any team conference, within the previous 60 days.

▶Physicians or other qualified health care professionals who may report evaluation and management services should report their time spent in a team conference with the patient and/or family present using evaluation and management (E/M) codes (and time as the key controlling factor for code selection when counseling and/or coordination of care dominates the service). These introductory guidelines do not apply to services reported using E/M codes (see E/M services guidelines). However, the individual must be directly involved with the patient, providing face-to-face services outside of the conference visit with other physicians, qualified health care professionals, or agencies.◀

Reporting participants shall document their participation in the team conference as well as their contributed information and subsequent treatment recommendations.

No more than one individual from the same specialty may report 99366-99368 at the same encounter.

▶Individuals should not report 99366-99368 when their participation in the medical team conference is part of a facility or organizational service contractually provided by the organization or facility.

The team conference starts at the beginning of the review of an individual patient and ends at the conclusion of the review. Time related to record keeping and report generation is not reported. The reporting participant shall be present for all time reported. The time reported is not limited to the time that the participant is communicating to the other team members or patient and/or family. Time reported for medical team conferences may not be used in the determination of time for other services such as care plan oversight (99374-99380), home, domiciliary, or rest home care plan oversight (99339-99340), prolonged services (99354-99359), psychotherapy, or any E/M service. For team conferences where the patient is present for any part of the duration of the conference, nonphysician qualified health care professionals (eg, speech-language pathologists, physical therapists, occupational therapists, social workers, dietitians) report the team conference face-to-face code 99366.◀

Medical Team Conference, Direct (Face-to-Face) Contact With Patient and/or Family

99366   **Medical team conference** with interdisciplinary team of health care professionals, face-to-face with patient and/or family, 30 minutes or more, participation by nonphysician qualified health care professional

➔ *CPT Changes: An Insider's View* 2008

(Team conference services of less than 30 minutes duration are not reported separately)

(For team conference services by a physician with patient and/or family present, see Evaluation and Management services)

▶(Do not report 99366 during the same month with 99487-99489)◀

▶(Do not report 99366 when performed during the service time of codes 99495 or 99496)◀

Medical Team Conference, Without Direct (Face-to-Face) Contact With Patient and/or Family

99367   **Medical team conference** with interdisciplinary team of health care professionals, patient and/or family not present, 30 minutes or more; participation by physician

➔ *CPT Changes: An Insider's View* 2008

99368   participation by nonphysician qualified health care professional

➔ *CPT Changes: An Insider's View* 2008

(Team conference services of less than 30 minutes duration are not reported separately)

▶(Do not report 99367, 99368 during the same month with 99487-99489)◀

▶(Do not report 99367, 99368 when performed during the service time of codes 99495 or 99496)◀

Care Plan Oversight Services

▶Care plan oversight services are reported separately from codes for office/outpatient, hospital, home, nursing facility or domiciliary, or non-face-to-face services. The complexity and approximate time of the care plan oversight services provided within a 30-day period determine code selection. Only one individual may report services for a given period of time, to reflect the sole or predominant supervisory role with a particular patient. These codes should not be reported for supervision of patients in nursing facilities or under the care of home health agencies unless they require recurrent supervision of therapy.◀

The work involved in providing very low intensity or infrequent supervision services is included in the pre- and post-encounter work for home, office/outpatient and nursing facility or domiciliary visit codes.

▶(For care plan oversight services of patients in the home, domiciliary, or rest home [eg, assisted living facility], see 99339, 99340, and for hospice agency, see 99377, 99378)◀

(Do not report 99374-99380 for time reported with 98966-98969, 99441-99444)

▶(Do not report 99374-99378 during the same month with 99487-99489)◀

▶(Do not report 99374-99380 when performed during the service time of codes 99495 or 99496)◀

▲ **99374**   **Supervision** of a patient under care of home health agency (patient not present) in home, domiciliary or equivalent environment (eg, Alzheimer's facility) requiring complex and multidisciplinary care modalities involving regular development and/or revision of care plans by that individual, review of subsequent reports of patient status, review of related laboratory and other studies, communication (including telephone calls) for purposes of assessment or care decisions with health care professional(s), family member(s), surrogate decision maker(s) (eg, legal guardian) and/or key caregiver(s) involved in patient's care, integration of new information into the medical treatment plan and/or adjustment of medical therapy, within a calendar month; 15-29 minutes

➔ *CPT Assistant* Summer 94:9, Nov 97:8-9, May 05:1, Dec 06:4, Mar 07:11, Mar 08:6, Sep 08:3, Jul 09:5, 10; *CPT Changes: An Insider's View* 2002, 2013

▲ **99375**   30 minutes or more
> *CPT Assistant* Summer 94:9, Nov 97:8-9, Dec 06:4,
Mar 07:11, Mar 08:6, Sep 08:3, Jul 09:5, 10; *CPT Changes:
An Insider's View* 2013

▲ **99377**   **Supervision** of a hospice patient (patient not present)
requiring complex and multidisciplinary care modalities
involving regular development and/or revision of care
plans by that individual, review of subsequent reports of
patient status, review of related laboratory and other
studies, communication (including telephone calls) for
purposes of assessment or care decisions with health
care professional(s), family member(s), surrogate decision
maker(s) (eg, legal guardian) and/or key caregiver(s)
involved in patient's care, integration of new information
into the medical treatment plan and/or adjustment of
medical therapy, within a calendar month; 15-29 minutes
> *CPT Assistant* Nov 97:8-9, Dec 06:4, Mar 07:11, Sep 08:3,
Jul 09:5, 10; *CPT Changes: An Insider's View* 2001, 2002, 2013

▲ **99378**   30 minutes or more
> *CPT Assistant* Nov 97:8-9, Dec 06:4, Mar 07:11, Mar 08:6,
Sep 08:3, Jul 09:5, 10; *CPT Changes: An Insider's View* 2013

▲ **99379**   **Supervision** of a nursing facility patient (patient not
present) requiring complex and multidisciplinary care
modalities involving regular development and/or revision
of care plans by that individual, review of subsequent
reports of patient status, review of related laboratory and
other studies, communication (including telephone calls)
for purposes of assessment or care decisions with health
care professional(s), family member(s), surrogate decision
maker(s) (eg, legal guardian) and/or key caregiver(s)
involved in patient's care, integration of new information
into the medical treatment plan and/or adjustment of
medical therapy, within a calendar month; 15-29 minutes
> *CPT Assistant* Dec 06:4, Mar 08:6, Sep 08:3, Jul 09:5; *CPT
Changes: An Insider's View* 2002, 2013

▲ **99380**   30 minutes or more
> *CPT Assistant* Nov 97:8-9, Dec 06:4, Mar 08:6, Sep 08:3,
Jul 09:5; *CPT Changes: An Insider's View* 2013

Preventive Medicine Services

The following codes are used to report the preventive
medicine evaluation and management of infants,
children, adolescents, and adults.

The extent and focus of the services will largely depend
on the age of the patient.

►If an abnormality is encountered or a preexisting
problem is addressed in the process of performing this
preventive medicine evaluation and management service,
and if the problem or abnormality is significant enough
to require additional work to perform the key
components of a problem-oriented E/M service, then the
appropriate Office/Outpatient code 99201-99215 should

also be reported. Modifier 25 should be added to the
Office/Outpatient code to indicate that a significant,
separately identifiable evaluation and management service
was provided on the same day as the preventive medicine
service. The appropriate preventive medicine service is
additionally reported.◄

An insignificant or trivial problem/abnormality that is
encountered in the process of performing the preventive
medicine evaluation and management service and which
does not require additional work and the performance of
the key components of a problem-oriented E/M service
should not be reported.

The "comprehensive" nature of the Preventive Medicine
Services codes 99381-99397 reflects an age and gender
appropriate history/exam and is **not** synonymous with
the "comprehensive" examination required in Evaluation
and Management codes 99201-99350.

Codes 99381-99397 include counseling/anticipatory
guidance/risk factor reduction interventions which are
provided at the time of the initial or periodic
comprehensive preventive medicine examination. (Refer
to codes 99401-99412 for reporting those counseling/
anticipatory guidance/risk factor reduction interventions
that are provided at an encounter separate from the
preventive medicine examination.)

Vaccine/toxoid products, immunization administrations,
ancillary studies involving laboratory, radiology, other
procedures, or screening tests (eg, vision, hearing,
developmental) identified with a specific CPT code are
reported separately. For immunization administration and
vaccine risk/benefit counseling, see 90460, 90461,
90471-90474. For vaccine/toxoid products, see 90476-
90749.

New Patient

99381   **Initial comprehensive preventive medicine**
evaluation and management of an individual including an
age and gender appropriate history, examination,
counseling/anticipatory guidance/risk factor reduction
interventions, and the ordering of laboratory/diagnostic
procedures, new patient; infant (age younger than 1 year)
> *CPT Assistant* Winter 91:11, Spring 93:14, 34, Spring 95:1,
Aug 97:1, Jul 98:9, Sep 98:5, Nov 98:3-4, May 02:1, May 05:1,
Aug 05:15, Oct 06:15, Mar 09:3, Jul 09:7, Aug 09:5; *CPT
Changes: An Insider's View* 2002, 2009

99382   early childhood (age 1 through 4 years)
> *CPT Assistant* Winter 91:11, Spring 93:14, 34, Spring 95:1,
Aug 97:1, Jul 98:9, Sep 98:5, Nov 98:3-4, May 02:1,
Aug 05:15, Oct 06:15, Jul 09:5, Aug 09:5; *CPT Changes: An
Insider's View* 2009

99383   late childhood (age 5 through 11 years)
> *CPT Assistant* Winter 91:11, Spring 93:14, 34, Spring 95:1,
Aug 97:1, Jul 98:9, Sep 98:5, Nov 98:3-4, May 02:1,
Aug 05:15, Oct 06:15, Jul 09:7, Aug 09:5; *CPT Changes: An
Insider's View* 2009

99384 adolescent (age 12 through 17 years)

> *CPT Assistant* Winter 91:11, Spring 93:14, 34, Spring 95:1, Aug 97:1, Jul 98:9, Sep 98:5, Nov 98:3-4, May 02:1, Aug 05:15, Oct 06:15, Jul 09:7, Aug 09:5; *CPT Changes: An Insider's View* 2009

99385 18-39 years

> *CPT Assistant* Winter 91:11, Spring 93:14, 34, Spring 95:1, Aug 97:7, Jul 98:9, Sep 98:5, Nov 98:3-4, May 02:1, Aug 05:15, Oct 06:15, Jul 09:5, Aug 09:5; *CPT Changes: An Insider's View* 2009

99386 40-64 years

> *CPT Assistant* Winter 91:11, Spring 93:14, 34, Spring 95:1, Aug 97:1, Jul 98:9, Sep 98:5, Nov 98:3-4, May 02:1, Aug 05:15, Oct 06:15, Jul 09:7, Aug 09:5; *CPT Changes: An Insider's View* 2009

99387 65 years and older

> *CPT Assistant* Winter 91:11, Spring 93:14, 34, Spring 95:1, Aug 97:1, Jul 98:9, Sep 98:5, Nov 98:3-4, May 02:1, Aug 05:15, Oct 06:15, Jul 09:7, Aug 09:5; *CPT Changes: An Insider's View* 2009

Established Patient

99391 Periodic comprehensive preventive medicine reevaluation and management of an individual including an age and gender appropriate history, examination, counseling/anticipatory guidance/risk factor reduction interventions, and the ordering of laboratory/diagnostic procedures, established patient; infant (age younger than 1 year)

> *CPT Assistant* Winter 91:11, Spring 93:14, 34, Spring 95:1, Aug 97:1, Jul 98:9, Sep 98:5, Nov 98:3-4, May 02:1, May 05:1, Aug 05:15, Oct 06:15, Mar 09:3, Jul 09:7, Aug 09:5; *CPT Changes: An Insider's View* 2002, 2009

99392 early childhood (age 1 through 4 years)

> *CPT Assistant* Winter 91:11, Spring 93:14, 34, Spring 95:1, Aug 97:1, Jul 98:9, Sep 98:5, Nov 98:3-4, May 02:1, Aug 05:15, Oct 06:15, Jul 09:7; *CPT Changes: An Insider's View* 2009

99393 late childhood (age 5 through 11 years)

> *CPT Assistant* Winter 91:11, Spring 93:14, 34, Spring 95:1, Aug 97:1, Jul 98:9, Sep 98:5, Nov 98:3-4, May 02:1, Aug 05:15, Oct 06:15, Jul 09:7; *CPT Changes: An Insider's View* 2009

99394 adolescent (age 12 through 17 years)

> *CPT Assistant* Winter 91:11, Spring 93:14, 34, Spring 95:1, Aug 97:1, Jul 98:9, Sep 98:5, Nov 98:3-4, May 02:1, Aug 05:15, Oct 06:15, Jul 09:7; *CPT Changes: An Insider's View* 2009

99395 18-39 years

> *CPT Assistant* Winter 91:11, Spring 93:14, 34, Spring 95:1, Aug 97:1, Jul 98:9, Sep 98:5, Nov 98:3-4, May 02:1, Aug 05:15, Oct 06:15, Mar 08:3, Jul 09:7; *CPT Changes: An Insider's View* 2009

99396 40-64 years

> *CPT Assistant* Winter 91:11, Spring 93:14, 34, Spring 95:1, Aug 97:1, Jul 98:9, Sep 98:5, Nov 98:3-4, May 02:1, Aug 05:15, Oct 06:15, Jul 09:7, Mar 12:4; *CPT Changes: An Insider's View* 2009

99397 65 years and older

> *CPT Assistant* Winter 91:11, Spring 93:14, 34, Spring 95:1, Aug 97:1, Jul 98:9, Sep 98:5, Nov 98:3-4, May 02:1, Aug 05:15, Oct 06:15, Jul 09:7; *CPT Changes: An Insider's View* 2009

Counseling Risk Factor Reduction and Behavior Change Intervention

New or Established Patient

These codes are used to report services provided face-to-face by a physician or other qualified health care professional for the purpose of promoting health and preventing illness or injury. They are distinct from evaluation and management (E/M) services that may be reported separately when performed. Risk factor reduction services are used for persons without a specific illness for which the counseling might otherwise be used as part of treatment.

Preventive medicine counseling and risk factor reduction interventions will vary with age and should address such issues as family problems, diet and exercise, substance use, sexual practices, injury prevention, dental health, and diagnostic and laboratory test results available at the time of the encounter.

Behavior change interventions are for persons who have a behavior that is often considered an illness itself, such as tobacco use and addiction, substance abuse/misuse, or obesity. Behavior change services may be reported when performed as part of the treatment of condition(s) related to or potentially exacerbated by the behavior or when performed to change the harmful behavior that has not yet resulted in illness. Any E/M services reported on the same day must be distinct, and time spent providing these services may not be used as a basis for the E/M code selection. Behavior change services involve specific validated interventions of assessing readiness for change and barriers to change, advising a change in behavior, assisting by providing specific suggested actions and motivational counseling, and arranging for services and follow-up.

For counseling groups of patients with symptoms or established illness, use 99078.

▶Health and Behavior Assessment/Intervention services (96150-96155) should not be reported on the same day as codes 99401-99412.◄

Preventive Medicine, Individual Counseling

99401 Preventive medicine counseling and/or risk factor reduction intervention(s) provided to an individual (separate procedure); approximately 15 minutes

> *CPT Assistant* Aug 97:1, Jan 98:12, May 05:1, Aug 07:9, Oct 10:3, Dec 10:3

99402   approximately 30 minutes
> *CPT Assistant* Aug 97:1, Jan 98:12, May 05:1, Oct 10:3, Dec 10:3

99403   approximately 45 minutes
> *CPT Assistant* Aug 97:1, Jan 98:12, May 05:1, Oct 10:3, Dec 10:3

99404   approximately 60 minutes
> *CPT Assistant* Aug 97:1, Jan 98:12, May 05:1, Oct 10:3, Dec 10:3

Behavior Change Interventions, Individual

99406   Smoking and tobacco use cessation counseling visit; intermediate, greater than 3 minutes up to 10 minutes
> *CPT Assistant* Jan 08:1, Sep 09:11, Oct 10:3, Dec 10:3; *CPT Changes: An Insider's View* 2008

99407   intensive, greater than 10 minutes
> *CPT Assistant* Jan 08:1, Sep 09:11, Oct 10:3, Dec 10:3; *CPT Changes: An Insider's View* 2008

(Do not report 99407 in conjunction with 99406)

99408   Alcohol and/or substance (other than tobacco) abuse structured screening (eg, AUDIT, DAST), and brief intervention (SBI) services; 15 to 30 minutes
> *CPT Assistant* Oct 10:3, Dec 10:3; *CPT Changes: An Insider's View* 2008

(Do not report services of less than 15 minutes with 99408)

99409   greater than 30 minutes
> *CPT Assistant* Oct 10:3, Dec 10:3; *CPT Changes: An Insider's View* 2008

(Do not report 99409 in conjunction with 99408)

(Do not report 99408, 99409 in conjunction with 99420)

(Use 99408, 99409 only for initial screening and brief intervention)

Preventive Medicine, Group Counseling

99411   **Preventive medicine counseling** and/or risk factor reduction intervention(s) provided to individuals in a group setting (separate procedure); approximately 30 minutes
> *CPT Assistant* Aug 97:1, Jan 98:12, Sep 98:5, May 05:1, Oct 10:3, Dec 10:3

99412   approximately 60 minutes
> *CPT Assistant* Aug 97:1, Jan 98:12, Sep 98:5, May 05:1, Aug 07:9, Oct 10:3, Dec 10:3

Other Preventive Medicine Services

99420   **Administration and interpretation** of health risk assessment instrument (eg, health hazard appraisal)
> *CPT Assistant* May 05:1, Oct 10:3, Dec 10:3

99429   **Unlisted preventive** medicine service
> *CPT Assistant* Sep 98:5, May 05:1, Oct 10:3, Dec 10:3

(99431 has been deleted. To report, use 99460)

(99432 has been deleted. To report, use 99461)

(99433 has been deleted. To report, use 99462)

(99435 has been deleted. To report, use 99463)

(99436 has been deleted. To report, use 99464)

(99440 has been deleted. To report, use 99465)

Non-Face-to-Face Services

Telephone Services

►Telephone services are non-face-to-face evaluation and management (E/M) services provided to a patient using the telephone by a physician or other qualified health care professional, who may report evaluation and management services. These codes are used to report episodes of patient care initiated by an established patient or guardian of an established patient. If the telephone service ends with a decision to see the patient within 24 hours or next available urgent visit appointment, the code is not reported; rather the encounter is considered part of the preservice work of the subsequent E/M service, procedure, and visit. Likewise if the telephone call refers to an E/M service performed and reported by that individual within the previous seven days (either requested or unsolicited patient follow-up) or within the postoperative period of the previously completed procedure, then the service(s) are considered part of that previous E/M service or procedure. (Do not report 99441-99443 if reporting 99441-99444 performed in the previous seven days.)◄

> ►(For telephone services provided by a qualified nonphysician health care professional who may not report evaluation and management services [eg, speech-language pathologists, physical therapists, occupational therapists, social workers, dietitians], see 98966-98968)◄

▲ **99441**   Telephone evaluation and management service by a physician or other qualified health care professional who may report evaluation and management services provided to an established patient, parent, or guardian not originating from a related E/M service provided within the previous 7 days nor leading to an E/M service or procedure within the next 24 hours or soonest available appointment; 5-10 minutes of medical discussion
> *CPT Assistant* Mar 08:6; *CPT Changes: An Insider's View* 2008, 2013

▲ **99442**   11-20 minutes of medical discussion
> *CPT Assistant* Mar 08:6; *CPT Changes: An Insider's View* 2008, 2013

▲ **99443**   21-30 minutes of medical discussion
> *CPT Assistant* Mar 08:6; *CPT Changes: An Insider's View* 2008, 2013

(Do not report 99441-99443 when using 99339-99340, 99374-99380 for the same call[s])

▲=Revised code   ●=New code   ► ◄=Contains new or revised text   ⊘=Modifier 51 exempt

(Do not report 99441-99443 for anticoagulation management when reporting 99363, 99364)

►(Do not report 99441-99443 during the same month with 99487-99489)◄

►(Do not report 99441-99443 when performed during the service time of codes 99495 or 99496)◄

On-Line Medical Evaluation

An on-line electronic medical evaluation is a non-face-to-face evaluation and management (E/M) service by a physician to a patient using Internet resources in response to a patient's on-line inquiry. Reportable services involve the physician's personal timely response to the patient's inquiry and must involve permanent storage (electronic or hard copy) of the encounter. This service is reported only once for the same episode of care during a seven-day period, although multiple physicians could report their exchange with the same patient. If the on-line medical evaluation refers to an E/M service previously performed and reported by the physician within the previous seven days (either physician requested or unsolicited patient follow-up) or within the postoperative period of the previously completed procedure, then the service(s) are considered covered by the previous E/M service or procedure. A reportable service encompasses the sum of communication (eg, related telephone calls, prescription provision, laboratory orders) pertaining to the on-line patient encounter.

(For an on-line medical evaluation provided by a qualified nonphysician health care professional, use 98969)

▲ **99444**   Online evaluation and management service provided by a physician or other qualified health care professional who may report an evaluation and management services provided to an established patient or guardian, not originating from a related E/M service provided within the previous 7 days, using the Internet or similar electronic communications network

➔ *CPT Changes: An Insider's View* 2008, 2013

(Do not report 99444 when using 99339, 99340, 99374-99380 for the same communication[s])

(Do not report 99444 for anticoagulation management when reporting 99363, 99364)

►(Do not report 99444 during the same month with 99487-99489)◄

►(Do not report 99444 when performed during the service time of codes 99495 or 99496)◄

Special Evaluation and Management Services

The following codes are used to report evaluations performed to establish baseline information prior to life or disability insurance certificates being issued. This service is performed in the office or other setting, and applies to both new and established patients. When using

these codes, no active management of the problem(s) is undertaken during the encounter.

If other evaluation and management services and/or procedures are performed on the same date, the appropriate E/M or procedure code(s) should be reported in addition to these codes.

Basic Life and/or Disability Evaluation Services

99450   **Basic life** and/or disability examination that includes:

- **Measurement of height, weight, and blood pressure;**
- **Completion of a medical history following a life insurance pro forma;**
- **Collection of blood sample and/or urinalysis complying with "chain of custody" protocols; and**
- **Completion of necessary documentation/ certificates.**

➔ *CPT Assistant* Summer 95:14, Sep 98:5, May 05:1

Work Related or Medical Disability Evaluation Services

99455   **Work related** or medical disability examination by the treating physician that includes:

- **Completion of a medical history commensurate with the patient's condition;**
- **Performance of an examination commensurate with the patient's condition;**
- **Formulation of a diagnosis, assessment of capabilities and stability, and calculation of impairment;**
- **Development of future medical treatment plan; and**
- **Completion of necessary documentation/ certificates and report.**

➔ *CPT Assistant* Summer 95:14, Sep 98:5, May 05:1

99456   **Work related** or medical disability examination by other than the treating physician that includes:

- **Completion of a medical history commensurate with the patient's condition;**
- **Performance of an examination commensurate with the patient's condition;**
- **Formulation of a diagnosis, assessment of capabilities and stability, and calculation of impairment;**
- **Development of future medical treatment plan; and**
- **Completion of necessary documentation/ certificates and report.**

➔ *CPT Assistant* Summer 95:14, Sep 98:5

(Do not report 99455, 99456 in conjunction with 99080 for the completion of Workman's Compensation forms)

Newborn Care Services

The following codes are used to report the services provided to newborns (birth through the first 28 days) in several different settings. Use of the normal newborn codes is limited to the initial care of the newborn in the first days after birth prior to home discharge.

Evaluation and Management (E/M) services for the newborn include maternal and/or fetal and newborn history, newborn physical examination(s), ordering of diagnostic tests and treatments, meetings with the family, and documentation in the medical record.

When delivery room attendance services (99464) or delivery room resuscitation services (99465) are required, report these in addition to normal newborn services Evaluation and Management codes.

▶For E/M services provided to newborns who are other than normal, see codes for hospital inpatient services (99221-99233) and neonatal intensive and critical care services (99466-99469, 99477-99480). When normal newborn services are provided by the same individual on the same date that the newborn later becomes ill and receives additional intensive or critical care services, report the appropriate E/M code with modifier 25 for these services in addition to the normal newborn code.◀

Procedures (eg, 54150, newborn circumcision) are not included with the normal newborn codes, and when performed, should be reported in addition to the newborn services.

When newborns are seen in follow-up after the date of discharge in the office or outpatient setting, see 99201-99215, 99381, 99391 as appropriate.

99460   Initial hospital or birthing center care, per day, for evaluation and management of normal newborn infant
➔ *CPT Changes: An Insider's View* 2009

99461   Initial care, per day, for evaluation and management of normal newborn infant seen in other than hospital or birthing center
➔ *CPT Changes: An Insider's View* 2009

99462   Subsequent hospital care, per day, for evaluation and management of normal newborn
➔ *CPT Changes: An Insider's View* 2009

99463   Initial hospital or birthing center care, per day, for evaluation and management of normal newborn infant admitted and discharged on the same date
➔ *CPT Changes: An Insider's View* 2009

(For newborn hospital discharge services provided on a date subsequent to the admission date, see 99238, 99239)

Delivery/Birthing Room Attendance and Resuscitation Services

▲ **99464**   Attendance at delivery (when requested by the delivering physician or other qualified health care professional) and initial stabilization of newborn
➔ *CPT Changes: An Insider's View* 2009, 2013

(99464 may be reported in conjunction with 99460, 99468, 99477)

(Do not report 99464 in conjunction with 99465)

99465   Delivery/birthing room resuscitation, provision of positive pressure ventilation and/or chest compressions in the presence of acute inadequate ventilation and/or cardiac output
➔ *CPT Changes: An Insider's View* 2009

(99465 may be reported in conjunction with 99460, 99468, 99477)

(Do not report 99465 in conjunction with 99464)

(Procedures that are performed as a necessary part of the resuscitation [eg, intubation, vascular lines] are reported separately in addition to 99465. In order to report these procedures, they must be performed as a necessary component of the resuscitation and not as a convenience before admission to the neonatal intensive care unit)

Inpatient Neonatal Intensive Care Services and Pediatric and Neonatal Critical Care Services

Pediatric Critical Care Patient Transport

▶Codes 99466, 99467 are used to report the physical attendance and direct face-to-face care by a physician during the interfacility transport of a critically ill or critically injured pediatric patient 24 months of age or younger. Codes 99485, 99486 are used to report the control physician's non-face-to-face supervision of interfacility transport of a critically ill or critically injured pediatric patient 24 months of age or younger. These codes are not reported together for the same patient by the same physician. For the purpose of reporting 99466 and 99467, face-to-face care begins when the physician assumes primary responsibility of the pediatric patient at the referring facility, and ends when the receiving facility accepts responsibility for the pediatric patient's care. Only the time the physician spends in direct face-to-face contact with the patient during the transport should be reported. Pediatric patient transport services involving less than 30 minutes of face-to-face physician care should not be reported using 99466, 99467. Procedure(s) or service(s) performed by other members of the transporting team may not be reported by the supervising physician.

Codes 99485, 99486 are used to report control physician's non-face-to-face supervision of interfacility pediatric critical care transport, which includes all two-way communication between the control physician and the specialized transport team prior to transport, at the referring facility and during transport of the patient back to the receiving facility. The "control" physician is the physician directing transport services. These codes do not include pretransport communication between the control physician and the referring facility before or following patient transport. These codes are only reported for patients 24 months of age or younger who are critically ill or critically injured. The control physician provides treatment advice to a specialized transport team who are present and delivering the hands-on patient care. The control physician does not report any services provided by the specialized transport team. The control physician's non-face-to-face time begins with the first contact by the control physician with the specialized transport team and ends when the patient's care is handed over to the receiving facility team. Refer to 99466 and 99467 for face-to-face transport care of the critically ill/injured patient. Time spent with the individual patient's transport team and reviewing data submissions should be recorded. Code 99485 is used to report the first 16-45 minutes of direction on a given date and should only be used once even if time spent by the physician is discontinuous. Do not report services of 15 minutes or less or any time when another physician is reporting 99466, 99467. Do not report 99485 or 99486 in conjunction with 99466, 99467 when performed by the same physician.◄

For the definition of the critically injured pediatric patient, see the **Neonatal and Pediatric Critical Care Services** section.

►The non-face-to-face direction of emergency care to a patient's transporting staff by a physician located in a hospital or other facility by two-way communication is not considered direct face-to-face care and should not be reported with 99466, 99467. Physician-directed non-face-to-face emergency care through outside voice communication to transporting staff personnel is reported with 99288 or 99485, 99486 based upon the age and clinical condition of the patient.◄

Emergency department services (99281-99285), initial hospital care (99221-99223), critical care (99291, 99292), initial date neonatal intensive (99477) or critical care (99468) are only reported after the patient has been admitted to the emergency department, the inpatient floor, or the critical care unit of the receiving facility. If inpatient critical care services are reported in the referring facility prior to transfer to the receiving hospital, use the critical care codes (99291, 99292).

►Services provided by the specialized transport team during non-face-to-face transport supervision are not reported by the control physician.◄

Code 99466 is used to report the first 30 to 74 minutes of direct face-to-face time with the transport pediatric patient and should be reported only once on a given date. Code 99467 is used to report each additional 30 minutes provided on a given date. Face-to-face services of less than 30 minutes should not be reported with these codes.

►Code 99485 is used to report the first 30 minutes of non-face-to-face supervision of an interfacility transport of a critically ill or critically injured pediatric patient and should be reported only once per date of service. Code 99486 is used to report each additional 30 minutes beyond the initial 30 minutes. Non-face-to-face interfacility transport of 15 minutes or less is not reported.◄

(For total body cooling of neonates, see 0260T, 0261T)

▲ **99466**   **Critical care** face-to-face services during an interfacility transport of critically ill or critically injured pediatric patient, 24 months of age or younger; first 30-74 minutes of hands-on care during transport

➡ *CPT Assistant* Sep 11:3; *CPT Changes: An Insider's View* 2009, 2013

+▲ **99467**   each additional 30 minutes (List separately in addition to code for primary service)

➡ *CPT Assistant* Sep 11:3; *CPT Changes: An Insider's View* 2009, 2013

(Use 99467 in conjunction with 99466)

(Critical care of less than 30 minutes total duration should be reported with the appropriate E/M code)

#● **99485**   Supervision by a control physician of interfacility transport care of the critically ill or critically injured pediatric patient, 24 months of age or younger, includes two-way communication with transport team before transport, at the referring facility and during the transport, including data interpretation and report; first 30 minutes

➡ *CPT Changes: An Insider's View* 2013

#+● **99486**   each additional 30 minutes (List separately in addition to code for primary procedure)

➡ *CPT Changes: An Insider's View* 2013

►(Use 99486 in conjunction with 99485)◄

►(For physician direction of emergency medical systems supervision for a pediatric patient older than 24 months of age, or at any age if not critically ill or injured, use 99288)◄

►(Do not report 99485, 99486 with any other services reported by the control physician for the same period)◄

►(Do not report 99485, 99486 in conjunction with 99466, 99467 when performed by the same physician)◄

Inpatient Neonatal and Pediatric Critical Care

The same definitions for critical care services apply for the adult, child, and neonate.

►Codes 99468, 99469 are used to report the services of directing the inpatient care of a critically ill neonate or infant 28 days of age or younger. They represent care starting with the date of admission (99468) to a critical care unit and subsequent day(s) (99469) that the neonate remains critical. These codes may be reported only by a single individual and only once per day, per patient, per hospital stay in a given facility. If readmitted to the neonatal critical care unit during the same day, report the subsequent day(s) code 99469 for the first day of readmission to critical care, and 99469 for each day of critical care following readmission.

The initial day neonatal critical care code (99468) can be used in addition to 99464 or 99465 as appropriate, when the physician or other qualified health care professional is present for the delivery (99464) or resuscitation (99465) is required. Other procedures performed as a necessary part of the resuscitation (eg, endotracheal intubation [31500]) are also reported separately when performed as part of the pre-admission delivery room care. In order to report these procedures separately, they must be performed as a necessary component of the resuscitation and not simply as a convenience before admission to the neonatal intensive care unit.

Codes 99471-99476 are used to report direction of the inpatient care of a critically ill infant or young child from 29 days of postnatal age through less than 6 years of age. They represent care starting with the date of admission (99471, 99475) to all subsequent day(s) (99472, 99476) the infant or child remains critical. These codes may be reported only by a single individual and only once per day, per patient in a given setting. Services for the critically ill or critically injured child 6 years of age or older would be reported with the time based critical care codes (99291, 99292). Report 99471, 99475 only once per hospital stay in a given facility. If readmitted to the pediatric critical care unit during the same stay, report 99472 or 99476 for the first day of readmission to critical care and 99472 for each day of critical care following readmission.◄

The pediatric and neonatal critical care codes include those procedures listed for the critical care codes (99291, 99292). In addition, the following procedures are also included (and are not separately reported by professionals, but may be reported by facilities) in the pediatric and neonatal critical care service codes (99468-99472, 99475, 99476) and the intensive care services codes (99477-99480):

Any services performed that are not included in these listings may be reported separately. Facilities may report the included services separately.

Invasive or non-invasive electronic monitoring of vital signs

Vascular access procedures

  Peripheral vessel catheterization (36000)

  Other arterial catheters (36140, 36620)

  Umbilical venous catheters (36510)

  Central vessel catheterization (36555)

  Vascular access procedures (36400, 36405, 36406)

  Vascular punctures (36420, 36600)

  Umbilical arterial catheters (36660)

Airway and ventilation management

  Endotracheal intubation (31500)

  Ventilatory management (94002-94004)

  Bedside pulmonary function testing (94375)

  Surfactant administration (94610)

  Continuous positive airway pressure (CPAP) (94660)

Monitoring or interpretation of blood gases or oxygen saturation (94760-94762)

Car Seat Evaluation (94780-94781)

Transfusion of blood components (36430, 36440)

Oral or nasogastric tube placement (43752)

Suprapubic bladder aspiration (51100)

Bladder catheterization (51701, 51702)

Lumbar puncture (62270)

Any services performed which are not listed above may be reported separately.

When a neonate or infant is not critically ill but requires intensive observation, frequent interventions, and other intensive care services, the Continuing Intensive Care Services codes (99477-99480) should be used to report these services.

►To report critical care services provided in the outpatient setting (eg, emergency department or office) for neonates and pediatric patients of any age, see the Critical Care codes 99291, 99292. If the same individual provides critical care services for a neonatal or pediatric patient less than 6 years of age in both the outpatient and inpatient settings on the same day, report only the appropriate Neonatal or Pediatric Critical Care codes 99468-99476 for all critical care services provided on that day. Critical care services provided by a second individual of a different specialty not reporting a per-day neonatal or pediatric critical care code can be reported with 99291, 99292.

When critical care services are provided to neonates or pediatric patients less than 6 years of age at two separate institutions by an individual from a different group on the same date of service, the individual from the referring institution should report their critical care services with the time-based critical care codes (99291, 99292) and the receiving institution should report the appropriate initial day of care code 99468, 99471, 99475 for the same date of service.◄

Critical care services to a pediatric patient 6 years of age or older are reported with the time based critical care codes 99291, 99292.

►When the critically ill neonate or pediatric patient improves and is transferred to a lower level of care to another individual in another group within the same facility, the transferring individual does not report a per day critical care service. Subsequent hospital care (99231-99233) or time-based critical care services (99291-99292) is reported, as appropriate based upon the condition of the neonate or child. The receiving individual reports subsequent intensive care (99478-99480) or subsequent hospital care (99231-99233) services, as appropriate based upon the condition of the neonate or child.

When the neonate or infant becomes critically ill on a day when initial or subsequent intensive care services (99477-99480), hospital services (99221-99233), or normal newborn services (99460, 99461, 99462) have been performed by one individual and is transferred to a critical care level of care provided by a different individual in a different group, the transferring individual reports either the time-based critical care services performed (99291, 99292) for the time spent providing critical care to the patient, the intensive care service (99477-99480), hospital care services (99221-99233), or normal newborn service (99460, 99461, 99462) performed, but only one service. The receiving individual reports initial or subsequent inpatient neonatal or pediatric critical care (99468-99476), as appropriate based upon the patient's age and whether this is the first or subsequent admission to the critical care unit for the hospital stay.

When a newborn becomes critically ill on the same day they have already received normal newborn care (99460, 99461, 99462), and the same individual or group assumes critical care, report initial critical care service (99468) with modifier 25 in addition to the normal newborn code.

When a neonate, infant, or child requires initial critical care services on the same day the patient already has received hospital care or intensive care services by the same individual or group, only the initial critical care service code (99468, 99471, 99475) is reported.

Time-based critical care services (99291, 99292) are not reportable by the same individual or different individual within the same group when neonatal or pediatric critical care services (99468-99476) are reported for the same patient on the same day.

No individual may report remote real-time videoconferenced critical care (0188T, 0189T) when neonatal or pediatric intensive or critical care services (99468-99476) are reported.◄

99468 **Initial inpatient neonatal critical care,** per day, for the evaluation and management of a critically ill neonate, 28 days of age or younger
➔ *CPT Assistant* Nov 11:5; *CPT Changes: An Insider's View* 2009

99469 **Subsequent inpatient neonatal critical care,** per day, for the evaluation and management of a critically ill neonate, 28 days of age or younger
➔ *CPT Assistant* Nov 11:5; *CPT Changes: An Insider's View* 2009

99471 **Initial inpatient pediatric critical care,** per day, for the evaluation and management of a critically ill infant or young child, 29 days through 24 months of age
➔ *CPT Assistant* Nov 11:5; *CPT Changes: An Insider's View* 2009

99472 **Subsequent inpatient pediatric critical care,** per day, for the evaluation and management of a critically ill infant or young child, 29 days through 24 months of age
➔ *CPT Assistant* Nov 11:5; *CPT Changes: An Insider's View* 2009

99475 **Initial inpatient pediatric critical care,** per day, for the evaluation and management of a critically ill infant or young child, 2 through 5 years of age
➔ *CPT Changes: An Insider's View* 2009

99476 **Subsequent inpatient pediatric critical care,** per day, for the evaluation and management of a critically ill infant or young child, 2 through 5 years of age
➔ *CPT Changes: An Insider's View* 2009

Initial and Continuing Intensive Care Services

►Code 99477 represents the initial day of inpatient care for the child who is not critically ill but requires intensive observation, frequent interventions, and other intensive care services. Codes 99478-99480 are used to report the subsequent day services of directing the continuing intensive care of the low birth weight (LBW 1500-2500 grams) present body weight infant, very low birth weight (VLBW less than 1500 grams) present body weight infant, or normal (2501-5000 grams) present body weight newborn who does not meet the definition of critically ill but continues to require intensive observation, frequent interventions, and other intensive care services. These services are for infants and neonates who are not critically ill but continue to require intensive cardiac and respiratory monitoring, continuous and/or frequent vital sign monitoring, heat maintenance, enteral and/or parenteral nutritional adjustments, laboratory and oxygen monitoring, and constant observation by the health care team under direct supervision of the physician or other qualified health care professional. Codes 99477-99480 may be reported by a single individual and only once per day, per patient in a given facility. If readmitted to the intensive care unit during the same hospital stay, report 99478-99480 for the first day of intensive care and for each successive day that the child requires intensive care services.

These codes include the same procedures that are outlined in the **Neonatal and Pediatric Critical Care**

Services section and these services should not be separately reported.

The initial day neonatal intensive care code (99477) can be used in addition to 99464 or 99465 as appropriate, when the physician or other qualified health care professional is present for the delivery (99464) or resuscitation (99465) is required. In this situation, report 99477 with modifier 25. Other procedures performed as a necessary part of the resuscitation (eg, endotracheal intubation [31500]) are also reported separately when performed as part of the pre-admission delivery room care. In order to report these procedures separately, they must be performed as a necessary component of the resuscitation and not simply as a convenience before admission to the neonatal intensive care unit.

The same procedures are included as bundled services with the neonatal intensive care codes as those listed for the neonatal (99468, 99469) and pediatric (99471-99476) critical care codes.

When the neonate or infant improves after the initial day and no longer requires intensive care services and is transferred to a lower level of care, the transferring individual does not report a per day intensive care service. Subsequent hospital care (99231-99233) or subsequent normal newborn care (99460, 99462) is reported as appropriate based upon the condition of the neonate or infant. If the transfer to a lower level of care occurs on the same day as initial intensive care services were provided by the transferring individual, 99477 may be reported.

When the neonate or infant is transferred after the initial day within the same facility to the care of another individual in a different group, both individuals report subsequent hospital care (99231-99233) services. The receiving individual reports subsequent hospital care (99231-99233) or subsequent normal newborn care (99462).

When the neonate or infant becomes critically ill on a day when initial or subsequent intensive care services (99477-99480) have been reported by one individual and is transferred to a critical care level of care provided by a different individual from a different group, the transferring individual reports either the time-based critical care services performed (99291, 99292) for the time spent providing critical care to the patient or the initial or subsequent intensive care (99477-99480) service, but not both. The receiving individual reports initial or subsequent inpatient neonatal or pediatric critical care (99468-99476) based upon the patient's age and whether this is the first or subsequent admission to critical care for the same hospital stay.

When the neonate or infant becomes critically ill on a day when initial or subsequent intensive care services (99477-99480) have been performed by the same individual or group, report only initial or subsequent inpatient neonatal or pediatric critical care (99468-99476) based upon the patient's age and whether this is the first or subsequent admission to critical care for the same hospital stay.◄

For the subsequent care of the sick neonate younger than 28 days of age but more than 5000 grams who does not require intensive or critical care services, use codes 99231-99233.

99477   **Initial hospital care,** per day, for the evaluation and management of the neonate, 28 days of age or younger, who requires intensive observation, frequent interventions, and other intensive care services

➔ *CPT Assistant* Jan 08:8, Jul 08:10, Mar 09:3, Nov 11:5; *CPT Changes: An Insider's View* 2008

(For the initiation of inpatient care of the normal newborn, use 99460)

(For the initiation of care of the critically ill neonate, use 99468)

(For initiation of inpatient hospital care of the ill neonate not requiring intensive observation, frequent interventions, and other intensive care services, see 99221-99223)

99478   **Subsequent intensive care,** per day, for the evaluation and management of the recovering very low birth weight infant (present body weight less than 1500 grams)

➔ *CPT Changes: An Insider's View* 2009

99479   **Subsequent intensive care,** per day, for the evaluation and management of the recovering low birth weight infant (present body weight of 1500-2500 grams)

➔ *CPT Changes: An Insider's View* 2009

99480   **Subsequent intensive care,** per day, for the evaluation and management of the recovering infant (present body weight of 2501-5000 grams)

➔ *CPT Changes: An Insider's View* 2009

99485   Code is out of numerical sequence. See 99466-99486

99486   Code is out of numerical sequence. See 99466-99486

►Complex Chronic Care Coordination Services◄

►Complex chronic care coordination services are patient-centered management and support services provided by physicians, other qualified health care professionals, and clinical staff to an individual who resides at home or in a domiciliary, rest home, or assisted living facility. These services typically involve clinical staff implementing a care plan directed by the physician or other qualified health care professional. These services address the coordination of care by multiple disciplines and community service agencies. The reporting individual provides or oversees the management and/or coordination of services, as needed, for all medical conditions, psychosocial needs, and activities of daily living.

Patients who require complex chronic care coordination services may be identified by algorithms that utilize reported conditions and services (eg, predictive modeling risk score or repeat admissions or emergency department use) or by clinician judgment. Typical patients have 1 or more chronic continuous or episodic health conditions expected to last at least 12 months, or until the death of the patient, that place the patient at significant risk of death, acute exacerbation/decompensation, or functional decline. Because of the complex nature of their diseases and morbidities, these patients commonly require the coordination of a number of specialties and services. Patients may have medical and psychiatric behavioral co-morbidities (eg, dementia and chronic obstructive pulmonary disease or substance abuse and diabetes) that complicate their care. Social support weaknesses or access to care difficulties may cause a need for these services. Medical, functional, and/or psychosocial problems that require medical decision making of moderate or high complexity and extensive clinical staff support are expected. Medical decision making as defined in the Evaluation and Management (E/M) guidelines is not only applied to the face-to-face services but is determined by the nature of the problems addressed by the reporting individual during the month. A plan of care should be documented and shared with the patient and/or caregiver.

Codes 99487-99489 are reported only **once** per calendar month and include all non-face-to-face complex chronic care coordination services and none or 1 face-to-face office or other outpatient, home, or domiciliary visit. Codes 99487-99489 may only be reported by the single physician or other qualified health care professional who assumes the care coordination role with a particular patient for the calendar month.

Code selection is as follows:

Code 99487 is reported when, during the calendar month, there is no face-to-face visit with the physician or other qualified health care professional and at least 31 minutes of clinical staff time is spent in care coordination activities. Code 99488 is reported when, during the calendar month, there is a face-to-face visit with the physician or other qualified health care professional and at least 31 minutes of clinical staff time is spent in care coordination activities.

The face-to-face and non-face-to-face time spent by the clinical staff in communicating with the patient and/or family, caregivers, other professionals and agencies; revising, documenting and implementing the care plan; or teaching self-management is used in determining the complex chronic care coordination clinical staff time for the month. **Note:** Do not count any clinical staff time on the date of the first visit or on a day when the physician or qualified health care professional reports an E/M service (office or other outpatient services 99211-99215; domiciliary; rest home services 99334-99337; home services 99347-99350).

Care coordination activities performed by clinical staff may include:

- communication (with patient, family members, guardian or caretaker, surrogate decision makers, and/or other professionals) regarding aspects of care;
- communication with home health agencies and other community services utilized by the patient;
- collection of health outcomes data and registry documentation;
- patient and/or family/caretaker education to support self-management, independent living, and activities of daily living;
- assessment and support for treatment regimen adherence and medication management;
- identification of available community and health resources;
- facilitating access to care and services needed by the patient and/or family;
- development and maintenance of a comprehensive care plan.

If a face-to-face visit was provided during the month by the physician or other qualified health care professional, report 99488. Additional E/M services beyond the first visit may be reported separately by the same physician or other qualified health care professional during the same calendar month. Complex care coordination services include care plan oversight services (99339, 99340, 99374-99378), prolonged services without direct patient contact (99358, 99359), anticoagulant management (99363, 99364), medical team conferences (99366-99368), education and training (98960-98962, 99071, 99078), telephone services (98966-98968, 99441-99443), on-line medical evaluation (98969, 99444), preparation of special reports (99080), analysis of data (99090, 99091), transitional care management services (99495, 99496), medication therapy management services (99605-99607), and if performed, these services may not be reported separately during the month for which 99487-99489 are reported. All other services may be reported. Do not report 99487-99489 if reporting ESRD services (90951-90970) during the same month. If the complex chronic care coordination services are performed within the postoperative period of a reported surgery, the same individual may not report 99487-99489.

Complex chronic care coordination can be reported in any calendar month during which the clinical staff time requirements are met. If care coordination resumes after a discharge during a new month, start a new period or report transitional care management services (99495, 99496) as appropriate. If discharge occurs in the same month, continue the reporting period or report transitional care management services. Do not report 99487-99489 for any post-discharge complex chronic care coordination services for any days within 30 days of discharge, if reporting 99495, 99496.◄

Total Duration of Staff Care Coordination Services	Code(s)
Less than 30 minutes	Not reported separately
31 to 74 minutes (31 minutes - 1 hr. 14 min.)	99487 or 99488 X 1
75 - 104 minutes (1 hr. 15 min. - 1 hr. 44 min.)	99487 or 99488 X 1 and 99489 X 1
105 minutes or more (1 hr. 45 min. or more)	99487 or 99488 X 1 and 99489 X 2 or more for each additional 30 minutes

● **99487** Complex chronic care coordination services; first hour of clinical staff time directed by a physician or other qualified health care professional with no face-to-face visit, per calendar month
→ *CPT Changes: An Insider's View* 2013

● **99488** first hour of clinical staff time directed by a physician or other qualified health care professional with one face-to-face visit, per calendar month
→ *CPT Changes: An Insider's View* 2013

+● **99489** each additional 30 minutes of clinical staff time directed by a physician or other qualified health care professional, per calendar month (List separately in addition to code for primary procedure)
→ *CPT Changes: An Insider's View* 2013

►(Report 99489 in conjunction with 99487, 99488)◄

►(Do not report 99487-99489 during the same month with 90951-90970, 98960-98962, 98966-98969, 99071, 99078, 99080, 99090, 99091, 99339, 99340, 99358, 99359, 99363, 99364, 99366-99368, 99374-99378, 99441-99444, 99495, 99496, 99605-99607)◄

[handwritten: Clinical staff require chronic care coordinator   Co-morbidity]

—— *Coding Tip* ——

Time of care coordination with the emergency department is reportable using 99487-99489, but time while the patient is inpatient or admitted as observation is not.

If the physician personally performs the clinical staff activities, his or her time may be counted toward the required clinical staff time to meet the elements of the code.

►Transitional Care Management Services◄

►Codes 99495 and 99496 are used to report transitional care management services (TCM). These services are for an established patient whose medical and/or psychosocial problems require moderate or high complexity medical decision making during transitions in care from an inpatient hospital setting (including acute hospital,

rehabilitation hospital, long-term acute care hospital), partial hospital, observation status in a hospital, or skilled nursing facility/nursing facility, to the patient's community setting (home, domiciliary, rest home, or assisted living). TCM commences upon the date of discharge and continues for the next 29 days.

TCM is comprised of one face-to-face visit within the specified time frames, in combination with non- face-to-face services that may be performed by the physician or other qualified health care professional and/or licensed clinical staff under his or her direction.

Non-face-to-face services provided by clinical staff, under the direction of the physician or other qualified health care professional, may include:

- communication (with patient, family members, guardian or caretaker, surrogate decision makers, and/or other professionals) regarding aspects of care;
- communication with home health agencies and other community services utilized by the patient;
- patient and/or family/caretaker education to support self-management, independent living, and activities of daily living;
- assessment and support for treatment regimen adherence and medication management;
- identification of available community and health resources;
- facilitating access to care and services needed by the patient and/or family.

Non-face-to-face services provided by the physician or other qualified health care provider may include:

- obtaining and reviewing the discharge information (eg, discharge summary, as available, or continuity of care documents);
- reviewing need for or follow-up on pending diagnostic tests and treatments;
- interaction with other qualified health care professionals who will assume or reassume care of the patient's system-specific problems;
- education of patient, family, guardian, and/or caregiver;
- establishment or reestablishment of referrals and arranging for needed community resources;
- assistance in scheduling any required follow-up with community providers and services.

TCM requires a face-to-face visit, initial patient contact, and medication reconciliation within specified time frames. The first face-to-face visit is part of the TCM service and not reported separately. Additional E/M services after the first face-to-face visit may be reported separately. TCM requires an interactive contact with the patient or caregiver, as appropriate, within two business days of discharge. The contact may be direct (face-to-face), telephonic, or by electronic means. Medication reconciliation and management must occur no later than the date of the face-to-face visit.

These services address any needed coordination of care performed by multiple disciplines and community service agencies. The reporting individual provides or oversees the management and/or coordination of services, as needed, for all medical conditions, psychosocial needs, and activities of daily living support by providing first contact and continuous access.

Medical decision making and the date of the first face-to-face visit are used to select and report the appropriate TCM code. For 99496, the face-to-face visit must occur within 7 calendar days of the date of discharge, and medical decision making must be of high complexity. For 99495, the face-to-face visit must occur within 14 calendar days of the date of discharge, and medical decision making must be of at least moderate complexity.

Type of Medical Decision Making	Face-to-face visit within 7 days	Face to face visit within 8 to 14 days
Moderate Complexity	99495	99495
High Complexity	99496	99495

Medical decision making is defined by the E/M Services Guidelines. The medical decision making over the service period reported is used to define the medical decision making of TCM. Documentation includes the timing of the initial post-discharge communication with the patient or caregivers, date of the face-to-face visit, and the complexity of medical decision making.

Only one individual may report these services and only once per patient within 30 days of discharge. Another TCM may not be reported by the same individual or group for any subsequent discharge(s) within the 30 days. The same individual may report hospital or observation discharge services and TCM. The same individual should not report TCM services provided in the postoperative period.

A physician or other qualified health care professional who reports codes 99495, 99496 may not report care plan oversight services (99339, 99340, 99374-99380), prolonged services without direct patient contact (99358, 99359), anticoagulant management (99363, 99364), medical team conferences (99366-99368), education and training (98960-98962, 99071, 99078), telephone services (98966-98968, 99441-99443), end stage renal disease services (90951-90970), online medical evaluation services (98969, 99444), preparation of special reports (99080), analysis of data (99090, 99091), complex chronic care coordination services (99487-99489), or medication therapy management services (99605-99607) during the time period covered by the transitional care management services codes.◄

● **99495** **Transitional Care Management Services** with the following required elements:

- Communication (direct contact, telephone, electronic) with the patient and/or caregiver within 2 business days of discharge
- Medical decision making of at least moderate complexity during the service period
- Face-to-face visit, within 14 calendar days of discharge

➔ *CPT Changes: An Insider's View* 2013

● **99496** **Transitional Care Management Services** with the following required elements:

- Communication (direct contact, telephone, electronic) with the patient and/or caregiver within 2 business days of discharge
- Medical decision making of high complexity during the service period
- Face-to-face visit, within 7 calendar days of discharge

➔ *CPT Changes: An Insider's View* 2013

►(Do not report 90951-90970, 98960-98962, 98966-98969, 99071, 99078, 99080, 99090, 99091, 99339, 99340, 99358, 99359, 99363, 99364, 99366-99368, 99374-99380, 99441-99444, 99487-99489, 99605-99607 when performed during the service time of codes 99495 or 99496)◄

─── *Coding Tip* ───

If another individual provides TCM services within the post operative period of a surgical package, modifier 54 is not required.

The required contact with the patient or caregiver, as appropriate, may be by the physician or qualified health care professional or clinical staff. Within two business days of discharge is Monday through Friday except holidays without respect to normal practice hours or date of notification of discharge. The contact must include capacity for prompt interactive communication addressing patient status and needs beyond scheduling follow-up care. If two or more separate attempts are made in a timely manner, but are unsuccessful and other transitional care management criteria are met, the service may be reported.

Other Evaluation and Management Services

99499 **Unlisted evaluation and management** service

➔ *CPT Assistant* Apr 96:11, Mar 05:11, May 05:1, Jan 06:46, Sep 06:8, Jan 07:30, May 11:7, Apr 12:10, Jul 12:10, 11

Anesthesia Guidelines

Anesthesia

Anesthesia Guidelines

Services involving administration of anesthesia are reported by the use of the anesthesia five-digit procedure code (00100-01999) plus modifier codes (defined under "Anesthesia Modifiers" later in these Guidelines).

The reporting of anesthesia services is appropriate by or under the responsible supervision of a physician. These services may include but are not limited to general, regional, supplementation of local anesthesia, or other supportive services in order to afford the patient the anesthesia care deemed optimal by the anesthesiologist during any procedure. These services include the usual preoperative and postoperative visits, the anesthesia care during the procedure, the administration of fluids and/or blood and the usual monitoring services (eg, ECG, temperature, blood pressure, oximetry, capnography, and mass spectrometry). Unusual forms of monitoring (eg, intra-arterial, central venous, and Swan-Ganz) are not included.

Items used by all physicians in reporting their services are presented in the **Introduction.** Some of the commonalities are repeated in this section for the convenience of those physicians referring to this section on **Anesthesia.** Other definitions and items unique to anesthesia are also listed.

To report moderate (conscious) sedation provided by a physician also performing the service for which conscious sedation is being provided, see codes 99143-99145.

For the procedures listed in Appendix G, when a second physician other than the health care professional performing the diagnostic or therapeutic services provides moderate (conscious) sedation in the facility setting (eg, hospital, outpatient hospital/ambulatory surgery center, skilled nursing facility), the second physician reports the associated moderate sedation procedure/service 99148-99150; when these services are performed by the second physician in the nonfacility setting (eg, physician office, freestanding imaging center), codes 99148-99150 would not be reported. Moderate sedation does not include minimal sedation (anxiolysis), deep sedation, or monitored anesthesia care (00100-01999).

To report regional or general anesthesia provided by a physician also performing the services for which the anesthesia is being provided, see modifier 47 in Appendix A.

Time Reporting

Time for anesthesia procedures may be reported as is customary in the local area. Anesthesia time begins when the anesthesiologist begins to prepare the patient for the induction of anesthesia in the operating room (or in an equivalent area) and ends when the anesthesiologist is no longer in personal attendance, that is, when the patient may be safely placed under postoperative supervision.

►Anesthesia Services◄

►Services rendered in the office, home, or hospital; consultation; and other medical services are listed in the **Evaluation and Management Services** section, beginning on page 11 (99201-99499). "Special Services and Reporting" (99000-99091) are listed in the **Medicine** section.◄

►Supplied Materials◄

►Supplies and materials provided (eg, sterile trays, drugs) over and above those usually included with the office visit or other services rendered may be listed separately. Drugs, tray supplies, and materials provided should be listed and identified with 99070 or the appropriate supply code.◄

Separate or Multiple Procedures

When multiple surgical procedures are performed during a single anesthetic administration, the anesthesia code representing the most complex procedure is reported. The time reported is the combined total for all procedures.

Special Report

A service that is rarely provided, unusual, variable, or new may require a special report. Pertinent information should include an adequate definition or description of the nature, extent, and need for the procedure and the time, effort, and equipment necessary to provide the service.

Anesthesia Modifiers

All anesthesia services are reported by use of the anesthesia five-digit procedure code (00100-01999) plus the addition of a physical status modifier. The use of other optional modifiers may be appropriate.

Physical Status Modifiers

Physical Status modifiers are represented by the initial letter 'P' followed by a single digit from 1 to 6 as defined in the following list:

P1: A normal healthy patient

P2: A patient with mild systemic disease

P3: A patient with severe systemic disease

P4: A patient with severe systemic disease that is a constant threat to life

P5: A moribund patient who is not expected to survive without the operation

P6: A declared brain-dead patient whose organs are being removed for donor purposes

These six levels are consistent with the American Society of Anesthesiologists (ASA) ranking of patient physical status. Physical status is included in the CPT codebook to distinguish among various levels of complexity of the anesthesia service provided.

Example: 00100-P1

Qualifying Circumstances

More than one qualifying circumstance may be selected.

Many anesthesia services are provided under particularly difficult circumstances, depending on factors such as extraordinary condition of patient, notable operative conditions, and/or unusual risk factors. This section includes a list of important qualifying circumstances that significantly affect the character of the anesthesia service provided. These procedures would not be reported alone but would be reported as additional procedure numbers qualifying an anesthesia procedure or service.

+ 99100   Anesthesia for patient of extreme age, younger than 1 year and older than 70 (List separately in addition to code for primary anesthesia procedure)

                   (For procedure performed on infants younger than 1 year of age at time of surgery, see 00326, 00561, 00834, 00836)

+ 99116   Anesthesia complicated by utilization of total body hypothermia (List separately in addition to code for primary anesthesia procedure)

+ 99135   Anesthesia complicated by utilization of controlled hypotension (List separately in addition to code for primary anesthesia procedure)

+ 99140   Anesthesia complicated by emergency conditions (specify) (List separately in addition to code for primary anesthesia procedure)

                   (An emergency is defined as existing when delay in treatment of the patient would lead to a significant increase in the threat to life or body part)

Anesthesia

Head

00100 Anesthesia for procedures on salivary glands, including biopsy
→ *CPT Assistant* Feb 97:4, Nov 99:6, Feb 06:9, Mar 06:15, Nov 07:8, Oct 11:3, Jul 12:13
→ *Clinical Examples in Radiology* Summer 11:2

00102 Anesthesia for procedures involving plastic repair of cleft lip
→ *CPT Assistant* Nov 99:6; *CPT Changes: An Insider's View* 2000

00103 Anesthesia for reconstructive procedures of eyelid (eg, blepharoplasty, ptosis surgery)
→ *CPT Assistant* Nov 99:6; *CPT Changes: An Insider's View* 2000

00104 Anesthesia for electroconvulsive therapy

00120 Anesthesia for procedures on external, middle, and inner ear including biopsy; not otherwise specified

00124   otoscopy
→ *CPT Assistant* Nov 99:7

00126   tympanotomy

00140 Anesthesia for procedures on eye; not otherwise specified

00142   lens surgery

00144   corneal transplant

00145   vitreoretinal surgery
→ *CPT Changes: An Insider's View* 2001

00147   iridectomy

00148   ophthalmoscopy

00160 Anesthesia for procedures on nose and accessory sinuses; not otherwise specified

00162   radical surgery

00164   biopsy, soft tissue

00170 Anesthesia for intraoral procedures, including biopsy; not otherwise specified

00172   repair of cleft palate

00174   excision of retropharyngeal tumor

00176   radical surgery

00190 Anesthesia for procedures on facial bones or skull; not otherwise specified
→ *CPT Changes: An Insider's View* 2001

00192   radical surgery (including prognathism)

00210 Anesthesia for intracranial procedures; not otherwise specified

00211   craniotomy or craniectomy for evacuation of hematoma
→ *CPT Changes: An Insider's View* 2009

00212   subdural taps

00214   burr holes, including ventriculography
→ *CPT Assistant* Nov 99:7; *CPT Changes: An Insider's View* 2000

00215   cranioplasty or elevation of depressed skull fracture, extradural (simple or compound)
→ *CPT Changes: An Insider's View* 2001

00216   vascular procedures

00218   procedures in sitting position

00220   cerebrospinal fluid shunting procedures

00222   electrocoagulation of intracranial nerve
→ *CPT Assistant* Jul 12:13

Neck

00300 Anesthesia for all procedures on the integumentary system, muscles and nerves of head, neck, and posterior trunk, not otherwise specified
→ *CPT Assistant* Nov 99:7, Mar 06:15, Oct 11:3, Jul 12:13

00320 Anesthesia for all procedures on esophagus, thyroid, larynx, trachea and lymphatic system of neck; not otherwise specified, age 1 year or older
→ *CPT Changes: An Insider's View* 2003

00322   needle biopsy of thyroid

(For procedures on cervical spine and cord, see 00600, 00604, 00670)

00326 Anesthesia for all procedures on the larynx and trachea in children younger than 1 year of age
→ *CPT Changes: An Insider's View* 2003

(Do not report 00326 in conjunction with 99100)

00350 Anesthesia for procedures on major vessels of neck; not otherwise specified

00352   simple ligation
→ *CPT Assistant* Nov 07:8, Jul 12:13

(For arteriography, use 01916)

Thorax (Chest Wall and Shoulder Girdle)

00400 Anesthesia for procedures on the integumentary system on the extremities, anterior trunk and perineum; not otherwise specified
→ *CPT Assistant* Mar 06:15, Nov 07:8, Oct 11:3, Jul 12:13

00402   reconstructive procedures on breast (eg, reduction or augmentation mammoplasty, muscle flaps)

00404   radical or modified radical procedures on breast

00406   radical or modified radical procedures on breast with internal mammary node dissection

00410   electrical conversion of arrhythmias

00450   Anesthesia for procedures on clavicle and scapula; not otherwise specified

00452   radical surgery

00454   biopsy of clavicle

00470   Anesthesia for partial rib resection; not otherwise specified

00472   thoracoplasty (any type)

00474   radical procedures (eg, pectus excavatum)
→ *CPT Assistant* Nov 07:8, Jul 12:13

Intrathoracic

00500   Anesthesia for all procedures on esophagus
→ *CPT Assistant* Mar 06:15, Nov 07:8, Oct 11:3, Jul 12:13

00520   Anesthesia for closed chest procedures; (including bronchoscopy) not otherwise specified
→ *CPT Assistant* Nov 99:7; *CPT Changes: An Insider's View* 2000

00522   needle biopsy of pleura

00524   pneumocentesis

00528   mediastinoscopy and diagnostic thoracoscopy not utilizing 1 lung ventilation
→ *CPT Assistant* Nov 99:7; *CPT Changes: An Insider's View* 2000, 2003, 2004

(For tracheobronchial reconstruction, use 00539)

00529   mediastinoscopy and diagnostic thoracoscopy utilizing 1 lung ventilation
→ *CPT Assistant* Jun 04:3; *CPT Changes: An Insider's View* 2004

00530   Anesthesia for permanent transvenous pacemaker insertion
→ *CPT Changes: An Insider's View* 2001

00532   Anesthesia for access to central venous circulation

00534   Anesthesia for transvenous insertion or replacement of pacing cardioverter-defibrillator
→ *CPT Changes: An Insider's View* 2001

(For transthoracic approach, use 00560)

00537   Anesthesia for cardiac electrophysiologic procedures including radiofrequency ablation
→ *CPT Changes: An Insider's View* 2001

00539   Anesthesia for tracheobronchial reconstruction
→ *CPT Changes: An Insider's View* 2003

00540   Anesthesia for thoracotomy procedures involving lungs, pleura, diaphragm, and mediastinum (including surgical thoracoscopy); not otherwise specified

00541   utilizing 1 lung ventilation
→ *CPT Changes: An Insider's View* 2003

(For thoracic spine and cord anesthesia procedures via an anterior transthoracic approach, see 00625-00626)

00542   decortication

00546   pulmonary resection with thoracoplasty

00548   intrathoracic procedures on the trachea and bronchi
→ *CPT Assistant* Nov 97:10

00550   Anesthesia for sternal debridement
→ *CPT Changes: An Insider's View* 2001

00560   Anesthesia for procedures on heart, pericardial sac, and great vessels of chest; without pump oxygenator
→ *CPT Changes: An Insider's View* 2002

00561   with pump oxygenator, younger than 1 year of age
→ *CPT Changes: An Insider's View* 2005

(Do not report 00561 in conjunction with 99100, 99116, and 99135)

00562   with pump oxygenator, age 1 year or older, for all non-coronary bypass procedures (eg, valve procedures) or for re-operation for coronary bypass more than 1 month after original operation
→ *CPT Changes: An Insider's View* 2009

00563   with pump oxygenator with hypothermic circulatory arrest
→ *CPT Changes: An Insider's View* 2001

00566   Anesthesia for direct coronary artery bypass grafting; without pump oxygenator
→ *CPT Changes: An Insider's View* 2001, 2009

00567   with pump oxygenator
→ *CPT Changes: An Insider's View* 2009

00580   Anesthesia for heart transplant or heart/lung transplant
→ *CPT Assistant* Nov 07:8, Jul 12:13

Spine and Spinal Cord

00600   Anesthesia for procedures on cervical spine and cord; not otherwise specified
→ *CPT Assistant* Mar 06:15, May 07:9, Nov 07:8, Oct 11:3, Jul 12:13

(For percutaneous image-guided spine and spinal cord anesthesia procedures, see 01935, 01936)

00604   procedures with patient in the sitting position
→ *CPT Changes: An Insider's View* 2001

00620   Anesthesia for procedures on thoracic spine and cord; not otherwise specified
→ *CPT Assistant* Mar 07:9

00622   thoracolumbar sympathectomy
→ *CPT Assistant* Mar 07:9

00625   Anesthesia for procedures on the thoracic spine and cord, via an anterior transthoracic approach; not utilizing 1 lung ventilation
→ *CPT Assistant* Mar 07:9; *CPT Changes: An Insider's View* 2007

Anesthesia

00626 utilizing 1 lung ventilation

➡ *CPT Assistant* Mar 07:9; *CPT Changes: An Insider's View* 2007

(For anesthesia for thoracotomy procedures other than spinal, see 00540-00541)

00630 Anesthesia for procedures in lumbar region; not otherwise specified

00632 lumbar sympathectomy

00634 chemonucleolysis

00635 diagnostic or therapeutic lumbar puncture

➡ *CPT Changes: An Insider's View* 2001

00640 Anesthesia for manipulation of the spine or for closed procedures on the cervical, thoracic or lumbar spine

➡ *CPT Changes: An Insider's View* 2003

00670 Anesthesia for extensive spine and spinal cord procedures (eg, spinal instrumentation or vascular procedures)

➡ *CPT Assistant* Nov 07:8, Jul 12:13; *CPT Changes: An Insider's View* 2001

Upper Abdomen

00700 Anesthesia for procedures on upper anterior abdominal wall; not otherwise specified

➡ *CPT Assistant* Mar 06:15, Nov 07:8, Oct 11:3, Jul 12:13

00702 percutaneous liver biopsy

00730 Anesthesia for procedures on upper posterior abdominal wall

00740 Anesthesia for upper gastrointestinal endoscopic procedures, endoscope introduced proximal to duodenum

➡ *CPT Assistant* Nov 99:7; *CPT Changes: An Insider's View* 2000

00750 Anesthesia for hernia repairs in upper abdomen; not otherwise specified

00752 lumbar and ventral (incisional) hernias and/or wound dehiscence

00754 omphalocele

00756 transabdominal repair of diaphragmatic hernia

00770 Anesthesia for all procedures on major abdominal blood vessels

00790 Anesthesia for intraperitoneal procedures in upper abdomen including laparoscopy; not otherwise specified

00792 partial hepatectomy or management of liver hemorrhage (excluding liver biopsy)

➡ *CPT Changes: An Insider's View* 2001

00794 pancreatectomy, partial or total (eg, Whipple procedure)

00796 liver transplant (recipient)

(For harvesting of liver, use 01990)

00797 gastric restrictive procedure for morbid obesity

➡ *CPT Assistant* Nov 07:8, Jul 12:13; *CPT Changes: An Insider's View* 2002

Lower Abdomen

00800 Anesthesia for procedures on lower anterior abdominal wall; not otherwise specified

➡ *CPT Assistant* Mar 06:15, Nov 07:8, Oct 11:3, Jul 12:13

00802 panniculectomy

00810 Anesthesia for lower intestinal endoscopic procedures, endoscope introduced distal to duodenum

➡ *CPT Assistant* Nov 99:7; *CPT Changes: An Insider's View* 2000

00820 Anesthesia for procedures on lower posterior abdominal wall

00830 Anesthesia for hernia repairs in lower abdomen; not otherwise specified

00832 ventral and incisional hernias

(For hernia repairs in the infant 1 year of age or younger, see 00834, 00836)

00834 Anesthesia for hernia repairs in the lower abdomen not otherwise specified, younger than 1 year of age

➡ *CPT Changes: An Insider's View* 2003

(Do not report 00834 in conjunction with 99100)

00836 Anesthesia for hernia repairs in the lower abdomen not otherwise specified, infants younger than 37 weeks gestational age at birth and younger than 50 weeks gestational age at time of surgery

➡ *CPT Changes: An Insider's View* 2003

(Do not report 00836 in conjunction with 99100)

00840 Anesthesia for intraperitoneal procedures in lower abdomen including laparoscopy; not otherwise specified

00842 amniocentesis

00844 abdominoperineal resection

00846 radical hysterectomy

00848 pelvic exenteration

00851 tubal ligation/transection

➡ *CPT Changes: An Insider's View* 2002

00860 Anesthesia for extraperitoneal procedures in lower abdomen, including urinary tract; not otherwise specified

00862 renal procedures, including upper one-third of ureter, or donor nephrectomy

00864 total cystectomy

00865 radical prostatectomy (suprapubic, retropubic)

00866 adrenalectomy

00868 renal transplant (recipient)

(For donor nephrectomy, use 00862)

(For harvesting kidney from brain-dead patient, use 01990)

00870   cystolithotomy

00872   Anesthesia for lithotripsy, extracorporeal shock wave; with water bath

00873   without water bath

00880   Anesthesia for procedures on major lower abdominal vessels; not otherwise specified

00882   inferior vena cava ligation

Perineum

(For perineal procedures on integumentary system, muscles and nerves, see 00300, 00400)

00902   Anesthesia for; anorectal procedure

    ➲ *CPT Assistant* Mar 06:15, Oct 11:3, Jul 12:13; *CPT Changes: An Insider's View* 2001

00904   radical perineal procedure

00906   vulvectomy

00908   perineal prostatectomy

00910   Anesthesia for transurethral procedures (including urethrocystoscopy); not otherwise specified

00912   transurethral resection of bladder tumor(s)

00914   transurethral resection of prostate

00916   post-transurethral resection bleeding

00918   with fragmentation, manipulation and/or removal of ureteral calculus

    ➲ *CPT Assistant* Nov 99:8, Apr 09:8; *CPT Changes: An Insider's View* 2000

00920   Anesthesia for procedures on male genitalia (including open urethral procedures); not otherwise specified

    ➲ *CPT Changes: An Insider's View* 2001

00921   vasectomy, unilateral or bilateral

    ➲ *CPT Changes: An Insider's View* 2003

00922   seminal vesicles

00924   undescended testis, unilateral or bilateral

00926   radical orchiectomy, inguinal

00928   radical orchiectomy, abdominal

00930   orchiopexy, unilateral or bilateral

00932   complete amputation of penis

00934   radical amputation of penis with bilateral inguinal lymphadenectomy

00936   radical amputation of penis with bilateral inguinal and iliac lymphadenectomy

00938   insertion of penile prosthesis (perineal approach)

00940   Anesthesia for vaginal procedures (including biopsy of labia, vagina, cervix or endometrium); not otherwise specified

00942   colpotomy, vaginectomy, colporrhaphy, and open urethral procedures

    ➲ *CPT Changes: An Insider's View* 2001, 2002

00944   vaginal hysterectomy

00948   cervical cerclage

00950   culdoscopy

00952   hysteroscopy and/or hysterosalpingography

    ➲ *CPT Assistant* Nov 99:8, Jul 12:13; *CPT Changes: An Insider's View* 2000

Pelvis (Except Hip)

01112   Anesthesia for bone marrow aspiration and/or biopsy, anterior or posterior iliac crest

    ➲ *CPT Assistant* Mar 06:15, Oct 11:3, Jul 12:13; *CPT Changes: An Insider's View* 2001

01120   Anesthesia for procedures on bony pelvis

01130   Anesthesia for body cast application or revision

01140   Anesthesia for interpelviabdominal (hindquarter) amputation

01150   Anesthesia for radical procedures for tumor of pelvis, except hindquarter amputation

01160   Anesthesia for closed procedures involving symphysis pubis or sacroiliac joint

01170   Anesthesia for open procedures involving symphysis pubis or sacroiliac joint

01173   Anesthesia for open repair of fracture disruption of pelvis or column fracture involving acetabulum

    ➲ *CPT Assistant* Jun 04:3-4; *CPT Changes: An Insider's View* 2004

01180   Anesthesia for obturator neurectomy; extrapelvic

01190   intrapelvic

    ➲ *CPT Assistant* Nov 07:8, Jul 12:13

Upper Leg (Except Knee)

01200   Anesthesia for all closed procedures involving hip joint

    ➲ *CPT Assistant* Mar 06:15, Nov 07:8, Jul 12:13

01202   Anesthesia for arthroscopic procedures of hip joint

01210   Anesthesia for open procedures involving hip joint; not otherwise specified

01212   hip disarticulation

01214   total hip arthroplasty

    ➲ *CPT Changes: An Insider's View* 2001, 2002

01215   revision of total hip arthroplasty

    ➲ *CPT Changes: An Insider's View* 2001, 2002

01220   Anesthesia for all closed procedures involving upper two-thirds of femur

01230   Anesthesia for open procedures involving upper two-thirds of femur; not otherwise specified

---

Anesthesia

Anesthesia

01232   amputation

01234   radical resection

01250   Anesthesia for all procedures on nerves, muscles, tendons, fascia, and bursae of upper leg

01260   Anesthesia for all procedures involving veins of upper leg, including exploration

01270   Anesthesia for procedures involving arteries of upper leg, including bypass graft; not otherwise specified

01272   femoral artery ligation

01274   femoral artery embolectomy
➜ *CPT Assistant* Nov 07:8, Jul 12:13

Knee and Popliteal Area

01320   Anesthesia for all procedures on nerves, muscles, tendons, fascia, and bursae of knee and/or popliteal area
➜ *CPT Assistant* Mar 06:15, Nov 07:8, Oct 11:3, Jul 12:13

01340   Anesthesia for all closed procedures on lower one-third of femur

01360   Anesthesia for all open procedures on lower one-third of femur

01380   Anesthesia for all closed procedures on knee joint

01382   Anesthesia for diagnostic arthroscopic procedures of knee joint
➜ *CPT Changes: An Insider's View* 2003

01390   Anesthesia for all closed procedures on upper ends of tibia, fibula, and/or patella

01392   Anesthesia for all open procedures on upper ends of tibia, fibula, and/or patella

01400   Anesthesia for open or surgical arthroscopic procedures on knee joint; not otherwise specified
➜ *CPT Changes: An Insider's View* 2003

01402   total knee arthroplasty
➜ *CPT Changes: An Insider's View* 2002

01404   disarticulation at knee

01420   Anesthesia for all cast applications, removal, or repair involving knee joint

01430   Anesthesia for procedures on veins of knee and popliteal area; not otherwise specified

01432   arteriovenous fistula

01440   Anesthesia for procedures on arteries of knee and popliteal area; not otherwise specified

01442   popliteal thromboendarterectomy, with or without patch graft

01444   popliteal excision and graft or repair for occlusion or aneurysm
➜ *CPT Assistant* Nov 07:8, Jul 12:13

Lower Leg (Below Knee, Includes Ankle and Foot)

01462   Anesthesia for all closed procedures on lower leg, ankle, and foot
➜ *CPT Assistant* Mar 06:15, Nov 07:8, Oct 11:3, Jul 12:13

01464   Anesthesia for arthroscopic procedures of ankle and/or foot
➜ *CPT Changes: An Insider's View* 2003

01470   Anesthesia for procedures on nerves, muscles, tendons, and fascia of lower leg, ankle, and foot; not otherwise specified

01472   repair of ruptured Achilles tendon, with or without graft

01474   gastrocnemius recession (eg, Strayer procedure)

01480   Anesthesia for open procedures on bones of lower leg, ankle, and foot; not otherwise specified

01482   radical resection (including below knee amputation)
➜ *CPT Changes: An Insider's View* 2001

01484   osteotomy or osteoplasty of tibia and/or fibula

01486   total ankle replacement

01490   Anesthesia for lower leg cast application, removal, or repair

01500   Anesthesia for procedures on arteries of lower leg, including bypass graft; not otherwise specified

01502   embolectomy, direct or with catheter

01520   Anesthesia for procedures on veins of lower leg; not otherwise specified

01522   venous thrombectomy, direct or with catheter
➜ *CPT Assistant* Nov 07:8, Jul 12:13

Shoulder and Axilla

Includes humeral head and neck, sternoclavicular joint, acromioclavicular joint, and shoulder joint.

01610   Anesthesia for all procedures on nerves, muscles, tendons, fascia, and bursae of shoulder and axilla
➜ *CPT Assistant* Mar 06:15, Nov 07:8, Oct 11:3, Jul 12:13

01620   Anesthesia for all closed procedures on humeral head and neck, sternoclavicular joint, acromioclavicular joint, and shoulder joint

01622   Anesthesia for diagnostic arthroscopic procedures of shoulder joint
➜ *CPT Changes: An Insider's View* 2003

01630   Anesthesia for open or surgical arthroscopic procedures on humeral head and neck, sternoclavicular joint, acromioclavicular joint, and shoulder joint; not otherwise specified
➜ *CPT Changes: An Insider's View* 2003

(01632 has been deleted. To report, see 01630, 01638)

01634   shoulder disarticulation

01636   interthoracoscapular (forequarter) amputation

01638   total shoulder replacement

01650   Anesthesia for procedures on arteries of shoulder and axilla; not otherwise specified

01652   axillary-brachial aneurysm

01654   bypass graft

01656   axillary-femoral bypass graft

01670   Anesthesia for all procedures on veins of shoulder and axilla

01680   Anesthesia for shoulder cast application, removal or repair; not otherwise specified

01682   shoulder spica
        ➔ *CPT Assistant* Nov 07:8, Jul 12:13

Upper Arm and Elbow

01710   Anesthesia for procedures on nerves, muscles, tendons, fascia, and bursae of upper arm and elbow; not otherwise specified
        ➔ *CPT Assistant* Mar 06:15, Nov 07:8, Oct 11:3, Jul 12:13

01712   tenotomy, elbow to shoulder, open

01714   tenoplasty, elbow to shoulder

01716   tenodesis, rupture of long tendon of biceps

01730   Anesthesia for all closed procedures on humerus and elbow

01732   Ancsthesia for diagnostic arthroscopic procedures of elbow joint
        ➔ *CPT Changes: An Insider's View* 2003

01740   Anesthesia for open or surgical arthroscopic procedures of the elbow; not otherwise specified
        ➔ *CPT Changes: An Insider's View* 2003

01742   osteotomy of humerus

01744   repair of nonunion or malunion of humerus

01756   radical procedures

01758   excision of cyst or tumor of humerus

01760   total elbow replacement

01770   Anesthesia for procedures on arteries of upper arm and elbow; not otherwise specified

01772   embolectomy

01780   Anesthesia for procedures on veins of upper arm and elbow; not otherwise specified

01782   phleborrhaphy
        ➔ *CPT Assistant* Nov 07:8, Jul 12:13

Forearm, Wrist, and Hand

01810   Anesthesia for all procedures on nerves, muscles, tendons, fascia, and bursae of forearm, wrist, and hand
        ➔ *CPT Assistant* Mar 06:15, Nov 07:8, Oct 11:3, Jul 12:13

01820   Anesthesia for all closed procedures on radius, ulna, wrist, or hand bones

01829   Anesthesia for diagnostic arthroscopic procedures on the wrist
        ➔ *CPT Changes: An Insider's View* 2003

01830   Anesthesia for open or surgical arthroscopic/endoscopic procedures on distal radius, distal ulna, wrist, or hand joints; not otherwise specified
        ➔ *CPT Changes: An Insider's View* 2003

01832   total wrist replacement

01840   Anesthesia for procedures on arteries of forearm, wrist, and hand; not otherwise specified

01842   embolectomy

01844   Anesthesia for vascular shunt, or shunt revision, any type (eg, dialysis)

01850   Anesthesia for procedures on veins of forearm, wrist, and hand; not otherwise specified

01852   phleborrhaphy

01860   Anesthesia for forearm, wrist, or hand cast application, removal, or repair
        ➔ *CPT Assistant* Nov 07:8, Jul 12:13

Radiological Procedures

01916   Anesthesia for diagnostic arteriography/venography
        ➔ *CPT Assistant* Nov 07:8, Oct 11:3, Jul 12:13; *CPT Changes: An Insider's View* 2002

        (Do not report 01916 in conjunction with therapeutic codes 01924-01926, 01930-01933)

01920   Anesthesia for cardiac catheterization including coronary angiography and ventriculography (not to include Swan-Ganz catheter)

01922   Anesthesia for non-invasive imaging or radiation therapy

01924   Anesthesia for therapeutic interventional radiological procedures involving the arterial system; not otherwise specified
        ➔ *CPT Changes: An Insider's View* 2002

01925   carotid or coronary
        ➔ *CPT Changes: An Insider's View* 2002

01926   intracranial, intracardiac, or aortic
        ➔ *CPT Changes: An Insider's View* 2002

01930   Anesthesia for therapeutic interventional radiological procedures involving the venous/lymphatic system (not to include access to the central circulation); not otherwise specified
        ➔ *CPT Changes: An Insider's View* 2002

Anesthesia

01931 intrahepatic or portal circulation (eg, transvenous intrahepatic portosystemic shunt[s] [TIPS])

➔ *CPT Assistant* Apr 08:3; *CPT Changes: An Insider's View* 2002, 2008

01932 intrathoracic or jugular

➔ *CPT Changes: An Insider's View* 2002

01933 intracranial

➔ *CPT Changes: An Insider's View* 2002

01935 Anesthesia for percutaneous image guided procedures on the spine and spinal cord; diagnostic

➔ *CPT Assistant* Apr 08:3; *CPT Changes: An Insider's View* 2008

01936 therapeutic

➔ *CPT Assistant* Apr 08:3, Jul 12:13; *CPT Changes: An Insider's View* 2008

Burn Excisions or Debridement

01951 Anesthesia for second- and third-degree burn excision or debridement with or without skin grafting, any site, for total body surface area (TBSA) treated during anesthesia and surgery; less than 4% total body surface area

➔ *CPT Assistant* Mar 06:15, Oct 11:3, Jul 12:13; *CPT Changes: An Insider's View* 2001, 2002

01952 between 4% and 9% of total body surface area

➔ *CPT Changes: An Insider's View* 2001, 2002

+ 01953 each additional 9% total body surface area or part thereof (List separately in addition to code for primary procedure)

➔ *CPT Assistant* Jun 11:13, Jul 12:13; *CPT Changes: An Insider's View* 2001

(Use 01953 in conjunction with 01952)

Obstetric

01958 Anesthesia for external cephalic version procedure

➔ *CPT Assistant* Jun 04:5-6, Oct 11:3, Jul 12:13; *CPT Changes: An Insider's View* 2004

01960 Anesthesia for vaginal delivery only

➔ *CPT Assistant* Dec 01:3; *CPT Changes: An Insider's View* 2002

01961 Anesthesia for cesarean delivery only

➔ *CPT Changes: An Insider's View* 2002, 2003

01962 Anesthesia for urgent hysterectomy following delivery

➔ *CPT Changes: An Insider's View* 2002, 2003

01963 Anesthesia for cesarean hysterectomy without any labor analgesia/anesthesia care

➔ *CPT Changes: An Insider's View* 2002, 2003

01965 Anesthesia for incomplete or missed abortion procedures

➔ *CPT Changes: An Insider's View* 2006

01966 Anesthesia for induced abortion procedures

➔ *CPT Changes: An Insider's View* 2006

01967 Neuraxial labor analgesia/anesthesia for planned vaginal delivery (this includes any repeat subarachnoid needle placement and drug injection and/or any necessary replacement of an epidural catheter during labor)

➔ *CPT Assistant* Dec 01:3; *CPT Changes: An Insider's View* 2002

+ 01968 Anesthesia for cesarean delivery following neuraxial labor analgesia/anesthesia (List separately in addition to code for primary procedure performed)

➔ *CPT Assistant* Dec 01:3, Jun 11:13; *CPT Changes: An Insider's View* 2002, 2003

(Use 01968 in conjunction with 01967)

+ 01969 Anesthesia for cesarean hysterectomy following neuraxial labor analgesia/anesthesia (List separately in addition to code for primary procedure performed)

➔ *CPT Assistant* Dec 01:3, Jun 11:13, Jul 12:13; *CPT Changes: An Insider's View* 2002, 2003

(Use 01969 in conjunction with 01967)

Other Procedures

01990 Physiological support for harvesting of organ(s) from brain-dead patient

➔ *CPT Assistant* Mar 06:15, Nov 07:8, Oct 11:3, Jul 12:13

▲ **01991** Anesthesia for diagnostic or therapeutic nerve blocks and injections (when block or injection is performed by a different physician or other qualified health care professional); other than the prone position

➔ *CPT Changes: An Insider's View* 2003, 2013

▲ **01992** prone position

➔ *CPT Changes: An Insider's View* 2003, 2013

(Do not report 01991 or 01992 in conjunction with 99143-99150)

(When regional intravenous administration of local anesthetic agent or other medication in the upper or lower extremity is used as the anesthetic for a surgical procedure, report the appropriate anesthesia code. To report a Bier block for pain management, use 64999)

(For intra-arterial or intravenous therapy for pain management, see 96373, 96374)

01996 Daily hospital management of epidural or subarachnoid continuous drug administration

➔ *CPT Assistant* Feb 97:5, Nov 97:10, May 99:6, Jul 12:5; *CPT Changes: An Insider's View* 2003

(Report code 01996 for daily hospital management of continuous epidural or subarachnoid drug administration performed after insertion of an epidural or subarachnoid catheter)

01999 Unlisted anesthesia procedure(s)

➔ *CPT Assistant* Feb 97:4, Feb 06:9, Mar 06:15, Jan 07:30, Nov 07:8, Oct 11:3, Jul 12:13

➔ *Clinical Examples in Radiology* Summer 11:2

Surgery Guidelines

Surgery

Surgery Guidelines

►Guidelines to direct general reporting of services are presented in the **Introduction.** Some of the commonalities are repeated here for the convenience of those referring to this section on **Surgery.** Other definitions and items unique to Surgery are also listed.◄

►Services◄

►Services rendered in the office, home, or hospital, consultations, and other medical services are listed in the **Evaluation and Management Services** section (99201-99499), beginning on page 11. "Special Services and Reports" (99000-99091) are listed in the **Medicine** section.◄

►CPT Surgical Package Definition◄

►By their very nature, the services to any patient are variable. The CPT codes that represent a readily identifiable surgical procedure thereby include, on a procedure-by-procedure basis, a variety of services. In defining the specific services "included" in a given CPT surgical code, the following services are always included in addition to the operation per se:

■ Local infiltration, metacarpal/metatarsal/digital block or topical anesthesia

■ Subsequent to the decision for surgery, one related Evaluation and Management (E/M) encounter on the date immediately prior to or on the date of procedure (including history and physical)

■ Immediate postoperative care, including dictating operative notes, talking with the family and other physicians or other qualified health care professionals

■ Writing orders

■ Evaluating the patient in the postanesthesia recovery area

■ Typical postoperative follow-up care◄

Follow-Up Care for Diagnostic Procedures

Follow-up care for diagnostic procedures (eg, endoscopy, arthroscopy, injection procedures for radiography) includes only that care related to recovery from the diagnostic procedure itself. Care of the condition for which the diagnostic procedure was performed or of

other concomitant conditions is not included and may be listed separately.

Follow-Up Care for Therapeutic Surgical Procedures

Follow-up care for therapeutic surgical procedures includes only that care which is usually a part of the surgical service. Complications, exacerbations, recurrence, or the presence of other diseases or injuries requiring additional services should be separately reported.

►Supplied Materials◄

►Supplies and materials (eg, sterile trays/drugs), over and above those usually included with the procedure(s) rendered are reported separately. List drugs, trays, supplies, and materials provided. Identify as 99070 or specific supply code.◄

Reporting More Than One Procedure/Service

►When more than one procedure/service is performed on the same date, same session or during a post-operative period (subject to the "surgical package" concept), several CPT modifiers may apply (see Appendix A for definition).◄

Separate Procedure

Some of the procedures or services listed in the CPT codebook that are commonly carried out as an integral component of a total service or procedure have been identified by the inclusion of the term "separate procedure." The codes designated as "separate procedure" should not be reported in addition to the code for the total procedure or service of which it is considered an integral component.

However, when a procedure or service that is designated as a "separate procedure" is carried out independently or considered to be unrelated or distinct from other procedures/services provided at that time, it may be reported by itself, or in addition to other procedures/ services by appending modifier 59 to the specific "separate procedure" code to indicate that the procedure

⊙=Moderate sedation ✚=Add-on code ✗=FDA approval pending #=Resequenced code ○=Recycled/reinstated code ➲➲=See p xiii for details is not considered to be a component of another procedure, but is a distinct, independent procedure. This may represent a different session, different procedure or surgery, different site or organ system, separate incision/excision, separate lesion, or separate injury (or area of injury in extensive injuries).

Unlisted Service or Procedure

A service or procedure may be provided that is not listed in this edition of the CPT codebook. When reporting such a service, the appropriate "Unlisted Procedure" code may be used to indicate the service, identifying it by "Special Report" as discussed in the section below. The "Unlisted Procedures" and accompanying codes for **Surgery** are as follows:

15999	Unlisted procedure, excision pressure ulcer
17999	Unlisted procedure, skin, mucous membrane and subcutaneous tissue
19499	Unlisted procedure, breast
20999	Unlisted procedure, musculoskeletal system, general
21089	Unlisted maxillofacial prosthetic procedure
21299	Unlisted craniofacial and maxillofacial procedure
21499	Unlisted musculoskeletal procedure, head
21899	Unlisted procedure, neck or thorax
22899	Unlisted procedure, spine
22999	Unlisted procedure, abdomen, musculoskeletal system
23929	Unlisted procedure, shoulder
24999	Unlisted procedure, humerus or elbow
25999	Unlisted procedure, forearm or wrist
26989	Unlisted procedure, hands or fingers
27299	Unlisted procedure, pelvis or hip joint
27599	Unlisted procedure, femur or knee
27899	Unlisted procedure, leg or ankle
28899	Unlisted procedure, foot or toes
29799	Unlisted procedure, casting or strapping
29999	Unlisted procedure, arthroscopy
30999	Unlisted procedure, nose
31299	Unlisted procedure, accessory sinuses
31599	Unlisted procedure, larynx
31899	Unlisted procedure, trachea, bronchi
32999	Unlisted procedure, lungs and pleura
33999	Unlisted procedure, cardiac surgery
36299	Unlisted procedure, vascular injection
37501	Unlisted vascular endoscopy procedure

37799	Unlisted procedure, vascular surgery
38129	Unlisted laparoscopy procedure, spleen
38589	Unlisted laparoscopy procedure, lymphatic system
38999	Unlisted procedure, hemic or lymphatic system
39499	Unlisted procedure, mediastinum
39599	Unlisted procedure, diaphragm
40799	Unlisted procedure, lips
40899	Unlisted procedure, vestibule of mouth
41599	Unlisted procedure, tongue, floor of mouth
41899	Unlisted procedure, dentoalveolar structures
42299	Unlisted procedure, palate, uvula
42699	Unlisted procedure, salivary glands or ducts
42999	Unlisted procedure, pharynx, adenoids, or tonsils
43289	Unlisted laparoscopy procedure, esophagus
43499	Unlisted procedure, esophagus
43659	Unlisted laparoscopy procedure, stomach
43999	Unlisted procedure, stomach
44238	Unlisted laparoscopy procedure, intestine (except rectum)
44799	Unlisted procedure, intestine
44899	Unlisted procedure, Meckel's diverticulum and the mesentery
44979	Unlisted laparoscopy procedure, appendix
45499	Unlisted laparoscopy procedure, rectum
45999	Unlisted procedure, rectum
46999	Unlisted procedure, anus
47379	Unlisted laparoscopic procedure, liver
47399	Unlisted procedure, liver
47579	Unlisted laparoscopy procedure, biliary tract
47999	Unlisted procedure, biliary tract
48999	Unlisted procedure, pancreas
49329	Unlisted laparoscopy procedure, abdomen, peritoneum and omentum
49659	Unlisted laparoscopy procedure, hernioplasty, herniorrhaphy, herniotomy
49999	Unlisted procedure, abdomen, peritoneum and omentum
50549	Unlisted laparoscopy procedure, renal
50949	Unlisted laparoscopy procedure, ureter
51999	Unlisted laparoscopy procedure, bladder
53899	Unlisted procedure, urinary system
54699	Unlisted laparoscopy procedure, testis
55559	Unlisted laparoscopy procedure, spermatic cord
55899	Unlisted procedure, male genital system

Surgery

58578	Unlisted laparoscopy procedure, uterus
58579	Unlisted hysteroscopy procedure, uterus
58679	Unlisted laparoscopy procedure, oviduct, ovary
58999	Unlisted procedure, female genital system (nonobstetrical)
59897	Unlisted fetal invasive procedure, including ultrasound guidance, when performed
59898	Unlisted laparoscopy procedure, maternity care and delivery
59899	Unlisted procedure, maternity care and delivery
60659	Unlisted laparoscopy procedure, endocrine system
60699	Unlisted procedure, endocrine system
64999	Unlisted procedure, nervous system
66999	Unlisted procedure, anterior segment of eye
67299	Unlisted procedure, posterior segment
67399	Unlisted procedure, ocular muscle
67599	Unlisted procedure, orbit
67999	Unlisted procedure, eyelids
68399	Unlisted procedure, conjunctiva
68899	Unlisted procedure, lacrimal system
69399	Unlisted procedure, external ear
69799	Unlisted procedure, middle ear
69949	Unlisted procedure, inner ear
69979	Unlisted procedure, temporal bone, middle fossa approach

Special Report

A service that is rarely provided, unusual, variable, or new may require a special report. Pertinent information should include an adequate definition or description of the nature, extent, and need for the procedure, and the time, effort, and equipment necessary to provide the service.

Surgical Destruction

Surgical destruction is a part of a surgical procedure and different methods of destruction are not ordinarily listed separately unless the technique substantially alters the standard management of a problem or condition. Exceptions under special circumstances are provided for by separate code numbers.

Surgery

The following is a listing of headings and subheadings that appear within the Integumentary System section of the CPT codebook. The subheadings or subsections denoted with asterisks (*) below have special instructions unique to that section. Where these are indicated, special "notes" or guidelines will be presented preceding those procedural terminology listings, referring to that subsection specifically.

Integumentary

Surgery

General

10021   Fine needle aspiration; without imaging guidance
→ *CPT Assistant* Aug 02:10, Mar 05:11; *CPT Changes: An Insider's View* 2002
→ *Clinical Examples in Radiology* Fall 08:4, Fall 10:3, 8

10022   with imaging guidance
→ *CPT Assistant* Nov 02:1, Jun 07:10; *CPT Changes: An Insider's View* 2002
→ *Clinical Examples in Radiology* Summer 05:1, 6, Summer 08:5, Fall 08:2, 3, 4, Fall 10:3, 8

(For placement of percutaneous localization clip during breast biopsy, use 19295)

(For radiological supervision and interpretation, see 76942, 77002, 77012, 77021)

(For percutaneous needle biopsy other than fine needle aspiration, see 20206 for muscle, 32400 for pleura, 32405 for lung or mediastinum, 42400 for salivary gland, 47000 for liver, 48102 for pancreas, 49180 for abdominal or retroperitoneal mass, 50200 for kidney, 54500 for testis, 54800 for epididymis, 60100 for thyroid, 62267 for nucleus pulposus, intervertebral disc, or paravertebral tissue, 62269 for spinal cord)

(For evaluation of fine needle aspirate, see 88172, 88173)

Integumentary System

Skin, Subcutaneous, and Accessory Structures

Incision and Drainage

(For excision, see 11400, et seq)

10040   Acne surgery (eg, marsupialization, opening or removal of multiple milia, comedones, cysts, pustules)
→ *CPT Assistant* Fall 92:10, Feb 08:8

10060   Incision and drainage of abscess (eg, carbuncle, suppurative hidradenitis, cutaneous or subcutaneous abscess, cyst, furuncle, or paronychia); simple or single

10061   complicated or multiple

10080   Incision and drainage of pilonidal cyst; simple
→ *CPT Assistant* Fall 92:13, Dec 06:15, May 07:5

10081   complicated
→ *CPT Assistant* Fall 92:13, Dec 06:15, May 07:5

(For excision of pilonidal cyst, see 11770-11772)

10120   Incision and removal of foreign body, subcutaneous tissues; simple

10121   complicated
→ *CPT Assistant* Spring 91:7, Dec 06:15

(To report wound exploration due to penetrating trauma without laparotomy or thoracotomy, see 20100-20103, as appropriate)

(To report debridement associated with open fracture(s) and/or dislocation(s), use 11010-11012, as appropriate)

10140   Incision and drainage of hematoma, seroma or fluid collection
→ *CPT Changes: An Insider's View* 2002

(If imaging guidance is performed, see 76942, 77012, 77021)

10160   Puncture aspiration of abscess, hematoma, bulla, or cyst
→ *CPT Changes: An Insider's View* 2002
→ *Clinical Examples in Radiology* Fall 09:8

(If imaging guidance is performed, see 76942, 77012, 77021)

10180   Incision and drainage, complex, postoperative wound infection

(For secondary closure of surgical wound, see 12020, 12021, 13160)

Debridement

Wound debridements (11042-11047) are reported by depth of tissue that is removed and by surface area of the wound. These services may be reported for injuries, infections, wounds and chronic ulcers. When performing debridement of a single wound, report depth using the deepest level of tissue removed. In multiple wounds, sum the surface area of those wounds that are at the same depth, but do not combine sums from different depths. For example: When bone is debrided from a 4 sq cm heel ulcer and from a 10 sq cm ischial ulcer, report the work with a single code, 11044. When subcutaneous tissue is debrided from a 16 sq cm dehisced abdominal wound and a 10 sq cm thigh wound, report the work with 11042 for the first 20 sq cm and 11045 for the second 6 sq cm. If all four wounds were debrided on the same day, use modifier 59 with either 11042, or 11044 as appropriate.

(For dermabrasions, see 15780-15783)

(For nail debridement, see 11720-11721)

(For burn(s), see 16000-16035)

(For pressure ulcers, see 15920-15999)

Integumentary

Integumentary

—— *Coding Tip* ——————

Use of Depth and Surface Area For Reporting Debridement of Wounds

When performing debridement of a single wound, report depth using the deepest level of tissue removed. In multiple wounds, sum the surface area of those wounds that are at the same depth, but do not combine sums from different depths.

CPT Coding Guidelines, Debridement

11000   Debridement of extensive eczematous or infected skin; up to 10% of body surface

➔ *CPT Assistant* May 99:10

(For abdominal wall or genitalia debridement for necrotizing soft tissue infection, see 11004-11006)

+ 11001   each additional 10% of the body surface, or part thereof (List separately in addition to code for primary procedure)

➔ *CPT Assistant* May 99:10; *CPT Changes: An Insider's View* 2009

(Use 11001 in conjunction with 11000)

11004   Debridement of skin, subcutaneous tissue, muscle and fascia for necrotizing soft tissue infection; external genitalia and perineum

➔ *CPT Assistant* Jan 12:6; *CPT Changes: An Insider's View* 2005

11005   abdominal wall, with or without fascial closure

➔ *CPT Assistant* Jan 12:6; *CPT Changes: An Insider's View* 2005

Debridement of Abdominal Wall
11005

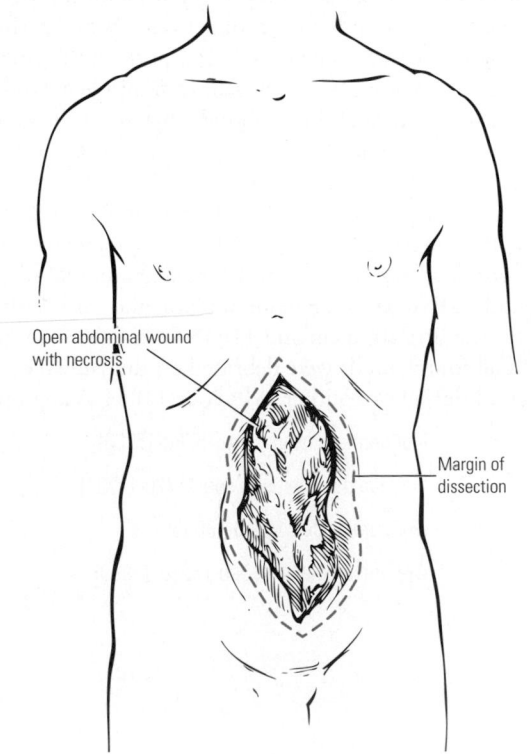

Open abdominal wound with necrosis

Margin of dissection

11006   external genitalia, perineum and abdominal wall, with or without fascial closure

➔ *CPT Assistant* Jan 12:6; *CPT Changes: An Insider's View* 2005

(If orchiectomy is performed, use 54520)

(If testicular transplantation is performed, use 54680)

+ 11008   Removal of prosthetic material or mesh, abdominal wall for infection (eg, for chronic or recurrent mesh infection or necrotizing soft tissue infection) (List separately in addition to code for primary procedure)

➔ *CPT Assistant* Jan 12:6; *CPT Changes: An Insider's View* 2005, 2008

(Use 11008 in conjunction with 10180, 11004-11006)

(Do not report 11008 in conjunction with 11000-11001, 11010-11044)

(Report skin grafts or flaps separately when performed for closure at the same session as 11004-11008)

(When insertion of mesh is used for closure, use 49568)

11010   Debridement including removal of foreign material at the site of an open fracture and/or an open dislocation (eg, excisional debridement); skin and subcutaneous tissues

➔ *CPT Assistant* Mar 97:2, Apr 97:10, Aug 97:6, Oct 03:10, May 11:3; *CPT Changes: An Insider's View* 2011

11011   skin, subcutaneous tissue, muscle fascia, and muscle

➔ *CPT Assistant* Mar 97:2, Apr 97:10, Aug 97:6, May 11:3; *CPT Changes: An Insider's View* 2011

11012   skin, subcutaneous tissue, muscle fascia, muscle, and bone

➔ *CPT Assistant* Mar 97:2, Apr 97:10, Aug 97:6, Oct 03:10, May 11:3; *CPT Changes: An Insider's View* 2011

(11040, 11041 have been deleted)

(For debridement of skin, ie, epidermis and/or dermis only, see 97597, 97598)

(For active wound care management, see 97597, 97598)

(For debridement of burn wounds, see 16020-16030)

11042   Debridement, subcutaneous tissue (includes epidermis and dermis, if performed); first 20 sq cm or less

➔ *CPT Assistant* Winter 92:10, May 96:6, Feb 97:7, Aug 97:6, Jun 05:1, 10, Oct 07:15, Nov 10:9, May 11:3, Sep 11:11, Jan 12:6, Mar 12:3; *CPT Changes: An Insider's View* 2011

(For debridement of skin [ie, epidermis and/or dermis only], see 97597, 97598)

#+ 11045   each additional 20 sq cm, or part thereof (List separately in addition to code for primary procedure)

➔ *CPT Assistant* May 11:3, Sep 11:11, Jan 12:6, Mar 12:3; *CPT Changes: An Insider's View* 2011

(Use 11045 in conjunction with 11042)

11043   Debridement, muscle and/or fascia (includes epidermis, dermis, and subcutaneous tissue, if performed); first 20 sq cm or less

➔ *CPT Assistant* May 96:6, Feb 97:7, Apr 97:11, Aug 97:6, Dec 99:10, Jun 05:1, 10, Oct 07:15, Nov 10:9, May 11:3, Sep 11:11, Jan 12:6, Mar 12:3; *CPT Changes: An Insider's View* 2011

#+ **11046** each additional 20 sq cm, or part thereof (List separately in addition to code for primary procedure)

> ➜ *CPT Assistant* May 11:3, Sep 11:11, Jan 12:6, Mar 12:3; *CPT Changes: An Insider's View* 2011

(Use 11046 in conjunction with 11043)

11044 Debridement, bone (includes epidermis, dermis, subcutaneous tissue, muscle and/or fascia, if performed); first 20 sq cm or less

> ➜ *CPT Assistant* Fall 93:21, Mar 96:10, May 96:6, Feb 97:7, Apr 97:11, Aug 97:6, Jun 05:1, 10, Oct 07:15, Nov 10:9, May 11:3, Sep 11:11, Jan 12:6, Mar 12:3; *CPT Changes: An Insider's View* 2011

11045 Code is out of numerical sequence. See 11000-11047

11046 Code is out of numerical sequence. See 11000-11047

+ **11047** each additional 20 sq cm, or part thereof (List separately in addition to code for primary procedure)

> ➜ *CPT Assistant* May 11:3, Sep 11:11, Jan 12:6, Mar 12:3; *CPT Changes: An Insider's View* 2011

(Do not report 11042-11047 in conjunction with 97597-97602 for the same wound)

(Use 11047 in conjunction with 11044)

Paring or Cutting

(To report destruction, see 17000-17004)

11055 Paring or cutting of benign hyperkeratotic lesion (eg, corn or callus); single lesion

> ➜ *CPT Assistant* Nov 97:11, Jan 99:11

11056 2 to 4 lesions

> ➜ *CPT Assistant* Nov 97:11, Jan 99:11, Sep 10:9

11057 more than 4 lesions

> ➜ *CPT Assistant* Nov 97:11, Jan 99:11, May 99:10

Biopsy

During certain surgical procedures in the integumentary system, such as excision, destruction, or shave removals, the removed tissue is often submitted for pathologic examination. The obtaining of tissue for pathology during the course of these procedures is a routine component of such procedures. This obtaining of tissue is not considered a separate biopsy procedure and is not separately reported. The use of a biopsy procedure code (eg, 11100, 11101) indicates that the procedure to obtain tissue for pathologic examination was performed independently, or was unrelated or distinct from other procedures/services provided at that time. Such biopsies are not considered components of other procedures when performed on different lesions or different sites on the same date, and are to be reported separately.

(For biopsy of conjunctiva, use 68100; eyelid, use 67810)

11100 Biopsy of skin, subcutaneous tissue and/or mucous membrane (including simple closure), unless otherwise listed; single lesion

> ➜ *CPT Assistant* Fall 94:20, Mar 97:12, Jun 97:12, Apr 00:7, Nov 02:6, Jul 04:5, Oct 04:4, Nov 06:1, Feb 08:1; *CPT Changes: An Insider's View* 2004

+ **11101** each separate/additional lesion (List separately in addition to code for primary procedure)

> ➜ *CPT Assistant* Fall 94:20, Apr 00:6, 7, Nov 02:6, Jul 04:5, Oct 04:4, Nov 06:1, Feb 08:1

(Use 11101 in conjunction with 11100)

Removal of Skin Tags

Removal by scissoring or any sharp method, ligature strangulation, electrosurgical destruction or combination of treatment modalities, including chemical destruction or electrocauterization of wound, with or without local anesthesia.

11200 Removal of skin tags, multiple fibrocutaneous tags, any area; up to and including 15 lesions

> ➜ *CPT Assistant* Winter 90:3, Nov 97:11-12, Nov 02:11, Aug 09:7, Jun 11:13

+ **11201** each additional 10 lesions, or part thereof (List separately in addition to code for primary procedure)

> ➜ *CPT Assistant* Winter 90:3, Nov 97:11-12, Nov 02:11, Jun 11:13; *CPT Changes: An Insider's View* 2009

(Use 11201 in conjunction with 11200)

Removal of Skin Tags
11200,11201

Skin tags

Scissor excision of skin tag

Integumentary

Shaving of Epidermal or Dermal Lesions

Shaving is the sharp removal by transverse incision or horizontal slicing to remove epidermal and dermal lesions without a full-thickness dermal excision. This includes local anesthesia, chemical or electrocauterization of the wound. The wound does not require suture closure.

11300 Shaving of epidermal or dermal lesion, single lesion, trunk, arms or legs; lesion diameter 0.5 cm or less

➡ *CPT Assistant* Feb 00:11, Nov 02:11, Feb 08:1

11301 lesion diameter 0.6 to 1.0 cm

➡ *CPT Assistant* Feb 00:11, Feb 08:1

11302 lesion diameter 1.1 to 2.0 cm

➡ *CPT Assistant* Feb 00:11, Feb 08:1

11303 lesion diameter over 2.0 cm

➡ *CPT Assistant* Feb 00:11, Feb 08:1

11305 Shaving of epidermal or dermal lesion, single lesion, scalp, neck, hands, feet, genitalia; lesion diameter 0.5 cm or less

➡ *CPT Assistant* Feb 00:11, Feb 08:1

11306 lesion diameter 0.6 to 1.0 cm

➡ *CPT Assistant* Feb 00:11, Feb 08:1

11307 lesion diameter 1.1 to 2.0 cm

➡ *CPT Assistant* Feb 00:11, Feb 08:1

11308 lesion diameter over 2.0 cm

➡ *CPT Assistant* Feb 00:11, Feb 08:1

11310 Shaving of epidermal or dermal lesion, single lesion, face, ears, eyelids, nose, lips, mucous membrane; lesion diameter 0.5 cm or less

➡ *CPT Assistant* Feb 00:11, Feb 08:1

11311 lesion diameter 0.6 to 1.0 cm

➡ *CPT Assistant* Feb 00:11, Feb 08:1

11312 lesion diameter 1.1 to 2.0 cm

➡ *CPT Assistant* Feb 00:11, Feb 08:1

11313 lesion diameter over 2.0 cm

➡ *CPT Assistant* Feb 00:11, Feb 08:1

Measuring and Coding the Removal of a Lesion

Measuring lesion removal.

A. Example: excision, malignant lesion of the back, 1.0 cm. Code 11606.

B. Example: Excision of benign lesion of the neck, 1.0 cm by 2.0 cm. Code 11423.

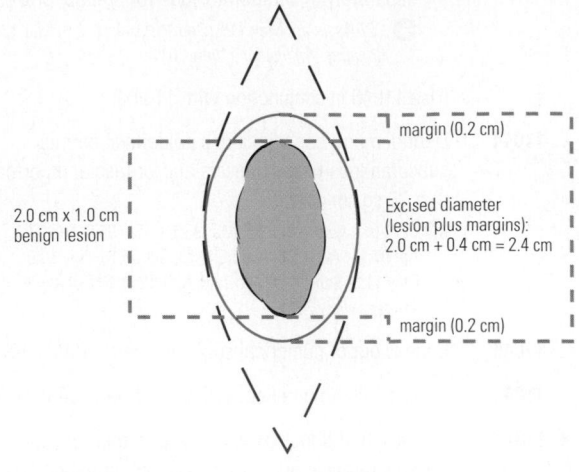

C. Example: Excision, malignant lesion of the nose, 0.9 cm. Code 11642.

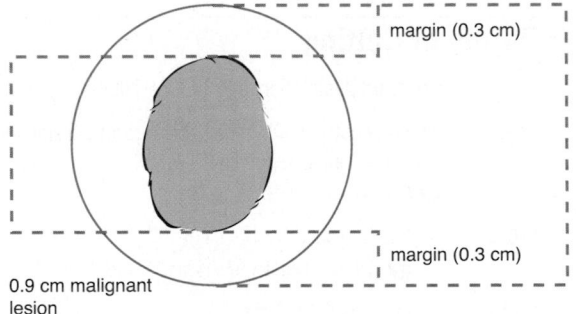

Excision—Benign Lesions

Excision (including simple closure) of benign lesions of skin (eg, neoplasm, cicatricial, fibrous, inflammatory, congenital, cystic lesions), includes local anesthesia. See appropriate size and area below. For shave removal, see 11300 et seq, and for electrosurgical and other methods see 17000 et seq.

▶Excision is defined as full-thickness (through the dermis) removal of a lesion, including margins, and includes simple (non-layered) closure when performed. Report separately each benign lesion excised. Code selection is determined by measuring the greatest clinical diameter of the apparent lesion plus that margin required for complete excision (lesion diameter plus the most narrow margins required equals the excised diameter). The margins refer to the most narrow margin required to adequately excise the lesion, based on individual judgment. The measurement of lesion plus margin is made prior to excision. The excised diameter is the same whether the surgical defect is repaired in a linear fashion, or reconstructed (eg, with a skin graft).◀

The closure of defects created by incision, excision, or trauma may require intermediate or complex closure. Repair by intermediate or complex closure should be reported separately. For excision of benign lesions requiring more than simple closure, ie, requiring intermediate or complex closure, report 11400-11446 in addition to appropriate intermediate (12031-12057) or complex closure (13100-13153) codes. For reconstructive closure, see 15002-15261, 15570-15770. For excision performed in conjunction with adjacent tissue transfer, report only the adjacent tissue transfer code (14000-14302). Excision of lesion (11400-11446) is not separately reportable with adjacent tissue transfer. See pages 64-65 for the definition of *intermediate* or *complex* closure.

11400   Excision, benign lesion including margins, except skin tag (unless listed elsewhere), trunk, arms or legs; excised diameter 0.5 cm or less
> *CPT Assistant* Summer 92:22, Fall 93:7, Fall 95:3, May 96:11, Aug 00:5, Nov 02:5, 7, Aug 06:10, Jul 08:5, Apr 10:3, Jul 10:10, Jan 11:9, May 12:13; *CPT Changes: An Insider's View* 2003

11401   excised diameter 0.6 to 1.0 cm
> *CPT Assistant* Summer 92:22, Fall 93:7, Fall 95:3, May 96:11, Nov 02:5, 7, Jul 10:10, Jan 11:9, May 12:13; *CPT Changes: An Insider's View* 2003

11402   excised diameter 1.1 to 2.0 cm
> *CPT Assistant* Summer 92:22, Fall 93:7, Fall 95:3, May 96:11, Nov 02:5, 7, Jul 10:10, Jan 11:9, May 12:13; *CPT Changes: An Insider's View* 2003

11403   excised diameter 2.1 to 3.0 cm
> *CPT Assistant* Summer 92:22, Fall 93:7, Fall 95:3, May 96:11, Nov 02:5, 7, Jul 10:10, Jan 11:9, May 12:13; *CPT Changes: An Insider's View* 2003

11404   excised diameter 3.1 to 4.0 cm
> *CPT Assistant* Summer 92:22, Fall 93:7, Fall 95:3, May 96:11, Nov 02:5, 7, Jul 10:10, Jan 11:9, May 12:13; *CPT Changes: An Insider's View* 2003

11406   excised diameter over 4.0 cm
> *CPT Assistant* Summer 92:22, Fall 93:7, Fall 95:3, May 96:11, Nov 02:5, 7, Jul 10:10, Jan 11:9, May 12:13; *CPT Changes: An Insider's View* 2003

(For unusual or complicated excision, add modifier 22)

11420   Excision, benign lesion including margins, except skin tag (unless listed elsewhere), scalp, neck, hands, feet, genitalia; excised diameter 0.5 cm or less
> *CPT Assistant* Summer 92:22, Fall 95:3, Jul 08:5, Jul 10:10, May 12:13; *CPT Changes: An Insider's View* 2003

11421   excised diameter 0.6 to 1.0 cm
> *CPT Assistant* Summer 92:22, Fall 95:3, May 96:11, Jul 10:10, May 12:13; *CPT Changes: An Insider's View* 2003

11422   excised diameter 1.1 to 2.0 cm
> *CPT Assistant* Summer 92:22, Fall 95:3, May 96:11, Aug 00:5, Jul 10:10, Mar 12:4, May 12:13; *CPT Changes: An Insider's View* 2003

11423   excised diameter 2.1 to 3.0 cm
> *CPT Assistant* Summer 92:22, Fall 95:3, May 96:11, Jul 10:10, May 12:13; *CPT Changes: An Insider's View* 2003

11424   excised diameter 3.1 to 4.0 cm
> *CPT Assistant* Summer 92:22, Fall 95:3, May 96:11, Jul 10:10, May 12:13; *CPT Changes: An Insider's View* 2003

11426   excised diameter over 4.0 cm
> *CPT Assistant* Summer 92:22, Fall 95:3, May 96:11, Jul 10:10, May 12:13; *CPT Changes: An Insider's View* 2003

(For unusual or complicated excision, add modifier 22)

11440   Excision, other benign lesion including margins, except skin tag (unless listed elsewhere), face, ears, eyelids, nose, lips, mucous membrane; excised diameter 0.5 cm or less
> *CPT Assistant* Summer 92:22, Fall 95:3, May 96:11, Jul 08:5, Jul 10:10, May 12:13; *CPT Changes: An Insider's View* 2003

11441   excised diameter 0.6 to 1.0 cm
> *CPT Assistant* Summer 92:22, Fall 95:3, May 96:11, Jul 10:10, May 12:13; *CPT Changes: An Insider's View* 2003

11442   excised diameter 1.1 to 2.0 cm
> *CPT Assistant* Summer 92:22, Fall 95:3, May 96:11, Aug 00:5, Jun 08:14, Jul 10:10, May 12:13; *CPT Changes: An Insider's View* 2003

11443   excised diameter 2.1 to 3.0 cm
> *CPT Assistant* Summer 92:22, Fall 95:3, May 96:11, Jul 10:10, May 12:13; *CPT Changes: An Insider's View* 2003

11444   excised diameter 3.1 to 4.0 cm
> *CPT Assistant* Summer 92:22, Fall 95:3, May 96:11, Jul 10:10, May 12:13; *CPT Changes: An Insider's View* 2003

11446   excised diameter over 4.0 cm
> *CPT Assistant* Summer 92:22, Fall 95:3, May 96:11, Aug 06:10, Jul 08:5, Apr 10:3, Jul 10:10, May 12:13; *CPT Changes: An Insider's View* 2003

(For unusual or complicated excision, add modifier 22)

(For eyelids involving more than skin, see also 67800 et seq)

11450   Excision of skin and subcutaneous tissue for hidradenitis, axillary; with simple or intermediate repair
> *CPT Assistant* May 12:13

11451   with complex repair
> *CPT Assistant* May 12:13

11462   Excision of skin and subcutaneous tissue for hidradenitis, inguinal; with simple or intermediate repair
> *CPT Assistant* May 12:13

11463   with complex repair
> *CPT Assistant* May 12:13

11470   Excision of skin and subcutaneous tissue for hidradenitis, perianal, perineal, or umbilical; with simple or intermediate repair
> *CPT Assistant* May 12:13

11471   with complex repair
> *CPT Assistant* May 12:13

(When skin graft or flap is used for closure, use appropriate procedure code in addition)

(For bilateral procedure, add modifier 50)

Excision—Malignant Lesions

Excision (including simple closure) of malignant lesions of skin (eg, basal cell carcinoma, squamous cell carcinoma, melanoma) includes local anesthesia. (See appropriate size and body area below.) For destruction of malignant lesions of skin, see destruction codes 17260-17286.

Excision is defined as full-thickness (through the dermis) removal of a lesion including margins, and includes simple (non-layered) closure when performed. Report separately each malignant lesion excised. Code selection is determined by measuring the greatest clinical diameter of the apparent lesion plus that margin required for complete excision (lesion diameter plus the most narrow margins required equals the excised diameter). The margins refer to the most narrow margin required to adequately excise the lesion, based on the physician's judgment. The measurement of lesion plus margin is made prior to excision. The excised diameter is the same whether the surgical defect is repaired in a linear fashion, or reconstructed (eg, with a skin graft).

The closure of defects created by incision, excision, or trauma may require intermediate or complex closure. Repair by intermediate or complex closure should be reported separately. For excision of malignant lesions requiring more than simple closure, ie, requiring intermediate or complex closure, report 11600-11646 in addition to appropriate intermediate (12031-12057) or complex closure (13100-13153) codes. For reconstructive closure, see 15002-15261, 15570-15770. For excision performed in conjunction with adjacent tissue transfer, report only the adjacent tissue transfer code (14000-14302). Excision of lesion (11600-11646) is not separately reportable with adjacent tissue transfer. See pages 64-65 for the definition of *intermediate* or *complex* closure.

When frozen section pathology shows the margins of excision were not adequate, an additional excision may be necessary for complete tumor removal. Use only one code to report the additional excision and re-excision(s) based on the final widest excised diameter required for complete tumor removal at the same operative session. To report a re-excision procedure performed to widen margins at a subsequent operative session, see codes 11600-11646, as appropriate. Append modifier 58 if the re-excision procedure is performed during the postoperative period of the primary excision procedure.

11600 Excision, malignant lesion including margins, trunk, arms, or legs; excised diameter 0.5 cm or less

➔ *CPT Assistant* Fall 95:3, May 96:11, Nov 02:5, Oct 04:4, Feb 08:8, Feb 10:3, Apr 10:3, May 12:13, Jul 12:12; *CPT Changes: An Insider's View* 2003

Measuring and Coding the Removal of a Lesion
11600

Example: Excision, malignant lesion, 0.4 cm. Code 11600.

0.2 cm lesion

margin (0.1 cm)   margin (0.1 cm)

Excised diameter (lesion plus margins): 0.2 cm + 0.2 cm = 0.4 cm

11601 excised diameter 0.6 to 1.0 cm

➔ *CPT Assistant* Fall 95:3, May 96:11, Nov 02:5, Feb 10:3, Mar 12:7, May 12:13, Jul 12:12; *CPT Changes: An Insider's View* 2003

11602 excised diameter 1.1 to 2.0 cm

➔ *CPT Assistant* Fall 95:3, May 96:11, Nov 02:5, Feb 08:8, Feb 10:3, Apr 10:3, Mar 12:7, May 12:13, Jul 12:12; *CPT Changes: An Insider's View* 2003

11603 excised diameter 2.1 to 3.0 cm

➔ *CPT Assistant* Fall 95:3, May 96:11, Nov 02:5, Feb 08:8, Feb 10:3, May 12:13, Jul 12:12; *CPT Changes: An Insider's View* 2003

11604 excised diameter 3.1 to 4.0 cm

➔ *CPT Assistant* Fall 95:3, May 96:11, Nov 02:5, Feb 08:8, Feb 10:3, May 12:13, Jul 12:12; *CPT Changes: An Insider's View* 2003

11606 excised diameter over 4.0 cm

➔ *CPT Assistant* Fall 91:6, Fall 95:3, May 96:11, Nov 02:5, Feb 08:8, Feb 10:3, May 12:13, Jul 12:12; *CPT Changes: An Insider's View* 2003

11620 Excision, malignant lesion including margins, scalp, neck, hands, feet, genitalia; excised diameter 0.5 cm or less

➔ *CPT Assistant* Fall 95:3, Nov 02:5, Oct 04:4, Feb 08:8, Feb 10:3, May 12:13, Jul 12:12; *CPT Changes: An Insider's View* 2003

11621 excised diameter 0.6 to 1.0 cm

➔ *CPT Assistant* Fall 95:3, May 96:11, Nov 02:5, Feb 08:8, Feb 10:3, May 12:13; *CPT Changes: An Insider's View* 2003

11622 excised diameter 1.1 to 2.0 cm

➔ *CPT Assistant* Fall 95:3, May 96:11, Nov 02:5, Feb 08:8, Feb 10:3, May 12:13; *CPT Changes: An Insider's View* 2003

11623 excised diameter 2.1 to 3.0 cm

➔ *CPT Assistant* Fall 95:3, May 96:11, Nov 02:5, Feb 08:8, Feb 10:3, May 12:13; *CPT Changes: An Insider's View* 2003

11624   excised diameter 3.1 to 4.0 cm
➔ *CPT Assistant* Fall 95:3, May 96:11, Nov 02:5, Feb 08:8, Feb 10:3, May 12:13; *CPT Changes: An Insider's View* 2003

11626   excised diameter over 4.0 cm
➔ *CPT Assistant* Fall 95:3, May 96:11, Nov 02:5, Feb 08:8, Feb 10:3, May 12:13; *CPT Changes: An Insider's View* 2003

11640   Excision, malignant lesion including margins, face, ears, eyelids, nose, lips; excised diameter 0.5 cm or less
➔ *CPT Assistant* Fall 95:3, May 96:11, Nov 02:5, Oct 04:4, Feb 08:8, Feb 10:3, May 12:13; *CPT Changes: An Insider's View* 2003

11641   excised diameter 0.6 to 1.0 cm
➔ *CPT Assistant* Fall 95:3, May 96:11, Feb 08:8, Feb 10:3, May 12:13; *CPT Changes: An Insider's View* 2003

11642   excised diameter 1.1 to 2.0 cm
➔ *CPT Assistant* Fall 95:3, May 96:11, Feb 08:8, Feb 10:3, May 12:13; *CPT Changes: An Insider's View* 2003

11643   excised diameter 2.1 to 3.0 cm
➔ *CPT Assistant* Fall 95:3, May 96:11, Feb 08:8, Feb 10:3, May 12:13; *CPT Changes: An Insider's View* 2003

11644   excised diameter 3.1 to 4.0 cm
➔ *CPT Assistant* Fall 95:3, May 96:11, Feb 08:8, Feb 10:3, May 12:13; *CPT Changes: An Insider's View* 2003

11646   excised diameter over 4.0 cm
➔ *CPT Assistant* Fall 95:3, May 96:11, Feb 08:8, Feb 10:3, Apr 10:3, May 12:13; *CPT Changes: An Insider's View* 2003

(For eyelids involving more than skin, see also 67800 et seq)

Nails

(For drainage of paronychia or onychia, see 10060, 10061)

11719   Trimming of nondystrophic nails, any number
➔ *CPT Assistant* Nov 97:12, Dec 02:4

Lateral Nail View
11719-11765

11720   Debridement of nail(s) by any method(s); 1 to 5
➔ *CPT Assistant* Nov 96:3, Dec 02:4

11721   6 or more
➔ *CPT Assistant* Nov 96:3, Dec 02:4

11730   Avulsion of nail plate, partial or complete, simple; single
➔ *CPT Assistant* Mar 96:10, Dec 02:4, Dec 03:11

+ 11732   each additional nail plate (List separately in addition to code for primary procedure)
➔ *CPT Assistant* Dec 02:4

(Use 11732 in conjunction with 11730)

11740   Evacuation of subungual hematoma
➔ *CPT Assistant* Dec 02:4

11750   Excision of nail and nail matrix, partial or complete (eg, ingrown or deformed nail), for permanent removal;
➔ *CPT Assistant* Dec 02:4

11752   with amputation of tuft of distal phalanx
➔ *CPT Assistant* Dec 02:4

(For skin graft, if used, use 15050)

11755   Biopsy of nail unit (eg, plate, bed, matrix, hyponychium, proximal and lateral nail folds) (separate procedure)
➔ *CPT Assistant* Mar 96:11, Dec 02:4, Oct 04:14; *CPT Changes: An Insider's View* 2002

11760   Repair of nail bed
➔ *CPT Assistant* Dec 02:4

11762   Reconstruction of nail bed with graft
➔ *CPT Assistant* Dec 02:4

11765   Wedge excision of skin of nail fold (eg, for ingrown toenail)
➔ *CPT Assistant* Dec 02:4

Dorsal Nail View
11719-11765

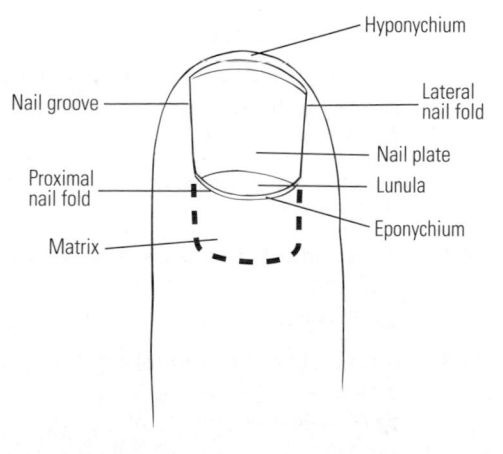

Pilonidal Cyst

11770   Excision of pilonidal cyst or sinus; simple

11771   extensive

11772   complicated

(For incision of pilonidal cyst, see 10080, 10081)

Integumentary

Integumentary

Introduction

11900   Injection, intralesional; up to and including 7 lesions
  → *CPT Assistant* Sep 96:5, May 98:10, Nov 99:8, Feb 00:11, Sep 04:12

11901   more than 7 lesions
  → *CPT Assistant* Sep 96:5, May 98:10, Nov 99:8, Feb 00:11, Sep 04:12

(11900, 11901 are not to be used for preoperative local anesthetic injection)

(For veins, see 36470, 36471)

(For intralesional chemotherapy administration, see 96405, 96406)

11920   Tattooing, intradermal introduction of insoluble opaque pigments to correct color defects of skin, including micropigmentation; 6.0 sq cm or less

11921   6.1 to 20.0 sq cm

+ 11922   each additional 20.0 sq cm, or part thereof (List separately in addition to code for primary procedure)
  → *CPT Changes: An Insider's View* 2009

(Use 11922 in conjunction with 11921)

11950   Subcutaneous injection of filling material (eg, collagen); 1 cc or less
  → *CPT Assistant* Jun 12:15

11951   1.1 to 5.0 cc
  → *CPT Assistant* Jun 12:15

11952   5.1 to 10.0 cc
  → *CPT Assistant* Jun 12:15

11954   over 10.0 cc
  → *CPT Assistant* Jun 12:15

11960   Insertion of tissue expander(s) for other than breast, including subsequent expansion
  → *CPT Assistant* Winter 91:2

(For breast reconstruction with tissue expander(s), use 19357)

11970   Replacement of tissue expander with permanent prosthesis
  → *CPT Assistant* Aug 05:1

11971   Removal of tissue expander(s) without insertion of prosthesis
  → *CPT Assistant* Jun 05:11

(11975 has been deleted. To report insertion of non-biodegradable drug delivery implant for contraception, use 11981)

11976   Removal, implantable contraceptive capsules

(11977 has been deleted. To report removal of implantable contraceptive capsules with subsequent insertion of non-biodegradable drug delivery implant, use 11976 and 11981)

11980   Subcutaneous hormone pellet implantation (implantation of estradiol and/or testosterone pellets beneath the skin)
  → *CPT Assistant* Nov 99:8; *CPT Changes: An Insider's View* 2000

11981   Insertion, non-biodegradable drug delivery implant
  → *CPT Assistant* Apr 11:12; *CPT Changes: An Insider's View* 2002

11982   Removal, non-biodegradable drug delivery implant
  → *CPT Changes: An Insider's View* 2002

11983   Removal with reinsertion, non-biodegradable drug delivery implant
  → *CPT Changes: An Insider's View* 2002

Repair (Closure)

Use the codes in this section to designate wound closure utilizing sutures, staples, or tissue adhesives (eg, 2-cyanoacrylate), either singly or in combination with each other, or in combination with adhesive strips. Wound closure utilizing adhesive strips as the sole repair material should be coded using the appropriate E/M code.

Definitions

The repair of wounds may be classified as Simple, Intermediate, or Complex.

Simple repair is used when the wound is superficial; eg, involving primarily epidermis or dermis, or subcutaneous tissues without significant involvement of deeper structures, and requires simple one layer closure. This includes local anesthesia and chemical or electrocauterization of wounds not closed.

Intermediate repair includes the repair of wounds that, in addition to the above, require layered closure of one or more of the deeper layers of subcutaneous tissue and superficial (non-muscle) fascia, in addition to the skin (epidermal and dermal) closure. Single-layer closure of heavily contaminated wounds that have required extensive cleaning or removal of particulate matter also constitutes intermediate repair.

Complex repair includes the repair of wounds requiring more than layered closure, viz., scar revision, debridement (eg, traumatic lacerations or avulsions), extensive undermining, stents or retention sutures. Necessary preparation includes creation of a limited defect for repairs or the debridement of complicated lacerations or avulsions. Complex repair does not include excision of benign (11400-11446) or malignant (11600-11646) lesions, excisional preparation of a wound bed (15002-15005) or debridement of an open fracture or open dislocation.

Instructions for listing services at time of wound repair:

1. The repaired wound(s) should be measured and recorded in centimeters, whether curved, angular, or stellate.

2. When multiple wounds are repaired, add together the lengths of those in the same classification (see above) and from all anatomic sites that are grouped together into the same code descriptor. For example, add together the lengths of intermediate repairs to the trunk and extremities. Do not add lengths of repairs from different

groupings of anatomic sites (eg, face and extremities). Also, do not add together lengths of different classifications (eg, intermediate and complex repairs).

When more than one classification of wounds is repaired, list the more complicated as the primary procedure and the less complicated as the secondary procedure, using modifier 59.

3. Decontamination and/or debridement: Debridement is considered a separate procedure only when gross contamination requires prolonged cleansing, when appreciable amounts of devitalized or contaminated tissue are removed, or when debridement is carried out separately without immediate primary closure.

> (For extensive debridement of soft tissue and/or bone, not associated with open fracture(s) and/or dislocation(s) resulting from penetrating and/or blunt trauma, see 11042-11047.)

> (For extensive debridement of subcutaneous tissue, muscle fascia, muscle, and/or bone associated with open fracture(s) and/or dislocation(s), see 11010-11012.)

4. Involvement of nerves, blood vessels and tendons: Report under appropriate system (Nervous, Cardiovascular, Musculoskeletal) for repair of these structures. The repair of these associated wounds is included in the primary procedure unless it qualifies as a complex repair, in which case modifier 59 applies.

Simple ligation of vessels in an open wound is considered as part of any wound closure.

Simple "exploration" of nerves, blood vessels or tendons exposed in an open wound is also considered part of the essential treatment of the wound and is not a separate procedure unless appreciable dissection is required. If the wound requires enlargement, extension of dissection (to determine penetration), debridement, removal of foreign body(s), ligation or coagulation of minor subcutaneous and/or muscular blood vessel(s) of the subcutaneous tissue, muscle fascia, and/or muscle, not requiring thoracotomy or laparotomy, use codes 20100-20103, as appropriate.

Repair—Simple

Sum of lengths of repairs for each group of anatomic sites.

12001   Simple repair of superficial wounds of scalp, neck, axillae, external genitalia, trunk and/or extremities (including hands and feet); 2.5 cm or less
> CPT Assistant Jun 96:7, Feb 98:11, Jan 00:11, Feb 00:10, Apr 00:8, Jul 00:10, Jan 02:10, Feb 07:10, Feb 08:8

12002   2.6 cm to 7.5 cm
> CPT Assistant Feb 00:10, Jan 02:10, Feb 08:8

12004   7.6 cm to 12.5 cm
> CPT Assistant Feb 00:10, Jan 02:10, Feb 08:8

12005   12.6 cm to 20.0 cm
> CPT Assistant Feb 00:10, Jan 02:10, Feb 08:8

12006   20.1 cm to 30.0 cm
> CPT Assistant Feb 98:11, Feb 00:10, Jan 02:10, Feb 08:8

12007   over 30.0 cm
> CPT Assistant Feb 00:10, Jan 02:10, Feb 08:8

12011   Simple repair of superficial wounds of face, ears, eyelids, nose, lips and/or mucous membranes; 2.5 cm or less
> CPT Assistant Feb 00:10, May 00:8, Jan 02:10, Feb 08:8

12013   2.6 cm to 5.0 cm
> CPT Assistant Feb 00:10, Jan 02:10, Feb 08:8

12014   5.1 cm to 7.5 cm
> CPT Assistant Feb 00:10, Jan 02:10, Feb 08:8

12015   7.6 cm to 12.5 cm
> CPT Assistant Feb 00:10, Jan 02:10, Feb 08:8

12016   12.6 cm to 20.0 cm
> CPT Assistant Feb 00:10, Jan 02:10, Feb 08:8

12017   20.1 cm to 30.0 cm
> CPT Assistant Feb 00:10, Jan 02:10, Feb 08:8

12018   over 30.0 cm
> CPT Assistant Feb 00:10, Jan 02:10, Feb 07:10, Feb 08:8

12020   Treatment of superficial wound dehiscence; simple closure
> CPT Assistant Feb 00:10, Jan 02:10, Feb 08:8

12021   with packing
> CPT Assistant Feb 00:10, Jan 02:10, Feb 08:8

(For extensive or complicated secondary wound closure, use 13160)

Repair—Intermediate

Sum of lengths of repairs for each group of anatomic sites.

12031   Repair, intermediate, wounds of scalp, axillae, trunk and/or extremities (excluding hands and feet); 2.5 cm or less
> CPT Assistant Sep 97:11, Feb 00:10, Apr 00:8, Jan 02:10, Aug 06:1, Feb 07:10, Apr 10:3; CPT Changes: An Insider's View 2009

12032   2.6 cm to 7.5 cm
> CPT Assistant May 96:6, Jun 96:8, Feb 00:10, Jan 02:10, Feb 07:10; CPT Changes: An Insider's View 2009

12034   7.6 cm to 12.5 cm
> CPT Assistant Fall 91:6, Feb 00:10, Jan 02:10, Feb 07:10; CPT Changes: An Insider's View 2009

12035   12.6 cm to 20.0 cm
> CPT Assistant Feb 00:10, Jan 02:10, Feb 07:10; CPT Changes: An Insider's View 2009

12036   20.1 cm to 30.0 cm
> CPT Assistant Feb 00:10, Jan 02:10, Feb 07:10; CPT Changes: An Insider's View 2009

12037   over 30.0 cm
> CPT Assistant Feb 00:10, Jan 02:10, Feb 07:10; CPT Changes: An Insider's View 2009

12041 Repair, intermediate, wounds of neck, hands, feet and/or external genitalia; 2.5 cm or less

➔ *CPT Assistant* Sep 97:11, Feb 00:10, Apr 00:8, Jan 02:10, Feb 07:10; *CPT Changes: An Insider's View* 2009

12042 2.6 cm to 7.5 cm

➔ *CPT Assistant* Feb 00:10, Apr 00:9, Jan 02:10, Feb 07:10; *CPT Changes: An Insider's View* 2009

12044 7.6 cm to 12.5 cm

➔ *CPT Assistant* Feb 00:10, Jan 02:10, Feb 07:10; *CPT Changes: An Insider's View* 2009

12045 12.6 cm to 20.0 cm

➔ *CPT Assistant* Feb 00:10, Jan 02:10, Feb 07:10; *CPT Changes: An Insider's View* 2009

12046 20.1 cm to 30.0 cm

➔ *CPT Assistant* Feb 00:10, Jan 02:10, Feb 07:10; *CPT Changes: An Insider's View* 2009

12047 over 30.0 cm

➔ *CPT Assistant* Feb 00:10, Jan 02:10, Feb 07:10; *CPT Changes: An Insider's View* 2009

12051 Repair, intermediate, wounds of face, ears, eyelids, nose, lips and/or mucous membranes; 2.5 cm or less

➔ *CPT Assistant* Sep 97:11, Feb 00:10, Apr 00:8, Jan 02:10, Feb 07:10; *CPT Changes: An Insider's View* 2009

12052 2.6 cm to 5.0 cm

➔ *CPT Assistant* Feb 00:10, Aug 00:9, Jan 02:10, Feb 07:10, Jul 08:5; *CPT Changes: An Insider's View* 2009

12053 5.1 cm to 7.5 cm

➔ *CPT Assistant* Feb 00:10, Jan 02:10, Feb 07:10; *CPT Changes: An Insider's View* 2009

12054 7.6 cm to 12.5 cm

➔ *CPT Assistant* Feb 00:10, Jan 02:10, Feb 07:10; *CPT Changes: An Insider's View* 2009

12055 12.6 cm to 20.0 cm

➔ *CPT Assistant* Feb 00:10, Jan 02:10, Feb 07:10; *CPT Changes: An Insider's View* 2009

12056 20.1 cm to 30.0 cm

➔ *CPT Assistant* Feb 00:10, Jan 02:10, Feb 07:10; *CPT Changes: An Insider's View* 2009

12057 over 30.0 cm

➔ *CPT Assistant* Feb 00:10, Jan 02:10, Feb 07:10, Apr 10:3; *CPT Changes: An Insider's View* 2009

Repair—Complex

Reconstructive procedures, complicated wound closure. Sum of lengths of repairs for each group of anatomic sites.

(For full thickness repair of lip or eyelid, see respective anatomical subsections)

13100 Repair, complex, trunk; 1.1 cm to 2.5 cm

➔ *CPT Assistant* Sep 97:11, Dec 98:5, Nov 99:9-10, Feb 00:10, Apr 00:8, Feb 10:3, Apr 10:3, May 11:4, Jan 12:8

(For 1.0 cm or less, see simple or intermediate repairs)

13101 2.6 cm to 7.5 cm

➔ *CPT Assistant* Dec 98:5, Nov 99:9-10, Feb 00:10, Apr 00:9, Feb 10:3, May 11:4, Jan 12:8

+ 13102 each additional 5 cm or less (List separately in addition to code for primary procedure)

➔ *CPT Assistant* Nov 99:9-10, Feb 00:10, Apr 00:9, Feb 10:3, May 11:4, Jan 12:8; *CPT Changes: An Insider's View* 2000

(Use 13102 in conjunction with 13101)

13120 Repair, complex, scalp, arms, and/or legs; 1.1 cm to 2.5 cm

➔ *CPT Assistant* Sep 97:11, Apr 99:11, Nov 99:9-10, Feb 00:10, Apr 00:8, Feb 10:3, May 11:4, Jan 12:8

(For 1.0 cm or less, see simple or intermediate repairs)

13121 2.6 cm to 7.5 cm

➔ *CPT Assistant* Dec 98:5, Nov 99:9-10, Feb 00:10, Feb 10:3, Apr 10:3, May 11:4, Jan 12:8

+ 13122 each additional 5 cm or less (List separately in addition to code for primary procedure)

➔ *CPT Assistant* Nov 99:10, Feb 10:3, May 11:4, Jan 12:8; *CPT Changes: An Insider's View* 2000

(Use 13122 in conjunction with 13121)

13131 Repair, complex, forehead, cheeks, chin, mouth, neck, axillae, genitalia, hands and/or feet; 1.1 cm to 2.5 cm

➔ *CPT Assistant* Fall 93:7, Sep 97:11, Dec 98:5, Nov 99:10, Feb 00:10, Apr 00:8, Feb 10:3, May 11:4, Jan 12:8

(For 1.0 cm or less, see simple or intermediate repairs)

13132 2.6 cm to 7.5 cm

➔ *CPT Assistant* Fall 93:7, Dec 98:5, Nov 99:10, Dec 99:10, Feb 00:10, Apr 00:9, Aug 00:9, Feb 10:3, May 11:4, Jan 12:8

+ 13133 each additional 5 cm or less (List separately in addition to code for primary procedure)

➔ *CPT Assistant* Fall 93:7, Feb 00:10, Apr 00:9, Feb 10:3, May 11:4, Jan 12:8; *CPT Changes: An Insider's View* 2000

(Use 13133 in conjunction with 13132)

13150 Repair, complex, eyelids, nose, ears and/or lips; 1.0 cm or less

➔ *CPT Assistant* Sep 97:11, Dec 98:5, Nov 99:10, Feb 00:10, Apr 00:8, Feb 10:3, May 11:4, Jan 12:8

(See also 40650-40654, 67961-67975)

13151 1.1 cm to 2.5 cm

➔ *CPT Assistant* Dec 98:5, Nov 99:10, Feb 00:10, Feb 10:3, May 11:4, Jan 12:8

13152 2.6 cm to 7.5 cm

➔ *CPT Assistant* Dec 98:5, Nov 99:10, Feb 00:10, Feb 10:3, May 11:4, Jan 12:8

+ 13153 each additional 5 cm or less (List separately in addition to code for primary procedure)

➔ *CPT Assistant* Nov 99:10, Feb 00:10, Feb 10:3, Apr 10:3, May 11:4, Jan 12:8; *CPT Changes: An Insider's View* 2000

(Use 13153 in conjunction with 13152)

13160 Secondary closure of surgical wound or dehiscence, extensive or complicated

➔ *CPT Assistant* Sep 97:11, Dec 98:5, Apr 00:8, May 11:4

(For packing or simple secondary wound closure, see 12020, 12021)

⊙=Moderate sedation ✛=Add-on code ✗=FDA approval pending #=Resequenced code O=Recycled/reinstated code ➔➔=See p xiii for details

Adjacent Tissue Transfer or Rearrangement

For full thickness repair of lip or eyelid, see respective anatomical subsections.

Codes 14000-14302 are used for excision (including lesion) and/or repair by adjacent tissue transfer or rearrangement (eg, Z-plasty, W-plasty, V-Y plasty, rotation flap, random island flap, advancement flap). When applied in repairing lacerations, the procedures listed must be performed by the surgeon to accomplish the repair. They do not apply to direct closure or rearrangement of traumatic wounds incidentally resulting in these configurations. Undermining alone of adjacent tissues to achieve closure, without additional incisions, does not constitute adjacent tissue transfer, see complex repair codes 13100-13160. The excision of a benign lesion (11400-11446) or a malignant lesion (11600-11646) is not separately reportable with codes 14000-14302.

Skin graft necessary to close secondary defect is considered an additional procedure. For purposes of code selection, the term "defect" includes the primary and secondary defects. The primary defect resulting from the excision and the secondary defect resulting from flap design to perform the reconstruction are measured together to determine the code.

14000   Adjacent tissue transfer or rearrangement, trunk; defect 10 sq cm or less

> *CPT Assistant* Sep 96:11, Jul 99:3, Jul 00:10, Jan 06:47, Dec 06:15, Jul 08:5, Mar 10:4, Apr 10:3, Jan 12:8, May 12:13

14001   defect 10.1 sq cm to 30.0 sq cm

> *CPT Assistant* Aug 98:8, Jul 99:3, Jan 06:47, Dec 06:15, Jul 08:5, Mar 10:4, Jan 12:8, May 12:13

14020   Adjacent tissue transfer or rearrangement, scalp, arms and/or legs; defect 10 sq cm or less

> *CPT Assistant* Jul 99:3, Jan 06:47, Dec 06:15, Jul 08:5, Mar 10:4, Jan 12:8, May 12:13

14021   defect 10.1 sq cm to 30.0 sq cm

> *CPT Assistant* Jul 99:3, Jan 06:47, Dec 06:15, Jul 08:5, Mar 10:4, Jan 12:8, May 12:13

14040   Adjacent tissue transfer or rearrangement, forehead, cheeks, chin, mouth, neck, axillae, genitalia, hands and/or feet; defect 10 sq cm or less

> *CPT Assistant* Jul 99:3, Jul 00:10, Jan 06:47, Dec 06:15, Jul 08:5, Mar 10:4, Jan 12:8, May 12:13

14041   defect 10.1 sq cm to 30.0 sq cm

> *CPT Assistant* Jul 99:3, Jan 06:47, Dec 06:15, Jul 08:5, Mar 10:4, Jan 12:8, May 12:13

14060   Adjacent tissue transfer or rearrangement, eyelids, nose, ears and/or lips; defect 10 sq cm or less

> *CPT Assistant* Fall 93:7, Jul 99:3, Jan 06:47, Dec 06:15, Jul 08:5, Mar 10:4, Jan 12:8, May 12:13

14061   defect 10.1 sq cm to 30.0 sq cm

> *CPT Assistant* Jul 99:3, Jan 06:47, Dec 06:15, Jul 08:5, Mar 10:4, Jan 12:8, May 12:13

(For eyelid, full thickness, see 67961 et seq)

Adjacent Tissue Repairs
14000-14061

Repair of primary and secondary defects requires assignment of a code based upon the location and the approximate description (as demonstrated below) of the area required.

A. Advancement Flap

Area 1: 1.0 cm x 1.0 cm = 1.0 sq cm
Area 2: 1.0 cm x 2.0 cm = 2.0 sq cm
(Area 1) + (Area 2) = 1.0 sq cm + 2.0 sq cm = 3.0 sq cm

B. Rotation Flap

Area 1: 1.0 cm x 1.0 cm = 1.0 sq cm
Area 2: 2.5 cm x 1.2 cm = 3.0 sq cm
(Area 1) + (Area 2) = 1.0 sq cm + 3.0 sq cm = 4.0 sq cm

(14300 has been deleted. To report, see 14301, 14302)

14301   Adjacent tissue transfer or rearrangement, any area; defect 30.1 sq cm to 60.0 sq cm

> *CPT Assistant* May 12:13; *CPT Changes: An Insider's View* 2010

+ 14302   each additional 30.0 sq cm, or part thereof (List separately in addition to code for primary procedure)

➔ *CPT Assistant* May 12:13; *CPT Changes: An Insider's View* 2010

(Use 14302 in conjunction with 14301)

14350   Filleted finger or toe flap, including preparation of recipient site

➔ *CPT Assistant* Jan 06:47, Jul 08:5, Mar 10:4, May 12:13

Skin Replacement Surgery

▶Skin replacement surgery consists of *surgical preparation* and topical placement of an *autograft* (including tissue cultured autograft) or *skin substitute graft* (ie, homograft, allograft, xenograft). The graft is anchored using the individual's choice of fixation. When services are performed in the office, routine dressing supplies are not reported separately.◀

The following definition should be applied to those codes that reference "100 sq cm or 1% of body area of infants and children" when determining the involvement of body size: The measurement of 100 sq cm is applicable to adults and children 10 years of age and older; and percentages of body surface area apply to infants and children younger than 10 years of age. The measurements apply to the size of the recipient area.

Procedures involving wrist and/or ankle are reported with codes that include arm or leg in the descriptor.

When a primary procedure requires a skin substitute or skin autograft for definitive skin closure (eg, orbitectomy, radical mastectomy, deep tumor removal), use 15100-15278 in conjunction with primary procedure.

For biological implant for soft tissue reinforcement, use 15777 in conjunction with primary procedure.

The supply of skin substitute graft(s) should be reported separately in conjunction with 15271-15278.

Definitions

Surgical preparation codes 15002-15005 for skin replacement surgery describe the initial services related to preparing a clean and viable wound surface for placement of an autograft, flap, skin substitute graft or for negative pressure wound therapy. In some cases, closure may be possible using adjacent tissue transfer (14000-14061) or complex repair (13100-13153). In all cases, appreciable nonviable tissue is removed to treat a burn, traumatic wound or a necrotizing infection. The clean wound bed may also be created by incisional release of a scar contracture resulting in a surface defect from separation of tissues. The intent is to heal the wound by primary intention, or by the use of negative pressure wound therapy. Patient conditions may require the closure or application of graft, flap, or skin substitute to be delayed, but in all cases the intent is to include these treatments or negative pressure wound therapy to heal the wound. Do

not report 15002-15005 for removal of nonviable tissue/debris in a chronic wound (eg, venous or diabetic) when the wound is left to heal by secondary intention. See active wound management codes (97597, 97598) and debridement codes (11042-11047) for this service. For necrotizing soft tissue infections in specific anatomic locations, see 11004-11008.

Select the appropriate code from 15002-15005 based upon location and size of the resultant defect. For multiple wounds, sum the surface area of all wounds from all anatomic sites that are grouped together into the same code descriptor. For example, sum the surface area of all wounds on the trunk and arms. Do not sum wounds from different groupings of anatomic sites (eg, face and arms). Use 15002 or 15004, as appropriate, for excisions and incisional releases resulting in wounds up to and including 100 sq cm of surface area. Use 15003 or 15005 for each additional 100 sq cm or part thereof. For example: Surgical preparation of a 20 sq cm wound on the right hand and a 15 sq cm wound on the left hand would be reported with a single code, 15004. Surgical preparation of a 75 sq cm wound on the right thigh and a 75 sq cm wound on the left thigh would be reported with 15002 for the first 100 sq cm and 15003 for the second 50 sq cm. If all four wounds required surgical preparation on the same day, use modifier 59 with 15002, and 15004.

Autografts/tissue cultured autografts include the harvest and/or application of an autologous skin graft. Repair of donor site requiring skin graft or local flaps is reported separately. Removal of current graft and/or simple cleansing of the wound is included, when performed. Do not report 97602. Debridement is considered a separate procedure only when gross contamination requires prolonged cleansing, when appreciable amounts of devitalized or contaminated tissue are removed, or when debridement is carried out separately without immediate primary closure.

Select the appropriate code from 15040-15261 based upon type of autograft and location and size of the defect. The measurements apply to the size of the recipient area. For multiple wounds, sum the surface area of all wounds from all anatomic sites that are grouped together into the same code descriptor. For example, sum the surface area of all wounds on the trunk and arms. Do not sum wounds from different groupings of anatomic sites (eg, face and arms).

Skin substitute grafts include non-autologous human skin (dermal or epidermal, cellular and acellular) grafts (eg, homograft, allograft), non-human skin substitute grafts (ie, xenograft), and biological products that form a sheet scaffolding for skin growth. These codes are not to be reported for application of non-graft wound dressings (eg, gel, ointment, foam, liquid) or injected skin substitutes. Removal of current graft and/or simple cleansing of the wound is included, when performed. Do not report 97602. Debridement is considered a separate procedure only when gross contamination requires prolonged cleansing, when appreciable amounts of devitalized or contaminated tissue are removed, or when debridement is carried out separately without immediate primary closure.

Select the appropriate code from 15271-15278 based upon location and size of the defect. For multiple wounds, sum the surface area of all wounds from all anatomic sites that are grouped together into the same code descriptor. For example, sum the surface area of all wounds on the trunk and arms. Do not sum wounds from different groupings of anatomic sites (eg, face and arms).

Surgical Preparation

15002 Surgical preparation or creation of recipient site by excision of open wounds, burn eschar, or scar (including subcutaneous tissues), or incisional release of scar contracture, trunk, arms, legs; first 100 sq cm or 1% of body area of infants and children

➡️ *CPT Assistant* Jan 12:6; *CPT Changes: An Insider's View* 2007

(For linear scar revision, see 13100-13153)

+ 15003   each additional 100 sq cm, or part thereof, or each additional 1% of body area of infants and children (List separately in addition to code for primary procedure)

➡️ *CPT Assistant* Jan 12:6; *CPT Changes: An Insider's View* 2007, 2009

(Use 15003 in conjunction with 15002)

15004 Surgical preparation or creation of recipient site by excision of open wounds, burn eschar, or scar (including subcutaneous tissues), or incisional release of scar contracture, face, scalp, eyelids, mouth, neck, ears, orbits, genitalia, hands, feet and/or multiple digits; first 100 sq cm or 1% of body area of infants and children

➡️ *CPT Assistant* Jan 12:6; *CPT Changes: An Insider's View* 2007

+ 15005   each additional 100 sq cm, or part thereof, or each additional 1% of body area of infants and children (List separately in addition to code for primary procedure)

➡️ *CPT Assistant* Jan 12:6; *CPT Changes: An Insider's View* 2007, 2009

(Use 15005 in conjunction with 15004)

Autografts/Tissue Cultured Autograft

15040 Harvest of skin for tissue cultured skin autograft, 100 sq cm or less

➡️ *CPT Assistant* Aug 06:10, Oct 06:1, Feb 08:3, Apr 10:3, Jan 12:6; *CPT Changes: An Insider's View* 2006

15050 Pinch graft, single or multiple, to cover small ulcer, tip of digit, or other minimal open area (except on face), up to defect size 2 cm diameter

➡️ *CPT Assistant* Apr 97:4, Sep 97:2, Nov 98:6, Jan 12:6

15100 Split-thickness autograft, trunk, arms, legs; first 100 sq cm or less, or 1% of body area of infants and children (except 15050)

➡️ *CPT Assistant* Fall 93:7, Apr 97:4, Aug 97:6, Sep 97:3, Nov 98:6, Sep 02:3, Oct 06:1, Feb 08:3, Mar 11:9, Jan 12:6; *CPT Changes: An Insider's View* 2002, 2006

+ 15101   each additional 100 sq cm, or each additional 1% of body area of infants and children, or part thereof (List separately in addition to code for primary procedure)

➡️ *CPT Assistant* Apr 97:4, Nov 98:6, Sep 02:3, Feb 08:3, Mar 11:9, Jan 12:6; *CPT Changes: An Insider's View* 2002

(Use 15101 in conjunction with 15100)

15110 Epidermal autograft, trunk, arms, legs; first 100 sq cm or less, or 1% of body area of infants and children

➡️ *CPT Assistant* Feb 08:3, Mar 11:9, Jan 12:6; *CPT Changes: An Insider's View* 2006

+ 15111   each additional 100 sq cm, or each additional 1% of body area of infants and children, or part thereof (List separately in addition to code for primary procedure)

➡️ *CPT Assistant* Feb 08:3, Mar 11:9, Jan 12:6; *CPT Changes: An Insider's View* 2006

(Use 15111 in conjunction with 15110)

15115 Epidermal autograft, face, scalp, eyelids, mouth, neck, ears, orbits, genitalia, hands, feet, and/or multiple digits; first 100 sq cm or less, or 1% of body area of infants and children

➡️ *CPT Assistant* Feb 08:3, Mar 11:9, Jan 12:6; *CPT Changes: An Insider's View* 2006

+ 15116   each additional 100 sq cm, or each additional 1% of body area of infants and children, or part thereof (List separately in addition to code for primary procedure)

➡️ *CPT Assistant* Feb 08:3, Mar 11:9, Jan 12:6; *CPT Changes: An Insider's View* 2006

(Use 15116 in conjunction with 15115)

15120 Split-thickness autograft, face, scalp, eyelids, mouth, neck, ears, orbits, genitalia, hands, feet, and/or multiple digits; first 100 sq cm or less, or 1% of body area of infants and children (except 15050)

➡️ *CPT Assistant* Apr 97:4, Aug 97:6, Sep 97:3, Nov 98:6, Jan 99:4, Sep 02:3, Feb 08:3, Jul 08:5, Mar 11:9, Jan 12:6; *CPT Changes: An Insider's View* 2002, 2006

+ 15121   each additional 100 sq cm, or each additional 1% of body area of infants and children, or part thereof (List separately in addition to code for primary procedure)

➡️ *CPT Assistant* Apr 97:4, Aug 97:6, Sep 97:3, Nov 98:6, Jan 99:4, Sep 02:3, Feb 08:3, Mar 11:9, Jan 12:6; *CPT Changes: An Insider's View* 2002

(Use 15121 in conjunction with 15120)

(For eyelids, see also 67961-67975)

15130 Dermal autograft, trunk, arms, legs; first 100 sq cm or less, or 1% of body area of infants and children

➡️ *CPT Assistant* Feb 08:3, Mar 11:9, Jan 12:6; *CPT Changes: An Insider's View* 2006

Integumentary

+ 15131 each additional 100 sq cm, or each additional 1% of body area of infants and children, or part thereof (List separately in addition to code for primary procedure)

➔ *CPT Assistant* Feb 08:3, Mar 11:9, Jan 12:6; *CPT Changes: An Insider's View* 2006

(Use 15131 in conjunction with 15130)

15135 Dermal autograft, face, scalp, eyelids, mouth, neck, ears, orbits, genitalia, hands, feet, and/or multiple digits; first 100 sq cm or less, or 1% of body area of infants and children

➔ *CPT Assistant* Feb 08:3, Mar 11:9, Jan 12:6; *CPT Changes: An Insider's View* 2006

+ 15136 each additional 100 sq cm, or each additional 1% of body area of infants and children, or part thereof (List separately in addition to code for primary procedure)

➔ *CPT Assistant* Mar 11:9, Jan 12:6; *CPT Changes: An Insider's View* 2006

(Use 15136 in conjunction with 15135)

15150 Tissue cultured skin autograft, trunk, arms, legs; first 25 sq cm or less

➔ *CPT Assistant* Oct 06:1, Feb 08:3, Mar 11:9, Jan 12:6; *CPT Changes: An Insider's View* 2006, 2012

+ 15151 additional 1 sq cm to 75 sq cm (List separately in addition to code for primary procedure)

➔ *CPT Assistant* Oct 06:1, Feb 08:3, Mar 11:9, Jan 12:6; *CPT Changes: An Insider's View* 2006, 2012

(Do not report 15151 more than once per session)

(Use 15151 in conjunction with 15150)

+ 15152 each additional 100 sq cm, or each additional 1% of body area of infants and children, or part thereof (List separately in addition to code for primary procedure)

➔ *CPT Assistant* Oct 06:1, Feb 08:3, Mar 11:9, Jan 12:6; *CPT Changes: An Insider's View* 2006, 2012

(Use 15152 in conjunction with 15151)

15155 Tissue cultured skin autograft, face, scalp, eyelids, mouth, neck, ears, orbits, genitalia, hands, feet, and/or multiple digits; first 25 sq cm or less

➔ *CPT Assistant* Oct 06:1, Feb 08:3, Mar 11:9, Jan 12:6; *CPT Changes: An Insider's View* 2006, 2012

+ 15156 additional 1 sq cm to 75 sq cm (List separately in addition to code for primary procedure)

➔ *CPT Assistant* Oct 06:1, Feb 08:3, Mar 11:9, Jan 12:6; *CPT Changes: An Insider's View* 2006, 2012

(Do not report 15156 more than once per session)

(Use 15156 in conjunction with 15155)

+ 15157 each additional 100 sq cm, or each additional 1% of body area of infants and children, or part thereof (List separately in addition to code for primary procedure)

➔ *CPT Assistant* Oct 06:1, Feb 08:3, Apr 10:3, Mar 11:9, Jan 12:6; *CPT Changes: An Insider's View* 2006, 2012

(Use 15157 in conjunction with 15156)

(15170-15176 have been deleted. To report, see 15271-15278)

15200 Full thickness graft, free, including direct closure of donor site, trunk; 20 sq cm or less

➔ *CPT Assistant* Aug 96:11, Aug 97:6, Sep 97:3, Feb 08:3, Mar 08:14, Jan 12:6; *CPT Changes: An Insider's View* 2002

+ 15201 each additional 20 sq cm, or part thereof (List separately in addition to code for primary procedure)

➔ *CPT Assistant* Apr 97:4, Aug 97:6, Sep 97:3, Feb 08:3, Mar 08:14, Jan 12:6; *CPT Changes: An Insider's View* 2002, 2009

(Use 15201 in conjunction with 15200)

15220 Full thickness graft, free, including direct closure of donor site, scalp, arms, and/or legs; 20 sq cm or less

➔ *CPT Assistant* Apr 97:4, Aug 97:6, Sep 97:3, Aug 98:9, Feb 08:3, Mar 08:14, Jan 12:6; *CPT Changes: An Insider's View* 2002

+ 15221 each additional 20 sq cm, or part thereof (List separately in addition to code for primary procedure)

➔ *CPT Assistant* Apr 97:4, Aug 97:6, Sep 97:3, Aug 98:9, Feb 08:3, Mar 08:14, Jan 12:6; *CPT Changes: An Insider's View* 2002, 2009

(Use 15221 in conjunction with 15220)

15240 Full thickness graft, free, including direct closure of donor site, forehead, cheeks, chin, mouth, neck, axillae, genitalia, hands, and/or feet; 20 sq cm or less

➔ *CPT Assistant* Apr 97:4, Aug 97:6, Sep 97:3, Nov 00:10, Feb 08:3, Mar 08:14, Jan 12:6; *CPT Changes: An Insider's View* 2002

(For finger tip graft, use 15050)

(For repair of syndactyly, fingers, see 26560-26562)

+ 15241 each additional 20 sq cm, or part thereof (List separately in addition to code for primary procedure)

➔ *CPT Assistant* Apr 97:4, Aug 97:6, Sep 97:3, Feb 08:3, Mar 08:14, Jan 12:6; *CPT Changes: An Insider's View* 2002, 2009

(Use 15241 in conjunction with 15240)

15260 Full thickness graft, free, including direct closure of donor site, nose, ears, eyelids, and/or lips; 20 sq cm or less

➔ *CPT Assistant* Fall 91:7, Fall 93:7, Apr 97:4, Aug 97:6, Sep 97:3, Jul 99:3, Feb 08:3, Mar 08:14, Jan 12:6; *CPT Changes: An Insider's View* 2002

+ 15261 each additional 20 sq cm, or part thereof (List separately in addition to code for primary procedure)

➔ *CPT Assistant* Fall 91:7, Apr 97:4, Aug 97:6, Sep 97:3, Feb 08:3, Mar 08:14, Apr 10:3, Jan 12:6; *CPT Changes: An Insider's View* 2002, 2009

(Use 15261 in conjunction with 15260)

(For eyelids, see also 67961-67975)

(Repair of donor site requiring skin graft or local flaps is considered a separate procedure)

Skin Substitute Grafts

The supply of skin substitute graft(s) should be reported separately in conjunction with 15271-15278. For biologic implant for soft tissue reinforcement, use 15777 in conjunction with code for primary procedure.

15271   Application of skin substitute graft to trunk, arms, legs, total wound surface area up to 100 sq cm; first 25 sq cm or less wound surface area

➔ *CPT Assistant Jan 12:6; CPT Changes: An Insider's View 2012*

+ 15272   each additional 25 sq cm wound surface area, or part thereof (List separately in addition to code for primary procedure)

➔ *CPT Assistant Jan 12:6; CPT Changes: An Insider's View 2012*

(Use 15272 in conjunction with 15271)

(For total wound surface area greater than or equal to 100 sq cm, see 15273, 15274)

(Do not report 15271, 15272 in conjunction with 15273, 15274)

15273   Application of skin substitute graft to trunk, arms, legs, total wound surface area greater than or equal to 100 sq cm; first 100 sq cm wound surface area, or 1% of body area of infants and children

➔ *CPT Assistant Jan 12:6; CPT Changes: An Insider's View 2012*

+ 15274   each additional 100 sq cm wound surface area, or part thereof, or each additional 1% of body area of infants and children, or part thereof (List separately in addition to code for primary procedure)

➔ *CPT Assistant Jan 12:6; CPT Changes: An Insider's View 2012*

(Use 15274 in conjunction with 15273)

(For total wound surface area up to 100 sq cm, see 15271, 15272)

15275   Application of skin substitute graft to face, scalp, eyelids, mouth, neck, ears, orbits, genitalia, hands, feet, and/or multiple digits, total wound surface area up to 100 sq cm; first 25 sq cm or less wound surface area

➔ *CPT Assistant Jan 12:6; CPT Changes: An Insider's View 2012*

+ 15276   each additional 25 sq cm wound surface area, or part thereof (List separately in addition to code for primary procedure)

➔ *CPT Assistant Jan 12:6; CPT Changes: An Insider's View 2012*

(Use 15276 in conjunction with 15275)

(For total wound surface area greater than or equal to 100 sq cm, see 15277, 15278)

(Do not report 15275, 15276 in conjunction with 15277, 15278)

15277   Application of skin substitute graft to face, scalp, eyelids, mouth, neck, ears, orbits, genitalia, hands, feet, and/or multiple digits, total wound surface area greater than or equal to 100 sq cm; first 100 sq cm wound surface area, or 1% of body area of infants and children

➔ *CPT Assistant Jan 12:6; CPT Changes: An Insider's View 2012*

+ 15278   each additional 100 sq cm wound surface area, or part thereof, or each additional 1% of body area of infants and children, or part thereof (List separately in addition to code for primary procedure)

➔ *CPT Assistant Jan 12:6; CPT Changes: An Insider's View 2012*

(Use 15278 in conjunction with 15277)

(For total wound surface area up to 100 sq cm, see 15275, 15276)

(Do not report 15271-15278 in conjunction with 97602)

(15300, 15301 have been deleted. To report, see 15271-15274)

(15320, 15321 have been deleted. To report, see 15275-15278)

(15330, 15331 have been deleted. To report, see 15271-15274)

(15335, 15336 have been deleted. To report, see 15275-15278)

(15340, 15341 have been deleted. To report, see 15271-15278)

(15360, 15361 have been deleted. To report, see 15271-15274)

(15365, 15366 have been deleted. To report, see 15275-15278)

(15400, 15401 have been deleted. To report, see 15271-15274)

(15420, 15421 have been deleted. To report, see 15275-15278)

(15430, 15431 have been deleted. To report, see 15271-15278)

Flaps (Skin and/or Deep Tissues)

The regions listed refer to the recipient area (not the donor site) when a flap is being attached in a transfer or to a final site.

The regions listed refer to a donor site when a tube is formed for later transfer or when a "delay" of flap occurs prior to the transfer. Codes 15732-15738 are described by donor site of the muscle, myocutaneous, or fasciocutaneous flap.

Codes 15570-15738 do not include extensive immobilization (eg, large plaster casts and other immobilizing devices are considered additional separate procedures).

A repair of a donor site requiring a skin graft or local flaps is considered an additional separate procedure.

(For microvascular flaps, see 15756-15758)

(For flaps without inclusion of a vascular pedicle, see 15570-15576)

(For adjacent tissue transfer flaps, see 14000-14302)

▲=Revised code   ●=New code   ▶◀=Contains new or revised text   ⊘=Modifier 51 exempt

Integumentary

15570 Formation of direct or tubed pedicle, with or without transfer; trunk
> *CPT Assistant* Nov 02:7, Mar 10:4, Apr 10:3

15572 scalp, arms, or legs

15574 forehead, cheeks, chin, mouth, neck, axillae, genitalia, hands or feet

15576 eyelids, nose, ears, lips, or intraoral

15600 Delay of flap or sectioning of flap (division and inset); at trunk
> *CPT Assistant* Nov 99:10, Mar 10:4

15610 at scalp, arms, or legs

15620 at forehead, cheeks, chin, neck, axillae, genitalia, hands, or feet

15630 at eyelids, nose, ears, or lips

15650 Transfer, intermediate, of any pedicle flap (eg, abdomen to wrist, Walking tube), any location

(For eyelids, nose, ears, or lips, see also anatomical area)

(For revision, defatting or rearranging of transferred pedicle flap or skin graft, see 13100-14302)

15731 Forehead flap with preservation of vascular pedicle (eg, axial pattern flap, paramedian forehead flap)
> *CPT Changes: An Insider's View* 2007

(For muscle, myocutaneous, or fasciocutaneous flap of the head or neck, use 15732)

Axial Pattern Forehead Flap
15731

Reconstruction of a nasal defect with a forehead flap based on the left supratrochlear vessels

Donor defect

Forehead flap

15732 Muscle, myocutaneous, or fasciocutaneous flap; head and neck (eg, temporalis, masseter muscle, sternocleidomastoid, levator scapulae)
> *CPT Changes: An Insider's View* 2002

(For forehead flap with preservation of vascular pedicle, use 15731)

15734 trunk

15736 upper extremity

15738 lower extremity
> *CPT Assistant* Sep 03:15, Apr 10:3

Other Flaps and Grafts

▶Code 15740 describes a cutaneous flap, transposed into a nearby but not immediately adjacent defect, with a pedicle that incorporates an anatomically named axial vessel into its design. The flap is typically transferred through a tunnel underneath the skin and sutured into its new position. The donor site is closed directly.◀

Neurovascular pedicle procedures are reported with 15750. This code includes not only skin but also a functional motor or sensory nerve(s). The flap serves to reinnervate a damaged portion of the body dependent on touch or movement (eg, thumb).

Repair of donor site requiring skin graft or local flaps should be reported as an additional procedure.

▶For random island flaps, V-Y subcutaneous flaps, advancement flaps, and other flaps from adjacent areas without clearly defined anatomically named axial vessels, see 14000-14302.◀

▲ **15740** Flap; island pedicle requiring identification and dissection of an anatomically named axial vessel
> *CPT Assistant* Mar 04:11, Sep 04:12, Oct 04:15, Apr 10:3; *CPT Changes: An Insider's View* 2013

15750 neurovascular pedicle

15756 Free muscle or myocutaneous flap with microvascular anastomosis
> *CPT Assistant* Apr 97:5, Nov 97:12, Nov 98:6; *CPT Changes: An Insider's View* 2003

(Do not report code 69990 in addition to code 15756)

15757 Free skin flap with microvascular anastomosis
> *CPT Assistant* Apr 97:5, Nov 98:6

(Do not report code 69990 in addition to code 15757)

15758 Free fascial flap with microvascular anastomosis
> *CPT Assistant* Apr 97:5, Nov 98:6

(Do not report code 69990 in addition to code 15758)

15760 Graft; composite (eg, full thickness of external ear or nasal ala), including primary closure, donor area
> *CPT Assistant* Sep 97:3

15770   derma-fat-fascia
> *CPT Assistant* Sep 97:3, Apr 10:3

15775   Punch graft for hair transplant; 1 to 15 punch grafts
> *CPT Assistant* Sep 97:3

15776   more than 15 punch grafts
> *CPT Assistant* Sep 97:3

(For strip transplant, use 15220)

+ 15777   Implantation of biologic implant (eg, acellular dermal matrix) for soft tissue reinforcement (eg, breast, trunk) (List separately in addition to code for primary procedure)
> *CPT Assistant* Jan 12:10; *CPT Changes: An Insider's View* 2012

(For bilateral breast procedure, report 15777 with modifier 50)

(For implantation of mesh or other prosthesis for open incisional or ventral hernia repair, use 49568 in conjunction with 49560-49566)

(For insertion of mesh or other prosthesis for closure of a necrotizing soft tissue infection wound, use 49568 in conjunction with 11004-11006)

(For topical application of skin substitute graft to a wound surface, see 15271-15278)

(For repair of anorectal fistula with plug (eg, porcine small intestine submucosa [SIS]), use 46707)

(For insertion of mesh or other prosthesis for repair of pelvic floor defect, use 57267)

(The supply of biologic implant should be reported separately in conjunction with 15777)

Other Procedures

15780   Dermabrasion; total face (eg, for acne scarring, fine wrinkling, rhytids, general keratosis)
> *CPT Assistant* Apr 03:27

15781   segmental, face

15782   regional, other than face

15783   superficial, any site (eg, tattoo removal)
> *CPT Assistant* Apr 03:27

15786   Abrasion; single lesion (eg, keratosis, scar)

+ 15787   each additional 4 lesions or less (List separately in addition to code for primary procedure)

(Use 15787 in conjunction with 15786)

15788   Chemical peel, facial; epidermal

15789   dermal

15792   Chemical peel, nonfacial; epidermal

15793   dermal

15819   Cervicoplasty

15820   Blepharoplasty, lower eyelid;
> *CPT Assistant* Feb 04:11, May 04:12, Feb 05:16

15821   with extensive herniated fat pad
> *CPT Assistant* Feb 04:11, May 04.12, Feb 05:16

15822   Blepharoplasty, upper eyelid;
> *CPT Assistant* Feb 04:11, May 04:12, Feb 05:16

15823   with excessive skin weighting down lid
> *CPT Assistant* Sep 00:7, Feb 04:11, May 04:12, Feb 05:16, Aug 11:8

(For bilateral blepharoplasty, add modifier 50)

15824   Rhytidectomy; forehead

(For repair of brow ptosis, use 67900)

15825   neck with platysmal tightening (platysmal flap, P-flap)

15826   glabellar frown lines

15828   cheek, chin, and neck

15829   superficial musculoaponeurotic system (SMAS) flap

(For bilateral rhytidectomy, add modifier 50)

15830   Excision, excessive skin and subcutaneous tissue (includes lipectomy); abdomen, infraumbilical panniculectomy
> *CPT Changes: An Insider's View* 2007

(Do not report 15830 in conjunction with 12031-12037, 13100-13102, 14000, 14001, 14302)

15832   thigh

15833   leg

15834   hip

15835   buttock

15836   arm

15837   forearm or hand

15838   submental fat pad

15839   other area

(For bilateral procedure, add modifier 50)

15840   Graft for facial nerve paralysis; free fascia graft (including obtaining fascia)

(For bilateral procedure, add modifier 50)

15841   free muscle graft (including obtaining graft)

15842   free muscle flap by microsurgical technique
> *CPT Changes: An Insider's View* 2001

(Do not report code 69990 in addition to code 15842)

Integumentary

15845   regional muscle transfer

(For intravenous fluorescein examination of blood flow in graft or flap, use 15860)

(For nerve transfers, decompression, or repair, see 64831-64876, 64905, 64907, 69720, 69725, 69740, 69745, 69955)

+ 15847   Excision, excessive skin and subcutaneous tissue (includes lipectomy), abdomen (eg, abdominoplasty) (includes umbilical transposition and fascial plication) (List separately in addition to code for primary procedure)
➔ *CPT Changes: An Insider's View* 2007

(Use 15847 in conjunction with 15830)

(For abdominal wall hernia repair, see 49491-49587)

(To report other abdominoplasty, use 17999)

15850   Removal of sutures under anesthesia (other than local), same surgeon
➔ *CPT Assistant* Spring 93:34, Nov 97:22

15851   Removal of sutures under anesthesia (other than local), other surgeon
➔ *CPT Assistant* Spring 93:34, Nov 97:22

15852   Dressing change (for other than burns) under anesthesia (other than local)

15860   Intravenous injection of agent (eg, fluorescein) to test vascular flow in flap or graft
➔ *CPT Changes: An Insider's View* 2002

15876   Suction assisted lipectomy; head and neck

15877   trunk
➔ *CPT Assistant* Oct 99:10, Feb 05:14

15878   upper extremity

15879   lower extremity

Pressure Ulcers (Decubitus Ulcers)

15920   Excision, coccygeal pressure ulcer, with coccygectomy; with primary suture

15922   with flap closure

15931   Excision, sacral pressure ulcer, with primary suture;

15933   with ostectomy

15934   Excision, sacral pressure ulcer, with skin flap closure;

15935   with ostectomy

15936   Excision, sacral pressure ulcer, in preparation for muscle or myocutaneous flap or skin graft closure;
➔ *CPT Assistant* Nov 98:6-7

15937   with ostectomy

(For repair of defect using muscle or myocutaneous flap, use code(s) 15734 and/or 15738 in addition to 15936, 15937. For repair of defect using split skin graft, use codes 15100 and/or 15101 in addition to 15936, 15937)

15940   Excision, ischial pressure ulcer, with primary suture;

15941   with ostectomy (ischiectomy)

15944   Excision, ischial pressure ulcer, with skin flap closure;

15945   with ostectomy

15946   Excision, ischial pressure ulcer, with ostectomy, in preparation for muscle or myocutaneous flap or skin graft closure
➔ *CPT Assistant* Nov 98:6-7, Jun 02:10, Jan 03:23

(For repair of defect using muscle or myocutaneous flap, use code(s) 15734 and/or 15738 in addition to 15946. For repair of defect using split skin graft, use codes 15100 and/or 15101 in addition to 15946)

15950   Excision, trochanteric pressure ulcer, with primary suture;

15951   with ostectomy

15952   Excision, trochanteric pressure ulcer, with skin flap closure;

15953   with ostectomy

15956   Excision, trochanteric pressure ulcer, in preparation for muscle or myocutaneous flap or skin graft closure;
➔ *CPT Assistant* Nov 98:6-7

15958   with ostectomy
➔ *CPT Assistant* Nov 98:6-7

(For repair of defect using muscle or myocutaneous flap, use code(s) 15734 and/or 15738 in addition to 15956, 15958. For repair of defect using split skin graft, use codes 15100 and/or 15101 in addition to 15956, 15958)

15999   Unlisted procedure, excision pressure ulcer

(For free skin graft to close ulcer or donor site, see 15002 et seq)

Burns, Local Treatment

Procedures 16000-16036 refer to local treatment of burned surface only. Codes 16020-16030 include the application of materials (eg, dressings) not described in codes 15100-15278.

List percentage of body surface involved and depth of burn.

For necessary related medical services (eg, hospital visits, detention) in management of burned patients, see appropriate services in **Evaluation and Management** and **Medicine** sections.

For the application of skin grafts or skin substitutes, see codes 15100-15777.

16000   Initial treatment, first degree burn, when no more than local treatment is required
➔ *CPT Assistant* Aug 97:6

Calculation of Total Body Surface Area (TBSA) Burn
16000

Calculation of the percentage of a body burned is achieved by dividing the total body surface area into 9% or multiples of 9% segments. In the infant or child, the "rule" deviates because of the large surface area of the child's head.

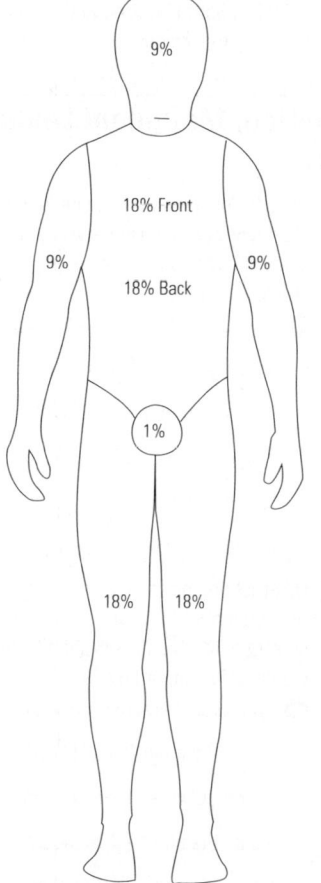

16020   Dressings and/or debridement of partial-thickness burns, initial or subsequent; small (less than 5% total body surface area)

> *CPT Assistant* Aug 97:6; *CPT Changes: An Insider's View* 2006

16025   medium (eg, whole face or whole extremity, or 5% to 10% total body surface area)

> *CPT Assistant* Aug 97:6, Jun 08:14; *CPT Changes: An Insider's View* 2006

16030   large (eg, more than 1 extremity, or greater than 10% total body surface area)

> *CPT Assistant* Aug 97:6, Jun 08:14; *CPT Changes: An Insider's View* 2006

16035   Escharotomy; initial incision

> *CPT Assistant* Aug 97:6; *CPT Changes: An Insider's View* 2001

+ 16036   each additional incision (List separately in addition to code for primary procedure)

> *CPT Changes: An Insider's View* 2001

(Use 16036 in conjunction with 16035)

(For debridement, curettement of burn wound, see 16020-16030)

Destruction

Destruction means the ablation of benign, premalignant or malignant tissues by any method, with or without curettement, including local anesthesia, and not usually requiring closure.

Any method includes electrosurgery, cryosurgery, laser and chemical treatment. Lesions include condylomata, papillomata, molluscum contagiosum, herpetic lesions, warts (ie, common, plantar, flat), milia, or other benign, premalignant (eg, actinic keratoses), or malignant lesions.

> (For destruction of lesion(s) in specific anatomic sites, see 40820, 46900-46917, 46924, 54050-54057, 54065, 56501, 56515, 57061, 57065, 67850, 68135)
>
> (For laser treatment for inflammatory skin disease, see 96920-96922)
>
> (For paring or cutting of benign hyperkeratotic lesions (eg, corns or calluses), see 11055-11057)
>
> (For sharp removal or electrosurgical destruction of skin tags and fibrocutaneous tags, see 11200, 11201)
>
> (For cryotherapy of acne, use 17340)
>
> (For initiation or follow-up care of topical chemotherapy (eg, 5-FU or similar agents), see appropriate office visits)
>
> (For shaving of epidermal or dermal lesions, see 11300-11313)

Destruction, Benign or Premalignant Lesions

17000   Destruction (eg, laser surgery, electrosurgery, cryosurgery, chemosurgery, surgical curettement), premalignant lesions (eg, actinic keratoses); first lesion

> *CPT Assistant* Winter 90:3, Nov 97:12, Jun 99:10, May 06:19, Feb 07:10, Aug 09:7, Mar 10:10, Mar 12:7, May 12:13; *CPT Changes: An Insider's View* 2002, 2007

+ 17003   second through 14 lesions, each (List separately in addition to code for first lesion)

> *CPT Assistant* Nov 97:12, Jun 99:10, May 06:19, Feb 07:10, Aug 09:7, Mar 10:10

(Use 17003 in conjunction with 17000)

(For destruction of common or plantar warts, see 17110, 17111)

Integumentary

⊘ **17004**   Destruction (eg, laser surgery, electrosurgery, cryosurgery, chemosurgery, surgical curettement), premalignant lesions (eg, actinic keratoses), 15 or more lesions

➜ *CPT Assistant* Nov 97:12, Nov 98:7, Jun 99:10, Mar 03:21, Feb 07:10, Aug 09:7, Mar 10:10; *CPT Changes: An Insider's View* 2002, 2007

(Do not report 17004 in conjunction with 17000-17003)

Destruction, Benign or Premalignant Lesions
17004

The lesions, seen as rough scaling patches scattered over the face, scalp, and ears, are destroyed by cryosurgery or other surgical means.

Ice field

Cryo probe (spray nozzle)

17106   Destruction of cutaneous vascular proliferative lesions (eg, laser technique); less than 10 sq cm

➜ *CPT Assistant* Winter 90:3, Apr 07:11, Jun 08:14, Aug 09:7

17107   10.0 to 50.0 sq cm

➜ *CPT Assistant* Winter 90:3, Apr 07:11, Jun 08:14, Aug 09:7

17108   over 50.0 sq cm

➜ *CPT Assistant* Winter 90:3, Apr 07:11, Jun 08:14, Aug 09:7

17110   Destruction (eg, laser surgery, electrosurgery, cryosurgery, chemosurgery, surgical curettement), of benign lesions other than skin tags or cutaneous vascular proliferative lesions; up to 14 lesions

➜ *CPT Assistant* Nov 97:13, Feb 07:10, Apr 07:11, Nov 08:10, Aug 09:7; *CPT Changes: An Insider's View* 2002, 2007, 2008

17111   15 or more lesions

➜ *CPT Assistant* Nov 97:13, Feb 07:10, Apr 07:11, Nov 08:10, Aug 09:7

17250   Chemical cauterization of granulation tissue (proud flesh, sinus or fistula)

➜ *CPT Assistant* May 12:13

(17250 is not to be used with removal or excision codes for the same lesion)

Destruction, Malignant Lesions, Any Method

17260   Destruction, malignant lesion (eg, laser surgery, electrosurgery, cryosurgery, chemosurgery, surgical curettement), trunk, arms or legs; lesion diameter 0.5 cm or less

➜ *CPT Assistant* May 12:13; *CPT Changes: An Insider's View* 2002

17261   lesion diameter 0.6 to 1.0 cm

17262   lesion diameter 1.1 to 2.0 cm

17263   lesion diameter 2.1 to 3.0 cm

17264   lesion diameter 3.1 to 4.0 cm

17266   lesion diameter over 4.0 cm

17270   Destruction, malignant lesion (eg, laser surgery, electrosurgery, cryosurgery, chemosurgery, surgical curettement), scalp, neck, hands, feet, genitalia; lesion diameter 0.5 cm or less

➜ *CPT Changes: An Insider's View* 2002

17271   lesion diameter 0.6 to 1.0 cm

17272   lesion diameter 1.1 to 2.0 cm

17273   lesion diameter 2.1 to 3.0 cm

17274   lesion diameter 3.1 to 4.0 cm

17276   lesion diameter over 4.0 cm

17280   Destruction, malignant lesion (eg, laser surgery, electrosurgery, cryosurgery, chemosurgery, surgical curettement), face, ears, eyelids, nose, lips, mucous membrane; lesion diameter 0.5 cm or less

➜ *CPT Changes: An Insider's View* 2002

17281   lesion diameter 0.6 to 1.0 cm

17282   lesion diameter 1.1 to 2.0 cm

17283   lesion diameter 2.1 to 3.0 cm

17284   lesion diameter 3.1 to 4.0 cm

17286   lesion diameter over 4.0 cm

Mohs Micrographic Surgery

►Mohs micrographic surgery is a technique for the removal of complex or ill-defined skin cancer with histologic examination of 100% of the surgical margins. It requires the integration of an individual functioning in two separate and distinct capacities: surgeon and pathologist. If either of these responsibilities is delegated to another physician or other qualified health care professional who reports the services separately, these codes should not be reported. The Mohs surgeon removes the tumor tissue and maps and divides the tumor specimen into pieces, and each piece is embedded into an individual tissue block for histopathologic examination. Thus a tissue block in Mohs surgery is defined as an individual tissue piece embedded in a mounting medium for sectioning.◄

If repair is performed, use separate repair, flap, or graft codes. If a biopsy of a suspected skin cancer is performed on the same day as Mohs surgery because there was no prior pathology confirmation of a diagnosis, then report diagnostic skin biopsy (11100, 11101) and frozen section pathology (88331) with modifier 59 to distinguish from the subsequent definitive surgical procedure of Mohs surgery.

> (If additional special pathology procedures, stains or immunostains are required, use 88311-88314, 88342)

> (Do not report 88314 in conjunction with 17311-17315 for routine frozen section stain (eg, hematoxylin and eosin, toluidine blue) performed during Mohs surgery. When a nonroutine histochemical stain on frozen tissue is utilized, report 88314 with modifier 59)

> (Do not report 88302-88309 on the same specimen as part of the Mohs surgery)

17311 Mohs micrographic technique, including removal of all gross tumor, surgical excision of tissue specimens, mapping, color coding of specimens, microscopic examination of specimens by the surgeon, and histopathologic preparation including routine stain(s) (eg, hematoxylin and eosin, toluidine blue), head, neck, hands, feet, genitalia, or any location with surgery directly involving muscle, cartilage, bone, tendon, major nerves, or vessels; first stage, up to 5 tissue blocks
> ➔ *CPT Changes: An Insider's View* 2007

+ 17312 each additional stage after the first stage, up to 5 tissue blocks (List separately in addition to code for primary procedure)
> ➔ *CPT Changes: An Insider's View* 2007

> (Use 17312 in conjunction with 17311)

17313 Mohs micrographic technique, including removal of all gross tumor, surgical excision of tissue specimens, mapping, color coding of specimens, microscopic examination of specimens by the surgeon, and histopathologic preparation including routine stain(s) (eg, hematoxylin and eosin, toluidine blue), of the trunk, arms, or legs; first stage, up to 5 tissue blocks
> ➔ *CPT Changes: An Insider's View* 2007

+ 17314 each additional stage after the first stage, up to 5 tissue blocks (List separately in addition to code for primary procedure)
> ➔ *CPT Changes: An Insider's View* 2007

> (Use 17314 in conjunction with 17313)

+ 17315 Mohs micrographic technique, including removal of all gross tumor, surgical excision of tissue specimens, mapping, color coding of specimens, microscopic examination of specimens by the surgeon, and histopathologic preparation including routine stain(s) (eg, hematoxylin and eosin, toluidine blue), each additional block after the first 5 tissue blocks, any stage (List separately in addition to code for primary procedure)
> ➔ *CPT Assistant* May 12:13; *CPT Changes: An Insider's View* 2007

> (Use 17315 in conjunction with 17311-17314)

Other Procedures

17340 Cryotherapy (CO_2 slush, liquid N_2) for acne
> ➔ *CPT Assistant* May 12:13

17360 Chemical exfoliation for acne (eg, acne paste, acid)

17380 Electrolysis epilation, each 30 minutes

> (For actinotherapy, use 96900)

17999 Unlisted procedure, skin, mucous membrane and subcutaneous tissue
> ➔ *CPT Assistant* Dec 98:9, May 99:11, Jun 05:11, Nov 08:10, Mar 11:9, May 12:13
> ➔ *Clinical Examples in Radiology* Winter 10:15

Breast

Incision

19000 Puncture aspiration of cyst of breast;
> ➔ *CPT Assistant* Fall 94:18, Apr 05:6, Nov 08:10

+ 19001 each additional cyst (List separately in addition to code for primary procedure)
> ➔ *CPT Assistant* Fall 94:18, Apr 05:6

> (Use 19001 in conjunction with 19000)

> (If imaging guidance is performed, see 76942, 77021, 77031, 77032)

19020 Mastotomy with exploration or drainage of abscess, deep
> ➔ *CPT Assistant* Apr 05:6

19030 Injection procedure only for mammary ductogram or galactogram
> ➔ *CPT Assistant* Jul 04:8, Apr 05:6

> (For radiological supervision and interpretation, see 77053, 77054)

Integumentary

Excision

Excisional breast surgery includes certain biopsy procedures, the removal of cysts or other benign or malignant tumors or lesions, and the surgical treatment of breast and chest wall malignancies. Biopsy procedures may be percutaneous or open, and they involve the removal of differing amounts of tissue for diagnosis.

Breast biopsies are reported using codes 19100-19103. The open excision of breast lesions (eg, lesions of the breast ducts, cysts, benign or malignant tumors), without specific attention to adequate surgical margins, with or without the preoperative placement of radiological markers, is reported using codes 19110-19126. Partial mastectomy procedures (eg, lumpectomy, tylectomy, quadrantectomy, or segmentectomy) describe open excisions of breast tissue with specific attention to adequate surgical margins.

Partial mastectomy procedures are reported using codes 19301 or 19302 as appropriate. Documentation for partial mastectomy procedures includes attention to the removal of adequate surgical margins surrounding the breast mass or lesion.

Total mastectomy procedures include simple mastectomy, complete mastectomy, subcutaneous mastectomy, modified radical mastectomy, radical mastectomy, and more extended procedures (eg, Urban type operation). Total mastectomy procedures are reported using codes 19303-19307 as appropriate.

Excisions or resections of chest wall tumors including ribs, with or without reconstruction, with or without mediastinal lymphadenectomy, are reported using codes 19260, 19271, or 19272. Codes 19260-19272 are not restricted to breast tumors and are used to report resections of chest wall tumors originating from any chest wall component. (For excision of lung or pleura, see 32310 et seq)

(To report bilateral procedure, report modifier 50 with the procedure code)

19100   Biopsy of breast; percutaneous, needle core, not using imaging guidance (separate procedure)
> *CPT Assistant* Spring 93:35, Fall 94:18, Apr 96:8, Mar 97:4, Nov 97:24, Nov 98:7, Jan 01:10, May 02:18, Apr 05:6, Dec 06:10, Nov 08:10; *CPT Changes: An Insider's View* 2001
> *Clinical Examples in Radiology* Fall 10:3

(For fine needle aspiration, use 10021)

(For image guided breast biopsy, see 19102, 19103, 10022)

19101   open, incisional
> *CPT Assistant* Spring 93:35, Fall 94:19, Nov 97:24, Jan 01:8, May 02:18, Apr 05:6; *CPT Changes: An Insider's View* 2001

19102   percutaneous, needle core, using imaging guidance
> *CPT Assistant* Jan 01:10, May 02:18, Apr 05:6, Nov 08:10, Mar 10:9; *CPT Changes: An Insider's View* 2001
> *Clinical Examples in Radiology* Summer 05:1, 2, Fall 08:3, Fall 10:3

(For placement of percutaneous localization clip, use 19295)

19103   percutaneous, automated vacuum assisted or rotating biopsy device, using imaging guidance
> *CPT Assistant* Jan 01:10, May 02:18, Apr 03:7, Apr 05:6, Nov 08:10, Mar 10:9; *CPT Changes: An Insider's View* 2001
> *Clinical Examples in Radiology* Fall 08:3, Fall 10:1-3

(For imaging guidance performed in conjunction with 19102, 19103, see 76942, 77012, 77021, 77031, 77032)

(For placement of percutaneous localization clip, use 19295)

19105   Ablation, cryosurgical, of fibroadenoma, including ultrasound guidance, each fibroadenoma
> *CPT Changes: An Insider's View* 2007

(Do not report 19105 in conjunction with 76940, 76942)

(For adjacent lesions treated with 1 cryoprobe insertion, report once)

19110   Nipple exploration, with or without excision of a solitary lactiferous duct or a papilloma lactiferous duct
> *CPT Assistant* Apr 05:6

19112   Excision of lactiferous duct fistula
> *CPT Assistant* Apr 05:6

19120   Excision of cyst, fibroadenoma, or other benign or malignant tumor, aberrant breast tissue, duct lesion, nipple or areolar lesion (except 19300), open, male or female, 1 or more lesions
> *CPT Assistant* Feb 96:9, Nov 97:14, Jan 01:8, May 01:10, Apr 05:6, 13; *CPT Changes: An Insider's View* 2001, 2007

19125   Excision of breast lesion identified by preoperative placement of radiological marker, open; single lesion
> *CPT Assistant* Fall 94:18, Mar 98:10, Jan 01:8, Apr 05:6, Mar 09:10; *CPT Changes: An Insider's View* 2001

+ 19126   each additional lesion separately identified by a preoperative radiological marker (List separately in addition to code for primary procedure)
> *CPT Assistant* Fall 94:18, Mar 98:10, Jan 01:8, Apr 05:6; *CPT Changes: An Insider's View* 2001

(Use 19126 in conjunction with 19125)

19260   Excision of chest wall tumor including ribs
> *CPT Assistant* Apr 05:6, 7, Apr 10:3

19271   Excision of chest wall tumor involving ribs, with plastic reconstruction; without mediastinal lymphadenectomy
> *CPT Assistant* Apr 05:6, 7

19272   with mediastinal lymphadenectomy
> *CPT Assistant* Apr 05:6, 7

►(Do not report 19260, 19271, 19272 in conjunction with 32100, 32503, 32504, 32551, 32554, 32555)◄

Introduction

19290   Preoperative placement of needle localization wire, breast;
→ *CPT Assistant* Fall 94:19, Apr 05:6
→ *Clinical Examples in Radiology* Fall 05:01, Summer 09:15

+ 19291   each additional lesion (List separately in addition to code for primary procedure)
→ *CPT Assistant* Fall 94:19, Apr 05:6

(Use 19291 in conjunction with 19290)

(For radiological supervision and interpretation, see 76942, 77031, 77032)

+ 19295   Image guided placement, metallic localization clip, percutaneous, during breast biopsy/aspiration (List separately in addition to code for primary procedure)
→ *CPT Assistant* Jan 01:10, Apr 05:6, Nov 08:10; *CPT Changes: An Insider's View* 2001, 2010
→ *Clinical Examples in Radiology* Fall 08:2, 3, Fall 10:3

(Use 19295 in conjunction with 10022, 19102, 19103)

19296   Placement of radiotherapy afterloading expandable catheter (single or multichannel) into the breast for interstitial radioelement application following partial mastectomy, includes imaging guidance; on date separate from partial mastectomy
→ *CPT Assistant* Apr 05:6-8, Nov 05:15, Apr 09:3, Dec 09:9, Mar 10:10; *CPT Changes: An Insider's View* 2005, 2009

+ 19297   concurrent with partial mastectomy (List separately in addition to code for primary procedure)
→ *CPT Assistant* Apr 05:6-8, Nov 05:15, Apr 09:3, Mar 10:10; *CPT Changes: An Insider's View* 2005, 2009

(Use 19297 in conjunction with 19301 or 19302)

⊙ 19298   Placement of radiotherapy afterloading brachytherapy catheters (multiple tube and button type) into the breast for interstitial radioelement application following (at the time of or subsequent to) partial mastectomy, includes imaging guidance
→ *CPT Assistant* Apr 05:6-7, 9, 16, Nov 05:15, Apr 09:3, Mar 10:10; *CPT Changes: An Insider's View* 2005

Mastectomy Procedures

19300   Mastectomy for gynecomastia
→ *CPT Assistant* Feb 07:4; *CPT Changes: An Insider's View* 2007

19301   Mastectomy, partial (eg, lumpectomy, tylectomy, quadrantectomy, segmentectomy);
→ *CPT Assistant* Feb 07:4, Dec 07:8, Sep 08:5, Mar 10:10; *CPT Changes: An Insider's View* 2007

19302   with axillary lymphadenectomy
→ *CPT Assistant* Feb 07:4, Dec 07:8, Sep 08:5, Mar 10:10; *CPT Changes: An Insider's View* 2007

(For placement of radiotherapy afterloading balloon/brachytherapy catheters, see 19296-19298)

19303   Mastectomy, simple, complete
→ *CPT Assistant* Feb 07:4; *CPT Changes: An Insider's View* 2007

(For immediate or delayed insertion of implant, see 19340, 19342)

(For gynecomastia, use 19300)

19304   Mastectomy, subcutaneous
→ *CPT Assistant* Feb 07:4, Dec 07:7, 8; *CPT Changes: An Insider's View* 2007

(For immediate or delayed insertion of implant, see 19340, 19342)

19305   Mastectomy, radical, including pectoral muscles, axillary lymph nodes
→ *CPT Assistant* Feb 07:4, Sep 08:5; *CPT Changes: An Insider's View* 2007

(For immediate or delayed insertion of implant, see 19340, 19342)

19306   Mastectomy, radical, including pectoral muscles, axillary and internal mammary lymph nodes (Urban type operation)
→ *CPT Assistant* Feb 07:4, Sep 08:5; *CPT Changes: An Insider's View* 2007

(For immediate or delayed insertion of implant, see 19340, 19342)

19307   Mastectomy, modified radical, including axillary lymph nodes, with or without pectoralis minor muscle, but excluding pectoralis major muscle
→ *CPT Assistant* Feb 07:4, Sep 08:5; *CPT Changes: An Insider's View* 2007

(For immediate or delayed insertion of implant, see 19340, 19342)

Repair and/or Reconstruction

(To report bilateral procedure, report modifier 50 with the procedure code)

(For biologic implant for soft tissue reinforcement, use 15777 in conjunction with primary procedure)

19316   Mastopexy
→ *CPT Assistant* Jan 03:7, Apr 05:6, Feb 12:11

19318   Reduction mammaplasty
→ *CPT Assistant* Jan 03:7, Apr 05:6

19324   Mammaplasty, augmentation; without prosthetic implant
→ *CPT Assistant* Apr 05:6

19325   with prosthetic implant
→ *CPT Assistant* Apr 05:6

(For flap or graft, use also appropriate number)

19328   Removal of intact mammary implant
→ *CPT Assistant* Apr 05:6

19330   Removal of mammary implant material
→ *CPT Assistant* Nov 01:11, Apr 05:6

19340   Immediate insertion of breast prosthesis following mastopexy, mastectomy or in reconstruction
→ *CPT Assistant* Aug 96:8, Apr 05:6, Aug 05:1, Mar 10:9

Integumentary

19342   Delayed insertion of breast prosthesis following mastopexy, mastectomy or in reconstruction
→ *CPT Assistant* Aug 96:8, Apr 05:6, Aug 05:1

(For supply of implant, use 99070)

(For preparation of custom breast implant, use 19396)

19350   Nipple/areola reconstruction
→ *CPT Assistant* Aug 96:11, Apr 05:6

19355   Correction of inverted nipples
→ *CPT Assistant* Apr 05:6

19357   Breast reconstruction, immediate or delayed, with tissue expander, including subsequent expansion
→ *CPT Assistant* Winter 91:2, Apr 05:6, Aug 05:1, Mar 10:9

19361   Breast reconstruction with latissimus dorsi flap, without prosthetic implant
→ *CPT Assistant* Apr 05:6, Aug 05:1, Mar 10:9; *CPT Changes: An Insider's View* 2007

(For insertion of prosthesis, use also 19340)

19364   Breast reconstruction with free flap
→ *CPT Assistant* Aug 96:8, Nov 98:7, Apr 05:6, Aug 05:1, Jun 10:8, Dec 11:14, Jul 12:12

(Do not report code 69990 in addition to code 19364)

(19364 includes harvesting of the flap, microvascular transfer, closure of the donor site, and inset shaping the flap into a breast)

19366   Breast reconstruction with other technique
→ *CPT Assistant* Aug 96:8, Nov 98:7, Apr 05:6, Dec 11:14

(For operating microscope, use 69990)

(For insertion of prosthesis, use also 19340 or 19342)

19367   Breast reconstruction with transverse rectus abdominis myocutaneous flap (TRAM), single pedicle, including closure of donor site;
→ *CPT Assistant* Nov 98:7, Apr 05:6, Aug 05:1

19368   with microvascular anastomosis (supercharging)
→ *CPT Assistant* Nov 98:7, Apr 05:6, Aug 05:1

(Do not report code 69990 in addition to code 19368)

19369   Breast reconstruction with transverse rectus abdominis myocutaneous flap (TRAM), double pedicle, including closure of donor site
→ *CPT Assistant* Oct 00:3, Apr 05:6, Aug 05:1

19370   Open periprosthetic capsulotomy, breast
→ *CPT Assistant* Aug 96:8, Apr 05:6

19371   Periprosthetic capsulectomy, breast
→ *CPT Assistant* Aug 96:8, Nov 01:11, Apr 05:6

19380   Revision of reconstructed breast
→ *CPT Assistant* Apr 05:6

19396   Preparation of moulage for custom breast implant
→ *CPT Assistant* Jan 03:7, Apr 05:6

Other Procedures

19499   Unlisted procedure, breast
→ *CPT Assistant* Apr 05:6, Dec 09:9
→ *Clinical Examples in Radiology* Fall 08:4, Summer 09:15

Surgery

The following is a listing of headings and subheadings that appear within the Musculoskeletal System section of the CPT codebook. The subheadings or subsections denoted with asterisks (*) below have special instructions unique to that section. Where these are indicated, special "notes" or guidelines will be presented preceding those procedural terminology listings, referring to that subsection specifically.

Musculoskeletal

Thoracic Vertebra—Superior View

Lumbar Vertebra—Superior View

Lumbar Vertebrae—Lateral View

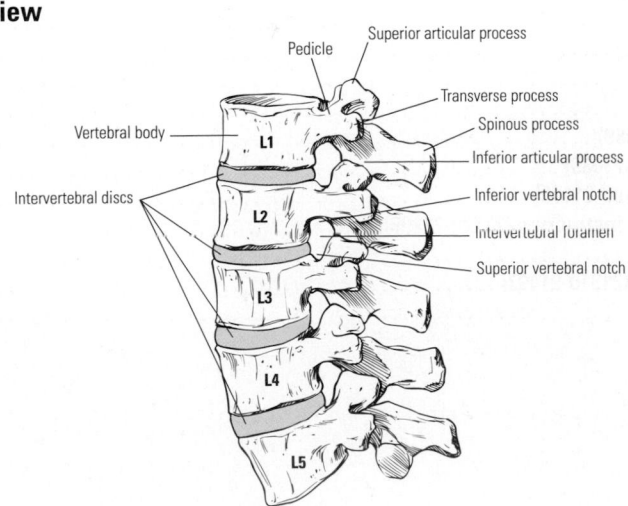

Musculoskeletal

Musculoskeletal

Musculoskeletal System

Cast and strapping procedures appear at the end of this section.

The services listed below include the application and removal of the first cast or traction device only. Subsequent replacement of cast and/or traction device may require an additional listing.

Definitions

The terms "closed treatment," "open treatment," and "percutaneous skeletal fixation" have been carefully chosen to accurately reflect current orthopaedic procedural treatments.

Closed treatment specifically means that the fracture site is not surgically opened (exposed to the external environment and directly visualized). This terminology is used to describe procedures that treat fractures by three methods: (1) without manipulation; (2) with manipulation; or (3) with or without traction.

Open treatment is used when the fractured bone is either: (1) surgically opened (exposed to the external environment) and the fracture (bone ends) visualized and internal fixation may be used; or (2) the fractured bone is opened remote from the fracture site in order to insert an intramedullary nail across the fracture site (the fracture site is not opened and visualized).

Percutaneous skeletal fixation describes fracture treatment which is neither open nor closed. In this procedure, the fracture fragments are not visualized, but fixation (eg, pins) is placed across the fracture site, usually under X-ray imaging.

The type of fracture (eg, open, compound, closed) does not have any coding correlation with the type of treatment (eg, closed, open, or percutaneous) provided.

The codes for treatment of fractures and joint injuries (dislocations) are categorized by the type of manipulation (reduction) and stabilization (fixation or immobilization). These codes can apply to either open (compound) or closed fractures or joint injuries.

Skeletal traction is the application of a force (distracting or traction force) to a limb segment through a wire, pin, screw, or clamp that is attached (eg, penetrates) to bone.

Skin traction is the application of a force (longitudinal) to a limb using felt or strapping applied directly to skin only.

External fixation is the usage of skeletal pins plus an attaching mechanism/device used for temporary or definitive treatment of acute or chronic bony deformity.

Codes for obtaining autogenous bone grafts, cartilage, tendon, fascia lata grafts or other tissues through separate incisions are to be used only when the graft is not already listed as part of the basic procedure.

►Re-reduction of a fracture and/or dislocation performed by the primary physician or other qualified health care professional may be identified by the addition of modifier 76 to the usual procedure number to indicate "Repeat Procedure or Service by Same Physician or Other Qualified Health Care Professional." (See Appendix A guidelines.)◄

Codes for external fixation are to be used only when external fixation is not already listed as part of the basic procedure.

All codes for suction irrigation have been deleted. To report, list only the primary surgical procedure performed (eg, sequestrectomy, deep incision).

Manipulation is used throughout the musculoskeletal fracture and dislocation subsections to specifically mean the attempted reduction or restoration of a fracture or joint dislocation to its normal anatomic alignment by the application of manually applied forces.

Excision of subcutaneous soft tissue tumors (including simple or intermediate repair) involves the simple or marginal resection of tumors confined to subcutaneous tissue below the skin but above the deep fascia. These tumors are usually benign and are resected without removing a significant amount of surrounding normal tissue. Code selection is based on the location and size of the tumor. Code selection is determined by measuring the greatest diameter of the tumor plus that margin required for complete excision of the tumor. The margins refer to the most narrow margin required to adequately excise the tumor, based on the physician's judgment. The measurement of the tumor plus margin is made at the time of the excision. Appreciable vessel exploration and/or neuroplasty should be reported separately. Extensive undermining or other techniques to close a defect created by skin excision may require a complex repair which should be reported separately. Dissection or elevation of tissue planes to permit resection of the tumor is included in the excision.

►***Excision of fascial or subfascial soft tissue tumors*** (including simple or intermediate repair) involves the resection of tumors confined to the tissue within or below the deep fascia, but not involving the bone. These tumors are usually benign, are often intramuscular, and are resected without removing a significant amount of surrounding normal tissue. Code selection is based on size and location of the tumor. Code selection is determined by measuring the greatest diameter of the tumor plus that margin required for complete excision of the tumor. The margins refer to the most narrow margin required to adequately excise the tumor, based on individual judgment. The measurement of the tumor plus margin is made at the time of the excision. Appreciable vessel exploration and/or neuroplasty should be reported separately. Extensive undermining or other techniques to close a defect created by skin excision may require a complex repair which should be reported separately. Dissection or elevation of tissue planes to permit resection of the tumor is included in the excision.◄

Digital (ie, fingers and toes) subfascial tumors are defined as those tumors involving the tendons, tendon sheaths, or joints of the digit. Tumors which simply abut but do not breach the tendon, tendon sheath, or joint capsule are considered subcutaneous soft tissue tumors.

▶*Radical resection of soft tissue tumors* (including simple or intermediate repair) involves the resection of the tumor with wide margins of normal tissue. Appreciable vessel exploration and/or neuroplasty repair or reconstruction (eg, adjacent tissue transfer[s], flap[s]) should be reported separately. Extensive undermining or other techniques to close a defect created by skin excision may require a complex repair which should be reported separately. Dissection or elevation of tissue planes to permit resection of the tumor is included in the excision. Although these tumors may be confined to a specific layer (eg, subcutaneous, subfascial), radical resection may involve removal of tissue from one or more layers. Radical resection of soft tissue tumors is most commonly used for malignant tumors or very aggressive benign tumors. Code selection is based on size and location of the tumor. Code selection is determined by measuring the greatest diameter of the tumor plus that margin required for complete excision of the tumor. The margins refer to the most narrow margin required to adequately excise the tumor, based on individual judgment. The measurement of the tumor plus margin is made at the time of the excision. For radical resection of tumors of cutaneous origin (eg, melanoma), see 11600-11646.◀

Radical resection of bone tumors (including simple or intermediate repair) involves the resection of the tumor with wide margins of normal tissue. Appreciable vessel exploration and/or neuroplasty and complex bone repair or reconstruction (eg, adjacent tissue transfer[s], flap[s]) should be reported separately. Extensive undermining or other techniques to close a defect created by skin excision may require a complex repair which should be reported separately. Dissection or elevation of tissue planes to permit resection of the tumor is included in the excision. It may require removal of the entire bone if tumor growth is extensive (eg, clavicle). Radical resection of bone tumors is usually performed for malignant tumors or very aggressive benign tumors. If surrounding soft tissue is removed during these procedures, the radical resection of soft tissue tumor codes should not be reported separately. Code selection is based solely on the location of the tumor, **not** on the size of the tumor or whether the tumor is benign or malignant, primary or metastatic.

General

Incision

(20000 has been deleted)

(For incision and drainage procedures, cutaneous/subcutaneous, see 10060, 10061)

20005 Incision and drainage of soft tissue abscess, subfascial (ie, involves the soft tissue below the deep fascia)
↪ *CPT Changes: An Insider's View* 2011

Wound Exploration—Trauma (eg, Penetrating Gunshot, Stab Wound)

20100-20103 relate to wound(s) resulting from penetrating trauma. These codes describe surgical exploration and enlargement of the wound, extension of dissection (to determine penetration), debridement, removal of foreign body(s), ligation or coagulation of minor subcutaneous and/or muscular blood vessel(s), of the subcutaneous tissue, muscle fascia, and/or muscle, not requiring thoracotomy or laparotomy. If a repair is done to major structure(s) or major blood vessel(s) requiring thoracotomy or laparotomy, then those specific code(s) would supersede the use of codes 20100-20103. To report simple, intermediate, or complex repair of wound(s) that do not require enlargement of the wound, extension of dissection, etc, as stated above, use specific Repair code(s) in the **Integumentary System** section.

20100 Exploration of penetrating wound (separate procedure); neck
↪ *CPT Assistant* Jun 96:7, Aug 96:10, Sep 06:13

20101 chest
↪ *CPT Assistant* Jun 96:7, Sep 06:13

20102 abdomen/flank/back
↪ *CPT Assistant* Jun 96:7, Sep 06:13

20103 extremity
↪ *CPT Assistant* Jun 96:7, Aug 96:10, Sep 06:13

Excision

20150 Excision of epiphyseal bar, with or without autogenous soft tissue graft obtained through same fascial incision

(For aspiration of bone marrow, use 38220)

20200 Biopsy, muscle; superficial

20205 deep

20206 Biopsy, muscle, percutaneous needle
↪ *Clinical Examples in Radiology* Summer 08:5, Fall 10:7

(If imaging guidance is performed, see 76942, 77012, 77021)

(For fine needle aspiration, use 10021 or 10022)

(For evaluation of fine needle aspirate, see 88172-88173)

(For excision of muscle tumor, deep, see specific anatomic section)

20220 Biopsy, bone, trocar, or needle; superficial (eg, ilium, sternum, spinous process, ribs)
↪ *CPT Assistant* Winter 92:17, Jul 98:4
↪ *Clinical Examples in Radiology* Summer 08:5, Fall 10:7

20225 deep (eg, vertebral body, femur)
↪ *CPT Assistant* Winter 92:17, Jul 98:4, Jun 12:10; *CPT Changes: An Insider's View* 2002
↪ *Clinical Examples in Radiology* Fall 10:8

(For bone marrow biopsy, use 38221)

(For radiologic supervision and interpretation, see 77002, 77012, 77021)

Musculoskeletal

20240 Biopsy, bone, open; superficial (eg, ilium, sternum, spinous process, ribs, trochanter of femur)
➲ *CPT Assistant* Winter 92:17, Jul 98:4, Aug 04:11, Aug 05:13; *CPT Changes: An Insider's View* 2004

20245 deep (eg, humerus, ischium, femur)
➲ *CPT Assistant* Winter 92:17, Jul 98:4

20250 Biopsy, vertebral body, open; thoracic
➲ *CPT Assistant* Winter 92:17, Jul 98:4

20251 lumbar or cervical
➲ *CPT Assistant* Winter 92:17, Jul 98:4

(For sequestrectomy, osteomyelitis or drainage of bone abscess, see anatomical area)

Introduction or Removal

(For injection procedure for arthrography, see anatomical area)

20500 Injection of sinus tract; therapeutic (separate procedure)

20501 diagnostic (sinogram)

(For radiological supervision and interpretation, use 76080)

(For contrast injection[s] and radiological assessment of gastrostomy, duodenostomy, jejunostomy, gastro-jejunostomy, or cecostomy [or other colonic] tube including fluoroscopic imaging guidance, use 49465)

20520 Removal of foreign body in muscle or tendon sheath; simple

20525 deep or complicated

20526 Injection, therapeutic (eg, local anesthetic, corticosteroid), carpal tunnel
➲ *CPT Assistant* Mar 02:7; *CPT Changes: An Insider's View* 2002

20527 Injection, enzyme (eg, collagenase), palmar fascial cord (ie, Dupuytren's contracture)
➲ *CPT Assistant* Jul 12:8, 14; *CPT Changes: An Insider's View* 2012

(For manipulation of palmar fascial cord (ie, Dupuytren's cord) post enzyme injection (eg, collagenase), use 26341)

20550 Injection(s); single tendon sheath, or ligament, aponeurosis (eg, plantar "fascia")
➲ *CPT Assistant* Jan 96:7, Jun 98:10, Mar 02:7, Aug 03:14, Sep 03:13, Dec 03:11, Jan 09:6, Jul 12:14; *CPT Changes: An Insider's View* 2002, 2003, 2004
➲ *Clinical Examples in Radiology* Winter 10:14

(For injection of Morton's neuroma, see 64455, 64632)

20551 single tendon origin/insertion
➲ *CPT Assistant* Mar 02:7, Sep 03:13; *CPT Changes: An Insider's View* 2002, 2004
➲ *Clinical Examples in Radiology* Fall 10:10, Winter 10:14

(Do not report 20550, 20551 in conjunction with 0232T)

(For injection(s) of platelet rich plasma, use 0232T)

20552 Injection(s); single or multiple trigger point(s), 1 or 2 muscle(s)
➲ *CPT Assistant* Mar 02:7, May 03:19, Sep 03:11, Feb 10:9, Feb 11:5, Jul 11:16, Apr 12:19; *CPT Changes: An Insider's View* 2002, 2003, 2004
➲ *Clinical Examples in Radiology* Winter 10:14, Fall 11:10

20553 single or multiple trigger point(s), 3 or more muscle(s)
➲ *CPT Assistant* Mar 02:7, May 03:19, Sep 03:11, Jun 08:8, Feb 10:9, Feb 11:5, Jul 11:16; *CPT Changes: An Insider's View* 2002, 2003
➲ *Clinical Examples in Radiology* Winter 10:14

(If imaging guidance is performed, see 76942, 77002, 77021)

Trigger Point Injection
20552, 20553

Insertion of needle into muscle trigger point for injection of therapeutic agent

Injection site

Cross section through the body wall at level of lumbar vertebra

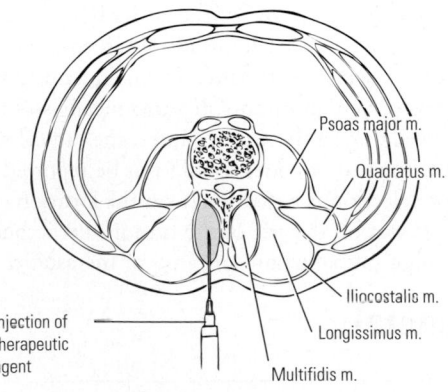

Psoas major m.

Quadratus m.

Iliocostalis m.

Longissimus m.

Injection of therapeutic agent

Multifidis m.

20555 Placement of needles or catheters into muscle and/or soft tissue for subsequent interstitial radioelement application (at the time of or subsequent to the procedure)
➲ *CPT Assistant* Feb 08:8; *CPT Changes: An Insider's View* 2008

(For placement of devices into the breast for interstitial radioelement application, see 19296-19298)

(For placement of needles, catheters, or devices into muscle or soft tissue of the head and neck, for interstitial radioelement application, use 41019)

(For placement of needles or catheters for interstitial radioelement application into prostate, use 55875)

(For placement of needles or catheters into the pelvic organs or genitalia [except prostate] for interstitial radioelement application, use 55920)

(For interstitial radioelement application, see 77776-77778, 77785-77787)

(For imaging guidance, see 76942, 77002, 77012, 77021)

20600   Arthrocentesis, aspiration and/or injection; small joint or bursa (eg, fingers, toes)
➔ *CPT Assistant* Dec 07:10; *CPT Changes: An Insider's View* 2003

20605   intermediate joint or bursa (eg, temporomandibular, acromioclavicular, wrist, elbow or ankle, olecranon bursa)
➔ *CPT Assistant* Dec 07:10; *CPT Changes: An Insider's View* 2003

20610   major joint or bursa (eg, shoulder, hip, knee joint, subacromial bursa)
➔ *CPT Assistant* Spring 92:8, Mar 01:10, Apr 04:15, Jul 06:1, Dec 07:10, Jul 08:9, Mar 12:6, Jun 12:14

(If imaging guidance is performed, see 76942, 77002, 77012, 77021)

Arthrocentesis, Aspiration, or Injection of Major Joint or Bursa
20610

Insertion of needle into major joint or bursa for injection of therapeutic or diagnostic agent, aspiration, or arthrocentesis

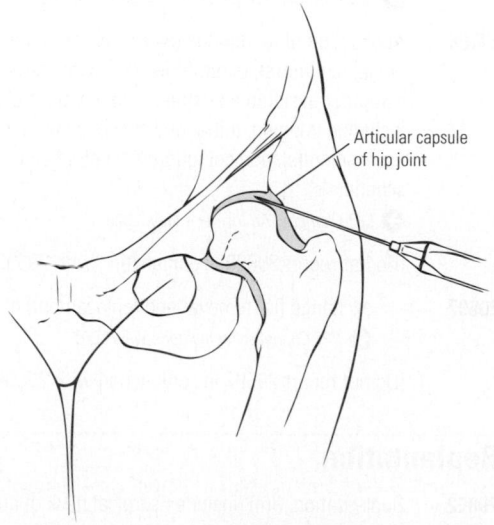

Articular capsule of hip joint

20612   Aspiration and/or injection of ganglion cyst(s) any location
➔ *CPT Changes: An Insider's View* 2003

(To report multiple ganglion cyst aspirations/injections, use 20612 and append modifier 59)

20615   Aspiration and injection for treatment of bone cyst

20650   Insertion of wire or pin with application of skeletal traction, including removal (separate procedure)

20660   Application of cranial tongs, caliper, or stereotactic frame, including removal (separate procedure)
➔ *CPT Assistant* Jun 96:10, Nov 97:14, Jan 06:46, Dec 06:10, Feb 08:8, Jul 08:10, Nov 09:6, Apr 12:11; *CPT Changes: An Insider's View* 2008

20661   Application of halo, including removal; cranial
➔ *CPT Assistant* Nov 97:14

20662   pelvic

20663   femoral

20664   Application of halo, including removal, cranial, 6 or more pins placed, for thin skull osteology (eg, pediatric patients, hydrocephalus, osteogenesis imperfecta)
➔ *CPT Assistant* Nov 97:14; *CPT Changes: An Insider's View* 2011

Halo Application for Thin Skull Osteology
20664

A cranial halo is placed on the head of a child whose skull is unusually thin due to congenital or developmental problems.

▲ **20665**   Removal of tongs or halo applied by another individual
➔ *CPT Assistant* Apr 12:12; *CPT Changes: An Insider's View* 2013

▲ =Revised code   ●=New code   ▶ ◀=Contains new or revised text   ⊘ =Modifier 51 exempt

Musculoskeletal

20670 Removal of implant; superficial (eg, buried wire, pin or rod) (separate procedure)

> *CPT Assistant* Dec 07:7, 8, Jun 09:7, Apr 12:17

20680 deep (eg, buried wire, pin, screw, metal band, nail, rod or plate)

> *CPT Assistant* Spring 92:11, Jun 09:7

20690 Application of a uniplane (pins or wires in 1 plane), unilateral, external fixation system

> *CPT Assistant* Winter 90:4, Winter 92:11, Fall 93:21, Oct 99:5, Jan 04:27, Jun 05:12, Oct 07:7, Jan 08:4, Feb 08:9, Jun 09:7; *CPT Changes: An Insider's View* 2008

Uniplane External Fixation System
20690

The following figures are examples of types of stabilization devices. Codes 20690 and 20692 describe the placement of types of external fixation devices. The method of stabilization depends upon fracture grade (degree of soft tissue injury/skin integrity disruption), type (eg, comminuted, spiral, impacted), and location (eg, extremity, pelvis).

Fracture

External fixation system

External fixation system

20692 Application of a multiplane (pins or wires in more than 1 plane), unilateral, external fixation system (eg, Ilizarov, Monticelli type)

> *CPT Assistant* Winter 90:4, Fall 93:21, Oct 99:5, Jul 00:11, Feb 08:9, Jun 09:7; *CPT Changes: An Insider's View* 2008

Multiplane External Fixation System
20692

The following figure is an example of a type of multiplane stabilization device. Codes 20690 and 20692 describe the placement of types of external fixation devices. The method of stabilization depends upon fracture grade (degree of soft tissue injury/skin integrity disruption), type (eg, comminuted, spiral, impacted), and location (eg, extremity, pelvis).

Defect

External fixation system

20693 Adjustment or revision of external fixation system requiring anesthesia (eg, new pin[s] or wire[s] and/or new ring[s] or bar[s])

> *CPT Assistant* Fall 93:21, Oct 99:5, Jul 00:11, Jun 09:7

20694 Removal, under anesthesia, of external fixation system

> *CPT Assistant* Winter 92:10, Fall 93:21, Oct 99:5, Jul 00:11

20696 Application of multiplane (pins or wires in more than 1 plane), unilateral, external fixation with stereotactic computer-assisted adjustment (eg, spatial frame), including imaging; initial and subsequent alignment(s), assessment(s), and computation(s) of adjustment schedule(s)

> *CPT Changes: An Insider's View* 2009

(Do not report 20696 in conjunction with 20692, 20697)

⊘ **20697** exchange (ie, removal and replacement) of strut, each

> *CPT Changes: An Insider's View* 2009

(Do not report 20697 in conjunction with 20692, 20696)

Replantation

20802 Replantation, arm (includes surgical neck of humerus through elbow joint), complete amputation

(To report replantation of incomplete arm amputation, see specific code[s] for repair of bone[s], ligament[s], tendon[s], nerve[s], or blood vessel[s] with modifier 52)

20805   Replantation, forearm (includes radius and ulna to radial carpal joint), complete amputation

(To report replantation of incomplete forearm amputation, see specific code[s] for repair of bone[s], ligament[s], tendon[s], nerve[s], or blood vessel[s] with modifier 52)

20808   Replantation, hand (includes hand through metacarpophalangeal joints), complete amputation

(To report replantation of incomplete hand amputation, see specific code[s] for repair of bone[s], ligament[s], tendon[s], nerve[s], or blood vessel[s] with modifier 52)

20816   Replantation, digit, excluding thumb (includes metacarpophalangeal joint to insertion of flexor sublimis tendon), complete amputation

➔ *CPT Assistant* Oct 96:11

(To report replantation of incomplete digit amputation, excluding thumb, see specific code[s] for repair of bone[s], ligament[s], tendon[s], nerve[s], or blood vessel[s] with modifier 52)

20822   Replantation, digit, excluding thumb (includes distal tip to sublimis tendon insertion), complete amputation

(To report replantation of incomplete digit amputation, excluding thumb, see specific code[s] for repair of bone[s], ligament[s], tendon[s], nerve[s], or blood vessel[s] with modifier 52)

20824   Replantation, thumb (includes carpometacarpal joint to MP joint), complete amputation

(To report replantation of incomplete thumb amputation, see specific code[s] for repair of bone[s], ligament[s], tendon[s], nerve[s], or blood vessel[s] with modifier 52)

20827   Replantation, thumb (includes distal tip to MP joint), complete amputation

(To report replantation of incomplete thumb amputation, see specific code[s] for repair of bone[s], ligament[s], tendon[s], nerve[s], or blood vessel[s] with modifier 52)

(To report replantation of complete leg amputation, see specific code[s] for repair of bone[s], ligament[s], tendon[s], nerve[s], or blood vessel[s] with modifier 52)

(To report replantation of incomplete leg amputation, see specific code[s] for repair of bone[s], ligament[s], tendon[s], nerve[s], or blood vessel[s] with modifier 52)

20838   Replantation, foot, complete amputation

(To report replantation of incomplete foot amputation, see specific code[s] for repair of bone[s], ligament[s], tendon[s], nerve[s], or blood vessel[s] with modifier 52)

Grafts (or Implants)

Codes for obtaining autogenous bone, cartilage, tendon, fascia lata grafts, or other tissues through separate skin/fascial incisions should be reported separately unless the code descriptor references the harvesting of the graft or implant (eg, includes obtaining graft).

Do not append modifier 62 to bone graft codes 20900-20938.

(For spinal surgery bone graft[s] see codes 20930-20938)

20900   Bone graft, any donor area; minor or small (eg, dowel or button)

➔ *CPT Assistant* Dec 00:15, Jul 11:18; *CPT Changes: An Insider's View* 2008

20902   major or large

➔ *CPT Assistant* Dec 00:15, Jul 11:18; *CPT Changes: An Insider's View* 2008

20910   Cartilage graft; costochondral

➔ *CPT Changes: An Insider's View* 2008

20912   nasal septum

➔ *CPT Changes: An Insider's View* 2008

(For ear cartilage, use 21235)

20920   Fascia lata graft; by stripper

➔ *CPT Assistant* Aug 99:5, Jan 05:8; *CPT Changes: An Insider's View* 2008

20922   by incision and area exposure, complex or sheet

➔ *CPT Assistant* Jan 05:8; *CPT Changes: An Insider's View* 2008

20924   Tendon graft, from a distance (eg, palmaris, toe extensor, plantaris)

➔ *CPT Changes: An Insider's View* 2008

20926   Tissue grafts, other (eg, paratenon, fat, dermis)

➔ *CPT Assistant* Summer 91:12, Aug 99:5, Nov 99:10, May 06:16, Jun 12:15; *CPT Changes: An Insider's View* 2008

(For injection(s) of platelet rich plasma, use 0232T)

+ 20930   Allograft, morselized, or placement of osteopromotive material, for spine surgery only (List separately in addition to code for primary procedure)

➔ *CPT Assistant* Feb 96:6, Mar 96:4, Sep 97:8, Nov 99:10, Feb 02:6, Jan 04:27, Dec 07:1, Feb 08:8, Nov 10:8, Jul 11:18, Dec 11:15, Apr 12:14, Jun 12:11; *CPT Changes: An Insider's View* 2008, 2011

▶(Use 20930 in conjunction with 22319, 22532, 22533, 22548-22558, 22590-22612, 22630, 22633, 22634, 22800-22812, 0195T, 0196T)◀

+ 20931   Allograft, structural, for spine surgery only (List separately in addition to code for primary procedure)

➔ *CPT Assistant* Feb 96:6, Feb 02:6, Feb 05:15, Feb 08:8, Nov 10:8, Jul 11:18, Sep 11:12, Dec 11:15, Apr 12:14, Jun 12:11; *CPT Changes: An Insider's View* 2008, 2011

▶(Use 20931 in conjunction with 22319, 22532-22533, 22548-22558, 22590-22612, 22630, 22633, 22634, 22800-22812)◀

+ 20936   Autograft for spine surgery only (includes harvesting the graft); local (eg, ribs, spinous process, or laminar fragments) obtained from same incision (List separately in addition to code for primary procedure)

➔ *CPT Assistant* Feb 96:6, Sep 97:8, Feb 02:6, Feb 08:8, Dec 11:15, Apr 12:14, Jun 12:11; *CPT Changes: An Insider's View* 2008

▶(Use 20936 in conjunction with 22319, 22532, 22533, 22548-22558, 22590-22612, 22630, 22633, 22634, 22800-22812, 0195T, 0196T)◀

+ 20937 morselized (through separate skin or fascial incision) (List separately in addition to code for primary procedure)

➔ *CPT Assistant* Feb 96:6, Sep 97:8, Dec 99:2, Feb 02:6, Feb 08:8, Dec 11:15, Apr 12:11, Jun 12:11; *CPT Changes: An Insider's View* 2008

▶(Use 20937 in conjunction with 22319, 22532, 22533, 22548-22558, 22590-22612, 22630, 22633, 22634, 22800-22812, 0195T, 0196T)◀

+ 20938 structural, bicortical or tricortical (through separate skin or fascial incision) (List separately in addition to code for primary procedure)

➔ *CPT Assistant* Feb 96:6, Mar 96:5, Sep 97:8, Feb 02:6, Feb 08:8, Jul 11:18, Dec 11:15, Apr 12:12, Apr 12:11, May 12:11, Jun 12:11; *CPT Changes: An Insider's View* 2008

▶(Use 20938 in conjunction with 22319, 22532, 22533, 22548-22558, 22590-22612, 22630, 22633, 22634, 22800-22812)◀

▶(For needle aspiration of bone marrow for the purpose of bone grafting, use 38220. Do not report 38220-38230 for bone marrow aspiration for platelet rich stem cell injection. For bone marrow aspiration for platelet rich stem cell injection, use 0232T)◀

Other Procedures

20950 Monitoring of interstitial fluid pressure (includes insertion of device, eg, wick catheter technique, needle manometer technique) in detection of muscle compartment syndrome

➔ *CPT Assistant* Sep 07:10

20955 Bone graft with microvascular anastomosis; fibula

➔ *CPT Assistant* Apr 97:4

20956 iliac crest

➔ *CPT Assistant* Apr 97:4

20957 metatarsal

➔ *CPT Assistant* Apr 97:4

20962 other than fibula, iliac crest, or metatarsal

➔ *CPT Assistant* Apr 97:4

(Do not report code 69990 in addition to codes 20955-20962)

20969 Free osteocutaneous flap with microvascular anastomosis; other than iliac crest, metatarsal, or great toe

➔ *CPT Assistant* Apr 97:4

20970 iliac crest

➔ *CPT Assistant* Apr 97:4

20972 metatarsal

➔ *CPT Assistant* Apr 97:4

20973 great toe with web space

➔ *CPT Assistant* Apr 97:4

(Do not report code 69990 in addition to codes 20969-20973)

(For great toe, wrap-around procedure, use 26551)

⊘ **20974** Electrical stimulation to aid bone healing; noninvasive (nonoperative)

➔ *CPT Assistant* Sep 96:11, Nov 00:8

⊘ **20975** invasive (operative)

➔ *CPT Assistant* Nov 00:8

20979 Low intensity ultrasound stimulation to aid bone healing, noninvasive (nonoperative)

➔ *CPT Assistant* Nov 99:10, Nov 00:8; *CPT Changes: An Insider's View* 2000

⊙ **20982** Ablation, bone tumor(s) (eg, osteoid osteoma, metastasis) radiofrequency, percutaneous, including computed tomographic guidance

➔ *CPT Changes: An Insider's View* 2004

(Do not report 20982 in conjunction with 77013)

+ 20985 Computer-assisted surgical navigational procedure for musculoskeletal procedures, image-less (List separately in addition to code for primary procedure)

➔ *CPT Assistant* Jul 11:12; *CPT Changes: An Insider's View* 2008, 2009

(Do not report 20985 in conjunction with 61781-61783)

(20986, 20987 have been deleted)

(For computer-assisted navigational procedures with image guidance based on pre-operative and intraoperatively obtained images, see 0054T, 0055T)

20999 Unlisted procedure, musculoskeletal system, general

➔ *CPT Assistant* Sep 03:13

Head

Skull, facial bones, and temporomandibular joint.

Incision

(For incision and drainage of superficial abscess and hematoma, see 10060, 10061)

(For incision and drainage of soft tissue abscess, use 20005)

(For removal of embedded foreign body from dentoalveolar structure, see 41805, 41806)

21010 Arthrotomy, temporomandibular joint

(To report bilateral procedure, report 21010 with modifier 50)

Excision

21011 Excision, tumor, soft tissue of face or scalp, subcutaneous; less than 2 cm

➔ *CPT Assistant* Feb 10:3, Apr 10:3; *CPT Changes: An Insider's View* 2010

Musculoskeletal

21012　　2 cm or greater

➔ *CPT Assistant* Feb 10:3, Apr 10:3; *CPT Changes: An Insider's View* 2010

21013　Excision, tumor, soft tissue of face and scalp, subfascial (eg, subgaleal, intramuscular); less than 2 cm

➔ *CPT Assistant* Feb 10:3, Apr 10:3; *CPT Changes: An Insider's View* 2010

21014　　2 cm or greater

➔ *CPT Assistant* Feb 10:3, Apr 10:3; *CPT Changes: An Insider's View* 2010

21015　Radical resection of tumor (eg, malignant neoplasm), soft tissue of face or scalp; less than 2 cm

➔ *CPT Assistant* Feb 10:3, Apr 10:3; *CPT Changes: An Insider's View* 2010

(To report excision of skull tumor for osteomyelitis, use 61501)

21016　　2 cm or greater

➔ *CPT Assistant* Feb 10:3, Apr 10:3; *CPT Changes: An Insider's View* 2010

21025　Excision of bone (eg, for osteomyelitis or bone abscess); mandible

➔ *CPT Assistant* Oct 11:10

21026　　facial bone(s)

21029　Removal by contouring of benign tumor of facial bone (eg, fibrous dysplasia)

21030　Excision of benign tumor or cyst of maxilla or zygoma by enucleation and curettage

➔ *CPT Assistant* Nov 03:9; *CPT Changes: An Insider's View* 2003

21031　Excision of torus mandibularis

21032　Excision of maxillary torus palatinus

21034　Excision of malignant tumor of maxilla or zygoma

➔ *CPT Assistant* Nov 03:9; *CPT Changes: An Insider's View* 2003

21040　Excision of benign tumor or cyst of mandible, by enucleation and/or curettage

➔ *CPT Assistant* Nov 03:9; *CPT Changes: An Insider's View* 2003

(For enucleation and/or curettage of benign cysts or tumors of mandible not requiring osteotomy, use 21040)

(For excision of benign tumor or cyst of mandible requiring osteotomy, see 21046-21047)

21044　Excision of malignant tumor of mandible;

21045　　radical resection

(For bone graft, use 21215)

21046　Excision of benign tumor or cyst of mandible; requiring intra-oral osteotomy (eg, locally aggressive or destructive lesion[s])

➔ *CPT Assistant* Nov 03:9; *CPT Changes: An Insider's View* 2003

21047　　requiring extra-oral osteotomy and partial mandibulectomy (eg, locally aggressive or destructive lesion[s])

➔ *CPT Assistant* Nov 03:9; *CPT Changes: An Insider's View* 2003

21048　Excision of benign tumor or cyst of maxilla; requiring intra-oral osteotomy (eg, locally aggressive or destructive lesion[s])

➔ *CPT Assistant* Nov 03:9; *CPT Changes: An Insider's View* 2003

21049　　requiring extra-oral osteotomy and partial maxillectomy (eg, locally aggressive or destructive lesion[s])

➔ *CPT Assistant* Nov 03:9; *CPT Changes: An Insider's View* 2003

21050　Condylectomy, temporomandibular joint (separate procedure)

(For bilateral procedures, report 21050 with modifier 50)

21060　Meniscectomy, partial or complete, temporomandibular joint (separate procedure)

(For bilateral procedures, report 21060 with modifier 50)

21070　Coronoidectomy (separate procedure)

(For bilateral procedures, report 21070 with modifier 50)

Manipulation

21073　Manipulation of temporomandibular joint(s) (TMJ), therapeutic, requiring an anesthesia service (ie, general or monitored anesthesia care)

➔ *CPT Assistant* Feb 08.9; *CPT Changes: An Insider's View* 2008

(For TMJ manipulation without an anesthesia service [ie, general or monitored anesthesia care], see 97140, 98925-98929, 98943)

(For closed treatment of temporomandibular dislocation, see 21480, 21485)

Head Prosthesis

▶Codes 21076-21089 describe professional services for the rehabilitation of patients with oral, facial, or other anatomical deficiencies by means of prostheses such as an artificial eye, ear, or nose or intraoral obturator to close a cleft. Codes 21076-21089 should only be used when the physician or other qualified health care professional actually designs and prepares the prosthesis (ie, not prepared by an outside laboratory).◀

(For application or removal of caliper or tongs, see 20660, 20665)

21076　Impression and custom preparation; surgical obturator prosthesis

21077　　orbital prosthesis

21079　　interim obturator prosthesis

➔ *CPT Assistant* Winter 90:5, Sep 06:13, Dec 06:10

21080　　definitive obturator prosthesis

➔ *CPT Assistant* Winter 90:5, Sep 06:13, Dec 06:10

21081　　mandibular resection prosthesis

➔ *CPT Assistant* Winter 90:5, Sep 06:13, Dec 06:10

21082　　palatal augmentation prosthesis

➔ *CPT Assistant* Winter 90:5, Sep 06:13, Dec 06:10

Musculoskeletal

21083 palatal lift prosthesis
➜ *CPT Assistant* Winter 90:5, Sep 06:13, Dec 06:10

21084 speech aid prosthesis
➜ *CPT Assistant* Winter 90:5, Sep 06:13, Dec 06:10

21085 oral surgical splint
➜ *CPT Assistant* Winter 90:5, Sep 06:13, Dec 06:10

21086 auricular prosthesis
➜ *CPT Assistant* Winter 90:5, Sep 06:13, Dec 06:10

21087 nasal prosthesis
➜ *CPT Assistant* Winter 90:5, Sep 06:13, Dec 06:10

21088 facial prosthesis
➜ *CPT Assistant* Winter 90:5, Sep 06:13, Dec 06:10

Other Procedures

21089 Unlisted maxillofacial prosthetic procedure
➜ *CPT Assistant* Winter 90:5, Sep 06:13, Dec 06:10

Introduction or Removal

21100 Application of halo type appliance for maxillofacial fixation, includes removal (separate procedure)

21110 Application of interdental fixation device for conditions other than fracture or dislocation, includes removal
➜ *CPT Assistant* Mar 97:10

►(For removal of interdental fixation by another individual, see 20670-20680)◄

21116 Injection procedure for temporomandibular joint arthrography

(For radiological supervision and interpretation, use 70332. Do not report 77002 in conjunction with 70332)

Repair, Revision, and/or Reconstruction

(For cranioplasty, see 21179, 21180 and 62116, 62120, 62140-62147)

21120 Genioplasty; augmentation (autograft, allograft, prosthetic material)

21121 sliding osteotomy, single piece

21122 sliding osteotomies, 2 or more osteotomies (eg, wedge excision or bone wedge reversal for asymmetrical chin)

21123 sliding, augmentation with interpositional bone grafts (includes obtaining autografts)

21125 Augmentation, mandibular body or angle; prosthetic material

21127 with bone graft, onlay or interpositional (includes obtaining autograft)

21137 Reduction forehead; contouring only

21138 contouring and application of prosthetic material or bone graft (includes obtaining autograft)

21139 contouring and setback of anterior frontal sinus wall

21141 Reconstruction midface, LeFort I; single piece, segment movement in any direction (eg, for Long Face Syndrome), without bone graft

21142 2 pieces, segment movement in any direction, without bone graft

21143 3 or more pieces, segment movement in any direction, without bone graft

21145 single piece, segment movement in any direction, requiring bone grafts (includes obtaining autografts)

21146 2 pieces, segment movement in any direction, requiring bone grafts (includes obtaining autografts) (eg, ungrafted unilateral alveolar cleft)

21147 3 or more pieces, segment movement in any direction, requiring bone grafts (includes obtaining autografts) (eg, ungrafted bilateral alveolar cleft or multiple osteotomies)

21150 Reconstruction midface, LeFort II; anterior intrusion (eg, Treacher-Collins Syndrome)

21151 any direction, requiring bone grafts (includes obtaining autografts)

21154 Reconstruction midface, LeFort III (extracranial), any type, requiring bone grafts (includes obtaining autografts); without LeFort I

21155 with LeFort I

21159 Reconstruction midface, LeFort III (extra and intracranial) with forehead advancement (eg, mono bloc), requiring bone grafts (includes obtaining autografts); without LeFort I

21160 with LeFort I

21172 Reconstruction superior-lateral orbital rim and lower forehead, advancement or alteration, with or without grafts (includes obtaining autografts)

(For frontal or parietal craniotomy performed for craniosynostosis, use 61556)

21175 Reconstruction, bifrontal, superior-lateral orbital rims and lower forehead, advancement or alteration (eg, plagiocephaly, trigonocephaly, brachycephaly), with or without grafts (includes obtaining autografts)

(For bifrontal craniotomy performed for craniosynostosis, use 61557)

21179 Reconstruction, entire or majority of forehead and/or supraorbital rims; with grafts (allograft or prosthetic material)

21180 with autograft (includes obtaining grafts)

(For extensive craniectomy for multiple suture craniosynostosis, use only 61558 or 61559)

21181 Reconstruction by contouring of benign tumor of cranial bones (eg, fibrous dysplasia), extracranial

Musculoskeletal

21182   Reconstruction of orbital walls, rims, forehead, nasoethmoid complex following intra- and extracranial excision of benign tumor of cranial bone (eg, fibrous dysplasia), with multiple autografts (includes obtaining grafts); total area of bone grafting less than 40 sq cm

21183   total area of bone grafting greater than 40 sq cm but less than 80 sq cm
> *CPT Changes: An Insider's View* 2002

21184   total area of bone grafting greater than 80 sq cm
> *CPT Changes: An Insider's View* 2002

(For excision of benign tumor of cranial bones, see 61563, 61564)

21188   Reconstruction midface, osteotomies (other than LeFort type) and bone grafts (includes obtaining autografts)

21193   Reconstruction of mandibular rami, horizontal, vertical, C, or L osteotomy; without bone graft
> *CPT Assistant* Apr 96:11

21194   with bone graft (includes obtaining graft)
> *CPT Assistant* Apr 96:11

21195   Reconstruction of mandibular rami and/or body, sagittal split; without internal rigid fixation
> *CPT Assistant* Apr 96:11

21196   with internal rigid fixation
> *CPT Assistant* Apr 96:11, Mar 97:11

Reconstruction of Mandibular Rami
21196

The mandibular ramus is reconstructed to lengthen, set back, or rotate the mandible.

Mandibular nerve

Rigid fixation screw

21198   Osteotomy, mandible, segmental;
> *CPT Changes: An Insider's View* 2001

21199   with genioglossus advancement
> *CPT Changes: An Insider's View* 2001

(To report total osteotomy of the maxilla, see 21141-21160)

21206   Osteotomy, maxilla, segmental (eg, Wassmund or Schuchard)

21208   Osteoplasty, facial bones; augmentation (autograft, allograft, or prosthetic implant)

21209   reduction

21210   Graft, bone; nasal, maxillary or malar areas (includes obtaining graft)

(For cleft palate repair, see 42200-42225)

21215   mandible (includes obtaining graft)

21230   Graft; rib cartilage, autogenous, to face, chin, nose or ear (includes obtaining graft)

21235   ear cartilage, autogenous, to nose or ear (includes obtaining graft)

(To report graft augmentation of facial bones, use 21208)

21240   Arthroplasty, temporomandibular joint, with or without autograft (includes obtaining graft)

21242   Arthroplasty, temporomandibular joint, with allograft

21243   Arthroplasty, temporomandibular joint, with prosthetic joint replacement

21244   Reconstruction of mandible, extraoral, with transosteal bone plate (eg, mandibular staple bone plate)

21245   Reconstruction of mandible or maxilla, subperiosteal implant; partial

21246   complete

21247   Reconstruction of mandibular condyle with bone and cartilage autografts (includes obtaining grafts) (eg, for hemifacial microsomia)

21248   Reconstruction of mandible or maxilla, endosteal implant (eg, blade, cylinder); partial

21249   complete

(To report midface reconstruction, see 21141-21160)

21255   Reconstruction of zygomatic arch and glenoid fossa with bone and cartilage (includes obtaining autografts)

21256   Reconstruction of orbit with osteotomies (extracranial) and with bone grafts (includes obtaining autografts) (eg, micro-ophthalmia)

21260   Periorbital osteotomies for orbital hypertelorism, with bone grafts; extracranial approach

21261   combined intra- and extracranial approach

21263   with forehead advancement

21267   Orbital repositioning, periorbital osteotomies, unilateral, with bone grafts; extracranial approach

21268   combined intra- and extracranial approach

21270   Malar augmentation, prosthetic material

(For malar augmentation with bone graft, use 21210)

21275   Secondary revision of orbitocraniofacial reconstruction

21280   Medial canthopexy (separate procedure)

(For medial canthoplasty, use 67950)

Musculoskeletal

21282	Lateral canthopexy
21295	Reduction of masseter muscle and bone (eg, for treatment of benign masseteric hypertrophy); extraoral approach
21296	intraoral approach

Other Procedures

21299	Unlisted craniofacial and maxillofacial procedure

Fracture and/or Dislocation

(For operative repair of skull fracture, see 62000-62010)

(To report closed treatment of skull fracture, use the appropriate Evaluation and Management code)

21310	Closed treatment of nasal bone fracture without manipulation
21315	Closed treatment of nasal bone fracture; without stabilization
21320	with stabilization
21325	Open treatment of nasal fracture; uncomplicated
21330	complicated, with internal and/or external skeletal fixation
21335	with concomitant open treatment of fractured septum
21336	Open treatment of nasal septal fracture, with or without stabilization
21337	Closed treatment of nasal septal fracture, with or without stabilization
21338	Open treatment of nasoethmoid fracture; without external fixation
21339	with external fixation
21340	Percutaneous treatment of nasoethmoid complex fracture, with splint, wire or headcap fixation, including repair of canthal ligaments and/or the nasolacrimal apparatus
21343	Open treatment of depressed frontal sinus fracture
21344	Open treatment of complicated (eg, comminuted or involving posterior wall) frontal sinus fracture, via coronal or multiple approaches
21345	Closed treatment of nasomaxillary complex fracture (LeFort II type), with interdental wire fixation or fixation of denture or splint
21346	Open treatment of nasomaxillary complex fracture (LeFort II type); with wiring and/or local fixation
21347	requiring multiple open approaches
21348	with bone grafting (includes obtaining graft)
21355	Percutaneous treatment of fracture of malar area, including zygomatic arch and malar tripod, with manipulation

21356	Open treatment of depressed zygomatic arch fracture (eg, Gillies approach)
21360	Open treatment of depressed malar fracture, including zygomatic arch and malar tripod
21365	Open treatment of complicated (eg, comminuted or involving cranial nerve foramina) fracture(s) of malar area, including zygomatic arch and malar tripod; with internal fixation and multiple surgical approaches
21366	with bone grafting (includes obtaining graft)
21385	Open treatment of orbital floor blowout fracture; transantral approach (Caldwell-Luc type operation)
21386	periorbital approach
21387	combined approach
21390	periorbital approach, with alloplastic or other implant
21395	periorbital approach with bone graft (includes obtaining graft)
21400	Closed treatment of fracture of orbit, except blowout; without manipulation
21401	with manipulation
21406	Open treatment of fracture of orbit, except blowout; without implant
21407	with implant
21408	with bone grafting (includes obtaining graft)
21421	Closed treatment of palatal or maxillary fracture (LeFort I type), with interdental wire fixation or fixation of denture or splint
21422	Open treatment of palatal or maxillary fracture (LeFort I type);
21423	complicated (comminuted or involving cranial nerve foramina), multiple approaches
21431	Closed treatment of craniofacial separation (LeFort III type) using interdental wire fixation of denture or splint
21432	Open treatment of craniofacial separation (LeFort III type); with wiring and/or internal fixation
21433	complicated (eg, comminuted or involving cranial nerve foramina), multiple surgical approaches
21435	complicated, utilizing internal and/or external fixation techniques (eg, head cap, halo device, and/or intermaxillary fixation)

(For removal of internal or external fixation device, use 20670)

21436	complicated, multiple surgical approaches, internal fixation, with bone grafting (includes obtaining graft)
21440	Closed treatment of mandibular or maxillary alveolar ridge fracture (separate procedure)
21445	Open treatment of mandibular or maxillary alveolar ridge fracture (separate procedure)
21450	Closed treatment of mandibular fracture; without manipulation

21451   with manipulation

21452   Percutaneous treatment of mandibular fracture, with external fixation

21453   Closed treatment of mandibular fracture with interdental fixation
➔ *CPT Assistant* Dec 07:7, 8

21454   Open treatment of mandibular fracture with external fixation

21461   Open treatment of mandibular fracture; without interdental fixation

21462   with interdental fixation

21465   Open treatment of mandibular condylar fracture

21470   Open treatment of complicated mandibular fracture by multiple surgical approaches including internal fixation, interdental fixation, and/or wiring of dentures or splints
➔ *CPT Assistant* Nov 02:10

21480   Closed treatment of temporomandibular dislocation; initial or subsequent

21485   complicated (eg, recurrent requiring intermaxillary fixation or splinting), initial or subsequent

21490   Open treatment of temporomandibular dislocation

(For interdental wire fixation, use 21497)

21495   Open treatment of hyoid fracture

(For laryngoplasty with open reduction of fracture, use 31584)

(To report treatment of closed fracture of larynx, use the applicable Evaluation and Management codes)

21497   Interdental wiring, for condition other than fracture
➔ *CPT Assistant* Mar 97:10

Other Procedures

21499   Unlisted musculoskeletal procedure, head

(For unlisted craniofacial or maxillofacial procedure, use 21299)

Neck (Soft Tissues) and Thorax

(For cervical spine and back, see 21920 et seq)

(For injection of fracture site or trigger point, use 20550)

Incision

(For incision and drainage of abscess or hematoma, superficial, see 10060, 10140)

21501   Incision and drainage, deep abscess or hematoma, soft tissues of neck or thorax;

(For posterior spine subfascial incision and drainage, see 22010-22015)

21502   with partial rib ostectomy

21510   Incision, deep, with opening of bone cortex (eg, for osteomyelitis or bone abscess), thorax

Excision

(For bone biopsy, see 20220-20251)

21550   Biopsy, soft tissue of neck or thorax

(For needle biopsy of soft tissue, use 20206)

21552   Code is out of numerical sequence. See 21550-21632

21554   Code is out of numerical sequence. See 21550-21632

21555   Excision, tumor, soft tissue of neck or anterior thorax, subcutaneous; less than 3 cm
➔ *CPT Assistant* Oct 02:11; *CPT Changes: An Insider's View* 2010

21552   3 cm or greater
➔ *CPT Changes: An Insider's View* 2010

21556   Excision, tumor, soft tissue of neck or anterior thorax, subfascial (eg, intramuscular); less than 5 cm
➔ *CPT Changes: An Insider's View* 2010

21554   5 cm or greater
➔ *CPT Changes: An Insider's View* 2010

21557   Radical resection of tumor (eg, malignant neoplasm), soft tissue of neck or anterior thorax; less than 5 cm
➔ *CPT Assistant* Apr 10:3; *CPT Changes: An Insider's View* 2010

21558   5 cm or greater
➔ *CPT Changes: An Insider's View* 2010

21600   Excision of rib, partial
➔ *CPT Assistant* Jul 12:12

(For radical resection of chest wall and rib cage for tumor, use 19260)

(For radical debridement of chest wall and rib cage for injury, see 11044, 11047)

21610   Costotransversectomy (separate procedure)

21615   Excision first and/or cervical rib;

21616   with sympathectomy

21620   Ostectomy of sternum, partial

21627   Sternal debridement
➔ *CPT Assistant* May 11:3

(For debridement and closure, use 21750)

21630   Radical resection of sternum;

21632   with mediastinal lymphadenectomy

Repair, Revision, and/or Reconstruction

(For superficial wound, see **Integumentary System** section under Repair—Simple)

21685   Hyoid myotomy and suspension
➔ *CPT Assistant* Aug 04:11; *CPT Changes: An Insider's View* 2004

21700   Division of scalenus anticus; without resection of cervical rib

Musculoskeletal

21705 with resection of cervical rib

21720 Division of sternocleidomastoid for torticollis, open operation; without cast application

(For transection of spinal accessory and cervical nerves, see 63191, 64722)

21725 with cast application

21740 Reconstructive repair of pectus excavatum or carinatum; open
➜ *CPT Changes: An Insider's View* 2003

21742 minimally invasive approach (Nuss procedure), without thoracoscopy
➜ *CPT Changes: An Insider's View* 2003

21743 minimally invasive approach (Nuss procedure), with thoracoscopy
➜ *CPT Changes: An Insider's View* 2003

21750 Closure of median sternotomy separation with or without debridement (separate procedure)
➜ *CPT Assistant* May 11:3; *CPT Changes: An Insider's View* 2002

Fracture and/or Dislocation

21800 Closed treatment of rib fracture, uncomplicated, each

21805 Open treatment of rib fracture without fixation, each

21810 Treatment of rib fracture requiring external fixation (flail chest)

21820 Closed treatment of sternum fracture

21825 Open treatment of sternum fracture with or without skeletal fixation

(For sternoclavicular dislocation, see 23520-23532)

Other Procedures

21899 Unlisted procedure, neck or thorax

Back and Flank

Excision

21920 Biopsy, soft tissue of back or flank; superficial

21925 deep

(For needle biopsy of soft tissue, use 20206)

21930 Excision, tumor, soft tissue of back or flank, subcutaneous; less than 3 cm
➜ *CPT Changes: An Insider's View* 2010

21931 3 cm or greater
➜ *CPT Changes: An Insider's View* 2010

21932 Excision, tumor, soft tissue of back or flank, subfascial (eg, intramuscular); less than 5 cm
➜ *CPT Changes: An Insider's View* 2010

21933 5 cm or greater
➜ *CPT Changes: An Insider's View* 2010

21935 Radical resection of tumor (eg, malignant neoplasm), soft tissue of back or flank; less than 5 cm
➜ *CPT Changes: An Insider's View* 2010

21936 5 cm or greater
➜ *CPT Changes: An Insider's View* 2010

Spine (Vertebral Column)

Cervical, thoracic, and lumbar spine.

Within the spine section, bone grafting procedures are reported separately and in addition to arthrodesis. For bone grafts in other Musculoskeletal sections, see specific code(s) descriptor(s) and/or accompanying guidelines.

To report bone grafts performed after arthrodesis, see 20930-20938. Do not append modifier 62 to bone graft codes 20900-20938.

Example:

Posterior arthrodesis of L5-S1 for degenerative disc disease utilizing morselized autogenous iliac bone graft harvested through a separate fascial incision.

Report as 22612 and 20937.

Within the spine section, instrumentation is reported separately and in addition to arthrodesis. To report instrumentation procedures performed with definitive vertebral procedure(s), see 22840-22855. Instrumentation procedure codes 22840-22848 and 22851 are reported in addition to the definitive procedure(s). Modifier 62 may not be appended to the definitive or add-on spinal instrumentation procedure code(s) 22840-22848 and 22850-22852.

Example:

Posterior arthrodesis of L4-S1, utilizing morselized autogenous iliac bone graft harvested through separate fascial incision, and pedicle screw fixation.

Report as 22612, 22614, 22842, and 20937.

Vertebral procedures are sometimes followed by arthrodesis and in addition may include bone grafts and instrumentation.

When arthrodesis is performed in addition to another procedure, the arthrodesis should be reported in addition to the original procedure with modifier 51 (multiple procedures). Examples are after osteotomy, fracture care, vertebral corpectomy, and laminectomy. Bone grafts and instrumentation are never performed without arthrodesis.

Example:

Treatment of a burst fracture of L2 by corpectomy followed by arthrodesis of L1-L3, utilizing anterior instrumentation L1-L3 and structural allograft.

Report as 63090, 22558-51, 22585, 22845, and 20931.

When two surgeons work together as primary surgeons performing distinct part(s) of a single reportable procedure, each surgeon should report his/her distinct operative work by appending modifier 62 to the single

Musculoskeletal

definitive procedure code. If additional procedure(s) (including add-on procedure[s]) are performed during the same surgical session, separate code(s) may be reported by each co-surgeon, with modifier 62 appended (see Appendix A).

Example:

A 42-year-old male with a history of posttraumatic degenerative disc disease at L3-4 and L4-5 (internal disc disruption) underwent surgical repair. Surgeon A performed an anterior exposure of the spine with mobilization of the great vessels. Surgeon B performed anterior (minimal) discectomy and fusion at L3-4 and L4-5 using anterior interbody technique.

Report surgeon A: 22558 append modifier 62, 22585 append modifier 62

Report surgeon B: 22558 append modifier 62, 22585 append modifier 62, 20931

(Do not append modifier 62 to bone graft code 20931)

(For injection procedure for myelography, use 62284)

(For injection procedure for discography, see 62290, 62291)

(For injection procedure, chemonucleolysis, single or multiple levels, use 62292)

(For injection procedure for facet joints, see 64490-64495, 64633-64636)

(For needle or trocar biopsy, see 20220-20225)

Incision

22010   Incision and drainage, open, of deep abscess (subfascial), posterior spine; cervical, thoracic, or cervicothoracic
➔ *CPT Changes: An Insider's View* 2006

22015   lumbar, sacral, or lumbosacral
➔ *CPT Changes: An Insider's View* 2006

(Do not report 22015 in conjunction with 22010)

(Do not report 22015 in conjunction with instrumentation removal, 10180, 22850, 22852)

(For incision and drainage of abscess or hematoma, superficial, see 10060, 10140)

Excision

For the following codes, when two surgeons work together as primary surgeons performing distinct part(s) of partial vertebral body excision, each surgeon should report his/her distinct operative work by appending modifier 62 to the procedure code. In this situation, modifier 62 may be appended to the procedure code(s) 22100-22102, 22110-22114 and, as appropriate, to the associated additional vertebral segment add-on code(s) 22103, 22116 as long as both surgeons continue to work together as primary surgeons.

(For bone biopsy, see 20220-20251)

(To report soft tissue biopsy of back or flank, see 21920-21925)

(For needle biopsy of soft tissue, use 20206)

(To report excision of soft tissue tumor of back or flank, use 21930)

22100   Partial excision of posterior vertebral component (eg, spinous process, lamina or facet) for intrinsic bony lesion, single vertebral segment; cervical

22101   thoracic

22102   lumbar

(For insertion of posterior spinous process distraction devices, see 0171T, 0172T)

+ 22103   each additional segment (List separately in addition to code for primary procedure)
➔ *CPT Assistant* Feb 96:6

(Use 22103 in conjunction with 22100, 22101, 22102)

22110   Partial excision of vertebral body, for intrinsic bony lesion, without decompression of spinal cord or nerve root(s), single vertebral segment; cervical

22112   thoracic

22114   lumbar

+ 22116   each additional vertebral segment (List separately in addition to code for primary procedure)
➔ *CPT Assistant* Feb 96:6

(Use 22116 in conjunction with 22110, 22112, 22114)

(For complete or near complete resection of vertebral body, see vertebral corpectomy, 63081-63091)

(For spinal reconstruction with bone graft [autograft, allograft] and/or methylmethacrylate of cervical vertebral body, use 63081 and 22554 and 20931 or 20938)

(For spinal reconstruction with bone graft [autograft, allograft] and/or methylmethacrylate of thoracic vertebral body, use 63085 or 63087 and 22556 and 20931 or 20938)

(For spinal reconstruction with bone graft [autograft, allograft] and/or methylmethacrylate of lumbar vertebral body, use 63087 or 63090 and 22558 and 20931 or 20938)

(For spinal reconstruction following vertebral body resection, use 63082 or 63086 or 63088 or 63091, and 22585)

(For harvest of bone autograft for vertebral reconstruction, see 20931 or 20938)

(For cervical spinal reconstruction with prosthetic replacement of resected vertebral bodies, see codes 63081 and 22554 and 20931 or 20938 and 22851)

(For thoracic spinal reconstruction with prosthetic replacement of resected vertebral bodies, see codes 63085 or 63087 and 22556 and 20931 or 20938 and 22851)

Musculoskeletal

(For lumbar spinal reconstruction with prosthetic replacement of resected vertebral bodies, see codes 63087 or 63090 and 22558, and 20931 or 20938 and 22851)

(For osteotomy of spine, see 22210-22226)

Osteotomy

To report arthrodesis, see codes 22590-22632. (Report in addition to code[s] for the definitive procedure with modifier 51.)

To report instrumentation procedures, see 22840-22855. (Report in addition to code[s] for the definitive procedure[s].) Do not append modifier 62 to spinal instrumentation codes 22840-22848 and 22850-22852.

To report bone graft procedures, see 20930-20938. (Report in addition to code[s] for the definitive procedure[s].) Do not append modifier 62 to bone graft codes 20900-20938.

For the following codes, when two surgeons work together as primary surgeons performing distinct part(s) of an anterior spine osteotomy, each surgeon should report his/her distinct operative work by appending modifier 62 to the procedure code. In this situation, modifier 62 may be appended to the procedure code(s) 22210-22214, 22220-22224 and, as appropriate, to associated additional segment add-on code(s) 22216, 22226 as long as both surgeons continue to work together as primary surgeons.

Spinal osteotomy procedures are reported when a portion(s) of the vertebral segment(s) is cut and removed in preparation for re-aligning the spine as part of a spinal deformity correction. For excision of an intrinsic lesion of the vertebra without deformity correction, see 22100-22116. For decompression of the spinal cord and/or nerve roots, see 63001-63308.

The three columns are defined as anterior (anterior two-thirds of the vertebral body), middle (posterior third of the vertebral body and the pedicle), and posterior (articular facets, lamina, and spinous process).

22206 Osteotomy of spine, posterior or posterolateral approach, 3 columns, 1 vertebral segment (eg, pedicle/vertebral body subtraction); thoracic
→ *CPT Assistant* Feb 08:9; *CPT Changes: An Insider's View* 2008

(Do not report 22206 in conjunction with 22207)

22207 lumbar
→ *CPT Assistant* Feb 08:9; *CPT Changes: An Insider's View* 2008

(Do not report 22207 in conjunction with 22206)

+ 22208 each additional vertebral segment (List separately in addition to code for primary procedure)
→ *CPT Assistant* Feb 08:9; *CPT Changes: An Insider's View* 2008

(Use 22208 in conjunction with 22206, 22207)

(Do not report 22206, 22207, 22208 in conjunction with 22210-22226, 22830, 63001-63048, 63055-63066, 63075-63091, 63101-63103, when performed at the same level)

22210 Osteotomy of spine, posterior or posterolateral approach, 1 vertebral segment; cervical

22212 thoracic
→ *CPT Assistant* Dec 07:1

22214 lumbar
→ *CPT Assistant* Dec 07:1

+ 22216 each additional vertebral segment (List separately in addition to primary procedure)
→ *CPT Assistant* Dec 07:1

(Use 22216 in conjunction with 22210, 22212, 22214)

22220 Osteotomy of spine, including discectomy, anterior approach, single vertebral segment; cervical
→ *CPT Assistant* Feb 02:4

22222 thoracic
→ *CPT Assistant* Feb 02:4

22224 lumbar
→ *CPT Assistant* Feb 02:4

+ 22226 each additional vertebral segment (List separately in addition to code for primary procedure)
→ *CPT Assistant* Feb 96:6, Feb 02:4

(Use 22226 in conjunction with 22220, 22222, 22224)

(For vertebral corpectomy, see 63081-63091)

Fracture and/or Dislocation

To report arthrodesis, see codes 22590-22632. (Report in addition to code[s] for the definitive procedure with modifier 51.)

To report instrumentation procedures, see 22840-22855. (Report in addition to code[s] for the definitive procedure[s].) Do not append modifier 62 to spinal instrumentation codes 22840-22848 and 22850-22852.

To report bone graft procedures, see 20930-20938. (Report in addition to code[s] for the definitive procedure[s].) Do not append modifier 62 to bone graft codes 20900-20938.

For the following codes, when two surgeons work together as primary surgeons performing distinct part(s) of open fracture and/or dislocation procedure(s), each surgeon should report his/her distinct operative work by appending modifier 62 to the procedure code. In this situation, modifier 62 may be appended to the procedure code(s) 22318-22327 and, as appropriate, the associated additional fracture vertebrae or dislocated segment add-on code 22328 as long as both surgeons continue to work together as primary surgeons.

22305 Closed treatment of vertebral process fracture(s)

22310 Closed treatment of vertebral body fracture(s), without manipulation, requiring and including casting or bracing
➜ *CPT Assistant* Jun 12:10

22315 Closed treatment of vertebral fracture(s) and/or dislocation(s) requiring casting or bracing, with and including casting and/or bracing by manipulation or traction
➜ *CPT Assistant* Apr 12:11, Jun 12:10; *CPT Changes: An Insider's View* 2011

(For spinal subluxation, use 97140)

22318 Open treatment and/or reduction of odontoid fracture(s) and or dislocation(s) (including os odontoideum), anterior approach, including placement of internal fixation; without grafting
➜ *CPT Assistant* Nov 99:11, Apr 12:13; *CPT Changes: An Insider's View* 2000

22319 with grafting
➜ *CPT Assistant* Nov 99:11, Apr 12:16; *CPT Changes: An Insider's View* 2000

22325 Open treatment and/or reduction of vertebral fracture(s) and/or dislocation(s), posterior approach, 1 fractured vertebra or dislocated segment; lumbar
➜ *CPT Assistant* Sep 97:8, Jun 12:10

22326 cervical
➜ *CPT Assistant* Sep 97:8

22327 thoracic
➜ *CPT Assistant* Sep 97:8, Jun 12:10

+ 22328 each additional fractured vertebra or dislocated segment (List separately in addition to code for primary procedure)
➜ *CPT Assistant* Feb 96:6

(Use 22328 in conjunction with 22325-22327)

(For treatment of vertebral fracture by the anterior approach, see corpectomy 63081-63091, and appropriate arthrodesis, bone graft and instrument codes)

(For decompression of spine following fracture, see 63001-63091; for arthrodesis of spine following fracture, see 22548-22632)

Manipulation

(For spinal manipulation without anesthesia, use 97140)

22505 Manipulation of spine requiring anesthesia, any region
➜ *CPT Assistant* Mar 97:11, Jan 99:11

Vertebral Body, Embolization or Injection

⊙ **22520** Percutaneous vertebroplasty (bone biopsy included when performed), 1 vertebral body, unilateral or bilateral injection; thoracic
➜ *CPT Assistant* Mar 01:2, Oct 06:13, Jun 12:10; *CPT Changes: An Insider's View* 2001, 2010, 2012

⊙ **22521** lumbar
➜ *CPT Assistant* Mar 01:2, Oct 06:13, Jun 12:10; *CPT Changes: An Insider's View* 2001, 2010, 2012

⊙+▲ **22522** each additional thoracic or lumbar vertebral body (List separately in addition to code for primary procedure)
➜ *CPT Assistant* Mar 01:2, Oct 06:13, Jun 12:10; *CPT Changes: An Insider's View* 2001, 2012, 2013

(Do not report 22520-22522 in conjunction with 20225, 22310-22315, 22325, 22327 when performed at the same level as 22520-22522)

(Use 22522 in conjunction with 22520, 22521 as appropriate)

(For radiological supervision and interpretation, see 72291, 72292)

Percutaneous Vertebroplasty
22520

Augmentation of a vertebral fracture is achieved by percutaneous injections of polymethylmethacrylate under fluoroscopic guidance.

Spinal canal (vertebral foramen)

Fractured vertebral body

Needle (trocar)

Pedicle

Fractured vertebral body filled with bone cement

22523 Percutaneous vertebral augmentation, including cavity creation (fracture reduction and bone biopsy included when performed) using mechanical device, 1 vertebral body, unilateral or bilateral cannulation (eg, kyphoplasty); thoracic
➜ *CPT Assistant* Jun 12:10; *CPT Changes: An Insider's View* 2006
➜ *Clinical Examples in Radiology* Winter 06:14

22524 lumbar
➜ *CPT Assistant* Jun 12:10; *CPT Changes: An Insider's View* 2006
➜ *Clinical Examples in Radiology* Winter 06:14

+ 22525 each additional thoracic or lumbar vertebral body (List separately in addition to code for primary procedure)
➜ *CPT Assistant* Jun 12:10; *CPT Changes: An Insider's View* 2006
➜ *Clinical Examples in Radiology* Winter 06:14

(Do not report 22523-22525 in conjunction with 20225, 22310-22315, 22325, 22327 when performed at the same level as 22523-22525)

Musculoskeletal

(Use 22525 in conjunction with 22523, 22524)

(For radiological supervision and interpretation, see 72291, 72292)

⊙ **22526** Percutaneous intradiscal electrothermal annuloplasty, unilateral or bilateral including fluoroscopic guidance; single level
➔ *CPT Assistant* Sep 07:10, Nov 10:3, Jan 11:8; *CPT Changes: An Insider's View* 2007

⊙+ **22527** 1 or more additional levels (List separately in addition to code for primary procedure)
➔ *CPT Assistant* Sep 07:10, Nov 10:3, Jan 11:8; *CPT Changes: An Insider's View* 2007

(Use 22527 in conjunction with 22526)

(Do not report codes 22526, 22527 in conjunction with 77002, 77003)

(For percutaneous intradiscal annuloplasty using method other than electrothermal, use 22899)

Arthrodesis

Arthrodesis may be performed in the absence of other procedures and therefore when it is combined with another definitive procedure (eg, osteotomy, fracture care, vertebral corpectomy or laminectomy), modifier 51 is appropriate. However, arthrodesis codes 22585, 22614, and 22632 are considered add-on procedure codes and should not be used with modifier 51.

To report instrumentation procedures, see 22840-22855. (Codes 22840-22848, 22851 are reported in conjunction with code[s] for the definitive procedure[s]. When instrumentation reinsertion or removal is reported in conjunction with other definitive procedures including arthrodesis, decompression, and exploration of fusion, append modifier 51 to 22849, 22850, 22852, and 22855.) To report exploration of fusion, use 22830. (When exploration is reported in conjunction with other definitive procedures, including arthrodesis and decompression, append modifier 51 to 22830.) Do not append modifier 62 to spinal instrumentation codes 22840-22848 and 22850-22852.

To report bone graft procedures, see 20930-20938. (Report in addition to code[s] for the definitive procedure[s].) Do not append modifier 62 to bone graft codes 20900-20938.

Lateral Extracavitary Approach Technique

22532 Arthrodesis, lateral extracavitary technique, including minimal discectomy to prepare interspace (other than for decompression); thoracic
➔ *CPT Assistant* Apr 12:16; *CPT Changes: An Insider's View* 2004

22533 lumbar
➔ *CPT Assistant* Apr 12:16; *CPT Changes: An Insider's View* 2004

+ **22534** thoracic or lumbar, each additional vertebral segment (List separately in addition to code for primary procedure)
➔ *CPT Changes: An Insider's View* 2004

(Use 22534 in conjunction with 22532 and 22533)

Anterior or Anterolateral Approach Technique

Procedure codes 22554-22558 are for SINGLE interspace; for additional interspaces, use 22585. A vertebral interspace is the non-bony compartment between two adjacent vertebral bodies, which contains the intervertebral disc, and includes the nucleus pulposus, annulus fibrosus, and two cartilagenous endplates.

For the following codes, when two surgeons work together as primary surgeons performing distinct part(s) of an anterior interbody arthrodesis, each surgeon should report his/her distinct operative work by appending modifier 62 to the procedure code. In this situation, modifier 62 may be appended to the procedure code(s) 22548-22558 and, as appropriate, to the associated additional interspace add-on code 22585 as long as both surgeons continue to work together as primary surgeons.

22548 Arthrodesis, anterior transoral or extraoral technique, clivus-C1-C2 (atlas-axis), with or without excision of odontoid process
➔ *CPT Assistant* Spring 93:36, Feb 96:7, Sep 97:8, Sep 00:10, Feb 02:4, Apr 12:16

(For intervertebral disc excision by laminotomy or laminectomy, see 63020-63042)

Arthrodesis (Anterior Transoral Technique)
22548

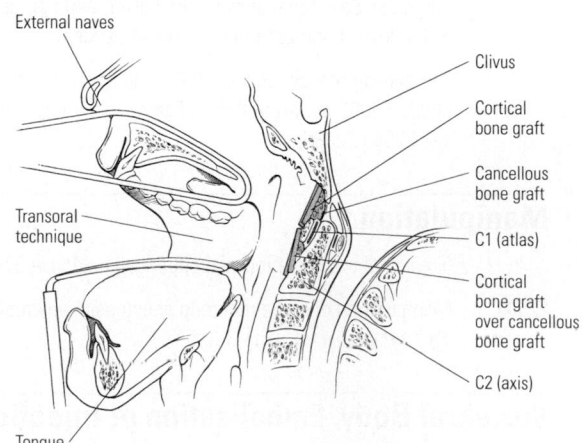

Musculoskeletal

22551   Arthrodesis, anterior interbody, including disc space preparation, discectomy, osteophytectomy and decompression of spinal cord and/or nerve roots; cervical below C2

➔ *CPT Assistant* Apr 12:16; *CPT Changes: An Insider's View* 2011

+ 22552   cervical below C2, each additional interspace (List separately in addition to code for separate procedure)

➔ *CPT Assistant* Apr 12:16; *CPT Changes: An Insider's View* 2011

(Use 22552 in conjunction with 22551)

22554   Arthrodesis, anterior interbody technique, including minimal discectomy to prepare interspace (other than for decompression); cervical below C2

➔ *CPT Assistant* Spring 93:36, Sep 97:8, Sep 00:10, Jan 01:12, Feb 02:4, Apr 12:16

►(Do not report 22554 in conjunction with 63075, even if performed by a separate individual. To report anterior cervical discectomy and interbody fusion at the same level during the same session, use 22551)◄

22556   thoracic

➔ *CPT Assistant* Spring 93:36, Jul 96:7, Sep 97:8, Sep 00:10, Feb 02:4, Apr 12:16

Anterior Approach for Cervical Fusion
22554

An example of an exposure technique used to reach anterior cervical vertebrae for spinal procedures (eg, discectomy, arthrodesis, spinal instrumentation)

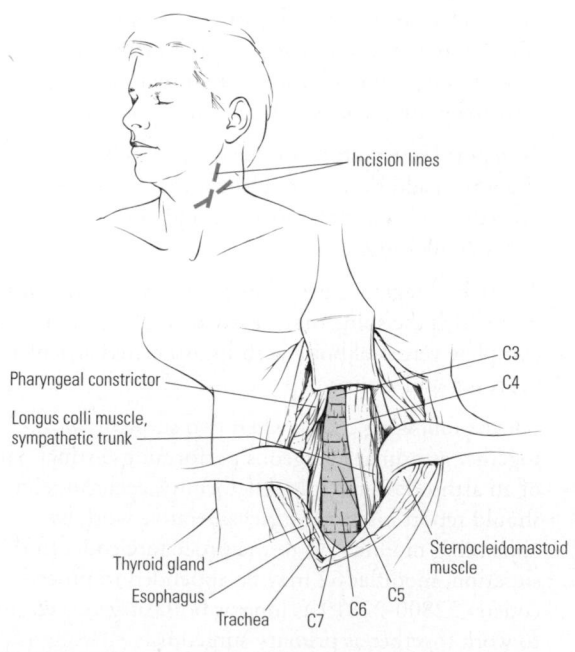

22558   lumbar

➔ *CPT Assistant* Spring 93:36, Mar 96:6, Jul 96:7, Sep 97:8, Sep 00:10, Feb 02:4, Oct 09:9, Apr 12:16

►(For arthrodesis using pre-sacral interbody technique, see 22586, 0195T)◄

Anterior Approach for Lumbar Fusion (Anterior Retroperitoneal Exposure)
22558

An example of an exposure technique used to reach anterior lumbar vertebrae for spinal procedures (eg, discectomy, arthrodesis, spinal instrumentation)

+ 22585   each additional interspace (List separately in addition to code for primary procedure)

➔ *CPT Assistant* Spring 93:36, Feb 96:6, Mar 96:6, Sep 97:8, Sep 00:10, Feb 02:4, Apr 08:11; *CPT Changes: An Insider's View* 2011

(Use 22585 in conjunction with 22554, 22556, 22558)

►(Do not report 22585 in conjunction with 63075, even if performed by a separate individual. To report anterior cervical discectomy and interbody fusion at the same level during the same session, use 22552)◄

● **22586**   Arthrodesis, pre-sacral interbody technique, including disc space preparation, discectomy, with posterior instrumentation, with image guidance, includes bone graft when performed, L5-S1 interspace

➔ *CPT Changes: An Insider's View* 2013

►(Do not report 22586 in conjunction with 20930-20938, 22840, 22848, 72275, 77002, 77003, 77011, 77012)◄

Posterior, Posterolateral or Lateral Transverse Process Technique

To report instrumentation procedures, see 22840-22855. (Report in addition to code[s] for the definitive procedure[s].) Do not append modifier 62 to spinal instrumentation codes 22840-22848 and 22850-22852.

To report bone graft procedures, see 20930-20938. (Report in addition to code[s] for the definitive procedure[s].) Do not append modifier 62 to bone graft codes 20900-20938.

A vertebral segment describes the basic constituent part into which the spine may be divided. It represents a single complete vertebral bone with its associated articular processes and laminae. A vertebral interspace is the non-bony compartment between two adjacent vertebral bodies which contains the intervertebral disc, and includes the nucleus pulposus, annulus fibrosus, and two cartilagenous endplates.

22590 Arthrodesis, posterior technique, craniocervical (occiput-C2)

> *CPT Assistant* Spring 93:36, Sep 97:8, Apr 12:16

22595 Arthrodesis, posterior technique, atlas-axis (C1-C2)

> *CPT Assistant* Spring 93:36, Sep 97:8, Apr 12:12

22600 Arthrodesis, posterior or posterolateral technique, single level; cervical below C2 segment

> *CPT Assistant* Spring 93:36, Sep 97:8, Nov 10:8, Apr 12:16, Jun 12:11

22610 thoracic (with lateral transverse technique, when performed)

> *CPT Assistant* Spring 93:36, Sep 97:8, Nov 10:8, Apr 12:16, Jun 12:10; *CPT Changes: An Insider's View* 2012

22612 lumbar (with lateral transverse technique, when performed)

> *CPT Assistant* Spring 93:36, Mar 96:7, Sep 97:8, 11, Apr 08:11, Jul 08:7, Oct 09:9, Nov 10:8, Dec 11:14, Jan 12:3, Apr 12:16, Jun 12:10; *CPT Changes: An Insider's View* 2012

(Do not report 22612 in conjunction with 22630 for the same interspace and segment, use 22633)

+ 22614 each additional vertebral segment (List separately in addition to code for primary procedure)

> *CPT Assistant* Feb 96:6, Mar 96:7, Nov 10:8, Jun 12:11

(Use 22614 in conjunction with 22600, 22610, 22612, 22630 or 22633 when performed at a different level. When performing a posterior or posterolateral technique for fusion/arthrodesis at an additional level, use 22614. When performing a posterior interbody fusion arthrodesis at an additional level, use 22632. When performing a combined posterior or posterolateral technique with posterior interbody arthrodesis at an additional level, use 22634)

(For facet joint fusion, see 0219T-0222T)

(For placement of a posterior intrafacet implant, see 0219T-0222T)

22630 Arthrodesis, posterior interbody technique, including laminectomy and/or discectomy to prepare interspace (other than for decompression), single interspace; lumbar

> *CPT Assistant* Spring 93:36, Sep 97:8, Nov 99:11, Dec 99:2, Jan 01:12, Oct 09:9, Nov 11:10, Dec 11:14, Jan 12:3, Apr 12:16, Jun 12:11; *CPT Changes: An Insider's View* 2000

(Do not report 22630 in conjunction with 22612 for the same interspace and segment, use 22633)

+ 22632 each additional interspace (List separately in addition to code for primary procedure)

> *CPT Assistant* Feb 96:6, Sep 97:8, Dec 99:2, Jun 12:11

(Use 22632 in conjunction with 22612, 22630, or 22633 when performed at a different level. When performing a posterior interbody fusion arthrodesis at an additional level, use 22632. When performing a posterior or posterolateral technique for fusion/arthrodesis at an additional level, use 22614. When performing a combined posterior or posterolateral technique with posterior interbody arthrodesis at an additional level, use 22634)

22633 Arthrodesis, combined posterior or posterolateral technique with posterior interbody technique including laminectomy and/or discectomy sufficient to prepare interspace (other than for decompression), single interspace and segment; lumbar

> *CPT Assistant* Dec 11:14, Jan 12:3, Jun 12:10; *CPT Changes: An Insider's View* 2012

(Do not report with 22612 or 22630 at the same level)

+ 22634 each additional interspace and segment (List separately in addition to code for primary procedure)

> *CPT Assistant* Dec 11:14, Jan 12:3, Jun 12:10; *CPT Changes: An Insider's View* 2012

(Use 22634 in conjunction with 22633)

Spine Deformity (eg, Scoliosis, Kyphosis)

To report instrumentation procedures, see 22840-22855. (Report in addition to code[s] for the definitive procedure[s].) Do not append modifier 62 to spinal instrumentation codes 22840-22848 and 22850-22852.

To report bone graft procedures, see 20930-20938. (Report in addition to code[s] for the definitive procedure[s].) Do not append modifier 62 to bone graft codes 20900-20938.

A vertebral segment describes the basic constituent part into which the spine may be divided. It represents a single complete vertebral bone with its associated articular processes and laminae.

For the following codes, when two surgeons work together as primary surgeons performing distinct part(s) of an arthrodesis for spinal deformity, each surgeon should report his/her distinct operative work by appending modifier 62 to the procedure code. In this situation, modifier 62 may be appended to procedure code(s) 22800-22819 as long as both surgeons continue to work together as primary surgeons.

22800 Arthrodesis, posterior, for spinal deformity, with or without cast; up to 6 vertebral segments

> *CPT Assistant* Apr 12:16

22802 7 to 12 vertebral segments

> *CPT Assistant* Mar 96:10, Apr 12:16

22804   13 or more vertebral segments
→ *CPT Assistant* Apr 12:16

22808   Arthrodesis, anterior, for spinal deformity, with or without cast; 2 to 3 vertebral segments
→ *CPT Assistant* Feb 02:4, Apr 12:16

22810   4 to 7 vertebral segments
→ *CPT Assistant* Mar 96:10, Sep 97:8, Feb 02:4, Apr 12:16

22812   8 or more vertebral segments
→ *CPT Assistant* Feb 02:4, Apr 12:16

22818   Kyphectomy, circumferential exposure of spine and resection of vertebral segment(s) (including body and posterior elements); single or 2 segments
→ *CPT Assistant* Nov 97:14

22819   3 or more segments
→ *CPT Assistant* Nov 97:14

(To report arthrodesis, see 22800-22804 and add modifier 51)

Exploration

To report instrumentation procedures, see 22840-22855. (Codes 22840-22848 and 22851 are reported in conjunction with code[s] for the definitive procedure[s]. When instrumentation reinsertion or removal is reported in conjunction with other definitive procedures including arthrodesis, decompression, and exploration of fusion, append modifier 51 to 22849, 22850, 22852 and 22855.) Code 22849 should not be reported with 22850, 22852, and 22855 at the same spinal levels. To report exploration of fusion, see 22830. (When exploration is reported in conjunction with other definitive procedures, including arthrodesis and decompression, append modifier 51 to 22830.)

(To report bone graft procedures, see 20930-20938)

22830   Exploration of spinal fusion
→ *CPT Assistant* Sep 97:11, Mar 10:9

Spinal Instrumentation

Segmental instrumentation is defined as fixation at each end of the construct and at least one additional interposed bony attachment.

Non-segmental instrumentation is defined as fixation at each end of the construct and may span several vertebral segments without attachment to the intervening segments.

Insertion of spinal instrumentation is reported separately and in addition to arthrodesis. Instrumentation procedure codes 22840-22848 and 22851 are reported in addition to the definitive procedure(s). Do not append modifier 62 to spinal instrumentation codes 22840-22848 and 22850-22852.

To report bone graft procedures, see 20930-20938. (Report in addition to code[s] for definitive procedure[s].) Do not append modifier 62 to bone graft codes 20900-20938.

A vertebral segment describes the basic constituent part into which the spine may be divided. It represents a single complete vertebral bone with its associated articular processes and laminae. A vertebral interspace is the non-bony compartment between two adjacent vertebral bodies, which contains the intervertebral disc, and includes the nucleus pulposus, annulus fibrosus, and two cartilagenous endplates.

Codes 22849, 22850, 22852, and 22855 are subject to modifier 51 if reported with other definitive procedure(s), including arthrodesis, decompression, and exploration of fusion. Code 22849 should not be reported in conjunction with 22850, 22852, and 22855 at the same spinal levels. Only the appropriate insertion code (22840-22848) should be reported when previously placed spinal instrumentation is being removed or revised during the same session where new instrumentation is inserted at levels including all or part of the previously instrumented segments. Do not report the reinsertion (22849) or removal (22850, 22852, 22855) procedures in addition to the insertion of the new instrumentation (22840-22848).

+ **22840**   Posterior non-segmental instrumentation (eg, Harrington rod technique, pedicle fixation across 1 interspace, atlantoaxial transarticular screw fixation, sublaminar wiring at C1, facet screw fixation) (List separately in addition to code for primary procedure)
→ *CPT Assistant* Feb 96:6, Jul 96:10, Sep 97:8, Nov 99:12, Feb 02:6, Nov 10:8, Jan 11:9, Dec 11:15, Apr 12:12, Jun 12:11; *CPT Changes: An Insider's View* 2000, 2008

▶(Use 22840 in conjunction with 22100-22102, 22110-22114, 22206, 22207, 22210-22214, 22220-22224, 22305-22327, 22532, 22533, 22548-22558, 22590-22612, 22630, 22633, 22634, 22800-22812, 63001-63030, 63040-63042, 63045-63047, 63050-63056, 63064, 63075, 63077, 63081, 63085, 63087, 63090, 63101, 63102, 63170-63290, 63300-63307)◀

(For insertion of posterior spinous process distraction devices, see 0171T, 0172T)

Musculoskeletal

Non-Segmental Spinal Instrumentation
22840

Fixation at each end of the construct

+ 22841 Internal spinal fixation by wiring of spinous processes (List separately in addition to code for primary procedure)

→ *CPT Assistant* Feb 96:6, Sep 97:8, Feb 02:6, Jun 12:11; *CPT Changes: An Insider's View* 2008

►(Use 22841 in conjunction with 22100-22102, 22110-22114, 22206, 22207, 22210-22214, 22220-22224, 22305-22327, 22532, 22533, 22548-22558, 22590-22612, 22630, 22633, 22634, 22800-22812, 63001-63030, 63040-63042, 63045-63047, 63050-63056, 63064, 63075, 63077, 63081, 63085, 63087, 63090, 63101, 63102, 63170-63290, 63300-63307)◄

+ 22842 Posterior segmental instrumentation (eg, pedicle fixation, dual rods with multiple hooks and sublaminar wires); 3 to 6 vertebral segments (List separately in addition to code for primary procedure)

→ *CPT Assistant* Feb 96:6, Mar 96:7, Sep 97:8, Feb 02:6, Dec 11:15, Jun 12:11; *CPT Changes: An Insider's View* 2008

►(Use 22842 in conjunction with 22100-22102, 22110-22114, 22206, 22207, 22210-22214, 22220-22224, 22305-22327, 22532, 22533, 22548-22558, 22590-22612, 22630, 22633, 22634, 22800-22812, 63001-63030, 63040-63042, 63045-63047, 63050-63056, 63064, 63075, 63077, 63081, 63085, 63087, 63090, 63101, 63102, 63170-63290, 63300-63307)◄

+ 22843 7 to 12 vertebral segments (List separately in addition to code for primary procedure)

→ *CPT Assistant* Feb 96:6, Sep 97:8, Feb 02:6, Dec 11:15, Jun 12:11; *CPT Changes: An Insider's View* 2008

►(Use 22843 in conjunction with 22100-22102, 22110-22114, 22206, 22207, 22210-22214, 22220-22224, 22305-22327, 22532, 22533, 22548-22558, 22590-22612, 22630, 22633, 22634, 22800-22812, 63001-63030, 63040-63042, 63045-63047, 63050-63056, 63064, 63075, 63077, 63081, 63085, 63087, 63090, 63101, 63102, 63170-63290, 63300-63307)◄

+ 22844 13 or more vertebral segments (List separately in addition to code for primary procedure)

→ *CPT Assistant* Feb 96:6, Sep 97:8, Feb 02:6, Dec 11:15, Jun 12:11; *CPT Changes: An Insider's View* 2008

►(Use 22844 in conjunction with 22100-22102, 22110-22114, 22206, 22207, 22210-22214, 22220-22224, 22305-22327, 22532, 22533, 22548-22558, 22590-22612, 22630, 22633, 22634, 22800-22812, 63001-63030, 63040-63042, 63045-63047, 63050-63056, 63064, 63075, 63077, 63081, 63085, 63087, 63090, 63101, 63102, 63170-63290, 63300-63307)◄

Segmental Spinal Instrumentation
22842-22844

Fixation at each end of the construct and at least one additional interposed bony attachment

+ 22845 Anterior instrumentation; 2 to 3 vertebral segments (List separately in addition to code for primary procedure)

→ *CPT Assistant* Feb 96:6, Mar 96:10, Jul 96:7, 10, Sep 97:8, Feb 02:6, Jun 12:11; *CPT Changes: An Insider's View* 2008

►(Use 22845 in conjunction with 22100-22102, 22110-22114, 22206, 22207, 22210-22214, 22220-22224, 22305-22327, 22532, 22533, 22548-22558, 22590-22612, 22630, 22633, 22634, 22800-22812, 63001-63030, 63040-63042, 63045-63047, 63050-63056, 63064, 63075, 63077, 63081, 63085, 63087, 63090, 63101, 63102, 63170-63290, 63300-63307)◄

Musculoskeletal (side tab)

+ 22846   4 to 7 vertebral segments (List separately in addition to code for primary procedure)

→ *CPT Assistant* Feb 96:6, Sep 97:8, Feb 02:6, Jun 12:11; *CPT Changes: An Insider's View* 2008

▶(Use 22846 in conjunction with 22100-22102, 22110-22114, 22206, 22207, 22210-22214, 22220-22224, 22305-22327, 22532, 22533, 22548-22558, 22590-22612, 22630, 22633, 22634, 22800-22812, 63001-63030, 63040-63042, 63045-63047, 63050-63056, 63064, 63075, 63077, 63081, 63085, 63087, 63090, 63101, 63102, 63170-63290, 63300-63307)◀

+ 22847   8 or more vertebral segments (List separately in addition to code for primary procedure)

→ *CPT Assistant* Feb 96:6, Sep 97:8, Feb 02:6, Jun 12:11; *CPT Changes: An Insider's View* 2008

▶(Use 22847 in conjunction with 22100-22102, 22110-22114, 22206, 22207, 22210-22214, 22220-22224, 22305-22327, 22532, 22533, 22548-22558, 22590-22612, 22630, 22633, 22634, 22800-22812, 63001-63030, 63040-63042, 63045-63047, 63050-63056, 63064, 63075, 63077, 63081, 63085, 63087, 63090, 63101, 63102, 63170-63290, 63300-63307)◀

+ 22848   Pelvic fixation (attachment of caudal end of instrumentation to pelvic bony structures) other than sacrum (List separately in addition to code for primary procedure)

→ *CPT Assistant* Feb 96:6, Sep 97:8, Feb 02:6, Jun 12:11; *CPT Changes: An Insider's View* 2008

▶(Use 22848 in conjunction with 22100-22102, 22110-22114, 22206, 22207, 22210-22214, 22220-22224, 22305-22327, 22532, 22533, 22548-22558, 22590-22612, 22630, 22633, 22634, 22800-22812, 63001-63030, 63040-63042, 63045-63047, 63050-63056, 63064, 63075, 63077, 63081, 63085, 63087, 63090, 63101, 63102, 63170-63290, 63300-63307)◀

22849   Reinsertion of spinal fixation device

→ *CPT Assistant* Feb 96:6, Sep 97:8, Feb 02:6, Nov 02:3, Oct 11:10, Jun 12:11

22850   Removal of posterior nonsegmental instrumentation (eg, Harrington rod)

→ *CPT Assistant* Feb 96:6, Sep 97:8, Feb 02:6, Jun 12:11

+ 22851   Application of intervertebral biomechanical device(s) (eg, synthetic cage(s), methylmethacrylate) to vertebral defect or interspace (List separately in addition to code for primary procedure)

→ *CPT Assistant* Feb 96:6, Sep 97:8, Nov 99:12, Dec 99:2, May 00:11, Mar 01:2, Feb 02:6, Feb 05:14-15, Nov 10:8, Oct 11:10, Dec 11:15, Jun 12:11; *CPT Changes: An Insider's View* 2002, 2008, 2011

▶(Use 22851 in conjunction with 22100-22102, 22110-22114, 22206, 22207, 22210-22214, 22220-22224, 22305-22327, 22532, 22533, 22548-22558, 22590-22612, 22630, 22633, 22634, 22800-22812, 63001-63030, 63040-63042, 63045-63047, 63050-63056, 63064, 63075, 63077, 63081, 63085, 63087, 63090, 63101, 63102, 63170-63290, 63300-63307)◀

(For application of an intervertebral bone device/graft, see 20930-20938)

(For insertion of posterior spinous process distraction devices, see 0171T, 0172T)

Spinal Prosthetic Devices
22851

Application of prosthetic device

Methylmethacrylate replacement

22852   Removal of posterior segmental instrumentation

→ *CPT Assistant* Feb 96:6, Sep 97:8, Feb 02:6, May 06:16, Jun 12:11

22855   Removal of anterior instrumentation

→ *CPT Assistant* Feb 96:6, Sep 97:8, Feb 02:6, Nov 02:2, Jun 12:11

22856   Total disc arthroplasty (artificial disc), anterior approach, including discectomy with end plate preparation (includes osteophytectomy for nerve root or spinal cord decompression and microdissection), single interspace, cervical

→ *CPT Changes: An Insider's View* 2009

(Do not report 22856 in conjunction with 22554, 22845, 22851, 63075 when performed at the same level)

(Do not report 22856 in conjunction with 69990)

(For additional interspace cervical total disc arthroplasty, use 0092T)

22857   Total disc arthroplasty (artificial disc), anterior approach, including discectomy to prepare interspace (other than for decompression), single interspace, lumbar

→ *CPT Changes: An Insider's View* 2007, 2009

(Do not report 22857 in conjunction with 22558, 22845, 22851, 49010 when performed at the same level)

(For additional interspace, use Category III code 0163T)

22861   Revision including replacement of total disc arthroplasty (artificial disc), anterior approach, single interspace; cervical

→ *CPT Changes: An Insider's View* 2009

(Do not report 22861 in conjunction with 22845, 22851, 22864, 63075 when performed at the same level)

(Do not report 22861 in conjunction with 69990)

Musculoskeletal

(For additional interspace revision of cervical total disc arthroplasty, use 0098T)

22862   lumbar
> *CPT Assistant* Jun 07:1; *CPT Changes: An Insider's View* 2007, 2009

(Do not report 22862 in conjunction with 22558, 22845, 22851, 22865, 49010 when performed at the same level)

(For additional interspace, use Category III code 0165T)

22864   Removal of total disc arthroplasty (artificial disc), anterior approach, single interspace; cervical
> *CPT Changes: An Insider's View* 2009

(Do not report 22864 in conjunction with 22861, 69990)

(For additional interspace removal of cervical total disc arthroplasty, use 0095T)

22865   lumbar
> *CPT Assistant* Jun 07:1; *CPT Changes: An Insider's View* 2007, 2009

(Do not report 22865 in conjunction with 49010)

(For additional interspace, see Category III code 0164T)

(22856-22865 include fluoroscopy when performed)

(For decompression, see 63001-63048)

Other Procedures

22899   Unlisted procedure, spine
> *CPT Assistant* May 00:11, Sep 00:10, Jul 06:19, Feb 10:13, Nov 10:4, Jan 12:14

Abdomen

Excision

22900   Excision, tumor, soft tissue of abdominal wall, subfascial (eg, intramuscular); less than 5 cm
> *CPT Changes: An Insider's View* 2010

22901   5 cm or greater
> *CPT Changes: An Insider's View* 2010

22902   Excision, tumor, soft tissue of abdominal wall, subcutaneous; less than 3 cm
> *CPT Changes: An Insider's View* 2010

22903   3 cm or greater
> *CPT Changes: An Insider's View* 2010

22904   Radical resection of tumor (eg, malignant neoplasm), soft tissue of abdominal wall; less than 5 cm
> *CPT Changes: An Insider's View* 2010

22905   5 cm or greater
> *CPT Changes: An Insider's View* 2010

Other Procedures

22999   Unlisted procedure, abdomen, musculoskeletal system

Shoulder

The area known as the shoulder is made up of the clavicle, scapula, humerus head and neck, sternoclavicular joint, acromioclavicular joint, and shoulder joint.

Incision

23000   Removal of subdeltoid calcareous deposits, open
> *CPT Changes: An Insider's View* 2002, 2003

(For arthroscopic removal of bursal deposits, use 29999)

23020   Capsular contracture release (eg, Sever type procedure)

(For incision and drainage procedures, superficial, see 10040-10160)

23030   Incision and drainage, shoulder area; deep abscess or hematoma

23031   infected bursa

23035   Incision, bone cortex (eg, osteomyelitis or bone abscess), shoulder area

23040   Arthrotomy, glenohumeral joint, including exploration, drainage, or removal of foreign body
> *CPT Assistant* Nov 98:8

23044   Arthrotomy, acromioclavicular, sternoclavicular joint, including exploration, drainage, or removal of foreign body
> *CPT Assistant* Nov 98:8

Excision

23065   Biopsy, soft tissue of shoulder area; superficial

23066   deep

(For needle biopsy of soft tissue, use 20206)

23071   Code is out of numerical sequence. See 23065-23220

23073   Code is out of numerical sequence. See 23065-23220

23075   Excision, tumor, soft tissue of shoulder area, subcutaneous; less than 3 cm
> *CPT Assistant* Summer 92:22, Nov 98:8; *CPT Changes: An Insider's View* 2010

23071   3 cm or greater
> *CPT Changes: An Insider's View* 2010

23076   Excision, tumor, soft tissue of shoulder area, subfascial (eg, intramuscular); less than 5 cm
> *CPT Assistant* Summer 92:22, Oct 09:7; *CPT Changes: An Insider's View* 2010

23073   5 cm or greater
> *CPT Changes: An Insider's View* 2010

23077   Radical resection of tumor (eg, malignant neoplasm), soft tissue of shoulder area; less than 5 cm
> *CPT Changes: An Insider's View* 2010

23078   5 cm or greater
> *CPT Changes: An Insider's View* 2010

23100   Arthrotomy, glenohumeral joint, including biopsy
➔ *CPT Assistant* Nov 98:8

23101   Arthrotomy, acromioclavicular joint or sternoclavicular joint, including biopsy and/or excision of torn cartilage
➔ *CPT Assistant* Nov 98:8

23105   Arthrotomy; glenohumeral joint, with synovectomy, with or without biopsy
➔ *CPT Assistant* Nov 98:8

23106   sternoclavicular joint, with synovectomy, with or without biopsy

23107   Arthrotomy, glenohumeral joint, with joint exploration, with or without removal of loose or foreign body

23120   Claviculectomy; partial

(For arthroscopic procedure, use 29824)

23125   total

23130   Acromioplasty or acromionectomy, partial, with or without coracoacromial ligament release
➔ *CPT Assistant* Aug 01:11

23140   Excision or curettage of bone cyst or benign tumor of clavicle or scapula;

23145   with autograft (includes obtaining graft)

23146   with allograft

23150   Excision or curettage of bone cyst or benign tumor of proximal humerus;

23155   with autograft (includes obtaining graft)

23156   with allograft

23170   Sequestrectomy (eg, for osteomyelitis or bone abscess), clavicle

23172   Sequestrectomy (eg, for osteomyelitis or bone abscess), scapula

23174   Sequestrectomy (eg, for osteomyelitis or bone abscess), humeral head to surgical neck

23180   Partial excision (craterization, saucerization, or diaphysectomy) bone (eg, osteomyelitis), clavicle
➔ *CPT Assistant* Nov 98:9

23182   Partial excision (craterization, saucerization, or diaphysectomy) bone (eg, osteomyelitis), scapula
➔ *CPT Assistant* Nov 98:9

23184   Partial excision (craterization, saucerization, or diaphysectomy) bone (eg, osteomyelitis), proximal humerus
➔ *CPT Assistant* Nov 98:9

23190   Ostectomy of scapula, partial (eg, superior medial angle)

23195   Resection, humeral head

(For replacement with implant, use 23470)

23200   Radical resection of tumor; clavicle
➔ *CPT Changes: An Insider's View* 2010

23210   scapula
➔ *CPT Changes: An Insider's View* 2010

23220   Radical resection of tumor, proximal humerus
➔ *CPT Assistant* Nov 98:8; *CPT Changes: An Insider's View* 2010

(23221, 23222 have been deleted)

Introduction or Removal

(For arthrocentesis or needling of bursa, use 20610)

(For K-wire or pin insertion or removal, see 20650, 20670, 20680)

23330   Removal of foreign body, shoulder; subcutaneous
➔ *CPT Assistant* Aug 99:3

23331   deep (eg, Neer hemiarthroplasty removal)
➔ *CPT Assistant* Aug 99:3

23332   complicated (eg, total shoulder)
➔ *CPT Assistant* Jun 96:10, Nov 98:8, Aug 99:3

▶(Do not report 23331, 23332 in conjunction with 23473, 23474 if a prosthesis [ie, humeral and/or glenoid component(s)] is being removed and replaced in the same shoulder)◀

23350   Injection procedure for shoulder arthrography or enhanced CT/MRI shoulder arthrography
➔ *CPT Assistant* Jul 01:3; *CPT Changes: An Insider's View* 2002
➔ *Clinical Examples in Radiology* Spring 05:5, Spring 09:6, 7

(For radiographic arthrography, radiological supervision and interpretation, use 73040. Fluoroscopy [77002] is inclusive of radiographic arthrography)

(When fluoroscopic guided injection is performed for enhanced CT arthrography, use 23350, 77002, and 73201 or 73202)

(When fluoroscopic guided injection is performed for enhanced MR arthrography, use 23350, 77002, and 73222 or 73223)

(For enhanced CT or enhanced MRI arthrography, use 77002 and either 73201, 73202, 73222, or 73223)

(To report biopsy of the shoulder and joint, see 29805-29826)

Repair, Revision, and/or Reconstruction

23395   Muscle transfer, any type, shoulder or upper arm; single

23397   multiple

23400   Scapulopexy (eg, Sprengels deformity or for paralysis)

23405   Tenotomy, shoulder area; single tendon
➔ *CPT Assistant* Nov 98:8

23406   multiple tendons through same incision
➔ *CPT Assistant* Nov 98:8

23410   Repair of ruptured musculotendinous cuff (eg, rotator cuff) open; acute
➔ *CPT Assistant* Aug 01:11, Feb 02:11; *CPT Changes: An Insider's View* 2003

Musculoskeletal

23412   chronic
➔ *CPT Assistant* Feb 02:11

(For arthroscopic procedure, use 29827)

23415   Coracoacromial ligament release, with or without acromioplasty

(For arthroscopic procedure, use 29826)

23420   Reconstruction of complete shoulder (rotator) cuff avulsion, chronic (includes acromioplasty)
➔ *CPT Assistant* Feb 02:11, Oct 05:23

23430   Tenodesis of long tendon of biceps

(For arthroscopic biceps tenodesis, use 29828)

23440   Resection or transplantation of long tendon of biceps

23450   Capsulorrhaphy, anterior; Putti-Platt procedure or Magnuson type operation

(To report arthroscopic thermal capsulorrhaphy, use 29999)

23455   with labral repair (eg, Bankart procedure)
➔ *CPT Assistant* Nov 98:8

(For arthroscopic procedure, use 29806)

23460   Capsulorrhaphy, anterior, any type; with bone block

23462   with coracoid process transfer

(To report open thermal capsulorrhaphy, use 23929)

23465   Capsulorrhaphy, glenohumeral joint, posterior, with or without bone block
➔ *CPT Assistant* Nov 98:8

(For sternoclavicular and acromioclavicular reconstruction, see 23530, 23550)

23466   Capsulorrhaphy, glenohumeral joint, any type multi-directional instability
➔ *CPT Assistant* Nov 98:8

23470   Arthroplasty, glenohumeral joint; hemiarthroplasty
➔ *CPT Assistant* Nov 98:8

23472   total shoulder (glenoid and proximal humeral replacement (eg, total shoulder))
➔ *CPT Assistant* Jun 96:10, Nov 98:8

(For removal of total shoulder implants, see 23331, 23332)

(For osteotomy, proximal humerus, use 24400)

● **23473**   Revision of total shoulder arthroplasty, including allograft when performed; humeral **or** glenoid component
➔ *CPT Changes: An Insider's View* 2013

● **23474**   humeral **and** glenoid component
➔ *CPT Changes: An Insider's View* 2013

▶(Do not report 23473, 23474 in conjunction with 23331, 23332 if a prosthesis [ie, humeral and/or glenoid component(s)] is being removed and replaced in the same shoulder)◀

23480   Osteotomy, clavicle, with or without internal fixation;

23485   with bone graft for nonunion or malunion (includes obtaining graft and/or necessary fixation)

23490   Prophylactic treatment (nailing, pinning, plating or wiring) with or without methylmethacrylate; clavicle

23491   proximal humerus
➔ *CPT Assistant* Nov 98:8

Fracture and/or Dislocation

23500   Closed treatment of clavicular fracture; without manipulation

23505   with manipulation

23515   Open treatment of clavicular fracture, includes internal fixation, when performed
➔ *CPT Assistant* Jan 08:4; *CPT Changes: An Insider's View* 2008

23520   Closed treatment of sternoclavicular dislocation; without manipulation

23525   with manipulation

23530   Open treatment of sternoclavicular dislocation, acute or chronic;

23532   with fascial graft (includes obtaining graft)

23540   Closed treatment of acromioclavicular dislocation; without manipulation

23545   with manipulation

23550   Open treatment of acromioclavicular dislocation, acute or chronic;

23552   with fascial graft (includes obtaining graft)

23570   Closed treatment of scapular fracture; without manipulation

23575   with manipulation, with or without skeletal traction (with or without shoulder joint involvement)

23585   Open treatment of scapular fracture (body, glenoid or acromion) includes internal fixation, when performed
➔ *CPT Assistant* Oct 04:10; *CPT Changes: An Insider's View* 2009

23600   Closed treatment of proximal humeral (surgical or anatomical neck) fracture; without manipulation

23605   with manipulation, with or without skeletal traction

23615   Open treatment of proximal humeral (surgical or anatomical neck) fracture, includes internal fixation, when performed, includes repair of tuberosity(s), when performed;
➔ *CPT Assistant* Jan 08:4; *CPT Changes: An Insider's View* 2008

23616   with proximal humeral prosthetic replacement
➔ *CPT Changes: An Insider's View* 2008

23620   Closed treatment of greater humeral tuberosity fracture; without manipulation
➔ *CPT Assistant* Nov 98:8

23625   with manipulation

23630   Open treatment of greater humeral tuberosity fracture, includes internal fixation, when performed
> *CPT Assistant* Nov 98:8; *CPT Changes: An Insider's View* 2008

23650   Closed treatment of shoulder dislocation, with manipulation; without anesthesia

23655   requiring anesthesia

23660   Open treatment of acute shoulder dislocation
> *CPT Assistant* Feb 96:5

(Repairs for recurrent dislocations, see 23450-23466)

23665   Closed treatment of shoulder dislocation, with fracture of greater humeral tuberosity, with manipulation
> *CPT Assistant* Nov 98:8

23670   Open treatment of shoulder dislocation, with fracture of greater humeral tuberosity, includes internal fixation, when performed
> *CPT Assistant* Nov 98:8; *CPT Changes: An Insider's View* 2008

23675   Closed treatment of shoulder dislocation, with surgical or anatomical neck fracture, with manipulation

23680   Open treatment of shoulder dislocation, with surgical or anatomical neck fracture, includes internal fixation, when performed
> *CPT Changes: An Insider's View* 2008

Manipulation

23700   Manipulation under anesthesia, shoulder joint, including application of fixation apparatus (dislocation excluded)
> *CPT Assistant* Jan 99:10, Apr 05:14, May 09:8

Arthrodesis

23800   Arthrodesis, glenohumeral joint;
> *CPT Assistant* Nov 98:8

23802   with autogenous graft (includes obtaining graft)

Amputation

23900   Interthoracoscapular amputation (forequarter)

23920   Disarticulation of shoulder;

23921   secondary closure or scar revision

Other Procedures

23929   Unlisted procedure, shoulder

Humerus (Upper Arm) and Elbow

The elbow area includes the head and neck of the radius and olecranon process.

Incision

(For incision and drainage procedures, superficial, see 10040-10160)

23930   Incision and drainage, upper arm or elbow area; deep abscess or hematoma

23931   bursa
> *CPT Assistant* Nov 98:8

23935   Incision, deep, with opening of bone cortex (eg, for osteomyelitis or bone abscess), humerus or elbow

24000   Arthrotomy, elbow, including exploration, drainage, or removal of foreign body
> *CPT Assistant* Nov 98:8-9

24006   Arthrotomy of the elbow, with capsular excision for capsular release (separate procedure)

Excision

24065   Biopsy, soft tissue of upper arm or elbow area; superficial

24066   deep (subfascial or intramuscular)

(For needle biopsy of soft tissue, use 20206)

24071   Code is out of numerical sequence. See 24065-24155

24073   Code is out of numerical sequence. See 24065-24155

24075   Excision, tumor, soft tissue of upper arm or elbow area, subcutaneous; less than 3 cm
> *CPT Changes: An Insider's View* 2002, 2010

 # 24071   3 cm or greater
> *CPT Changes: An Insider's View* 2010

24076   Excision, tumor, soft tissue of upper arm or elbow area, subfascial (eg, intramuscular); less than 5 cm
> *CPT Changes: An Insider's View* 2010

 # 24073   5 cm or greater
> *CPT Changes: An Insider's View* 2010

24077   Radical resection of tumor (eg, malignant neoplasm), soft tissue of upper arm or elbow area; less than 5 cm
> *CPT Changes: An Insider's View* 2010

24079   5 cm or greater
> *CPT Changes: An Insider's View* 2010

24100   Arthrotomy, elbow; with synovial biopsy only

24101   with joint exploration, with or without biopsy, with or without removal of loose or foreign body

24102   with synovectomy

24105   Excision, olecranon bursa

24110   Excision or curettage of bone cyst or benign tumor, humerus;

24115   with autograft (includes obtaining graft)

24116   with allograft

24120   Excision or curettage of bone cyst or benign tumor of head or neck of radius or olecranon process;

24125   with autograft (includes obtaining graft)

24126   with allograft

24130   Excision, radial head

(For replacement with implant, use 24366)

Musculoskeletal

24134   Sequestrectomy (eg, for osteomyelitis or bone abscess), shaft or distal humerus

24136   Sequestrectomy (eg, for osteomyelitis or bone abscess), radial head or neck

24138   Sequestrectomy (eg, for osteomyelitis or bone abscess), olecranon process

24140   Partial excision (craterization, saucerization, or diaphysectomy) bone (eg, osteomyelitis), humerus
   ➡ *CPT Assistant* Nov 98:9

24145   Partial excision (craterization, saucerization, or diaphysectomy) bone (eg, osteomyelitis), radial head or neck
   ➡ *CPT Assistant* Nov 98:9

24147   Partial excision (craterization, saucerization, or diaphysectomy) bone (eg, osteomyelitis), olecranon process
   ➡ *CPT Assistant* Nov 98:9

24149   Radical resection of capsule, soft tissue, and heterotopic bone, elbow, with contracture release (separate procedure)
   ➡ *CPT Assistant* Nov 96:4

   (For capsular and soft tissue release only, use 24006)

24150   Radical resection of tumor, shaft or distal humerus
   ➡ *CPT Changes: An Insider's View* 2010

   (24151 has been deleted)

24152   Radical resection of tumor, radial head or neck
   ➡ *CPT Changes: An Insider's View* 2010

   (24153 has been deleted)

24155   Resection of elbow joint (arthrectomy)

Introduction or Removal

(For K-wire or pin insertion or removal, see 20650, 20670, 20680)

(For arthrocentesis or needling of bursa or joint, use 20605)

24160   Implant removal; elbow joint

   ▶(Do not report 24160 in conjunction with 24370 or 24371 if a prosthesis [ie, humeral and/or ulnar component(s)] is being removed and replaced in the same elbow)◀

24164   radial head

24200   Removal of foreign body, upper arm or elbow area; subcutaneous

24201   deep (subfascial or intramuscular)
   ➡ *CPT Assistant* Nov 98:8

24220   Injection procedure for elbow arthrography

(For radiological supervision and interpretation, use 73085. Do not report 77002 in conjunction with 73085)

(For injection for tennis elbow, use 20550)

Repair, Revision, and/or Reconstruction

24300   Manipulation, elbow, under anesthesia
   ➡ *CPT Changes: An Insider's View* 2002

   (For application of external fixation, see 20690 or 20692)

24301   Muscle or tendon transfer, any type, upper arm or elbow, single (excluding 24320-24331)

24305   Tendon lengthening, upper arm or elbow, each tendon
   ➡ *CPT Assistant* Nov 98:8

24310   Tenotomy, open, elbow to shoulder, each tendon
   ➡ *CPT Assistant* Nov 98:8

24320   Tenoplasty, with muscle transfer, with or without free graft, elbow to shoulder, single (Seddon-Brookes type procedure)

24330   Flexor-plasty, elbow (eg, Steindler type advancement);

24331   with extensor advancement

24332   Tenolysis, triceps
   ➡ *CPT Changes: An Insider's View* 2002

24340   Tenodesis of biceps tendon at elbow (separate procedure)

24341   Repair, tendon or muscle, upper arm or elbow, each tendon or muscle, primary or secondary (excludes rotator cuff)
   ➡ *CPT Assistant* Nov 96:4

24342   Reinsertion of ruptured biceps or triceps tendon, distal, with or without tendon graft
   ➡ *CPT Assistant* Nov 96:4

24343   Repair lateral collateral ligament, elbow, with local tissue
   ➡ *CPT Changes: An Insider's View* 2002

24344   Reconstruction lateral collateral ligament, elbow, with tendon graft (includes harvesting of graft)
   ➡ *CPT Changes: An Insider's View* 2002

24345   Repair medial collateral ligament, elbow, with local tissue
   ➡ *CPT Changes: An Insider's View* 2002

24346   Reconstruction medial collateral ligament, elbow, with tendon graft (includes harvesting of graft)
   ➡ *CPT Changes: An Insider's View* 2002

24357   Tenotomy, elbow, lateral or medial (eg, epicondylitis, tennis elbow, golfer's elbow); percutaneous
   ➡ *CPT Assistant* Jan 08:4; *CPT Changes: An Insider's View* 2008

24358   debridement, soft tissue and/or bone, open
   ➡ *CPT Assistant* Jan 08:4; *CPT Changes: An Insider's View* 2008

Musculoskeletal

24359 debridement, soft tissue and/or bone, open with tendon repair or reattachment

→ *CPT Assistant* Jan 08:4; *CPT Changes: An Insider's View* 2008

(Do not report 24357-24359 in conjunction with 29837, 29838)

24360 Arthroplasty, elbow; with membrane (eg, fascial)

→ *CPT Assistant* Nov 98:8

24361 with distal humeral prosthetic replacement

24362 with implant and fascia lata ligament reconstruction

24363 with distal humerus and proximal ulnar prosthetic replacement (eg, total elbow)

►(For revision of total elbow implant, see 24370, 24371)◄

24365 Arthroplasty, radial head;

24366 with implant

● **24370** Revision of total elbow arthroplasty, including allograft when performed; humeral **or** ulnar component

→ *CPT Changes: An Insider's View* 2013

● **24371** humeral **and** ulnar component

→ *CPT Changes: An Insider's View* 2013

►(Do not report 24370, 24371 in conjunction with 24160 if a prosthesis [ie, humeral and/or ulnar component(s)] is being removed and replaced in the same elbow)◄

24400 Osteotomy, humerus, with or without internal fixation

24410 Multiple osteotomies with realignment on intramedullary rod, humeral shaft (Sofield type procedure)

24420 Osteoplasty, humerus (eg, shortening or lengthening) (excluding 64876)

24430 Repair of nonunion or malunion, humerus; without graft (eg, compression technique)

24435 with iliac or other autograft (includes obtaining graft)

(For proximal radius and/or ulna, see 25400-25420)

24470 Hemiepiphyseal arrest (eg, cubitus varus or valgus, distal humerus)

24495 Decompression fasciotomy, forearm, with brachial artery exploration

24498 Prophylactic treatment (nailing, pinning, plating or wiring), with or without methylmethacrylate, humeral shaft

→ *CPT Assistant* Nov 98:8

Fracture and/or Dislocation

24500 Closed treatment of humeral shaft fracture; without manipulation

24505 with manipulation, with or without skeletal traction

24515 Open treatment of humeral shaft fracture with plate/screws, with or without cerclage

24516 Treatment of humeral shaft fracture, with insertion of intramedullary implant, with or without cerclage and/or locking screws

→ *CPT Assistant* Feb 96:4, Jun 09:7; *CPT Changes: An Insider's View* 2003

24530 Closed treatment of supracondylar or transcondylar humeral fracture, with or without intercondylar extension; without manipulation

24535 with manipulation, with or without skin or skeletal traction

24538 Percutaneous skeletal fixation of supracondylar or transcondylar humeral fracture, with or without intercondylar extension

→ *CPT Assistant* Winter 92:10

24545 Open treatment of humeral supracondylar or transcondylar fracture, includes internal fixation, when performed; without intercondylar extension

→ *CPT Changes: An Insider's View* 2008

24546 with intercondylar extension

→ *CPT Changes: An Insider's View* 2008

24560 Closed treatment of humeral epicondylar fracture, medial or lateral; without manipulation

24565 with manipulation

24566 Percutaneous skeletal fixation of humeral epicondylar fracture, medial or lateral, with manipulation

24575 Open treatment of humeral epicondylar fracture, medial or lateral, includes internal fixation, when performed

→ *CPT Changes: An Insider's View* 2008

24576 Closed treatment of humeral condylar fracture, medial or lateral; without manipulation

24577 with manipulation

24579 Open treatment of humeral condylar fracture, medial or lateral, includes internal fixation, when performed

→ *CPT Changes: An Insider's View* 2008

(To report closed treatment of fractures without manipulation, see 24530, 24560, 24576, 24650, 24670)

(To report closed treatment of fractures with manipulation, see 24535, 24565, 24577, 24675)

24582 Percutaneous skeletal fixation of humeral condylar fracture, medial or lateral, with manipulation

24586 Open treatment of periarticular fracture and/or dislocation of the elbow (fracture distal humerus and proximal ulna and/or proximal radius);

24587 with implant arthroplasty

(See also 24361)

24600 Treatment of closed elbow dislocation; without anesthesia

24605 requiring anesthesia

24615 Open treatment of acute or chronic elbow dislocation

Musculoskeletal

24620   Closed treatment of Monteggia type of fracture dislocation at elbow (fracture proximal end of ulna with dislocation of radial head), with manipulation

24635   Open treatment of Monteggia type of fracture dislocation at elbow (fracture proximal end of ulna with dislocation of radial head), includes internal fixation, when performed
➔ *CPT Changes: An Insider's View* 2008

24640   Closed treatment of radial head subluxation in child, nursemaid elbow, with manipulation

24650   Closed treatment of radial head or neck fracture; without manipulation

24655   with manipulation

24665   Open treatment of radial head or neck fracture, includes internal fixation or radial head excision, when performed;
➔ *CPT Changes: An Insider's View* 2008

24666   with radial head prosthetic replacement
➔ *CPT Changes: An Insider's View* 2008

24670   Closed treatment of ulnar fracture, proximal end (eg, olecranon or coronoid process[es]); without manipulation
➔ *CPT Changes: An Insider's View* 2008

24675   with manipulation
➔ *CPT Changes: An Insider's View* 2008

24685   Open treatment of ulnar fracture, proximal end (eg, olecranon or coronoid process[es]), includes internal fixation, when performed
➔ *CPT Changes: An Insider's View* 2008

(Do not report 24685 in conjunction with 24100-24102)

Arthrodesis

24800   Arthrodesis, elbow joint; local

24802   with autogenous graft (includes obtaining graft)

Amputation

24900   Amputation, arm through humerus; with primary closure

24920   open, circular (guillotine)

24925   secondary closure or scar revision

24930   re-amputation

24931   with implant

24935   Stump elongation, upper extremity

24940   Cineplasty, upper extremity, complete procedure

Other Procedures

24999   Unlisted procedure, humerus or elbow

Forearm and Wrist

Radius, ulna, carpal bones, and joints.

Incision

25000   Incision, extensor tendon sheath, wrist (eg, deQuervains disease)
➔ *CPT Assistant* Nov 98:8

(For decompression median nerve or for carpal tunnel syndrome, use 64721)

25001   Incision, flexor tendon sheath, wrist (eg, flexor carpi radialis)
➔ *CPT Changes: An Insider's View* 2002

25020   Decompression fasciotomy, forearm and/or wrist, flexor OR extensor compartment; without debridement of nonviable muscle and/or nerve
➔ *CPT Changes: An Insider's View* 2002

25023   with debridement of nonviable muscle and/or nerve

(For decompression fasciotomy with brachial artery exploration, use 24495)

(For incision and drainage procedures, superficial, see 10060-10160)

(For debridement, see also 11000-11044)

25024   Decompression fasciotomy, forearm and/or wrist, flexor AND extensor compartment; without debridement of nonviable muscle and/or nerve
➔ *CPT Changes: An Insider's View* 2002

25025   with debridement of nonviable muscle and/or nerve
➔ *CPT Changes: An Insider's View* 2002

25028   Incision and drainage, forearm and/or wrist; deep abscess or hematoma

25031   bursa
➔ *CPT Assistant* Nov 98:9

25035   Incision, deep, bone cortex, forearm and/or wrist (eg, osteomyelitis or bone abscess)

25040   Arthrotomy, radiocarpal or midcarpal joint, with exploration, drainage, or removal of foreign body

Excision

25065   Biopsy, soft tissue of forearm and/or wrist; superficial

25066   deep (subfascial or intramuscular)
➔ *CPT Assistant* Nov 98:8

(For needle biopsy of soft tissue, use 20206)

25071   Code is out of numerical sequence. See 25065-25240

25073   Code is out of numerical sequence. See 25065-25240

25075   Excision, tumor, soft tissue of forearm and/or wrist area, subcutaneous; less than 3 cm
➔ *CPT Changes: An Insider's View* 2002, 2010

25071   3 cm or greater
➔ *CPT Changes: An Insider's View* 2010

Musculoskeletal

25076   Excision, tumor, soft tissue of forearm and/or wrist area, subfascial (eg, intramuscular); less than 3 cm
→ *CPT Changes: An Insider's View* 2010

25073   3 cm or greater
→ *CPT Changes: An Insider's View* 2010

25077   Radical resection of tumor (eg, malignant neoplasm), soft tissue of forearm and/or wrist area; less than 3 cm
→ *CPT Changes: An Insider's View* 2010

25078   3 cm or greater
→ *CPT Changes: An Insider's View* 2010

25085   Capsulotomy, wrist (eg, contracture)

25100   Arthrotomy, wrist joint; with biopsy

25101   with joint exploration, with or without biopsy, with or without removal of loose or foreign body

25105   with synovectomy

25107   Arthrotomy, distal radioulnar joint including repair of triangular cartilage, complex

25109   Excision of tendon, forearm and/or wrist, flexor or extensor, each
→ *CPT Changes: An Insider's View* 2007

25110   Excision, lesion of tendon sheath, forearm and/or wrist

25111   Excision of ganglion, wrist (dorsal or volar); primary

25112   recurrent

(For hand or finger, use 26160)

25115   Radical excision of bursa, synovia of wrist, or forearm tendon sheaths (eg, tenosynovitis, fungus, Tbc, or other granulomas, rheumatoid arthritis); flexors
→ *CPT Assistant* Jun 12:15

25116   extensors, with or without transposition of dorsal retinaculum

(For finger synovectomies, use 26145)

25118   Synovectomy, extensor tendon sheath, wrist, single compartment;
→ *CPT Assistant* Apr 12:17

25119   with resection of distal ulna

25120   Excision or curettage of bone cyst or benign tumor of radius or ulna (excluding head or neck of radius and olecranon process);

(For head or neck of radius or olecranon process, see 24120-24126)

25125   with autograft (includes obtaining graft)

25126   with allograft

25130   Excision or curettage of bone cyst or benign tumor of carpal bones;

25135   with autograft (includes obtaining graft)

25136   with allograft

25145   Sequestrectomy (eg, for osteomyelitis or bone abscess), forearm and/or wrist

25150   Partial excision (craterization, saucerization, or diaphysectomy) of bone (eg, for osteomyelitis); ulna

25151   radius

(For head or neck of radius or olecranon process, see 24145, 24147)

25170   Radical resection of tumor, radius or ulna
→ *CPT Changes: An Insider's View* 2010

25210   Carpectomy; 1 bone

(For carpectomy with implant, see 25441-25445)

25215   all bones of proximal row

25230   Radial styloidectomy (separate procedure)

25240   Excision distal ulna partial or complete (eg, Darrach type or matched resection)

(For implant replacement, distal ulna, use 25442)

(For obtaining fascia for interposition, see 20920, 20922)

Introduction or Removal

(For K-wire, pin or rod insertion or removal, see 20650, 20670, 20680)

25246   Injection procedure for wrist arthrography

(For radiological supervision and interpretation, use 73115. Do not report 77002 in conjunction with 73115)

(For foreign body removal, superficial use 20520)

25248   Exploration with removal of deep foreign body, forearm or wrist

25250   Removal of wrist prosthesis; (separate procedure)

25251   complicated, including total wrist

25259   Manipulation, wrist, under anesthesia
→ *CPT Assistant* Jan 04:27, Jun 05:12; *CPT Changes: An Insider's View* 2002

(For application of external fixation, see 20690 or 20692)

Repair, Revision, and/or Reconstruction

25260   Repair, tendon or muscle, flexor, forearm and/or wrist; primary, single, each tendon or muscle

25263   secondary, single, each tendon or muscle

25265   secondary, with free graft (includes obtaining graft), each tendon or muscle

25270   Repair, tendon or muscle, extensor, forearm and/or wrist; primary, single, each tendon or muscle

25272   secondary, single, each tendon or muscle

25274   secondary, with free graft (includes obtaining graft), each tendon or muscle
→ *CPT Changes: An Insider's View* 2002

Musculoskeletal

25275   Repair, tendon sheath, extensor, forearm and/or wrist, with free graft (includes obtaining graft) (eg, for extensor carpi ulnaris subluxation)
> *CPT Changes: An Insider's View* 2002

25280   Lengthening or shortening of flexor or extensor tendon, forearm and/or wrist, single, each tendon

25290   Tenotomy, open, flexor or extensor tendon, forearm and/or wrist, single, each tendon

25295   Tenolysis, flexor or extensor tendon, forearm and/or wrist, single, each tendon
> *CPT Assistant* Apr 97:11, Aug 98:10

25300   Tenodesis at wrist; flexors of fingers

25301   extensors of fingers

25310   Tendon transplantation or transfer, flexor or extensor, forearm and/or wrist, single; each tendon
> *CPT Assistant* Jun 02:11

25312   with tendon graft(s) (includes obtaining graft), each tendon

25315   Flexor origin slide (eg, for cerebral palsy, Volkmann contracture), forearm and/or wrist;

25316   with tendon(s) transfer

25320   Capsulorrhaphy or reconstruction, wrist, open (eg, capsulodesis, ligament repair, tendon transfer or graft) (includes synovectomy, capsulotomy and open reduction) for carpal instability
> *CPT Changes: An Insider's View* 2003

25332   Arthroplasty, wrist, with or without interposition, with or without external or internal fixation
> *CPT Assistant* Nov 96:5, Jan 05:8

          (For obtaining fascia for interposition, see 20920, 20922)

          (For prosthetic replacement arthroplasty, see 25441-25446)

25335   Centralization of wrist on ulna (eg, radial club hand)

25337   Reconstruction for stabilization of unstable distal ulna or distal radioulnar joint, secondary by soft tissue stabilization (eg, tendon transfer, tendon graft or weave, or tenodesis) with or without open reduction of distal radioulnar joint

          (For harvesting of fascia lata graft, see 20920, 20922)

25350   Osteotomy, radius; distal third

25355   middle or proximal third

25360   Osteotomy; ulna

25365   radius AND ulna

25370   Multiple osteotomies, with realignment on intramedullary rod (Sofield type procedure); radius OR ulna

25375   radius AND ulna

25390   Osteoplasty, radius OR ulna; shortening

25391   lengthening with autograft

25392   Osteoplasty, radius AND ulna; shortening (excluding 64876)

25393   lengthening with autograft

25394   Osteoplasty, carpal bone, shortening
> *CPT Changes: An Insider's View* 2002

25400   Repair of nonunion or malunion, radius OR ulna; without graft (eg, compression technique)

25405   with autograft (includes obtaining graft)
> *CPT Changes: An Insider's View* 2002

25415   Repair of nonunion or malunion, radius AND ulna; without graft (eg, compression technique)

25420   with autograft (includes obtaining graft)
> *CPT Changes: An Insider's View* 2002

25425   Repair of defect with autograft; radius OR ulna

25426   radius AND ulna

25430   Insertion of vascular pedicle into carpal bone (eg, Hori procedure)
> *CPT Changes: An Insider's View* 2002

25431   Repair of nonunion of carpal bone (excluding carpal scaphoid (navicular)) (includes obtaining graft and necessary fixation), each bone
> *CPT Changes: An Insider's View* 2002

25440   Repair of nonunion, scaphoid carpal (navicular) bone, with or without radial styloidectomy (includes obtaining graft and necessary fixation)
> *CPT Changes: An Insider's View* 2002

25441   Arthroplasty with prosthetic replacement; distal radius
> *CPT Assistant* Jan 05:8-9

25442   distal ulna
> *CPT Assistant* Jan 05:8-9

25443   scaphoid carpal (navicular)
> *CPT Assistant* Jan 05:8-9; *CPT Changes: An Insider's View* 2002

25444   lunate
> *CPT Assistant* Jan 05:8,10

25445   trapezium
> *CPT Assistant* Jan 05:8,10

25446   distal radius and partial or entire carpus (total wrist)
> *CPT Assistant* Jan 05:8,11

25447   Arthroplasty, interposition, intercarpal or carpometacarpal joints
> *CPT Assistant* Nov 98:8, Jan 05:8, 11-12

          (For wrist arthroplasty, use 25332)

25449   Revision of arthroplasty, including removal of implant, wrist joint

25450   Epiphyseal arrest by epiphysiodesis or stapling; distal radius OR ulna

25455   distal radius AND ulna

25490   Prophylactic treatment (nailing, pinning, plating or wiring) with or without methylmethacrylate; radius

Musculoskeletal

| 25491 | ulna |
| 25492 | radius AND ulna |

Fracture and/or Dislocation

(For application of external fixation in addition to internal fixation, use 20690 and the appropriate internal fixation code)

25500 Closed treatment of radial shaft fracture; without manipulation

25505 with manipulation

25515 Open treatment of radial shaft fracture, includes internal fixation, when performed
➔ *CPT Changes: An Insider's View* 2008

25520 Closed treatment of radial shaft fracture and closed treatment of dislocation of distal radioulnar joint (Galeazzi fracture/dislocation)
➔ *CPT Changes: An Insider's View* 2002

25525 Open treatment of radial shaft fracture, includes internal fixation, when performed, and closed treatment of distal radioulnar joint dislocation (Galeazzi fracture/dislocation), includes percutaneous skeletal fixation, when performed
➔ *CPT Changes: An Insider's View* 2008

25526 Open treatment of radial shaft fracture, includes internal fixation, when performed, and open treatment of distal radioulnar joint dislocation (Galeazzi fracture/dislocation), includes internal fixation, when performed, includes repair of triangular fibrocartilage complex
➔ *CPT Changes: An Insider's View* 2002, 2008

25530 Closed treatment of ulnar shaft fracture; without manipulation
➔ *CPT Assistant* Apr 02:14

25535 with manipulation
➔ *CPT Assistant* Sep 10:7

25545 Open treatment of ulnar shaft fracture, includes internal fixation, when performed
➔ *CPT Assistant* Fall 93:23, Oct 99:5; *CPT Changes: An Insider's View* 2008

25560 Closed treatment of radial and ulnar shaft fractures; without manipulation

25565 with manipulation

25574 Open treatment of radial AND ulnar shaft fractures, with internal fixation, when performed; of radius OR ulna
➔ *CPT Assistant* Fall 93:23, Oct 99:5; *CPT Changes: An Insider's View* 2008

25575 of radius AND ulna
➔ *CPT Changes: An Insider's View* 2008

25600 Closed treatment of distal radial fracture (eg, Colles or Smith type) or epiphyseal separation, includes closed treatment of fracture of ulnar styloid, when performed; without manipulation
➔ *CPT Assistant* Oct 07:7; *CPT Changes: An Insider's View* 2007

25605 with manipulation
➔ *CPT Assistant* Oct 07:7

(Do not report 25600, 25605 in conjunction with 25650)

25606 Percutaneous skeletal fixation of distal radial fracture or epiphyseal separation
➔ *CPT Changes: An Insider's View* 2007

(Do not report 25606 in conjunction with 25650)

(For percutaneous treatment of ulnar styloid fracture, use 25651)

(For open treatment of ulnar styloid fracture, use 25652)

25607 Open treatment of distal radial extra-articular fracture or epiphyseal separation, with internal fixation
➔ *CPT Assistant* Oct 07:7; *CPT Changes: An Insider's View* 2007

(Do not report 25607 in conjunction with 25650)

(For percutaneous treatment of ulnar styloid fracture, use 25651)

(For open treatment of ulnar styloid fracture, use 25652)

25608 Open treatment of distal radial intra-articular fracture or epiphyseal separation; with internal fixation of 2 fragments
➔ *CPT Assistant* Oct 07:7; *CPT Changes: An Insider's View* 2007

(Do not report 25608 in conjunction with 25609)

25609 with internal fixation of 3 or more fragments
➔ *CPT Assistant* Oct 07:7; *CPT Changes: An Insider's View* 2007

(Do not report 25608, 25609 in conjunction with 25650)

(For percutaneous treatment of ulnar styloid fracture, use 25651)

(For open treatment of ulnar styloid fracture, use 25652)

25622 Closed treatment of carpal scaphoid (navicular) fracture; without manipulation

25624 with manipulation

25628 Open treatment of carpal scaphoid (navicular) fracture, includes internal fixation, when performed
➔ *CPT Changes: An Insider's View* 2008

25630 Closed treatment of carpal bone fracture (excluding carpal scaphoid [navicular]); without manipulation, each bone

25635 with manipulation, each bone

25645 Open treatment of carpal bone fracture (other than carpal scaphoid [navicular]), each bone
➔ *CPT Changes: An Insider's View* 2002

25650 Closed treatment of ulnar styloid fracture
➔ *CPT Assistant* Oct 07:7

(Do not report 25650 in conjunction with 25600, 25605, 25607-25609)

25651 Percutaneous skeletal fixation of ulnar styloid fracture
➔ *CPT Changes: An Insider's View* 2002

Musculoskeletal

25652 Open treatment of ulnar styloid fracture
→ *CPT Assistant* Oct 07:7; *CPT Changes: An Insider's View* 2002

25660 Closed treatment of radiocarpal or intercarpal dislocation, 1 or more bones, with manipulation

25670 Open treatment of radiocarpal or intercarpal dislocation, 1 or more bones

25671 Percutaneous skeletal fixation of distal radioulnar dislocation
→ *CPT Changes: An Insider's View* 2002

25675 Closed treatment of distal radioulnar dislocation with manipulation

25676 Open treatment of distal radioulnar dislocation, acute or chronic

25680 Closed treatment of trans-scaphoperilunar type of fracture dislocation, with manipulation

25685 Open treatment of trans-scaphoperilunar type of fracture dislocation

25690 Closed treatment of lunate dislocation, with manipulation

25695 Open treatment of lunate dislocation

Arthrodesis

25800 Arthrodesis, wrist; complete, without bone graft (includes radiocarpal and/or intercarpal and/or carpometacarpal joints)
→ *CPT Assistant* Nov 98:8

25805 with sliding graft

25810 with iliac or other autograft (includes obtaining graft)

25820 Arthrodesis, wrist; limited, without bone graft (eg, intercarpal or radiocarpal)
→ *CPT Assistant* Nov 98:8

25825 with autograft (includes obtaining graft)
→ *CPT Assistant* Jul 12:12

25830 Arthrodesis, distal radioulnar joint with segmental resection of ulna, with or without bone graft (eg, Sauve-Kapandji procedure)
→ *CPT Assistant* Nov 98:8

Amputation

25900 Amputation, forearm, through radius and ulna;

25905 open, circular (guillotine)

25907 secondary closure or scar revision

25909 re-amputation

25915 Krukenberg procedure

25920 Disarticulation through wrist;

25922 secondary closure or scar revision

25924 re-amputation

25927 Transmetacarpal amputation;

25929 secondary closure or scar revision

25931 re-amputation

Other Procedures

25999 Unlisted procedure, forearm or wrist

Hand and Fingers

Incision

26010 Drainage of finger abscess; simple

26011 complicated (eg, felon)

26020 Drainage of tendon sheath, digit and/or palm, each

26025 Drainage of palmar bursa; single, bursa
→ *CPT Assistant* Nov 98:8

26030 multiple bursa
→ *CPT Assistant* Nov 98:8

26034 Incision, bone cortex, hand or finger (eg, osteomyelitis or bone abscess)
→ *CPT Assistant* Nov 98:8

26035 Decompression fingers and/or hand, injection injury (eg, grease gun)

26037 Decompressive fasciotomy, hand (excludes 26035)

(For injection injury, use 26035)

26040 Fasciotomy, palmar (eg, Dupuytren's contracture); percutaneous
→ *CPT Assistant* Nov 98:8, Apr 10:10, Oct 10:10, Jun 11:13

26045 open, partial
→ *CPT Assistant* Jun 11:13

(For palmar fasciotomy by enzyme injection (eg, collagenase), see 20527, 26341)

(For fasciectomy, see 26121-26125)

26055 Tendon sheath incision (eg, for trigger finger)

26060 Tenotomy, percutaneous, single, each digit

26070 Arthrotomy, with exploration, drainage, or removal of loose or foreign body; carpometacarpal joint
→ *CPT Assistant* Nov 98:10

26075 metacarpophalangeal joint, each

26080 interphalangeal joint, each

Excision

26100 Arthrotomy with biopsy; carpometacarpal joint, each

26105 metacarpophalangeal joint, each

26110 interphalangeal joint, each

26111 Code is out of numerical sequence. See 26100-26262

26113 Code is out of numerical sequence. See 26100-26262

26115   Excision, tumor or vascular malformation, soft tissue of hand or finger, subcutaneous; less than 1.5 cm
➔ *CPT Changes: An Insider's View* 2002, 2010

 # 26111   1.5 cm or greater
➔ *CPT Changes: An Insider's View* 2010

26116   Excision, tumor, soft tissue, or vascular malformation, of hand or finger, subfascial (eg, intramuscular); less than 1.5 cm
➔ *CPT Assistant* Apr 10:3; *CPT Changes: An Insider's View* 2002, 2010

 # 26113   1.5 cm or greater
➔ *CPT Changes: An Insider's View* 2010

26117   Radical resection of tumor (eg, malignant neoplasm), soft tissue of hand or finger; less than 3 cm
➔ *CPT Changes: An Insider's View* 2010

26118   3 cm or greater
➔ *CPT Changes: An Insider's View* 2010

26121   Fasciectomy, palm only, with or without Z-plasty, other local tissue rearrangement, or skin grafting (includes obtaining graft)
➔ *CPT Assistant* Oct 10:10, Jun 11:13

26123   Fasciectomy, partial palmar with release of single digit including proximal interphalangeal joint, with or without Z-plasty, other local tissue rearrangement, or skin grafting (includes obtaining graft);
➔ *CPT Assistant* Jan 05:8, Oct 10:10, Jun 11:13

+ 26125   each additional digit (List separately in addition to code for primary procedure)
➔ *CPT Assistant* Jan 05:8, Oct 10:10, Jun 11:13

(Use 26125 in conjunction with 26123)

(For palmar fasciotomy by enzyme injection (eg, collagenase), see 20527, 26341)

(For fasciotomy, see 26040, 26045)

26130   Synovectomy, carpometacarpal joint

26135   Synovectomy, metacarpophalangeal joint including intrinsic release and extensor hood reconstruction, each digit

26140   Synovectomy, proximal interphalangeal joint, including extensor reconstruction, each interphalangeal joint

26145   Synovectomy, tendon sheath, radical (tenosynovectomy), flexor tendon, palm and/or finger, each tendon
➔ *CPT Assistant* Nov 98:8

(For tendon sheath synovectomies at wrist, see 25115, 25116)

26160   Excision of lesion of tendon sheath or joint capsule (eg, cyst, mucous cyst, or ganglion), hand or finger
➔ *CPT Changes: An Insider's View* 2002

(For wrist ganglion, see 25111, 25112)

(For trigger digit, use 26055)

26170   Excision of tendon, palm, flexor or extensor, single, each tendon
➔ *CPT Changes: An Insider's View* 2007

(Do not report 26170 in conjunction with 26390, 26415)

26180   Excision of tendon, finger, flexor or extensor, each tendon
➔ *CPT Assistant* Nov 98:8; *CPT Changes: An Insider's View* 2007

(Do not report 26180 in conjunction with 26390, 26415)

26185   Sesamoidectomy, thumb or finger (separate procedure)

26200   Excision or curettage of bone cyst or benign tumor of metacarpal;

26205   with autograft (includes obtaining graft)

26210   Excision or curettage of bone cyst or benign tumor of proximal, middle, or distal phalanx of finger;

26215   with autograft (includes obtaining graft)

26230   Partial excision (craterization, saucerization, or diaphysectomy) bone (eg, osteomyelitis); metacarpal

26235   proximal or middle phalanx of finger

26236   distal phalanx of finger

26250   Radical resection of tumor, metacarpal
➔ *CPT Assistant* Nov 98:8; *CPT Changes: An Insider's View* 2010

(26255 has been deleted)

26260   Radical resection of tumor, proximal or middle phalanx of finger
➔ *CPT Assistant* Nov 98:8; *CPT Changes: An Insider's View* 2010

(26261 has been deleted)

26262   Radical resection of tumor, distal phalanx of finger
➔ *CPT Assistant* Nov 98:8; *CPT Changes: An Insider's View* 2010

Introduction or Removal

26320   Removal of implant from finger or hand

(For removal of foreign body in hand or finger, see 20520, 20525)

Repair, Revision, and/or Reconstruction

26340   Manipulation, finger joint, under anesthesia, each joint
➔ *CPT Assistant* Nov 02:10; *CPT Changes: An Insider's View* 2002

(For application of external fixation, see 20690 or 20692)

26341   Manipulation, palmar fascial cord (ie, Dupuytren's cord), post enzyme injection (eg, collagenase), single cord
➔ *CPT Assistant* Jul 12:8, 14; *CPT Changes: An Insider's View* 2012

(For enzyme injection (eg, collagenase), palmar fascial cord (eg, Dupuytren's contracture), use 20527)

(Report custom orthotic fabrication/application separately)

26350   Repair or advancement, flexor tendon, not in zone 2 digital flexor tendon sheath (eg, no man's land); primary or secondary without free graft, each tendon
➔ *CPT Assistant* Nov 98:8; *CPT Changes: An Insider's View* 2002

Musculoskeletal

26352   secondary with free graft (includes obtaining graft), each tendon

26356   Repair or advancement, flexor tendon, in zone 2 digital flexor tendon sheath (eg, no man's land); primary, without free graft, each tendon
> *CPT Assistant* Nov 98:8, Dec 98:9, Dec 08:6; *CPT Changes: An Insider's View* 2002, 2004

26357   secondary, without free graft, each tendon
> *CPT Changes: An Insider's View* 2004

26358   secondary, with free graft (includes obtaining graft), each tendon

26370   Repair or advancement of profundus tendon, with intact superficialis tendon; primary, each tendon
> *CPT Assistant* Nov 98:8, Dec 08:6

26372   secondary with free graft (includes obtaining graft), each tendon
> *CPT Assistant* Nov 98:8

26373   secondary without free graft, each tendon
> *CPT Assistant* Nov 98:8

26390   Excision flexor tendon, with implantation of synthetic rod for delayed tendon graft, hand or finger, each rod
> *CPT Assistant* Nov 98:8; *CPT Changes: An Insider's View* 2002

26392   Removal of synthetic rod and insertion of flexor tendon graft, hand or finger (includes obtaining graft), each rod
> *CPT Assistant* Nov 98:8; *CPT Changes: An Insider's View* 2002

26410   Repair, extensor tendon, hand, primary or secondary; without free graft, each tendon
> *CPT Assistant* Nov 98:8

26412   with free graft (includes obtaining graft), each tendon
> *CPT Assistant* Nov 98:8

26415   Excision of extensor tendon, with implantation of synthetic rod for delayed tendon graft, hand or finger, each rod
> *CPT Assistant* Nov 98:8; *CPT Changes: An Insider's View* 2002

26416   Removal of synthetic rod and insertion of extensor tendon graft (includes obtaining graft), hand or finger, each rod
> *CPT Assistant* Nov 99:12; *CPT Changes: An Insider's View* 2000, 2002

26418   Repair, extensor tendon, finger, primary or secondary; without free graft, each tendon
> *CPT Assistant* Nov 98:8, Dec 99:10, Dec 00:14

26420   with free graft (includes obtaining graft) each tendon

26426   Repair of extensor tendon, central slip, secondary (eg, boutonniere deformity); using local tissue(s), including lateral band(s), each finger
> *CPT Assistant* Nov 98:8; *CPT Changes: An Insider's View* 2002

26428   with free graft (includes obtaining graft), each finger
> *CPT Changes: An Insider's View* 2002

26432   Closed treatment of distal extensor tendon insertion, with or without percutaneous pinning (eg, mallet finger)
> *CPT Assistant* Nov 98:8

26433   Repair of extensor tendon, distal insertion, primary or secondary; without graft (eg, mallet finger)
> *CPT Assistant* Nov 98:8

26434   with free graft (includes obtaining graft)

(For tenovaginotomy for trigger finger, use 26055)

26437   Realignment of extensor tendon, hand, each tendon
> *CPT Assistant* Nov 98:8

26440   Tenolysis, flexor tendon; palm OR finger, each tendon
> *CPT Assistant* Apr 02:18; *CPT Changes: An Insider's View* 2003

26442   palm AND finger, each tendon

26445   Tenolysis, extensor tendon, hand OR finger, each tendon
> *CPT Assistant* Nov 98:8, Dec 02:11, Mar 03:20; *CPT Changes: An Insider's View* 2002

26449   Tenolysis, complex, extensor tendon, finger, including forearm, each tendon
> *CPT Assistant* Nov 98:8

26450   Tenotomy, flexor, palm, open, each tendon
> *CPT Assistant* Nov 98:8

26455   Tenotomy, flexor, finger, open, each tendon
> *CPT Assistant* Nov 98:8

26460   Tenotomy, extensor, hand or finger, open, each tendon
> *CPT Assistant* Nov 98:8

26471   Tenodesis; of proximal interphalangeal joint, each joint
> *CPT Assistant* Nov 98:8

26474   of distal joint, each joint
> *CPT Assistant* Nov 98:8

26476   Lengthening of tendon, extensor, hand or finger, each tendon
> *CPT Assistant* Nov 98:8

26477   Shortening of tendon, extensor, hand or finger, each tendon
> *CPT Assistant* Nov 98:8

26478   Lengthening of tendon, flexor, hand or finger, each tendon
> *CPT Assistant* Nov 98:8

26479   Shortening of tendon, flexor, hand or finger, each tendon
> *CPT Assistant* Nov 98:8

26480   Transfer or transplant of tendon, carpometacarpal area or dorsum of hand; without free graft, each tendon
> *CPT Assistant* Nov 98:8

26483   with free tendon graft (includes obtaining graft), each tendon

26485   Transfer or transplant of tendon, palmar; without free tendon graft, each tendon
> *CPT Assistant* Nov 98:8

26489   with free tendon graft (includes obtaining graft), each tendon

26490   Opponensplasty; superficialis tendon transfer type, each tendon

26492   tendon transfer with graft (includes obtaining graft), each tendon

26494   hypothenar muscle transfer

26496   other methods

(For thumb fusion in opposition, use 26820)

26497   Transfer of tendon to restore intrinsic function; ring and small finger
➔ *CPT Assistant* Nov 98:8

26498   all 4 fingers

26499   Correction claw finger, other methods

26500   Reconstruction of tendon pulley, each tendon; with local tissues (separate procedure)
➔ *CPT Assistant* Nov 98:8

26502   with tendon or fascial graft (includes obtaining graft) (separate procedure)

26508   Release of thenar muscle(s) (eg, thumb contracture)
➔ *CPT Assistant* Nov 98:8

26510   Cross intrinsic transfer, each tendon
➔ *CPT Changes: An Insider's View* 2002

26516   Capsulodesis, metacarpophalangeal joint; single digit
➔ *CPT Assistant* Nov 98:8

26517   2 digits

26518   3 or 4 digits

26520   Capsulectomy or capsulotomy; metacarpophalangeal joint, each joint
➔ *CPT Assistant* Nov 98:8

26525   interphalangeal joint, each joint
➔ *CPT Assistant* Nov 98:8, Apr 02:18, Mar 03:20

(To report carpometacarpal joint arthroplasty, use 25447)

26530   Arthroplasty, metacarpophalangeal joint; each joint
➔ *CPT Assistant* Nov 98:8

26531   with prosthetic implant, each joint
➔ *CPT Assistant* Nov 98:8, Sep 11:12

26535   Arthroplasty, interphalangeal joint; each joint
➔ *CPT Assistant* Nov 98:8

26536   with prosthetic implant, each joint
➔ *CPT Assistant* Nov 98:8

26540   Repair of collateral ligament, metacarpophalangeal or interphalangeal joint
➔ *CPT Assistant* Nov 96:6

26541   Reconstruction, collateral ligament, metacarpophalangeal joint, single; with tendon or fascial graft (includes obtaining graft)
➔ *CPT Assistant* Jan 97:3

26542   with local tissue (eg, adductor advancement)
➔ *CPT Assistant* Jan 97:3

26545   Reconstruction, collateral ligament, interphalangeal joint, single, including graft, each joint

26546   Repair non-union, metacarpal or phalanx (includes obtaining bone graft with or without external or internal fixation)
➔ *CPT Assistant* Nov 96:6

26548   Repair and reconstruction, finger, volar plate, interphalangeal joint

26550   Pollicization of a digit

26551   Transfer, toe-to-hand with microvascular anastomosis; great toe wrap-around with bone graft
➔ *CPT Assistant* Nov 96:6, Apr 97:7, Jun 97:9, Nov 98:8, 10-11

(For great toe with web space, use 20973)

26553   other than great toe, single
➔ *CPT Assistant* Nov 96:6, Apr 97:7, Jun 97:9, Nov 98:8, 10-11

26554   other than great toe, double
➔ *CPT Assistant* Nov 96:6, Apr 97:7, Jun 97:9, Nov 98:8, 10-11

(Do not report code 69990 in addition to codes 26551-26554)

26555   Transfer, finger to another position without microvascular anastomosis
➔ *CPT Assistant* Nov 98:8, 10-11

26556   Transfer, free toe joint, with microvascular anastomosis
➔ *CPT Assistant* Nov 96:6, Apr 97:7, Jun 97:9, Nov 98:8

(Do not report code 69990 in addition to code 26556)

(To report great toe-to-hand transfer, use 20973)

26560   Repair of syndactyly (web finger) each web space; with skin flaps

26561   with skin flaps and grafts

26562   complex (eg, involving bone, nails)

26565   Osteotomy; metacarpal, each
➔ *CPT Assistant* Nov 98:9

26567   phalanx of finger, each
➔ *CPT Assistant* Apr 12:17

26568   Osteoplasty, lengthening, metacarpal or phalanx

26580   Repair cleft hand

26587   Reconstruction of polydactylous digit, soft tissue and bone
➔ *CPT Assistant* Oct 01:10, Aug 03:14, May 04:16; *CPT Changes: An Insider's View* 2002

(For excision of polydactylous digit, soft tissue only, use 11200)

26590   Repair macrodactylia, each digit
➔ *CPT Assistant* Oct 01:10, Aug 03:14, May 04:16; *CPT Changes: An Insider's View* 2002

26591   Repair, intrinsic muscles of hand, each muscle
➔ *CPT Assistant* May 98:11, Jul 98:11, Nov 98:8, 11

26593   Release, intrinsic muscles of hand, each muscle
➔ *CPT Assistant* Nov 98:8, 11

26596   Excision of constricting ring of finger, with multiple Z-plasties

Musculoskeletal

(To report release of scar contracture or graft repairs see 11042, 14040-14041, or 15120, 15240)

Fracture and/or Dislocation

26600 Closed treatment of metacarpal fracture, single; without manipulation, each bone

26605 with manipulation, each bone

26607 Closed treatment of metacarpal fracture, with manipulation, with external fixation, each bone
➔ *CPT Changes: An Insider's View* 2002

26608 Percutaneous skeletal fixation of metacarpal fracture, each bone

26615 Open treatment of metacarpal fracture, single, includes internal fixation, when performed, each bone
➔ *CPT Changes: An Insider's View* 2008

26641 Closed treatment of carpometacarpal dislocation, thumb, with manipulation

26645 Closed treatment of carpometacarpal fracture dislocation, thumb (Bennett fracture), with manipulation

26650 Percutaneous skeletal fixation of carpometacarpal fracture dislocation, thumb (Bennett fracture), with manipulation
➔ *CPT Changes: An Insider's View* 2008

26665 Open treatment of carpometacarpal fracture dislocation, thumb (Bennett fracture), includes internal fixation, when performed
➔ *CPT Changes: An Insider's View* 2008

26670 Closed treatment of carpometacarpal dislocation, other than thumb, with manipulation, each joint; without anesthesia
➔ *CPT Changes: An Insider's View* 2002

26675 requiring anesthesia

26676 Percutaneous skeletal fixation of carpometacarpal dislocation, other than thumb, with manipulation, each joint
➔ *CPT Changes: An Insider's View* 2002

26685 Open treatment of carpometacarpal dislocation, other than thumb; includes internal fixation, when performed, each joint
➔ *CPT Changes: An Insider's View* 2002, 2008

26686 complex, multiple, or delayed reduction

26700 Closed treatment of metacarpophalangeal dislocation, single, with manipulation; without anesthesia

26705 requiring anesthesia

26706 Percutaneous skeletal fixation of metacarpophalangeal dislocation, single, with manipulation

26715 Open treatment of metacarpophalangeal dislocation, single, includes internal fixation, when performed
➔ *CPT Changes: An Insider's View* 2008

26720 Closed treatment of phalangeal shaft fracture, proximal or middle phalanx, finger or thumb; without manipulation, each

26725 with manipulation, with or without skin or skeletal traction, each

26727 Percutaneous skeletal fixation of unstable phalangeal shaft fracture, proximal or middle phalanx, finger or thumb, with manipulation, each

26735 Open treatment of phalangeal shaft fracture, proximal or middle phalanx, finger or thumb, includes internal fixation, when performed, each
➔ *CPT Changes: An Insider's View* 2008

26740 Closed treatment of articular fracture, involving metacarpophalangeal or interphalangeal joint; without manipulation, each

26742 with manipulation, each

26746 Open treatment of articular fracture, involving metacarpophalangeal or interphalangeal joint, includes internal fixation, when performed, each
➔ *CPT Changes: An Insider's View* 2008

26750 Closed treatment of distal phalangeal fracture, finger or thumb; without manipulation, each

26755 with manipulation, each

26756 Percutaneous skeletal fixation of distal phalangeal fracture, finger or thumb, each

26765 Open treatment of distal phalangeal fracture, finger or thumb, includes internal fixation, when performed, each
➔ *CPT Changes: An Insider's View* 2008

26770 Closed treatment of interphalangeal joint dislocation, single, with manipulation; without anesthesia

26775 requiring anesthesia

26776 Percutaneous skeletal fixation of interphalangeal joint dislocation, single, with manipulation

26785 Open treatment of interphalangeal joint dislocation, includes internal fixation, when performed, single
➔ *CPT Changes: An Insider's View* 2008

Arthrodesis

26820 Fusion in opposition, thumb, with autogenous graft (includes obtaining graft)

26841 Arthrodesis, carpometacarpal joint, thumb, with or without internal fixation;

26842 with autograft (includes obtaining graft)

26843 Arthrodesis, carpometacarpal joint, digit, other than thumb, each;
➔ *CPT Changes: An Insider's View* 2002

26844 with autograft (includes obtaining graft)

26850 Arthrodesis, metacarpophalangeal joint, with or without internal fixation;

26852 with autograft (includes obtaining graft)

26860 Arthrodesis, interphalangeal joint, with or without internal fixation;

+ 26861 each additional interphalangeal joint (List separately in addition to code for primary procedure)

(Use 26861 in conjunction with 26860)

26862 with autograft (includes obtaining graft)

+ 26863 with autograft (includes obtaining graft), each additional joint (List separately in addition to code for primary procedure)

(Use 26863 in conjunction with 26862)

Amputation

(For hand through metacarpal bones, use 25927)

26910 Amputation, metacarpal, with finger or thumb (ray amputation), single, with or without interosseous transfer

(For repositioning, see 26550, 26555)

26951 Amputation, finger or thumb, primary or secondary, any joint or phalanx, single, including neurectomies; with direct closure

26952 with local advancement flaps (V-Y, hood)

(For repair of soft tissue defect requiring split or full thickness graft or other pedicle flaps, see 15050-15758)

Other Procedures

26989 Unlisted procedure, hands or fingers

Pelvis and Hip Joint

Including head and neck of femur.

Incision

(For incision and drainage procedures, superficial, see 10040-10160)

26990 Incision and drainage, pelvis or hip joint area; deep abscess or hematoma

26991 infected bursa

26992 Incision, bone cortex, pelvis and/or hip joint (eg, osteomyelitis or bone abscess)
➔ *CPT Assistant* Jan 02:10

27000 Tenotomy, adductor of hip, percutaneous (separate procedure)

27001 Tenotomy, adductor of hip, open

(To report bilateral procedure, report 27001 with modifier 50)

27003 Tenotomy, adductor, subcutaneous, open, with obturator neurectomy

(To report bilateral procedure, report 27003 with modifier 50)

27005 Tenotomy, hip flexor(s), open (separate procedure)

27006 Tenotomy, abductors and/or extensor(s) of hip, open (separate procedure)

27025 Fasciotomy, hip or thigh, any type

(To report bilateral procedure, report 27025 with modifier 50)

27027 Decompression fasciotomy(ies), pelvic (buttock) compartment(s) (eg, gluteus medius-minimus, gluteus maximus, iliopsoas, and/or tensor fascia lata muscle), unilateral
➔ *CPT Changes: An Insider's View* 2009

(To report bilateral procedure, report 27027 with modifier 50)

27030 Arthrotomy, hip, with drainage (eg, infection)
➔ *CPT Assistant* Nov 98:8

27033 Arthrotomy, hip, including exploration or removal of loose or foreign body
➔ *CPT Assistant* Spring 92:11

27035 Denervation, hip joint, intrapelvic or extrapelvic intra-articular branches of sciatic, femoral, or obturator nerves
➔ *CPT Assistant* Nov 98:8

(For obturator neurectomy, see 64763, 64766)

27036 Capsulectomy or capsulotomy, hip, with or without excision of heterotopic bone, with release of hip flexor muscles (ie, gluteus medius, gluteus minimus, tensor fascia latae, rectus femoris, sartorius, iliopsoas)
➔ *CPT Assistant* Jan 05:8

Excision

27040 Biopsy, soft tissue of pelvis and hip area; superficial

27041 deep, subfascial or intramuscular
➔ *CPT Assistant* Nov 98:8

(For needle biopsy of soft tissue, use 20206)

27043 Code is out of numerical sequence. See 27040-27080

27045 Code is out of numerical sequence. See 27040-27080

27047 Excision, tumor, soft tissue of pelvis and hip area, subcutaneous; less than 3 cm
➔ *CPT Assistant* Nov 98:8; *CPT Changes: An Insider's View* 2010

 # 27043 3 cm or greater
➔ *CPT Changes: An Insider's View* 2010

27048 Excision, tumor, soft tissue of pelvis and hip area, subfascial (eg, intramuscular); less than 5 cm
➔ *CPT Changes: An Insider's View* 2010

 # 27045 5 cm or greater
➔ *CPT Changes: An Insider's View* 2010

27049 Radical resection of tumor (eg, malignant neoplasm), soft tissue of pelvis and hip area; less than 5 cm
➔ *CPT Assistant* Nov 98:8; *CPT Changes: An Insider's View* 2010

 # 27059 5 cm or greater
➔ *CPT Changes: An Insider's View* 2010

27050 Arthrotomy, with biopsy; sacroiliac joint

▲=Revised code   ●=New code   ▶◀=Contains new or revised text   ⊘=Modifier 51 exempt

Musculoskeletal

27052   hip joint

27054   Arthrotomy with synovectomy, hip joint

27057   Decompression fasciotomy(ies), pelvic (buttock) compartment(s) (eg, gluteus medius-minimus, gluteus maximus, iliopsoas, and/or tensor fascia lata muscle) with debridement of nonviable muscle, unilateral
➤ *CPT Changes: An Insider's View* 2009

(To report bilateral procedure, report 27057 with modifier 50)

27059   Code is out of numerical sequence. See 27040-27080

27060   Excision; ischial bursa

27062   trochanteric bursa or calcification

(For arthrocentesis or needling of bursa, use 20610)

27065   Excision of bone cyst or benign tumor, wing of ilium, symphysis pubis, or greater trochanter of femur; superficial, includes autograft, when performed
➤ *CPT Changes: An Insider's View* 2011

27066   deep (subfascial), includes autograft, when performed
➤ *CPT Changes: An Insider's View* 2011

27067   with autograft requiring separate incision
➤ *CPT Changes: An Insider's View* 2011

27070   Partial excision, wing of ilium, symphysis pubis, or greater trochanter of femur, (craterization, saucerization) (eg, osteomyelitis or bone abscess); superficial
➤ *CPT Changes: An Insider's View* 2011

27071   deep (subfascial or intramuscular)
➤ *CPT Changes: An Insider's View* 2011

27075   Radical resection of tumor; wing of ilium, 1 pubic or ischial ramus or symphysis pubis
➤ *CPT Changes: An Insider's View* 2010

27076   ilium, including acetabulum, both pubic rami, or ischium and acetabulum
➤ *CPT Changes: An Insider's View* 2010

27077   innominate bone, total
➤ *CPT Changes: An Insider's View* 2010

27078   ischial tuberosity and greater trochanter of femur
➤ *CPT Changes: An Insider's View* 2010

(27079 has been deleted)

27080   Coccygectomy, primary

(For pressure (decubitus) ulcer, see 15920, 15922 and 15931-15958)

Introduction or Removal

27086   Removal of foreign body, pelvis or hip; subcutaneous tissue
➤ *CPT Assistant* Jul 98:8

27087   deep (subfascial or intramuscular)
➤ *CPT Assistant* Nov 98:8

27090   Removal of hip prosthesis; (separate procedure)

27091   complicated, including total hip prosthesis, methylmethacrylate with or without insertion of spacer

27093   Injection procedure for hip arthrography; without anesthesia
➤ *CPT Assistant* Jun 12:14
➤ *Clinical Examples in Radiology* Fall 07:7

(For radiological supervision and interpretation, use 73525. Do not report 77002 in conjunction with 73525)

27095   with anesthesia
➤ *CPT Assistant* Jun 12:14
➤ *Clinical Examples in Radiology* Fall 07:7

(For radiological supervision and interpretation, use 73525. Do not report 77002 in conjunction with 73525)

27096   Injection procedure for sacroiliac joint, anesthetic/steroid, with image guidance (fluoroscopy or CT) including arthrography when performed
➤ *CPT Assistant* Nov 99:12, Apr 03:8, Apr 04:15, Jul 08:9, Jan 12:3; *CPT Changes: An Insider's View* 2000, 2012
➤ *Clinical Examples in Radiology* Fall 11:10

(27096 is to be used only with CT or fluoroscopic imaging confirmation of intra-articular needle positioning)

(If CT or fluoroscopy imaging is not performed, use 20552)

(Code 27096 is a unilateral procedure. For bilateral procedure, use modifier 50)

Repair, Revision, and/or Reconstruction

27097   Release or recession, hamstring, proximal
➤ *CPT Assistant* Nov 98:8

27098   Transfer, adductor to ischium
➤ *CPT Assistant* Nov 98:8

27100   Transfer external oblique muscle to greater trochanter including fascial or tendon extension (graft)

27105   Transfer paraspinal muscle to hip (includes fascial or tendon extension graft)

27110   Transfer iliopsoas; to greater trochanter of femur
➤ *CPT Changes: An Insider's View* 2002

27111   to femoral neck

27120   Acetabuloplasty; (eg, Whitman, Colonna, Haygroves, or cup type)

27122   resection, femoral head (eg, Girdlestone procedure)

27125   Hemiarthroplasty, hip, partial (eg, femoral stem prosthesis, bipolar arthroplasty)
➤ *CPT Assistant* Spring 92:8, Feb 98:11, Nov 98:8

(For prosthetic replacement following fracture of the hip, use 27236)

Partial Hip Replacement With or Without Bipolar Prosthesis
27125

The femoral neck is excised so the physician can measure and then replace the femoral stem.

Bipolar prosthesis (Acetabular cup)

27130 Arthroplasty, acetabular and proximal femoral prosthetic replacement (total hip arthroplasty), with or without autograft or allograft
➔ *CPT Assistant* Spring 92:8, Jan 07:1, Dec 11:14; *CPT Changes: An Insider's View* 2002

Total Hip Replacement
27130

The femoral head is excised, osteophytes are removed, and acetabulum is reamed out before replacement is inserted in the femoral shaft.

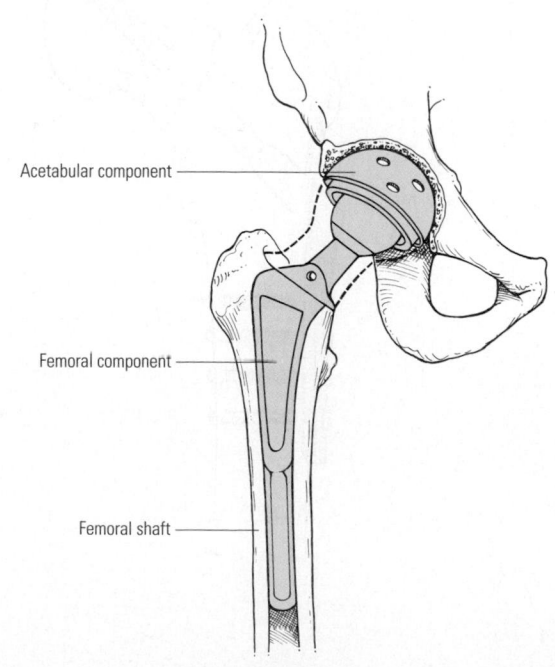

Acetabular component

Femoral component

Femoral shaft

27132 Conversion of previous hip surgery to total hip arthroplasty, with or without autograft or allograft
➔ *CPT Assistant* Spring 92:11, Dec 08:3; *CPT Changes: An Insider's View* 2002

27134 Revision of total hip arthroplasty; both components, with or without autograft or allograft
➔ *CPT Assistant* Spring 92:7, Dec 08:3

27137 acetabular component only, with or without autograft or allograft
➔ *CPT Assistant* Spring 92:7

27138 femoral component only, with or without allograft
➔ *CPT Assistant* Spring 92:7

27140 Osteotomy and transfer of greater trochanter of femur (separate procedure)
➔ *CPT Changes: An Insider's View* 2002

27146 Osteotomy, iliac, acetabular or innominate bone;
➔ *CPT Assistant* Feb 99:10

27147 with open reduction of hip

27151 with femoral osteotomy

27156 with femoral osteotomy and with open reduction of hip

27158 Osteotomy, pelvis, bilateral (eg, congenital malformation)

27161 Osteotomy, femoral neck (separate procedure)

27165 Osteotomy, intertrochanteric or subtrochanteric including internal or external fixation and/or cast
➔ *CPT Assistant* Spring 92:11

27170 Bone graft, femoral head, neck, intertrochanteric or subtrochanteric area (includes obtaining bone graft)
➔ *CPT Assistant* Spring 92:11

27175 Treatment of slipped femoral epiphysis; by traction, without reduction

27176 by single or multiple pinning, in situ

27177 Open treatment of slipped femoral epiphysis; single or multiple pinning or bone graft (includes obtaining graft)

27178 closed manipulation with single or multiple pinning

27179 osteoplasty of femoral neck (Heyman type procedure)

27181 osteotomy and internal fixation

27185 Epiphyseal arrest by epiphysiodesis or stapling, greater trochanter of femur
➔ *CPT Changes: An Insider's View* 2002

27187 Prophylactic treatment (nailing, pinning, plating or wiring) with or without methylmethacrylate, femoral neck and proximal femur

Fracture and/or Dislocation

27193 Closed treatment of pelvic ring fracture, dislocation, diastasis or subluxation; without manipulation

27194 with manipulation, requiring more than local anesthesia

27200 Closed treatment of coccygeal fracture

27202 Open treatment of coccygeal fracture

Musculoskeletal

▲=Revised code   ●=New code   ►◄=Contains new or revised text   ⊘=Modifier 51 exempt

27215 Open treatment of iliac spine(s), tuberosity avulsion, or iliac wing fracture(s), unilateral, for pelvic bone fracture patterns that do not disrupt the pelvic ring, includes internal fixation, when performed

➲ *CPT Changes: An Insider's View* 2009

(To report bilateral procedure, report 27215 with modifier 50)

27216 Percutaneous skeletal fixation of posterior pelvic bone fracture and/or dislocation, for fracture patterns that disrupt the pelvic ring, unilateral (includes ipsilateral ilium, sacroiliac joint and/or sacrum)

➲ *CPT Changes: An Insider's View* 2009

(To report bilateral procedure, report 27216 with modifier 50)

27217 Open treatment of anterior pelvic bone fracture and/or dislocation for fracture patterns that disrupt the pelvic ring, unilateral, includes internal fixation, when performed (includes pubic symphysis and/or ipsilateral superior/inferior rami)

➲ *CPT Changes: An Insider's View* 2009

(To report bilateral procedure, report 27217 with modifier 50)

27218 Open treatment of posterior pelvic bone fracture and/or dislocation, for fracture patterns that disrupt the pelvic ring, unilateral, includes internal fixation, when performed (includes ipsilateral ilium, sacroiliac joint and/or sacrum)

➲ *CPT Changes: An Insider's View* 2009

(To report bilateral procedure, report 27218 with modifier 50)

27220 Closed treatment of acetabulum (hip socket) fracture(s); without manipulation

27222 with manipulation, with or without skeletal traction

27226 Open treatment of posterior or anterior acetabular wall fracture, with internal fixation

27227 Open treatment of acetabular fracture(s) involving anterior or posterior (one) column, or a fracture running transversely across the acetabulum, with internal fixation

27228 Open treatment of acetabular fracture(s) involving anterior and posterior (two) columns, includes T-fracture and both column fracture with complete articular detachment, or single column or transverse fracture with associated acetabular wall fracture, with internal fixation

27230 Closed treatment of femoral fracture, proximal end, neck; without manipulation

27232 with manipulation, with or without skeletal traction

27235 Percutaneous skeletal fixation of femoral fracture, proximal end, neck

➲ *CPT Changes: An Insider's View* 2003

Percutaneous Treatment of Femoral Fracture
27235

Femoral fracture treatment without fracture exposure

Head of femur

Fracture site

Femoral shaft

27236 Open treatment of femoral fracture, proximal end, neck, internal fixation or prosthetic replacement

➲ *CPT Assistant* Spring 92:10, Feb 98:11, Jan 07:1; *CPT Changes: An Insider's View* 2000

Open Treatment of Femoral Fracture
27236

A. Femoral fracture treatment by internal fixation device (with fracture exposure)

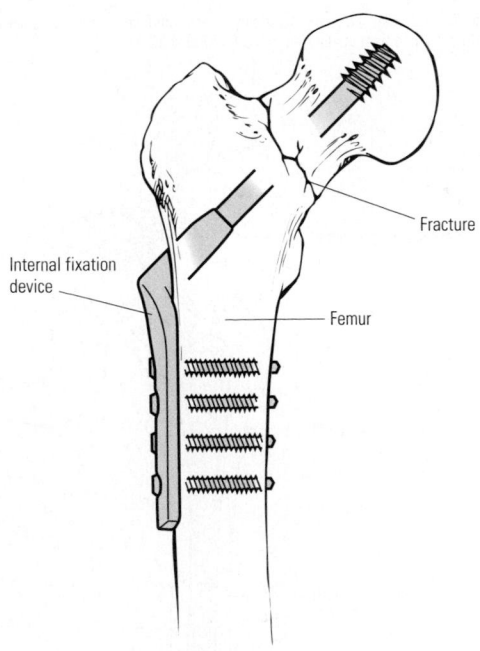

Fracture

Internal fixation device

Femur

Musculoskeletal

B. Femoral fracture treatment by prosthetic replacement

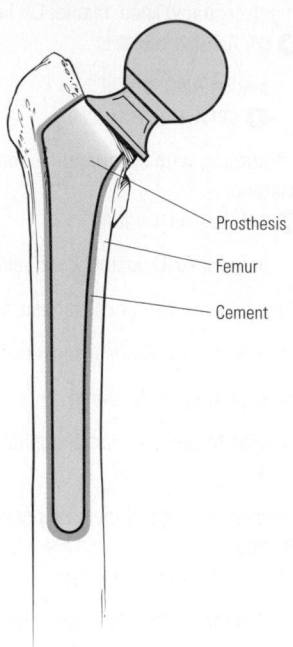

Prosthesis

Femur

Cement

27238   Closed treatment of intertrochanteric, peritrochanteric, or subtrochanteric femoral fracture; without manipulation
➔ *CPT Assistant* Summer 93:12

27240   with manipulation, with or without skin or skeletal traction
➔ *CPT Assistant* Summer 93:12

27244   Treatment of intertrochanteric, peritrochanteric, or subtrochanteric femoral fracture; with plate/screw type implant, with or without cerclage
➔ *CPT Assistant* Summer 93:12; *CPT Changes: An Insider's View* 2003

27245   with intramedullary implant, with or without interlocking screws and/or cerclage
➔ *CPT Assistant* Summer 93:12

27246   Closed treatment of greater trochanteric fracture, without manipulation

27248   Open treatment of greater trochanteric fracture, includes internal fixation, when performed
➔ *CPT Changes: An Insider's View* 2008

27250   Closed treatment of hip dislocation, traumatic; without anesthesia

27252   requiring anesthesia

27253   Open treatment of hip dislocation, traumatic, without internal fixation

27254   Open treatment of hip dislocation, traumatic, with acetabular wall and femoral head fracture, with or without internal or external fixation

(For treatment of acetabular fracture with fixation, see 27226, 27227)

27256   Treatment of spontaneous hip dislocation (developmental, including congenital or pathological), by abduction, splint or traction; without anesthesia, without manipulation

27257   with manipulation, requiring anesthesia

27258   Open treatment of spontaneous hip dislocation (developmental, including congenital or pathological), replacement of femoral head in acetabulum (including tenotomy, etc);

27259   with femoral shaft shortening

27265   Closed treatment of post hip arthroplasty dislocation; without anesthesia

27266   requiring regional or general anesthesia

27267   Closed treatment of femoral fracture, proximal end, head; without manipulation
➔ *CPT Assistant* Jan 08:4; *CPT Changes: An Insider's View* 2008

27268   with manipulation
➔ *CPT Assistant* Jan 08:4; *CPT Changes: An Insider's View* 2008

27269   Open treatment of femoral fracture, proximal end, head, includes internal fixation, when performed
➔ *CPT Assistant* Jan 08:4, Dec 08:3; *CPT Changes: An Insider's View* 2008

(Do not report 27269 in conjunction with 27033, 27253)

Manipulation

27275   Manipulation, hip joint, requiring general anesthesia

Arthrodesis

27280   Arthrodesis, sacroiliac joint (including obtaining graft)

(To report bilateral procedure, report 27280 with modifier 50)

27282   Arthrodesis, symphysis pubis (including obtaining graft)

27284   Arthrodesis, hip joint (including obtaining graft);

27286   with subtrochanteric osteotomy

Amputation

27290   Interpelviabdominal amputation (hindquarter amputation)

27295   Disarticulation of hip

Other Procedures

27299   Unlisted procedure, pelvis or hip joint
➔ *CPT Assistant* Jan 02:10, Dec 05:9, Dec 08:3

Musculoskeletal

Femur (Thigh Region) and Knee Joint

Including tibial plateaus.

Incision

(For incision and drainage of abscess or hematoma, superficial, see 10040-10160)

27301   Incision and drainage, deep abscess, bursa, or hematoma, thigh or knee region
→ *CPT Assistant* Nov 98:9, Dec 08:3

27303   Incision, deep, with opening of bone cortex, femur or knee (eg, osteomyelitis or bone abscess)
→ *CPT Assistant* Nov 98:8

27305   Fasciotomy, iliotibial (tenotomy), open

(For combined Ober-Yount fasciotomy, use 27025)

27306   Tenotomy, percutaneous, adductor or hamstring; single tendon (separate procedure)
→ *CPT Assistant* Nov 98:8

27307   multiple tendons
→ *CPT Assistant* Nov 98:8

27310   Arthrotomy, knee, with exploration, drainage, or removal of foreign body (eg, infection)
→ *CPT Assistant* Nov 98:8, Dec 08:3

Excision

27323   Biopsy, soft tissue of thigh or knee area; superficial
→ *CPT Assistant* Jun 97:12

27324   deep (subfascial or intramuscular)
→ *CPT Assistant* Mar 97:4, Nov 98:8

(For needle biopsy of soft tissue, use 20206)

27325   Neurectomy, hamstring muscle
→ *CPT Changes: An Insider's View* 2007

27326   Neurectomy, popliteal (gastrocnemius)
→ *CPT Changes: An Insider's View* 2007

27327   Excision, tumor, soft tissue of thigh or knee area, subcutaneous; less than 3 cm
→ *CPT Changes: An Insider's View* 2010

 # 27337   3 cm or greater
→ *CPT Changes: An Insider's View* 2010

27328   Excision, tumor, soft tissue of thigh or knee area, subfascial (eg, intramuscular); less than 5 cm
→ *CPT Changes: An Insider's View* 2010

 # 27339   5 cm or greater
→ *CPT Changes: An Insider's View* 2010

27329   Code is out of numerical sequence. See 27323-27365

27330   Arthrotomy, knee; with synovial biopsy only
→ *CPT Assistant* Mar 12:9

27331   including joint exploration, biopsy, or removal of loose or foreign bodies
→ *CPT Assistant* May 96:6, Nov 98:8

27332   Arthrotomy, with excision of semilunar cartilage (meniscectomy) knee; medial OR lateral
→ *CPT Assistant* Nov 98:8

27333   medial AND lateral
→ *CPT Assistant* Mar 12:9

27334   Arthrotomy, with synovectomy, knee; anterior OR posterior
→ *CPT Assistant* Nov 98:8

27335   anterior AND posterior including popliteal area

27337   Code is out of numerical sequence. See 27323-27365

27339   Code is out of numerical sequence. See 27323-27365

27340   Excision, prepatellar bursa

27345   Excision of synovial cyst of popliteal space (eg, Baker's cyst)

27347   Excision of lesion of meniscus or capsule (eg, cyst, ganglion), knee
→ *CPT Assistant* Nov 98:11

27350   Patellectomy or hemipatellectomy

27355   Excision or curettage of bone cyst or benign tumor of femur;

27356   with allograft

27357   with autograft (includes obtaining graft)
→ *CPT Assistant* Dec 02:11

+ 27358   with internal fixation (List in addition to code for primary procedure)

(Use 27358 in conjunction with 27355, 27356, or 27357)

27360   Partial excision (craterization, saucerization, or diaphysectomy) bone, femur, proximal tibia and/or fibula (eg, osteomyelitis or bone abscess)
→ *CPT Assistant* Nov 98:8

 # 27329   Radical resection of tumor (eg, malignant neoplasm), soft tissue of thigh or knee area; less than 5 cm
→ *CPT Changes: An Insider's View* 2010

27364   5 cm or greater
→ *CPT Changes: An Insider's View* 2010

27365   Radical resection of tumor, femur or knee
→ *CPT Changes: An Insider's View* 2010

(For radical resection of tumor, soft tissue of thigh or knee area, see 27329, 27364)

Introduction or Removal

27370   Injection procedure for knee arthrography

(For radiological supervision and interpretation, use 73580. Do not report 77002 in conjunction with 73580)

27372   Removal of foreign body, deep, thigh region or knee area

(For removal of knee prosthesis including "total knee," use 27488)

(For surgical arthroscopic knee procedures, see 29870-29887)

Repair, Revision, and/or Reconstruction

27380 Suture of infrapatellar tendon; primary

27381 secondary reconstruction, including fascial or tendon graft

27385 Suture of quadriceps or hamstring muscle rupture; primary

27386 secondary reconstruction, including fascial or tendon graft

27390 Tenotomy, open, hamstring, knee to hip; single tendon
➔ *CPT Assistant* Nov 98:8

27391 multiple tendons, 1 leg
➔ *CPT Assistant* Nov 98:8

27392 multiple tendons, bilateral
➔ *CPT Assistant* Nov 98:8

27393 Lengthening of hamstring tendon; single tendon
➔ *CPT Assistant* Nov 98:8

27394 multiple tendons, 1 leg
➔ *CPT Assistant* Nov 98:8

27395 multiple tendons, bilateral
➔ *CPT Assistant* Nov 98:8

27396 Transplant or transfer (with muscle redirection or rerouting), thigh (eg, extensor to flexor); single tendon
➔ *CPT Assistant* Nov 98:8; *CPT Changes: An Insider's View* 2009

27397 multiple tendons
➔ *CPT Assistant* Nov 98:8; *CPT Changes: An Insider's View* 2009

27400 Transfer, tendon or muscle, hamstrings to femur (eg, Egger's type procedure)
➔ *CPT Assistant* Nov 98:8

27403 Arthrotomy with meniscus repair, knee
➔ *CPT Assistant* Nov 98:8

(For arthroscopic repair, use 29882)

27405 Repair, primary, torn ligament and/or capsule, knee; collateral

27407 cruciate

(For cruciate ligament reconstruction, use 27427)

27409 collateral and cruciate ligaments

(For ligament reconstruction, see 27427-27429)

27412 Autologous chondrocyte implantation, knee
➔ *CPT Changes: An Insider's View* 2005

(Do not report 27412 in conjunction with 20926, 27331, 27570)

(For harvesting of chondrocytes, use 29870)

27415 Osteochondral allograft, knee, open
➔ *CPT Changes: An Insider's View* 2005

(For arthroscopic implant of osteochondral allograft, use 29867)

(Do not report 27415 in conjunction with 27416)

27416 Osteochondral autograft(s), knee, open (eg, mosaicplasty) (includes harvesting of autograft[s])
➔ *CPT Assistant* Jan 08:4; *CPT Changes: An Insider's View* 2008

(Do not report 27416 in conjunction with 27415, 29870, 29871, 29875, 29884 when performed at the same session and/or 29874, 29877, 29879, 29885-29887 when performed in the same compartment)

(For arthroscopic osteochondral autograft of knee, use 29866)

27418 Anterior tibial tubercleplasty (eg, Maquet type procedure)
➔ *CPT Assistant* Feb 10:13

27420 Reconstruction of dislocating patella; (eg, Hauser type procedure)

27422 with extensor realignment and/or muscle advancement or release (eg, Campbell, Goldwaite type procedure)
➔ *CPT Assistant* Mar 11:9

27424 with patellectomy

27425 Lateral retinacular release, open
➔ *CPT Assistant* Nov 00:11, Mar 11:9; *CPT Changes: An Insider's View* 2002, 2003

(For arthroscopic lateral release, use 29873)

27427 Ligamentous reconstruction (augmentation), knee; extra-articular
➔ *CPT Assistant* Nov 99:13; *CPT Changes: An Insider's View* 2000

27428 intra-articular (open)
➔ *CPT Assistant* Nov 99:13, Apr 09:8; *CPT Changes: An Insider's View* 2000

27429 intra-articular (open) and extra-articular
➔ *CPT Assistant* Nov 99:13, Apr 09:8; *CPT Changes: An Insider's View* 2000

(For primary repair of ligament(s) performed in conjunction with reconstruction, report 27405, 27407 or 27409 in conjunction with 27427, 27428 or 27429)

27430 Quadricepsplasty (eg, Bennett or Thompson type)

27435 Capsulotomy, posterior capsular release, knee
➔ *CPT Assistant* Nov 98:8

27437 Arthroplasty, patella; without prosthesis

27438 with prosthesis

27440 Arthroplasty, knee, tibial plateau;

27441 with debridement and partial synovectomy

27442 Arthroplasty, femoral condyles or tibial plateau(s), knee;
➔ *CPT Assistant* Nov 99:13

27443 with debridement and partial synovectomy

27445 Arthroplasty, knee, hinge prosthesis (eg, Walldius type)
➔ *CPT Assistant* Nov 98:8

27446 Arthroplasty, knee, condyle and plateau; medial OR lateral compartment

Musculoskeletal

27447 medial AND lateral compartments with or without patella resurfacing (total knee arthroplasty)

➔ *CPT Assistant* Jan 07:1; *CPT Changes: An Insider's View* 2002

(For revision of total knee arthroplasty, use 27487)

(For removal of total knee prosthesis, use 27488)

27448 Osteotomy, femur, shaft or supracondylar; without fixation

(To report bilateral procedure, report 27448 with modifier 50)

27450 with fixation

(To report bilateral procedure, report 27450 with modifier 50)

27454 Osteotomy, multiple, with realignment on intramedullary rod, femoral shaft (eg, Sofield type procedure)

➔ *CPT Assistant* Nov 98:8

27455 Osteotomy, proximal tibia, including fibular excision or osteotomy (includes correction of genu varus [bowleg] or genu valgus [knock-knee]); before epiphyseal closure

(To report bilateral procedure, report 27455 with modifier 50)

27457 after epiphyseal closure

(To report bilateral procedure, report 27457 with modifier 50)

27465 Osteoplasty, femur; shortening (excluding 64876)

27466 lengthening

27468 combined, lengthening and shortening with femoral segment transfer

27470 Repair, nonunion or malunion, femur, distal to head and neck; without graft (eg, compression technique)

27472 with iliac or other autogenous bone graft (includes obtaining graft)

27475 Arrest, epiphyseal, any method (eg, epiphysiodesis); distal femur

➔ *CPT Assistant* Nov 98:8

27477 tibia and fibula, proximal

27479 combined distal femur, proximal tibia and fibula

27485 Arrest, hemiepiphyseal, distal femur or proximal tibia or fibula (eg, genu varus or valgus)

➔ *CPT Assistant* Nov 98:8

27486 Revision of total knee arthroplasty, with or without allograft; 1 component

27487 femoral and entire tibial component

➔ *CPT Assistant* Nov 98:8

27488 Removal of prosthesis, including total knee prosthesis, methylmethacrylate with or without insertion of spacer, knee

➔ *CPT Assistant* Nov 98:8

27495 Prophylactic treatment (nailing, pinning, plating, or wiring) with or without methylmethacrylate, femur

27496 Decompression fasciotomy, thigh and/or knee, 1 compartment (flexor or extensor or adductor);

27497 with debridement of nonviable muscle and/or nerve

27498 Decompression fasciotomy, thigh and/or knee, multiple compartments;

27499 with debridement of nonviable muscle and/or nerve

Fracture and/or Dislocation

(For arthroscopic treatment of intercondylar spine[s] and tuberosity fracture[s] of the knee, see 29850, 29851)

(For arthroscopic treatment of tibial fracture, see 29855, 29856)

27500 Closed treatment of femoral shaft fracture, without manipulation

27501 Closed treatment of supracondylar or transcondylar femoral fracture with or without intercondylar extension, without manipulation

27502 Closed treatment of femoral shaft fracture, with manipulation, with or without skin or skeletal traction

➔ *CPT Assistant* Fall 93:22, Oct 99:5

27503 Closed treatment of supracondylar or transcondylar femoral fracture with or without intercondylar extension, with manipulation, with or without skin or skeletal traction

27506 Open treatment of femoral shaft fracture, with or without external fixation, with insertion of intramedullary implant, with or without cerclage and/or locking screws

➔ *CPT Assistant* Winter 92:10, Jun 09:7

27507 Open treatment of femoral shaft fracture with plate/screws, with or without cerclage

27508 Closed treatment of femoral fracture, distal end, medial or lateral condyle, without manipulation

27509 Percutaneous skeletal fixation of femoral fracture, distal end, medial or lateral condyle, or supracondylar or transcondylar, with or without intercondylar extension, or distal femoral epiphyseal separation

27510 Closed treatment of femoral fracture, distal end, medial or lateral condyle, with manipulation

27511 Open treatment of femoral supracondylar or transcondylar fracture without intercondylar extension, includes internal fixation, when performed

➔ *CPT Assistant* May 96:6; *CPT Changes: An Insider's View* 2008

27513 Open treatment of femoral supracondylar or transcondylar fracture with intercondylar extension, includes internal fixation, when performed

➔ *CPT Changes: An Insider's View* 2008

27514 Open treatment of femoral fracture, distal end, medial or lateral condyle, includes internal fixation, when performed

➔ *CPT Changes: An Insider's View* 2008

27516 Closed treatment of distal femoral epiphyseal separation; without manipulation

27517   with manipulation, with or without skin or skeletal traction

27519 Open treatment of distal femoral epiphyseal separation, includes internal fixation, when performed
➔ *CPT Changes: An Insider's View* 2008

27520 Closed treatment of patellar fracture, without manipulation

27524 Open treatment of patellar fracture, with internal fixation and/or partial or complete patellectomy and soft tissue repair

27530 Closed treatment of tibial fracture, proximal (plateau); without manipulation

27532   with or without manipulation, with skeletal traction

(For arthroscopic treatment, see 29855, 29856)

27535 Open treatment of tibial fracture, proximal (plateau); unicondylar, includes internal fixation, when performed
➔ *CPT Changes: An Insider's View* 2008

27536   bicondylar, with or without internal fixation

(For arthroscopic treatment, see 29855, 29856)

27538 Closed treatment of intercondylar spine(s) and/or tuberosity fracture(s) of knee, with or without manipulation

(For arthroscopic treatment, see 29850, 29851)

27540 Open treatment of intercondylar spine(s) and/or tuberosity fracture(s) of the knee, includes internal fixation, when performed
➔ *CPT Changes: An Insider's View* 2000

27550 Closed treatment of knee dislocation; without anesthesia

27552   requiring anesthesia

27556 Open treatment of knee dislocation, includes internal fixation, when performed; without primary ligamentous repair or augmentation/reconstruction
➔ *CPT Changes: An Insider's View* 2008

27557   with primary ligamentous repair
➔ *CPT Changes: An Insider's View* 2008

27558   with primary ligamentous repair, with augmentation/reconstruction
➔ *CPT Changes: An Insider's View* 2008

27560 Closed treatment of patellar dislocation; without anesthesia
➔ *CPT Assistant* Apr 02:15

(For recurrent dislocation, see 27420-27424)

27562   requiring anesthesia

27566 Open treatment of patellar dislocation, with or without partial or total patellectomy

Manipulation

27570 Manipulation of knee joint under general anesthesia (includes application of traction or other fixation devices)
➔ *CPT Assistant* Mar 11:9

Arthrodesis

27580 Arthrodesis, knee, any technique

Amputation

27590 Amputation, thigh, through femur, any level;

27591   immediate fitting technique including first cast

27592   open, circular (guillotine)

27594   secondary closure or scar revision

27596   re-amputation

27598 Disarticulation at knee

Other Procedures

27599 Unlisted procedure, femur or knee
➔ *CPT Assistant* Mar 08:14

Leg (Tibia and Fibula) and Ankle Joint

Incision

27600 Decompression fasciotomy, leg; anterior and/or lateral compartments only

27601   posterior compartment(s) only

27602   anterior and/or lateral, and posterior compartment(s)

(For incision and drainage procedures, superficial, see 10040-10160)

(For decompression fasciotomy with debridement, see 27892-27894)

27603 Incision and drainage, leg or ankle; deep abscess or hematoma

27604   infected bursa

27605 Tenotomy, percutaneous, Achilles tendon (separate procedure); local anesthesia

27606   general anesthesia

27607 Incision (eg, osteomyelitis or bone abscess), leg or ankle

27610 Arthrotomy, ankle, including exploration, drainage, or removal of foreign body
➔ *CPT Assistant* Nov 98:9

27612 Arthrotomy, posterior capsular release, ankle, with or without Achilles tendon lengthening
➔ *CPT Assistant* Nov 98:8

(See also 27685)

Excision

27613   Biopsy, soft tissue of leg or ankle area; superficial

27614   deep (subfascial or intramuscular)
> *CPT Assistant* Nov 98:8

(For needle biopsy of soft tissue, use 20206)

27615   Radical resection of tumor (eg, malignant neoplasm), soft tissue of leg or ankle area; less than 5 cm
> *CPT Changes: An Insider's View* 2010

27616   5 cm or greater
> *CPT Changes: An Insider's View* 2010

27618   Excision, tumor, soft tissue of leg or ankle area, subcutaneous; less than 3 cm
> *CPT Assistant* Apr 10:3; *CPT Changes: An Insider's View* 2010

 # 27632   3 cm or greater
> *CPT Changes: An Insider's View* 2010

27619   Excision, tumor, soft tissue of leg or ankle area, subfascial (eg, intramuscular); less than 5 cm
> *CPT Changes: An Insider's View* 2010

 # 27634   5 cm or greater
> *CPT Changes: An Insider's View* 2010

27620   Arthrotomy, ankle, with joint exploration, with or without biopsy, with or without removal of loose or foreign body

27625   Arthrotomy, with synovectomy, ankle;
> *CPT Assistant* Nov 98:8

27626   including tenosynovectomy

27630   Excision of lesion of tendon sheath or capsule (eg, cyst or ganglion), leg and/or ankle

27632   Code is out of numerical sequence. See 27613-27647

27634   Code is out of numerical sequence. See 27613-27647

27635   Excision or curettage of bone cyst or benign tumor, tibia or fibula;
> *CPT Assistant* Apr 12:17

27637   with autograft (includes obtaining graft)

27638   with allograft

27640   Partial excision (craterization, saucerization, or diaphysectomy), bone (eg, osteomyelitis); tibia
> *CPT Assistant* Apr 12:17; *CPT Changes: An Insider's View* 2010

(For exostosis excision, use 27635)

27641   fibula
> *CPT Changes: An Insider's View* 2010

(For exostosis excision, use 27635)

27645   Radical resection of tumor; tibia
> *CPT Changes: An Insider's View* 2010

27646   fibula
> *CPT Changes: An Insider's View* 2010

27647   talus or calcaneus
> *CPT Changes: An Insider's View* 2010

Introduction or Removal

27648   Injection procedure for ankle arthrography

(For radiological supervision and interpretation, use 73615. Do not report 77002 in conjunction with 73615)

(For ankle arthroscopy, see 29894-29898)

Repair, Revision, and/or Reconstruction

27650   Repair, primary, open or percutaneous, ruptured Achilles tendon;

27652   with graft (includes obtaining graft)

27654   Repair, secondary, Achilles tendon, with or without graft

27656   Repair, fascial defect of leg

27658   Repair, flexor tendon, leg; primary, without graft, each tendon
> *CPT Assistant* Nov 98:8

27659   secondary, with or without graft, each tendon

27664   Repair, extensor tendon, leg; primary, without graft, each tendon
> *CPT Assistant* Nov 98:8

27665   secondary, with or without graft, each tendon
> *CPT Assistant* Nov 98:8

27675   Repair, dislocating peroneal tendons; without fibular osteotomy

27676   with fibular osteotomy

27680   Tenolysis, flexor or extensor tendon, leg and/or ankle; single, each tendon
> *CPT Assistant* Nov 98:8

27681   multiple tendons (through separate incision[s])
> *CPT Assistant* Nov 98:8

27685   Lengthening or shortening of tendon, leg or ankle; single tendon (separate procedure)
> *CPT Assistant* Nov 98:8, Sep 09:11

27686   multiple tendons (through same incision), each
> *CPT Assistant* Nov 98:8, Sep 09:11

27687   Gastrocnemius recession (eg, Strayer procedure)

(Toe extensors are considered as a group to be a single tendon when transplanted into midfoot)

27690   Transfer or transplant of single tendon (with muscle redirection or rerouting); superficial (eg, anterior tibial extensors into midfoot)

27691   deep (eg, anterior tibial or posterior tibial through interosseous space, flexor digitorum longus, flexor hallucis longus, or peroneal tendon to midfoot or hindfoot)

+ 27692   each additional tendon (List separately in addition to code for primary procedure)

(Use 27692 in conjunction with 27690, 27691)

Musculoskeletal

27695   Repair, primary, disrupted ligament, ankle; collateral

27696   both collateral ligaments

27698   Repair, secondary, disrupted ligament, ankle, collateral (eg, Watson-Jones procedure)

27700   Arthroplasty, ankle;

27702   with implant (total ankle)

27703   revision, total ankle

27704   Removal of ankle implant

27705   Osteotomy; tibia

27707   fibula

27709   tibia and fibula

27712   multiple, with realignment on intramedullary rod (eg, Sofield type procedure)

(For osteotomy to correct genu varus [bowleg] or genu valgus [knock-knee], see 27455-27457)

27715   Osteoplasty, tibia and fibula, lengthening or shortening

27720   Repair of nonunion or malunion, tibia; without graft, (eg, compression technique)

27722   with sliding graft

27724   with iliac or other autograft (includes obtaining graft)
→ *CPT Assistant* May 12:11

27725   by synostosis, with fibula, any method

27726   Repair of fibula nonunion and/or malunion with internal fixation
→ *CPT Assistant* Jan 08:4, Apr 09:9; *CPT Changes: An Insider's View* 2008

(Do not report 27726 in conjunction with 27707)

27727   Repair of congenital pseudarthrosis, tibia

27730   Arrest, epiphyseal (epiphysiodesis), open; distal tibia
→ *CPT Assistant* Nov 98:8; *CPT Changes: An Insider's View* 2003

27732   distal fibula

27734   distal tibia and fibula

27740   Arrest, epiphyseal (epiphysiodesis), any method, combined, proximal and distal tibia and fibula;
→ *CPT Assistant* Nov 98:8

27742   and distal femur

(For epiphyseal arrest of proximal tibia and fibula, use 27477)

27745   Prophylactic treatment (nailing, pinning, plating or wiring) with or without methylmethacrylate, tibia

Fracture and/or Dislocation

27750   Closed treatment of tibial shaft fracture (with or without fibular fracture); without manipulation
→ *CPT Assistant* Winter 92:10, Fall 93:21, Mar 96:10

27752   with manipulation, with or without skeletal traction
→ *CPT Assistant* Winter 92:10, Fall 93:21, Feb 96:3, Mar 96:10

27756   Percutaneous skeletal fixation of tibial shaft fracture (with or without fibular fracture) (eg, pins or screws)
→ *CPT Assistant* Winter 92:10

27758   Open treatment of tibial shaft fracture (with or without fibular fracture), with plate/screws, with or without cerclage
→ *CPT Assistant* Winter 92:10, Mar 00:11

27759   Treatment of tibial shaft fracture (with or without fibular fracture) by intramedullary implant, with or without interlocking screws and/or cerclage
→ *CPT Assistant* Winter 92:10; *CPT Changes: An Insider's View* 2003

27760   Closed treatment of medial malleolus fracture; without manipulation

27762   with manipulation, with or without skin or skeletal traction

27766   Open treatment of medial malleolus fracture, includes internal fixation, when performed
→ *CPT Changes: An Insider's View* 2008

27767   Closed treatment of posterior malleolus fracture; without manipulation
→ *CPT Changes: An Insider's View* 2008

27768   with manipulation
→ *CPT Changes: An Insider's View* 2008

27769   Open treatment of posterior malleolus fracture, includes internal fixation, when performed
→ *CPT Changes: An Insider's View* 2008

(Do not report 27767-27769 in conjunction with 27808-27823)

27780   Closed treatment of proximal fibula or shaft fracture; without manipulation
→ *CPT Assistant* Winter 92:11

27781   with manipulation

27784   Open treatment of proximal fibula or shaft fracture, includes internal fixation, when performed
→ *CPT Assistant* Mar 00:11; *CPT Changes: An Insider's View* 2008

27786   Closed treatment of distal fibular fracture (lateral malleolus); without manipulation

27788   with manipulation

27792   Open treatment of distal fibular fracture (lateral malleolus), includes internal fixation, when performed
→ *CPT Changes: An Insider's View* 2008

(For treatment of tibia and fibula shaft fractures, see 27750-27759)

27808   Closed treatment of bimalleolar ankle fracture (eg, lateral and medial malleoli, or lateral and posterior malleoli or medial and posterior malleoli); without manipulation
→ *CPT Changes: An Insider's View* 2008

27810   with manipulation
→ *CPT Changes: An Insider's View* 2008

Musculoskeletal

27814 Open treatment of bimalleolar ankle fracture (eg, lateral and medial malleoli, or lateral and posterior malleoli, or medial and posterior malleoli), includes internal fixation, when performed
➔ *CPT Changes: An Insider's View* 2008

27816 Closed treatment of trimalleolar ankle fracture; without manipulation

27818   with manipulation

27822 Open treatment of trimalleolar ankle fracture, includes internal fixation, when performed, medial and/or lateral malleolus; without fixation of posterior lip
➔ *CPT Changes: An Insider's View* 2008

27823   with fixation of posterior lip
➔ *CPT Changes: An Insider's View* 2008

27824 Closed treatment of fracture of weight bearing articular portion of distal tibia (eg, pilon or tibial plafond), with or without anesthesia; without manipulation

27825   with skeletal traction and/or requiring manipulation

27826 Open treatment of fracture of weight bearing articular surface/portion of distal tibia (eg, pilon or tibial plafond), with internal fixation, when performed; of fibula only
➔ *CPT Changes: An Insider's View* 2008

27827   of tibia only
➔ *CPT Changes: An Insider's View* 2008

27828   of both tibia and fibula
➔ *CPT Changes: An Insider's View* 2008

27829 Open treatment of distal tibiofibular joint (syndesmosis) disruption, includes internal fixation, when performed
➔ *CPT Assistant* Winter 92:11, Mar 09:10; *CPT Changes: An Insider's View* 2008

27830 Closed treatment of proximal tibiofibular joint dislocation; without anesthesia

27831   requiring anesthesia

27832 Open treatment of proximal tibiofibular joint dislocation, includes internal fixation, when performed, or with excision of proximal fibula
➔ *CPT Changes: An Insider's View* 2008

27840 Closed treatment of ankle dislocation; without anesthesia

27842   requiring anesthesia, with or without percutaneous skeletal fixation

27846 Open treatment of ankle dislocation, with or without percutaneous skeletal fixation; without repair or internal fixation

27848   with repair or internal or external fixation

(For surgical or diagnostic arthroscopic procedures, see 29894-29898)

Manipulation

27860 Manipulation of ankle under general anesthesia (includes application of traction or other fixation apparatus)

Arthrodesis

27870 Arthrodesis, ankle, open
➔ *CPT Changes: An Insider's View* 2003

(For arthroscopic ankle arthrodesis, use 29899)

27871 Arthrodesis, tibiofibular joint, proximal or distal

Amputation

27880 Amputation, leg, through tibia and fibula;

27881   with immediate fitting technique including application of first cast

27882   open, circular (guillotine)

27884   secondary closure or scar revision

27886   re-amputation

27888 Amputation, ankle, through malleoli of tibia and fibula (eg, Syme, Pirogoff type procedures), with plastic closure and resection of nerves

27889 Ankle disarticulation

Other Procedures

27892 Decompression fasciotomy, leg; anterior and/or lateral compartments only, with debridement of nonviable muscle and/or nerve

(For decompression fasciotomy of the leg without debridement, use 27600)

27893   posterior compartment(s) only, with debridement of nonviable muscle and/or nerve

(For decompression fasciotomy of the leg without debridement, use 27601)

27894   anterior and/or lateral, and posterior compartment(s), with debridement of nonviable muscle and/or nerve

(For decompression fasciotomy of the leg without debridement, use 27602)

27899 Unlisted procedure, leg or ankle
➔ *CPT Assistant* Aug 00:11

Foot and Toes

Incision

(For incision and drainage procedures, superficial, see 10040-10160)

28001 Incision and drainage, bursa, foot
➔ *CPT Assistant* Nov 98:9

28002   Incision and drainage below fascia, with or without tendon sheath involvement, foot; single bursal space
  → *CPT Assistant* Nov 98:8

28003   multiple areas
  → *CPT Assistant* Nov 98:9

28005   Incision, bone cortex (eg, osteomyelitis or bone abscess), foot
  → *CPT Assistant* Nov 98:9

28008   Fasciotomy, foot and/or toe

   (See also 28060, 28062, 28250)

28010   Tenotomy, percutaneous, toe; single tendon
  → *CPT Assistant* Nov 98:8

28011   multiple tendons
  → *CPT Assistant* Nov 98:8

   (For open tenotomy, see 28230-28234)

28020   Arthrotomy, including exploration, drainage, or removal of loose or foreign body; intertarsal or tarsometatarsal joint

28022   metatarsophalangeal joint

28024   interphalangeal joint

28035   Release, tarsal tunnel (posterior tibial nerve decompression)
  → *CPT Assistant* Nov 98:8

   (For other nerve entrapments, see 64704, 64722)

Excision

28039   Code is out of numerical sequence. See 28043-28175

28041   Code is out of numerical sequence. See 28043-28175

28043   Excision, tumor, soft tissue of foot or toe, subcutaneous; less than 1.5 cm
  → *CPT Changes: An Insider's View* 2010

28039   1.5 cm or greater
  → *CPT Changes: An Insider's View* 2010

28045   Excision, tumor, soft tissue of foot or toe, subfascial (eg, intramuscular); less than 1.5 cm
  → *CPT Changes: An Insider's View* 2010

28041   1.5 cm or greater
  → *CPT Changes: An Insider's View* 2010

28046   Radical resection of tumor (eg, malignant neoplasm), soft tissue of foot or toe; less than 3 cm
  → *CPT Changes: An Insider's View* 2010

28047   3 cm or greater
  → *CPT Changes: An Insider's View* 2010

28050   Arthrotomy with biopsy; intertarsal or tarsometatarsal joint

28052   metatarsophalangeal joint

28054   interphalangeal joint

28055   Neurectomy, intrinsic musculature of foot
  → *CPT Changes: An Insider's View* 2007

28060   Fasciectomy, plantar fascia; partial (separate procedure)
  → *CPT Assistant* Mar 08:14

28062   radical (separate procedure)

   (For plantar fasciotomy, see 28008, 28250)

28070   Synovectomy; intertarsal or tarsometatarsal joint, each

28072   metatarsophalangeal joint, each

28080   Excision, interdigital (Morton) neuroma, single, each

28086   Synovectomy, tendon sheath, foot; flexor

28088   extensor

28090   Excision of lesion, tendon, tendon sheath, or capsule (including synovectomy) (eg, cyst or ganglion); foot
  → *CPT Assistant* Nov 98:8

28092   toe(s), each

28100   Excision or curettage of bone cyst or benign tumor, talus or calcaneus;

28102   with iliac or other autograft (includes obtaining graft)

28103   with allograft

28104   Excision or curettage of bone cyst or benign tumor, tarsal or metatarsal, except talus or calcaneus;
  → *CPT Changes: An Insider's View* 2002

28106   with iliac or other autograft (includes obtaining graft)

28107   with allograft

28108   Excision or curettage of bone cyst or benign tumor, phalanges of foot

   (For osteotomy, partial (eg, hallux valgus, Silver type procedure), use 28290)

28110   Ostectomy, partial excision, fifth metatarsal head (bunionette) (separate procedure)
  → *CPT Assistant* Oct 98:10, Sep 00:9, Oct 10:17, Dec 10:17

28111   Ostectomy, complete excision; first metatarsal head

28112   other metatarsal head (second, third or fourth)

28113   fifth metatarsal head

28114   all metatarsal heads, with partial proximal phalangectomy, excluding first metatarsal (eg, Clayton type procedure)

28116   Ostectomy, excision of tarsal coalition

28118   Ostectomy, calcaneus;
  → *CPT Assistant* May 11:9

28119   for spur, with or without plantar fascial release
  → *CPT Assistant* May 11:9

28120   Partial excision (craterization, saucerization, sequestrectomy, or diaphysectomy) bone (eg, osteomyelitis or bossing); talus or calcaneus
  → *CPT Assistant* May 11:9

Musculoskeletal

28122   tarsal or metatarsal bone, except talus or calcaneus
➔ *CPT Assistant* Nov 98:11

(For partial excision of talus or calcaneus, use 28120)

(For cheilectomy for hallux rigidus, use 28289)

28124   phalanx of toe

28126 Resection, partial or complete, phalangeal base, each toe
➔ *CPT Assistant* Nov 98:8

28130 Talectomy (astragalectomy)

(For calcanectomy, use 28118)

28140 Metatarsectomy

28150 Phalangectomy, toe, each toe
➔ *CPT Assistant* Nov 98:8

28153 Resection, condyle(s), distal end of phalanx, each toe
➔ *CPT Assistant* Nov 98:8, Dec 11:15

28160 Hemiphalangectomy or interphalangeal joint excision, toe, proximal end of phalanx, each
➔ *CPT Assistant* Nov 98:8

28171 Radical resection of tumor; tarsal (except talus or calcaneus)
➔ *CPT Changes: An Insider's View* 2010

28173   metatarsal
➔ *CPT Changes: An Insider's View* 2010

28175   phalanx of toe
➔ *CPT Changes: An Insider's View* 2010

(For talus or calcaneus, use 27647)

Introduction or Removal

28190 Removal of foreign body, foot; subcutaneous

28192   deep

28193   complicated

Repair, Revision, and/or Reconstruction

28200 Repair, tendon, flexor, foot; primary or secondary, without free graft, each tendon
➔ *CPT Assistant* Nov 98:8

28202   secondary with free graft, each tendon (includes obtaining graft)

28208 Repair, tendon, extensor, foot; primary or secondary, each tendon
➔ *CPT Assistant* Nov 98:8

28210   secondary with free graft, each tendon (includes obtaining graft)

28220 Tenolysis, flexor, foot; single tendon
➔ *CPT Assistant* Nov 98:8

28222   multiple tendons
➔ *CPT Assistant* Nov 98:8

28225 Tenolysis, extensor, foot; single tendon
➔ *CPT Assistant* Nov 98:8

28226   multiple tendons
➔ *CPT Assistant* Nov 98:8

28230 Tenotomy, open, tendon flexor; foot, single or multiple tendon(s) (separate procedure)
➔ *CPT Assistant* Nov 98:8

28232   toe, single tendon (separate procedure)
➔ *CPT Assistant* Nov 98:8

28234 Tenotomy, open, extensor, foot or toe, each tendon
➔ *CPT Assistant* Nov 98:8, Sep 10:9

(For tendon transfer to midfoot or hindfoot, see 27690, 27691)

28238 Reconstruction (advancement), posterior tibial tendon with excision of accessory tarsal navicular bone (eg, Kidner type procedure)
➔ *CPT Changes: An Insider's View* 2002

(For subcutaneous tenotomy, see 28010, 28011)

(For transfer or transplant of tendon with muscle redirection or rerouting, see 27690-27692)

(For extensor hallucis longus transfer with great toe IP fusion (Jones procedure), use 28760)

28240 Tenotomy, lengthening, or release, abductor hallucis muscle

28250 Division of plantar fascia and muscle (eg, Steindler stripping) (separate procedure)

28260 Capsulotomy, midfoot; medial release only (separate procedure)

28261   with tendon lengthening

28262   extensive, including posterior talotibial capsulotomy and tendon(s) lengthening (eg, resistant clubfoot deformity)

28264 Capsulotomy, midtarsal (eg, Heyman type procedure)

28270 Capsulotomy; metatarsophalangeal joint, with or without tenorrhaphy, each joint (separate procedure)
➔ *CPT Assistant* Sep 10:9, Sep 11:11

28272   interphalangeal joint, each joint (separate procedure)
➔ *CPT Assistant* Dec 02:11

28280 Syndactylization, toes (eg, webbing or Kelikian type procedure)
➔ *CPT Assistant* Nov 98:8

28285 Correction, hammertoe (eg, interphalangeal fusion, partial or total phalangectomy)
➔ *CPT Assistant* Nov 98:8, May 06:18, Sep 10:9, Sep 11:11

28286   Correction, cock-up fifth toe, with plastic skin closure (eg, Ruiz-Mora type procedure)

➔ *CPT Assistant* Nov 98:8

28288   Ostectomy, partial, exostectomy or condylectomy, metatarsal head, each metatarsal head

28289   Hallux rigidus correction with cheilectomy, debridement and capsular release of the first metatarsophalangeal joint

➔ *CPT Assistant* Nov 98:11, May 11:3

28290   Correction, hallux valgus (bunion), with or without sesamoidectomy; simple exostectomy (eg, Silver type procedure)

➔ *CPT Assistant* Dec 96:5, Nov 98:8, Jan 07:31, May 10:9

28292   Keller, McBride, or Mayo type procedure

➔ *CPT Assistant* Dec 96:5, Sep 00:9, Jan 07:31, May 10:9, Oct 10:12, Dec 10:12

28293   resection of joint with implant

➔ *CPT Assistant* Dec 96:6, Jan 07:31, May 10:9

Hallux Valgus Correction
28290

Simple resection of the medial eminence (Silver-type procedure)

Medial eminence of metatarsal bone

Before

After

Keller-Type Procedure
28292

Simple resection of the base of the proximal phalanx is accompanied by removal of the medial eminence. A hemi implant is optional.

Proximal phalanx

Medial eminence of metatarsal bone

Before

Kirschner wire holding joint

After

Keller-Mayo Procedure With Implant
28293

A total double stem implant is usually used.

Proximal phalanx

Medial eminence of metatarsal bone

Before

Implant in proximal phalanx

After

Musculoskeletal

28294	with tendon transplants (eg, Joplin type procedure)
	→ *CPT Assistant* Dec 96:6, Jan 07:31, May 10:9
28296	with metatarsal osteotomy (eg, Mitchell, Chevron, or concentric type procedures)
	→ *CPT Assistant* Dec 96:6, Jan 97:10, Jan 07:31, May 10:9
28297	Lapidus-type procedure
	→ *CPT Assistant* Dec 96:6, Jan 07:31, May 10:9
28298	by phalanx osteotomy
	→ *CPT Assistant* Dec 96:7, Jan 07:31, May 10:9
28299	by double osteotomy
	→ *CPT Assistant* Dec 96:7, Jan 07:31, May 10:9; *CPT Changes: An Insider's View* 2002

Joplin Procedure
28294

A tendon transplant is an important part of the procedure.

Extensor tendon of great toe

Medial eminence of metatarsal bone

Before

Fusion of proximal phalanx and metatarsal bone

Extensor tendon transplanted to head of metatarsal bone

After

Mitchell Procedure
28296

A complex, biplanar, double step-cut osteotomy through the neck of the first metatarsal is also known as the Mitchell Chevron (Austin) procedure.

Medial eminence of metatarsal bone

Osteotomy

Before

Wirelink

After

Lapidus-Type Procedure
28297

A metatarsocuneiform fusion of bones and a distal bunion repair to correct valgus deformity

Medial eminence of metatarsal bone

Before

Tenotomy

Arthrodesis of the first metatarsal and first cuneiform joint and the first and second metatarsal bases

After

Musculoskeletal

Phalanx Osteotomy
28298

The Akin procedure involves removal of a bony wedge from the base of the proximal phalanx to reorient the axis.

Proximal phalanx

Medial eminence of metatarsal bone

Before

Kirschner wire

After

Double Osteotomy
28299

A. This technique depicts a medial resection of the first metatarsal, osteotomy of the distal first metatarsal with correction of the hallux valgus, followed by an osteotomy of the proximal phalanx to correct additional angular deformity, with placement of appropriate internal fixation (eg, wire[s], pin[s], screw[s]).

PREOP

Angular deformity of proximal phalanx

Medial eminence of metatarsal bone

POSTOP

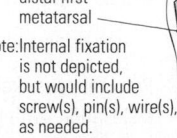

Osteotomy proximal phalanx

Osteotomy distal first metatarsal

Note: Internal fixation is not depicted, but would include screw(s), pin(s), wire(s), as needed.

B. This technique depicts hallux valgus correction (without the medial resection of the base of the proximal phalanx) with double osteotomy of the first metatarsal and placement of appropriate internal fixation (eg, wire[s], pin[s], screw[s]).

PREOP

Medial eminence of metatarsal bone

POSTOP

Double osteotomy of the metatarsal with internal fixation (eg, wire[s], pin[s], screw[s])

Note: Internal fixation depicted is for illustrative purpose only and does not suggest to limit choice of fixation options required.

28300	Osteotomy; calcaneus (eg, Dwyer or Chambers type procedure), with or without internal fixation
28302	talus
28304	Osteotomy, tarsal bones, other than calcaneus or talus; ➔ *CPT Assistant* Nov 98:8
28305	with autograft (includes obtaining graft) (eg, Fowler type)
28306	Osteotomy, with or without lengthening, shortening or angular correction, metatarsal; first metatarsal ➔ *CPT Assistant* Nov 98:8, Dec 99:7, Oct 10:12, Dec 10:12
28307	first metatarsal with autograft (other than first toe) ➔ *CPT Assistant* Nov 98:9
28308	other than first metatarsal, each
28309	multiple (eg, Swanson type cavus foot procedure) ➔ *CPT Assistant* Nov 98:8, Dec 99:7
28310	Osteotomy, shortening, angular or rotational correction; proximal phalanx, first toe (separate procedure)
28312	other phalanges, any toe
28313	Reconstruction, angular deformity of toe, soft tissue procedures only (eg, overlapping second toe, fifth toe, curly toes) ➔ *CPT Assistant* Nov 98:8
28315	Sesamoidectomy, first toe (separate procedure)
28320	Repair, nonunion or malunion; tarsal bones ➔ *CPT Assistant* Nov 98:9
28322	metatarsal, with or without bone graft (includes obtaining graft)
28340	Reconstruction, toe, macrodactyly; soft tissue resection
28341	requiring bone resection
28344	Reconstruction, toe(s); polydactyly
28345	syndactyly, with or without skin graft(s), each web
28360	Reconstruction, cleft foot

Fracture and/or Dislocation

28400	Closed treatment of calcaneal fracture; without manipulation
28405	with manipulation
28406	Percutaneous skeletal fixation of calcaneal fracture, with manipulation
28415	Open treatment of calcaneal fracture, includes internal fixation, when performed; ➔ *CPT Changes: An Insider's View* 2008
28420	with primary iliac or other autogenous bone graft (includes obtaining graft) ➔ *CPT Changes: An Insider's View* 2008
28430	Closed treatment of talus fracture; without manipulation
28435	with manipulation

Musculoskeletal

28436   Percutaneous skeletal fixation of talus fracture, with manipulation

28445   Open treatment of talus fracture, includes internal fixation, when performed
> *CPT Changes: An Insider's View* 2008

28446   Open osteochondral autograft, talus (includes obtaining graft[s])
> *CPT Assistant* Jan 08:4, Dec 08:6; *CPT Changes: An Insider's View* 2008

(Do not report 28446 in conjunction with 27705, 27707)

(For arthroscopic osteochondral talus graft, use 29892)

(For open osteochondral allograft or repairs with industrial grafts, use 28899)

28450   Treatment of tarsal bone fracture (except talus and calcaneus); without manipulation, each
> *CPT Assistant* Dec 01:7

28455   with manipulation, each

28456   Percutaneous skeletal fixation of tarsal bone fracture (except talus and calcaneus), with manipulation, each

28465   Open treatment of tarsal bone fracture (except talus and calcaneus), includes internal fixation, when performed, each
> *CPT Changes: An Insider's View* 2008

28470   Closed treatment of metatarsal fracture; without manipulation, each

28475   with manipulation, each

28476   Percutaneous skeletal fixation of metatarsal fracture, with manipulation, each

28485   Open treatment of metatarsal fracture, includes internal fixation, when performed, each
> *CPT Changes: An Insider's View* 2008

28490   Closed treatment of fracture great toe, phalanx or phalanges; without manipulation

28495   with manipulation

28496   Percutaneous skeletal fixation of fracture great toe, phalanx or phalanges, with manipulation

28505   Open treatment of fracture, great toe, phalanx or phalanges, includes internal fixation, when performed
> *CPT Changes: An Insider's View* 2008

28510   Closed treatment of fracture, phalanx or phalanges, other than great toe; without manipulation, each

28515   with manipulation, each

28525   Open treatment of fracture, phalanx or phalanges, other than great toe, includes internal fixation, when performed, each
> *CPT Changes: An Insider's View* 2008

28530   Closed treatment of sesamoid fracture

28531   Open treatment of sesamoid fracture, with or without internal fixation

28540   Closed treatment of tarsal bone dislocation, other than talotarsal; without anesthesia

28545   requiring anesthesia

28546   Percutaneous skeletal fixation of tarsal bone dislocation, other than talotarsal, with manipulation

28555   Open treatment of tarsal bone dislocation, includes internal fixation, when performed
> *CPT Changes: An Insider's View* 2008

28570   Closed treatment of talotarsal joint dislocation; without anesthesia

28575   requiring anesthesia

28576   Percutaneous skeletal fixation of talotarsal joint dislocation, with manipulation

28585   Open treatment of talotarsal joint dislocation, includes internal fixation, when performed
> *CPT Assistant* Sep 11:12; *CPT Changes: An Insider's View* 2008

28600   Closed treatment of tarsometatarsal joint dislocation; without anesthesia

28605   requiring anesthesia

28606   Percutaneous skeletal fixation of tarsometatarsal joint dislocation, with manipulation

28615   Open treatment of tarsometatarsal joint dislocation, includes internal fixation, when performed
> *CPT Changes: An Insider's View* 2008

28630   Closed treatment of metatarsophalangeal joint dislocation; without anesthesia

28635   requiring anesthesia

28636   Percutaneous skeletal fixation of metatarsophalangeal joint dislocation, with manipulation

28645   Open treatment of metatarsophalangeal joint dislocation, includes internal fixation, when performed
> *CPT Changes: An Insider's View* 2008

28660   Closed treatment of interphalangeal joint dislocation; without anesthesia

28665   requiring anesthesia

28666   Percutaneous skeletal fixation of interphalangeal joint dislocation, with manipulation

28675   Open treatment of interphalangeal joint dislocation, includes internal fixation, when performed
> *CPT Changes: An Insider's View* 2008

Arthrodesis

28705   Arthrodesis; pantalar

28715   triple

28725   subtalar
> *CPT Assistant* Sep 11:11

28730   Arthrodesis, midtarsal or tarsometatarsal, multiple or transverse;

Musculoskeletal

28735   with osteotomy (eg, flatfoot correction)

28737   Arthrodesis, with tendon lengthening and advancement, midtarsal, tarsal navicular-cuneiform (eg, Miller type procedure)
→ *CPT Changes: An Insider's View* 2002

28740   Arthrodesis, midtarsal or tarsometatarsal, single joint

28750   Arthrodesis, great toe; metatarsophalangeal joint
→ *CPT Assistant* Dec 96:7

28755   interphalangeal joint

28760   Arthrodesis, with extensor hallucis longus transfer to first metatarsal neck, great toe, interphalangeal joint (eg, Jones type procedure)
→ *CPT Assistant* Nov 98:8

(For hammertoe operation or interphalangeal fusion, use 28285)

Amputation

28800   Amputation, foot; midtarsal (eg, Chopart type procedure)

28805   transmetatarsal
→ *CPT Assistant* May 97:8

28810   Amputation, metatarsal, with toe, single

28820   Amputation, toe; metatarsophalangeal joint
→ *CPT Assistant* May 97:8

28825   interphalangeal joint

(For amputation of tuft of distal phalanx, use 11752)

Other Procedures

▲ **28890**   Extracorporeal shock wave, high energy, performed by a physician or other qualified health care professional, requiring anesthesia other than local, including ultrasound guidance, involving the plantar fascia
→ *CPT Assistant* Dec 05:10, Mar 06:1; *CPT Changes: An Insider's View* 2006, 2013

(For extracorporeal shock wave therapy involving musculoskeletal system not otherwise specified, see 0019T, 0101T, 0102T)

▶(For extracorporeal shock wave therapy involving integumentary system not otherwise specified, see 0299T, 0300T)◀

▶(Do not report 28890 in conjunction with 0299T, 0300T when treating the same area)◀

28899   Unlisted procedure, foot or toes
→ *CPT Assistant* Sep 11:12

Application of Casts and Strapping

▶The listed procedures apply when the cast application or strapping is a replacement procedure used during or after the period of follow-up care, or when the cast application or strapping is an initial service performed without a restorative treatment or procedure(s) to stabilize or protect a fracture, injury, or dislocation and/or to afford comfort to a patient. Restorative treatment or procedure(s) rendered by another individual following the application of the initial cast/splint/strap may be reported with a treatment of fracture and/or dislocation code.

An individual who applies the initial cast, strap, or splint and also assumes all of the subsequent fracture, dislocation, or injury care cannot use the application of casts and strapping codes as an initial service, since the first cast/splint or strap application is included in the treatment of fracture and/or dislocation codes. (See notes under Musculoskeletal System, page 92.) A temporary cast/splint/strap is not considered to be part of the preoperative care, and the use of the modifier 56 is not applicable. Additional evaluation and management services are reportable only if significant identifiable further services are provided at the time of the cast application or strapping.

If cast application or strapping is provided as an initial service (eg, casting of a sprained ankle or knee) in which no other procedure or treatment (eg, surgical repair, reduction of a fracture, or joint dislocation) is performed or is expected to be performed by an individual rendering the initial care only, use the casting, strapping, and/or supply code (99070) in addition to an evaluation and management code as appropriate.◀

Listed procedures include removal of cast or strapping.

(For orthotics management and training, see 97760-97762)

Body and Upper Extremity

Casts

29000   Application of halo type body cast (see 20661-20663 for insertion)
→ *CPT Assistant* Feb 96:3, 5, Apr 02:13

29010   Application of Risser jacket, localizer, body; only
→ *CPT Assistant* Feb 96:3, Apr 02:13

29015   including head
→ *CPT Assistant* Feb 96:3, Apr 02:13

29020   Application of turnbuckle jacket, body; only
→ *CPT Assistant* Feb 96:3, Apr 02:13

29025   including head
→ *CPT Assistant* Feb 96:3, Apr 02:13

29035   Application of body cast, shoulder to hips;
→ *CPT Assistant* Feb 96:3, Apr 02:13

29040   including head, Minerva type
→ *CPT Assistant* Feb 96:3, Apr 02:13

29044   including 1 thigh
→ *CPT Assistant* Feb 96:3, Apr 02:13

29046   including both thighs
→ *CPT Assistant* Feb 96:3, Apr 02:13

Musculoskeletal

29049   Application, cast; figure-of-eight
> *CPT Assistant* Feb 96:3, Apr 02:13; *CPT Changes: An Insider's View* 2002

29055   shoulder spica
> *CPT Assistant* Feb 96:3, Apr 02:13

29058   plaster Velpeau
> *CPT Assistant* Feb 96:3, Apr 02:13

29065   shoulder to hand (long arm)
> *CPT Assistant* Feb 96:3, Apr 02:13

29075   elbow to finger (short arm)
> *CPT Assistant* Feb 96:3-4, Apr 02:13

29085   hand and lower forearm (gauntlet)
> *CPT Assistant* Feb 96:3, Apr 02:13, Dec 02:11

29086   finger (eg, contracture)
> *CPT Assistant* Apr 02:13; *CPT Changes: An Insider's View* 2002

Splints

29105   Application of long arm splint (shoulder to hand)
> *CPT Assistant* Feb 96:3, Apr 02:13, May 09:8

29125   Application of short arm splint (forearm to hand); static
> *CPT Assistant* Feb 96:3-4, Apr 02:13

29126   dynamic
> *CPT Assistant* Feb 96:3, Apr 02:13

29130   Application of finger splint; static
> *CPT Assistant* Feb 96:3, Apr 02:13

29131   dynamic
> *CPT Assistant* Feb 96:3, Apr 02:13

Strapping—Any Age

29200   Strapping; thorax
> *CPT Assistant* Feb 96:3, Apr 02:13

(29220 has been deleted)

(To report low back strapping, use 29799)

29240   shoulder (eg, Velpeau)
> *CPT Assistant* Feb 96:3, Apr 02:13, Jun 10:8

29260   elbow or wrist
> *CPT Assistant* Feb 96:3, Apr 02:13

29280   hand or finger
> *CPT Assistant* Feb 96:3, Apr 02:13

Lower Extremity

Casts

29305   Application of hip spica cast; 1 leg
> *CPT Assistant* Feb 96:3, Apr 02:13

29325   1 and one-half spica or both legs
> *CPT Assistant* Feb 96:3, Apr 02:13

(For hip spica (body) cast, including thighs only, use 29046)

29345   Application of long leg cast (thigh to toes);
> *CPT Assistant* Feb 96:3, Apr 02:13, Sep 11:11

29355   walker or ambulatory type
> *CPT Assistant* Feb 96:3, Apr 02:13, Sep 11:11

29358   Application of long leg cast brace
> *CPT Assistant* Feb 96:3, Apr 02:13, Sep 11:11

29365   Application of cylinder cast (thigh to ankle)
> *CPT Assistant* Feb 96:3, Apr 02:13, Sep 11:11

29405   Application of short leg cast (below knee to toes);
> *CPT Assistant* Feb 96:3, Apr 02:13, Mar 03:17, Sep 11:11

29425   walking or ambulatory type
> *CPT Assistant* Feb 96:3, Apr 02:13, Sep 11:11

29435   Application of patellar tendon bearing (PTB) cast
> *CPT Assistant* Feb 96:3, Apr 02:13, Sep 11:11

29440   Adding walker to previously applied cast
> *CPT Assistant* Feb 96:3, Apr 02:13

29445   Application of rigid total contact leg cast
> *CPT Assistant* Feb 96:3, Apr 02:13, Sep 11:11

29450   Application of clubfoot cast with molding or manipulation, long or short leg
> *CPT Assistant* Feb 96:3, Apr 02:13

(To report bilateral procedure, use 29450 with modifier 50)

Splints

29505   Application of long leg splint (thigh to ankle or toes)
> *CPT Assistant* Feb 96:3, Apr 02:13, May 09:8

29515   Application of short leg splint (calf to foot)
> *CPT Assistant* Feb 96:3, Apr 02:13, Mar 03:18

Strapping—Any Age

29520   Strapping; hip
> *CPT Assistant* Feb 96:3, Apr 02:13

29530   knee
> *CPT Assistant* Feb 96:3, Apr 02:13, Jun 10:8, Aug 10:15

29540   ankle and/or foot
> *CPT Assistant* Feb 96:3, Apr 02:13, Mar 03:17, Jun 10:8, Aug 10:15; *CPT Changes: An Insider's View* 2003

(Do not report 29540 in conjunction with 29581, 29582)

29550   toes
> *CPT Assistant* Feb 96:3, Apr 02:13

Musculoskeletal

29580   Unna boot
            ➲ *CPT Assistant* Feb 96:3, Jul 99:10, Apr 02:13

            (Do not report 29580 in conjunction with 29581, 29582)

29581   Application of multi-layer compression system; leg
            (below knee), including ankle and foot
            ➲ *CPT Assistant* May 11:11; *CPT Changes: An Insider's View* 2010,
            2012

            ►(Do not report 29581 in conjunction with 29540, 29580,
            29582, 36475, 36478)◄

29582   thigh and leg, including ankle and foot, when
            performed
            ➲ *CPT Changes: An Insider's View* 2012

            ►(Do not report 29582 in conjunction with 29540, 29580,
            29581, 36475, 36478)◄

29583   upper arm and forearm
            ➲ *CPT Changes: An Insider's View* 2012

            ►(Do not report 29583 in conjunction with 29584)◄

29584   upper arm, forearm, hand, and fingers
            ➲ *CPT Changes: An Insider's View* 2012

            ►(Do not report 29584 in conjunction with 29583)◄

            ►(29590 has been deleted)◄

Removal or Repair

►Codes for cast removals should be employed only for
casts applied by another individual.◄

29700   Removal or bivalving; gauntlet, boot or body cast
            ➲ *CPT Assistant* Apr 02:13

29705   full arm or full leg cast
            ➲ *CPT Assistant* Apr 02:13

29710   shoulder or hip spica, Minerva, or Risser jacket, etc.
            ➲ *CPT Assistant* Apr 02:13

29715   turnbuckle jacket
            ➲ *CPT Assistant* Apr 02:13

29720   Repair of spica, body cast or jacket
            ➲ *CPT Assistant* Apr 02:13

29730   Windowing of cast
            ➲ *CPT Assistant* Apr 02:13

29740   Wedging of cast (except clubfoot casts)
            ➲ *CPT Assistant* Apr 02:13

29750   Wedging of clubfoot cast
            ➲ *CPT Assistant* Apr 02:13

            (To report bilateral procedure, use 29750 with modifier
            50)

Other Procedures

29799   Unlisted procedure, casting or strapping

Endoscopy/Arthroscopy

Surgical endoscopy/arthroscopy always includes a
diagnostic endoscopy/arthroscopy.

When arthroscopy is performed in conjunction with
arthrotomy, add modifier 51.

29800   Arthroscopy, temporomandibular joint, diagnostic, with or
            without synovial biopsy (separate procedure)

29804   Arthroscopy, temporomandibular joint, surgical

            (For open procedure, use 21010)

29805   Arthroscopy, shoulder, diagnostic, with or without
            synovial biopsy (separate procedure)
            ➲ *CPT Changes: An Insider's View* 2002

            (For open procedure, see 23065-23066, 23100-23101)

29806   Arthroscopy, shoulder, surgical; capsulorrhaphy
            ➲ *CPT Changes: An Insider's View* 2002

            (For open procedure, see 23450-23466)

            (To report thermal capsulorrhaphy, use 29999)

29807   repair of SLAP lesion
            ➲ *CPT Changes: An Insider's View* 2002

29819   with removal of loose body or foreign body
            ➲ *CPT Changes: An Insider's View* 2002

            (For open procedure, see 23040-23044, 23107)

29820   synovectomy, partial

            (For open procedure, see 23105)

29821   synovectomy, complete

            (For open procedure, see 23105)

29822   debridement, limited
            ➲ *CPT Assistant* May 01:9, Apr 12:17

            (For open procedure, see specific open shoulder
            procedure performed)

29823   debridement, extensive
            ➲ *CPT Assistant* Apr 12:17

            (For open procedure, see specific open shoulder
            procedure performed)

29824   distal claviculectomy including distal articular surface
            (Mumford procedure)
            ➲ *CPT Changes: An Insider's View* 2002

Musculoskeletal

Arthroscopy, Shoulder, Distal Claviculectomy (Mumford Procedure)
29824

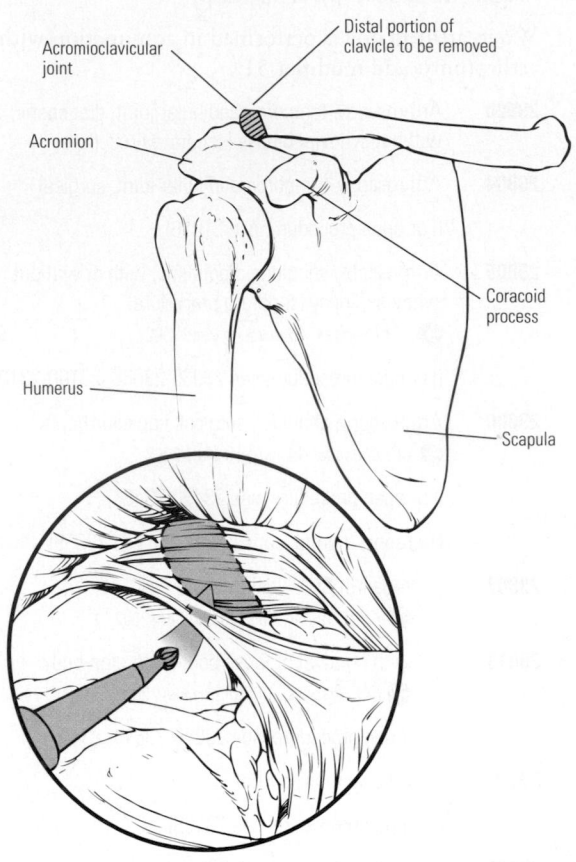

Acromioclavicular joint

Distal portion of clavicle to be removed

Acromion

Coracoid process

Humerus

Scapula

(For open procedure, use 23120)

29825 with lysis and resection of adhesions, with or without manipulation

(For open procedure, see specific open shoulder procedure performed)

+ 29826 decompression of subacromial space with partial acromioplasty, with coracoacromial ligament (ie, arch) release, when performed (List separately in addition to code for primary procedure)

➔ *CPT Assistant* May 01:9, Aug 02:10; *CPT Changes: An Insider's View* 2012

(For open procedure, use 23130 or 23415)

(Use 29826 in conjunction with 29806-29825, 29827, 29828)

29827 with rotator cuff repair

➔ *CPT Assistant* Mar 08:14; *CPT Changes: An Insider's View* 2003

(For open or mini-open rotator cuff repair, use 23412)

(When arthroscopic distal clavicle resection is performed at the same setting, use 29824 and append modifier 51)

29828 biceps tenodesis

➔ *CPT Assistant* Feb 08:9; *CPT Changes: An Insider's View* 2008

(Do not report 29828 in conjunction with 29805, 29820, 29822)

(For open biceps tenodesis, use 23430)

29830 Arthroscopy, elbow, diagnostic, with or without synovial biopsy (separate procedure)

29834 Arthroscopy, elbow, surgical; with removal of loose body or foreign body

29835 synovectomy, partial

29836 synovectomy, complete

29837 debridement, limited

29838 debridement, extensive

29840 Arthroscopy, wrist, diagnostic, with or without synovial biopsy (separate procedure)

29843 Arthroscopy, wrist, surgical; for infection, lavage and drainage

29844 synovectomy, partial

29845 synovectomy, complete

➔ *CPT Assistant* Dec 03:11

29846 excision and/or repair of triangular fibrocartilage and/or joint debridement

➔ *CPT Assistant* Dec 03:11

29847 internal fixation for fracture or instability

29848 Endoscopy, wrist, surgical, with release of transverse carpal ligament

➔ *CPT Assistant* Dec 99:7

(For open procedure, use 64721)

29850 Arthroscopically aided treatment of intercondylar spine(s) and/or tuberosity fracture(s) of the knee, with or without manipulation; without internal or external fixation (includes arthroscopy)

29851 with internal or external fixation (includes arthroscopy)

(For bone graft, use 20900, 20902)

29855 Arthroscopically aided treatment of tibial fracture, proximal (plateau); unicondylar, includes internal fixation, when performed (includes arthroscopy)

➔ *CPT Changes: An Insider's View* 2008

29856 bicondylar, includes internal fixation, when performed (includes arthroscopy)

➔ *CPT Changes: An Insider's View* 2008

(For bone graft, use 20900, 20902)

29860 Arthroscopy, hip, diagnostic with or without synovial biopsy (separate procedure)

➔ *CPT Assistant* Nov 97:15, Jul 98:8, Sep 11:6

Musculoskeletal

29861   Arthroscopy, hip, surgical; with removal of loose body or foreign body
➜ *CPT Assistant* Nov 97:15, Jul 98:8, Sep 11:5

29862   with debridement/shaving of articular cartilage (chondroplasty), abrasion arthroplasty, and/or resection of labrum
➜ *CPT Assistant* Nov 97:15, Jul 98:8, Sep 11:5

29863   with synovectomy
➜ *CPT Assistant* Nov 97:15, Jul 98:8, Sep 11:5

 # 29914   with femoroplasty (ie, treatment of cam lesion)
➜ *CPT Assistant* Sep 11:5; *CPT Changes: An Insider's View* 2011

 # 29915   with acetabuloplasty (ie, treatment of pincer lesion)
➜ *CPT Assistant* Sep 11:5; *CPT Changes: An Insider's View* 2011

(Do not report 29914, 29915 in conjunction with 29862, 29863)

 # 29916   with labral repair
➜ *CPT Assistant* Sep 11:5; *CPT Changes: An Insider's View* 2011

▶(Do not report 29916 in conjunction with 29915, 29862, 29863)◀

Arthroscopy of the Knee
29866-29887

Portal incisions are made on either side of the patellar tendon and compartments of the knee are examined using the arthroscope and a probe. Additional treatment is performed as needed.

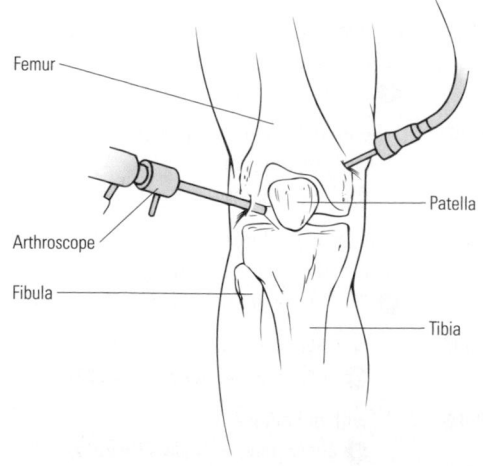

Femur
Patella
Arthroscope
Fibula
Tibia

29866   Arthroscopy, knee, surgical; osteochondral autograft(s) (eg, mosaicplasty) (includes harvesting of the autograft[s])
➜ *CPT Changes: An Insider's View* 2005, 2008

(Do not report 29866 in conjunction with 29870, 29871, 29875, 29884 when performed at the same session and/or 29874, 29877, 29879, 29885-29887 when performed in the same compartment)

(For open osteochondral autograft of knee, use 27416)

29867   osteochondral allograft (eg, mosaicplasty)
➜ *CPT Changes: An Insider's View* 2005

(Do not report 29867 in conjunction with 27570, 29870, 29871, 29875, 29884 when performed at the same session and/or 29874, 29877, 29879, 29885-29887 when performed in the same compartment)

(Do not report 29867 in conjunction with 27415)

29868   meniscal transplantation (includes arthrotomy for meniscal insertion), medial or lateral
➜ *CPT Changes: An Insider's View* 2005

(Do not report 29868 in conjunction with 29870, 29871, 29875, 29880, 29883, 29884 when performed at the same session or 29874, 29877, 29881, 29882 when performed in the same compartment)

29870   Arthroscopy, knee, diagnostic, with or without synovial biopsy (separate procedure)
➜ *CPT Assistant* Dec 07:10, Mar 11:9

(For open autologous chondrocyte implantation of the knee, use 27412)

29871   Arthroscopy, knee, surgical; for infection, lavage and drainage
➜ *CPT Assistant* Aug 01:6

(For implantation of osteochondral graft for treatment of articular surface defect, see 27412, 27415, 29866, 29867)

29873   with lateral release
➜ *CPT Assistant* Dec 07:10, Aug 09:11; *CPT Changes: An Insider's View* 2003

(For open lateral release, use 27425)

29874   for removal of loose body or foreign body (eg, osteochondritis dissecans fragmentation, chondral fragmentation)
➜ *CPT Assistant* Aug 01:6, Apr 03:12

29875   synovectomy, limited (eg, plica or shelf resection) (separate procedure)
➜ *CPT Assistant* Aug 01:6

29876   synovectomy, major, 2 or more compartments (eg, medial or lateral)
➜ *CPT Assistant* Aug 01:6

29877   debridement/shaving of articular cartilage (chondroplasty)
➜ *CPT Assistant* Feb 96:9, Jun 99:11, Aug 01:7, Apr 03:7, Apr 05:14, Dec 07:10

(When performed with arthroscopic meniscectomy, see 29880 or 29881)

29879   abrasion arthroplasty (includes chondroplasty where necessary) or multiple drilling or microfracture
➜ *CPT Assistant* Nov 99:13, Aug 01:7; *CPT Changes: An Insider's View* 2000

Musculoskeletal

29880 with meniscectomy (medial AND lateral, including any meniscal shaving) including debridement/shaving of articular cartilage (chondroplasty), same or separate compartment(s), when performed

→ *CPT Assistant* Jun 99:11, Aug 01:7, Jan 12:3; *CPT Changes: An Insider's View* 2012

29881 with meniscectomy (medial OR lateral, including any meniscal shaving) including debridement/shaving of articular cartilage (chondroplasty), same or separate compartment(s), when performed

→ *CPT Assistant* Feb 96:9, Jun 99:11, Aug 01:7, Oct 03:11, Apr 05:14, Dec 07:10, Jan 12:3; *CPT Changes: An Insider's View* 2012

29882 with meniscus repair (medial OR lateral)

→ *CPT Assistant* Aug 01:7, Sep 04:12, Dec 07:10, Dec 11:15

29883 with meniscus repair (medial AND lateral)

→ *CPT Assistant* Aug 01:7, Sep 04:12, Dec 07:10, Dec 11:15

(For meniscal transplantation, medial or lateral, knee, use 29868)

29884 with lysis of adhesions, with or without manipulation (separate procedure)

→ *CPT Assistant* Aug 01:7, Mar 11:9

29885 drilling for osteochondritis dissecans with bone grafting, with or without internal fixation (including debridement of base of lesion)

→ *CPT Assistant* Aug 01:7

29886 drilling for intact osteochondritis dissecans lesion

→ *CPT Assistant* Aug 01:12

29887 drilling for intact osteochondritis dissecans lesion with internal fixation

→ *CPT Assistant* Aug 01:12

29888 Arthroscopically aided anterior cruciate ligament repair/augmentation or reconstruction

→ *CPT Assistant* Oct 03:11, Dec 07:10

29889 Arthroscopically aided posterior cruciate ligament repair/augmentation or reconstruction

→ *CPT Assistant* Sep 96:9, Oct 98:11, Aug 01:8, Dec 07:10

(Procedures 29888 and 29889 should not be used with reconstruction procedures 27427-27429)

29891 Arthroscopy, ankle, surgical, excision of osteochondral defect of talus and/or tibia, including drilling of the defect

→ *CPT Assistant* Nov 97:15

29892 Arthroscopically aided repair of large osteochondritis dissecans lesion, talar dome fracture, or tibial plafond fracture, with or without internal fixation (includes arthroscopy)

→ *CPT Assistant* Nov 97:15, Dec 08:6

29893 Endoscopic plantar fasciotomy

→ *CPT Assistant* Nov 97:15

29894 Arthroscopy, ankle (tibiotalar and fibulotalar joints), surgical; with removal of loose body or foreign body

Arthroscopy of the Ankle
29894-29899

Incisions are made allowing the ankle to be examined using the arthroscope and a probe. Additional treatment is performed as needed.

29895 synovectomy, partial

29897 debridement, limited

29898 debridement, extensive

29899 with ankle arthrodesis

→ *CPT Changes: An Insider's View* 2003

(For open ankle arthrodesis, use 27870)

29900 Arthroscopy, metacarpophalangeal joint, diagnostic, includes synovial biopsy

→ *CPT Changes: An Insider's View* 2002

(Do not report 29900 with 29901, 29902)

29901 Arthroscopy, metacarpophalangeal joint, surgical; with debridement

→ *CPT Changes: An Insider's View* 2002

29902 with reduction of displaced ulnar collateral ligament (eg, Stenar lesion)

→ *CPT Changes: An Insider's View* 2002

29904 Arthroscopy, subtalar joint, surgical; with removal of loose body or foreign body

→ *CPT Changes: An Insider's View* 2008

29905 with synovectomy

→ *CPT Changes: An Insider's View* 2008

29906 with debridement

→ *CPT Changes: An Insider's View* 2008

29907 with subtalar arthrodesis

→ *CPT Changes: An Insider's View* 2008

29914 Code is out of numerical sequence. See 29800-29999

29915 Code is out of numerical sequence. See 29800-29999

29916 Code is out of numerical sequence. See 29800-29999

29999 Unlisted procedure, arthroscopy

→ *CPT Assistant* Aug 02:10, Sep 04:12, Nov 08:10, Mar 09:10, Dec 11:15, Apr 12:17; *CPT Changes: An Insider's View* 2002

Musculoskeletal

Surgery

Frontal
Ethnoid
Sphenoid
Maxillary

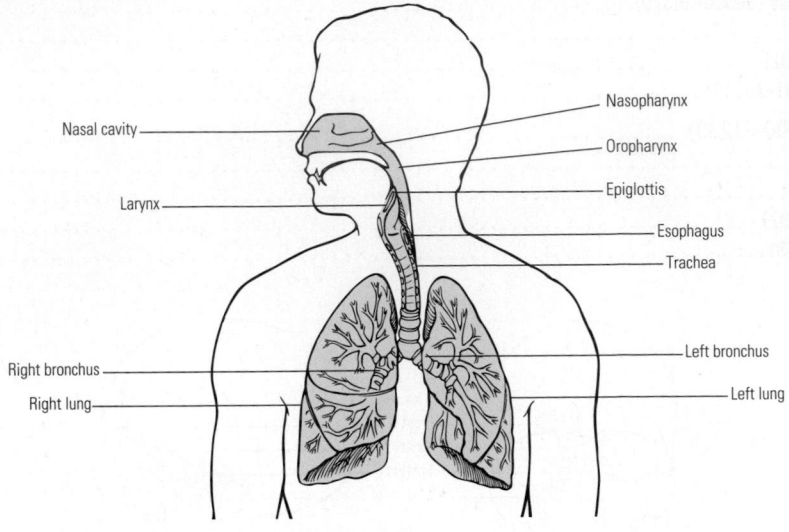

Nasal cavity

Larynx

Right bronchus

Right lung

Nasopharynx

Oropharynx

Epiglottis

Esophagus

Trachea

Left bronchus

Left lung

Respiratory

Respiratory System

Nose

Incision

30000   Drainage abscess or hematoma, nasal, internal approach

(For external approach, see 10060, 10140)

30020   Drainage abscess or hematoma, nasal septum

(For lateral rhinotomy, see specific application [eg, 30118, 30320])

Excision

30100   Biopsy, intranasal

(For biopsy skin of nose, see 11100, 11101)

30110   Excision, nasal polyp(s), simple

(30110 would normally be completed in an office setting)

(To report bilateral procedure, use 30110 with modifier 50)

30115   Excision, nasal polyp(s), extensive

(30115 would normally require the facilities available in a hospital setting)

(To report bilateral procedure, use 30115 with modifier 50)

30117   Excision or destruction (eg, laser), intranasal lesion; internal approach
> *CPT Changes: An Insider's View* 2002

30118   external approach (lateral rhinotomy)
> *CPT Changes: An Insider's View* 2002

30120   Excision or surgical planing of skin of nose for rhinophyma
> *CPT Assistant* May 07:9

30124   Excision dermoid cyst, nose; simple, skin, subcutaneous

30125   complex, under bone or cartilage

30130   Excision inferior turbinate, partial or complete, any method
> *CPT Assistant* Feb 98:11, Nov 98:11, Sep 01:10, May 03:5; *CPT Changes: An Insider's View* 2006

(For excision of superior or middle turbinate, use 30999)

30140   Submucous resection inferior turbinate, partial or complete, any method
> *CPT Assistant* Nov 98:11, Dec 02:10, Apr 03:26, May 03:5, Dec 04:18, Mar 08:14; *CPT Changes: An Insider's View* 2006

(Do not report 30130 or 30140 in conjunction with 30801, 30802, 30930)

(For submucous resection of superior or middle turbinate, use 30999)

(For endoscopic resection of concha bullosa of middle turbinate, use 31240)

(For submucous resection of nasal septum, use 30520)

30150   Rhinectomy; partial

30160   total

(For closure and/or reconstruction, primary or delayed, see **Integumentary System,**13150-13160, 14060-14302, 15120, 15121, 15260, 15261, 15760, 20900-20912)

Introduction

30200   Injection into turbinate(s), therapeutic
> *CPT Assistant* Dec 04:19

30210   Displacement therapy (Proetz type)

30220   Insertion, nasal septal prosthesis (button)

Removal of Foreign Body

30300   Removal foreign body, intranasal; office type procedure
> *CPT Assistant* Jan 12:13

30310   requiring general anesthesia

30320   by lateral rhinotomy

Repair

(For obtaining tissues for graft, see 20900-20926, 21210)

30400   Rhinoplasty, primary; lateral and alar cartilages and/or elevation of nasal tip

(For columellar reconstruction, see 13150 et seq)

30410   complete, external parts including bony pyramid, lateral and alar cartilages, and/or elevation of nasal tip

30420   including major septal repair

30430   Rhinoplasty, secondary; minor revision (small amount of nasal tip work)

30435   intermediate revision (bony work with osteotomies)

30450   major revision (nasal tip work and osteotomies)

30460   Rhinoplasty for nasal deformity secondary to congenital cleft lip and/or palate, including columellar lengthening; tip only

30462   tip, septum, osteotomies

30465   Repair of nasal vestibular stenosis (eg, spreader grafting, lateral nasal wall reconstruction)
> *CPT Changes: An Insider's View* 2001

(30465 excludes obtaining graft. For graft procedure, see 20900-20926, 21210)

(30465 is used to report a bilateral procedure. For unilateral procedure, use modifier 52)

Respiratory

Surgical Repair of Vestibular Stenosis
30465

An incision is made in the upper lateral cartilage and continued as an osteotomy of the medial aspect of the nasal bones. The spreader graft is placed to widen the nasal vestibule.

Nasal bone
Osteotomy site
Lateral nasal cartilage
Incision line
Greater alar cartilage
Spreader graft providing separation of upper lateral cartilage from septum

30520 Septoplasty or submucous resection, with or without cartilage scoring, contouring or replacement with graft
➜ *CPT Assistant* Oct 97:11, Dec 02:10, Mar 12:9

(For submucous resection of turbinates, use 30140)

30540 Repair choanal atresia; intranasal

30545 transpalatine

(Do not report modifier 63 in conjunction with 30540, 30545)

30560 Lysis intranasal synechia

30580 Repair fistula; oromaxillary (combine with 31030 if antrotomy is included)

30600 oronasal

30620 Septal or other intranasal dermatoplasty (does not include obtaining graft)

30630 Repair nasal septal perforations

Destruction

30801 Ablation, soft tissue of inferior turbinates, unilateral or bilateral, any method (eg, electrocautery, radiofrequency ablation, or tissue volume reduction); superficial
➜ *CPT Changes: An Insider's View* 2002, 2006, 2010

(For ablation of superior or middle turbinates, use 30999)

30802 intramural (ie, submucosal)
➜ *CPT Assistant* Mar 08:14, Sep 10:10; *CPT Changes: An Insider's View* 2010

(Do not report 30801 in conjunction with 30802)

(Do not report 30801, 30802, 30930 in conjunction with 30130 or 30140)

(For cautery performed for control of nasal hemorrhage, see 30901-30906)

Other Procedures

30901 Control nasal hemorrhage, anterior, simple (limited cautery and/or packing) any method

(To report bilateral procedure, use 30901 with modifier 50)

30903 Control nasal hemorrhage, anterior, complex (extensive cautery and/or packing) any method

(To report bilateral procedure, use 30903 with modifier 50)

30905 Control nasal hemorrhage, posterior, with posterior nasal packs and/or cautery, any method; initial
➜ *CPT Assistant* Sep 10:7; *CPT Changes: An Insider's View* 2002

30906 subsequent

30915 Ligation arteries; ethmoidal

30920 internal maxillary artery, transantral

(For ligation external carotid artery, use 37600)

30930 Fracture nasal inferior turbinate(s), therapeutic
➜ *CPT Assistant* Jul 01:11, Dec 02:10, Jul 03:15, Aug 03:14, Dec 04:18, Sep 10:10; *CPT Changes: An Insider's View* 2006

(Do not report 30801, 30802, 30930 in conjunction with 30130 or 30140)

(For fracture of superior or middle turbinate[s], use 30999)

30999 Unlisted procedure, nose

Accessory Sinuses

Incision

31000 Lavage by cannulation; maxillary sinus (antrum puncture or natural ostium)

(To report bilateral procedure, use 31000 with modifier 50)

31002 sphenoid sinus

31020 Sinusotomy, maxillary (antrotomy); intranasal

(To report bilateral procedure, use 31020 with modifier 50)

31030 radical (Caldwell-Luc) without removal of antrochoanal polyps

(To report bilateral procedure, use 31030 with modifier 50)

31032 radical (Caldwell-Luc) with removal of antrochoanal polyps

(To report bilateral procedure, use 31032 with modifier 50)

Respiratory

31040   Pterygomaxillary fossa surgery, any approach

(For transantral ligation of internal maxillary artery, use 30920)

31050   Sinusotomy, sphenoid, with or without biopsy;

31051   with mucosal stripping or removal of polyp(s)

31070   Sinusotomy frontal; external, simple (trephine operation)

(For frontal intranasal sinusotomy, use 31276)

Sinusotomy, Frontal
31070

A trephine is used to access the frontal sinus.

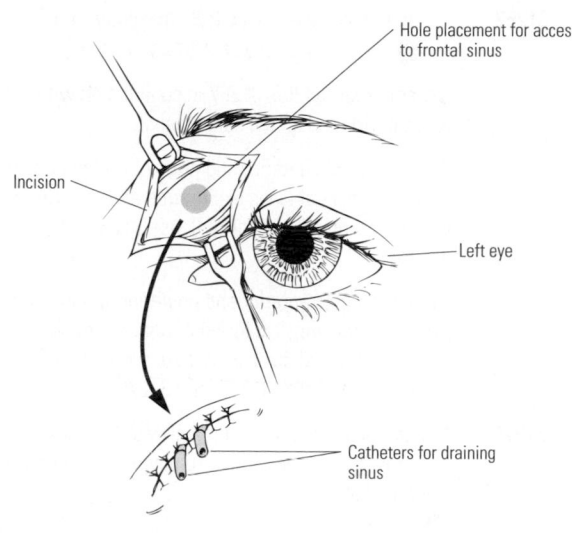

31075   transorbital, unilateral (for mucocele or osteoma, Lynch type)

31080   obliterative without osteoplastic flap, brow incision (includes ablation)

31081   obliterative, without osteoplastic flap, coronal incision (includes ablation)

31084   obliterative, with osteoplastic flap, brow incision

31085   obliterative, with osteoplastic flap, coronal incision

31086   nonobliterative, with osteoplastic flap, brow incision

31087   nonobliterative, with osteoplastic flap, coronal incision

31090   Sinusotomy, unilateral, 3 or more paranasal sinuses (frontal, maxillary, ethmoid, sphenoid)
   ➔ *CPT Assistant* Nov 97:15, Nov 98:11

Excision

31200   Ethmoidectomy; intranasal, anterior

31201   intranasal, total

31205   extranasal, total

31225   Maxillectomy; without orbital exenteration

31230   with orbital exenteration (en bloc)

(For orbital exenteration only, see 65110 et seq)

(For skin grafts, see 15120 et seq)

Endoscopy

A surgical sinus endoscopy includes a sinusotomy (when appropriate) and diagnostic endoscopy.

Codes 31295-31297 describe dilation of sinus ostia by displacement of tissue, any method, and include fluoroscopy if performed.

Codes 31233-31297 are used to report unilateral procedures unless otherwise specified.

Codes 31231-31235 for diagnostic evaluation refer to employing a nasal/sinus endoscope to inspect the interior of the nasal cavity and the middle and superior meatus, the turbinates, and the spheno-ethmoid recess. Any time a diagnostic evaluation is performed all these areas would be inspected and a separate code is not reported for each area.

Sinus Endoscopy
31231-31294

The physician uses an endoscope for visualizing and magnifying the internal structure of the sinuses.

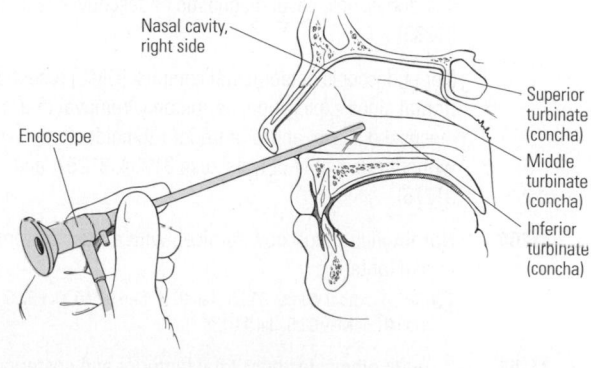

31231   Nasal endoscopy, diagnostic, unilateral or bilateral (separate procedure)
   ➔ *CPT Assistant* Winter 93:22, Jan 97:4

▲=Revised code   ●=New code   ▶◀=Contains new or revised text   ⊘=Modifier 51 exempt

Respiratory

31233 Nasal/sinus endoscopy, diagnostic with maxillary sinusoscopy (via inferior meatus or canine fossa puncture)

➔ *CPT Assistant* Winter 93:22, Jan 97:4, Jun 11:11

(Do not report 31233 in conjunction with 31295 when performed on the same sinus)

31235 Nasal/sinus endoscopy, diagnostic with sphenoid sinusoscopy (via puncture of sphenoidal face or cannulation of ostium)

➔ *CPT Assistant* Winter 93:22, Jan 97:4

(Do not report 31235 in conjunction with 31297 when performed on the same sinus)

31237 Nasal/sinus endoscopy, surgical; with biopsy, polypectomy or debridement (separate procedure)

➔ *CPT Assistant* Winter 93:23, Jan 97:4, Dec 01:6, May 03:5, Dec 11:13

31238 with control of nasal hemorrhage

➔ *CPT Assistant* Winter 93:23, Jan 97:4; *CPT Changes: An Insider's View* 2002

31239 with dacryocystorhinostomy

➔ *CPT Assistant* Winter 93:23, Jan 97:4

31240 with concha bullosa resection

➔ *CPT Assistant* Winter 93:23, Jan 97:4, May 03:5

(For endoscopic osteomeatal complex [OMC] resection with antrostomy and/or anterior ethmoidectomy, with or without removal of polyp[s], use 31254 and 31256)

(For endoscopic osteomeatal complex [OMC] resection with antrostomy, removal of antral mucosal disease, and/or anterior ethmoidectomy, with or without removal of polyp[s], use 31254 and 31267)

(For endoscopic frontal sinus exploration, osteomeatal complex [OMC] resection and/or anterior ethmoidectomy, with or without removal of polyp[s], use 31254 and 31276)

(For endoscopic frontal sinus exploration, osteomeatal complex [OMC] resection, antrostomy, and/or anterior ethmoidectomy, with or without removal of polyp[s], use 31254, 31256, and 31276)

(For endoscopic nasal diagnostic endoscopy, see 31231-31235)

(For endoscopic osteomeatal complex [OMC] resection, frontal sinus exploration, antrostomy, removal of antral mucosal disease, and/or anterior ethmoidectomy, with or without removal of polyp[s], use 31254, 31267, and 31276)

31254 Nasal/sinus endoscopy, surgical; with ethmoidectomy, partial (anterior)

➔ *CPT Assistant* Winter 93:23, Jan 97:4, Sep 97:10, Oct 97:5, Dec 01:6, May 03:5, Jul 11:13

31255 with ethmoidectomy, total (anterior and posterior)

➔ *CPT Assistant* Winter 93:23, Jan 97:4, Dec 02:10, May 03:5, Jul 11:13

31256 Nasal/sinus endoscopy, surgical, with maxillary antrostomy;

➔ *CPT Assistant* Winter 93:23, Jan 97:4, Jun 11:11, Jul 11:13

(For endoscopic anterior and posterior ethmoidectomy [APE] and antrostomy, with or without removal of polyp[s], use 31255 and 31256)

(For endoscopic anterior and posterior ethmoidectomy [APE], antrostomy and removal of antral mucosal disease, with or without removal of polyp[s], use 31255 and 31267)

(For endoscopic anterior and posterior ethmoidectomy [APE], and frontal sinus exploration, with or without removal of polyp[s], use 31255 and 31276)

31267 with removal of tissue from maxillary sinus

➔ *CPT Assistant* Jan 97:4, Dec 01:6, Jun 11:11, Jul 11:13

(Do not report 31256, 31267 in conjunction with 31295 when performed on the same sinus)

(For endoscopic anterior and posterior ethmoidectomy [APE], and frontal sinus exploration and antrostomy, with or without removal of polyp[s], use 31255, 31256, and 31276)

(For endoscopic anterior and posterior ethmoidectomy [APE], frontal sinus exploration, antrostomy, and removal of antral mucosal disease, with or without removal of polyp[s], use 31255, 31267, and 31276)

31276 Nasal/sinus endoscopy, surgical with frontal sinus exploration, with or without removal of tissue from frontal sinus

➔ *CPT Assistant* Winter 93:24, Jan 97:4, Jan 10:11, Jun 11:13

(Do not report 31276 in conjunction with 31296 when performed on the same sinus)

(For endoscopic anterior and posterior ethmoidectomy and sphenoidotomy [APS], with or without removal of polyp[s], use 31255, 31287 or 31288)

(For endoscopic anterior and posterior ethmoidectomy and sphenoidotomy [APS], and antrostomy, with or without removal of polyp[s], use 31255, 31256, and 31287 or 31288)

(For endoscopic anterior and posterior ethmoidectomy and sphenoidotomy [APS], antrostomy and removal of antral mucosal disease, with or without removal of polyp[s], use 31255, 31267, and 31287 or 31288)

(For endoscopic anterior and posterior ethmoidectomy and sphenoidotomy [APS], and frontal sinus exploration with or without removal of polyp[s], use 31255, 31287 or 31288, and 31276)

(For endoscopic anterior and posterior ethmoidectomy and sphenoidotomy [APS], with or without removal of polyp[s], with frontal sinus exploration and antrostomy, use 31255, 31256, 31287 or 31288, and 31276)

(For unilateral endoscopy of 2 or more sinuses, see 31231-31235)

Respiratory

(For endoscopic anterior and posterior ethmoidectomy and sphenoidotomy [APS], frontal sinus exploration, antrostomy and removal of antral mucosal disease, with or without removal of polyp[s], see 31255, 31267, 31287 or 31288 and 31276)

31287   Nasal/sinus endoscopy, surgical, with sphenoidotomy;
➔ *CPT Assistant* Winter 93:24, Jan 97:4, Jun 11:11

31288   with removal of tissue from the sphenoid sinus
➔ *CPT Assistant* Winter 93:24, Jan 97:4, Jun 11:11

(Do not report 31287, 31288 in conjunction with 31297 when performed on the same sinus)

31290   Nasal/sinus endoscopy, surgical, with repair of cerebrospinal fluid leak; ethmoid region
➔ *CPT Assistant* Winter 93:24, Jan 97:4, Jul 11:13

31291   sphenoid region
➔ *CPT Assistant* Winter 93:24, Jan 97:4, Jul 11:13

31292   Nasal/sinus endoscopy, surgical; with medial or inferior orbital wall decompression
➔ *CPT Assistant* Winter 93:24, Jan 97:4, Jul 11:13

31293   with medial orbital wall and inferior orbital wall decompression
➔ *CPT Assistant* Winter 93:24, Jan 97:4, Jul 11:13

31294   with optic nerve decompression
➔ *CPT Assistant* Winter 93:24, Jan 97:4, Jul 11:13

31295   Nasal/sinus endoscopy, surgical; with dilation of maxillary sinus ostium (eg, balloon dilation), transnasal or via canine fossa
➔ *CPT Assistant* Jun 11:11; *CPT Changes: An Insider's View* 2011

(Do not report 31295 in conjunction with 31233, 31256, 31267 when performed on the same sinus)

31296   with dilation of frontal sinus ostium (eg, balloon dilation)
➔ *CPT Assistant* Jun 11:11; *CPT Changes: An Insider's View* 2011

(Do not report 31296 in conjunction with 31276 when performed on the same sinus)

31297   with dilation of sphenoid sinus ostium (eg, balloon dilation)
➔ *CPT Assistant* Jun 11:11; *CPT Changes: An Insider's View* 2011

(Do not report 31297 in conjunction with 31235, 31287, 31288 when performed on the same sinus)

Other Procedures

(For hypophysectomy, transantral or transeptal approach, use 61548)

(For transcranial hypophysectomy, use 61546)

31299   Unlisted procedure, accessory sinuses
➔ *CPT Assistant* Jan 10:11, Jun 11:11

Larynx

Excision

31300   Laryngotomy (thyrotomy, laryngofissure); with removal of tumor or laryngocele, cordectomy

31320   diagnostic

31360   Laryngectomy; total, without radical neck dissection
➔ *CPT Assistant* Aug 10:4

31365   total, with radical neck dissection
➔ *CPT Assistant* Oct 01:10, Aug 10:4

31367   subtotal supraglottic, without radical neck dissection
➔ *CPT Assistant* Aug 10:4

31368   subtotal supraglottic, with radical neck dissection

31370   Partial laryngectomy (hemilaryngectomy); horizontal

31375   laterovertical

31380   anterovertical

31382   antero-latero-vertical

31390   Pharyngolaryngectomy, with radical neck dissection; without reconstruction

31395   with reconstruction

31400   Arytenoidectomy or arytenoidopexy, external approach

(For endoscopic arytenoidectomy, use 31560)

31420   Epiglottidectomy

Introduction

⊘ **31500**   Intubation, endotracheal, emergency procedure
➔ *CPT Assistant* Nov 99:32-33, Oct 03:2, Aug 04:8, Jul 06:4, Jul 07:1, Dec 09:10

31502   Tracheotomy tube change prior to establishment of fistula tract
➔ *CPT Assistant* Winter 90:6

Endoscopy

For endoscopic procedures, code appropriate endoscopy of each anatomic site examined. If using operating microscope, telescope, or both, use the applicable code only once per operative session.

31505   Laryngoscopy, indirect; diagnostic (separate procedure)
➔ *CPT Assistant* Nov 99:13; *CPT Changes: An Insider's View* 2000

31510   with biopsy
➔ *CPT Assistant* Nov 99:13

31511   with removal of foreign body
➔ *CPT Assistant* Nov 99:13

31512   with removal of lesion
➔ *CPT Assistant* Nov 99:13

31513   with vocal cord injection
➔ *CPT Assistant* Nov 99:13

Respiratory

▲=Revised code   ●=New code   ▶◀=Contains new or revised text   ⊘=Modifier 51 exempt

31515 Laryngoscopy direct, with or without tracheoscopy; for aspiration

31520 diagnostic, newborn

(Do not report modifier 63 in conjunction with 31520)

31525 diagnostic, except newborn
➔ *CPT Assistant* Aug 10:3

31526 diagnostic, with operating microscope or telescope
➔ *CPT Assistant* Nov 98:11-12; *CPT Changes: An Insider's View* 2006

(Do not report code 69990 in addition to code 31526)

31527 with insertion of obturator

31528 with dilation, initial
➔ *CPT Changes: An Insider's View* 2002

31529 with dilation, subsequent
➔ *CPT Changes: An Insider's View* 2002

31530 Laryngoscopy, direct, operative, with foreign body removal;

31531 with operating microscope or telescope
➔ *CPT Assistant* Nov 98:11-12; *CPT Changes: An Insider's View* 2006

(Do not report code 69990 in addition to code 31531)

31535 Laryngoscopy, direct, operative, with biopsy;

31536 with operating microscope or telescope
➔ *CPT Assistant* Nov 98:11-12; *CPT Changes: An Insider's View* 2006

(Do not report code 69990 in addition to code 31536)

31540 Laryngoscopy, direct, operative, with excision of tumor and/or stripping of vocal cords or epiglottis;

31541 with operating microscope or telescope
➔ *CPT Assistant* Nov 98:11-12; *CPT Changes: An Insider's View* 2006

(Do not report code 69990 in addition to code 31541)

31545 Laryngoscopy, direct, operative, with operating microscope or telescope, with submucosal removal of non-neoplastic lesion(s) of vocal cord; reconstruction with local tissue flap(s)
➔ *CPT Changes: An Insider's View* 2005

31546 reconstruction with graft(s) (includes obtaining autograft)
➔ *CPT Changes: An Insider's View* 2005

(Do not report 31546 in addition to 20926 for graft harvest)

(For reconstruction of vocal cord with allograft, use 31599)

(Do not report 31545 or 31546 in conjunction with 31540, 31541, 69990)

31560 Laryngoscopy, direct, operative, with arytenoidectomy;

31561 with operating microscope or telescope
➔ *CPT Assistant* Nov 98:11-12; *CPT Changes: An Insider's View* 2006

(Do not report code 69990 in addition to code 31561)

31570 Laryngoscopy, direct, with injection into vocal cord(s), therapeutic;

31571 with operating microscope or telescope
➔ *CPT Assistant* Nov 98:11-12; *CPT Changes: An Insider's View* 2006

(Do not report code 69990 in addition to code 31571)

31575 Laryngoscopy, flexible fiberoptic; diagnostic

31576 with biopsy

31577 with removal of foreign body

31578 with removal of lesion

(To report flexible fiberoptic endoscopic evaluation of swallowing, see 92612-92613)

(To report flexible fiberoptic endoscopic evaluation with sensory testing, see 92614-92615)

(To report flexible fiberoptic endoscopic evaluation of swallowing with sensory testing, see 92616-92617)

(For flexible fiberoptic laryngoscopy as part of flexible fiberoptic endoscopic evaluation of swallowing and/or laryngeal sensory testing by cine or video recording, see 92612-92617)

31579 Laryngoscopy, flexible or rigid fiberoptic, with stroboscopy

Repair

31580 Laryngoplasty; for laryngeal web, 2-stage, with keel insertion and removal

31582 for laryngeal stenosis, with graft or core mold, including tracheotomy

31584 with open reduction of fracture

31587 Laryngoplasty, cricoid split

31588 Laryngoplasty, not otherwise specified (eg, for burns, reconstruction after partial laryngectomy)
➔ *CPT Assistant* Aug 04:11

31590 Laryngeal reinnervation by neuromuscular pedicle

Destruction

31595 Section recurrent laryngeal nerve, therapeutic (separate procedure), unilateral

Other Procedures

31599 Unlisted procedure, larynx

Trachea and Bronchi

Incision

31600   Tracheostomy, planned (separate procedure);
➔ *CPT Assistant* Aug 10:5

31601   younger than 2 years

31603   Tracheostomy, emergency procedure; transtracheal

31605   cricothyroid membrane

31610   Tracheostomy, fenestration procedure with skin flaps

(For endotracheal intubation, use 31500)

(For tracheal aspiration under direct vision, use 31515)

31611   Construction of tracheoesophageal fistula and subsequent insertion of an alaryngeal speech prosthesis (eg, voice button, Blom-Singer prosthesis)

31612   Tracheal puncture, percutaneous with transtracheal aspiration and/or injection

31613   Tracheostoma revision; simple, without flap rotation

31614   complex, with flap rotation

Endoscopy

▶For endoscopy procedures, code appropriate endoscopy of each anatomic site examined. Surgical bronchoscopy always includes diagnostic bronchoscopy when performed by the same physician. Codes 31622-31649 include fluoroscopic guidance, when performed.◀

(For tracheoscopy, see laryngoscopy codes 31515-31578)

⊙ **31615**   Tracheobronchoscopy through established tracheostomy incision
➔ *CPT Assistant* Feb 10:6

⊙+ **31620**   Endobronchial ultrasound (EBUS) during bronchoscopic diagnostic or therapeutic intervention(s) (List separately in addition to code for primary procedure[s])
➔ *CPT Assistant* Aug 05:4, Nov 09:8; *CPT Changes: An Insider's View* 2005

(Use 31620 in conjunction with 31622-31646)

⊙ **31622**   Bronchoscopy, rigid or flexible, including fluoroscopic guidance, when performed; diagnostic, with cell washing, when performed (separate procedure)
➔ *CPT Assistant* Jul 96:11, Nov 98:12, Dec 98:8, Mar 99:3, Apr 00:10, Jun 01:10, Jan 02:10, Sep 04:8, 12, Aug 05:4, Dec 09:10, Feb 10:6, Apr 10:5, Feb 11:8; *CPT Changes: An Insider's View* 2004, 2010

⊙ **31623**   with brushing or protected brushings
➔ *CPT Assistant* Nov 98:12, Mar 99:3, Nov 99:13, Jan 02:10, Sep 04:8, Aug 05:4, May 08:15, Apr 10:5

⊙ **31624**   with bronchial alveolar lavage
➔ *CPT Assistant* Nov 98:12, Feb 99:9, Mar 99:3, 11, Jan 02:10, Sep 04:8, Aug 05:4, May 08:15, Feb 10:6, Apr 10:5

⊙ **31625**   with bronchial or endobronchial biopsy(s), single or multiple sites
➔ *CPT Assistant* Spring 91:2, Jan 02:10, Jun 02:10, Sep 03:15, Sep 04:9, Aug 05:4, Feb 10:6, Apr 10:5; *CPT Changes: An Insider's View* 2004

Bronchoscopy
31622-31646

A rigid or flexible bronchoscope is inserted through the oropharynx and vocal cords and beyond the trachea into the right or left bronchi.

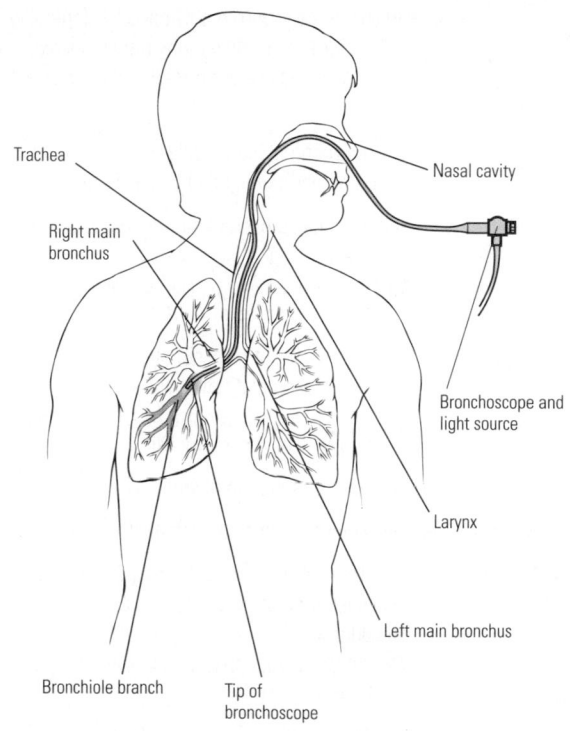

Trachea

Right main bronchus

Nasal cavity

Bronchoscope and light source

Larynx

Left main bronchus

Bronchiole branch   Tip of bronchoscope

⊙ **31626**   with placement of fiducial markers, single or multiple
➔ *CPT Assistant* Feb 10:6, Apr 10:5, Jan 11:6; *CPT Changes: An Insider's View* 2010

(Report supply of device separately)

⊙+ **31627**   with computer-assisted, image-guided navigation (List separately in addition to code for primary procedure[s])
➔ *CPT Assistant* Feb 10:6, Apr 10:5, Jan 11:6; *CPT Changes: An Insider's View* 2010

(31627 includes 3D reconstruction. Do not report 31627 in conjunction with 76376, 76377)

(Use 31627 in conjunction with 31615, 31622-31631, 31635, 31636, 31638-31643)

⊙ **31628**   with transbronchial lung biopsy(s), single lobe
➔ *CPT Assistant* Jun 01:10, Jan 02:10, Sep 04:9, Aug 05:4, May 08:15, Feb 10:6, Apr 10:5; *CPT Changes: An Insider's View* 2004

Respiratory

(31628 should be reported only once regardless of how many transbronchial lung biopsies are performed in a lobe)

(To report transbronchial lung biopsies performed on additional lobe, use 31632)

⊙ **31629** with transbronchial needle aspiration biopsy(s), trachea, main stem and/or lobar bronchus(i)

➔ *CPT Assistant* Apr 00:10, Jan 02:10, Sep 03:15, May 04:15, Jul 04:13, Aug 05:4, Nov 09:8, Feb 10:6, Apr 10:5, Apr 11:12; *CPT Changes: An Insider's View* 2004

(31629 should be reported only once for upper airway biopsies regardless of how many transbronchial needle aspiration biopsies are performed in the upper airway or in a lobe)

(To report transbronchial needle aspiration biopsies performed on additional lobe[s], use 31633)

31630 with tracheal/bronchial dilation or closed reduction of fracture

➔ *CPT Assistant* Jan 02:10, Aug 05:4, Feb 10:6, Apr 10:5; *CPT Changes: An Insider's View* 2005

31631 with placement of tracheal stent(s) (includes tracheal/bronchial dilation as required)

➔ *CPT Assistant* Jan 02:10, Aug 05:4, Feb 10:6, Apr 10:5; *CPT Changes: An Insider's View* 2005

(For placement of bronchial stent, see 31636, 31637)

(For revision of tracheal/bronchial stent, use 31638)

+ **31632** with transbronchial lung biopsy(s), each additional lobe (List separately in addition to code for primary procedure)

➔ *CPT Assistant* Jan 02:10, Sep 04:9, Aug 05:4; *CPT Changes: An Insider's View* 2004

(Use 31632 in conjunction with 31628)

(31632 should be reported only once regardless of how many transbronchial lung biopsies are performed in a lobe)

+ **31633** with transbronchial needle aspiration biopsy(s), each additional lobe (List separately in addition to code for primary procedure)

➔ *CPT Assistant* Jan 02:10, May 04:15, Jul 04:13, Sep 04:10, Aug 05:4, Nov 09:8, Apr 11:12; *CPT Changes: An Insider's View* 2004

(Use 31633 in conjunction with 31629)

(31633 should be reported only once regardless of how many transbronchial needle aspiration biopsies are performed in the trachea or the additional lobe)

⊙ **31634** with balloon occlusion, with assessment of air leak, with administration of occlusive substance (eg, fibrin glue), if performed

➔ *CPT Assistant* Jan 11:6; *CPT Changes: An Insider's View* 2011

▶(Do not report 31634 in conjunction with 31647, 31651 at the same session)◀

⊙ **31635** with removal of foreign body

➔ *CPT Assistant* Jan 02:10, Jun 02:10, Feb 10:6, Apr 10:5, Jan 11:6

▶(For removal of implanted bronchial valves, see 31648-31649)◀

31636 with placement of bronchial stent(s) (includes tracheal/bronchial dilation as required), initial bronchus

➔ *CPT Assistant* Aug 05:4, Apr 10:5; *CPT Changes: An Insider's View* 2005

+ **31637** each additional major bronchus stented (List separately in addition to code for primary procedure)

➔ *CPT Assistant* Aug 05:4; *CPT Changes: An Insider's View* 2005

(Use 31637 in conjunction with 31636)

31638 with revision of tracheal or bronchial stent inserted at previous session (includes tracheal/bronchial dilation as required)

➔ *CPT Assistant* Aug 05:4, Apr 10:5; *CPT Changes: An Insider's View* 2005

31640 with excision of tumor

➔ *CPT Assistant* Jan 02:10, Aug 05:4, Apr 10:5

31641 with destruction of tumor or relief of stenosis by any method other than excision (eg, laser therapy, cryotherapy)

➔ *CPT Assistant* Nov 99:13, Sep 00:5, Jan 02:10, Aug 05:4, Apr 10:5, Oct 11:11; *CPT Changes: An Insider's View* 2002, 2010

(For bronchoscopic photodynamic therapy, report 31641 in addition to 96570, 96571 as appropriate)

31643 with placement of catheter(s) for intracavitary radioelement application

➔ *CPT Assistant* Nov 98:12, Mar 99:3, Jan 02:10, Aug 05:4, Apr 09:3; *CPT Changes: An Insider's View* 2010

(For intracavitary radioelement application, see 77761-77763, 77785-77787)

⊙ **31645** with therapeutic aspiration of tracheobronchial tree, initial (eg, drainage of lung abscess)

➔ *CPT Assistant* Jan 02:10, Aug 05:4; *CPT Changes: An Insider's View* 2010

⊙ **31646** with therapeutic aspiration of tracheobronchial tree, subsequent

➔ *CPT Assistant* Jan 02:10, Aug 05:4; *CPT Changes: An Insider's View* 2010

(For catheter aspiration of tracheobronchial tree at bedside, use 31725)

⊙● **31647** with balloon occlusion, when performed, assessment of air leak, airway sizing, and insertion of bronchial valve(s), initial lobe

➔ *CPT Changes: An Insider's View* 2013

⊙● **31648** with removal of bronchial valve(s), initial lobe

➔ *CPT Changes: An Insider's View* 2013

▶(For removal and insertion of a bronchial valve at the same session, see 31647, 31648, and 31651)◀

Respiratory

31649 with removal of bronchial valve(s), each additional lobe (List separately in addition to code for primary procedure)

➔ *CPT Changes: An Insider's View* 2013

►(Use 31649 in conjunction with 31648)◄

31651 with balloon occlusion, when performed, assessment of air leak, airway sizing, and insertion of bronchial valve(s), each additional lobe (List separately in addition to code for primary procedure[s])

➔ *CPT Changes: An Insider's View* 2013

►(Use 31651 in conjunction with 31647)◄

►(31656 has been deleted. To report, use 31899)◄

►Bronchial Thermoplasty◄

31660 Bronchoscopy, rigid or flexible, including fluoroscopic guidance, when performed; with bronchial thermoplasty, 1 lobe

➔ *CPT Changes: An Insider's View* 2013

heat source

31661 with bronchial thermoplasty, 2 or more lobes

➔ *CPT Changes: An Insider's View* 2013

Introduction

(For endotracheal intubation, use 31500)

(For tracheal aspiration under direct vision, see 31515)

►(31715 has been deleted. To report, use 31899)◄

31717 Catheterization with bronchial brush biopsy

➔ *CPT Assistant* Feb 01:11

31720 Catheter aspiration (separate procedure); nasotracheal

31725 tracheobronchial with fiberscope, bedside

31730 Transtracheal (percutaneous) introduction of needle wire dilator/stent or indwelling tube for oxygen therapy

Excision, Repair

31750 Tracheoplasty; cervical

➔ *CPT Assistant* Jul 11:12

31755 tracheopharyngeal fistulization, each stage

31760 intrathoracic

31766 Carinal reconstruction

31770 Bronchoplasty; graft repair

31775 excision stenosis and anastomosis

(For lobectomy and bronchoplasty, use 32501)

31780 Excision tracheal stenosis and anastomosis; cervical

31781 cervicothoracic

31785 Excision of tracheal tumor or carcinoma; cervical

31786 thoracic

31800 Suture of tracheal wound or injury; cervical

31805 intrathoracic

31820 Surgical closure tracheostomy or fistula; without plastic repair

31825 with plastic repair

(For repair tracheoesophageal fistula, see 43305, 43312)

31830 Revision of tracheostomy scar

Other Procedures

31899 Unlisted procedure, trachea, bronchi

➔ *CPT Assistant* Jan 10:11

Lungs and Pleura

Pleural cavity or lung biopsy procedures may be accomplished using a percutaneous, thoracoscopic (Video-Assisted Thoracoscopic Surgery [VATS]), or thoracotomy approach. They involve the removal of differing amounts of tissue for diagnosis. A biopsy may be performed using different techniques such as incision or wedge. Lung resection procedures include diagnostic and therapeutic procedures, including the removal of blebs, bullae, cysts, and benign or malignant tumors or lesions. These procedures may involve the removal of small portions of the lung or even an entire lung. Additionally, lung resection procedures may require the removal of adjacent structures. Both diagnostic lung biopsies and therapeutic lung resections can be performed utilizing a wedge technique. However, a diagnostic biopsy of a lung nodule using a wedge technique requires only that a tissue sample be obtained without particular attention to resection margins. A therapeutic wedge resection requires attention to margins and complete resection even when the wedge resection is ultimately followed by a more extensive resection. In the case of a wedge resection in which intraoperative pathology consultation determines that a more extensive resection is required in the same anatomic location, it becomes classified as a diagnostic wedge resection (32507, 32668). When no more extensive resection is required, the same procedure is a therapeutic wedge resection (32505, 32666).

Pleural or lung biopsies or diagnostic wedge resections should be reported using codes 32096, 32097, 32098, 32400, 32405, 32507, 32607, 32608, 32609, or 32668. The open or thoracoscopic (VATS) therapeutic resection of lung mass or nodules via a wedge resection is reported using codes 32505, 32506, 32666, and 32667. More extensive anatomic lung resection procedures, which can be performed with either thoracotomy or thoracoscopic (VATS) approaches, include: segmentectomy, lobectomy, bilobectomy, and pneumonectomy.

Respiratory

When diagnostic biopsy(ies) of the lung are performed, regardless of the approach (ie, open or thoracoscopic [VATS]) or technique (eg, incisional resection, cautery resection, or stapled wedge), and the specimen is sent for intraoperative pathology consultation, and during that same operative session the surgeon uses these results to determine the extent of the necessary surgical resection that includes the anatomical location biopsied, only the most extensive procedure performed (eg, segmentectomy, lobectomy, thoracoscopic [VATS] lobectomy) should be reported.

The therapeutic wedge resection codes (32505, 32506, 32666, or 32667) should not be reported in addition to the more extensive lung procedure (eg, lobectomy) unless the therapeutic wedge resection was performed on a different lobe or on the contralateral lung, whether or not an intraoperative pathology consultation is used to determine the extent of lung resection. When a diagnostic wedge resection is followed by a more extensive procedure in the same anatomical location, report add-on codes 32507 or 32668 with the more extensive procedure(s). When a therapeutic wedge resection (32505, 32506, 32666, or 32667) is performed in a different lobe than the more extensive lung resection (eg, lobectomy), report the therapeutic wedge resection with modifier 59.

Incision

(32000 has been deleted. To report, use 32421)

(32002 has been deleted. To report, use 32422)

(32005 has been deleted. To report, use 32560)

(32019 has been deleted. To report, use 32550)

(32020 has been deleted. To report, use 32551)

32035 Thoracostomy; with rib resection for empyema

32036 with open flap drainage for empyema

(To report wound exploration due to penetrating trauma without thoractomy, use 20101)

(32095 has been deleted. To report, see 32096, 32097, 32098 for thoracotomy with biopsy of the lung or pleura)

32096 Thoracotomy, with diagnostic biopsy(ies) of lung infiltrate(s) (eg, wedge, incisional), unilateral
➔ CPT Changes: An Insider's View 2012

(Do not report 32096 more than once per lung)

(Do not report 32096 in conjunction with 32440, 32442, 32445, 32488)

32097 Thoracotomy, with diagnostic biopsy(ies) of lung nodule(s) or mass(es) (eg, wedge, incisional), unilateral
➔ CPT Changes: An Insider's View 2012

(Do not report 32097 more than once per lung)

(Do not report 32097 in conjunction with 32440, 32442, 32445, 32488)

32098 Thoracotomy, with biopsy(ies) of pleura
➔ CPT Changes: An Insider's View 2012

32100 Thoracotomy; with exploration
➔ CPT Assistant Mar 07:1; CPT Changes: An Insider's View 2012

(Do not report 32100 in conjunction with 19260, 19271, 19272, 32503, 32504)

32110 with control of traumatic hemorrhage and/or repair of lung tear
➔ CPT Changes: An Insider's View 2012

32120 for postoperative complications
➔ CPT Changes: An Insider's View 2012

32124 with open intrapleural pneumonolysis
➔ CPT Changes: An Insider's View 2012

32140 with cyst(s) removal, includes pleural procedure when performed
➔ CPT Changes: An Insider's View 2012

32141 with resection-plication of bullae, includes any pleural procedure when performed
➔ CPT Changes: An Insider's View 2012

(For lung volume reduction, use 32491)

32150 with removal of intrapleural foreign body or fibrin deposit
➔ CPT Changes: An Insider's View 2012

32151 with removal of intrapulmonary foreign body
➔ CPT Changes: An Insider's View 2012

32160 with cardiac massage
➔ CPT Changes: An Insider's View 2012

(For segmental or other resections of lung, see 32480-32504)

32200 Pneumonostomy; with open drainage of abscess or cyst
➔ CPT Assistant Nov 97:15

⊙ **32201** with percutaneous drainage of abscess or cyst
➔ CPT Assistant Nov 97:15-16, Mar 98:8

(For radiological supervision and interpretation, use 75989)

32215 Pleural scarification for repeat pneumothorax

32220 Decortication, pulmonary (separate procedure); total

32225 partial

Excision/Resection

32310 Pleurectomy, parietal (separate procedure)

32320 Decortication and parietal pleurectomy

32400 Biopsy, pleura; percutaneous needle
➔ CPT Assistant Fall 94:1-2
➔ Clinical Examples in Radiology Summer 08:5, 6

(If imaging guidance is performed, see 76942, 77002, 77012, 77021)

(For fine needle aspiration, use 10021 or 10022)

(32402 has been deleted. To report open biopsy of pleura, use 32098)

⊙ **32405**   Biopsy, lung or mediastinum, percutaneous needle
→ *CPT Assistant* Fall 94:1-2, Mar 97:4, Aug 02:10; *CPT Changes: An Insider's View* 2012
→ *Clinical Examples in Radiology* Summer 08:5, 6

(For open biopsy of lung, see 32096, 32097. For open biopsy of mediastinum, see 39000 or 39010. For thoracoscopic [VATS] biopsy of lung, pleura, pericardium, or mediastinal space structure, see 32604, 32606, 32607, 32608, 32609)

(For radiological supervision and interpretation, see 76942, 77002, 77012, 77021)

(For fine needle aspiration, use 10022)

Removal

►(32420 has been deleted. To report, use 32405)◄

►(32421 and 32422 have been deleted. To report, see 32554, 32555)◄

32440   Removal of lung, pneumonectomy;
→ *CPT Assistant* Fall 94:1; *CPT Changes: An Insider's View* 2012

32442   with resection of segment of trachea followed by broncho-tracheal anastomosis (sleeve pneumonectomy)
→ *CPT Assistant* Fall 94:1, 3; *CPT Changes: An Insider's View* 2012

32445   extrapleural
→ *CPT Assistant* Fall 94:1, 3; *CPT Changes: An Insider's View* 2012

(For extrapleural pneumonectomy, with empyemectomy, use 32445 and 32540)

(If lung resection is performed with chest wall tumor resection, report the appropriate chest wall tumor resection 19260-19272, in addition to lung resection 32440-32445)

32480   Removal of lung, other than pneumonectomy; single lobe (lobectomy)
→ *CPT Assistant* Spring 91:5, Fall 94:1, 4; *CPT Changes: An Insider's View* 2012

32482   2 lobes (bilobectomy)
→ *CPT Assistant* Fall 94:1, 4, Jan 07:31; *CPT Changes: An Insider's View* 2012

32484   single segment (segmentectomy)
→ *CPT Assistant* Fall 94:1, 4; *CPT Changes: An Insider's View* 2012

(For removal of lung with bronchoplasty, use 32501)

32486   with circumferential resection of segment of bronchus followed by broncho-bronchial anastomosis (sleeve lobectomy)
→ *CPT Assistant* Fall 94:1, 4; *CPT Changes: An Insider's View* 2012

32488   with all remaining lung following previous removal of a portion of lung (completion pneumonectomy)
→ *CPT Assistant* Fall 94:1, 4; *CPT Changes: An Insider's View* 2012

(For lobectomy or segmentectomy, with concomitant decortication, use 32320 and the appropriate removal of lung code)

32491   with resection-plication of emphysematous lung(s) (bullous or non-bullous) for lung volume reduction, sternal split or transthoracic approach, includes any pleural procedure, when performed
→ *CPT Assistant* Nov 96:7; *CPT Changes: An Insider's View* 2012

(32500 has been deleted. To report open wedge resection of lung, see 32505, 32506, 32507)

(If lung resection is performed with chest wall tumor resection, report the appropriate chest wall tumor resection 19260-19272, in addition to lung resection 32480, 32482, 32484, 32486, 32488, 32505, 32506, 32507)

+ 32501   Resection and repair of portion of bronchus (bronchoplasty) when performed at time of lobectomy or segmentectomy (List separately in addition to code for primary procedure)

(Use 32501 in conjunction with 32480, 32482, 32484)

(32501 is to be used when a portion of the bronchus to preserved lung is removed and requires plastic closure to preserve function of that preserved lung. It is not to be used for closure for the proximal end of a resected bronchus)

32503   Resection of apical lung tumor (eg, Pancoast tumor), including chest wall resection, rib(s) resection(s), neurovascular dissection, when performed; without chest wall reconstruction(s)
→ *CPT Changes: An Insider's View* 2006

32504   with chest wall reconstruction
→ *CPT Changes: An Insider's View* 2006

►(Do not report 32503, 32504 in conjunction with 19260, 19271, 19272, 32100, 32551, 32554, 32555)◄

32505   Thoracotomy; with therapeutic wedge resection (eg, mass, nodule), initial
→ *CPT Changes: An Insider's View* 2012

(Do not report 32505 in conjunction with 32440, 32442, 32445, 32488)

+ 32506   with therapeutic wedge resection (eg, mass or nodule), each additional resection, ipsilateral (List separately in addition to code for primary procedure)
→ *CPT Changes: An Insider's View* 2012

(Report 32506 only in conjunction with 32505)

(If lung resection is performed with chest wall tumor resection, report the appropriate chest wall tumor resection 19260-19272, in addition to lung resection 32480, 32482, 32484, 32486, 32488, 32505, 32506, 32507)

Respiratory

+ 32507   with diagnostic wedge resection followed by anatomic lung resection (List separately in addition to code for primary procedure)

→ *CPT Changes: An Insider's View* 2012

(Report 32507 in conjunction with 32440, 32442, 32445, 32480, 32482, 32484, 32486, 32488, 32503, 32504)

32540   Extrapleural enucleation of empyema (empyemectomy)

(For extrapleural enucleation of empyema [empyemectomy] with lobectomy, use 32540 and the appropriate removal of lung code)

Introduction and Removal

⊙ **32550**   Insertion of indwelling tunneled pleural catheter with cuff

→ *CPT Assistant* Jul 10:10; *CPT Changes: An Insider's View* 2008

►(Do not report 32550 in conjunction with 32554, 32555)◄

(If imaging guidance is performed, use 75989)

⊙ ▲ **32551**   Tube thoracostomy, includes connection to drainage system (eg, water seal), when performed, open (separate procedure)

→ *CPT Assistant* Feb 09:7, Sep 10:6, Aug 11:4; *CPT Changes: An Insider's View* 2008, 2013

→ *Clinical Examples in Radiology* Fall 09:7, 10:10

Thoracentesis
32554, 32555

Accumulated fluid or air is removed from the pleural space by puncturing space between the ribs. In 32555, a tube is inserted and a syringe attached to the catheter for the removal of fluid and/or air.

32552   Removal of indwelling tunneled pleural catheter with cuff

→ *CPT Assistant* Feb 10:6; *CPT Changes: An Insider's View* 2010

⊙ **32553**   Placement of interstitial device(s) for radiation therapy guidance (eg, fiducial markers, dosimeter), percutaneous, intra-thoracic, single or multiple

→ *CPT Assistant* Feb 10:6, 7; *CPT Changes: An Insider's View* 2010

(Report supply of device separately)

(For imaging guidance, see 76942, 77002, 77012, 77021)

(For percutaneous placement of interstitial device[s] for intra-abdominal, intrapelvic, and/or retroperitoneal radiation therapy guidance, use 49411)

● **32554**   Thoracentesis, needle or catheter, aspiration of the pleural space; without imaging guidance

→ *CPT Changes: An Insider's View* 2013

● **32555**   with imaging guidance

→ *CPT Changes: An Insider's View* 2013

● **32556**   Pleural drainage, percutaneous, with insertion of indwelling catheter; without imaging guidance

→ *CPT Changes: An Insider's View* 2013

● **32557**   with imaging guidance

→ *CPT Changes: An Insider's View* 2013

►(For insertion of indwelling tunneled pleural catheter with cuff, use 32550)◄

►(For open procedure, use 32551)◄

►(Do not report 32554-32557 in conjunction with 32550, 32551, 76942, 77002, 77012, 77021, 75989)◄

Destruction

The instillation of a fibrinolytic agent may be performed multiple times per day over the course of several days. Code 32561 should be reported only once on the initial day treatment. Code 32562 should be reported only once on each subsequent day of treatment.

32560   Instillation, via chest tube/catheter, agent for pleurodesis (eg, talc for recurrent or persistent pneumothorax)

→ *CPT Assistant* Feb 10:6; *CPT Changes: An Insider's View* 2008, 2010

(For chest tube insertion, use 32551)

32561   Instillation(s), via chest tube/catheter, agent for fibrinolysis (eg, fibrinolytic agent for break up of multiloculated effusion); initial day

→ *CPT Assistant* Feb 10:6; *CPT Changes: An Insider's View* 2010

(For chest tube insertion, use 32551)

32562   subsequent day

→ *CPT Assistant* Feb 10:6; *CPT Changes: An Insider's View* 2010

(For chest tube insertion, use 32551)

Thoracoscopy (Video-assisted thoracic surgery [VATS])

Surgical thoracoscopy (video-assisted thoracic surgery [VATS]) always includes diagnostic thoracoscopy.

Thoracoscopy
32601-32665

The inside of the chest cavity is examined through a fiberoptic endoscope.

Placement of endoscope

Endoscope

Pleural cavity

Lung

Heart

Schematic transverse section of thoracic region

32601   Thoracoscopy, diagnostic (separate procedure); lungs, pericardial sac, mediastinal or pleural space, without biopsy
➡️ *CPT Assistant* Fall 94:1, 4; *CPT Changes: An Insider's View* 2012

(32602 has been deleted. To report lung or pleural space biopsy[ies], see 32607, 32608, 32609)

(32603 has been deleted. To report diagnostic thoracoscopy, pericardial sac, without biopsy, use 32601)

32604   pericardial sac, with biopsy
➡️ *CPT Assistant* Fall 94:1, 4

(32605 has been deleted. To report diagnostic thoracoscopy within the mediastinal space, use 32601)

(For open pericardial bipsy, use 39010)

32606   mediastinal space, with biopsy
➡️ *CPT Assistant* Fall 94:1, 5

32607   Thoracoscopy; with diagnostic biopsy(ies) of lung infiltrate(s) (eg, wedge, incisional), unilateral
➡️ *CPT Changes: An Insider's View* 2012

(Do not report 32607 more than once per lung)

(Do not report 32607 in conjunction with 32440, 32442, 32445, 32488, 32671)

32608   with diagnostic biopsy(ies) of lung nodule(s) or mass(es) (eg, wedge, incisional), unilateral
➡️ *CPT Changes: An Insider's View* 2012

(Do not report 32608 more than once per lung)

(Do not report 32608 in conjunction with 32440, 32442, 32445, 32488, 32671)

32609   with biopsy(ies) of pleura
➡️ *CPT Changes: An Insider's View* 2012

32650   Thoracoscopy, surgical; with pleurodesis (eg, mechanical or chemical)
➡️ *CPT Assistant* Fall 94:1, 6; *CPT Changes: An Insider's View* 2002

32651   with partial pulmonary decortication
➡️ *CPT Assistant* Fall 94:1, 6

32652   with total pulmonary decortication, including intrapleural pneumonolysis
➡️ *CPT Assistant* Fall 94:1, 6

32653   with removal of intrapleural foreign body or fibrin deposit
➡️ *CPT Assistant* Fall 94:1, 6

32654   with control of traumatic hemorrhage
➡️ *CPT Assistant* Fall 94:1, 6

32655   with resection-plication of bullae, includes any pleural procedure when performed
➡️ *CPT Assistant* Fall 94:1, 6, Aug 05:15; *CPT Changes: An Insider's View* 2012

(For thoracoscopic [VATS] lung volume reduction surgery, use 32672)

32656   with parietal pleurectomy
➡️ *CPT Assistant* Fall 94:1, 6

(32657 has been deleted. To report thoracoscopic [VATS] wedge resection of lung, see 32666, 32667, 32668)

32658   with removal of clot or foreign body from pericardial sac
➡️ *CPT Assistant* Fall 94:1, 6

32659   with creation of pericardial window or partial resection of pericardial sac for drainage
➡️ *CPT Assistant* Fall 94:1, 6

(32660 has been deleted)

32661   with excision of pericardial cyst, tumor, or mass
➡️ *CPT Assistant* Fall 94:1, 6

32662   with excision of mediastinal cyst, tumor, or mass
➡️ *CPT Assistant* Fall 94:1, 6

32663   with lobectomy (single lobe)
➡️ *CPT Assistant* Fall 94:1, 6; *CPT Changes: An Insider's View* 2012

(For thoracoscopic [VATS] segmentectomy, use 32669)

32664   with thoracic sympathectomy
➡️ *CPT Assistant* Fall 94:1, Oct 99:10

32665   with esophagomyotomy (Heller type)
➡️ *CPT Assistant* Fall 94:1, 6

Respiratory

(For exploratory thoracoscopy, and exploratory thoracoscopy with biopsy, see 32601-32609)

32666   with therapeutic wedge resection (eg, mass, nodule), initial unilateral
➜ *CPT Changes: An Insider's View* 2012

(To report bilateral procedure, report 32666 with modifier 50)

(Do not report 32666 in conjunction with 32440, 32442, 32445, 32488, 32671)

+ 32667   with therapeutic wedge resection (eg, mass or nodule), each additional resection, ipsilateral (List separately in addition to code for primary procedure)
➜ *CPT Changes: An Insider's View* 2012

(Report 32667 only in conjunction with 32666)

(Do not report 32667 in conjunction with 32440, 32442, 32445, 32488, 32671)

+ 32668   with diagnostic wedge resection followed by anatomic lung resection (List separately in addition to code for primary procedure)
➜ *CPT Changes: An Insider's View* 2012

(Report 32668 in conjunction with 32440, 32442, 32445, 32480, 32482, 32484, 32486, 32488, 32503, 32504, 32663, 32669, 32670, 32671)

32669   with removal of a single lung segment (segmentectomy)
➜ *CPT Changes: An Insider's View* 2012

32670   with removal of two lobes (bilobectomy)
➜ *CPT Changes: An Insider's View* 2012

32671   with removal of lung (pneumonectomy)
➜ *CPT Changes: An Insider's View* 2012

32672   with resection-plication for emphysematous lung (bullous or non-bullous) for lung volume reduction (LVRS), unilateral includes any pleural procedure, when performed
➜ *CPT Changes: An Insider's View* 2012

32673   with resection of thymus, unilateral or bilateral
➜ *CPT Changes: An Insider's View* 2012

(For open thymectomy see 60520, 60521, 60522)

(For open excision mediastinal cyst, see 39200; for open excision mediastinal tumor, use 39220)

(For exploratory thoracoscopy, and exploratory thoracoscopy with biopsy, see 32601-32609)

+ 32674   with mediastinal and regional lymphadenectomy (List separately in addition to code for primary procedure)
➜ *CPT Changes: An Insider's View* 2012

(On the right, mediastinal lymph nodes include the paratracheal, subcarinal, paraesophageal, and inferior pulmonary ligament)

(On the left, mediastinal lymph nodes include the aortopulmonary window, subcarinal, paraesophageal, and inferior pulmonary ligament)

(Report 32674 in conjunction with 32440, 32442, 32445, 32480, 32482, 32484, 32486, 32488, 32503, 32504, 32505, 32663, 32666, 32667, 32669, 32670, 32671)

(To report mediastinal and regional lymphadenectomy via thoracotomy, use 38746)

►Stereotactic Radiation Therapy◄

►Thoracic stereotactic body radiation therapy (SRS/SBRT) is a distinct procedure which may involve collaboration between a surgeon and radiation oncologist. The surgeon identifies and delineates the target for therapy. The radiation oncologist reports the appropriate code(s) for clinical treatment planning, physics and dosimetry, treatment delivery and management from the Radiation Oncology section (see 77295, 77331, 77370, 77373, 77435). The same physician should not report target delineation services with radiation treatment management codes (77427-77499).

Target delineation involves specific determination of tumor borders to identify tumor volume and relationship with adjacent structures (eg, chest wall, intraparenchymal vasculature and atelectatic lung) and previously placed fiducial markers, when present. Target delineation also includes availability to identify and validate the thoracic target prior to treatment delivery when a fiducial-less tracking system is utilized.

Do not report target delineation more than once per entire course of treatment when the treatment requires greater than one session.◄

● **32701**   Thoracic target(s) delineation for stereotactic body radiation therapy (SRS/SBRT), (photon or particle beam), entire course of treatment
➜ *CPT Changes: An Insider's View* 2013

►(Do not report 32701 in conjunction with 77261-77799)◄

►(For placement of fiducial markers, see 31626, 32553)◄

Repair

32800   Repair lung hernia through chest wall

32810   Closure of chest wall following open flap drainage for empyema (Clagett type procedure)

32815   Open closure of major bronchial fistula

32820   Major reconstruction, chest wall (posttraumatic)

Lung Transplantation

Lung allotransplantation involves three distinct components of physician work:

1. ***Cadaver donor pneumonectomy(s)***, which include(s) harvesting the allograft and cold preservation of the allograft (perfusing with cold preservation solution and cold maintenance) (use 32850).

2. *Backbench work*:

Preparation of a cadaver donor single lung allograft prior to transplantation, including dissection of the allograft from surrounding soft tissues to prepare the pulmonary venous/atrial cuff, pulmonary artery, and bronchus unilaterally (use 32855).

Preparation of a cadaver donor double lung allograft prior to transplantation, including dissection of the allograft from surrounding soft tissues to prepare the pulmonary venous/atrial cuff, pulmonary artery, and bronchus bilaterally (use 32856).

3. *Recipient lung allotransplantation*, which includes transplantation of a single or double lung allograft and care of the recipient (see 32851-32854).

32850   Donor pneumonectomy(s) (including cold preservation), from cadaver donor

➔ *CPT Changes: An Insider's View* 2005

32851   Lung transplant, single; without cardiopulmonary bypass

32852   with cardiopulmonary bypass

32853   Lung transplant, double (bilateral sequential or en bloc); without cardiopulmonary bypass

32854   with cardiopulmonary bypass

32855   Backbench standard preparation of cadaver donor lung allograft prior to transplantation, including dissection of allograft from surrounding soft tissues to prepare pulmonary venous/atrial cuff, pulmonary artery, and bronchus; unilateral

➔ *CPT Changes: An Insider's View* 2005

32856   bilateral

➔ *CPT Changes: An Insider's View* 2005

▶(For repair or resection procedures on the donor lung, see 32491, 32505, 32506, 32507, 35216, 35276)◀

Surgical Collapse Therapy; Thoracoplasty

(See also 32503, 32504)

32900   Resection of ribs, extrapleural, all stages

32905   Thoracoplasty, Schede type or extrapleural (all stages);

32906   with closure of bronchopleural fistula

(For open closure of major bronchial fistula, use 32815)

(For resection of first rib for thoracic outlet compression, see 21615, 21616)

32940   Pneumonolysis, extraperiosteal, including filling or packing procedures

32960   Pneumothorax, therapeutic, intrapleural injection of air

Other Procedures

32997   Total lung lavage (unilateral)

➔ *CPT Assistant* Nov 98:13, Nov 99:14; *CPT Changes: An Insider's View* 2000, 2002

(For bronchoscopic bronchial alveolar lavage, use 31624)

32998   Ablation therapy for reduction or eradication of 1 or more pulmonary tumor(s) including pleura or chest wall when involved by tumor extension, percutaneous, radiofrequency, unilateral

➔ *CPT Changes: An Insider's View* 2007

(For imaging guidance and monitoring, see 76940, 77013, 77022)

32999   Unlisted procedure, lungs and pleura

➔ *CPT Assistant* Jan 02:11, Feb 02:11, Jul 08:10, Apr 10:10, Aug 11:9

➔ *Clinical Examples in Radiology* Spring 06:8-9

Notes

⊙=Moderate sedation ✚=Add-on code ✗=FDA approval pending #=Resequenced code ○=Recycled/reinstated code ➜➜=See p xiii for details

Surgery

Cardiovascular System* (33010-37799)...175

The following is a listing of headings and subheadings that appear within the Cardiovascular System section of the CPT codebook. The subheadings or subsections denoted with asterisks (*) below have special instructions unique to that section. Where these are indicated, special "notes" or guidelines will be presented preceding those procedural terminology listings, referring to that subsection specifically.

Cardiovascular 33010

Cardiovascular

Arteries   Veins

Cardiovascular

Brachiocephalic vein
Subclavian vein
Superior vena cava
Upper arm cephalic vein
Brachial artery
Brachial vein
Basilic vein
Radial artery
Lower arm cephalic vein
Ulnar artery

Cervical lymph nodes
Right lymphatic duct
Thoracic lymph nodes
Axillary lymph nodes
Supratrochlear lymph nodes
Mesenteric lymph nodes
Iliac lymph nodes
Inguinal lymph nodes
Left lymphatic duct
Heart
Thoracic duct
Spleen
Cisterna chyli
Lumbar lymph nodes
Popliteal lymph nodes

Cardiovascular

Cardiovascular System

Selective vascular catheterizations should be coded to include introduction and all lesser order selective catheterizations used in the approach (eg, the description for a selective right middle cerebral artery catheterization includes the introduction and placement catheterization of the right common and internal carotid arteries).

Additional second and/or third order arterial catheterizations within the same family of arteries supplied by a single first order artery should be expressed by 36218 or 36248. Additional first order or higher catheterizations in vascular families supplied by a first order vessel different from a previously selected and coded family should be separately coded using the conventions described above.

> (For monitoring, operation of pump and other nonsurgical services, see 99190-99192, 99291, 99292, 99354-99360)

> (For other medical or laboratory related services, see appropriate section)

> (For radiological supervision and interpretation, see 75600-75978)

Heart and Pericardium

Pericardium

> (For thoracoscopic (VATS) pericardial procedures, see 32601, 32604, 32658, 32659, 32661)

⊙ **33010**   Pericardiocentesis; initial

> (For radiological supervision and interpretation, use 76930)

⊙ **33011**   subsequent
> ➔ *CPT Assistant* Sep 10:7

> (For radiological supervision and interpretation, use 76930)

33015   Tube pericardiostomy

33020   Pericardiotomy for removal of clot or foreign body (primary procedure)

33025   Creation of pericardial window or partial resection for drainage

> (For thoracoscopic (VATS) pericardial window, use 32659)

33030   Pericardiectomy, subtotal or complete; without cardiopulmonary bypass

33031   with cardiopulmonary bypass

33050   Resection of pericardial cyst or tumor
> ➔ *CPT Changes: An Insider's View* 2012

> (For open pericardial biopsy, use 39010)

> (For thoracoscopic (VATS) resection of pericardial cyst, tumor or mass, use 32661)

Cardiac Tumor

33120   Excision of intracardiac tumor, resection with cardiopulmonary bypass
> ➔ *CPT Assistant* Mar 07:1

33130   Resection of external cardiac tumor
> ➔ *CPT Assistant* Mar 07:1

Transmyocardial Revascularization

33140   Transmyocardial laser revascularization, by thoracotomy; (separate procedure)
> ➔ *CPT Assistant* Nov 99:14, Nov 00:5, Apr 01:7; *CPT Changes: An Insider's View* 2000, 2001, 2002

+ **33141**   performed at the time of other open cardiac procedure(s) (List separately in addition to code for primary procedure)
> ➔ *CPT Assistant* Apr 01:7; *CPT Changes: An Insider's View* 2001

> (Use 33141 in conjunction with 33400-33496, 33510-33536, 33542)

Pacemaker or Pacing Cardioverter-Defibrillator

A pacemaker system includes a pulse generator containing electronics, a battery, and one or more electrodes (leads). Pulse generators are placed in a subcutaneous "pocket" created in either a subclavicular site or underneath the abdominal muscles just below the ribcage. Electrodes may be inserted through a vein (transvenous) or they may be placed on the surface of the heart (epicardial). The epicardial location of electrodes requires a thoracotomy for electrode insertion.

A single chamber pacemaker system includes a pulse generator and one electrode inserted in either the atrium or ventricle. A dual chamber pacemaker system includes a pulse generator and one electrode inserted in the right atrium and one electrode inserted in the right ventricle. In certain circumstances, an additional electrode may be required to achieve pacing of the left ventricle (bi-ventricular pacing). In this event, transvenous (cardiac vein) placement of the electrode should be separately reported using code 33224 or 33225. Epicardial placement of the electrode should be separately reported using 33202-33203.

Like a pacemaker system, a pacing cardioverter-defibrillator (ICD) system includes a pulse generator and electrodes, although pacing cardioverter-defibrillators may require multiple leads, even when only a single chamber is being paced. A pacing cardioverter-defibrillator system may be inserted in a single chamber (pacing in the ventricle) or in dual chambers (pacing in atrium and ventricle). These devices use a combination of antitachycardia pacing, low-energy cardioversion or defibrillating shocks to treat ventricular tachycardia or ventricular fibrillation.

Cardiovascular

Pacing cardioverter-defibrillator pulse generators may be implanted in a subcutaneous infraclavicular pocket or in an abdominal pocket. Removal of a pacing cardioverter-defibrillator pulse generator requires opening of the existing subcutaneous pocket and disconnection of the pulse generator from its electrode(s). A thoracotomy (or laparotomy in the case of abdominally placed pulse generators) is not required to remove the pulse generator.

The electrodes (leads) of a pacing cardioverter-defibrillator system are positioned in the heart via the venous system (transvenously), in most circumstances. In certain circumstances, an additional electrode may be required to achieve pacing of the left ventricle (bi-ventricular pacing). In this event, transvenous (cardiac vein) placement of the electrode should be separately reported using code 33224 or 33225. Epicardial placement of the electrode should be separately reported using 33202-33203.

Electrode positioning on the epicardial surface of the heart requires a thoracotomy, or thoracoscopic placement of the leads. Removal of electrode(s) may first be attempted by transvenous extraction (33234, 33235, or 33244). However, if transvenous extraction is unsuccessful, a thoracotomy may be required to remove the electrodes (33238 or 33243). Use 33212, 33213, 33221, 33230, 33231, 33240 as appropriate in addition to the thoracotomy or endoscopic epicardial lead placement codes (33202 or 33203) to report the insertion of the generator if done by the same physician during the same session.

When the "battery" of a pacemaker or pacing cardioverter-defibrillator is changed, it is actually the pulse generator that is changed. Removal of pacemaker or pacing cardioverter-defibrillator pulse generator only is reported with 33233 or 33241. Removal of a pacemaker or pacing cardioverter-defibrillator pulse generator with insertion of a new pulse generator without any replacement or insertion of a lead(s) is reported with 33227-33229 and 33262-33264. Insertion of a new pulse generator, when existing leads are already in place and when no prior pulse generator is removed, is reported with 33212, 33213, 33221, 33230, 33231, 33240. When a pulse generator insertion involves the insertion or replacement of one or more lead(s), use the system codes 33206-33208 for pacemaker or 33249 for pacing cardioverter-defibrillator. Removal of a pulse generator (33233 or 33241) or extraction of transvenous leads (33234, 33235 or 33244) should be reported separately. An exception involves a pacemaker upgrade from single to dual system which includes removal of pulse generator, replacement of new pulse generator, and insertion of new lead, reported with 33214.

Repositioning of a pacemaker electrode, pacing cardioverter-defibrillator electrode(s), or a left ventricular pacing electrode is reported using 33215 or 33226, as appropriate.

The pacemaker and pacing cardioverter-defibrillator device evaluation codes 93279-93299 may not be reported in conjunction with pulse generator and lead insertion or revision codes 33206-33249. Defibrillator threshold testing (DFT) during pacing cardioverter-defibrillator insertion or replacement may be separately reported using 93640, 93641.

Radiological supervision and interpretation related to the pacemaker or pacing cardioverter-defibrillator procedure is included in 33206-33249. To report fluoroscopic guidance for diagnostic lead evaluation without lead insertion, replacement, or revision procedures, use 76000.

The following definitions apply to 33206-33249.

Single lead: a pacemaker or pacing cardioverter-defibrillator with pacing and sensing function in only one chamber of the heart.

Dual lead: a pacemaker or pacing cardioverter-defibrillator with pacing and sensing function in only two chambers of the heart.

Multiple lead: a pacemaker or pacing cardioverter-defibrillator with pacing and sensing function in three or more chambers of the heart.

33202 Insertion of epicardial electrode(s); open incision (eg, thoracotomy, median sternotomy, subxiphoid approach)
➔ *CPT Assistant* Jun 12:5; *CPT Changes: An Insider's View* 2007

33203 endoscopic approach (eg, thoracoscopy, pericardioscopy)
➔ *CPT Assistant* Jun 12:4; *CPT Changes: An Insider's View* 2007

(When epicardial lead placement is performed with insertion of the generator, report 33202, 33203 in conjunction with 33212, 33213, 33221, 33230, 33231, 33240)

⊙ **33206** Insertion of new or replacement of permanent pacemaker with transvenous electrode(s); atrial
➔ *CPT Assistant* Summer 94:10, 17, Oct 96:9, Nov 99:15, Jun 08:14, Jun 12:3; *CPT Changes: An Insider's View* 2012

⊙ **33207** ventricular
➔ *CPT Assistant* Summer 94:10, 17, Oct 96:9, Nov 99:15, Jun 08:14, Jun 12:3; *CPT Changes: An Insider's View* 2012

⊙ **33208** atrial and ventricular
➔ *CPT Assistant* Summer 94:10, 17, Jul 96:10, Nov 99:15, Jun 08:14, Jun 12:3; *CPT Changes: An Insider's View* 2012

	System	
▶Transvenous Procedure	Pacemaker	Implantable Cardioverter-Defibrillator
Insert transvenous single lead only without pulse generator	33216	33216
Insert transvenous dual leads without pulse generator	33217	33217
Insert transvenous multiple leads without pulse generator	33217 + 33224	33217 + 33224
Initial pulse generator insertion only with existing single lead	33212	33240
Initial pulse generator insertion only with existing dual leads	33213	33230
Initial pulse generator insertion only with existing multiple leads	33221	33231
Initial pulse generator insertion or replacement plus insertion of transvenous single lead	33206 (atrial) or 33207 (ventricular)	33249
Initial pulse generator insertion or replacement plus insertion of transvenous dual leads	33208	33249
Initial pulse generator insertion or replacement plus insertion of transvenous multiple leads	33208 + 33225	33249 + 33225
Upgrade single chamber system to dual chamber system	33214 (includes removal of existing pulse generator)	33241 + 33249
Removal pulse generator only (without replacement)	33233	33241
Removal pulse generator with replacement pulse generator only single lead system (transvenous)	33227	33262
Removal pulse generator with replacement pulse generator only dual lead system (transvenous)	33228	33263
Removal pulse generator with replacement pulse generator only multiple lead system (transvenous)	33229	33264
Removal transvenous electrode only single lead system	33234	33244
Removal transvenous electrode only dual lead system	33235	33244
Removal and replacement of pulse generator and transvenous electrodes	33233 + (33234 or 33235) + (33206 or 33207 or 33208) and 33225, when appropriate	33241 + 33244 + 33249 and 33225, when appropriate
Conversion of existing system to bi-ventricular system (addition of LV lead and removal of current pulse generator with insertion of new pulse generator with bi-ventricular pacing capabilities	33225 + 33228 or 33229	33225 + 33263 or 33264◀

(Codes 33206-33208 include subcutaneous insertion of the pulse generator and transvenous placement of electrode[s])

(For removal and replacement of pacemaker pulse generator and transvenous electrode(s), use 33233 in conjunction with either 33234 or 33235 and 33206-33208)

(Do not report 33206-33208 in conjunction with 33227-33229)

⊙ **33210**   Insertion or replacement of temporary transvenous single chamber cardiac electrode or pacemaker catheter (separate procedure)

➔ *CPT Assistant* Summer 94:10, 17, Mar 07:1, Aug 11:4, Jun 12:3

Temporary Pacemaker
33210

The pacemaker pulse generator with the electrodes transvenously placed

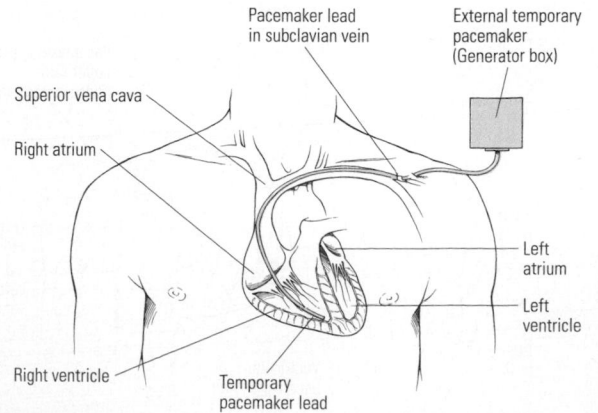

Pacemaker lead in subclavian vein

External temporary pacemaker (Generator box)

Superior vena cava

Right atrium

Left atrium

Left ventricle

Right ventricle

Temporary pacemaker lead

Cardiovascular

⊙ **33211** Insertion or replacement of temporary transvenous dual chamber pacing electrodes (separate procedure)

➔ *CPT Assistant* Summer 94:10, 17, Mar 07:1, Aug 11:4, Jun 12:3

⊙ **33212** Insertion of pacemaker pulse generator only; with existing single lead

➔ *CPT Assistant* Summer 94:10, 18, Fall 94:24, May 04:15, Jun 08:14, Jun 12:3; *CPT Changes: An Insider's View* 2012

⊙ **33213** with existing dual leads

➔ *CPT Assistant* Summer 94:10, 18, Oct 96:10, Feb 98:11, Jun 12:3; *CPT Changes: An Insider's View* 2012

\#⊙ **33221** with existing multiple leads

➔ *CPT Assistant* Jun 12:3; *CPT Changes: An Insider's View* 2012

(Do not report 33212, 33213, 33221 in conjunction with 33233 for removal and replacement of the pacemaker pulse generator. Use 33227-33229, as appropriate, when pulse generator replacement is indicated)

(When epicardial lead placement is performed with insertion of generator, report 33202, 33203 in conjunction with 33212, 33213, 33221)

Implanted Pacemaker
33212-33214

A. In 33212, a pacemaker pulse generator is inserted with an existing single lead.

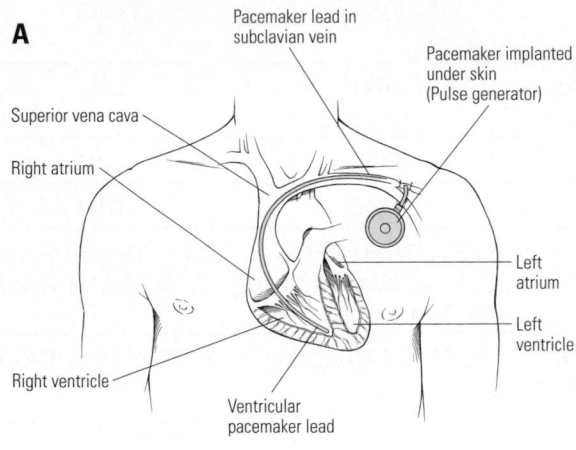

B. In 33213, a pacemaker pulse generator is inserted or replaced in two chambers. In 33214, an upgrade to an existing pacemaker system is done.

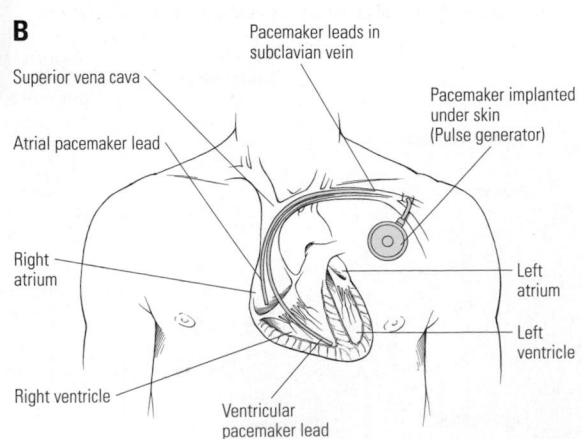

⊙ **33214** Upgrade of implanted pacemaker system, conversion of single chamber system to dual chamber system (includes removal of previously placed pulse generator, testing of existing lead, insertion of new lead, insertion of new pulse generator)

➔ *CPT Assistant* Summer 94:10, 18, Fall 94:24, Jun 08:14, Jun 12:3

(Do not report 33214 in conjunction with 33227-33229)

33215 Repositioning of previously implanted transvenous pacemaker or pacing cardioverter-defibrillator (right atrial or right ventricular) electrode

➔ *CPT Assistant* Jun 12:3; *CPT Changes: An Insider's View* 2003

⊙ **33216** Insertion of a single transvenous electrode, permanent pacemaker or cardioverter-defibrillator

➔ *CPT Assistant* Summer 94:10, 18, Jul 96:10, Nov 99:15-16; *CPT Changes: An Insider's View* 2000, 2003, 2010

⊙ **33217** Insertion of 2 transvenous electrodes, permanent pacemaker or cardioverter-defibrillator

➔ *CPT Assistant* Summer 94:10, 18, Jul 96:10, Nov 99:15-16, Jul 00:5, Apr 09:8, Jun 12:3; *CPT Changes: An Insider's View* 2000, 2010

(Do not report 33216-33217 in conjunction with 33214)

(For insertion or replacement of a cardiac venous system lead, see 33224, 33225)

⊙ **33218** Repair of single transvenous electrode, permanent pacemaker or pacing cardioverter-defibrillator

➔ *CPT Assistant* Summer 94:10, 19, Oct 96:9, Nov 99:15-16, Jun 12:3; *CPT Changes: An Insider's View* 2000, 2012

(For repair of single permanent pacemaker or pacing cardioverter-defibrillator electrode with replacement of pulse generator, see 33227-33229 or 33262-33264 and 33218)

⊙ **33220** Repair of 2 transvenous electrodes for permanent pacemaker or pacing cardioverter-defibrillator

➔ *CPT Assistant* Summer 94:10, 19, Oct 96:9, Nov 99:15-16, Jun 08:14, Jun 12:3; *CPT Changes: An Insider's View* 2000, 2012

(For repair of 2 transvenous electrodes for permanent pacemaker or pacing cardioverter-defibrillator with replacement of pulse generator, use 33220 in conjunction with 33228, 33229, 33263, 33264)

33221 Code is out of numerical sequence. See 33202-33249

⊙ **33222** Revision or relocation of skin pocket for pacemaker

➔ *CPT Assistant* Spring 94:30, Summer 94:10, Nov 99:15-16, Jun 08:14, Jun 12:3; *CPT Changes: An Insider's View* 2000

⊙ **33223** Revision of skin pocket for cardioverter-defibrillator

➔ *CPT Assistant* Summer 94:10, 19, Nov 99:15-16, Jun 08:14, Jun 12:3; *CPT Changes: An Insider's View* 2000, 2010

33224 Insertion of pacing electrode, cardiac venous system, for left ventricular pacing, with attachment to previously placed pacemaker or pacing cardioverter-defibrillator pulse generator (including revision of pocket, removal, insertion, and/or replacement of existing generator)

➔ *CPT Assistant* Dec 07:16, Jun 12:3; *CPT Changes: An Insider's View* 2003, 2012

(When epicardial electrode placement is performed, report 33224 in conjunction with 33202, 33203)

Biventricular Pacing
33224-33226

Insertion or repositioning of venous pacing electrode

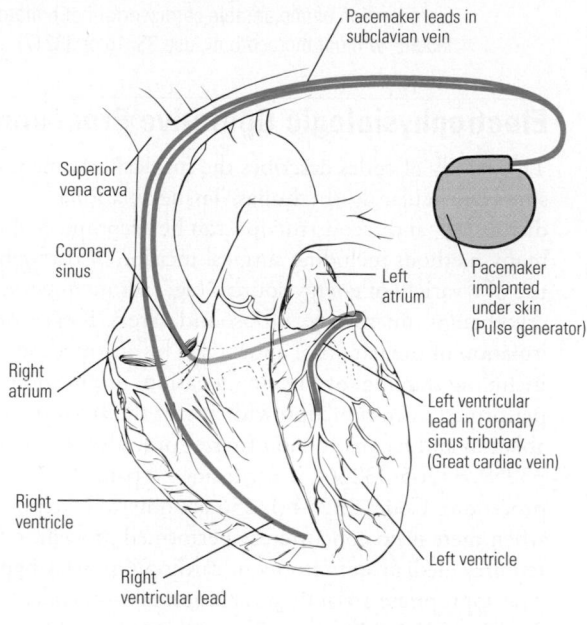

Pacemaker leads in subclavian vein

Superior vena cava

Coronary sinus

Left atrium

Pacemaker implanted under skin (Pulse generator)

Right atrium

Left ventricular lead in coronary sinus tributary (Great cardiac vein)

Right ventricle

Left ventricle

Right ventricular lead

+▲ 33225 Insertion of pacing electrode, cardiac venous system, for left ventricular pacing, at time of insertion of pacing cardioverter-defibrillator or pacemaker pulse generator (eg, for upgrade to dual chamber system) (List separately in addition to code for primary procedure)

➔ *CPT Assistant* Dec 07:16, Jun 12:3; *CPT Changes: An Insider's View* 2003, 2012, 2013

▶(Use 33225 in conjunction with 33206, 33207, 33208, 33212, 33213, 33214, 33216, 33217, 33221, 33228, 33229, 33230, 33231, 33233, 33234, 33235, 33240, 33249, 33263, 33264)◀

▶(Use 33225 in conjunction with 33222 only with pacemaker pulse generator pocket relocation and with 33223 only with pacing cardioverter-defibrillator [ICD] pocket relocation)◀

33226 Repositioning of previously implanted cardiac venous system (left ventricular) electrode (including removal, insertion and/or replacement of existing generator)

➔ *CPT Assistant* Jun 12:3; *CPT Changes: An Insider's View* 2003, 2012

33227 Code is out of numerical sequence. See 33202-33249

33228 Code is out of numerical sequence. See 33202-33249

33229 Code is out of numerical sequence. See 33202-33249

33230 Code is out of numerical sequence. See 33202-33249

33231 Code is out of numerical sequence. See 33202-33249

⊙ 33233 Removal of permanent pacemaker pulse generator only

➔ *CPT Assistant* Summer 94:10, 19, Fall 94:24, Oct 96:10, Jun 12:3; *CPT Changes: An Insider's View* 2000, 2012

#⊙ 33227 Removal of permanent pacemaker pulse generator with replacement of pacemaker pulse generator; single lead system

➔ *CPT Assistant* Jun 12:3; *CPT Changes: An Insider's View* 2012

#⊙ 33228 dual lead system

➔ *CPT Assistant* Jun 12:3; *CPT Changes: An Insider's View* 2012

#⊙ 33229 multiple lead system

➔ *CPT Assistant* Jun 12:3; *CPT Changes: An Insider's View* 2012

(Do not report 33227-33229 in conjunction with 33233)

(For removal and replacement of pacemaker pulse generator and transvenous electrode[s], use 33233 in conjunction with either 33234 or 33235 and 33206-33208)

⊙ 33234 Removal of transvenous pacemaker electrode(s); single lead system, atrial or ventricular

➔ *CPT Assistant* Summer 94:10, 19, Nov 99:16, Jun 12:3; *CPT Changes: An Insider's View* 2000

⊙ 33235 dual lead system

➔ *CPT Assistant* Summer 94:10, 19, Nov 99:16, Jun 12:3; *CPT Changes: An Insider's View* 2000

33236 Removal of permanent epicardial pacemaker and electrodes by thoracotomy; single lead system, atrial or ventricular

➔ *CPT Assistant* Summer 94:10, 19, Nov 99:16, Jun 12:3; *CPT Changes: An Insider's View* 2000

33237 dual lead system

➔ *CPT Assistant* Summer 94:10, 19, Nov 99:16, Jun 12:3; *CPT Changes: An Insider's View* 2000

33238 Removal of permanent transvenous electrode(s) by thoracotomy

➔ *CPT Assistant* Summer 94:10, 19, Nov 99:16, Jun 12:3; *CPT Changes: An Insider's View* 2000

⊙ 33240 Insertion of pacing cardioverter-defibrillator pulse generator only; with existing single lead

➔ *CPT Assistant* Summer 94:40, Jun 96:10, Nov 99:16-17, Jul 00:5, Apr 04:6, Jun 08:14, Jun 12:3; *CPT Changes: An Insider's View* 2000, 2012

(Use 33240, as appropriate, in addition to the epicardial lead placement codes to report the insertion of the generator when done by the same physician during the same session)

#⊙ 33230 with existing dual leads

➔ *CPT Assistant* Jun 12:3; *CPT Changes: An Insider's View* 2012

#⊙ 33231 with existing multiple leads

➔ *CPT Assistant* Jun 12:3; *CPT Changes: An Insider's View* 2012

(Do not report 33230, 33231, 33240 in conjunction with 33241 for removal and replacement of the pacing cardioverter-defibrillator pulse generator. Use 33262-33264, as appropriate, when pulse generator replacement is indicated)

(When epicardial lead placement is performed with insertion of generator, report 33202, 33203 in conjunction with 33230, 33231, 33240)

▲=Revised code   ●=New code   ▶ ◀=Contains new or revised text   ⊘=Modifier 51 exempt

Cardiovascular

⊙ **33241** Removal of pacing cardioverter-defibrillator pulse generator only

→ *CPT Assistant* Summer 94:40, Nov 99:16-17, Jun 12:3; *CPT Changes: An Insider's View* 2000, 2012

(For removal and replacement of a pacing cardioverter-defibrillator pulse generator and electrode(s), use 33241 in conjunction with either 33243 or 33244 and 33249)

#⊙ **33262** Removal of pacing cardioverter-defibrillator pulse generator with replacement of pacing cardioverter-defibrillator pulse generator; single lead system

→ *CPT Assistant* Jun 12:3; *CPT Changes: An Insider's View* 2012

#⊙ **33263** dual lead system

→ *CPT Assistant* Jun 12:3; *CPT Changes: An Insider's View* 2012

#⊙ **33264** multiple lead system

→ *CPT Assistant* Jun 12:3; *CPT Changes: An Insider's View* 2012

(Do not report 33262-33264 in conjunction with 33241)

(For removal of electrode[s] by thoracotomy in conjunction with pulse generator removal or replacement, use 33243 in conjunction with 33241, 33262-33264)

(For removal of electrode[s] by transvenous extraction in conjunction with pulse generator removal or replacement, use 33244 in conjunction with 33241, 33262-33264)

(For repair of implantable cardioverter-defibrillator pulse generator and/or leads, see 33218, 33220)

—— *Coding Tip* ——

Reporting for Electrode Removal and Lead Placement

Removal of electrode(s) may first be attempted by transvenous extraction (code 33244). However, if transvenous extraction is unsuccessful, a thoracotomy may be required to remove the electrodes (code 33243). Use codes 33212, 33213, 33240 as appropriate in addition to the thoracotomy or endoscopic epicardial lead placement codes to report the insertion of the generator if done by the same physician during the same session.

CPT Coding Guidelines, Pacemaker or Pacing Cardioverter-Defibrillator

33243 Removal of single or dual chamber pacing cardioverter-defibrillator electrode(s); by thoracotomy

→ *CPT Assistant* Summer 94:40, Nov 99:16-17, Jun 12:3; *CPT Changes: An Insider's View* 2000

⊙ **33244** by transvenous extraction

→ *CPT Assistant* Summer 94:40, Nov 99:16-17, Jul 00:5, Jun 12:3; *CPT Changes: An Insider's View* 2000, 2012

⊙ **33249** Insertion or replacement of permanent pacing cardioverter-defibrillator system with transvenous lead(s), single or dual chamber

→ *CPT Assistant* Summer 94:21, Nov 99:16-17, Apr 04:6, May 08:14, Jun 08:14, Jun 12:3; *CPT Changes: An Insider's View* 2000, 2012

(For removal and replacement of a pacing cardioverter-defibrillator system [pulse generator and electrodes], report 33241 in conjunction with either 33243 or 33244 and 33249)

(For insertion of implantable cardioverter-defibrillator lead(s), without thoracotomy, use 33216 or 33217)

Electrophysiologic Operative Procedures

This family of codes describes the surgical treatment of supraventricular dysrhythmias. Tissue ablation, disruption, and reconstruction can be accomplished by many methods including surgical incision or through the use of a variety of energy sources (eg, radiofrequency, cryotherapy, microwave, ultrasound, laser). If excision or isolation of the left atrial appendage by any method, including stapling, oversewing, ligation, or plication, is performed in conjunction with any of the atrial tissue ablation and reconstruction (maze) procedures (33254-33259, 33265-33266), it is considered part of the procedure. Codes 33254-33256 are only to be reported when there is no concurrently performed procedure that requires median sternotomy or cardiopulmonary bypass. The appropriate atrial tissue ablation add-on code, 33257, 33258, 33259 should be reported in addition to an open cardiac procedure requiring sternotomy or cardiopulmonary bypass if performed concurrently.

Definitions

Limited operative ablation and reconstruction includes:

Surgical isolation of triggers of supraventricular dysrhythmias by operative ablation that isolates the pulmonary veins or other anatomically defined triggers in the left or right atrium.

Extensive operative ablation and reconstruction includes:

1. The services included in "*limited*"

2. Additional ablation of atrial tissue to eliminate sustained supraventricular dysrhythmias. This must include operative ablation that involves either the right atrium, the atrial septum, or left atrium in continuity with the atrioventricular annulus.

Incision

33250 Operative ablation of supraventricular arrhythmogenic focus or pathway (eg, Wolff-Parkinson-White, atrioventricular node re-entry), tract(s) and/or focus (foci); without cardiopulmonary bypass

→ *CPT Assistant* Summer 94:16, Nov 99:17-18; *CPT Changes: An Insider's View* 2000, 2002

(For intraoperative pacing and mapping by a separate provider, use 93631)

33251 with cardiopulmonary bypass

→ *CPT Assistant* Summer 94:16, Nov 99:17-18; *CPT Changes: An Insider's View* 2000

Cardiovascular

Reporting Restriction for Operative Tissue Ablation

Codes 33254-33256 are only to be reported when there is no concurrently performed procedure that requires median sternotomy or cardiopulmonary bypass.

CPT Coding Guidelines, Electrophysiologic Operative Procedures

33254 Operative tissue ablation and reconstruction of atria, limited (eg, modified maze procedure)
➔ *CPT Assistant* Mar 07:1; *CPT Changes: An Insider's View* 2007

33255 Operative tissue ablation and reconstruction of atria, extensive (eg, maze procedure); without cardiopulmonary bypass
➔ *CPT Assistant* Mar 07:1; *CPT Changes: An Insider's View* 2007

33256 with cardiopulmonary bypass
➔ *CPT Assistant* Mar 07:1; *CPT Changes: An Insider's View* 2007

(Do not report 33254-33256 in conjunction with 32100, 32551, 33120, 33130, 33210, 33211, 33400-33507, 33510-33523, 33533-33548, 33600-33853, 33860-33864, 33910-33920)

+ 33257 Operative tissue ablation and reconstruction of atria, performed at the time of other cardiac procedure(s), limited (eg, modified maze procedure) (List separately in addition to code for primary procedure)
➔ *CPT Changes: An Insider's View* 2008

(Use 33257 in conjunction with 33120-33130, 33250-33251, 33261, 33300-33335, 33400-33496, 33500-33507, 33510-33516, 33533-33548, 33600-33619, 33641-33697, 33702-33732, 33735-33767, 33770-33814, 33840-33877, 33910-33922, 33925-33926, 33935, 33945, 33975-33980)

+ 33258 Operative tissue ablation and reconstruction of atria, performed at the time of other cardiac procedure(s), extensive (eg, maze procedure), without cardiopulmonary bypass (List separately in addition to code for primary procedure)
➔ *CPT Changes: An Insider's View* 2008

(Use 33258 in conjunction with 33130, 33250, 33300, 33310, 33320, 33321, 33330, 33332, 33401, 33414-33417, 33420, 33470-33472, 33501-33503, 33510-33516, 33533-33536, 33690, 33735, 33737, 33800-33813, 33840-33852, 33915, 33925 when the procedure is performed without cardiopulmonary bypass)

+ 33259 Operative tissue ablation and reconstruction of atria, performed at the time of other cardiac procedure(s), extensive (eg, maze procedure), with cardiopulmonary bypass (List separately in addition to code for primary procedure)
➔ *CPT Changes: An Insider's View* 2008

(Use 33259 in conjunction with 33120, 33251, 33261, 33305, 33315, 33322, 33335, 33400, 33403-33413, 33422-33468, 33474-33478, 33496, 33500, 33504-33507, 33510-33516, 33533-33548, 33600-33688, 33692-33722, 33730, 33732, 33736, 33750-33767, 33770-33781, 33786-33788, 33814, 33853, 33860-33877, 33910, 33916-33922, 33926, 33935, 33945, 33975-33980 when the procedure is performed with cardiopulmonary bypass)

(Do not report 33257, 33258 and 33259 in conjunction with 32551, 33210, 33211, 33254-33256, 33265, 33266)

33261 Operative ablation of ventricular arrhythmogenic focus with cardiopulmonary bypass
➔ *CPT Assistant* Summer 94:16

33262 Code is out of numerical sequence. See 33202-33264

33263 Code is out of numerical sequence. See 33202-33264

33264 Code is out of numerical sequence. See 33202-33264

Endoscopy

33265 Endoscopy, surgical; operative tissue ablation and reconstruction of atria, limited (eg, modified maze procedure), without cardiopulmonary bypass
➔ *CPT Assistant* Mar 07:1; *CPT Changes: An Insider's View* 2007

33266 operative tissue ablation and reconstruction of atria, extensive (eg, maze procedure), without cardiopulmonary bypass
➔ *CPT Assistant* Mar 07:1; *CPT Changes: An Insider's View* 2007

(Do not report 33265-33266 in conjunction with 32551, 33210, 33211)

Patient-Activated Event Recorder

33282 Implantation of patient activated cardiac event recorder
➔ *CPT Assistant* Nov 99:17-18, Jul 00:5, Jun 08:14; *CPT Changes: An Insider's View* 2000

(Initial implantation includes programming. For subsequent electronic analysis and/or reprogramming, use 93285, 93291, 93298)

33284 Removal of an implantable, patient-activated cardiac event recorder
➔ *CPT Assistant* Nov 99:17-18, Jul 00:5; *CPT Changes: An Insider's View* 2000

►Heart (Including Valves) and Great Vessels◄

►Patients receiving major cardiac procedures may require simultaneous cardiopulmonary bypass insertion of cannulae into the venous and arterial vasculatures with support of circulation and oxygenation by a heart-lung machine. Most services are described by codes in dyad arrangements to allow distinct reporting of procedures with or without cardiopulmonary bypass. Cardiopulmonary bypass is distinct from support of cardiac output using devices (eg, ventricular assist or intra-aortic balloon). For cardiac assist services see 33960-33983, 33990-33993.◄

33300   Repair of cardiac wound; without bypass

33305   with cardiopulmonary bypass

33310   Cardiotomy, exploratory (includes removal of foreign body, atrial or ventricular thrombus); without bypass
➜ *CPT Changes: An Insider's View* 2004

33315   with cardiopulmonary bypass
➜ *CPT Assistant* Oct 10:12, Dec 10:12

(Do not report removal of thrombus [33310-33315] in conjunction with other cardiac procedures unless a separate incision in the heart is required to remove the atrial or ventricular thrombus)

(If removal of thrombus with cardiopulmonary bypass [33315] is reported in conjunction with 33120, 33130, 33420-33430, 33460-33468, 33496, 33542, 33545, 33641-33647, 33670, 33681, 33975-33980 which requires a separate heart incision, report 33315 with modifier 59)

33320   Suture repair of aorta or great vessels; without shunt or cardiopulmonary bypass
➜ *CPT Assistant* Fall 91:7

33321   with shunt bypass
➜ *CPT Assistant* Fall 91:7

33322   with cardiopulmonary bypass
➜ *CPT Assistant* Fall 91:7

33330   Insertion of graft, aorta or great vessels; without shunt, or cardiopulmonary bypass

33332   with shunt bypass

33335   with cardiopulmonary bypass

Cardiac Valves

(For multiple valve procedures, see 33400-33478 and add modifier 51 to the secondary valve procedure code)

Aortic Valve

►Codes 33361-33365, 0318T are used to report transcatheter aortic valve replacement (TAVR)/transcatheter aortic valve implantation (TAVI). TAVR/TAVI requires two physician operators and all components of the procedure are reported using modifier 62.

Codes 33361-33365, 0318T include the work, when performed, of percutaneous access, placing the access sheath, balloon aortic valvuloplasty, advancing the valve delivery system into position, repositioning the valve as needed, deploying the valve, temporary pacemaker insertion for rapid pacing (33210), and closure of the arteriotomy when performed. Codes 33361-33365, 0318T include open arterial or cardiac approach.

Angiography, radiological supervision, and interpretation performed to guide TAVR/TAVI (eg, guiding valve placement, documenting completion of the intervention, assessing the vascular access site for closure) are included in these codes.

Diagnostic left heart catheterization codes (93452, 93453, 93458-93461) and the supravalvular aortography code (93567) should **not** be used with TAVR/TAVI services (33361-33365, 0318T) to report:

1. Contrast injections, angiography, roadmapping, and/or fluoroscopic guidance for the TAVR/TAVI,

2. Aorta/left ventricular outflow tract measurement for the TAVR/TAVI, or

3. Post-TAVR/TAVI aortic or left ventricular angiography, as this work is captured in the TAVR/TAVI services codes (33361-33365, 0318T).

Diagnostic coronary angiography performed at the time of TAVR/TAVI may be separately reportable if:

1. No prior catheter-based coronary angiography study is available and a full diagnostic study is performed, or

2. A prior study is available, but as documented in the medical record:

   a. The patient's condition with respect to the clinical indication has changed since the prior study, or

   b. There is inadequate visualization of the anatomy and/or pathology, or

   c. There is a clinical change during the procedure that requires new evaluation.

   d. For same session/same day diagnostic coronary angiography services, report the appropriate diagnostic cardiac catheterization code(s) appended with modifier 59 indicating separate and distinct procedural service from TAVR/TAVI.

Diagnostic coronary angiography performed at a separate session from an interventional procedure may be separately reportable.

Other cardiac catheterization services are reported separately when performed for diagnostic purposes not intrinsic to TAVR/TAVI.

Percutaneous coronary interventional procedures are reported separately, when performed.

When transcatheter ventricular support is required in conjunction with TAVR/TAVI, the appropriate code should be reported with the appropriate ventricular assist device (VAD) procedure code (33990-33993, 33975, 33976, 33999) or balloon pump insertion code (33967, 33970, 33973).

The TAVR/TAVI cardiovascular access and delivery procedures are reported with 33361-33365, 0318T. When cardiopulmonary bypass is performed in conjunction with TAVR/TAVI, codes 33361-33365, 0318T should be reported with the appropriate add-on code for percutaneous peripheral bypass (33367), open peripheral bypass (33368), or central bypass (33369).◄

● **33361**   Transcatheter aortic valve replacement (TAVR/TAVI) with prosthetic valve; percutaneous femoral artery approach
➜ *CPT Changes: An Insider's View* 2013

● **33362**   open femoral artery approach
➜ *CPT Changes: An Insider's View* 2013

● **33363**   open axillary artery approach
➜ *CPT Changes: An Insider's View* 2013

● **33364**   open iliac artery approach
➜ *CPT Changes: An Insider's View* 2013

● **33365**   transaortic approach (eg, median sternotomy, mediastinotomy)
➜ *CPT Changes: An Insider's View* 2013

►(Use 0318T for transapical approach [eg, left thoracotomy])◄

+● **33367**   cardiopulmonary bypass support with percutaneous peripheral arterial and venous cannulation (eg, femoral vessels) (List separately in addition to code for primary procedure)
➜ *CPT Changes: An Insider's View* 2013

►(Use 33367 in conjunction with 33361-33365, 0318T)◄

►(Do not report 33367 in conjunction with 33368, 33369)◄

+● **33368**   cardiopulmonary bypass support with open peripheral arterial and venous cannulation (eg, femoral, iliac, axillary vessels) (List separately in addition to code for primary procedure)
➜ *CPT Changes: An Insider's View* 2013

►(Use 33368 in conjunction with 33361-33365, 0318T)◄

►(Do not report 33368 in conjunction with 33367, 33369)◄

+● **33369**   cardiopulmonary bypass support with central arterial and venous cannulation (eg, aorta, right atrium, pulmonary artery) (List separately in addition to code for primary procedure)
➜ *CPT Changes: An Insider's View* 2013

►(Use 33369 in conjunction with 33361-33365, 0318T)◄

►(Do not report 33369 in conjunction with 33367, 33368)◄

33400   Valvuloplasty, aortic valve; open, with cardiopulmonary bypass
➜ *CPT Assistant* Feb 05:14, Mar 07:1

33401   open, with inflow occlusion
➜ *CPT Assistant* Feb 05:14

33403   using transventricular dilation, with cardiopulmonary bypass
➜ *CPT Assistant* Feb 05:14

(Do not report modifier 63 in conjunction with 33401, 33403)

33404   Construction of apical-aortic conduit
➜ *CPT Assistant* Jan 04:28, Feb 05:14

33405   Replacement, aortic valve, with cardiopulmonary bypass; with prosthetic valve other than homograft or stentless valve
➜ *CPT Assistant* Nov 99:18, Feb 05:14, Aug 11:3; *CPT Changes: An Insider's View* 2000

33406   with allograft valve (freehand)
➜ *CPT Assistant* Nov 99:18, Feb 05:14, Aug 11:3; *CPT Changes: An Insider's View* 2002

(For aortic valve valvotomy, [commissurotomy] with inflow occlusion, use 33401)

(For aortic valve valvotomy, [commissurotomy] with cardiopulmonary bypass, use 33403)

33410   with stentless tissue valve
➜ *CPT Assistant* Nov 99:18, Feb 05:14, Aug 11:3; *CPT Changes: An Insider's View* 2000

33411   Replacement, aortic valve; with aortic annulus enlargement, noncoronary sinus
➜ *CPT Assistant* Feb 05:14, Aug 11:3; *CPT Changes: An Insider's View* 2011

33412   with transventricular aortic annulus enlargement (Konno procedure)
➜ *CPT Assistant* Feb 05:14, Aug 11:3

33413   by translocation of autologous pulmonary valve with allograft replacement of pulmonary valve (Ross procedure)
➜ *CPT Assistant* Feb 05:14, Aug 11:3; *CPT Changes: An Insider's View* 2002

33414   Repair of left ventricular outflow tract obstruction by patch enlargement of the outflow tract
➜ *CPT Assistant* Feb 05:14

33415   Resection or incision of subvalvular tissue for discrete subvalvular aortic stenosis
➜ *CPT Assistant* Feb 05:14

33416   Ventriculomyotomy (-myectomy) for idiopathic hypertrophic subaortic stenosis (eg, asymmetric septal hypertrophy)
➜ *CPT Assistant* Feb 05:14

33417   Aortoplasty (gusset) for supravalvular stenosis
➜ *CPT Assistant* Feb 05:14

Cardiovascular

Mitral Valve

33420   Valvotomy, mitral valve; closed heart
     CPT Assistant Feb 05:14

33422   open heart, with cardiopulmonary bypass
       CPT Assistant Feb 05:14

33425   Valvuloplasty, mitral valve, with cardiopulmonary bypass;
     CPT Assistant May 03:19, Feb 05:14

33426   with prosthetic ring
       CPT Assistant Feb 05:14

33427   radical reconstruction, with or without ring
       CPT Assistant Feb 05:14

33430   Replacement, mitral valve, with cardiopulmonary bypass
     CPT Assistant Feb 05:14

Tricuspid Valve

33460   Valvectomy, tricuspid valve, with cardiopulmonary bypass
     CPT Assistant Feb 05:14

33463   Valvuloplasty, tricuspid valve; without ring insertion
     CPT Assistant Feb 05:14

33464   with ring insertion
       CPT Assistant Feb 05:14

33465   Replacement, tricuspid valve, with cardiopulmonary bypass
     CPT Assistant Feb 05:14

33468   Tricuspid valve repositioning and plication for Ebstein anomaly
     CPT Assistant Feb 05:14

Pulmonary Valve

33470   Valvotomy, pulmonary valve, closed heart; transventricular
     CPT Assistant Feb 05:14

     (Do not report modifier 63 in conjunction with 33470)

33471   via pulmonary artery
       CPT Assistant Feb 05:14

     (To report percutaneous valvuloplasty of pulmonary valve, use 92990)

33472   Valvotomy, pulmonary valve, open heart; with inflow occlusion
     CPT Assistant Feb 05:14

     (Do not report modifier 63 in conjunction with 33472)

33474   with cardiopulmonary bypass
       CPT Assistant Feb 05:14

33475   Replacement, pulmonary valve
     CPT Assistant Feb 05:14

33476   Right ventricular resection for infundibular stenosis, with or without commissurotomy
     CPT Assistant Feb 05:14

33478   Outflow tract augmentation (gusset), with or without commissurotomy or infundibular resection
     CPT Assistant Feb 05:14

     (Use 33478 in conjunction with 33768 when a cavopulmonary anastomosis to a second superior vena cava is performed)

Other Valvular Procedures

33496   Repair of non-structural prosthetic valve dysfunction with cardiopulmonary bypass (separate procedure)
     CPT Assistant Nov 97:16, Feb 05:14

     (For reoperation, use 33530 in addition to 33496)

Coronary Artery Anomalies

Basic procedures include endarterectomy or angioplasty.

33500   Repair of coronary arteriovenous or arteriocardiac chamber fistula; with cardiopulmonary bypass

33501   without cardiopulmonary bypass

33502   Repair of anomalous coronary artery from pulmonary artery origin; by ligation
     CPT Changes: An Insider's View 2006

33503   by graft, without cardiopulmonary bypass

     (Do not report modifier 63 in conjunction with 33502, 33503)

33504   by graft, with cardiopulmonary bypass

33505   with construction of intrapulmonary artery tunnel (Takeuchi procedure)

33506   by translocation from pulmonary artery to aorta

     (Do not report modifier 63 in conjunction with 33505, 33506)

33507   Repair of anomalous (eg, intramural) aortic origin of coronary artery by unroofing or translocation
     CPT Assistant Mar 07:1; *CPT Changes: An Insider's View* 2006

Endoscopy

Surgical vascular endoscopy always includes diagnostic endoscopy.

+ 33508   Endoscopy, surgical, including video-assisted harvest of vein(s) for coronary artery bypass procedure (List separately in addition to code for primary procedure)
     CPT Changes: An Insider's View 2003

     (Use 33508 in conjunction with 33510-33523)

     (For open harvest of upper extremity vein procedure, use 35500)

Cardiovascular

Venous Grafting Only for Coronary Artery Bypass

The following codes are used to report coronary artery bypass procedures using venous grafts only. These codes should NOT be used to report the performance of coronary artery bypass procedures using arterial grafts and venous grafts during the same procedure. See 33517-33523 and 33533-33536 for reporting combined arterial-venous grafts.

►Procurement of the saphenous vein graft is included in the description of the work for 33510-33516 and should not be reported as a separate service or co-surgery. To report harvesting of an upper extremity vein, use 35500 in addition to the bypass procedure. To report harvesting of a femoropopliteal vein segment, report 35572 in addition to the bypass procedure. When surgical assistant performs graft procurement, add modifier 80 to 33510-33516. For percutaneous ventricular assist device insertion, removal, repositioning, see 33990-33993.◄

Coronary Artery Bypass—Venous Grafting Only
33510-33516

A. Use 33510 to report a single coronary venous graft.

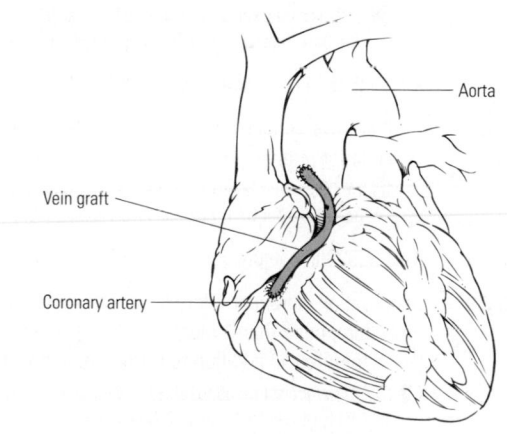

B. Report 33512 when 3 coronary venous grafts are performed.

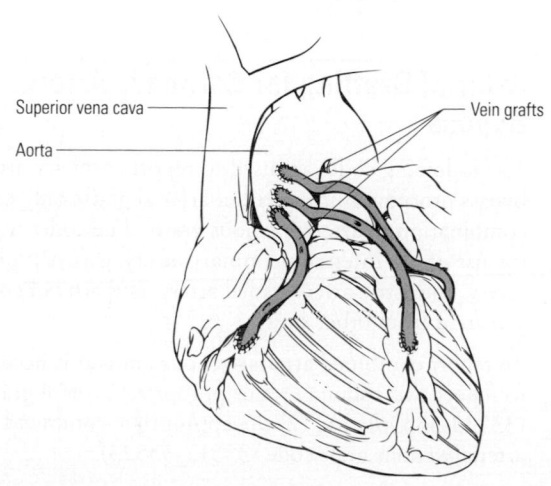

33510   Coronary artery bypass, vein only; single coronary venous graft

  ➔ *CPT Assistant* Fall 91:5, Winter 92:12, Jul 99:11, Apr 01:7, Feb 05:14, Jan 07:7, Mar 07:1

33511   2 coronary venous grafts

  ➔ *CPT Assistant* Fall 91:5, Winter 92:12, Jul 99:11, Apr 01:7, Feb 05:14, Jan 07:7, Mar 07:1

33512   3 coronary venous grafts

  ➔ *CPT Assistant* Fall 91:5, Winter 92:12, Apr 01:7, Feb 05:14, Jan 07:7, Mar 07:1

33513   4 coronary venous grafts

  ➔ *CPT Assistant* Fall 91:5, Winter 92:12, Apr 01:7, Feb 05:14, Jan 07:7, Mar 07:1

33514   5 coronary venous grafts

  ➔ *CPT Assistant* Fall 91:5, Winter 92:12, Apr 01:7, Feb 05:14, Jan 07:7, Mar 07:1

33516   6 or more coronary venous grafts

  ➔ *CPT Assistant* Fall 91:5, Winter 92:12, Jul 99:11, Apr 01:7, Feb 05:14, Jan 07:7, Mar 07:1

Combined Arterial-Venous Grafting for Coronary Bypass

The following codes are used to report coronary artery bypass procedures using venous grafts and arterial grafts during the same procedure. These codes may NOT be used alone.

To report combined arterial-venous grafts it is necessary to report two codes: (1) the appropriate combined arterial-venous graft code (33517-33523); and (2) the appropriate arterial graft code (33533-33536).

►Procurement of the saphenous vein graft is included in the description of the work for 33517-33523 and should not be reported as a separate service or co-surgery. Procurement of the artery for grafting is included in the description of the work for 33533-33536 and should not be reported as a separate service or co-surgery, except when an upper extremity artery (eg, radial artery) is procured. To report harvesting of an upper extremity artery, use 35600 in addition to the bypass procedure. To report harvesting of an upper extremity vein, use 35500 in addition to the bypass procedure. To report harvesting of a femoropopliteal vein segment, report 35572 in addition to the bypass procedure. When surgical assistant performs arterial and/or venous graft procurement, add modifier 80 to 33517-33523, 33533-33536, as appropriate. For percutaneous ventricular assist device insertion, removal, repositioning, see 33990-33993.◄

Coronary Artery Bypass—Combined Arterial-Venous Grafting
33517-33530

Both venous and arterial grafts are used in these bypass procedures. The appropriate arterial graft codes (33533-33536) must also be reported in conjunction with codes 33517-33530.

Coronary Artery Bypass—Sequential Combined Arterial-Venous Grafting
33517-33530

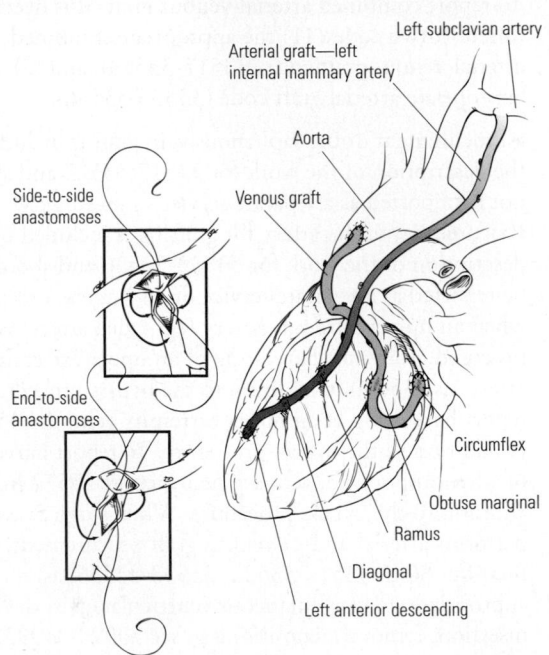

Note: To determine the number of bypass grafts in a coronary artery bypass (CABG), count the number of distal anastomoses (contact point[s]) where the bypass graft artery or vein is sutured to the diseased coronary artery(s).

+ 33517   Coronary artery bypass, using venous graft(s) and arterial graft(s); single vein graft (List separately in addition to code for primary procedure)

> *CPT Assistant* Fall 91:5, Winter 92:13, Nov 99:18, Apr 01:7, Feb 05:14; *CPT Changes: An Insider's View* 2000, 2008

(Use 33517 in conjunction with 33533-33536)

+ 33518   2 venous grafts (List separately in addition to code for primary procedure)

> *CPT Assistant* Fall 91:5, Winter 92:13, Apr 01:7, Feb 05:14, Jan 07:7, Mar 07:1; *CPT Changes: An Insider's View* 2008

(Use 33518 in conjunction with 33533-33536)

+ 33519   3 venous grafts (List separately in addition to code for primary procedure)

> *CPT Assistant* Fall 91:5, Winter 92:13, Apr 01:7, Feb 05:14, Jan 07:7, Mar 07:1; *CPT Changes: An Insider's View* 2008

(Use 33519 in conjunction with 33533-33536)

+ 33521   4 venous grafts (List separately in addition to code for primary procedure)

> *CPT Assistant* Fall 91:5, Winter 92:13, Apr 01:7, Feb 05:14, Jan 07:7, Mar 07:1; *CPT Changes: An Insider's View* 2008

(Use 33521 in conjunction with 33533-33536)

+ 33522   5 venous grafts (List separately in addition to code for primary procedure)

> *CPT Assistant* Fall 91:5, Winter 92:13, Apr 01:7, Feb 05:14, Jan 07:7, Mar 07:1; *CPT Changes: An Insider's View* 2008

(Use 33522 in conjunction with 33533-33536)

+ 33523   6 or more venous grafts (List separately in addition to code for primary procedure)

> *CPT Assistant* Fall 91:5, Winter 92:13, Apr 01:7, Feb 05:14, Jan 07:7, Mar 07:1; *CPT Changes: An Insider's View* 2008

(Use 33523 in conjunction with 33533-33536)

+ 33530   Reoperation, coronary artery bypass procedure or valve procedure, more than 1 month after original operation (List separately in addition to code for primary procedure)

> *CPT Assistant* Winter 90:6, Fall 91:5, Winter 92:13, Apr 01:7, Jul 01:11, Feb 05:13-14, Jan 07:7, Feb 11:8

(Use 33530 in conjunction with 33400-33496; 33510-33536, 33863)

Arterial Grafting for Coronary Artery Bypass

The following codes are used to report coronary artery bypass procedures using either arterial grafts only or a combination of arterial-venous grafts. The codes include the use of the internal mammary artery, gastroepiploic artery, epigastric artery, radial artery, and arterial conduits procured from other sites.

To report combined arterial-venous grafts it is necessary to report two codes: (1) the appropriate arterial graft code (33533-33536); and (2) the appropriate combined arterial-venous graft code (33517-33523).

Cardiovascular

►Procurement of the artery for grafting is included in the description of the work for 33533-33536 and should not be reported as a separate service or co-surgery, except when an upper extremity artery (eg, radial artery) is procured. To report harvesting of an upper extremity artery, use 35600 in addition to the bypass procedure. To report harvesting of an upper extremity vein, use 35500 in addition to the bypass procedure. To report harvesting of a femoropopliteal vein segment, report 35572 in addition to the bypass procedure. When surgical assistant performs arterial and/or venous graft procurement, add modifier 80 to 33517-33523, 33533-33536, as appropriate. For percutaneous ventricular assist device insertion, removal, repositioning, see 33990-33993.◄

33533   Coronary artery bypass, using arterial graft(s); single arterial graft
> *CPT Assistant* Winter 92:12, Nov 99:18, Apr 01:7, Feb 05:14, Jan 07:7, Mar 07:1; *CPT Changes: An Insider's View* 2000

33534   2 coronary arterial grafts
> *CPT Assistant* Winter 92:12, Apr 01:7, Feb 05:14, Jan 07:7, Mar 07:1

33535   3 coronary arterial grafts
> *CPT Assistant* Winter 92:12, Apr 01:7, Feb 05:14, Jan 07:7, Mar 07:1

33536   4 or more coronary arterial grafts
> *CPT Assistant* Winter 92:12, Apr 01:7, Feb 05:14, Jan 07:7, Mar 07:1

33542   Myocardial resection (eg, ventricular aneurysmectomy)
> *CPT Assistant* Winter 92:12, Mar 07:1

33545   Repair of postinfarction ventricular septal defect, with or without myocardial resection
> *CPT Assistant* Winter 92:12, Mar 07:1

33548   Surgical ventricular restoration procedure, includes prosthetic patch, when performed (eg, ventricular remodeling, SVR, SAVER, Dor procedures)
> *CPT Assistant* Nov 06:21, Dec 06:10, Mar 07:1; *CPT Changes: An Insider's View* 2006

(Do not report 33548 in conjunction with 32551, 33210, 33211, 33310, 33315)

(For Batista procedure or pachopexy, use 33999)

Coronary Endarterectomy

+ **33572**   Coronary endarterectomy, open, any method, of left anterior descending, circumflex, or right coronary artery performed in conjunction with coronary artery bypass graft procedure, each vessel (List separately in addition to primary procedure)

(Use 33572 in conjunction with 33510-33516, 33533-33536)

Single Ventricle and Other Complex Cardiac Anomalies

33600   Closure of atrioventricular valve (mitral or tricuspid) by suture or patch
> *CPT Assistant* Mar 07:1

33602   Closure of semilunar valve (aortic or pulmonary) by suture or patch

33606   Anastomosis of pulmonary artery to aorta (Damus-Kaye-Stansel procedure)

33608   Repair of complex cardiac anomaly other than pulmonary atresia with ventricular septal defect by construction or replacement of conduit from right or left ventricle to pulmonary artery

(For repair of pulmonary artery arborization anomalies by unifocalization, see 33925-33926)

33610   Repair of complex cardiac anomalies (eg, single ventricle with subaortic obstruction) by surgical enlargement of ventricular septal defect
> *CPT Changes: An Insider's View* 2002

(Do not report modifier 63 in conjunction with 33610)

33611   Repair of double outlet right ventricle with intraventricular tunnel repair;

(Do not report modifier 63 in conjunction with 33611)

33612   with repair of right ventricular outflow tract obstruction

33615   Repair of complex cardiac anomalies (eg, tricuspid atresia) by closure of atrial septal defect and anastomosis of atria or vena cava to pulmonary artery (simple Fontan procedure)

33617   Repair of complex cardiac anomalies (eg, single ventricle) by modified Fontan procedure

(Use 33617 in conjunction with 33768 when a cavopulmonary anastomosis to a second superior vena cava is performed)

33619   Repair of single ventricle with aortic outflow obstruction and aortic arch hypoplasia (hypoplastic left heart syndrome) (eg, Norwood procedure)
> *CPT Assistant* Mar 07:1, Apr 11:6, May 12:14

(Do not report modifier 63 in conjunction with 33619)

33620   Application of right and left pulmonary artery bands (eg, hybrid approach stage 1)
> *CPT Assistant* Apr 11:3, May 12:14; *CPT Changes: An Insider's View* 2011

(For banding of the main pulmonary artery related to septal defect, use 33690)

Cardiovascular

33621 Transthoracic insertion of catheter for stent placement with catheter removal and closure (eg, hybrid approach stage 1)

➜ *CPT Assistant* Apr 11:3; *CPT Changes: An Insider's View* 2011

(For placement of stent, use 37207)

(Report both 33620, 33621 if performed in same session)

Initial Hybrid Palliation
33621

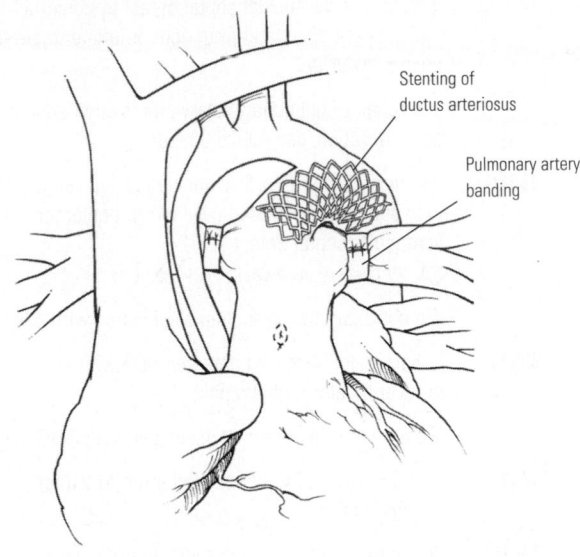

Initial Hybrid Palliation, Stage I

Stenting of ductus arteriosus

Pulmonary artery banding

33622 Reconstruction of complex cardiac anomaly (eg, single ventricle or hypoplastic left heart) with palliation of single ventricle with aortic outflow obstruction and aortic arch hypoplasia, creation of cavopulmonary anastomosis, and removal of right and left pulmonary bands (eg, hybrid approach stage 2, Norwood, bidirectional Glenn, pulmonary artery debanding)

➜ *CPT Assistant* Apr 11:3, May 12:14; *CPT Changes: An Insider's View* 2011

(Do not report 33622 in conjunction with 33619, 33767, 33822, 33840, 33845, 33851, 33853, 33917)

(For bilateral, bidirectional Glenn procedure, use 33622 in conjunction with 33768)

Septal Defect

33641 Repair atrial septal defect, secundum, with cardiopulmonary bypass, with or without patch

➜ *CPT Assistant* Mar 07:1, Dec 10:12

33645 Direct or patch closure, sinus venosus, with or without anomalous pulmonary venous drainage

(Do not report 33645 in conjunction with 33724, 33726)

33647 Repair of atrial septal defect and ventricular septal defect, with direct or patch closure

Hybrid Reconstruction
33622

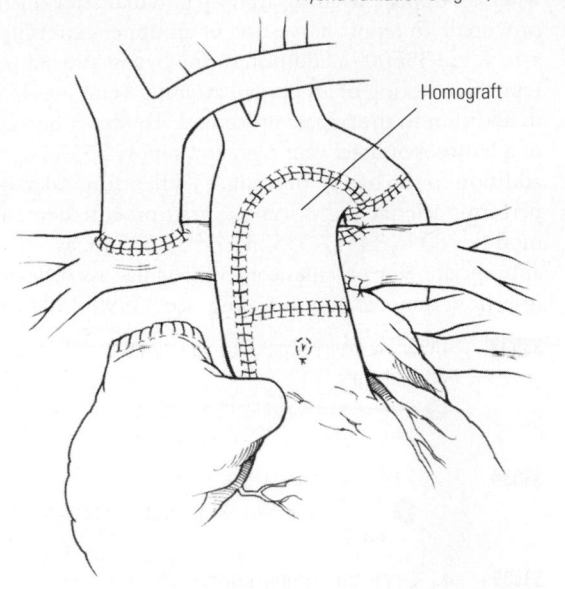

Hybrid Palliation Stage II, Reconstructi

Homograft

(Do not report modifier 63 in conjunction with 33647)

(For repair of tricuspid atresia (eg, Fontan, Gago procedures), use 33615)

33660 Repair of incomplete or partial atrioventricular canal (ostium primum atrial septal defect), with or without atrioventricular valve repair

33665 Repair of intermediate or transitional atrioventricular canal, with or without atrioventricular valve repair

33670 Repair of complete atrioventricular canal, with or without prosthetic valve

(Do not report modifier 63 in conjunction with 33670)

33675 Closure of multiple ventricular septal defects;

➜ *CPT Assistant* Mar 07:1; *CPT Changes: An Insider's View* 2007

33676 with pulmonary valvotomy or infundibular resection (acyanotic)

➜ *CPT Assistant* Mar 07:1; *CPT Changes: An Insider's View* 2007

33677 with removal of pulmonary artery band, with or without gusset

➜ *CPT Assistant* Mar 07:1; *CPT Changes: An Insider's View* 2007

►(Do not report 33675-33677 in conjunction with 32100, 32551, 32554, 32555, 33210, 33681, 33684, 33688)◄

(For percutaneous closure, use 93581)

33681 Closure of single ventricular septal defect, with or without patch;

➜ *CPT Assistant* Mar 07:1; *CPT Changes: An Insider's View* 2007

33684   with pulmonary valvotomy or infundibular resection (acyanotic)

33688   with removal of pulmonary artery band, with or without gusset

(For pulmonary vein repair requiring creation of atrial septal defect, use 33724)

33690   Banding of pulmonary artery

➔ *CPT Assistant* Apr 11:4, May 12:14

(For right and left pulmonary artery banding in a single ventricle [eg, hybrid approach stage 1], use 33620)

(Do not report modifier 63 in conjunction with 33690)

33692   Complete repair tetralogy of Fallot without pulmonary atresia;

33694   with transannular patch

(Do not report modifier 63 in conjunction with 33694)

(For ligation and takedown of a systemic-to-pulmonary artery shunt, performed in conjunction with a congenital heart procedure; see 33924)

33697   Complete repair tetralogy of Fallot with pulmonary atresia including construction of conduit from right ventricle to pulmonary artery and closure of ventricular septal defect

➔ *CPT Assistant* Mar 07:1

(For ligation and takedown of a systemic-to-pulmonary artery shunt, performed in conjunction with a congenital heart procedure; see 33924)

Sinus of Valsalva

33702   Repair sinus of Valsalva fistula, with cardiopulmonary bypass;

➔ *CPT Assistant* Mar 07:1

33710   with repair of ventricular septal defect

33720   Repair sinus of Valsalva aneurysm, with cardiopulmonary bypass

33722   Closure of aortico-left ventricular tunnel

➔ *CPT Assistant* Mar 07:1

Venous Anomalies

33724   Repair of isolated partial anomalous pulmonary venous return (eg, Scimitar Syndrome)

➔ *CPT Assistant* Mar 07:1; *CPT Changes: An Insider's View* 2007

(Do not report 33724 in conjunction with 32551, 33210, 33211)

33726   Repair of pulmonary venous stenosis

➔ *CPT Assistant* Mar 07:1; *CPT Changes: An Insider's View* 2007

(Do not report 33726 in conjunction with 32551, 33210, 33211)

33730   Complete repair of anomalous pulmonary venous return (supracardiac, intracardiac, or infracardiac types)

➔ *CPT Assistant* Mar 07:1

(Do not report modifier 63 in conjunction with 33730)

(For partial anomalous pulmonary venous return, use 33724; for repair of pulmonary venous stenosis, use 33726)

33732   Repair of cor triatriatum or supravalvular mitral ring by resection of left atrial membrane

➔ *CPT Assistant* Mar 07:1

(Do not report modifier 63 in conjunction with 33732)

Shunting Procedures

33735   Atrial septectomy or septostomy; closed heart (Blalock-Hanlon type operation)

➔ *CPT Assistant* Mar 07:1

33736   open heart with cardiopulmonary bypass

(Do not report modifier 63 in conjunction with 33735, 33736)

33737   open heart, with inflow occlusion

(For transvenous method cardiac catheterization balloon atrial septectomy or septostomy (Rashkind type), use 92992)

(For blade method cardiac catheterization atrial septectomy or septostomy (Sang-Park septostomy), use 92993)

33750   Shunt; subclavian to pulmonary artery (Blalock-Taussig type operation)

33755   ascending aorta to pulmonary artery (Waterston type operation)

33762   descending aorta to pulmonary artery (Potts-Smith type operation)

(Do not report modifier 63 in conjunction with 33750, 33755, 33762)

33764   central, with prosthetic graft

33766   superior vena cava to pulmonary artery for flow to 1 lung (classical Glenn procedure)

33767   superior vena cava to pulmonary artery for flow to both lungs (bidirectional Glenn procedure)

➔ *CPT Assistant* Apr 11:6

+ 33768   Anastomosis, cavopulmonary, second superior vena cava (List separately in addition to primary procedure)

➔ *CPT Assistant* Mar 07:1, Apr 11:6; *CPT Changes: An Insider's View* 2006

(Use 33768 in conjunction with 33478, 33617, 33622, 33767)

(Do not report 33768 in conjunction with 32551, 33210, 33211)

Cardiovascular

Transposition of the Great Vessels

33770 Repair of transposition of the great arteries with ventricular septal defect and subpulmonary stenosis; without surgical enlargement of ventricular septal defect
➔ *CPT Assistant* Mar 07:1

33771 with surgical enlargement of ventricular septal defect

33774 Repair of transposition of the great arteries, atrial baffle procedure (eg, Mustard or Senning type) with cardiopulmonary bypass;

33775 with removal of pulmonary band

33776 with closure of ventricular septal defect

33777 with repair of subpulmonic obstruction

33778 Repair of transposition of the great arteries, aortic pulmonary artery reconstruction (eg, Jatene type);

(Do not report modifier 63 in conjunction with 33778)

33779 with removal of pulmonary band

33780 with closure of ventricular septal defect

33781 with repair of subpulmonic obstruction
➔ *CPT Assistant* Mar 07:1

33782 Aortic root translocation with ventricular septal defect and pulmonary stenosis repair (ie, Nikaidoh procedure); without coronary ostium reimplantation
➔ *CPT Changes: An Insider's View* 2010

(Do not report 33782 in conjunction with 33412, 33413, 33608, 33681, 33770, 33771, 33778, 33780, 33920)

33783 with reimplantation of 1 or both coronary ostia
➔ *CPT Changes: An Insider's View* 2010

Truncus Arteriosus

33786 Total repair, truncus arteriosus (Rastelli type operation)
➔ *CPT Assistant* Mar 07:1

(Do not report modifier 63 in conjunction with 33786)

33788 Reimplantation of an anomalous pulmonary artery
➔ *CPT Assistant* Mar 07:1

(For pulmonary artery band, use 33690)

Aortic Anomalies

33800 Aortic suspension (aortopexy) for tracheal decompression (eg, for tracheomalacia) (separate procedure)
➔ *CPT Assistant* Mar 07:1

33802 Division of aberrant vessel (vascular ring);

33803 with reanastomosis

33813 Obliteration of aortopulmonary septal defect; without cardiopulmonary bypass

33814 with cardiopulmonary bypass

33820 Repair of patent ductus arteriosus; by ligation
➔ *CPT Assistant* Mar 07:1

Patent Ductus Arteriosus
33820

The tissues surrounding the ductus are dissected away and then several heavy ligatures are passed around the ductus and tied off on both ends.

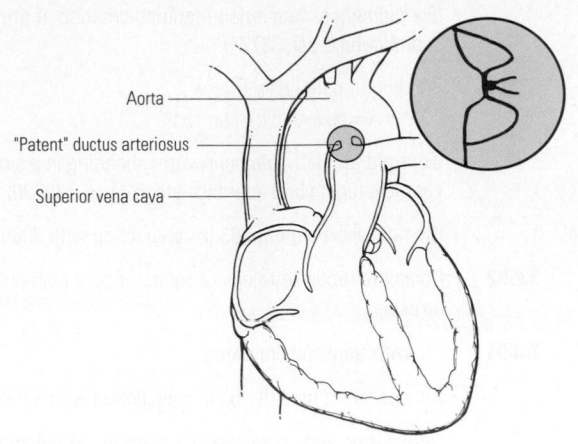

Aorta

"Patent" ductus arteriosus

Superior vena cava

33822 by division, younger than 18 years
➔ *CPT Assistant* Mar 07:1, Apr 11:6

33824 by division, 18 years and older

33840 Excision of coarctation of aorta, with or without associated patent ductus arteriosus; with direct anastomosis
➔ *CPT Assistant* Apr 11:6

33845 with graft
➔ *CPT Assistant* Apr 11:6

33851 repair using either left subclavian artery or prosthetic material as gusset for enlargement
➔ *CPT Assistant* Apr 11:6

33852 Repair of hypoplastic or interrupted aortic arch using autogenous or prosthetic material; without cardiopulmonary bypass

33853 with cardiopulmonary bypass
➔ *CPT Assistant* Mar 07:1, Apr 11:6

(For repair of hypoplastic left heart syndrome (eg, Norwood type), via excision of coarctation of aorta, use 33619)

Thoracic Aortic Aneurysm

33860 Ascending aorta graft, with cardiopulmonary bypass, includes valve suspension, when performed
➔ *CPT Assistant* Mar 07:1, Aug 11:3; *CPT Changes: An Insider's View* 2011

(33861 has been deleted. To report, use 33864)

33863 Ascending aorta graft, with cardiopulmonary bypass, with aortic root replacement using valved conduit and coronary reconstruction (eg, Bentall)
➔ *CPT Assistant* Feb 05:14, Mar 07:1, Aug 11:3; *CPT Changes: An Insider's View* 2011

Cardiovascular

(Do not report 33863 in conjunction with 33405, 33406, 33410, 33411, 33412, 33413, 33860)

33864   Ascending aorta graft, with cardiopulmonary bypass with valve suspension, with coronary reconstruction and valve-sparing aortic root remodeling (eg, David Procedure, Yacoub Procedure)

➜ *CPT Assistant* Aug 11:3; *CPT Changes: An Insider's View* 2008, 2011

(Do not report 33864 in conjunction with 33400, 33860-33863)

Aortic Root Remodeling: Coronary Arteries Reimplanted
33864

Valve sparing aortic root replacement. (code 33864)

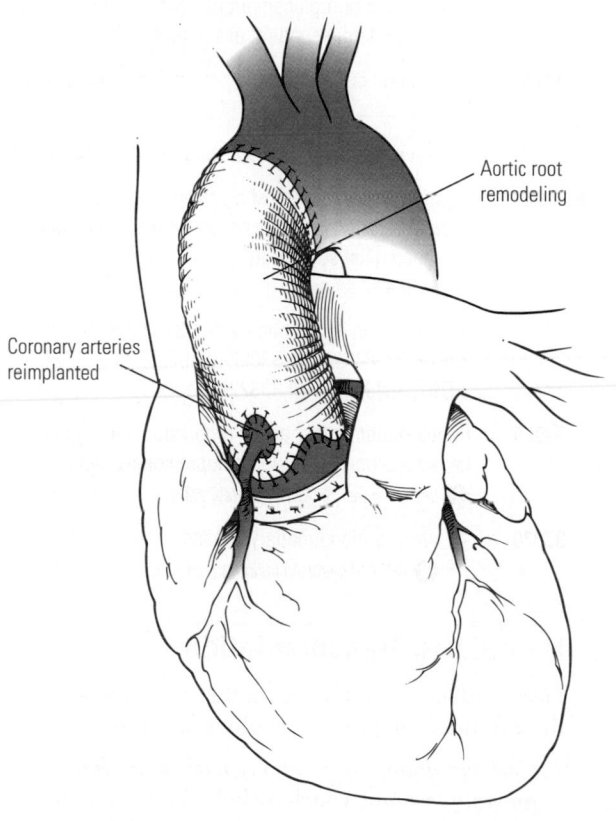

Aortic root remodeling

Coronary arteries reimplanted

33870   Transverse arch graft, with cardiopulmonary bypass

33875   Descending thoracic aorta graft, with or without bypass

33877   Repair of thoracoabdominal aortic aneurysm with graft, with or without cardiopulmonary bypass

Endovascular Repair of Descending Thoracic Aorta

Codes 33880-33891 represent a family of procedures to report placement of an endovascular graft for repair of the descending thoracic aorta. These codes include all device introduction, manipulation, positioning, and deployment. All balloon angioplasty and/or stent deployment within the target treatment zone for the endoprosthesis, either before or after endograft deployment, are not separately reportable. Open arterial exposure and associated closure of the arteriotomy sites (eg, 34812, 34820, 34833, 34834), introduction of guidewires and catheters (eg, 36140, 36200-36218), and extensive repair or replacement of an artery (eg, 35226, 35286) should be additionally reported. Transposition of subclavian artery to carotid, and carotid-carotid bypass performed in conjunction with endovascular repair of the descending thoracic aorta (eg, 33889, 33891) should be separately reported. The primary codes, 33880 and 33881, include placement of all distal extensions, if required, in the distal thoracic aorta, while proximal extensions, if needed, are reported separately.

For fluoroscopic guidance in conjunction with endovascular repair of the thoracic aorta, see codes 75956-75959 as appropriate. Codes 75956 and 75957 include all angiography of the thoracic aorta and its branches for diagnostic imaging prior to deployment of the primary endovascular devices (including all routine components of modular devices), fluoroscopic guidance in the delivery of the endovascular components, and intraprocedural arterial angiography (eg, confirm position, detect endoleak, evaluate runoff). Code 75958 includes the analogous services for placement of each proximal thoracic endovascular extension. Code 75959 includes the analogous services for placement of a distal thoracic endovascular extension(s) placed during a procedure after the primary repair.

Other interventional procedures performed at the time of endovascular repair of the descending thoracic aorta should be additionally reported (eg, innominate, carotid, subclavian, visceral, or iliac artery transluminal angioplasty or stenting, arterial embolization, intravascular ultrasound) when performed before or after deployment of the aortic prostheses.

(For transcatheter placement of wireless physiologic sensor in aneurysmal sac, use 34806)

(For analysis, interpretation, and report of implanted wireless pressure sensor in aneurysmal sac, use 93982)

33880   Endovascular repair of descending thoracic aorta (eg, aneurysm, pseudoaneurysm, dissection, penetrating ulcer, intramural hematoma, or traumatic disruption); involving coverage of left subclavian artery origin, initial endoprosthesis plus descending thoracic aortic extension(s), if required, to level of celiac artery origin

➜ *CPT Changes: An Insider's View* 2006

➜ *Clinical Examples in Radiology* Winter 06:14

Cardiovascular

(For radiological supervision and interpretation, use 75956 in conjunction with 33880)

33881   not involving coverage of left subclavian artery origin, initial endoprosthesis plus descending thoracic aortic extension(s), if required, to level of celiac artery origin
→ *CPT Changes: An Insider's View* 2006
→ *Clinical Examples in Radiology* Winter 06:14

(For radiological supervision and interpretation, use 75957 in conjunction with 33881)

33883   Placement of proximal extension prosthesis for endovascular repair of descending thoracic aorta (eg, aneurysm, pseudoaneurysm, dissection, penetrating ulcer, intramural hematoma, or traumatic disruption); initial extension
→ *CPT Changes: An Insider's View* 2006
→ *Clinical Examples in Radiology* Winter 06:14

(For radiological supervision and interpretation, use 75958 in conjunction with 33883)

(Do not report 33881, 33883 when extension placement converts repair to cover left subclavian origin. Use only 33880)

+ 33884   each additional proximal extension (List separately in addition to code for primary procedure)
→ *CPT Changes: An Insider's View* 2006
→ *Clinical Examples in Radiology* Winter 06:14

(Use 33884 in conjunction with 33883)

(For radiological supervision and interpretation, use 75958 in conjunction with 33884)

33886   Placement of distal extension prosthesis(s) delayed after endovascular repair of descending thoracic aorta
→ *CPT Changes: An Insider's View* 2006
→ *Clinical Examples in Radiology* Winter 06:14

(Do not report 33886 in conjunction with 33880, 33881)

(Report 33886 once, regardless of number of modules deployed)

(For radiological supervision and interpretation, use 75959 in conjunction with 33886)

33889   Open subclavian to carotid artery transposition performed in conjunction with endovascular repair of descending thoracic aorta, by neck incision, unilateral
→ *CPT Changes: An Insider's View* 2006
→ *Clinical Examples in Radiology* Winter 06:15

(Do not report 33889 in conjunction with 35694)

33891   Bypass graft, with other than vein, transcervical retropharyngeal carotid-carotid, performed in conjunction with endovascular repair of descending thoracic aorta, by neck incision
→ *CPT Changes: An Insider's View* 2006
→ *Clinical Examples in Radiology* Winter 06:15

(Do not report 33891 in conjunction with 35509, 35601)

Pulmonary Artery

33910   Pulmonary artery embolectomy; with cardiopulmonary bypass
→ *CPT Assistant* Mar 07:1

33915   without cardiopulmonary bypass
→ *CPT Assistant* Mar 07:1

33916   Pulmonary endarterectomy, with or without embolectomy, with cardiopulmonary bypass
→ *CPT Assistant* Mar 07:1

33917   Repair of pulmonary artery stenosis by reconstruction with patch or graft
→ *CPT Assistant* Mar 07:1, Apr 11:6

33920   Repair of pulmonary atresia with ventricular septal defect, by construction or replacement of conduit from right or left ventricle to pulmonary artery
→ *CPT Assistant* Mar 07:1

(For repair of other complex cardiac anomalies by construction or replacement of right or left ventricle to pulmonary artery conduit, use 33608)

33922   Transection of pulmonary artery with cardiopulmonary bypass

(Do not report modifier 63 in conjunction with 33922)

+ 33924   Ligation and takedown of a systemic-to-pulmonary artery shunt, performed in conjunction with a congenital heart procedure (List separately in addition to code for primary procedure)

(Use 33924 in conjunction with 33470-33475, 33600-33619, 33684-33688, 33692-33697, 33735-33767, 33770-33781, 33786, 33920-33922)

33925   Repair of pulmonary artery arborization anomalies by unifocalization; without cardiopulmonary bypass
→ *CPT Changes: An Insider's View* 2006

33926   with cardiopulmonary bypass
→ *CPT Changes: An Insider's View* 2006

Heart/Lung Transplantation

Heart with or without lung allotransplantation involves three distinct components of physician work:

1. *Cadaver donor cardiectomy with or without pneumonectomy,* which includes harvesting the allograft and cold preservation of the allograft (perfusing with cold preservation solution and cold maintenance) (see 33930, 33940).

2. *Backbench work:*

   Preparation of a cadaver donor heart and lung allograft prior to transplantation, including dissection of the allograft from surrounding soft tissues to prepare the aorta, superior vena cava, inferior vena cava, and trachea for implantation (use 33933).

Preparation of a cadaver donor heart allograft prior to transplantation, including dissection of the allograft from surrounding soft tissues to prepare aorta, superior vena cava, inferior vena cava, pulmonary artery, and left atrium for implantation (use 33944).

3. ***Recipient heart with or without lung allotransplantation,*** which includes transplantation of allograft and care of the recipient (see 33935, 33945).

> (For implantation of a total replacement heart system (artificial heart) with recipient cardiectomy or heart replacement system components, see Category III codes 0051T-0053T)

33930   Donor cardiectomy-pneumonectomy (including cold preservation)
> ➔ *CPT Changes: An Insider's View* 2005

33933   Backbench standard preparation of cadaver donor heart/lung allograft prior to transplantation, including dissection of allograft from surrounding soft tissues to prepare aorta, superior vena cava, inferior vena cava, and trachea for implantation
> ➔ *CPT Changes: An Insider's View* 2005

33935   Heart-lung transplant with recipient cardiectomy-pneumonectomy

33940   Donor cardiectomy (including cold preservation)
> ➔ *CPT Assistant* Apr 05:10-11; *CPT Changes: An Insider's View* 2005

33944   Backbench standard preparation of cadaver donor heart allograft prior to transplantation, including dissection of allograft from surrounding soft tissues to prepare aorta, superior vena cava, inferior vena cava, pulmonary artery, and left atrium for implantation
> ➔ *CPT Changes: An Insider's View* 2005

> (For repair or resection procedures on the donor heart, see 33300, 33310, 33320, 33400, 33463, 33464, 33510, 33641, 35216, 35276 or 35685)

33945   Heart transplant, with or without recipient cardiectomy
> ➔ *CPT Assistant* Fall 92:20

Cardiac Assist

▶The insertion of a ventricular assist device (VAD) can be performed via percutaneous (33990, 33991) or transthoracic (33975, 33976, 33979) approach. The location of the ventricular assist device may be intracorporeal or extracorporeal.

For surgical insertion of cannula(s) for prolonged extracorporeal circulation for cardiopulmonary insufficiency (ECMO), use 36822.

Open arterial exposure when necessary to facilitate percutaneous ventricular assist device insertion (33990, 33991), may be reported separately (34812). Extensive repair or replacement of an artery may be additionally reported (eg, 35226 or 35286).

Removal of a ventricular assist device (33977, 33978, 33980, 33992) includes removal of the entire device, including the cannulas. Removal of a percutaneous ventricular assist device at the same session as insertion is not separately reportable. For removal of a percutaneous ventricular assist device at a separate and distinct session, but on the same day as insertion, report 33992 appended with modifier 59 indicating a distinct procedural service.

Repositioning of a percutaneous ventricular assist device at the same session as insertion is not separately reportable. Repositioning of percutaneous ventricular assist device not necessitating imaging guidance is not a reportable service. For repositioning of a percutaneous ventricular assist device necessitating imaging guidance at a separate and distinct session, but on the same day as insertion, report 33993 with modifier 59 indicating a distinct procedural service.◀

Replacement of a ventricular assist device pump (ie, 33981-33983) includes the removal of the pump and insertion of a new pump, connection, de-airing, and initiation of the new pump.

▶Replacement of the entire implantable ventricular assist device system, ie, pump(s) and cannulas, is reported using the insertion codes (ie, 33975, 33976, 33979). Removal (ie, 33977, 33978, 33980) of the ventricular assist device system being replaced is not separately reported. Replacement of a percutaneous ventricular assist device is reported using implantation codes (ie, 33990, 33991). Removal (ie, 33992) is not reported separately.◀

33960   Prolonged extracorporeal circulation for cardiopulmonary insufficiency; initial day
> ➔ *CPT Changes: An Insider's View* 2012

⊘ **33961**   each subsequent day
> ➔ *CPT Changes: An Insider's View* 2012

> (Do not report modifier 63 in conjunction with 33960, 33961)

> (For insertion of cannula for prolonged extracorporeal circulation, use 36822)

33967   Insertion of intra-aortic balloon assist device, percutaneous
> ➔ *CPT Assistant* Feb 02:2, Nov 11:8; *CPT Changes: An Insider's View* 2002

33968   Removal of intra-aortic balloon assist device, percutaneous
> ➔ *CPT Assistant* Nov 99:19, Jan 00:10, Nov 11:8; *CPT Changes: An Insider's View* 2000

33970   Insertion of intra-aortic balloon assist device through the femoral artery, open approach
> ➔ *CPT Assistant* Nov 99:19, Nov 11:8; *CPT Changes: An Insider's View* 2000

33971   Removal of intra-aortic balloon assist device including repair of femoral artery, with or without graft
> ➔ *CPT Assistant* Nov 11:8

Cardiovascular

33973 Insertion of intra-aortic balloon assist device through the ascending aorta

➜ *CPT Assistant* Nov 11:8

33974 Removal of intra-aortic balloon assist device from the ascending aorta, including repair of the ascending aorta, with or without graft

➜ *CPT Assistant* Nov 11:8

33975 Insertion of ventricular assist device; extracorporeal, single ventricle

➜ *CPT Assistant* February 92:2, Jan 04:28, Nov 09:10, Jan 10:11, Apr 10:6; *CPT Changes: An Insider's View* 2002

33976 extracorporeal, biventricular

➜ *CPT Assistant* Feb 02:2, Nov 09:10, Jan 10:11, Apr 10:6; *CPT Changes: An Insider's View* 2002

33977 Removal of ventricular assist device; extracorporeal, single ventricle

➜ *CPT Assistant* Feb 02:2, Nov 09:10, Jan 10:11, Apr 10:6; *CPT Changes: An Insider's View* 2002

33978 extracorporeal, biventricular

➜ *CPT Assistant* Feb 02:2, Nov 09:10, Jan 10:11, Apr 10:6; *CPT Changes: An Insider's View* 2002

33979 Insertion of ventricular assist device, implantable intracorporeal, single ventricle

➜ *CPT Assistant* Feb 02:3, Jan 04:28, Nov 09:10, Jan 10:11, Apr 10:6; *CPT Changes: An Insider's View* 2002

33980 Removal of ventricular assist device, implantable intracorporeal, single ventricle

➜ *CPT Assistant* Feb 02:3, Nov 09:10, Apr 10:6; *CPT Changes: An Insider's View* 2002

33981 Replacement of extracorporeal ventricular assist device, single or biventricular, pump(s), single or each pump

➜ *CPT Assistant* Apr 10:6; *CPT Changes: An Insider's View* 2010

33982 Replacement of ventricular assist device pump(s); implantable intracorporeal, single ventricle, without cardiopulmonary bypass

➜ *CPT Assistant* Apr 10:6; *CPT Changes: An Insider's View* 2010

33983 implantable intracorporeal, single ventricle, with cardiopulmonary bypass

➜ *CPT Assistant* Apr 10:6; *CPT Changes: An Insider's View* 2010

⊙● **33990** Insertion of ventricular assist device, percutaneous including radiological supervision and interpretation; arterial access only

➜ *CPT Changes: An Insider's View* 2013

⊙● **33991** both arterial and venous access, with transseptal puncture

➜ *CPT Changes: An Insider's View* 2013

⊙● **33992** Removal of percutaneous ventricular assist device at separate and distinct session from insertion

➜ *CPT Changes: An Insider's View* 2013

Insertion of Implantable Single Ventricle Assist Device
33979

⊙● **33993** Repositioning of percutaneous ventricular assist device with imaging guidance at separate and distinct session from insertion

➜ *CPT Changes: An Insider's View* 2013

Other Procedures

33999 Unlisted procedure, cardiac surgery

➜ *CPT Assistant* Oct 99:11, Jan 04:7, Mar 07:1, Nov 09:10, Jan 10:11, Apr 10:6

Arteries and Veins

Primary vascular procedure listings include establishing both inflow and outflow by whatever procedures necessary. Also included is that portion of the operative arteriogram performed by the surgeon, as indicated. Sympathectomy, when done, is included in the listed aortic procedures. For unlisted vascular procedure, use 37799.

Cardiovascular

Embolectomy/Thrombectomy

Arterial, With or Without Catheter

34001   Embolectomy or thrombectomy, with or without catheter;
carotid, subclavian or innominate artery, by neck incision

34051   innominate, subclavian artery, by thoracic incision

34101   axillary, brachial, innominate, subclavian artery, by
arm incision

34111   radial or ulnar artery, by arm incision

34151   renal, celiac, mesentery, aortoiliac artery, by
abdominal incision

34201   femoropopliteal, aortoiliac artery, by leg incision
➡ *CPT Assistant* Aug 11:9

34203   popliteal-tibio-peroneal artery, by leg incision

Venous, Direct or With Catheter

34401   Thrombectomy, direct or with catheter; vena cava, iliac
vein, by abdominal incision

34421   vena cava, iliac, femoropopliteal vein, by leg incision
➡ *CPT Assistant* Spring 94:30

34451   vena cava, iliac, femoropopliteal vein, by abdominal
and leg incision

34471   subclavian vein, by neck incision

34490   axillary and subclavian vein, by arm incision

Venous Reconstruction

34501   Valvuloplasty, femoral vein

34502   Reconstruction of vena cava, any method

34510   Venous valve transposition, any vein donor

34520   Cross-over vein graft to venous system

34530   Saphenopopliteal vein anastomosis

Endovascular Repair of Abdominal Aortic Aneurysm

Codes 34800-34826 represent a family of component
procedures to report placement of an endovascular graft
for abdominal aortic aneurysm repair. These codes
describe open femoral or iliac artery exposure, device
manipulation and deployment, and closure of the
arteriotomy sites. Balloon angioplasty and/or stent
deployment within the target treatment zone for the
endoprosthesis, either before or after endograft
deployment, are not separately reportable. Introduction
of guidewires and catheters should be reported separately
(eg, 36200, 36245-36248, 36140). Extensive repair or
replacement of an artery should be additionally reported
(eg, 35226 or 35286).

For fluoroscopic guidance in conjunction with
endovascular aneurysm repair, see code 75952 or 75953,
as appropriate. Code 75952 includes angiography of the
aorta and its branches for diagnostic imaging prior to
deployment of the endovascular device (including all
routine components of modular devices), fluoroscopic
guidance in the delivery of the endovascular components,
and intraprocedural arterial angiography (eg, confirm
position, detect endoleak, evaluate runoff). Code 75953
includes the analogous services for placement of
additional extension prostheses (not for routine
components of modular devices).

Other interventional procedures performed at the time of
endovascular abdominal aortic aneurysm repair should be
additionally reported (eg, renal transluminal angioplasty,
arterial embolization, intravascular ultrasound, balloon
angioplasty or stenting of native artery[s] outside the
endoprosthesis target zone, when done before or after
deployment of graft).

(For transcatheter placement of wireless physiologic
sensor in aneurysmal sac, use 34806)

(For analysis, interpretation and report of implanted
wireless pressure sensor in aneurysmal sac, use 93982)

34800   Endovascular repair of infrarenal abdominal aortic
aneurysm or dissection; using aorto-aortic tube
prosthesis
➡ *CPT Assistant* Dec 00:1, 4, Sep 02:3, Feb 03:2, Nov 03:5,
Dec 04:18, Apr 12:3; *CPT Changes: An Insider's View* 2001

34802   using modular bifurcated prosthesis (1 docking limb)
➡ *CPT Assistant* Dec 00:1, 4, Sep 02:3, Feb 03:2, Dec 04:18,
Apr 12:3; *CPT Changes: An Insider's View* 2001

Endovascular Repair of Abdominal Aortic Aneurysm
34802

Using fluoroscopic guidance, a "compressed" prosthesis is introduced through arteries
in the groin and advanced into position with the aneurysm. Once in the aorta, the
prosthesis is expanded.

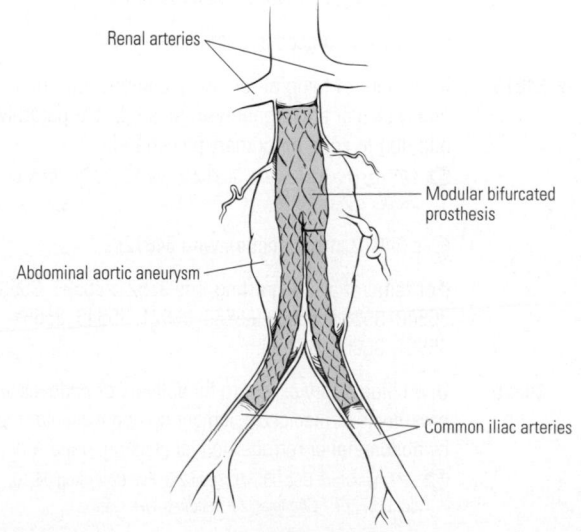

Renal arteries

Modular bifurcated
prosthesis

Abdominal aortic aneurysm

Common iliac arteries

Cardiovascular

34803   using modular bifurcated prosthesis (2 docking limbs)

> *CPT Assistant* Apr 12:3; *CPT Changes: An Insider's View* 2005

(For endovascular repair of abdominal aortic aneurysm or dissection involving visceral vessels using a fenestrated modular bifurcated prosthesis (2 docking limbs), use Category III codes 0078T, 0079T)

34804   using unibody bifurcated prosthesis

> *CPT Assistant* Dec 00:5, Sep 02:3, Feb 03:2, Apr 12:3; *CPT Changes: An Insider's View* 2001

34805   using aorto-uniiliac or aorto-unifemoral prosthesis

> *CPT Assistant* Jun 04:9, Dec 04:18, Apr 12:3; *CPT Changes: An Insider's View* 2004

(For radiological supervision and interpretation, use 75952 in conjunction with 34800-34805)

+ 34806   Transcatheter placement of wireless physiologic sensor in aneurysmal sac during endovascular repair, including radiological supervision and interpretation, instrument calibration, and collection of pressure data (List separately in addition to code for primary procedure)

> *CPT Assistant* Apr 12:3; *CPT Changes: An Insider's View* 2008, 2009

(Use 34806 in conjunction with 33880, 33881, 33886, 34800-34805, 34825, 34900)

(Do not report 34806 in conjunction with 93982)

+ 34808   Endovascular placement of iliac artery occlusion device (List separately in addition to code for primary procedure)

> *CPT Assistant* Dec 00:6, Sep 02:3, Apr 12:3; *CPT Changes: An Insider's View* 2001

(Use 34808 in conjunction with 34800, 34805, 34813, 34825, 34826)

(For open arterial exposure, report 34812, 34820, 34833, 34834 as appropriate, in addition to 34800-34808)

34812   Open femoral artery exposure for delivery of endovascular prosthesis, by groin incision, unilateral

> *CPT Assistant* Dec 00:6, Sep 02:3, Feb 03:2, Mar 04:10, Jul 06:7; *CPT Changes: An Insider's View* 2001, 2003

(For bilateral procedure, use modifier 50)

+ 34813   Placement of femoral-femoral prosthetic graft during endovascular aortic aneurysm repair (List separately in addition to code for primary procedure)

> *CPT Assistant* Dec 00:6, Sep 02:3, Apr 12:3; *CPT Changes: An Insider's View* 2001

(Use 34813 in conjunction with 34812)

(For femoral artery grafting, see 35521, 35533, 35539, 35540, 35556, 35558, 35566, 35621, 35646, 35654-35661, 35666, 35700)

34820   Open iliac artery exposure for delivery of endovascular prosthesis or iliac occlusion during endovascular therapy, by abdominal or retroperitoneal incision, unilateral

> *CPT Assistant* Dec 00:7-8, Sep 02:3, Feb 03:4, Aug 04:10, Jul 06:7; *CPT Changes: An Insider's View* 2001

(For bilateral procedure, use modifier 50)

34825   Placement of proximal or distal extension prosthesis for endovascular repair of infrarenal abdominal aortic or iliac aneurysm, false aneurysm, or dissection; initial vessel

> *CPT Assistant* Dec 00:5, Sep 02:3, Feb 03:3, Apr 12:3; *CPT Changes: An Insider's View* 2001, 2003

+ 34826   each additional vessel (List separately in addition to code for primary procedure)

> *CPT Assistant* Dec 00:6, Sep 02:3, Feb 03:3, Apr 12:3; *CPT Changes: An Insider's View* 2001

(Use 34826 in conjunction with 34825)

(Use 34825, 34826 in addition to 34800-34805, 34900 as appropriate)

(For radiological supervision and interpretation, use 75953)

34830   Open repair of infrarenal aortic aneurysm or dissection, plus repair of associated arterial trauma, following unsuccessful endovascular repair; tube prosthesis

> *CPT Assistant* Dec 00:6, Sep 02:3, Oct 08:10; *CPT Changes: An Insider's View* 2001

34831   aorto-bi-iliac prosthesis

> *CPT Assistant* Dec 00:6, Sep 02:3, Oct 08:10; *CPT Changes: An Insider's View* 2001

34832   aorto-bifemoral prosthesis

> *CPT Assistant* Dec 00:6, Sep 02:3, Oct 08:10; *CPT Changes: An Insider's View* 2001

34833   Open iliac artery exposure with creation of conduit for delivery of aortic or iliac endovascular prosthesis, by abdominal or retroperitoneal incision, unilateral

> *CPT Assistant* Feb 03:4, Aug 04:10, Jul 06:7; *CPT Changes: An Insider's View* 2003, 2006
> *Clinical Examples in Radiology* Winter 06:19

(Do not report 34833 in addition to 34820)

(For bilateral procedure, use modifier 50)

34834   Open brachial artery exposure to assist in the deployment of aortic or iliac endovascular prosthesis by arm incision, unilateral

> *CPT Assistant* Feb 03:4, Jul 06:7; *CPT Changes: An Insider's View* 2003, 2006
> *Clinical Examples in Radiology* Winter 06:19

(For bilateral procedure, use modifier 50)

Endovascular Repair of Iliac Aneurysm

Code 34900 represents a procedure to report introduction, positioning, and deployment of an endovascular graft for treatment of aneurysm, pseudoaneurysm, or arteriovenous malformation or trauma of the iliac artery (common, hypogastric, external). All balloon angioplasty and/or stent deployments within the target treatment zone for the endoprosthesis, either before or after endograft deployment, are included in the work of 34900 and are not separately reportable. Open femoral or iliac artery exposure (eg, 34812, 34820), introduction of guidewires and catheters (eg, 36200, 36245-36248), and extensive repair or replacement of an artery (eg, 35206-35286) should be additionally reported.

For fluoroscopic guidance in conjunction with endovascular iliac aneurysm repair, see code 75954. Code 75954 includes angiography of the aorta and iliac arteries for diagnostic imaging prior to deployment of the endovascular device (including all routine components), fluoroscopic guidance in the delivery of the endovascular components, and intraprocedural arterial angiography to confirm appropriate position of the graft, detect endoleaks, and evaluate the status of the runoff vessels (eg, evaluation for dissection, stenosis, thrombosis, distal embolization, or iatrogenic injury).

Other interventional procedures performed at the time of endovascular iliac aneurysm repair should be additionally reported (eg, transluminal angioplasty outside the aneurysm target zone, arterial embolization, intravascular ultrasound).

34900 Endovascular repair of iliac artery (eg, aneurysm, pseudoaneurysm, arteriovenous malformation, trauma) using ilio-iliac tube endoprosthesis

> *CPT Assistant* February 93:2, Apr 12:3; *CPT Changes: An Insider's View* 2003, 2011

(For endovascular repair of iliac artery bifurcation [eg, aneurysm, pseudoaneurysm, arteriovenous malformation, trauma] using bifurcated endoprosthesis, use 0254T)

(For radiological supervision and interpretation, use 75954)

(For placement of extension prosthesis during endovascular iliac artery repair, use 34825)

(For bilateral procedure, use modifier 50)

Direct Repair of Aneurysm or Excision (Partial or Total) and Graft Insertion for Aneurysm, Pseudoaneurysm, Ruptured Aneurysm, and Associated Occlusive Disease

Procedures 35001-35152 include preparation of artery for anastomosis including endarterectomy.

(For direct repairs associated with occlusive disease only, see 35201-35286)

(For intracranial aneurysm, see 61700 et seq)

(For endovascular repair of abdominal aortic aneurysm, see 34800-34826)

(For endovascular repair of iliac artery aneurysm, see 34900)

(For thoracic aortic aneurysm, see 33860-33875)

(For endovascular repair of descending thoracic aorta, involving coverage of left subclavian artery origin, use 33880)

35001 Direct repair of aneurysm, pseudoaneurysm, or excision (partial or total) and graft insertion, with or without patch graft; for aneurysm and associated occlusive disease, carotid, subclavian artery, by neck incision

> *CPT Changes: An Insider's View* 2002

35002 for ruptured aneurysm, carotid, subclavian artery, by neck incision

35005 for aneurysm, pseudoaneurysm, and associated occlusive disease, vertebral artery

> *CPT Changes: An Insider's View* 2002

35011 for aneurysm and associated occlusive disease, axillary-brachial artery, by arm incision

35013 for ruptured aneurysm, axillary-brachial artery, by arm incision

35021 for aneurysm, pseudoaneurysm, and associated occlusive disease, innominate, subclavian artery, by thoracic incision

> *CPT Changes: An Insider's View* 2002

35022 for ruptured aneurysm, innominate, subclavian artery, by thoracic incision

35045 for aneurysm, pseudoaneurysm, and associated occlusive disease, radial or ulnar artery

> *CPT Changes: An Insider's View* 2002

35081 for aneurysm, pseudoaneurysm, and associated occlusive disease, abdominal aorta

> *CPT Assistant* Dec 00:2, Dec 01:7; *CPT Changes: An Insider's View* 2002

35082 for ruptured aneurysm, abdominal aorta

35091 for aneurysm, pseudoaneurysm, and associated occlusive disease, abdominal aorta involving visceral vessels (mesenteric, celiac, renal)

> *CPT Assistant* Dec 00:2; *CPT Changes: An Insider's View* 2002

35092 for ruptured aneurysm, abdominal aorta involving visceral vessels (mesenteric, celiac, renal)

35102 for aneurysm, pseudoaneurysm, and associated occlusive disease, abdominal aorta involving iliac vessels (common, hypogastric, external)

> *CPT Changes: An Insider's View* 2002

35103 for ruptured aneurysm, abdominal aorta involving iliac vessels (common, hypogastric, external)

35111 for aneurysm, pseudoaneurysm, and associated occlusive disease, splenic artery

> *CPT Changes: An Insider's View* 2002

35112 for ruptured aneurysm, splenic artery

35121 for aneurysm, pseudoaneurysm, and associated occlusive disease, hepatic, celiac, renal, or mesenteric artery

> *CPT Changes: An Insider's View* 2002

35122 for ruptured aneurysm, hepatic, celiac, renal, or mesenteric artery

Cardiovascular

35131   for aneurysm, pseudoaneurysm, and associated occlusive disease, iliac artery (common, hypogastric, external)
> *CPT Assistant* Feb 03:2; *CPT Changes: An Insider's View* 2002

35132   for ruptured aneurysm, iliac artery (common, hypogastric, external)

35141   for aneurysm, pseudoaneurysm, and associated occlusive disease, common femoral artery (profunda femoris, superficial femoral)
> *CPT Changes: An Insider's View* 2002

35142   for ruptured aneurysm, common femoral artery (profunda femoris, superficial femoral)

35151   for aneurysm, pseudoaneurysm, and associated occlusive disease, popliteal artery
> *CPT Changes: An Insider's View* 2002

35152   for ruptured aneurysm, popliteal artery

Repair Arteriovenous Fistula

35180   Repair, congenital arteriovenous fistula; head and neck
> *CPT Assistant* Aug 11:9

35182   thorax and abdomen
> *CPT Assistant* Apr 11:9

35184   extremities
> *CPT Assistant* Apr 11:9

35188   Repair, acquired or traumatic arteriovenous fistula; head and neck
> *CPT Assistant* Apr 11:9

35189   thorax and abdomen
> *CPT Assistant* Apr 11:9

35190   extremities
> *CPT Assistant* Aug 11:9

Repair Blood Vessel Other Than for Fistula, With or Without Patch Angioplasty

(For AV fistula repair, see 35180-35190)

35201   Repair blood vessel, direct; neck

35206   upper extremity
> *CPT Assistant* Oct 00:3, Nov 03:5, Apr 12:4

35207   hand, finger

35211   intrathoracic, with bypass

35216   intrathoracic, without bypass
> *CPT Assistant* Apr 05:10-11

35221   intra-abdominal

35226   lower extremity
> *CPT Assistant* Apr 12:8, 9

35231   Repair blood vessel with vein graft; neck

35236   upper extremity
> *CPT Assistant* Oct 04:8

35241   intrathoracic, with bypass

35246   intrathoracic, without bypass

35251   intra-abdominal

35256   lower extremity

35261   Repair blood vessel with graft other than vein; neck

35266   upper extremity

35271   intrathoracic, with bypass

35276   intrathoracic, without bypass

35281   intra-abdominal

35286   lower extremity

Thromboendarterectomy

(For coronary artery, see 33510-33536 and 33572)

(35301-35372 include harvest of saphenous or upper extremity vein when performed)

35301   Thromboendarterectomy, including patch graft, if performed; carotid, vertebral, subclavian, by neck incision
> *CPT Assistant* Jan 07:7, Sep 10:7; *CPT Changes: An Insider's View* 2007

35302   superficial femoral artery
> *CPT Assistant* Jan 07:7, May 07:9; *CPT Changes: An Insider's View* 2007

35303   popliteal artery
> *CPT Assistant* Jan 07:7, May 07:9; *CPT Changes: An Insider's View* 2007

(Do not report 35302, 35303 in conjunction with 35500, 37225, 37227)

35304   tibioperoneal trunk artery
> *CPT Assistant* Jan 07:7, May 07:9; *CPT Changes: An Insider's View* 2007

35305   tibial or peroneal artery, initial vessel
> *CPT Assistant* May 07:9; *CPT Changes: An Insider's View* 2007

+ 35306   each additional tibial or peroneal artery (List separately in addition to code for primary procedure)
> *CPT Assistant* Jan 07:7, May 07:9; *CPT Changes: An Insider's View* 2007

(Use 35306 in conjunction with 35305)

(Do not report 35304, 35305, 35306 in conjunction with 35500, 37229, 37231, 37233, 37235)

35311   subclavian, innominate, by thoracic incision

35321   axillary-brachial

35331   abdominal aorta

35341   mesenteric, celiac, or renal

35351   iliac

35355   iliofemoral

35361   combined aortoiliac

Cardiovascular

35363   combined aortoiliofemoral

35371   common femoral
> *CPT Assistant* Jan 07:7

35372   deep (profunda) femoral
> *CPT Assistant* Jan 07:7

Thromboendarterectomy
35371-35372

The common femoral artery (35371) or the deep (profunda) femoral artery (35372) is incised and the plaque and lining are removed, enlarging the diameter of the artery.

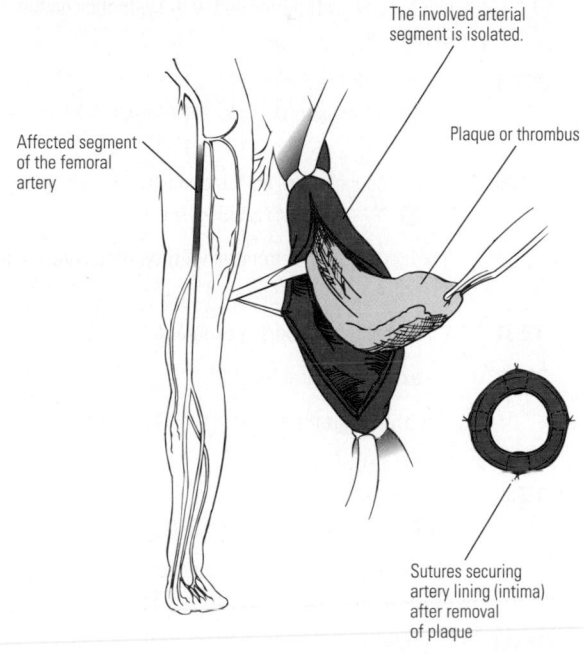

The involved arterial segment is isolated.

Affected segment of the femoral artery

Plaque or thrombus

Sutures securing artery lining (intima) after removal of plaque

+ **35390**   Reoperation, carotid, thromboendarterectomy, more than 1 month after original operation (List separately in addition to code for primary procedure)
> *CPT Assistant* Nov 97:16

(Use 35390 in conjunction with 35301)

Angioscopy

+ **35400**   Angioscopy (non-coronary vessels or grafts) during therapeutic intervention (List separately in addition to code for primary procedure)
> *CPT Assistant* Nov 97:16

Transluminal Angioplasty

If done as part of another operation, use modifier 51 or use modifier 52.

(For radiological supervision and interpretation, see 75962-75968 and 75978)

Open

35450   Transluminal balloon angioplasty, open; renal or other visceral artery
> *CPT Assistant* Feb 97:2-3

35452   aortic
> *CPT Assistant* Feb 97:2-3

(35454, 35456 have been deleted. To report, see 37220-37227)

35458   brachiocephalic trunk or branches, each vessel
> *CPT Assistant* Feb 97:2-3, May 01:11

(35459 has been deleted. To report, see 37228-37235)

35460   venous
> *CPT Assistant* Feb 97:2-3

Percutaneous

Codes for catheter placement and the radiologic supervision and interpretation should also be reported, in addition to the code(s) for the therapeutic aspect of the procedure.

(35470 has been deleted. To report, see 37228-37235)

⊙ **35471**   Transluminal balloon angioplasty, percutaneous; renal or visceral artery
> *CPT Assistant* Aug 96:3, Feb 97:2-3; *CPT Changes: An Insider's View* 2011
> *Clinical Examples in Radiology* Fall 11:3

⊙ **35472**   aortic
> *CPT Assistant* Aug 96:3, Feb 97:2-3

(35473, 35474 have been deleted. To report, see 37220-37227)

⊙ **35475**   brachiocephalic trunk or branches, each vessel
> *CPT Assistant* Aug 96:3, Feb 97:2-3, May 01:4, Sep 08:10
> *Clinical Examples in Radiology* Winter 10:9

⊙ **35476**   venous
> *CPT Assistant* Aug 96:3, Feb 97:2-3, May 01:4, Dec 03:2, Dec 11:16, Apr 12:5
> *Clinical Examples in Radiology* Spring 05:8-10, Spring 07:1-3, Winter 10:7, Spring 12:6

(For radiological supervision and interpretation, use 75978)

(35480 has been deleted. To report, see 0234T, 0235T)

(35481 has been deleted. To report, use 0236T)

(35482 has been deleted. To report, use 0238T)

(35483 has been deleted. To report, see 37225, 37227)

(35484 has been deleted. To report, use 0237T)

(35485 has been deleted. To report, see 37229, 37231, 37233, 37235)

(35490 has been deleted. To report, see 0234T, 0235T)

(35491 has been deleted. To report, use 0236T)

(35492 has been deleted. To report, use 0238T)

(35493 has been deleted. To report, see 37225, 37227)

(35494 has been deleted. To report, use 0237T)

(35495 has been deleted. To report, see 37229, 37231, 37233, 37235)

Cardiovascular

Bypass Graft

Vein

Procurement of the saphenous vein graft is included in the description of the work for 35501-35587 and should not be reported as a separate service or co-surgery. To report harvesting of an upper extremity vein, use 35500 in addition to the bypass procedure. To report harvesting of a femoropopliteal vein segment, use 35572 in addition to the bypass procedure. To report harvesting and construction of an autogenous composite graft of two segments from two distant locations, report 35682 in addition to the bypass procedure, for autogenous composite of three or more segments from distant sites, report 35683.

+ **35500** Harvest of upper extremity vein, 1 segment, for lower extremity or coronary artery bypass procedure (List separately in addition to code for primary procedure)

➜ *CPT Assistant* Nov 98:13, Mar 99:6, Nov 99:19, Jan 07:7, Apr 12:4; *CPT Changes: An Insider's View* 2000

(Use 35500 in conjunction with 33510-33536, 35556, 35566, 35570, 35571, 35583-35587)

(For harvest of more than one vein segment, see 35682, 35683)

(For endoscopic procedure, use 33508)

35501 Bypass graft, with vein; common carotid-ipsilateral internal carotid

➜ *CPT Assistant* Apr 99:11; *CPT Changes: An Insider's View* 2007

35506 carotid-subclavian or subclavian-carotid

➜ *CPT Assistant* Oct 04:6, Jan 07:7; *CPT Changes: An Insider's View* 2007

35508 carotid-vertebral

35509 carotid-contralateral carotid

➜ *CPT Assistant* Jan 07:7, May 07:9; *CPT Changes: An Insider's View* 2007

35510 carotid-brachial

➜ *CPT Assistant* Oct 04:6, Nov 07:8; *CPT Changes: An Insider's View* 2004

35511 subclavian-subclavian

35512 subclavian-brachial

➜ *CPT Assistant* Oct 04:7; *CPT Changes: An Insider's View* 2004

35515 subclavian-vertebral

35516 subclavian-axillary

35518 axillary-axillary

➜ *CPT Assistant* Oct 04:9

35521 axillary-femoral

(For bypass graft performed with synthetic graft, use 35621)

35522 axillary-brachial

➜ *CPT Assistant* Oct 04:9; *CPT Changes: An Insider's View* 2004

35523 brachial-ulnar or -radial

➜ *CPT Changes: An Insider's View* 2008

(Do not report 35523 in conjunction with 35206, 35500, 35525, 36838)

(For bypass graft performed with synthetic conduit, use 37799)

35525 brachial-brachial

➜ *CPT Assistant* Oct 04:10; *CPT Changes: An Insider's View* 2004

35526 aortosubclavian, aortoinnominate, or aortocarotid

➜ *CPT Changes: An Insider's View* 2011

(For bypass graft performed with synthetic graft, use 35626)

35531 aortoceliac or aortomesenteric

35533 axillary-femoral-femoral

(For bypass graft performed with synthetic graft, use 35654)

35535 hepatorenal

➜ *CPT Changes: An Insider's View* 2009

(Do not report 35535 in conjunction with 35221, 35251, 35281, 35500, 35536, 35560, 35631, 35636)

35536 splenorenal

➜ *CPT Assistant* Jun 99:10

35537 aortoiliac

➜ *CPT Assistant* Jan 07:7; *CPT Changes: An Insider's View* 2007

(For bypass graft performed with synthetic graft, use 35637)

(Do not report 35537 in conjunction with 35538)

35538 aortobi-iliac

➜ *CPT Assistant* Jan 07:7; *CPT Changes: An Insider's View* 2007

(For bypass graft performed with synthetic graft, use 35638)

(Do not report 35538 in conjunction with 35537)

35539   aortofemoral
➔ *CPT Assistant* Jan 07:7; *CPT Changes: An Insider's View* 2007

(For bypass graft performed with synthetic graft, use 35647)

(Do not report 35539 in conjunction with 35540)

35540   aortobifemoral
➔ *CPT Assistant* Jan 07:7; *CPT Changes: An Insider's View* 2007

(For bypass graft performed with synthetic graft, use 35646)

(Do not report 35540 in conjunction with 35539)

(35548 has been deleted. To report, see 35537, 35539, 35565)

(35549 has been deleted. To report, see 35537, 35538, 35539, 35540, 35565)

(35551 has been deleted. To report, see 35539, 35540, 35556, 35583)

35556   femoral-popliteal
➔ *CPT Assistant* Fall 92:20, May 97:10, Jan 07:7, Nov 07:8

35558   femoral-femoral

35560   aortorenal
➔ *CPT Assistant* Jun 99:10

35563   ilioiliac

35565   iliofemoral
➔ *CPT Assistant* Oct 04:8

35566   femoral-anterior tibial, posterior tibial, peroneal artery or other distal vessels
➔ *CPT Assistant* Jan 07:7, Nov 07:8

35570   tibial-tibial, peroneal-tibial, or tibial/peroneal trunk-tibial
➔ *CPT Assistant* Apr 12:4; *CPT Changes: An Insider's View* 2009

(Do not report 35570 in conjunction with 35256, 35286)

35571   popliteal-tibial, -peroneal artery or other distal vessels
➔ *CPT Assistant* Jan 07:7, Nov 07:8

+ 35572   Harvest of femoropopliteal vein, 1 segment, for vascular reconstruction procedure (eg, aortic, vena caval, coronary, peripheral artery) (List separately in addition to code for primary procedure)
➔ *CPT Assistant* Jan 07:28; *CPT Changes: An Insider's View* 2003

(Use 35572 in conjunction with 33510-33516, 33517-33523, 33533-33536, 34502, 34520, 35001, 35002, 35011-35022, 35102, 35103, 35121-35152, 35231-35256, 35501-35587, 35879-35907)

(For bilateral procedure, use modifier 50)

Bypass Graft, Vein
35571

The physician creates a bypass around the popliteal artery, using a harvested vein that is sutured to the tibial artery.

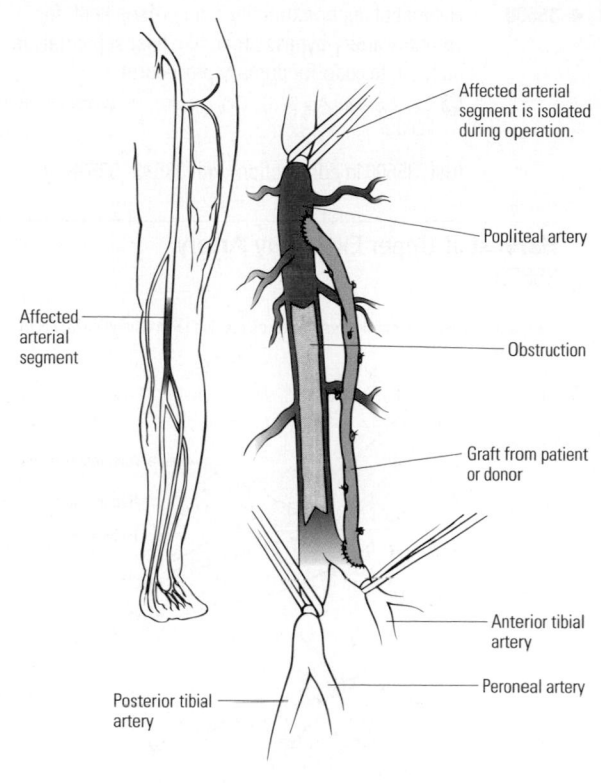

Affected arterial segment is isolated during operation.

Popliteal artery

Affected arterial segment

Obstruction

Graft from patient or donor

Anterior tibial artery

Peroneal artery

Posterior tibial artery

In-Situ Vein

(To report aortobifemoral bypass using synthetic conduit, and femoral-popliteal bypass with vein conduit in-situ, use 35646 and 35583. To report aorto[uni]femoral bypass with synthetic conduit, and femoral-popliteal bypass with vein conduit in-situ, use 35647 and 35583. To report aortofemoral bypass using vein conduit, and femoral-popliteal bypass with vein conduit in-situ, use 35539 and 35583)

35583   In-situ vein bypass; femoral-popliteal
➔ *CPT Assistant* Jan 07:7, Nov 07:8

35585   femoral-anterior tibial, posterior tibial, or peroneal artery
➔ *CPT Assistant* Jan 07:7, Nov 07:8

35587   popliteal-tibial, peroneal
➔ *CPT Assistant* Apr 99:11, Jan 07:7, Nov 07:8

Cardiovascular

Other Than Vein

(For arterial transposition and/or reimplantation, see 35691-35695)

+ **35600** Harvest of upper extremity artery, 1 segment, for coronary artery bypass procedure (List separately in addition to code for primary procedure)
→ *CPT Assistant* Apr 07:12; *CPT Changes: An Insider's View* 2001, 2008

(Use 35600 in conjunction with 33533–33536)

Harvest of Upper Extremity Artery
35600

Open procurement of a radial artery to secure conduit for construction of a coronary artery bypass graft

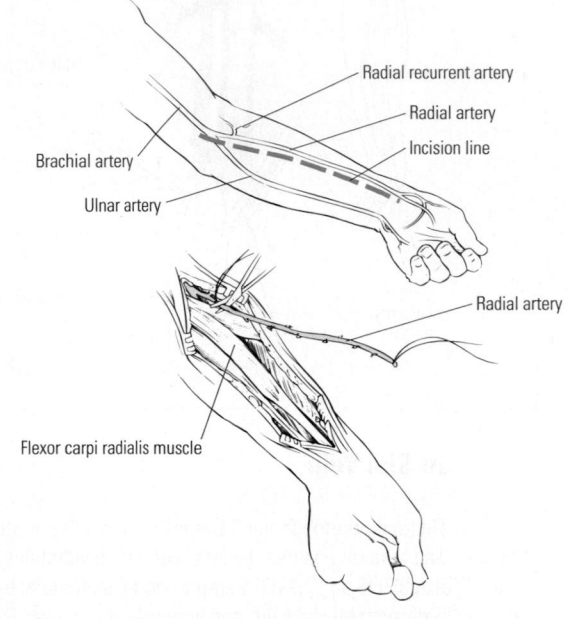

- Radial recurrent artery
- Radial artery
- Incision line
- Brachial artery
- Ulnar artery
- Radial artery
- Flexor carpi radialis muscle

35601 Bypass graft, with other than vein; common carotid-ipsilateral internal carotid
→ *CPT Assistant* Jul 06:7, Jan 07:7; *CPT Changes: An Insider's View* 2007

35606 carotid-subclavian

(For open transcervical common carotid-common carotid bypass performed in conjunction with endovascular repair of descending thoracic aorta, use 33891)

(For open subclavian to carotid artery transposition performed in conjunction with endovascular thoracic aneurysm repair by neck incision, use 33889)

35612 subclavian-subclavian

35616 subclavian-axillary

35621 axillary-femoral
→ *CPT Assistant* Jan 07:7

35623 axillary-popliteal or -tibial

35626 aortosubclavian, aortoinnominate, or aortocarotid
→ *CPT Changes: An Insider's View* 2011

35631 aortoceliac, aortomesenteric, aortorenal

35632 ilio-celiac
→ *CPT Changes: An Insider's View* 2009

(Do not report 35632 in conjunction with 35221, 35251, 35281, 35531, 35631)

35633 ilio-mesenteric
→ *CPT Changes: An Insider's View* 2009

(Do not report 35633 in conjunction with 35221, 35251, 35281, 35531, 35631)

35634 iliorenal
→ *CPT Changes: An Insider's View* 2009

(Do not report 35634 in conjunction with 35221, 35251, 35281, 35560, 35536, 35631)

35636 splenorenal (splenic to renal arterial anastomosis)

35637 aortoiliac
→ *CPT Assistant* Jan 07:7; *CPT Changes: An Insider's View* 2007

(Do not report 35637 in conjunction with 35638, 35646)

35638 aortobi-iliac
→ *CPT Assistant* Jan 07:7; *CPT Changes: An Insider's View* 2007

(Do not report 35638 in conjunction with 35637, 35646)

(For open placement of aortobi-iliac prosthesis following unsuccessful endovascular repair, use 34831)

35642 carotid-vertebral

35645 subclavian-vertebral

35646 aortobifemoral
→ *CPT Assistant* Jan 07:7; *CPT Changes: An Insider's View* 2002

(For bypass graft performed with vein graft, use 35540)

(For open placement of aortobifemoral prosthesis following unsuccessful endovascular repair, use 34832)

35647 aortofemoral
→ *CPT Assistant* Jan 07:7; *CPT Changes: An Insider's View* 2002

(For bypass graft performed with vein graft, use 35539)

35650 axillary-axillary

(35651 has been deleted. To report, see 35646, 35647, 35656)

35654 axillary-femoral-femoral
→ *CPT Assistant* Jan 07:7

35656 femoral-popliteal
→ *CPT Assistant* Nov 07:8

35661 femoral-femoral
→ *CPT Assistant* Dec 04:6, Jan 07:7

35663	ilioiliac
35665	iliofemoral

➔ *CPT Assistant* Jan 07:7

35666	femoral-anterior tibial, posterior tibial, or peroneal artery

➔ *CPT Assistant* Nov 07:8

35671	popliteal-tibial or -peroneal artery

Composite Grafts

Codes 35682-35683 are used to report harvest and anastomosis of multiple vein segments from distant sites for use as arterial bypass graft conduits. These codes are intended for use when the two or more vein segments are harvested from a limb other than that undergoing bypass.

+ 35681   Bypass graft; composite, prosthetic and vein (List separately in addition to code for primary procedure)

➔ *CPT Assistant* Nov 98:13-14, Mar 99:6, Apr 99:11

(Do not report 35681 in addition to 35682, 35683)

+ 35682   autogenous composite, 2 segments of veins from 2 locations (List separately in addition to code for primary procedure)

➔ *CPT Assistant* Nov 98:13-14, Mar 99:6, Apr 99:11, Sep 02:4

(Use 35682 in conjunction with 35556, 35566, 35570, 35571, 35583-35587)

(Do not report 35682 in addition to 35681, 35683)

+ 35683   autogenous composite, 3 or more segments of vein from 2 or more locations (List separately in addition to code for primary procedure)

➔ *CPT Assistant* Nov 98:13-14, Mar 99:6, Apr 99:11, Sep 02:4

(Use 35683 in conjunction with 35556, 35566, 35570, 35571, 35583-35587)

(Do not report 35683 in addition to 35681, 35682)

Adjuvant Techniques

Adjuvant (additional) technique(s) may be required at the time a bypass graft is created to improve patency of the lower extremity autogenous or synthetic bypass graft (eg, femoral-popliteal, femoral-tibial, or popliteal-tibial arteries). Code 35685 should be reported in addition to the primary synthetic bypass graft procedure, when an interposition of venous tissue (vein patch or cuff) is placed at the anastomosis between the synthetic bypass conduit and the involved artery (includes harvest).

Code 35686 should be reported in addition to the primary bypass graft procedure, when autogenous vein is used to create a fistula between the tibial or peroneal artery and vein at or beyond the distal bypass anastomosis site of the involved artery.

(For composite graft(s), see 35681-35683)

+ 35685   Placement of vein patch or cuff at distal anastomosis of bypass graft, synthetic conduit (List separately in addition to code for primary procedure)

➔ *CPT Assistant* Sep 02:3; *CPT Changes: An Insider's View* 2002

(Use 35685 in conjunction with 35656, 35666, or 35671)

+ 35686   Creation of distal arteriovenous fistula during lower extremity bypass surgery (non-hemodialysis) (List separately in addition to code for primary procedure)

➔ *CPT Assistant* Sep 02:3, Apr 12:4; *CPT Changes: An Insider's View* 2002

(Use 35686 in conjunction with 35556, 35566, 35570, 35571, 35583-35587, 35623, 35656, 35666, 35671)

Arterial Transposition

35691	Transposition and/or reimplantation; vertebral to carotid artery
35693	vertebral to subclavian artery
35694	subclavian to carotid artery

(For open subclavian to carotid artery transposition performed in conjunction with endovascular repair of descending thoracic aorta, use 33889)

35695	carotid to subclavian artery

+ 35697   Reimplantation, visceral artery to infrarenal aortic prosthesis, each artery (List separately in addition to code for primary procedure)

➔ *CPT Changes: An Insider's View* 2004

(Do not report 35697 in conjunction with 33877)

Excision, Exploration, Repair, Revision

+ 35700   Reoperation, femoral-popliteal or femoral (popliteal)-anterior tibial, posterior tibial, peroneal artery, or other distal vessels, more than 1 month after original operation (List separately in addition to code for primary procedure)

➔ *CPT Assistant* Apr 12:4

(Use 35700 in conjunction with 35556, 35566, 35570, 35571, 35583, 35585, 35587, 35656, 35666, 35671)

35701	Exploration (not followed by surgical repair), with or without lysis of artery; carotid artery
35721	femoral artery

➔ *CPT Assistant* Jun 96:8

35741	popliteal artery
35761	other vessels
35800	Exploration for postoperative hemorrhage, thrombosis or infection; neck
35820	chest
35840	abdomen

➔ *CPT Assistant* May 97:8

Cardiovascular

35860   extremity
➔ *CPT Assistant* Fall 92:21

35870   Repair of graft-enteric fistula

35875   Thrombectomy of arterial or venous graft (other than hemodialysis graft or fistula);
➔ *CPT Assistant* Nov 98:14, Feb 99:6, Mar 99:6, Apr 00:10

35876   with revision of arterial or venous graft
➔ *CPT Assistant* Nov 98:14

(For thrombectomy of hemodialysis graft or fistula, see 36831, 36833)

Codes 35879 and 35881 describe open revision of graft-threatening stenoses of lower extremity arterial bypass graft(s) (previously constructed with autogenous vein conduit) using vein patch angioplasty or segmental vein interposition techniques. For thrombectomy with revision of any non-coronary arterial or venous graft, including those of the lower extremity, (other than hemodialysis graft or fistula), use 35876. For direct repair (other than for fistula) of a lower extremity blood vessel (with or without patch angioplasty), use 35226. For repair (other than for fistula) of a lower extremity blood vessel using a vein graft, use 35256.

35879   Revision, lower extremity arterial bypass, without thrombectomy, open; with vein patch angioplasty
➔ *CPT Assistant* Nov 99:19; *CPT Changes: An Insider's View* 2000

35881   with segmental vein interposition
➔ *CPT Assistant* Nov 99:19; *CPT Changes: An Insider's View* 2000

(For revision of femoral anastomosis of synthetic arterial bypass graft, see 35883, 35884)

(For excision of infected graft, see 35901-35907 and appropriate revascularization code)

35883   Revision, femoral anastomosis of synthetic arterial bypass graft in groin, open; with nonautogenous patch graft (eg, Dacron, ePTFE, bovine pericardium)
➔ *CPT Assistant* Jan 07:7; *CPT Changes: An Insider's View* 2007

(For bilateral procedure, use modifier 50)

(Do not report 35883 in conjunction with 35700, 35875, 35876, 35884)

35884   with autogenous vein patch graft
➔ *CPT Assistant* Jan 07:7; *CPT Changes: An Insider's View* 2007

(For bilateral procedure, use modifier 50)

(Do not report 35884 in conjunction with 35700, 35875, 35876, 35883)

35901   Excision of infected graft; neck

35903   extremity

35905   thorax

35907   abdomen

Vascular Injection Procedures

Listed services for injection procedures include necessary local anesthesia, introduction of needles or catheter, injection of contrast media with or without automatic power injection, and/or necessary pre- and postinjection care specifically related to the injection procedure.

Selective vascular catheterization should be coded to include introduction and all lesser order selective catheterization used in the approach (eg, the description for a selective right middle cerebral artery catheterization includes the introduction and placement catheterization of the right common and internal carotid arteries).

Additional second and/or third order arterial catheterization within the same family of arteries or veins supplied by a single first order vessel should be expressed by 36012, 36218, or 36248.

Additional first order or higher catheterization in vascular families supplied by a first order vessel different from a previously selected and coded family should be separately coded using the conventions described above.

(For radiological supervision and interpretation, see **Radiology)**

(For injection procedures in conjunction with cardiac catheterization, see 93452-93461, 93563-93568)

(For chemotherapy of malignant disease, see 96401-96549)

Intravenous

An intracatheter is a sheathed combination of needle and short catheter.

36000   Introduction of needle or intracatheter, vein
➔ *CPT Assistant* Summer 95:2, Apr 98:1, 3, 7, Jul 98:1, Apr 03:26, Oct 03:2, Jul 06:4, Feb 07:10, Jul 07:1, Dec 08:7

36002   Injection procedures (eg, thrombin) for percutaneous treatment of extremity pseudoaneurysm
➔ *CPT Changes: An Insider's View* 2002

(For imaging guidance, see 76942, 77002, 77012, 77021)

(For ultrasound guided compression repair of pseudoaneurysms, use 76936)

(Do not report 36002 for vascular sealant of an arteriotomy site)

36005   Injection procedure for extremity venography (including introduction of needle or intracatheter)
➔ *CPT Changes: An Insider's View* 2002

(For radiological supervision and interpretation, see 75820, 75822)

⊙▲ **36010**   Introduction of catheter, superior or inferior vena cava
➔ *CPT Assistant* Aug 96:2, Apr 98:7, Sep 00:11, May 01:10, Jul 03:12, Oct 08:11, Jan 09:7, Apr 12:4; *CPT Changes: An Insider's View* 2013
➔ *Clinical Examples in Radiology* Winter 05:5-6, Spring 08:7-8, Winter 12:3

Cardiovascular

Injection Procedure (eg, Thrombin) for Percutaneous Treatment of Extremity Pseudoaneurysm
36002

Needle

Pseudoaneurysm

Thrombin injection

Artery

36011   Selective catheter placement, venous system; first order branch (eg, renal vein, jugular vein)
→ *CPT Assistant* Aug 96:11, Apr 98:7, Jul 03:12, Dec 03:2, Apr 12:5
→ *Clinical Examples in Radiology* Winter 12:3

36012   second order, or more selective, branch (eg, left adrenal vein, petrosal sinus)
→ *CPT Assistant* Aug 96:11, Sep 98:7, Jul 03:12, Apr 12:5
→ *Clinical Examples in Radiology* Winter 12:3

36013   Introduction of catheter, right heart or main pulmonary artery
→ *CPT Assistant* Aug 96:11, Oct 08:11, Jan 09:7

36014   Selective catheter placement, left or right pulmonary artery
→ *CPT Assistant* Aug 96:11, Apr 98:7

36015   Selective catheter placement, segmental or subsegmental pulmonary artery
→ *CPT Assistant* Aug 96:11, Sep 00:11, Mar 12:10

(For insertion of flow directed catheter (eg, Swan-Ganz), use 93503)

(For venous catheterization for selective organ blood sampling, use 36500)

Intra-Arterial—Intra-Aortic

(For radiological supervision and interpretation, see **Radiology**)

36100   Introduction of needle or intracatheter, carotid or vertebral artery
→ *CPT Assistant* Aug 96:11

(For bilateral procedure, report 36100 with modifier 50)

36120   Introduction of needle or intracatheter; retrograde brachial artery
→ *CPT Assistant* Fall 93:16, Aug 96:3, Jun 09:10

⊙▲ **36140**   extremity artery
→ *CPT Assistant* Fall 93:16, Aug 96:3, Nov 99:32-33, Oct 03:2, Jul 06:4, 7, Jul 07:1, Dec 07:10, 11, Jun 09:10, Jul 11:5; *CPT Changes: An Insider's View* 2013

(For insertion of arteriovenous cannula, see 36810-36821)

(36145 has been deleted. To report see 36147, 36148)

Diagnostic Studies of Arteriovenous (AV) Shunts for Dialysis: For diagnostic studies, the arteriovenous (AV) dialysis shunt (AV shunt) is defined as beginning with the arterial anastomosis and extending to the right atrium. This definition includes all upper and lower extremity AV shunts (arteriovenous fistulae [AVF] and arteriovenous grafts [AVG]). Code 36147 includes the work of directly accessing and imaging the entire AV shunt. Antegrade and/or retrograde punctures of the AV shunt are typically used for imaging, and contrast may be injected directly through a needle or through a catheter placed into the AV shunt. Occasionally the catheter needs to be advanced further into the shunt to adequately visualize the arterial anastomosis or the central veins, and all manipulation of the catheter for diagnostic imaging of the AV shunt is included in 36147. Advancement of the catheter to the vena cava to adequately image that segment of the AV shunt is included in 36147 and is not separately reported. Advancement of the catheter tip through the arterial anastomosis to adequately visualize the anastomosis is also considered integral to the work of 36147 and is not separately reported.

Ultrasound guidance for puncture of the AV shunt is not included in 36147. Particularly in the case of new or failing AVF, ultrasound may be necessary to safely and effectively puncture the AV access for evaluation, and this may be reported separately with 76937 if all the appropriate elements for reporting 76937 are performed.

Cardiovascular

Evaluation of the peri-anastomotic portion of the inflow is considered an integral part of the dialysis fistulagram and is included in the work of 36147. The peri-anastomotic portion of the vessel at the arterial anastomosis includes the short segment of the artery immediately adjacent to the anastomosis, the anastomosis itself, and the portion of the vessel or graft immediately distal to the anastomosis.

The arterial inflow to the AV access is considered a separate vessel. If a more proximal inflow problem separate from the peri-anastomotic segment is suspected and additional catheter work and imaging must be done for adequate evaluation, this work is not included in 36147. If a catheter is selectively advanced from the AV shunt puncture into the inflow artery, an additional catheterization code may be reported. In the typical case of an upper extremity AV shunt, 36215 is used to report this work, and includes placement of the catheter retrograde into the inflow artery and into the aorta if necessary (ie, 36200 may not be also reported since that work is included in the work defined by 36215).

Interventions for Arteriovenous (AV) Shunts Created for Dialysis (AV Grafts and AV Fistulae): For the purposes of coding interventional procedures in arteriovenous (AV) shunts created for dialysis (both arteriovenous fistulae [AVF] and arteriovenous grafts [AVG]), the AV shunt is artificially divided into two vessel segments. The first segment is peripheral and extends from the peri-arterial anastomosis through the axillary vein (or entire cephalic vein in the case of cephalic venous outflow). The second segment includes the veins central to the axillary and cephalic veins, including the subclavian and innominate veins through the vena cava. Interventions performed in a single segment, regardless of the number of lesions treated, are coded as a single intervention.

The AV shunt is considered to be venous and most interventions are coded with the venous intervention codes (ie, angioplasty is reported with venous angioplasty codes 35476, 75978). Codes 35476 and 75978 would be reported once to describe all angioplasty work performed in one segment of the AV dialysis shunt, regardless of the number of distinct lesions treated within that segment, the number of times the balloon is inflated, or the number of balloon catheters required to open all lesions.

There is an exception to the use of venous interventional codes. When there is a stenosis at the arterial anastomosis, it typically extends across the anastomosis and involves the artery just proximal to and at the anastomosis as well as the outflow vessel or graft. This segment is called the peri-anastomotic (or juxta-anastomotic) region, and even though the stenosis can involve multiple vessels, it is typically a single lesion with a single etiology crossing the anastomosis, and treatment to open this lesion crosses from the artery into the vein or venous graft. An intervention treated in this peri-anastomotic segment is coded as an arterial intervention (35475, 75962). Since

the entire segment of the AV shunt from the peri-arterial anastomosis through the axillary vein is considered a single vessel for coding of interventions, the arterial angioplasty codes include the work of opening the peri-anastomotic stenosis, as well as all other stenoses treated within this segment of the vessel. Codes 35475 and 75962 are reported once to describe all work done to angioplasty any lesion from the peri-arterial anastomosis through the axillary vein in procedures that involve angioplasty of the peri-arterial anastomosis of the AV shunt. In these special instances, venous angioplasty codes would not be reported additionally for this first or most peripheral shunt segment, even if balloon angioplasty is performed on segments of the AV dialysis shunt that are purely venous anatomy within this specific vessel segment.

It is never appropriate to report removal of the arterial plug during a declot/thrombectomy procedure as an arterial or venous angioplasty (35475, 35476). Removal of the arterial plug is included in the work of a fistula thrombectomy (36870), even if a balloon catheter is used to mechanically dislodge the resistant thrombus.

The central veins (eg, subclavian, innominate, and cava) are considered an additional, separate venous vessel segment for purposes of interventional coding for AV dialysis shunt interventions. If one or more central venous stenoses are treated with angioplasty, this is reported as a single venous angioplasty (35476, 75978), regardless of the number of discrete lesions treated within this segment, and also independent of the number of balloon inflations or number of balloon catheters or sizes required. This additional work should be clearly documented in the patient record and in the recorded images.

The codes for stents placed in AV dialysis accesses are generic for intravascular work and not specific for arterial or venous anatomy. However, the same rules used for angioplasty apply to stent placements for AV dialysis shunts with respect to the number of interventions reported for each patient. Stent codes (37205, 75960) are reported once to describe all work of stenting lesions within the defined AV dialysis shunt segment from the peri-arterial anastomosis through the axillary and cephalic veins, regardless of the number of stents placed or the number of discrete lesions treated within that vessel segment. If additional stenting is required for central venous stenosis, this may be reported as an additional stent placement (37206, 75960), describing all the work of stent placement within the central venous segment.

The work of catheterizing all the veins in the dialysis AV shunt is included in 36147 (and, if appropriate, 36148). Selective catheterization of the inferior/superior vena cava and central veins cannot be separately reported when performed from a direct puncture of the AVF/AVG.

Cardiovascular

However, if additional venous side branches off of the conduit, known as accessory veins, are separately catheterized for intervention such as embolization of a large competing accessory vein, this additional work may be separately reported using the appropriate selective venous catheterization codes (36011 and 36012). The embolization may be reported using 37204, 75894.

⊙ **36147**   Introduction of needle and/or catheter, arteriovenous shunt created for dialysis (graft/fistula); initial access with complete radiological evaluation of dialysis access, including fluoroscopy, image documentation and report (includes access of shunt, injection[s] of contrast, and all necessary imaging from the arterial anastomosis and adjacent artery through entire venous outflow including the inferior or superior vena cava)

➡ *CPT Assistant* Mar 10:3, Dec 11:15, Apr 12:5; *CPT Changes: An Insider's View* 2010

➡ *Clinical Examples in Radiology* Summer 10:12, Winter 10:7, Spring 12:4

(If 36147 indicates the need for a therapeutic intervention requiring a second catheterization of the shunt, use 36148)

(Do not report 36147 in conjunction with 75791)

⊙+ **36148**   additional access for therapeutic intervention (List separately in addition to code for primary procedure)

➡ *CPT Assistant* Mar 10:3, Apr 12:5; *CPT Changes: An Insider's View* 2010

➡ *Clinical Examples in Radiology* Winter 10:8

(Use 36148 in conjunction with 36147)

36160   Introduction of needle or intracatheter, aortic, translumbar

➡ *CPT Assistant* Aug 96:3

▶ *Diagnostic Studies of Cervicocerebral Arteries:* Codes 36221-36228 describe non-selective and selective arterial catheter placement and diagnostic imaging of the aortic arch, carotid, and vertebral arteries. Codes 36221-36226 include the work of accessing the vessel, placement of catheter(s), contrast injection(s), fluoroscopy, radiological supervision and interpretation, and closure of the arteriotomy by pressure, or application of an arterial closure device. Codes 36221-36228 describe arterial contrast injections with arterial, capillary, and venous phase imaging, when performed.

Code 36227 is an add-on code to report unilateral selective arterial catheter placement and diagnostic imaging of the ipsilateral external carotid circulation and includes all the work of accessing the additional vessel, placement of catheter(s), contrast injection(s), fluoroscopy, radiological supervision and interpretation. Code 36227 is reported in conjunction with 36222, 36223, or 36224.

Code 36228 is an add-on code to report unilateral selective arterial catheter placement and diagnostic imaging of the initial and each additional intracranial branch of the internal carotid or vertebral arteries. Code 36228 is reported in conjunction with 36224 or 36226.

This includes any additional second or third order catheter selective placement in the same primary branch of the internal carotid, vertebral, or basilar artery and includes all the work of accessing the additional vessel, placement of catheter(s), contrast injection(s), fluoroscopy, radiological supervision and interpretation. It is not reported more than twice per side regardless of the number of additional branches selectively catheterized.

Codes 36221-36226 are built on progressive hierarchies with more intensive services inclusive of less intensive services. The code inclusive of all of the services provided for that vessel should be reported (ie, use the code inclusive of the most intensive services provided). Only one code in the range 36222-36224 may be reported for each ipsilateral carotid territory. Only one code in the range 36225-36226 may be reported for each ipsilateral vertebral territory.

Code 36221 is reported for non-selective arterial catheter placement in the thoracic aorta and diagnostic imaging of the aortic arch and great vessel origins. Codes 36222-36228 are reported for unilateral artery catheterization. Do not report 36221 in conjunction with 36222-36226 as these selective codes include the work of 36221 when performed.

Do not report 36222, 36223, or 36224 together for ipsilateral angiography. Instead, select the code that represents the most comprehensive service using the following hierarchy of complexity (listed in descending order of complexity): 36224>36223>36222.

Do not report 36225 and 36226 together for ipsilateral angiography. Select the code that represents the more comprehensive service using the following hierarchy of complexity (listed in descending order of complexity): 36226>36225.

When bilateral carotid and/or vertebral arterial catheterization and imaging is performed, add modifier 50 to codes 36222-36228 if the same procedure is performed on both sides. For example, bilateral extracranial carotid angiography with selective catheterization of each common carotid artery would be reported with 36222 and modifier 50. However, when different territory(ies) is studied in the same session on both sides of the body, modifiers may be required to report the imaging performed. Use modifier 59 to denote that different carotid and/or vertebral arteries are being studied. For example, when selective right internal carotid artery catheterization accompanied by right extracranial and intracranial carotid angiography is followed by selective left common carotid artery catheterization with left extracranial carotid angiography, use 36224 to report the right side and 36222-59 to report the left side.

Diagnostic angiography of the cervicocerebral vessels may be followed by an interventional procedure at the same session. Interventional procedures may be separately reportable using standard coding conventions.

Cardiovascular

Do not report 75774 as part of diagnostic angiography of the extracranial and intracranial cervicocerebral vessels. It may be appropriate to report 75774 for diagnostic angiography of upper extremities and other vascular beds performed in the same session.

Report 76376 or 76377 for 3D rendering when performed in conjunction with 36221-36228.

Report 76937 for ultrasound guidance for vascular access, when performed in conjunction with 36221-36228.◄

⊙ **36200**   Introduction of catheter, aorta

➔ *CPT Assistant* Fall 93:16, Aug 96:3, Jul 06:7, Dec 07:10, 14, Apr 08:11, Dec 09:13, Jul 11:5, Oct 11:9, Apr 12:4; *CPT Changes: An Insider's View* 2012

➔ *Clinical Examples in Radiology* Spring 12:6

►(For non-selective angiography of the extracranial carotid and/or cerebral vessels and cervicocerebral arch, when performed, use 36221)◄

36215   Selective catheter placement, arterial system; each first order thoracic or brachiocephalic branch, within a vascular family

➔ *CPT Assistant* Fall 93:15, Aug 96:3, Nov 97:16, Apr 98:9, Sep 00:11, Oct 00:4, Feb 03:3, Apr 12:4

➔ *Clinical Examples in Radiology* Spring 12:4

(For catheter placement for coronary angiography, see 93454-93461)

36216   initial second order thoracic or brachiocephalic branch, within a vascular family

➔ *CPT Assistant* Fall 93:15, Aug 96:3, Oct 00:4, Dec 07:10, Dec 11:12, Apr 12:4

36217   initial third order or more selective thoracic or brachiocephalic branch, within a vascular family

➔ *CPT Assistant* Fall 93:15, Aug 96:3, Oct 00:4, Dec 07:10, Dec 11:12, Apr 12:5

➔ *Clinical Examples in Radiology* Summer 07:1, 2

+ **36218**   additional second order, third order, and beyond, thoracic or brachiocephalic branch, within a vascular family (List in addition to code for initial second or third order vessel as appropriate)

➔ *CPT Assistant* Fall 93:15, Aug 96:3, Oct 00:4, Jul 06:7, Dec 07:10, Apr 12:5

(Use 36218 in conjunction with 36216, 36217)

►(For angiography, see 36147, 36222-36228, 75600-75774, 75791)◄

►(For angioplasty, see 35471, 35472, 35475)◄

(For transcatheter therapies, see 37200-37208, 61624, 61626)

►(When coronary artery, arterial conduit [eg, internal mammary, inferior epigastric or free radical artery] or venous bypass graft angiography is performed in conjunction with cardiac catheterization, see the appropriate cardiac catheterization, injection procedure, and imaging supervision code[s] [93455, 93457, 93459, 93461, 93530-93533, 93564] in the **Medicine** section. When internal mammary artery angiography only is performed without a concomitant cardiac catheterization, use 36216 or 36217 as appropriate)◄

⊙● **36221**   Non-selective catheter placement, thoracic aorta, with angiography of the extracranial carotid, vertebral, and/or intracranial vessels, unilateral or bilateral, and all associated radiological supervision and interpretation, includes angiography of the cervicocerebral arch, when performed

➔ *CPT Changes: An Insider's View* 2013

►(Do not report 36221 with 36222-36226)◄

⊙● **36222**   Selective catheter placement, common carotid or innominate artery, unilateral, any approach, with angiography of the ipsilateral extracranial carotid circulation and all associated radiological supervision and interpretation, includes angiography of the cervicocerebral arch, when performed

➔ *CPT Changes: An Insider's View* 2013

⊙● **36223**   Selective catheter placement, common carotid or innominate artery, unilateral, any approach, with angiography of the ipsilateral intracranial carotid circulation and all associated radiological supervision and interpretation, includes angiography of the extracranial carotid and cervicocerebral arch, when performed

➔ *CPT Changes: An Insider's View* 2013

⊙● **36224**   Selective catheter placement, internal carotid artery, unilateral, with angiography of the ipsilateral intracranial carotid circulation and all associated radiological supervision and interpretation, includes angiography of the extracranial carotid and cervicocerebral arch, when performed

➔ *CPT Changes: An Insider's View* 2013

⊙● **36225**   Selective catheter placement, subclavian or innominate artery, unilateral, with angiography of the ipsilateral vertebral circulation and all associated radiological supervision and interpretation, includes angiography of the cervicocerebral arch, when performed

➔ *CPT Changes: An Insider's View* 2013

⊙● **36226**   Selective catheter placement, vertebral artery, unilateral, with angiography of the ipsilateral vertebral circulation and all associated radiological supervision and interpretation, includes angiography of the cervicocerebral arch, when performed

➔ *CPT Changes: An Insider's View* 2013

⊙+● **36227**   Selective catheter placement, external carotid artery, unilateral, with angiography of the ipsilateral external carotid circulation and all associated radiological supervision and interpretation (List separately in addition to code for primary procedure)

➔ *CPT Changes: An Insider's View* 2013

►(Use 36227 in conjunction with 36222, 36223, or 36224)◄

Cardiovascular

⊙+● **36228** Selective catheter placement, each intracranial branch of the internal carotid or vertebral arteries, unilateral, with angiography of the selected vessel circulation and all associated radiological supervision and interpretation (eg, middle cerebral artery, posterior inferior cerebellar artery) (List separately in addition to code for primary procedure)

> *CPT Changes: An Insider's View* 2013

►(Use 36228 in conjunction with 36224 or 36226)◄

►(Do not report 36228 more than twice per side)◄

Angiography, Carotid Artery
36222-36228

A radiologic contrast study is performed on the carotid artery vascular family.

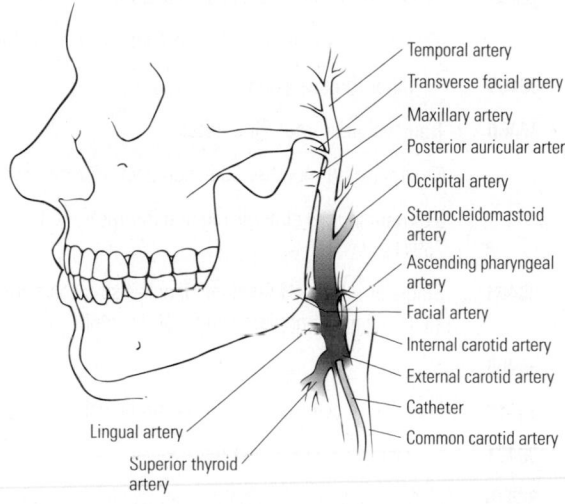

- Temporal artery
- Transverse facial artery
- Maxillary artery
- Posterior auricular artery
- Occipital artery
- Sternocleidomastoid artery
- Ascending pharyngeal artery
- Facial artery
- Internal carotid artery
- External carotid artery
- Catheter
- Common carotid artery
- Lingual artery
- Superior thyroid artery

⊙ **36245** Selective catheter placement, arterial system; each first order abdominal, pelvic, or lower extremity artery branch, within a vascular family

> *CPT Assistant* Fall 93:15, Aug 96:3, Jan 01:14, Jan 07:7, Dec 07:10, Jul 11:5, Oct 11:9, Apr 12:4; *CPT Changes: An Insider's View* 2012

> *Clinical Examples in Radiology* Summer 08:1-3, Fall 11:3

⊙ **36246** initial second order abdominal, pelvic, or lower extremity artery branch, within a vascular family

> *CPT Assistant* Fall 93:15, Aug 96:3, Jan 01:14, Jan 07:7, Dec 07:10, 11, Jul 11:5, Oct 11:9, Apr 12:4; *CPT Changes: An Insider's View* 2012

⊙ **36247** initial third order or more selective abdominal, pelvic, or lower extremity artery branch, within a vascular family

> *CPT Assistant* Fall 93:15, Aug 96:3, Jan 01:14, Jan 07:7, Dec 07:10, Jul 11:5, Apr 12:4; *CPT Changes: An Insider's View* 2012

> *Clinical Examples in Radiology* Summer 08:1-3, Winter 08:1

⊙+ **36248** additional second order, third order, and beyond, abdominal, pelvic, or lower extremity artery branch, within a vascular family (List in addition to code for initial second or third order vessel as appropriate)

> *CPT Assistant* Fall 93:15, Aug 96:3, Apr 98:1, 7, Oct 00:4, Jan 01:14, Jan 07:7, Jul 11:5, Apr 12:4; *CPT Changes: An Insider's View* 2012

> *Clinical Examples in Radiology* Winter 10:7

(Use 36248 in conjunction with 36246, 36247)

⊙ **36251** Selective catheter placement (first-order), main renal artery and any accessory renal artery(s) for renal angiography, including arterial puncture and catheter placement(s), fluoroscopy, contrast injection(s), image postprocessing, permanent recording of images, and radiological supervision and interpretation, including pressure gradient measurements when performed, and flush aortogram when performed; unilateral

> *CPT Assistant* Apr 12:6; *CPT Changes: An Insider's View* 2012

> *Clinical Examples in Radiology* Fall 11:2

⊙ **36252** bilateral

> *CPT Assistant* Apr 12:6; *CPT Changes: An Insider's View* 2012

> *Clinical Examples in Radiology* Fall 11:2

⊙ **36253** Superselective catheter placement (one or more second order or higher renal artery branches) renal artery and any accessory renal artery(s) for renal angiography, including arterial puncture, catheterization, fluoroscopy, contrast injection(s), image postprocessing, permanent recording of images, and radiological supervision and interpretation, including pressure gradient measurements when performed, and flush aortogram when performed; unilateral

> *CPT Assistant* Apr 12:6; *CPT Changes: An Insider's View* 2012

> *Clinical Examples in Radiology* Fall 11:2

(Do not report 36253 in conjunction with 36251 when performed for the same kidney)

⊙ **36254** bilateral

> *CPT Assistant* Apr 12:6; *CPT Changes: An Insider's View* 2012

> *Clinical Examples in Radiology* Fall 11:2

(Do not report 36254 in conjunction with 36252)

(Placement of closure device at the vascular access site is not separately reported with 36251-36254)

36260 Insertion of implantable intra-arterial infusion pump (eg, for chemotherapy of liver)

> *CPT Assistant* Fall 95:5

36261 Revision of implanted intra-arterial infusion pump

36262 Removal of implanted intra-arterial infusion pump

36299 Unlisted procedure, vascular injection

Cardiovascular

Venous

Venipuncture, needle or catheter for diagnostic study or intravenous therapy, percutaneous. These codes are also used to report the therapy as specified. For collection of a specimen from an established catheter, use 36592. For collection of a specimen from a completely implantable venous access device, use 36591.

▲ 36400   Venipuncture, younger than age 3 years, necessitating the skill of a physician or other qualified health care professional, not to be used for routine venipuncture; femoral or jugular vein

     ➔ *CPT Assistant* Jul 06:4, Jul 07:1, Dec 08:7; *CPT Changes: An Insider's View* 2002, 2004, 2013

▲ 36405   scalp vein

     ➔ *CPT Assistant* Jul 06:4, Jul 07:1, Dec 08:7; *CPT Changes: An Insider's View* 2013

▲ 36406   other vein

     ➔ *CPT Assistant* Jul 06:4, Jul 07:1; *CPT Changes: An Insider's View* 2013

▲ 36410   Venipuncture, age 3 years or older, necessitating the skill of a physician or other qualified health care professional (separate procedure), for diagnostic or therapeutic purposes (not to be used for routine venipuncture)

     ➔ *CPT Assistant* Jun 96:10, May 01:11, Aug 02:2, Oct 03:10, Feb 07:10, Jul 07:1, Dec 08:7; *CPT Changes: An Insider's View* 2004, 2013

     ➔ *Clinical Examples in Radiology* Spring 09:8

--- *Coding Tip* ---

Instructions for Use of the CPT Codebook

When advanced practice nurses and physician assistants are working with physicians they are considered as working in the exact same specialty and exact same subspecialties as the physician. A "physician or other qualified health care professional" is an individual who is qualified by education, training, licensure/regulation (when applicable), and facility privileging (when applicable) who performs a professional service within his or her scope of practice and independently reports that professional services. These professionals are distinct from "clinical staff." A clinical staff member is a person who works under the supervision of a physician or other qualified health care professional, and who is allowed by law, regulation and facility policy to perform or assist in the performance of a specific professional service, but does not individually report that professional service. Other policies may also affect who may report specific services.

CPT Coding Guidelines, Introduction, Instructions for Use of the CPT Codebook

36415   Collection of venous blood by venipuncture

     ➔ *CPT Assistant* Jun 96:10, Mar 98:10, Oct 99:11, Aug 00:2, Feb 07:10, Jul 07:1, Dec 08:7; *CPT Changes: An Insider's View* 2003

(Do not report modifier 63 in conjunction with 36415)

36416   Collection of capillary blood specimen (eg, finger, heel, ear stick)

     ➔ *CPT Changes: An Insider's View* 2003

36420   Venipuncture, cutdown; younger than age 1 year

     ➔ *CPT Assistant* Nov 99:32-33, Aug 00:2, Oct 03:2, Jul 06:4

(Do not report modifier 63 in conjunction with 36420)

36425   Clinical Examples in Radiology Summer 08:1
     age 1 or over

     ➔ *Clinical Examples in Radiology* Summer 08:1

36430   Transfusion, blood or blood components

     ➔ *CPT Assistant* Aug 97:18, Nov 99:32-33, Aug 00:2, Mar 01:10, Oct 03:2, Jul 06:4, Jul 07:1

36440   Push transfusion, blood, 2 years or younger

     ➔ *CPT Assistant* Aug 00:2, Oct 03:2, Jul 06:4, Jul 07:1

36450   Exchange transfusion, blood; newborn

(Do not report modifier 63 in conjunction with 36450)

36455   other than newborn

36460   Transfusion, intrauterine, fetal

(Do not report modifier 63 in conjunction with 36460)

(For radiological supervision and interpretation, use 76941)

36468   Single or multiple injections of sclerosing solutions, spider veins (telangiectasia); limb or trunk

36469   face

36470   Injection of sclerosing solution; single vein

36471   multiple veins, same leg

36475   Endovenous ablation therapy of incompetent vein, extremity, inclusive of all imaging guidance and monitoring, percutaneous, radiofrequency; first vein treated

     ➔ *CPT Assistant* Jul 10:11; *CPT Changes: An Insider's View* 2005

     ➔ *Clinical Examples in Radiology* Fall 08:10

+ 36476   second and subsequent veins treated in a single extremity, each through separate access sites (List separately in addition to code for primary procedure)

     ➔ *CPT Assistant* Jul 10:11; *CPT Changes: An Insider's View* 2005

(Use 36476 in conjunction with 36475)

(Do not report 36475, 36476 in conjunction with 29581, 29582, 36000-36005, 36410, 36425, 36478, 36479, 37204, 75894, 76000, 76001, 76937, 76942, 76998, 77022, 93970, 93971)

36478   Endovenous ablation therapy of incompetent vein, extremity, inclusive of all imaging guidance and monitoring, percutaneous, laser; first vein treated

     ➔ *CPT Assistant* Jul 12:12; *CPT Changes: An Insider's View* 2005

Cardiovascular

+ 36479   second and subsequent veins treated in a single extremity, each through separate access sites (List separately in addition to code for primary procedure)

➡ *CPT Assistant* Jul 10:11, Jul 12:12; *CPT Changes: An Insider's View* 2005

(Use 36479 in conjunction with 36478)

(Do not report 36478, 36479 in conjunction with 29581, 29582, 36000-36005, 36410, 36425, 36475, 36476, 37204, 75894, 76000, 76001, 76937, 76942, 76998, 77022, 93970, 93971)

⊙ **36481**   Percutaneous portal vein catheterization by any method

➡ *CPT Assistant* Oct 96:1, Mar 02:10, Dec 03:2; *CPT Changes: An Insider's View* 2010

(For radiological supervision and interpretation, see 75885, 75887)

36500   Venous catheterization for selective organ blood sampling

(For catheterization in superior or inferior vena cava, use 36010)

(For radiological supervision and interpretation, use 75893)

36510   Catheterization of umbilical vein for diagnosis or therapy, newborn

➡ *CPT Assistant* Nov 99:5-6, Aug 00:2, Oct 03:2, Jul 06:4, Jul 07:1

(Do not report modifier 63 in conjunction with 36510)

36511   Therapeutic apheresis; for white blood cells

➡ *CPT Changes: An Insider's View* 2003

36512   for red blood cells

➡ *CPT Changes: An Insider's View* 2003

36513   for platelets

➡ *CPT Changes: An Insider's View* 2003

36514   for plasma pheresis

➡ *CPT Changes: An Insider's View* 2003

36515   with extracorporeal immunoadsorption and plasma reinfusion

➡ *CPT Changes: An Insider's View* 2003

36516   with extracorporeal selective adsorption or selective filtration and plasma reinfusion

➡ *CPT Changes: An Insider's View* 2003

▶(For professional evaluation, use modifier 26)◀

36522   Photopheresis, extracorporeal

➡ *CPT Assistant* Fall 93:25, Jun 09:3, Sep 09:3, Aug 10:12

Central Venous Access Procedures

To qualify as a central venous access catheter or device, the tip of the catheter/device must terminate in the subclavian, brachiocephalic (innominate) or iliac veins, the superior or inferior vena cava, or the right atrium. The venous access device may be either centrally inserted (jugular, subclavian, femoral vein or inferior vena cava catheter entry site) or peripherally inserted (eg, basilic or cephalic vein). The device may be accessed for use either via exposed catheter (external to the skin), via a subcutaneous port or via a subcutaneous pump.

The procedures involving these types of devices fall into five categories:

1. ***Insertion*** (placement of catheter through a newly established venous access)

2. ***Repair*** (fixing device without replacement of either catheter or port/pump, other than pharmacologic or mechanical correction of intracatheter or pericatheter occlusion [see 36595 or 36596])

3. ***Partial replacement*** of only the catheter component associated with a port/pump device, but not entire device

4. ***Complete replacement*** of entire device via same venous access site (complete exchange)

5. ***Removal*** of entire device.

There is no coding distinction between venous access achieved percutaneously versus by cutdown or based on catheter size.

For the repair, partial (catheter only) replacement, complete replacement, or removal of both catheters (placed from separate venous access sites) of a multi-catheter device, with or without subcutaneous ports/pumps, use the appropriate code describing the service with a frequency of two.

If an existing central venous access device is removed and a new one placed via a separate venous access site, appropriate codes for both procedures (removal of old, if code exists, and insertion of new device) should be reported.

When imaging is used for these procedures, either for gaining access to the venous entry site or for manipulating the catheter into final central position, use 76937, 77001.

(For refilling and maintenance of an implantable pump or reservoir for intravenous or intra-arterial drug delivery, use 96522)

Cardiovascular

The Central Venous Access Procedures Table

	Non-tunneled	Tunneled Without Port or Pump	Central Tunneled	Tunneled With Port	Tunneled With Pump	Peripheral	<5 years	≥5 years	Any Age
Insertion									
Catheter	36555						36555		
	36556							36556	
		36557	36557				36557		
		36558	36558					36558	
	36568 (w/o port or pump)					36568 (w/o port or pump)	36568 (w/o port or pump)		
	36569 (w/o port or pump)					36569 (w/o port or pump)		36569 (w/o port or pump)	
Device			36560	36560			36560		
			36561	36561				36561	
			36563		36563				36563
		36565	36565						36565
			36566	36566					
	36570 (w port)			36570 (w port)		36570 (w port)	36570 (w port)		
	36571 (w port)			36571 (w port)		36571 (w port)		36571 (w port)	
Repair									
Catheter	36575 (w/o port or pump)	36575 (w/o port or pump)	36575 (w/o port or pump)			36575 (w/o port or pump)			36575
Device	36576 (w port or pump)					36576 (w port or pump)			36576
Partial Replacement - Central Venous Access Device (Catheter only)									
			36578	36578	36578	36578			36578
Complete Replacement - Central Venous Access Device (Through Same Venous Access Site)									
Catheter	36580 (w/o port or pump)								36580
		36581	36581						36581
	36584 (w/o port or pump)					36584 (w/o port or pump)			36584
Device			36582	36582					36582
			36583		36583				36583
				36585 (w port)		36585 (w port)			36585
Removal									
Catheter		36589							36589
Device			36590	36590	36590	36590			36590
Removal of Obstructive Material from Device									
	36595 (pericatheter)	36595 (pericatheter)	36595 (pericatheter)	36595 (pericatheter)	36595 (pericatheter)	36595 (pericatheter)			36595 (pericatheter)
	36596 (intraluminal)	36596 (intraluminal)	36596 (intraluminal)	36596 (intraluminal)	36596 (intraluminal)	36596 (intraluminal)			36596 (intraluminal)
Repositioning of Catheter									
	36597	36597	36597	36597	36597	36597	36597	36597	36597

Cardiovascular

Insertion of Central Venous Access Device

⊙ **36555**   Insertion of non-tunneled centrally inserted central venous catheter; younger than 5 years of age

➔ *CPT Assistant* Dec 04:7, Jul 06:4, Jul 07:1, Jun 08:8; *CPT Changes: An Insider's View* 2004

➔ *Clinical Examples in Radiology* Summer 06:8-9, Spring 09:10, Winter 09:9

(For peripherally inserted non-tunneled central venous catheter, younger than 5 years of age, use 36568)

36556   age 5 years or older

➔ *CPT Assistant* Dec 04:7, Jun 08:8; *CPT Changes: An Insider's View* 2004

➔ *Clinical Examples in Radiology* Summer 06:8-9, Spring 08:7, 8, Spring 09:10, Winter 09:8, 9

(For peripherally inserted non-tunneled central venous catheter, age 5 years or older, use 36569)

⊙ **36557**   Insertion of tunneled centrally inserted central venous catheter, without subcutaneous port or pump; younger than 5 years of age

➔ *CPT Assistant* Dec 04:7, Jun 08:8; *CPT Changes: An Insider's View* 2004

➔ *Clinical Examples in Radiology* Spring 09:10, Winter 09:9

⊙ **36558**   age 5 years or older

➔ *CPT Assistant* Dec 04:7, Jun 08:8; *CPT Changes: An Insider's View* 2004

➔ *Clinical Examples in Radiology* Spring 09:10, Winter 09:9

(For peripherally inserted central venous catheter with port, 5 years or older, use 36571)

Insertion of Non-Tunneled Centrally Inserted Central Venous Catheter
36555

During placement of a central venous catheter, a short tract is developed as the catheter is advanced from the skin entry site to the point of venous cannulation. The catheter tip must reside in the subclavian, innominate or iliac veins, the inferior or superior vena cava, or right atrium to be considered a "central venous" catheter.

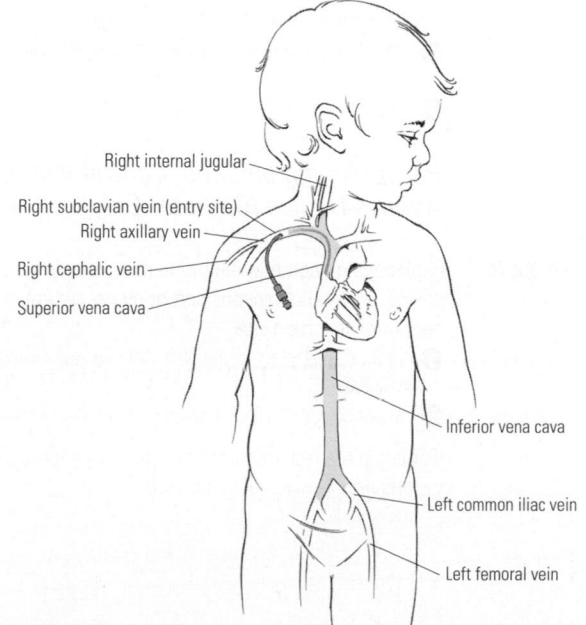

Insertion of Non-Tunneled Centrally Inserted Central Venous Catheter
36556

During placement of a central venous catheter, a short tract is developed as the catheter is advanced from the skin entry site to the point of venous cannulation. The catheter tip must reside in the subclavian, innominate or iliac veins, the inferior or superior vena cava, or right atrium, to be considered a "central venous" catheter.

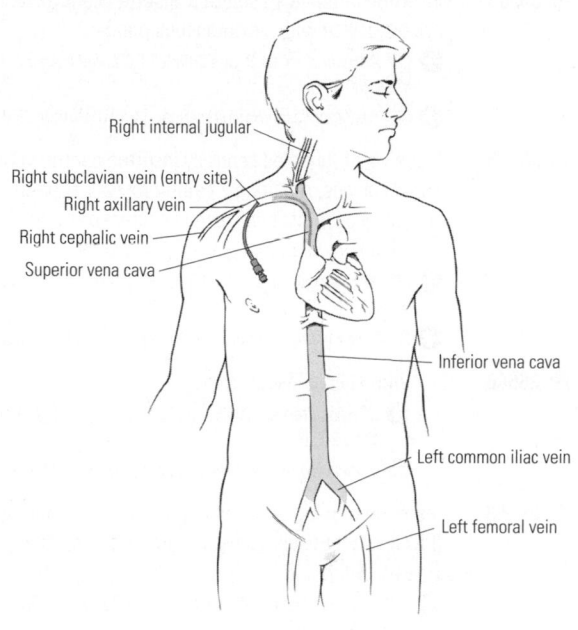

Insertion of Tunneled Central Venous Catheter
36557-36558

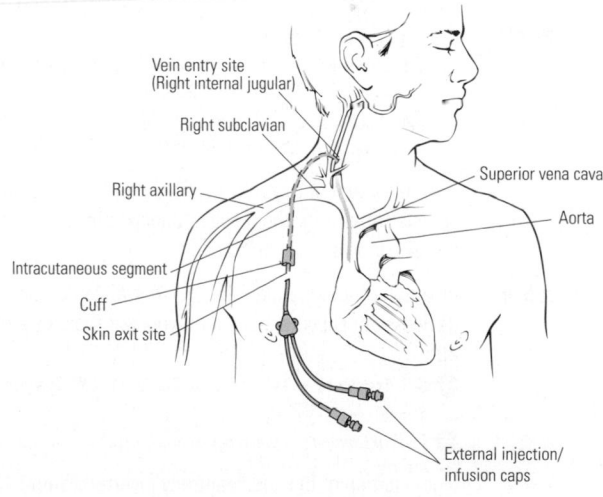

⊙ **36560**   Insertion of tunneled centrally inserted central venous access device, with subcutaneous port; younger than 5 years of age

➔ *CPT Assistant* Dec 04:7, Jun 08:8, Dec 09:11; *CPT Changes: An Insider's View* 2004

➔ *Clinical Examples in Radiology* Spring 09:10, Winter 09:9

(For peripherally inserted central venous access device with subcutaneous port, younger than 5 years of age, use 36570)

Cardiovascular

⊙ **36561** age 5 years or older

→ *CPT Assistant* Dec 04:7, Jun 08:8, Dec 09:11; *CPT Changes: An Insider's View* 2004

→ *Clinical Examples in Radiology* Spring 09:10, Winter 09:9

(For peripherally inserted central venous catheter with subcutaneous port, 5 years or older, use 36571)

⊙ **36563** Insertion of tunneled centrally inserted central venous access device with subcutaneous pump

→ *CPT Assistant* Dec 04:8, Jun 08:8; *CPT Changes: An Insider's View* 2004

→ *Clinical Examples in Radiology* Spring 09:10, Winter 09:9

⊙ **36565** Insertion of tunneled centrally inserted central venous access device, requiring 2 catheters via 2 separate venous access sites; without subcutaneous port or pump (eg, Tesio type catheter)

→ *CPT Assistant* Dec 04:8, Jun 08:8; *CPT Changes: An Insider's View* 2004

→ *Clinical Examples in Radiology* Spring 09:10, Winter 09:9

⊙ **36566** with subcutaneous port(s)

→ *CPT Assistant* Dec 04:8, Jun 08:8; *CPT Changes: An Insider's View* 2004

→ *Clinical Examples in Radiology* Spring 09:10, Winter 09:9

⊙ **36568** Insertion of peripherally inserted central venous catheter (PICC), without subcutaneous port or pump; younger than 5 years of age

→ *CPT Assistant* Oct 04:14, Dec 04:8, May 05:13, Jun 08:8; *CPT Changes: An Insider's View* 2004

→ *Clinical Examples in Radiology* Spring 09:10, Winter 09:9

(For placement of centrally inserted non-tunneled central venous catheter, without subcutaneous port or pump, younger than 5 years of age, use 36555)

36569 age 5 years or older

→ *CPT Assistant* Oct 04:14, Dec 04:8, May 05:13, Jun 08:8; *CPT Changes: An Insider's View* 2004

→ *Clinical Examples in Radiology* 2004_Inaugural 04:1-2, Spring 08:7, Fall 08:5, 6, Spring 09:10, Winter 09:9

(For placement of centrally inserted non-tunneled central venous catheter, without subcutaneous port or pump, age 5 years or older, use 36556)

⊙ **36570** Insertion of peripherally inserted central venous access device, with subcutaneous port; younger than 5 years of age

→ *CPT Assistant* Dec 04:8, Jun 08:8, Dec 09:11; *CPT Changes: An Insider's View* 2004

→ *Clinical Examples in Radiology* Spring 09:10, Winter 09:9

(For insertion of tunneled centrally inserted central venous access device with subcutaneous port, younger than 5 years of age, use 36560)

⊙ **36571** age 5 years or older

→ *CPT Assistant* Dec 04:9, Jun 08:8, Dec 09:11; *CPT Changes: An Insider's View* 2004

→ *Clinical Examples in Radiology* Spring 09:10, Winter 09:9

(For insertion of tunneled centrally inserted central venous access device with subcutaneous port, age 5 years or older, use 36561)

Implantable Venous Access Port

36570-36571, 36576, 36578

Noncoring needle

Venous access port

Central vein

Repair of Central Venous Access Device

(For mechanical removal of pericatheter obstructive material, use 36595)

(For mechanical removal of intracatheter obstructive material, use 36596)

36575 Repair of tunneled or non-tunneled central venous access catheter, without subcutaneous port or pump, central or peripheral insertion site

→ *CPT Changes: An Insider's View* 2004

→ *Clinical Examples in Radiology* Spring 09:10, Summer 10:11

⊙ **36576** Repair of central venous access device, with subcutaneous port or pump, central or peripheral insertion site

→ *CPT Assistant* Dec 04:9, Jun 08:8; *CPT Changes: An Insider's View* 2004

→ *Clinical Examples in Radiology* Spring 09:10

Partial Replacement of Central Venous Access Device (Catheter Only)

⊙ **36578** Replacement, catheter only, of central venous access device, with subcutaneous port or pump, central or peripheral insertion site

→ *CPT Assistant* Dec 04:10, Jun 08:8; *CPT Changes: An Insider's View* 2004

→ *Clinical Examples in Radiology* Spring 09:10, Winter 09:9

(For complete replacement of entire device through same venous access, use 36582 or 36583)

Cardiovascular

Complete Replacement of Central Venous Access Device Through Same Venous Access Site

36580 Replacement, complete, of a non-tunneled centrally inserted central venous catheter, without subcutaneous port or pump, through same venous access
➡ *CPT Assistant* Dec 04:10, Jun 08:8; *CPT Changes: An Insider's View* 2004
➡ *Clinical Examples in Radiology* Spring 09:10, Winter 09:9

⊙ **36581** Replacement, complete, of a tunneled centrally inserted central venous catheter, without subcutaneous port or pump, through same venous access
➡ *CPT Assistant* Dec 04:10, Jun 08:8; *CPT Changes: An Insider's View* 2004
➡ *Clinical Examples in Radiology* Spring 09:10, Winter 09:9

⊙ **36582** Replacement, complete, of a tunneled centrally inserted central venous access device, with subcutaneous port, through same venous access
➡ *CPT Assistant* Dec 04:10, Jun 08:8; *CPT Changes: An Insider's View* 2004
➡ *Clinical Examples in Radiology* Spring 09:10, Winter 09:9

⊙ **36583** Replacement, complete, of a tunneled centrally inserted central venous access device, with subcutaneous pump, through same venous access
➡ *CPT Assistant* Dec 04:10-11, Jun 08:8; *CPT Changes: An Insider's View* 2004
➡ *Clinical Examples in Radiology* Spring 09:10, Winter 09:9

36584 Replacement, complete, of a peripherally inserted central venous catheter (PICC), without subcutaneous port or pump, through same venous access
➡ *CPT Assistant* Dec 04:11, Jun 08:8; *CPT Changes: An Insider's View* 2004
➡ *Clinical Examples in Radiology* Spring 09:10, Winter 09:9

⊙ **36585** Replacement, complete, of a peripherally inserted central venous access device, with subcutaneous port, through same venous access
➡ *CPT Assistant* Dec 04:11, Jun 08:8; *CPT Changes: An Insider's View* 2004
➡ *Clinical Examples in Radiology* Spring 09:10, Winter 09:9

Removal of Central Venous Access Device

36589 Removal of tunneled central venous catheter, without subcutaneous port or pump
➡ *CPT Assistant* Dec 04:11, Jun 08:8; *CPT Changes: An Insider's View* 2004

⊙ **36590** Removal of tunneled central venous access device, with subcutaneous port or pump, central or peripheral insertion
➡ *CPT Assistant* Dec 04:11, Jun 08:8, Jul 10:10; *CPT Changes: An Insider's View* 2004
➡ *Clinical Examples in Radiology* Spring 08:7

(Do not report 36589 or 36590 for removal of non-tunneled central venous catheters)

Other Central Venous Access Procedures

36591 Collection of blood specimen from a completely implantable venous access device
➡ *CPT Assistant* Apr 08:9, Jul 11:16; *CPT Changes: An Insider's View* 2008

(Do not report 36591 in conjunction with other services except a laboratory service)

(For collection of venous blood specimen by venipuncture, use 36415)

(For collection of capillary blood specimen, use 36416)

36592 Collection of blood specimen using established central or peripheral catheter, venous, not otherwise specified
➡ *CPT Assistant* Apr 08:9, Jul 11:16; *CPT Changes: An Insider's View* 2008

(For blood collection from an established arterial catheter, use 37799)

(Do not report 36592 in conjunction with other services except a laboratory service)

36593 Declotting by thrombolytic agent of implanted vascular access device or catheter
➡ *CPT Assistant* Apr 08:9, Dec 09:11, Aug 11:9; *CPT Changes: An Insider's View* 2008

36595 Mechanical removal of pericatheter obstructive material (eg, fibrin sheath) from central venous device via separate venous access
➡ *CPT Assistant* Dec 04:9, 12; *CPT Changes: An Insider's View* 2004

(Do not report 36595 in conjunction with 36593)

(For venous catheterization, see 36010-36012)

(For radiological supervision and interpretation, use 75901)

36596 Mechanical removal of intraluminal (intracatheter) obstructive material from central venous device through device lumen
➡ *CPT Assistant* Dec 04:9, 12; *CPT Changes: An Insider's View* 2004

(Do not report 36596 in conjunction with 36593)

(For venous catheterization, see 36010-36012)

(For radiological supervision and interpretation, use 75902)

36597 Repositioning of previously placed central venous catheter under fluoroscopic guidance
➡ *CPT Assistant* Dec 04:12; *CPT Changes: An Insider's View* 2004

(For fluoroscopic guidance, use 76000)

36598 Contrast injection(s) for radiologic evaluation of existing central venous access device, including fluoroscopy, image documentation and report

➜ *CPT Changes: An Insider's View* 2006

➜ *Clinical Examples in Radiology* Winter 06:15, Spring 08:7

(Do not report 36598 in conjunction with 76000)

(Do not report 36598 in conjunction with 36595, 36596)

(For complete diagnostic studies, see 75820, 75825, 75827)

Arterial

36600 Arterial puncture, withdrawal of blood for diagnosis

➜ *CPT Assistant* Fall 95:7, Aug 00:2, Oct 03:2, Jul 05:11, Jul 06:4, Feb 07:10, Jul 07:1

⊘ **36620** Arterial catheterization or cannulation for sampling, monitoring or transfusion (separate procedure); percutaneous

➜ *CPT Assistant* Fall 95:7, Apr 98:3, Nov 99:32-33, Aug 00:2, Oct 03:2, Jul 06:4, Jul 07:1

36625 cutdown

➜ *CPT Assistant* Fall 95:7

36640 Arterial catheterization for prolonged infusion therapy (chemotherapy), cutdown

➜ *CPT Assistant* Fall 95:7

(See also 96420-96425)

(For arterial catheterization for occlusion therapy, see 75894)

36660 Catheterization, umbilical artery, newborn, for diagnosis or therapy

➜ *CPT Assistant* Fall 95:8, Oct 03:2, Jul 06:4, Jul 07:1; *CPT Changes: An Insider's View* 2008

(Do not report modifier 63 in conjunction with 36660)

Intraosseous

36680 Placement of needle for intraosseous infusion

Hemodialysis Access, Intervascular Cannulation for Extracorporeal Circulation, or Shunt Insertion

36800 Insertion of cannula for hemodialysis, other purpose (separate procedure); vein to vein

➜ *CPT Assistant* Fall 93:3

36810 arteriovenous, external (Scribner type)

➜ *CPT Assistant* Fall 93:3, May 97:10

36815 arteriovenous, external revision, or closure

➜ *CPT Assistant* Fall 93:3

36818 Arteriovenous anastomosis, open; by upper arm cephalic vein transposition

➜ *CPT Assistant* Jul 05:9; *CPT Changes: An Insider's View* 2005

(Do not report 36818 in conjunction with 36819, 36820, 36821, 36830 during a unilateral upper extremity procedure. For bilateral upper extremity open arteriovenous anastomoses performed at the same operative session, use modifier 50 or 59 as appropriate)

36819 by upper arm basilic vein transposition

➜ *CPT Assistant* Nov 99:20, Jul 05:9; *CPT Changes: An Insider's View* 2000, 2002

(Do not report 36819 in conjunction with 36818, 36820, 36821, 36830 during a unilateral upper extremity procedure. For bilateral upper extremity open arteriovenous anastomoses performed at the same operative session, use modifier 50 or 59 as appropriate)

36820 by forearm vein transposition

➜ *CPT Assistant* Fall 93:4, Jul 05:9; *CPT Changes: An Insider's View* 2002

36821 direct, any site (eg, Cimino type) (separate procedure)

➜ *CPT Assistant* Fall 93:3, Feb 97:2, Nov 99:20, Jul 05:9; *CPT Changes: An Insider's View* 2000

Arteriovenous Anastomosis, Direct
36821

A section of artery and a neighboring vein are joined, allowing blood to flow down the artery and into the vein for the purpose of increasing blood flow, usually in hemodialysis.

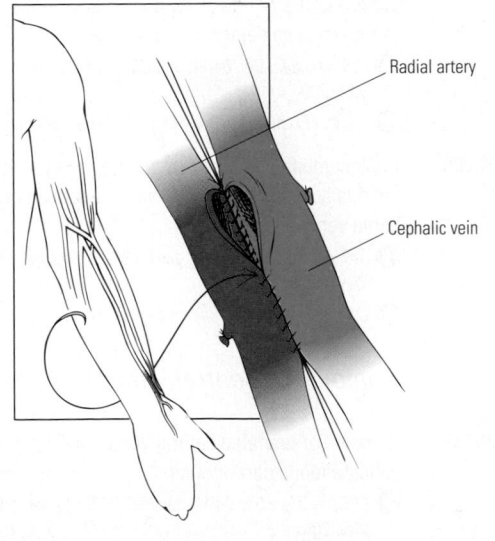

Radial artery

Cephalic vein

36822 Insertion of cannula(s) for prolonged extracorporeal circulation for cardiopulmonary insufficiency (ECMO) (separate procedure)

➜ *CPT Assistant* Feb 97:11

Cardiovascular

Insertion of Cannulas for Prolonged Extracorporeal Circulation Membrane Oxygenation (ECMO)
36822

The patient's venous blood is shunted and oxygenated outside of the body, bypassing the lungs. The treated blood is returned to body tissues through the femoral artery.

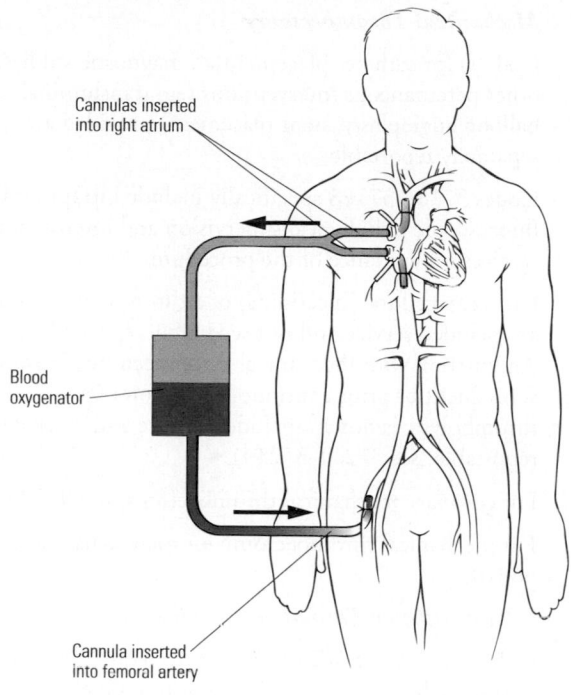

Cannulas inserted into right atrium

Blood oxygenator

Cannula inserted into femoral artery

(For maintenance of prolonged extracorporeal circulation, see 33960, 33961)

36823 Insertion of arterial and venous cannula(s) for isolated extracorporeal circulation including regional chemotherapy perfusion to an extremity, with or without hyperthermia, with removal of cannula(s) and repair of arteriotomy and venotomy sites

➔ *CPT Assistant* Nov 98:14-15; *CPT Changes: An Insider's View* 2002

(36823 includes chemotherapy perfusion supported by a membrane oxygenator/perfusion pump. Do not report 96409-96425 in conjunction with 36823)

36825 Creation of arteriovenous fistula by other than direct arteriovenous anastomosis (separate procedure); autogenous graft

➔ *CPT Assistant* Fall 93:3, Feb 97:2, Jul 05:9

(For direct arteriovenous anastomosis, use 36821)

36830 nonautogenous graft (eg, biological collagen, thermoplastic graft)

➔ *CPT Assistant* Fall 93:3, Feb 97:2, Jul 05:9; *CPT Changes: An Insider's View* 2003

(For direct arteriovenous anastomosis, use 36821)

Arteriovenous Fistula
36825-36830

A donor's vein (36825) or a synthetic vein (36830) is used to connect an artery and vein.

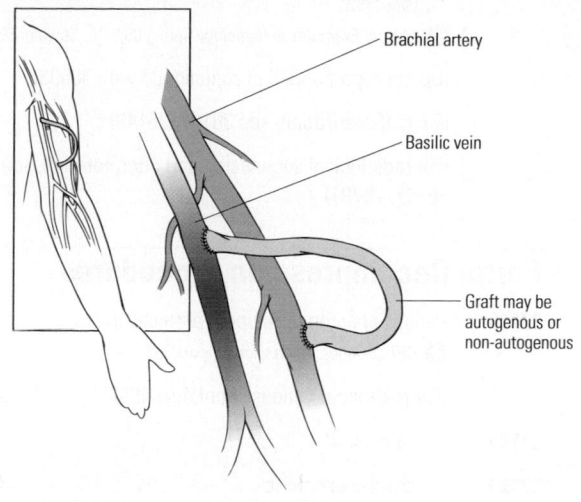

Brachial artery

Basilic vein

Graft may be autogenous or non-autogenous

36831 Thrombectomy, open, arteriovenous fistula without revision, autogenous or nonautogenous dialysis graft (separate procedure)

➔ *CPT Assistant* Nov 98:14-15, Feb 99:6, Mar 99:6, Apr 99:11, *CPT Changes: An Insider's View* 2001

36832 Revision, open, arteriovenous fistula; without thrombectomy, autogenous or nonautogenous dialysis graft (separate procedure)

➔ *CPT Assistant* Fall 93:3, Feb 97:2, Nov 98:15, Feb 99:6, Mar 99:6, Apr 99:11, Nov 99:20-21; *CPT Changes: An Insider's View* 2000, 2001

36833 with thrombectomy, autogenous or nonautogenous dialysis graft (separate procedure)

➔ *CPT Assistant* Nov 98:15, Feb 99:6, Apr 99:11

(36834 has been deleted. To report an arteriovenous access fistula or graft revision, use 36832)

36835 Insertion of Thomas shunt (separate procedure)

36838 Distal revascularization and interval ligation (DRIL), upper extremity hemodialysis access (steal syndrome)

➔ *CPT Changes: An Insider's View* 2004

(Do not report 36838 in conjunction with 35512, 35522, 35523, 36832, 37607, 37618)

36860 External cannula declotting (separate procedure); without balloon catheter

➔ *CPT Assistant* Fall 93:3, Feb 97:2, Nov 98:15, Feb 99:6, May 01:3

36861 with balloon catheter

➔ *CPT Assistant* Fall 93:3, Feb 97:2, May 01:3

(If imaging guidance is performed, use 76000)

Cardiovascular

⊙ **36870** Thrombectomy, percutaneous, arteriovenous fistula, autogenous or nonautogenous graft (includes mechanical thrombus extraction and intra-graft thrombolysis)

➔ *CPT Assistant* May 01:3, Dec 11:16; *CPT Changes: An Insider's View* 2001

➔ *Clinical Examples in Radiology* Spring 05:8-10, Summer 06:7, 12

(Do not report 36870 in conjunction with 36593)

(For catheterization, see 36147, 36148)

(For radiological supervision and interpretation, see 36147, 75791)

Portal Decompression Procedures

37140 Venous anastomosis, open; portocaval

➔ *CPT Changes: An Insider's View* 2003

(For peritoneal-venous shunt, use 49425)

37145 renoportal

37160 caval-mesenteric

37180 splenorenal, proximal

37181 splenorenal, distal (selective decompression of esophagogastric varices, any technique)

(For percutaneous procedure, use 37182)

37182 Insertion of transvenous intrahepatic portosystemic shunt(s) (TIPS) (includes venous access, hepatic and portal vein catheterization, portography with hemodynamic evaluation, intrahepatic tract formation/dilatation, stent placement and all associated imaging guidance and documentation)

➔ *CPT Assistant* Dec 03:2; *CPT Changes: An Insider's View* 2003

➔ *Clinical Examples in Radiology* Summer 10:2

(Do not report 75885 or 75887 in conjunction with 37182)

(For open procedure, use 37140)

⊙ **37183** Revision of transvenous intrahepatic portosystemic shunt(s) (TIPS) (includes venous access, hepatic and portal vein catheterization, portography with hemodynamic evaluation, intrahepatic tract recanulization/dilatation, stent placement and all associated imaging guidance and documentation)

➔ *CPT Assistant* Dec 03:2; *CPT Changes: An Insider's View* 2003, 2010

➔ *Clinical Examples in Radiology* Fall 09:9, Summer 10:3

(Do not report 75885 or 75887 in conjunction with 37183)

(For repair of arteriovenous aneurysm, use 36832)

Transcatheter Procedures

Codes for catheter placement and the radiologic supervision and interpretation should also be reported, in addition to the code(s) for the therapeutic aspect of the procedure.

Mechanical Thrombectomy

Code(s) for catheter placement(s), diagnostic studies, and other percutaneous interventions (eg, transluminal balloon angioplasty, stent placement) provided are separately reportable.

Codes 37184-37188 specifically include intraprocedural fluoroscopic radiological supervision and interpretation services for guidance of the procedure.

▶Intraprocedural injection(s) of a thrombolytic agent is an included service and not separately reportable in conjunction with mechanical thrombectomy. However, subsequent or prior continuous infusion of a thrombolytic is not an included service and is separately reportable (see 37211-37214).◀

For coronary mechanical thrombectomy, use 92973.

For mechanical thrombectomy for dialysis fistula, use 36870.

▶Transcatheter Thrombolytic Infusion◀

▶Codes 37211 or 37212 are used to report the initial day of transcatheter thrombolytic infusion(s) including follow-up arteriography/venography, and catheter position change or exchange, when performed. To report bilateral thrombolytic infusion through a separate access site(s), use modifier 50 in conjunction with 37211, 37212. Code 37213 is used to report continued transcatheter thrombolytic infusion(s) on subsequent day(s), other than initial day and final day of treatment. Code 37214 is used to report final day of transcatheter thrombolytic infusion(s). When initiation and completion of thrombolysis occur on the same day, report only 37211 or 37212.

Code(s) for catheter placement(s), diagnostic studies, and other percutaneous interventions (eg, transluminal balloon angioplasty, stent placement) provided may be separately reportable.

Codes 37211-37214 include fluoroscopic guidance and associated radiological supervision and interpretation.

Ongoing evaluation and management services on the day of the procedure related to thrombolysis are included in 37211-37214. If a significant, separately identifiable E/M service is performed by the same physician on the same day of the procedure, report the appropriate level of E/M service and append modifier 25.

Ultrasound guidance for vascular access is not included in 37211-37214. Code 76937 may be reported separately when performed if all the required elements are performed.◀

Cardiovascular

Arterial Mechanical Thrombectomy

Arterial mechanical thrombectomy may be performed as a "primary" transcatheter procedure with pretreatment planning, performance of the procedure, and postprocedure evaluation focused on providing this service. Typically, the diagnosis of thrombus has been made prior to the procedure, and a mechanical thrombectomy is planned preoperatively. Primary mechanical thrombectomy is reported per vascular family using 37184 for the initial vessel treated and 37185 for second or all subsequent vessel(s) within the same vascular family. To report mechanical thrombectomy of an additional vascular family treated through a separate access site, use modifier 51 in conjunction with 37184-37185.

Primary mechanical thrombectomy may precede or follow another percutaneous intervention. Most commonly primary mechanical thrombectomy will precede another percutaneous intervention with the decision regarding the need for other services not made until after mechanical thrombectomy has been performed. Occasionally, the performance of primary mechanical thrombectomy may follow another percutaneous intervention.

Do **NOT** report 37184-37185 for mechanical thrombectomy performed for the retrieval of short segments of thrombus or embolus evident during other percutaneous interventional procedures. See 37186 for these procedures.

Arterial mechanical thrombectomy is considered a "secondary" transcatheter procedure for removal or retrieval of short segments of thrombus or embolus when performed either before or after another percutaneous intervention (eg, percutaneous transluminal balloon angioplasty, stent placement). Secondary mechanical thrombectomy is reported using 37186. Do **NOT** report 37186 in conjunction with 37184-37185.

Venous Mechanical Thrombectomy

Use 37187 to report the initial application of venous mechanical thrombectomy. To report bilateral venous mechanical thrombectomy performed through a separate access site(s), use modifier 50 in conjunction with 37187. For repeat treatment on a subsequent day during a course of thrombolytic therapy, use 37188.

Arterial Mechanical Thrombectomy

⊙ **37184**   Primary percutaneous transluminal mechanical thrombectomy, noncoronary, arterial or arterial bypass graft, including fluoroscopic guidance and intraprocedural pharmacological thrombolytic injection(s); initial vessel
  ➔ *CPT Assistant* Nov 11:11; *CPT Changes: An Insider's View* 2006
  ➔ *Clinical Examples in Radiology* Winter 06:15, Summer 10:4

(Do not report 37184 in conjunction with 76000, 76001, 96374, 99143-99150)

⊙+ **37185**   second and all subsequent vessel(s) within the same vascular family (List separately in addition to code for primary mechanical thrombectomy procedure)
  ➔ *CPT Assistant* Nov 11:11; *CPT Changes: An Insider's View* 2006
  ➔ *Clinical Examples in Radiology* Winter 06:15

(Do not report 37185 in conjunction with 76000, 76001, 96375)

⊙+ **37186**   Secondary percutaneous transluminal thrombectomy (eg, nonprimary mechanical, snare basket, suction technique), noncoronary, arterial or arterial bypass graft, including fluoroscopic guidance and intraprocedural pharmacological thrombolytic injections, provided in conjunction with another percutaneous intervention other than primary mechanical thrombectomy (List separately in addition to code for primary procedure)
  ➔ *CPT Assistant* Jul 11:11, Nov 11:9; *CPT Changes: An Insider's View* 2006
  ➔ *Clinical Examples in Radiology* Winter 06:15

(Do not report 37186 in conjunction with 76000, 76001, 96375)

Venous Mechanical Thrombectomy

⊙ **37187**   Percutaneous transluminal mechanical thrombectomy, vein(s), including intraprocedural pharmacological thrombolytic injections and fluoroscopic guidance
  ➔ *CPT Assistant* Nov 11:11; *CPT Changes: An Insider's View* 2006
  ➔ *Clinical Examples in Radiology* Winter 06:15, Winter 12:3

(Do not report 37187 in conjunction with 76000, 76001, 96375)

⊙ **37188**   Percutaneous transluminal mechanical thrombectomy, vein(s), including intraprocedural pharmacological thrombolytic injections and fluoroscopic guidance, repeat treatment on subsequent day during course of thrombolytic therapy
  ➔ *CPT Assistant* Nov 11:11; *CPT Changes: An Insider's View* 2006
  ➔ *Clinical Examples in Radiology* Winter 06:15, Winter 12:3

(Do not report 37188 in conjunction with 76000, 76001, 96375)

Other Procedures

⊙ **37191**   Insertion of intravascular vena cava filter, endovascular approach including vascular access, vessel selection, and radiological supervision and interpretation, intraprocedural roadmapping, and imaging guidance (ultrasound and fluoroscopy), when performed
  ➔ *CPT Assistant* Apr 12:8; *CPT Changes: An Insider's View* 2012
  ➔ *Clinical Examples in Radiology* Winter 12:1

(For open surgical interruption of the inferior vena cava through a laparotomy or retroperitoneal exposure, use 37619)

Cardiovascular

Vena Cava Filter
37191

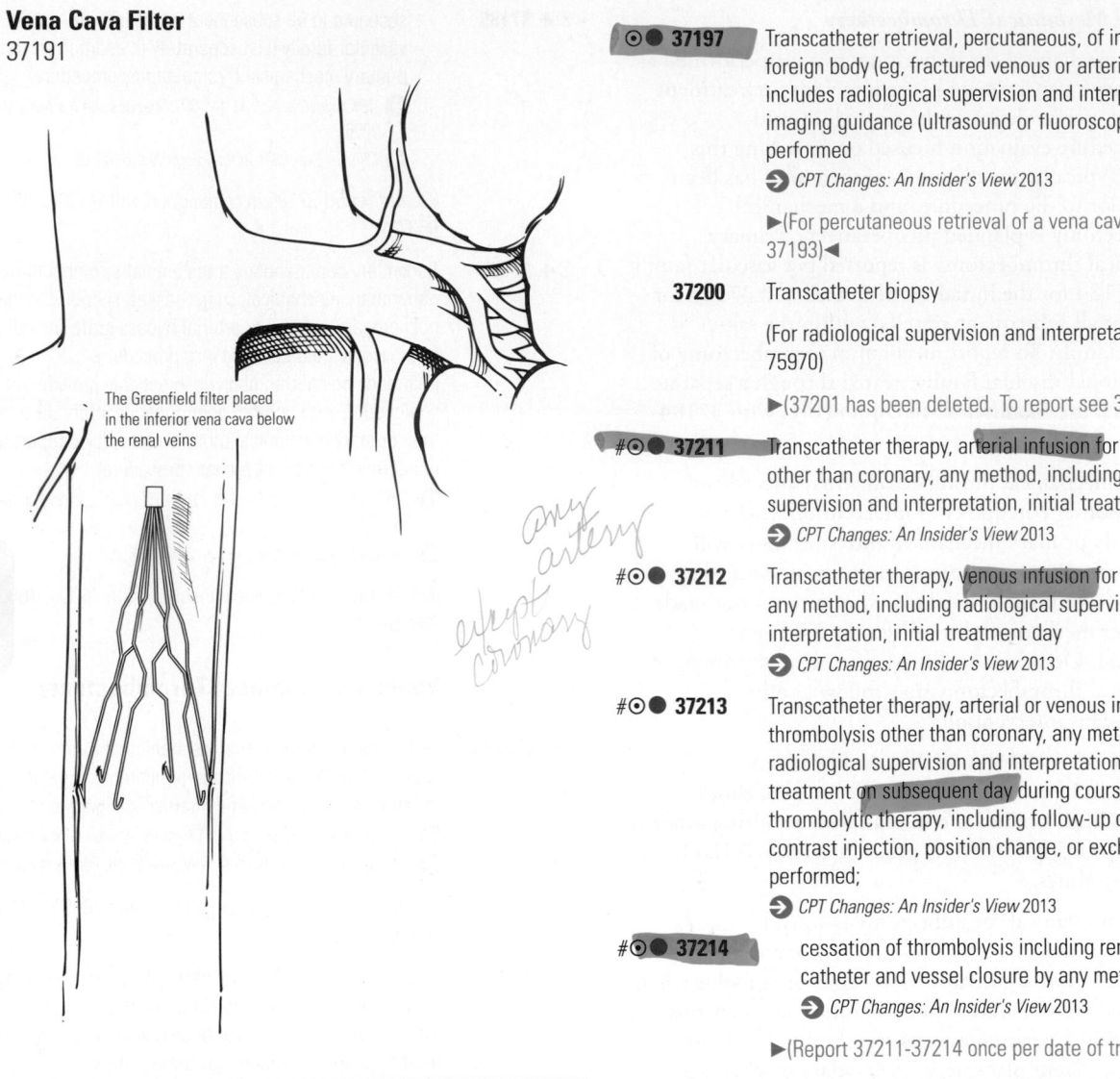

The Greenfield filter placed in the inferior vena cava below the renal veins

⊙ **37192** Repositioning of intravascular vena cava filter, endovascular approach including vascular access, vessel selection, and radiological supervision and interpretation, intraprocedural roadmapping, and imaging guidance (ultrasound and fluoroscopy), when performed
➔ *CPT Assistant* Apr 12:8; *CPT Changes: An Insider's View* 2012
➔ *Clinical Examples in Radiology* Winter 12:2

(Do not report 37192 in conjunction with 37191)

⊙ **37193** Retrieval (removal) of intravascular vena cava filter, endovascular approach including vascular access, vessel selection, and radiological supervision and interpretation, intraprocedural roadmapping, and imaging guidance (ultrasound and fluoroscopy), when performed
➔ *CPT Assistant* Apr 12:8; *CPT Changes: An Insider's View* 2012
➔ *Clinical Examples in Radiology* Winter 12:2

►(Do not report 37193 in conjunction with 37197)◄

37195 Thrombolysis, cerebral, by intravenous infusion
➔ *CPT Assistant* Nov 97:16

⊙● **37197** Transcatheter retrieval, percutaneous, of intravascular foreign body (eg, fractured venous or arterial catheter), includes radiological supervision and interpretation, and imaging guidance (ultrasound or fluoroscopy), when performed
➔ *CPT Changes: An Insider's View* 2013

►(For percutaneous retrieval of a vena cava filter, use 37193)◄

37200 Transcatheter biopsy

(For radiological supervision and interpretation, use 75970)

►(37201 has been deleted. To report see 37211-37214)◄

#⊙● **37211** Transcatheter therapy, arterial infusion for thrombolysis other than coronary, any method, including radiological supervision and interpretation, initial treatment day
➔ *CPT Changes: An Insider's View* 2013

#⊙● **37212** Transcatheter therapy, venous infusion for thrombolysis, any method, including radiological supervision and interpretation, initial treatment day
➔ *CPT Changes: An Insider's View* 2013

#⊙● **37213** Transcatheter therapy, arterial or venous infusion for thrombolysis other than coronary, any method, including radiological supervision and interpretation, continued treatment on subsequent day during course of thrombolytic therapy, including follow-up catheter contrast injection, position change, or exchange, when performed;
➔ *CPT Changes: An Insider's View* 2013

#⊙● **37214** cessation of thrombolysis including removal of catheter and vessel closure by any method
➔ *CPT Changes: An Insider's View* 2013

►(Report 37211-37214 once per date of treatment)◄

►(For declotting by thrombolytic agent of implanted vascular access device or catheter, use 36593)◄

37202 Transcatheter therapy, infusion other than for thrombolysis, any type (eg, spasmolytic, vasoconstrictive)
➔ *CPT Assistant* Oct 96:11, Jan 98:11, Apr 98:3, 9, Aug 11:9

(For thrombolysis of coronary vessels, see 92975, 92977)

(For radiological supervision and interpretation, use 75896)

►(37203 has been deleted. To report, use 37197)◄

(For removal of a vena cava filter, use 37193)

37204   Transcatheter occlusion or embolization (eg, for tumor destruction, to achieve hemostasis, to occlude a vascular malformation), percutaneous, any method, non-central nervous system, non-head or neck

→ *CPT Assistant* Sep 98:2, Oct 98:10, Feb 08:5, Apr 12:5

→ *Clinical Examples in Radiology* Winter 07:1, Summer 08:1, Winter 08:4, Fall 11:3

(See also 61624, 61626)

(For radiological supervision and interpretation, use 75894)

(For uterine fibroid embolization [uterine artery embolization performed to treat uterine fibroids], use 37210)

(For obstetrical and gynecologic embolization procedures other than uterine fibroid embolization [eg, embolization to treat obstetrical or postpartum hemorrhage], use 37204)

37205   Transcatheter placement of an intravascular stent(s) (except coronary, carotid, vertebral, iliac, and lower extremity arteries), percutaneous; initial vessel

→ *CPT Assistant* Fall 93:18, Feb 97:2, May 01:4, Feb 03:3, Dec 03:2, Jul 11:16, Apr 12:5; *CPT Changes: An Insider's View* 2005, 2011

→ *Clinical Examples in Radiology* Winter 06:19

(For radiological supervision and interpretation, use 75960)

(For transcatheter placement of intravascular cervical carotid artery stent(s), see 37215, 37216)

(For transcatheter placement of intracranial stents, use 61635)

►(For transcatherter coronary stent placement, see 92928-92944)◄

(For transcatheter stent placement of extracranial vertebral or intrathoracic carotid artery stent(s), see Category III codes 0075T, 0076T)

(For stent placement in iliac, femoral, popliteal, and tibial/peroneal arteries, see 37221, 37223, 37226, 37227, 37230, 37231, 37234, 37235)

+ 37206   each additional vessel (List separately in addition to code for primary procedure)

→ *CPT Assistant* Fall 93:18, Feb 97:2, Feb 03:3; *CPT Changes: An Insider's View* 2011

(Use 37206 in conjunction with 37205)

(For radiological supervision and interpretation, use 75960)

37207   Transcatheter placement of an intravascular stent(s) (except coronary, carotid, vertebral, iliac and lower extremity arteries), open; initial vessel

→ *CPT Assistant* Feb 97:2, Feb 03:3, Apr 11:3; *CPT Changes: An Insider's View* 2011

(For stent placement in iliac, femoral, popliteal, and tibial/peroneal arteries, see 37221, 37223, 37226, 37227, 37230, 37231, 37234, 37235)

+ 37208   each additional vessel (List separately in addition to code for primary procedure)

→ *CPT Assistant* Feb 97:2, Feb 03:3; *CPT Changes: An Insider's View* 2011

(Use 37208 in conjunction with 37207)

(For radiological supervision and interpretation, use 75960)

(For catheterizations, see 36215-36248)

►(For transcatheter placement of intracoronary stent[s], see 92928-92944)◄

►(37209 has been deleted. For exchange of a previously placed intravascular catheter during thrombolytic therapy, see 37211-37214)◄

⊙ **37210**   Uterine fibroid embolization (UFE, embolization of the uterine arteries to treat uterine fibroids, leiomyomata), percutaneous approach inclusive of vascular access, vessel selection, embolization, and all radiological supervision and interpretation, intraprocedural roadmapping, and imaging guidance necessary to complete the procedure

→ *CPT Assistant* Jan 07:7, Feb 08:5; *CPT Changes: An Insider's View* 2007

→ *Clinical Examples in Radiology* Winter 07:2, Winter 08:4

(37210 includes all catheterizations and intraprocedural imaging required for a UFE procedure to confirm the presence of previously known fibroids and to roadmap vascular anatomy to enable appropriate therapy)

(Do not report 37210 in conjunction with 36200, 36245-36248, 37204, 75894, 75898)

(For all other non-central nervous system (CNS) embolization procedures, use 37204)

37211   Code is out of numerical sequence. See 37191-37216

37212   Code is out of numerical sequence. See 37191-37216

37213   Code is out of numerical sequence. See 37191-37216

37214   Code is out of numerical sequence. See 37191-37216

⊙ **37215**   Transcatheter placement of intravascular stent(s), cervical carotid artery, percutaneous; with distal embolic protection

→ *CPT Assistant* May 05:7; *CPT Changes: An Insider's View* 2005

⊙ **37216**   without distal embolic protection

→ *CPT Assistant* May 05:7; *CPT Changes: An Insider's View* 2005

(37215 and 37216 include all ipsilateral selective carotid catheterization, all diagnostic imaging for ipsilateral, cervical and cerebral carotid arteriography, and all related radiological supervision and interpretation. When ipsilateral carotid arteriogram (including imaging and selective catheterization) confirms the need for carotid stenting, 37215 and 37216 are inclusive of these services. If carotid stenting is not indicated, then the appropriate codes for carotid catheterization and imaging should be reported in lieu of 37215 and 37216)

Cardiovascular

▶(Do not report 37215, 37216 in conjunction with 36222-36224 for the treated carotid artery)◀

(For transcatheter placement of extracranial vertebral or intrathoracic carotid artery stent(s), see Category III codes 0075T, 0076T)

(For percutaneous transcatheter placement of intravascular stents other than coronary, carotid, or vertebral, see 37205, 37206)

Endovascular Revascularization (Open or Percutaneous, Transcatheter)

Codes 37220-37235 are to be used to describe lower extremity endovascular revascularization services performed for occlusive disease. These lower extremity codes are built on progressive hierarchies with more intensive services inclusive of lesser intensive services. The code inclusive of all of the services provided for that vessel should be reported (ie, use the code inclusive of the most intensive services provided). Only one code from this family (37220-37235) should be reported for each lower extremity vessel treated.

These lower extremity endovascular revascularization codes all include the work of accessing and selectively catheterizing the vessel, traversing the lesion, radiological supervision and interpretation directly related to the intervention(s) performed, embolic protection if used, closure of the arteriotomy by pressure and application of an arterial closure device or standard closure of the puncture by suture, and imaging performed to document completion of the intervention in addition to the intervention(s) performed. Extensive repair or replacement of an artery may be additionally reported (eg, 35226 or 35286). These codes describe endovascular procedures performed percutaneously and/or through an open surgical exposure. These codes include balloon angioplasty (eg, low-profile, cutting balloon, cryoplasty), atherectomy (eg, directional, rotational, laser), and stenting (eg, balloon-expandable, self-expanding, bare metal, covered, drug-eluting). Each code in this family (37220-37235) includes balloon angioplasty, when performed.

These codes describe revascularization therapies (ie, transluminal angioplasty, atherectomy, and stent placement) provided in three arterial vascular territories: iliac, femoral/popliteal, and tibial/peroneal.

▶When treating multiple vessels within a territory, report each additional vessel using an add-on code, as applicable. Select the base code that represents the most complex service using the following hierarchy of complexity (in descending order of complexity): atherectomy and stent>atherectomy>stent>angioplasty. When treating multiple lesions within the same vessel, report one service that reflects the combined procedures, whether done on one lesion or different lesions, using the same hierarchy.◀

1. *Iliac Vascular Territory*—The iliac territory is divided into 3 vessels: common iliac, internal iliac, and external iliac.

2. *Femoral/Popliteal Vascular Territory*—The entire femoral/popliteal territory in 1 lower extremity is considered a single vessel for CPT reporting specifically for the endovascular lower extremity revascularization codes 37224-37227.

3. *Tibial/Peroneal Territory*—The tibial/peroneal territory is divided into 3 vessels: anterior tibial, posterior tibial, and peroneal arteries.

There are specific coding guidelines for each of the 3 vascular territories.

1. *Iliac Vascular Territory*—A single primary code is used for the initial iliac artery treated in each leg (37220 or 37221). If other iliac vessels are also treated in that leg, these interventions are reported with the appropriate add-on code(s) (37222, 37223). Up to 2 add-on codes can be used in a unilateral iliac vascular territory since there are 3 vessels which could be treated. Add-on codes are used for different vessels, not distinct lesions within the same vessel.

2. *Femoral/Popliteal Territory*—A single interventional code is used no matter what combination of angioplasty/stent/atherectomy is applied to all segments, including the common, deep and superficial femoral arteries as well as the popliteal artery (37224, 37225, 37226, or 37227). There are no add-on codes for additional vessels treated within the femoral/popliteal territory. Because only 1 service is reported when 2 lesions are treated in this territory, report the most complex service (eg, use 37227 if a stent is placed for 1 lesion and an atherectomy is performed on a second lesion)

3. *Tibial/Peroneal Territory*—A single primary code is used for the initial tibial/peroneal artery treated in each leg (37228, 37229, 37230, or 37231). If other tibial/peroneal vessels are also treated in the same leg, these interventions are reported with the appropriate add-on code(s) (37232-37235). Up to 2 add-on codes could be used to describe services provided in a single leg since there are 3 tibial/peroneal vessels which could be treated. Add-on codes are used for different vessels, not distinct lesions within the same vessel. The common tibio-peroneal trunk is considered part of the tibial/peroneal territory, but is not considered a separate, fourth segment of vessel in the tibio-peroneal family for CPT reporting of endovascular lower extremity interventions. For instance, if lesions in the common tibio-peroneal trunk are treated in conjunction with lesions in the posterior tibial artery, a single code would be reported for treatment of this segment.

⊙=Moderate sedation   ✚=Add-on code   ⟋=FDA approval pending   #=Resequenced code   ○=Recycled/reinstated code   ➲➲=See p xiii for details

When treating multiple territories in the same leg, one primary lower extremity revascularization code is used for each territory treated. When second or third vessel(s) are treated in the iliac and/or tibial/peroneal territories, add-on code(s) are used to report the additional service(s). When more than one stent is placed in the same vessel, the code should be reported only once.

When multiple vessels in multiple territories in a single leg are treated at the same setting, the primary code for the treatment in the initial vessel in each vascular territory is reported. Add-on code(s) are reported when second and third iliac or tibial/peroneal arteries are treated in addition to the initial vessel in that vascular territory.

If a lesion extends across the margins of one vessel vascular territory into another, but can be opened with a single therapy, this intervention should be reported with a single code despite treating more than one vessel and/or vascular territory. For instance, if a stenosis extends from the common iliac artery into the proximal external iliac artery, and a single stent is placed to open the entire lesion, this therapy should be coded as a single stent placement in the iliac artery (37221). In this example, a code for an additional vessel treatment would not be used (do not report both 37221 and 37223).

For bifurcation lesions distal to the common iliac origins which require therapy of 2 distinct branches of the iliac or tibial/peroneal vascular territories, a primary code and an add-on code would be used to describe the intervention. In the femoral/popliteal territory, all branches are included in the primary code, so treatment of a bifurcation lesion would be reported as a single code.

When the same territor(ies) of both legs are treated in the same session, modifiers may be required to describe the interventions. Use modifier 59 to denote that different legs are being treated, even if the mode of therapy is different.

Mechanical thrombectomy and/or thrombolysis in the lower extremity vessels are sometimes necessary to aid in restoring flow to areas of occlusive disease, and are reported separately.

⊙ **37220**   Revascularization, endovascular, open or percutaneous, iliac artery, unilateral, initial vessel; with transluminal angioplasty

➲ *CPT Assistant* Jul 11:3, Oct 11:9; *CPT Changes: An Insider's View* 2011

➲ *Clinical Examples in Radiology* Winter 11:3

⊙ **37221**   with transluminal stent placement(s), includes angioplasty within the same vessel, when performed

➲ *CPT Assistant* Jul 11:3, Oct 11:9; *CPT Changes: An Insider's View* 2011

➲ *Clinical Examples in Radiology* Winter 11:2

Transluminal Balloon Angioplasty
37220 and 37222

A balloon catheter is passed into the iliac artery and inflated to stretch the blood vessel to a larger diameter.

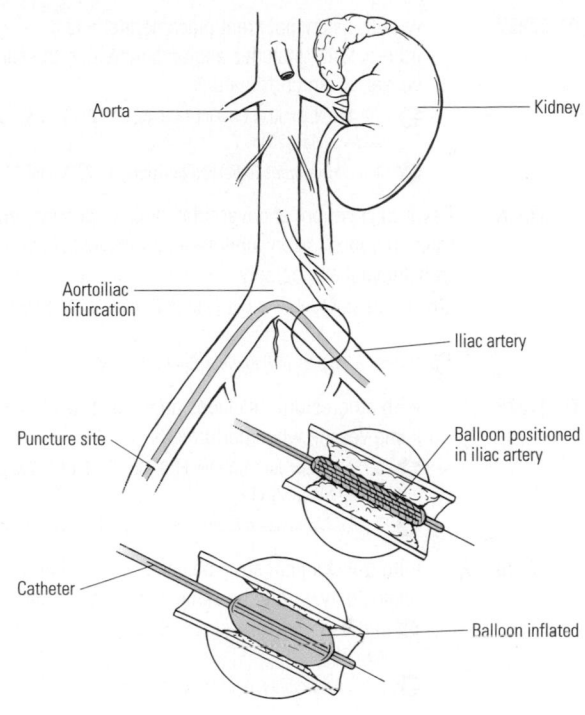

⊙+ **37222**   Revascularization, endovascular, open or percutaneous, iliac artery, each additional ipsilateral iliac vessel; with transluminal angioplasty (List separately in addition to code for primary procedure)

➲ *CPT Assistant* Jul 11:3, Oct 11:9; *CPT Changes: An Insider's View* 2011

➲ *Clinical Examples in Radiology* Winter 11:2

(Use 37222 in conjunction with 37220, 37221)

⊙+ **37223**   with transluminal stent placement(s), includes angioplasty within the same vessel, when performed (List separately in addition to code for primary procedure)

➲ *CPT Assistant* Jul 11:3, Oct 11:9, Apr 12:8; *CPT Changes: An Insider's View* 2011

➲ *Clinical Examples in Radiology* Winter 11:3

(Use 37223 in conjunction with 37221)

⊙ **37224**   Revascularization, endovascular, open or percutaneous, femoral, popliteal artery(s), unilateral; with transluminal angioplasty

➲ *CPT Assistant* Jul 11:3, Oct 11:9, Dec 11:15; *CPT Changes: An Insider's View* 2011

➲ *Clinical Examples in Radiology* Summer 11:10, Winter 11:3

⊙ **37225**   with atherectomy, includes angioplasty within the same vessel, when performed

➲ *CPT Assistant* Jul 11:3, Oct 11:9, Nov 11:9; *CPT Changes: An Insider's View* 2011

➲ *Clinical Examples in Radiology* Spring 11:3, Winter 11:3

Cardiovascular

⊙ **37226**   with transluminal stent placement(s), includes angioplasty within the same vessel, when performed

➜ *CPT Assistant* Jul 11:3, Oct 11:9, Dec 11:15; *CPT Changes: An Insider's View* 2011

➜ *Clinical Examples in Radiology* Winter 11:2

⊙ **37227**   with transluminal stent placement(s) and atherectomy, includes angioplasty within the same vessel, when performed

➜ *CPT Assistant* Jul 11:3, Oct 11:9, Nov 11:9; *CPT Changes: An Insider's View* 2011

➜ *Clinical Examples in Radiology* Spring 11:2, Winter 11:3

⊙ **37228**   Revascularization, endovascular, open or percutaneous, tibial, peroneal artery, unilateral, initial vessel; with transluminal angioplasty

➜ *CPT Assistant* Jul 11:3, Oct 11:9; *CPT Changes: An Insider's View* 2011

➜ *Clinical Examples in Radiology* Spring 11:2, Winter 11:2

⊙ **37229**   with atherectomy, includes angioplasty within the same vessel, when performed

➜ *CPT Assistant* Jul 11:3, Oct 11:9, Nov 11:9; *CPT Changes: An Insider's View* 2011

➜ *Clinical Examples in Radiology* Spring 11:3, Winter 11:3

⊙ **37230**   with transluminal stent placement(s), includes angioplasty within the same vessel, when performed

➜ *CPT Assistant* Jul 11:3, Oct 11:9; *CPT Changes: An Insider's View* 2011

➜ *Clinical Examples in Radiology* Winter 11:3

⊙ **37231**   with transluminal stent placement(s) and atherectomy, includes angioplasty within the same vessel, when performed

➜ *CPT Assistant* Jul 11:3, Oct 11:9, Nov 11:9; *CPT Changes: An Insider's View* 2011

➜ *Clinical Examples in Radiology* Spring 11:3, Winter 11:3

⊙✚ **37232**   Revascularization, endovascular, open or percutaneous, tibial/peroneal artery, unilateral, each additional vessel; with transluminal angioplasty (List separately in addition to code for primary procedure)

➜ *CPT Assistant* Jul 11:3, Oct 11:9, Apr 12:8; *CPT Changes: An Insider's View* 2011

➜ *Clinical Examples in Radiology* Winter 11:3

(Use 37232 in conjunction with 37228-37231)

⊙✚ **37233**   with atherectomy, includes angioplasty within the same vessel, when performed (List separately in addition to code for primary procedure)

➜ *CPT Assistant* Jul 11:3, Oct 11:9, Nov 11:9, Apr 12:8; *CPT Changes: An Insider's View* 2011

➜ *Clinical Examples in Radiology* Spring 11:3, Winter 11:3

(Use 37233 in conjunction with 37229, 37231)

⊙✚ **37234**   with transluminal stent placement(s), includes angioplasty within the same vessel, when performed (List separately in addition to code for primary procedure)

➜ *CPT Assistant* Jul 11:3, Oct 11:9, Apr 12:9; *CPT Changes: An Insider's View* 2011

➜ *Clinical Examples in Radiology* Spring 11:11, Winter 11:3

(Use 37234 in conjunction with 37229, 37230, 37231)

⊙✚ **37235**   with transluminal stent placement(s) and atherectomy, includes angioplasty within the same vessel, when performed (List separately in addition to code for primary procedure)

➜ *CPT Assistant* Jul 11:3, Oct 11:9, Nov 11:9; *CPT Changes: An Insider's View* 2011

➜ *Clinical Examples in Radiology* Spring 11:3, Winter 11:3

(Use 37235 in conjunction with 37231)

Iliac and Lower Extremity Arterial Anatomy Territory
37220-37235

Intravascular Ultrasound Services

Intravascular ultrasound services include all transducer manipulations and repositioning within the specific vessel being examined, both before and after therapeutic intervention (eg, stent placement).

Vascular access for intravascular ultrasound performed during a therapeutic intervention is not reported separately.

⊙=Moderate sedation   ✚=Add-on code   ✎=FDA approval pending   #=Resequenced code   ○=Recycled/reinstated code   ➜➜=See p xiii for details

+ 37250   Intravascular ultrasound (non-coronary vessel) during diagnostic evaluation and/or therapeutic intervention; initial vessel (List separately in addition to code for primary procedure)

➔ *CPT Assistant* Nov 96:7, Nov 97:17, Nov 99:20; *CPT Changes: An Insider's View* 2000

➔ *Clinical Examples in Radiology* Winter 12:3

+ 37251   each additional vessel (List separately in addition to code for primary procedure)

➔ *CPT Assistant* Nov 96:7, Nov 97:17, Nov 99:20; *CPT Changes: An Insider's View* 2000

➔ *Clinical Examples in Radiology* Winter 12:3

(Use 37251 in conjunction with 37250)

(For catheterizations, see 36215-36248)

(For transcatheter therapies, see 37200-37208, 61624, 61626)

(For radiological supervision and interpretation see 75945, 75946)

Endoscopy

Surgical vascular endoscopy always includes diagnostic endoscopy.

37500   Vascular endoscopy, surgical, with ligation of perforator veins, subfascial (SEPS)

➔ *CPT Assistant* Jul 10:6; *CPT Changes: An Insider's View* 2003

(For open procedure, use 37760)

37501   Unlisted vascular endoscopy procedure

➔ *CPT Changes: An Insider's View* 2003

Ligation

(For phleborraphy and arteriorraphy, see 35201-35286)

37565   Ligation, internal jugular vein

37600   Ligation; external carotid artery

37605   internal or common carotid artery

37606   internal or common carotid artery, with gradual occlusion, as with Selverstone or Crutchfield clamp

(For transcatheter permanent arterial occlusion or embolization, see 61624-61626)

(For endovascular temporary arterial balloon occlusion, use 61623)

(For ligation treatment of intracranial aneurysm, use 61703)

37607   Ligation or banding of angioaccess arteriovenous fistula

37609   Ligation or biopsy, temporal artery

37615   Ligation, major artery (eg, post-traumatic, rupture); neck

37616   chest

37617   abdomen

37618   extremity

37619   Ligation of inferior vena cava

➔ *CPT Assistant* Apr 12:8; *CPT Changes: An Insider's View* 2012

(For endovascular delivery of an inferior vena cava filter, use 37191)

(37620 has been deleted. To report, see 37191 for endovascular placement of intravascular filter or 37619 for open surgical ligation of the inferior vena cava)

37650   Ligation of femoral vein

(For bilateral procedure, report 37650 with modifier 50)

37660   Ligation of common iliac vein

37700   Ligation and division of long saphenous vein at saphenofemoral junction, or distal interruptions

➔ *CPT Assistant* Aug 96:10

(Do not report 37700 in conjunction with 37718, 37722)

(For bilateral procedure, report 37700 with modifier 50)

Ligation and Division of Long Saphenous Vein
37700

The physician ligates sections of the saphenous vein along the leg.

Femoral vein

Great saphenous vein

37718   Ligation, division, and stripping, short saphenous vein

➔ *CPT Changes: An Insider's View* 2006

(For bilateral procedure, use modifier 50)

(Do not report 37718 in conjunction with 37735, 37780)

37722   Ligation, division, and stripping, long (greater) saphenous veins from saphenofemoral junction to knee or below

➔ *CPT Changes: An Insider's View* 2006

(For ligation and stripping of the short saphenous vein, use 37718)

(For bilateral procedure, report 37722 with modifier 50)

(Do not report 37722 in conjunction with 37700, 37735)

(For ligation, division, and stripping of the greater saphenous vein, use 37722. For ligation, division, and stripping of the short saphenous vein, use 37718)

37735   Ligation and division and complete stripping of long or short saphenous veins with radical excision of ulcer and skin graft and/or interruption of communicating veins of lower leg, with excision of deep fascia

(Do not report 37735 in conjunction with 37700, 37718, 37722, 37780)

(For bilateral procedure, report 37735 with modifier 50)

37760   Ligation of perforator veins, subfascial, radical (Linton type), including skin graft, when performed, 1 leg
➔ *CPT Assistant* Jul 10:6; *CPT Changes: An Insider's View* 2003, 2010

(For endoscopic procedure, use 37500)

37761   Ligation of perforator vein(s), subfascial, open, including ultrasound guidance, when performed, 1 leg
➔ *CPT Assistant* Jul 10:6; *CPT Changes: An Insider's View* 2010

(For bilateral procedure, report 37761 with modifier 50)

(Do not report 37760, 37761 in conjunction with 76937, 76942, 76998, 93971)

(For endoscopic ligation of subfascial perforator veins, use 37500)

37765   Stab phlebectomy of varicose veins, 1 extremity; 10-20 stab incisions
➔ *CPT Assistant* Aug 04:6, Nov 10:9; *CPT Changes: An Insider's View* 2004

(For less than 10 incisions, use 37799)

(For more than 20 incisions, use 37766)

37766   more than 20 incisions
➔ *CPT Assistant* Aug 04:6; *CPT Changes: An Insider's View* 2004

37780   Ligation and division of short saphenous vein at saphenopopliteal junction (separate procedure)
➔ *CPT Assistant* Aug 96:10

(For bilateral procedure, report 37780 with modifier 50)

37785   Ligation, division, and/or excision of varicose vein cluster(s), 1 leg
➔ *CPT Assistant* Aug 04:5, Nov 10:9; *CPT Changes: An Insider's View* 2004

(For bilateral procedure, report 37785 with modifier 50)

Other Procedures

37788   Penile revascularization, artery, with or without vein graft

37790   Penile venous occlusive procedure

37799   Unlisted procedure, vascular surgery
➔ *CPT Assistant* Spring 93:12, Fall 93:3, Feb 97:10, Sep 97:10, May 01:11, Oct 04:16, Nov 10:9, Aug 11:9

Hemic and Lymphatic Systems

Spleen

Excision

38100   Splenectomy; total (separate procedure)
➔ *CPT Assistant* Summer 93:10, July 93:9

38101   partial (separate procedure)
➔ *CPT Assistant* Summer 93:10

+ 38102   total, en bloc for extensive disease, in conjunction with other procedure (List in addition to code for primary procedure)
➔ *CPT Assistant* Summer 93:10

Repair

38115   Repair of ruptured spleen (splenorrhaphy) with or without partial splenectomy
➔ *CPT Assistant* Summer 93:10

Laparoscopy

Surgical laparoscopy always includes diagnostic laparoscopy. To report a diagnostic laparoscopy (peritoneoscopy) (separate procedure), use 49320.

38120   Laparoscopy, surgical, splenectomy
➔ *CPT Assistant* Nov 99:20-21, Mar 00:8; *CPT Changes: An Insider's View* 2000

38129   Unlisted laparoscopy procedure, spleen
➔ *CPT Assistant* Nov 99:20-21, Mar 00:8; *CPT Changes: An Insider's View* 2000

Introduction

38200   Injection procedure for splenoportography

(For radiological supervision and interpretation, use 75810)

General

Bone Marrow or Stem Cell Services/ Procedures

Codes 38207-38215 describe various steps used to preserve, prepare and purify bone marrow/stem cells prior to transplantation or reinfusion. Each code may be reported only once per day regardless of the quantity of bone marrow/stem cells manipulated.

38204   Management of recipient hematopoietic progenitor cell donor search and cell acquisition
➔ *CPT Changes: An Insider's View* 2003

38205   Blood-derived hematopoietic progenitor cell harvesting for transplantation, per collection; allogeneic
➔ *CPT Changes: An Insider's View* 2003, 2012

Cardiovascular

38206   autologous

→ *CPT Changes: An Insider's View* 2003

38207   Transplant preparation of hematopoietic progenitor cells; cryopreservation and storage

→ *CPT Assistant* Jul 03:9, Jun 09:3; *CPT Changes: An Insider's View* 2003

(For diagnostic cryopreservation and storage, use 88240)

38208   thawing of previously frozen harvest, without washing, per donor

→ *CPT Assistant* Jul 03:9, Jun 09:3; *CPT Changes: An Insider's View* 2003, 2004, 2012

(For diagnostic thawing and expansion of frozen cells, use 88241)

38209   thawing of previously frozen harvest, with washing, per donor

→ *CPT Changes: An Insider's View* 2003, 2004, 2012

38210   specific cell depletion within harvest, T-cell depletion

→ *CPT Changes: An Insider's View* 2003

38211   tumor cell depletion

→ *CPT Changes: An Insider's View* 2003

38212   red blood cell removal

→ *CPT Changes: An Insider's View* 2003

38213   platelet depletion

→ *CPT Changes: An Insider's View* 2003

38214   plasma (volume) depletion

→ *CPT Changes: An Insider's View* 2003

38215   cell concentration in plasma, mononuclear, or buffy coat layer

→ *CPT Changes: An Insider's View* 2003

(Do not report 38207-38215 in conjunction with 88182, 88184-88189)

38220   Bone marrow; aspiration only

→ *CPT Assistant* Jan 04:26, Jun 07:10, Apr 12:15, May 12:11; *CPT Changes: An Insider's View* 2002, 2003

▶(For needle aspiration of bone marrow for the purpose of bone grafting, use 38220)◀

▶(Do not report 38220-38230 for bone marrow aspiration for platelet rich stem cell injection. For bone marrow aspiration for platelet rich stem cell injection, use 0232T)◀

38221   biopsy, needle or trocar

→ *CPT Changes: An Insider's View* 2002, 2003

(For bone marrow biopsy interpretation, use 88305)

38230   Bone marrow harvesting for transplantation; allogeneic

→ *CPT Assistant* Apr 96:1, Jun 09:3, May 12:11; *CPT Changes: An Insider's View* 2012

38232   autologous

→ *CPT Changes: An Insider's View* 2012

(For autologous and allogeneic blood-derived peripheral stem cell harvesting for transplantation, see 38205-38206)

▶(For bone marrow aspiration, use 38220)◀

Bone Marrow Harvesting for Transplantation
38230

A biopsy needle is inserted into the marrow cavity of the iliac crest and bone marrow is removed from the donor.

Placement of biopsy needle — Posterior iliac spine

Biopsy needle — Bone marrow

▶Transplantation and Post-Transplantation Cellular Infusions◀

▶Hematopoietic cell transplantation (HCT) refers to the infusion of hematopoietic progenitor cells (HPC) obtained from bone marrow, peripheral blood apheresis, and/or umbilical cord blood. These procedure codes (38240-38243) include physician monitoring of multiple physiologic parameters, physician verification of cell processing, evaluation of the patient during as well as immediately before and after the HPC/lymphocyte infusion, physician presence during the HPC/lymphocyte infusion with associated direct physician supervision of clinical staff, and management of uncomplicated adverse events (eg, nausea, urticaria) during the infusion, which is not separately reportable.

HCT may be autologous (when the HPC donor and recipient are the same person) or allogeneic (when the HPC donor and recipient are not the same person). Code 38241 is used to report any autologous transplant while 38240 is used to report an allogeneic transplant. In some cases allogeneic transplants involve more than one donor

Cardiovascular

and cells from each donor are infused sequentially whereby one unit of 38240 is reported for each donor infused. Code 38242 is used to report a donor lymphocyte infusion. Code 38243 is used to report a HPC boost from the original allogeneic HPC donor. A lymphocyte infusion or HPC boost can occur days, months or even years after the initial hematopoietic cell transplant. The lymphocyte infusion is used to treat relapse, infection, or post-transplant lymphoproliferative syndrome. HPC boost represents an infusion of hematopoietic progenitor cells from the original donor that is being used to treat a relapse or post-transplant cytopenia(s). Codes 38240, 38242, and 38243 should not be reported together on the same date of service.

If a separately identifiable evaluation and management service is performed on the same date of service, the appropriate E/M service code, including office or other outpatient services, established (99211-99215), hospital observation services (99217-99220, 99224-99226), hospital inpatient services (99221-99223, 99231-99239), and inpatient neonatal and pediatric critical care (99471, 99472, 99475, 99476) may be reported, using modifier 25, in addition to 38240, 38242, or 38243. Post-transplant infusion management of adverse reactions is reported separately using the appropriate E/M, prolonged service or critical care code(s). In accordance with place of service and facility reporting guidelines, the fluid used to administer the cells and other infusions for incidental hydration (eg, 96360, 96361) are not separately reportable. Similarly, infusion(s) of any medication(s) concurrently with the transplant infusion are not separately reportable. However, hydration or administration of medications (eg, antibiotics, narcotics) unrelated to the transplant are separately reportable using modifier 59.◄

▲ **38240**   Hematopoietic progenitor cell (HPC); allogeneic transplantation per donor
   ➡ *CPT Assistant* Apr 96:2, Nov 98:15, Nov 99:21, Jun 09:3; *CPT Changes: An Insider's View* 2000, 2012, 2013

▲ **38241**   autologous transplantation
   ➡ *CPT Assistant* Apr 96:2, Nov 98:15, Nov 99:21, Jun 09:3; *CPT Changes: An Insider's View* 2000, 2013

#● **38243**   HPC boost
   ➡ *CPT Changes: An Insider's View* 2013

▲ **38242**   Allogeneic lymphocyte infusions
   ➡ *CPT Changes: An Insider's View* 2003, 2013

(For bone marrow aspiration, use 38220)

►(For modification, treatment, and processing of hematopoietic progenitor cell specimens for transplantation, see 38210-38215)◄

►(For cryopreservation, freezing, and storage of hematopoietic progenitor cells for transplantation, use 38207)◄

►(For thawing and expansion of hematopoietic progenitor cells for transplantation, see 38208, 38209)◄

►(For compatibility studies, see 81379-81383, 86812-86822)◄

38243   Code is out of numerical sequence. See 38240-38242

Lymph Nodes and Lymphatic Channels

Incision

38300   Drainage of lymph node abscess or lymphadenitis; simple

38305   extensive

38308   Lymphangiotomy or other operations on lymphatic channels

38380   Suture and/or ligation of thoracic duct; cervical approach

38381   thoracic approach

38382   abdominal approach

Excision

(For injection for sentinel node identification, use 38792)

38500   Biopsy or excision of lymph node(s); open, superficial
   ➡ *CPT Assistant* Jun 97:5, Jul 99:7, Oct 05:23, Dec 07:8, Sep 08:5, Jan 09:7, Jun 12:15; *CPT Changes: An Insider's View* 2001

(Do not report 38500 with 38700-38780)

38505   by needle, superficial (eg, cervical, inguinal, axillary)
   ➡ *CPT Assistant* Jul 99:6, Jan 09:7

(If imaging guidance is performed, see 76942, 77012, 77021)

(For fine needle aspiration, use 10021 or 10022)

(For evaluation of fine needle aspirate, see 88172, 88173)

38510   open, deep cervical node(s)
   ➡ *CPT Assistant* May 98:10, Jul 99:6, Jun 12:15; *CPT Changes: An Insider's View* 2001

38520   open, deep cervical node(s) with excision scalene fat pad
   ➡ *CPT Assistant* May 98:10, Jul 99:6; *CPT Changes: An Insider's View* 2001

38525   open, deep axillary node(s)
   ➡ *CPT Assistant* May 98:10, Jul 99:7, Oct 05:23, Dec 07:8, Sep 08:5; *CPT Changes: An Insider's View* 2001

38530   open, internal mammary node(s)
   ➡ *CPT Assistant* May 98:10, Jul 99:6, Aug 10:6; *CPT Changes: An Insider's View* 2001

(Do not report 38530 with 38720-38746)

(For percutaneous needle biopsy, retroperitoneal lymph node or mass, use 49180. For fine needle aspiration, use 10022)

38542   Dissection, deep jugular node(s)
   ➡ *CPT Assistant* Jul 99:7, Aug 10:6

(For radical cervical neck dissection, use 38720)

Cardiovascular

38550 Excision of cystic hygroma, axillary or cervical; without deep neurovascular dissection

38555   with deep neurovascular dissection

Limited Lymphadenectomy for Staging

38562 Limited lymphadenectomy for staging (separate procedure); pelvic and para-aortic
→ *CPT Assistant* Mar 01:10

(When combined with prostatectomy, use 55812 or 55842)

(When combined with insertion of radioactive substance into prostate, use 55862)

38564   retroperitoneal (aortic and/or splenic)

Laparoscopy

Surgical laparoscopy always includes diagnostic laparoscopy. To report a diagnostic laparoscopy (peritoneoscopy) (separate procedure), use 49320.

38570 Laparoscopy, surgical; with retroperitoneal lymph node sampling (biopsy), single or multiple
→ *CPT Assistant* Nov 99:21, Mar 00:8; *CPT Changes: An Insider's View* 2000

38571   with bilateral total pelvic lymphadenectomy
→ *CPT Assistant* Nov 99:21, Mar 00:8; *CPT Changes: An Insider's View* 2000

38572   with bilateral total pelvic lymphadenectomy and peri-aortic lymph node sampling (biopsy), single or multiple
→ *CPT Assistant* Nov 99:21; *CPT Changes: An Insider's View* 2000

(For drainage of lymphocele to peritoneal cavity, use 49323)

38589 Unlisted laparoscopy procedure, lymphatic system
→ *CPT Assistant* Nov 99:21, Mar 00:8; *CPT Changes: An Insider's View* 2000

Radical Lymphadenectomy (Radical Resection of Lymph Nodes)

(For limited pelvic and retroperitoneal lymphadenectomies, see 38562, 38564)

38700 Suprahyoid lymphadenectomy
→ *CPT Assistant* Aug 02:8, Aug 10:3

(For bilateral procedure, report 38700 with modifier 50)

38720 Cervical lymphadenectomy (complete)
→ *CPT Assistant* Oct 01:10, Aug 02:8, Aug 10:4

(For bilateral procedure, report 38720 with modifier 50)

38724 Cervical lymphadenectomy (modified radical neck dissection)
→ *CPT Assistant* Jan 01:13, Aug 02:8, Aug 10:4

38740 Axillary lymphadenectomy; superficial

38745   complete

+ 38746 Thoracic lymphadenectomy by thoracotomy, mediastinal and regional lymphadenectomy (List separately in addition to code for primary procedure)
→ *CPT Changes: An Insider's View* 2012

(On the right, mediastinal lymph nodes include the paratracheal, subcarinal, paraesophageal, and inferior pulmonary ligament)

(On the left, mediastinal lymph nodes include the aortopulmonary window, subcarinal, paraesophageal, and inferior pulmonary ligament)

(Report 38746 in conjunction with 32440, 32442, 32445, 32480, 32482, 32484, 32486, 32488, 32503, 32504, 32505)

(To report mediastinal and regional lymphadenectomy via thoracoscopy [VATS], see 32674)

+ 38747 Abdominal lymphadenectomy, regional, including celiac, gastric, portal, peripancreatic, with or without para-aortic and vena caval nodes (List separately in addition to code for primary procedure)
→ *CPT Assistant* Nov 98:15

38760 Inguinofemoral lymphadenectomy, superficial, including Cloquets node (separate procedure)

(For bilateral procedure, report 38760 with modifier 50)

38765 Inguinofemoral lymphadenectomy, superficial, in continuity with pelvic lymphadenectomy, including external iliac, hypogastric, and obturator nodes (separate procedure)

(For bilateral procedure, report 38765 with modifier 50)

38770 Pelvic lymphadenectomy, including external iliac, hypogastric, and obturator nodes (separate procedure)

(For bilateral procedure, report 38770 with modifier 50)

38780 Retroperitoneal transabdominal lymphadenectomy, extensive, including pelvic, aortic, and renal nodes (separate procedure)

(For excision and repair of lymphedematous skin and subcutaneous tissue, see 15004-15005, 15570-15650)

Introduction

38790 Injection procedure; lymphangiography
→ *CPT Assistant* Jul 99:6

(For bilateral procedure, report 38790 with modifier 50)

(For radiological supervision and interpretation, see 75801-75807)

38792   radioactive tracer for identification of sentinel node
→ *CPT Assistant* Nov 98:15, Jul 99:6, Dec 99:8, Sep 08:5; *CPT Changes: An Insider's View* 2008, 2012

(For excision of sentinel node, see 38500-38542)

Cardiovascular

(For nuclear medicine lymphatics and lymph gland imaging, use 78195)

(For intraoperative identification (eg, mapping) of sentinel lymph node(s) including injection of non-radioactive dye, see 38900)

38794   Cannulation, thoracic duct

Other Procedures

+ **38900**   Intraoperative identification (eg, mapping) of sentinel lymph node(s) includes injection of non-radioactive dye, when performed (List separately in addition to code for primary procedure)
➔ CPT Changes: An Insider's View 2011

(Use 38900 in conjunction with 19302, 19307, 38500, 38510, 38520, 38525, 38530, 38542, 38740, 38745)

(For injection of radioactive tracer for identification of sentinel node, use 38792)

38999   Unlisted procedure, hemic or lymphatic system
➔ CPT Assistant May 98:10

Mediastinum and Diaphragm

Mediastinum

Incision

39000   Mediastinotomy with exploration, drainage, removal of foreign body, or biopsy; cervical approach

39010   transthoracic approach, including either transthoracic or median sternotomy

(For VATS pericardial biopsy, use 32604)

Excision/Resection

39200   Resection of mediastinal cyst
➔ CPT Changes: An Insider's View 2012

39220   Resection of mediastinal tumor
➔ CPT Changes: An Insider's View 2012

(For substernal thyroidectomy, use 60270)

(For thymectomy, use 60520)

(For thoracoscopic [VATS] resection of mediastinal cyst, tumor, or mass, use 32662)

Endoscopy

39400   Mediastinoscopy, includes biopsy(ies), when performed
➔ CPT Changes: An Insider's View 2012

Other Procedures

39499   Unlisted procedure, mediastinum

Diaphragm

Repair

(For transabdominal repair of diaphragmatic [esophageal hiatal] hernia, use 43325)

(For laparoscopic repair of diaphragmatic [esophageal hiatal] hernias and fundoplication, see 43280, 43281, 43282)

39501   Repair, laceration of diaphragm, any approach
➔ CPT Assistant Nov 00:3

(39502 has been deleted. To report transabdominal paraesophageal hiatal hernia repair with fundoplasty, vagotomy, and/or pyloroplasty when performed, see 43332, 43333, 43335, 43337)

(For laparoscopic paraesophageal hernia repair, see 43281, 43282)

39503   Repair, neonatal diaphragmatic hernia, with or without chest tube insertion and with or without creation of ventral hernia
➔ CPT Assistant Feb 12:3

(Do not report modifier 63 in conjunction with 39503)

(39520 has been deleted. To report transthoracic diaphragmatic [esophageal hiatal] hernia repair, see 43334, 43335)

(For laparoscopic paraesophageal hernia repair, see 43281, 43282)

(39530 has been deleted. To report thoracoabdominal diaphragmatic [esophageal hiatal] hernia repair, see 43336, 43337)?

(39531 has been deleted. To report thoracoabdominal diaphragmatic [esophageal hiatal] hernia repair, see 43336, 43337)

39540   Repair, diaphragmatic hernia (other than neonatal), traumatic; acute
➔ CPT Assistant Nov 00:9, Jun 08:3

39541   chronic

39545   Imbrication of diaphragm for eventration, transthoracic or transabdominal, paralytic or nonparalytic
➔ CPT Assistant Nov 00:3

39560   Resection, diaphragm; with simple repair (eg, primary suture)
➔ CPT Assistant Nov 99:21, Nov 00:3; CPT Changes: An Insider's View 2000

39561   with complex repair (eg, prosthetic material, local muscle flap)
➔ CPT Assistant Nov 99:21, Nov 00:3; CPT Changes: An Insider's View 2000

Other Procedures

39599   Unlisted procedure, diaphragm

Surgery

Digestive

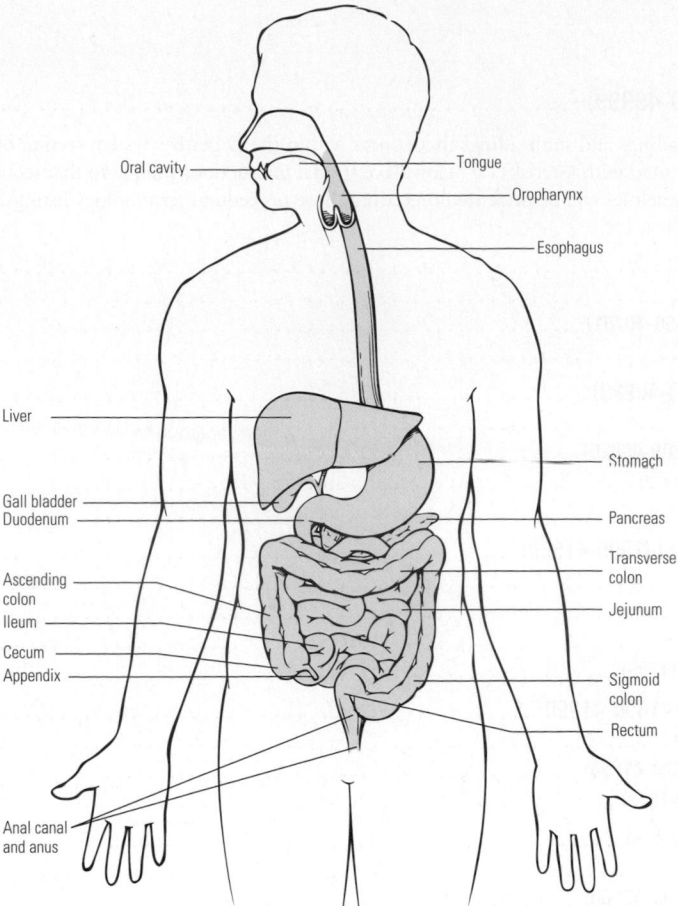

Oral cavity
Tongue
Oropharynx
Esophagus
Liver
Stomach
Gall bladder
Duodenum
Pancreas
Ascending colon
Transverse colon
Ileum
Jejunum
Cecum
Appendix
Sigmoid colon
Rectum
Anal canal and anus

Esophagus (43020-43499) **239**
  Incision (43020-43045) 239
  Excision (43100-43135) 239
  Endoscopy* (43200-43273) 240
  Laparoscopy* (43279-43289) 243
  Repair (43300-43425) 243
  Manipulation (43450-43460) 245
  Other Procedures (43496-43499) 245

Stomach (43500-43999) **245**
  Incision (43500-43520) 245
  Excision (43605-43641) 245
  Laparoscopy* (43644-43659) 246
  Introduction (43752-43761) 246
  Bariatric Surgery* (43770-43775) 247
    Laparoscopy* (43770-43775) **247**
  Other Procedures (43800-43999) 248

Intestines (Except Rectum) (44005-44799) **249**
  Incision (44005-44055) 249
  Excision* (44100-44160) 249
  Laparoscopy* (44180-44238) 251
    Incision (44180) **251**
    Enterostomy—External Fistulization of Intestines (44186-44188) **251**
    Excision (44202-44213) **251**
    Repair (44227) **252**
    Other Procedures (44238) **252**

Digestive

Digestive

Digestive System

Lips

(For procedures on skin of lips, see 10040 et seq)

Excision

40490   Biopsy of lip

40500   Vermilionectomy (lip shave), with mucosal advancement

40510   Excision of lip; transverse wedge excision with primary closure

40520   V-excision with primary direct linear closure

(For excision of mucous lesions, see 40810-40816)

40525   full thickness, reconstruction with local flap (eg, Estlander or fan)

40527   full thickness, reconstruction with cross lip flap (Abbe-Estlander)

40530   Resection of lip, more than one-fourth, without reconstruction

(For reconstruction, see 13131 et seq)

Repair (Cheiloplasty)

40650   Repair lip, full thickness; vermilion only
➜ *CPT Assistant* Jul 00:10

40652   up to half vertical height
➜ *CPT Assistant* Jul 00:10

40654   over one-half vertical height, or complex

40700   Plastic repair of cleft lip/nasal deformity; primary, partial or complete, unilateral

40701   primary bilateral, 1-stage procedure

40702   primary bilateral, 1 of 2 stages

40720   secondary, by recreation of defect and reclosure

(For bilateral procedure, report 40720 with modifier 50)

(To report rhinoplasty only for nasal deformity secondary to congenital cleft lip, see 30460, 30462)

(For repair of cleft lip, with cross lip pedicle flap (Abbe-Estlander type), use 40527)

40761   with cross lip pedicle flap (Abbe-Estlander type), including sectioning and inserting of pedicle

(For repair cleft palate, see 42200 et seq)

(For other reconstructive procedures, see 14060, 14061, 15120-15261, 15574, 15576, 15630)

Other Procedures

40799   Unlisted procedure, lips

Vestibule of Mouth

The vestibule is the part of the oral cavity outside the dentoalveolar structures; it includes the mucosal and submucosal tissue of lips and cheeks.

Incision

40800   Drainage of abscess, cyst, hematoma, vestibule of mouth; simple

40801   complicated

40804   Removal of embedded foreign body, vestibule of mouth; simple

40805   complicated

40806   Incision of labial frenum (frenotomy)

Excision, Destruction

40808   Biopsy, vestibule of mouth

40810   Excision of lesion of mucosa and submucosa, vestibule of mouth; without repair

40812   with simple repair

40814   with complex repair

40816   complex, with excision of underlying muscle

40818   Excision of mucosa of vestibule of mouth as donor graft

40819   Excision of frenum, labial or buccal (frenumectomy, frenulectomy, frenectomy)

40820   Destruction of lesion or scar of vestibule of mouth by physical methods (eg, laser, thermal, cryo, chemical)

Repair

40830   Closure of laceration, vestibule of mouth; 2.5 cm or less

40831   over 2.5 cm or complex

40840   Vestibuloplasty; anterior

40842   posterior, unilateral

40843   posterior, bilateral

40844   entire arch

40845   complex (including ridge extension, muscle repositioning)

(For skin grafts, see 15002 et seq)

Other Procedures

40899   Unlisted procedure, vestibule of mouth

Tongue and Floor of Mouth

Incision

41000 Intraoral incision and drainage of abscess, cyst, or hematoma of tongue or floor of mouth; lingual

41005 sublingual, superficial

41006 sublingual, deep, supramylohyoid

41007 submental space

41008 submandibular space

41009 masticator space

41010 Incision of lingual frenum (frenotomy)

41015 Extraoral incision and drainage of abscess, cyst, or hematoma of floor of mouth; sublingual

41016 submental

41017 submandibular

41018 masticator space

(For frenoplasty, use 41520)

41019 Placement of needles, catheters, or other device(s) into the head and/or neck region (percutaneous, transoral, or transnasal) for subsequent interstitial radioelement application
➔ *CPT Changes: An Insider's View* 2008

(For imaging guidance, see 76942, 77002, 77012, 77021)

(For stereotactic insertion of intracranial brachytherapy radiation sources, use 61770)

(For interstitial radioelement application, see 77776-77787)

Excision

41100 Biopsy of tongue; anterior two-thirds

41105 posterior one-third

41108 Biopsy of floor of mouth

41110 Excision of lesion of tongue without closure

41112 Excision of lesion of tongue with closure; anterior two-thirds

41113 posterior one-third

41114 with local tongue flap

(Do not report 41114 in conjunction with 41112 or 41113)

41115 Excision of lingual frenum (frenectomy)

41116 Excision, lesion of floor of mouth

41120 Glossectomy; less than one-half tongue
➔ *CPT Assistant* Aug 10:10

41130 hemiglossectomy
➔ *CPT Assistant* Aug 10:5

41135 partial, with unilateral radical neck dissection
➔ *CPT Assistant* Aug 10:5

41140 complete or total, with or without tracheostomy, without radical neck dissection
➔ *CPT Assistant* Aug 10:5

41145 complete or total, with or without tracheostomy, with unilateral radical neck dissection
➔ *CPT Assistant* Aug 10:5

41150 composite procedure with resection floor of mouth and mandibular resection, without radical neck dissection
➔ *CPT Assistant* Aug 10:5

41153 composite procedure with resection floor of mouth, with suprahyoid neck dissection
➔ *CPT Assistant* Aug 10:3

41155 composite procedure with resection floor of mouth, mandibular resection, and radical neck dissection (Commando type)
➔ *CPT Assistant* Jan 01:13, Aug 10:3

Repair

41250 Repair of laceration 2.5 cm or less; floor of mouth and/or anterior two-thirds of tongue

41251 posterior one-third of tongue

41252 Repair of laceration of tongue, floor of mouth, over 2.6 cm or complex

Other Procedures

41500 Fixation of tongue, mechanical, other than suture (eg, K-wire)
➔ *CPT Assistant* Aug 10:11

41510 Suture of tongue to lip for micrognathia (Douglas type procedure)
➔ *CPT Assistant* Aug 10:11

41512 Tongue base suspension, permanent suture technique
➔ *CPT Assistant* Aug 10:11; *CPT Changes: An Insider's View* 2009

(For fixation of tongue, mechanical, other than suture, use 41500)

(For suture of tongue to lip for micrognathia, use 41510)

41520 Frenoplasty (surgical revision of frenum, eg, with Z-plasty)

(For frenotomy, see 40806, 41010)

41530 Submucosal ablation of the tongue base, radiofrequency, 1 or more sites, per session
➔ *CPT Assistant* Aug 10:10; *CPT Changes: An Insider's View* 2009

41599 Unlisted procedure, tongue, floor of mouth
➔ *CPT Assistant* Dec 00:14
➔ *Clinical Examples in Radiology* Fall 09:11

Dentoalveolar Structures

Incision

41800　Drainage of abscess, cyst, hematoma from dentoalveolar structures

41805　Removal of embedded foreign body from dentoalveolar structures; soft tissues

41806　　bone

Excision, Destruction

41820　Gingivectomy, excision gingiva, each quadrant

41821　Operculectomy, excision pericoronal tissues

41822　Excision of fibrous tuberosities, dentoalveolar structures

41823　Excision of osseous tuberosities, dentoalveolar structures

41825　Excision of lesion or tumor (except listed above), dentoalveolar structures; without repair

41826　　with simple repair

41827　　with complex repair

　　(For nonexcisional destruction, use 41850)

41828　Excision of hyperplastic alveolar mucosa, each quadrant (specify)

41830　Alveolectomy, including curettage of osteitis or sequestrectomy

41850　Destruction of lesion (except excision), dentoalveolar structures

Other Procedures

41870　Periodontal mucosal grafting

41872　Gingivoplasty, each quadrant (specify)

41874　Alveoloplasty, each quadrant (specify)

　　(For closure of lacerations, see 40830, 40831)

　　(For segmental osteotomy, use 21206)

　　(For reduction of fractures, see 21421-21490)

41899　Unlisted procedure, dentoalveolar structures

Palate and Uvula

Incision

42000　Drainage of abscess of palate, uvula

Excision, Destruction

42100　Biopsy of palate, uvula

42104　Excision, lesion of palate, uvula; without closure

42106　　with simple primary closure

42107　　with local flap closure

　　(For skin graft, see 14040-14302)

　　(For mucosal graft, use 40818)

42120　Resection of palate or extensive resection of lesion

　　(For reconstruction of palate with extraoral tissue, see 14040-14302, 15050, 15120, 15240, 15576)

42140　Uvulectomy, excision of uvula

42145　Palatopharyngoplasty (eg, uvulopalatopharyngoplasty, uvulopharyngoplasty)
　　➔ *CPT Assistant* Dec 04:19

　　(For removal of exostosis of the bony palate, see 21031, 21032)

42160　Destruction of lesion, palate or uvula (thermal, cryo or chemical)
　　➔ *CPT Assistant* Apr 10:10

Repair

42180　Repair, laceration of palate; up to 2 cm

42182　　over 2 cm or complex

42200　Palatoplasty for cleft palate, soft and/or hard palate only

42205　Palatoplasty for cleft palate, with closure of alveolar ridge; soft tissue only

42210　　with bone graft to alveolar ridge (includes obtaining graft)

42215　Palatoplasty for cleft palate; major revision

42220　　secondary lengthening procedure

42225　　attachment pharyngeal flap

42226　Lengthening of palate, and pharyngeal flap

42227　Lengthening of palate, with island flap

42235　Repair of anterior palate, including vomer flap

　　(For repair of oronasal fistula, use 30600)

42260　Repair of nasolabial fistula

　　(For repair of cleft lip, see 40700 et seq)

42280　Maxillary impression for palatal prosthesis

42281　Insertion of pin-retained palatal prosthesis

Other Procedures

42299　Unlisted procedure, palate, uvula
　　➔ *CPT Assistant* Dec 04:19, Apr 10:10, Nov 10:9

Salivary Gland and Ducts

Incision

42300　Drainage of abscess; parotid, simple

42305　　parotid, complicated

42310 Drainage of abscess; submaxillary or sublingual, intraoral
→ *CPT Changes: An Insider's View* 2003

42320 submaxillary, external

42330 Sialolithotomy; submandibular (submaxillary), sublingual or parotid, uncomplicated, intraoral

42335 submandibular (submaxillary), complicated, intraoral

42340 parotid, extraoral or complicated intraoral

Excision

42400 Biopsy of salivary gland; needle

(For fine needle aspiration, see 10021, 10022)

(For evaluation of fine needle aspirate, see 88172, 88173)

(If imaging guidance is performed, see 76942, 77002, 77012, 77021)

42405 incisional

(If imaging guidance is performed, see 76942, 77002, 77012, 77021)

42408 Excision of sublingual salivary cyst (ranula)

42409 Marsupialization of sublingual salivary cyst (ranula)

42410 Excision of parotid tumor or parotid gland; lateral lobe, without nerve dissection

42415 lateral lobe, with dissection and preservation of facial nerve

42420 total, with dissection and preservation of facial nerve
→ *CPT Assistant* Aug 10:4

42425 total, en bloc removal with sacrifice of facial nerve

42426 total, with unilateral radical neck dissection

(For suture or grafting of facial nerve, see 64864, 64865, 69740, 69745)

42440 Excision of submandibular (submaxillary) gland

42450 Excision of sublingual gland

Repair

42500 Plastic repair of salivary duct, sialodochoplasty; primary or simple

42505 secondary or complicated

42507 Parotid duct diversion, bilateral (Wilke type procedure);

42508 with excision of 1 submandibular gland

42509 with excision of both submandibular glands

42510 with ligation of both submandibular (Wharton's) ducts

Other Procedures

42550 Injection procedure for sialography
→ *Clinical Examples in Radiology* Fall 09:9

(For radiological supervision and interpretation, use 70390)

42600 Closure salivary fistula

42650 Dilation salivary duct

42660 Dilation and catheterization of salivary duct, with or without injection

42665 Ligation salivary duct, intraoral

42699 Unlisted procedure, salivary glands or ducts

Pharynx, Adenoids, and Tonsils

Incision

42700 Incision and drainage abscess; peritonsillar

42720 retropharyngeal or parapharyngeal, intraoral approach

42725 retropharyngeal or parapharyngeal, external approach

Excision, Destruction

42800 Biopsy; oropharynx

42802 hypopharynx

42804 nasopharynx, visible lesion, simple

42806 nasopharynx, survey for unknown primary lesion

(For laryngoscopic biopsy, see 31510, 31535, 31536)

42808 Excision or destruction of lesion of pharynx, any method

42809 Removal of foreign body from pharynx

42810 Excision branchial cleft cyst or vestige, confined to skin and subcutaneous tissues

42815 Excision branchial cleft cyst, vestige, or fistula, extending beneath subcutaneous tissues and/or into pharynx

42820 Tonsillectomy and adenoidectomy; younger than age 12
→ *CPT Assistant* Feb 98:11, Mar 08:15, May 08:14

42821 age 12 or over
→ *CPT Assistant* Aug 97:18, Feb 98:11, Mar 08:15, May 08:14

42825 Tonsillectomy, primary or secondary; younger than age 12
→ *CPT Assistant* Aug 97:18, Feb 98:11, Mar 08:15

42826 age 12 or over
→ *CPT Assistant* Aug 97:18, Feb 98:11, Mar 08:15, Apr 10:10

42830 Adenoidectomy, primary; younger than age 12

42831 age 12 or over

42835 Adenoidectomy, secondary; younger than age 12

42836 age 12 or over
→ *CPT Assistant* Feb 98:11, Nov 10:9

42842 Radical resection of tonsil, tonsillar pillars, and/or retromolar trigone; without closure
→ *CPT Assistant* Aug 10:6

42844 closure with local flap (eg, tongue, buccal)
→ *CPT Assistant* Aug 10:6

42845   closure with other flap
➔ *CPT Assistant* Aug 10:6

(For closure with other flap(s), use appropriate number for flap(s))

(When combined with radical neck dissection, use also 38720)

42860   Excision of tonsil tags

42870   Excision or destruction lingual tonsil, any method (separate procedure)

(For resection of the nasopharynx [eg, juvenile angiofibroma] by bicoronal and/or transzygomatic approach, see 61586 and 61600)

42890   Limited pharyngectomy

42892   Resection of lateral pharyngeal wall or pyriform sinus, direct closure by advancement of lateral and posterior pharyngeal walls
➔ *CPT Assistant* Aug 10:6

(When combined with radical neck dissection, use also 38720)

42894   Resection of pharyngeal wall requiring closure with myocutaneous or fasciocutaneous flap or free muscle, skin, or fascial flap with microvascular anastamosis
➔ *CPT Assistant* Nov 07:8, Aug 10:6; *CPT Changes: An Insider's View* 2010

(When combined with radical neck dissection, use also 38720)

(For limited pharyngectomy with radical neck dissection, use 38720 with 42890)

(For flap used for reconstruction, see 15732, 15734, 15756, 15757, 15758)

Repair

42900   Suture pharynx for wound or injury

42950   Pharyngoplasty (plastic or reconstructive operation on pharynx)

(For pharyngeal flap, use 42225)

42953   Pharyngoesophageal repair

(For closure with myocutaneous or other flap, use appropriate number in addition)

Other Procedures

42955   Pharyngostomy (fistulization of pharynx, external for feeding)

42960   Control oropharyngeal hemorrhage, primary or secondary (eg, post-tonsillectomy); simple

42961   complicated, requiring hospitalization

42962   with secondary surgical intervention

42970   Control of nasopharyngeal hemorrhage, primary or secondary (eg, postadenoidectomy); simple, with posterior nasal packs, with or without anterior packs and/or cautery
➔ *CPT Changes: An Insider's View* 2002

42971   complicated, requiring hospitalization

42972   with secondary surgical intervention

42999   Unlisted procedure, pharynx, adenoids, or tonsils

Esophagus

Incision

(For esophageal intubation with laparotomy, use 43510)

43020   Esophagotomy, cervical approach, with removal of foreign body

43030   Cricopharyngeal myotomy

43045   Esophagotomy, thoracic approach, with removal of foreign body

Excision

(For gastrointestinal reconstruction for previous esophagectomy, see 43360, 43361)

43100   Excision of lesion, esophagus, with primary repair; cervical approach

43101   thoracic or abdominal approach
➔ *CPT Assistant* Aug 10:4

(For wide excision of malignant lesion of cervical esophagus, with total laryngectomy without radical neck dissection, see 43107, 43116, 43124, and 31360)

(For wide excision of malignant lesion of cervical esophagus, with total laryngectomy with radical neck dissection, see 43107, 43116, 43124, and 31365)

43107   Total or near total esophagectomy, without thoracotomy; with pharyngogastrostomy or cervical esophagogastrostomy, with or without pyloroplasty (transhiatal)
➔ *CPT Assistant* Aug 10:4

43108   with colon interposition or small intestine reconstruction, including intestine mobilization, preparation and anastomosis(es)
➔ *CPT Changes: An Insider's View* 2002

43112   Total or near total esophagectomy, with thoracotomy; with pharyngogastrostomy or cervical esophagogastrostomy, with or without pyloroplasty

43113   with colon interposition or small intestine reconstruction, including intestine mobilization, preparation, and anastomosis(es)
➔ *CPT Changes: An Insider's View* 2002

Digestive

43116 Partial esophagectomy, cervical, with free intestinal graft, including microvascular anastomosis, obtaining the graft and intestinal reconstruction
  → *CPT Assistant* Nov 97:17, Nov 98:16, Aug 10:4

  (Do not report 43116 in conjunction with 69990)

  (Report 43116 with the modifier 52 appended if intestinal or free jejunal graft with microvascular anastomosis is performed by another physician)

  (For free jejunal graft with microvascular anastomosis performed by another physician, use 43496)

43117 Partial esophagectomy, distal two-thirds, with thoracotomy and separate abdominal incision, with or without proximal gastrectomy; with thoracic esophagogastrostomy, with or without pyloroplasty (Ivor Lewis)

43118   with colon interposition or small intestine reconstruction, including intestine mobilization, preparation, and anastomosis(es)
  → *CPT Changes: An Insider's View* 2002

  (For total esophagectomy with gastropharyngostomy, see 43107, 43124)

  (For esophagogastrectomy (lower third) and vagotomy, use 43122)

43121 Partial esophagectomy, distal two-thirds, with thoracotomy only, with or without proximal gastrectomy, with thoracic esophagogastrostomy, with or without pyloroplasty

43122 Partial esophagectomy, thoracoabdominal or abdominal approach, with or without proximal gastrectomy; with esophagogastrostomy, with or without pyloroplasty

43123   with colon interposition or small intestine reconstruction, including intestine mobilization, preparation, and anastomosis(es)
  → *CPT Changes: An Insider's View* 2002

43124 Total or partial esophagectomy, without reconstruction (any approach), with cervical esophagostomy

43130 Diverticulectomy of hypopharynx or esophagus, with or without myotomy; cervical approach
  → *CPT Assistant* Oct 10:12, Dec 10:12

43135   thoracic approach
  → *CPT Assistant* Oct 10:12, Dec 10:12

Endoscopy

For endoscopic procedures, code appropriate endoscopy of each anatomic site examined.

Surgical endoscopy always includes diagnostic endoscopy.

⊙ **43200** Esophagoscopy, rigid or flexible; diagnostic, with or without collection of specimen(s) by brushing or washing (separate procedure)
  → *CPT Assistant* Spring 91:7, Spring 94:1, Jun 98:10, Nov 99:21, Sep 03:3, Oct 08:6; *CPT Changes: An Insider's View* 2000

⊙ **43201**   with directed submucosal injection(s), any substance
  → *CPT Assistant* Jun 10:4; *CPT Changes: An Insider's View* 2003

  (For injection sclerosis of esophageal varices, use 43204)

⊙ **43202**   with biopsy, single or multiple
  → *CPT Assistant* Spring 94:1, Oct 08:6

⊙ **43204**   with injection sclerosis of esophageal varices
  → *CPT Assistant* Spring 94:1, Oct 08:6, Jun 10:5

⊙ **43205**   with band ligation of esophageal varices
  → *CPT Assistant* Spring 94:1, Oct 08:6

⊙● **43206**   with optical endomicroscopy
  → *CPT Changes: An Insider's View* 2013

►(Report supply of contrast agent separately)◄

►(Do not report 43206 in conjunction with 88375)◄

⊙ **43215**   with removal of foreign body
  → *CPT Assistant* Spring 94:1, Oct 08:6

  (For radiological supervision and interpretation, use 74235)

⊙ **43216**   with removal of tumor(s), polyp(s), or other lesion(s) by hot biopsy forceps or bipolar cautery
  → *CPT Assistant* Spring 94:1, Oct 08:6

⊙ **43217**   with removal of tumor(s), polyp(s), or other lesion(s) by snare technique
  → *CPT Assistant* Spring 94:1, Oct 08:6

⊙ **43219**   with insertion of plastic tube or stent
  → *CPT Assistant* Spring 94:2, Oct 08:6

⊙ **43220**   with balloon dilation (less than 30 mm diameter)
  → *CPT Assistant* Spring 94:2, Jan 97:10, May 05:3, Oct 08:6

  (If imaging guidance is performed, use 74360)

  (For endoscopic dilation with balloon 30 mm diameter or larger, use 43458)

  (For dilation without visualization, use 43450-43453)

  (For diagnostic fiberoptic esophagogastroscopy, use 43200, 43235)

  (For fiberoptic esophagogastroscopy with biopsy or collection of specimen, use 43200, 43202, 43235, 43239)

  (For fiberoptic esophagogastroscopy with removal of foreign body, use 43215, 43247)

  (For fiberoptic esophagogastroscopy with removal of polyp(s), use 43217, 43251)

⊙ **43226**   with insertion of guide wire followed by dilation over guide wire
  → *CPT Assistant* Spring 94:2

  (For radiological supervision and interpretation, use 74360)

⊙ **43227**   with control of bleeding (eg, injection, bipolar cautery, unipolar cautery, laser, heater probe, stapler, plasma coagulator)
  → *CPT Assistant* Spring 94:2, Oct 08:6, Jun 10:4; *CPT Changes: An Insider's View* 2002

⊙ **43228**   with ablation of tumor(s), polyp(s), or other lesion(s), not amenable to removal by hot biopsy forceps, bipolar cautery or snare technique
➔ *CPT Assistant* Spring 94:2, Nov 98:21, Oct 08:6

(For esophagoscopic photodynamic therapy, report 43228 in addition to 96570, 96571 as appropriate)

⊙ **43231**   with endoscopic ultrasound examination
➔ *CPT Assistant* Oct 01:4, May 04:6, Oct 08:6, Mar 09:8; *CPT Changes: An Insider's View* 2001

(Do not report 43231 in conjunction with 76975)

⊙ **43232**   with transendoscopic ultrasound-guided intramural or transmural fine needle aspiration/biopsy(s)
➔ *CPT Assistant* Oct 01:4, Mar 04:11, May 04:6, Oct 08:6, Mar 09:8; *CPT Changes: An Insider's View* 2001

(Do not report 43232 in conjunction with 76942, 76975)

(For interpretation of specimen, see 88172-88173)

▶(43234 has been deleted. To report, use 43235)◀

⊙ **43235**   Upper gastrointestinal endoscopy including esophagus, stomach, and either the duodenum and/or jejunum as appropriate; diagnostic, with or without collection of specimen(s) by brushing or washing (separate procedure)
➔ *CPT Assistant* Spring 94:4, Dec 97:11, Jun 03:11, Sep 03:3, Oct 08:6, May 09:8

Upper Gastrointestinal Endoscopy
43235

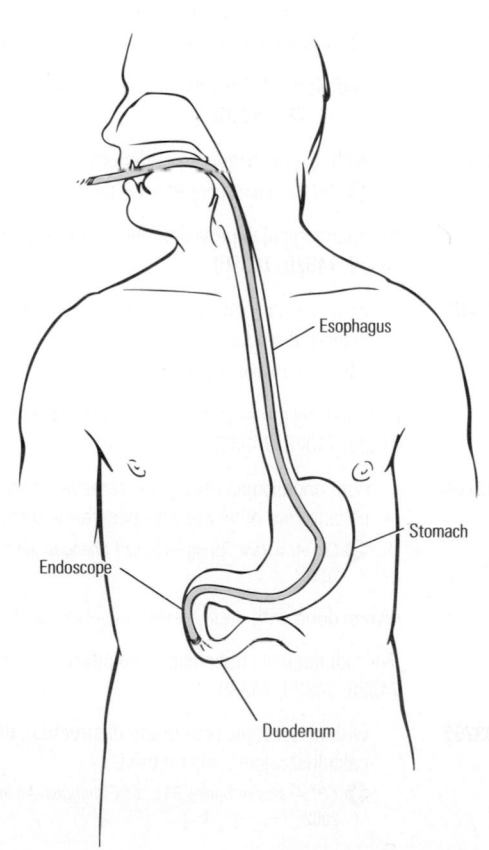

⊙ **43236**   with directed submucosal injection(s), any substance
➔ *CPT Assistant* Jun 10:4; *CPT Changes: An Insider's View* 2003

(For injection sclerosis of esophageal and/or gastric varices, use 43243)

⊙ **43237**   with endoscopic ultrasound examination limited to the esophagus
➔ *CPT Changes: An Insider's View* 2004

(Do not report 43237 in conjunction with 76942, 76975)

⊙ **43238**   with transendoscopic ultrasound-guided intramural or transmural fine needle aspiration/biopsy(s), esophagus (includes endoscopic ultrasound examination limited to the esophagus)
➔ *CPT Changes: An Insider's View* 2004

(Do not report 43238 in conjunction with 76942 or 76975)

⊙ **43239**   with biopsy, single or multiple
➔ *CPT Assistant* Spring 94:4, Apr 98:14, Feb 99:11, Oct 01:4, Nov 07:9

⊙ **43240**   with transmural drainage of pseudocyst
➔ *CPT Assistant* Oct 01:4; *CPT Changes: An Insider's View* 2001

⊙ **43241**   with transendoscopic intraluminal tube or catheter placement
➔ *CPT Assistant* Spring 94:4, Nov 01:7, Apr 09:3; *CPT Changes: An Insider's View* 2001

⊙ **43242**   with transendoscopic ultrasound-guided intramural or transmural fine needle aspiration/biopsy(s) (includes endoscopic ultrasound examination of the esophagus, stomach, and either the duodenum and/or jejunum as appropriate)
➔ *CPT Assistant* Oct 01:4, Mar 09:8; *CPT Changes: An Insider's View* 2001, 2004

(Do not report 43242 in conjunction with 76942, 76975)

(For transendoscopic fine needle aspiration/biopsy limited to esophagus, use 43238)

(For interpretation of specimen, see 88172-88173)

⊙ **43243**   with injection sclerosis of esophageal and/or gastric varices
➔ *CPT Assistant* Spring 94:4, Jun 10:5

⊙ **43244**   with band ligation of esophageal and/or gastric varices
➔ *CPT Assistant* Spring 94:4, Jun 11:13

⊙ **43245**   with dilation of gastric outlet for obstruction (eg, balloon, guide wire, bougie)
➔ *CPT Assistant* Spring 94:4, Oct 01:4, Jan 04:26; *CPT Changes: An Insider's View* 2002, 2003

(Do not report 43245 in conjunction with 43256)

⊙ **43246**   with directed placement of percutaneous gastrostomy tube
➔ *CPT Assistant* Spring 94:4, Feb 97:10, Mar 10:10

(For nonendoscopic percutaneous placement of gastrostomy tube, see 49440)

⊙ **43247** with removal of foreign body
→ *CPT Assistant* Spring 94:4

(For radiological supervision and interpretation, use 74235)

⊙ **43248** with insertion of guide wire followed by dilation of esophagus over guide wire
→ *CPT Assistant* Spring 94:4, Dec 97:11, Oct 08:6

⊙ **43249** with balloon dilation of esophagus (less than 30 mm diameter)
→ *CPT Assistant* May 05:3

⊙ **43250** with removal of tumor(s), polyp(s), or other lesion(s) by hot biopsy forceps or bipolar cautery
→ *CPT Assistant* Spring 94:4, Feb 99:11, Nov 07:9

⊙ **43251** with removal of tumor(s), polyp(s), or other lesion(s) by snare technique
→ *CPT Assistant* Spring 94:4, Oct 04:12, Nov 07:9, Jun 11:13

⊙ **43252** with optical endomicroscopy
→ *CPT Changes: An Insider's View* 2013

►(Report supply of contrast agent separately)◄

►Do not report 43252 in conjunction with 88375◄

►(For biopsy specimen pathology, use 88305)◄

⊙ **43255** with control of bleeding, any method
→ *CPT Assistant* Spring 94:4, Jun 10:4

⊙ **43256** with transendoscopic stent placement (includes predilation)
→ *CPT Changes: An Insider's View* 2001

⊙ **43257** with delivery of thermal energy to the muscle of lower esophageal sphincter and/or gastric cardia, for treatment of gastroesophageal reflux disease
→ *CPT Assistant* May 05:3; *CPT Changes: An Insider's View* 2005

⊙ **43258** with ablation of tumor(s), polyp(s), or other lesion(s) not amenable to removal by hot biopsy forceps, bipolar cautery or snare technique
→ *CPT Assistant* Spring 94:4

(For injection sclerosis of esophageal varices, use 43204, 43243)

⊙ **43259** with endoscopic ultrasound examination, including the esophagus, stomach, and either the duodenum and/or jejunum as appropriate
→ *CPT Assistant* Spring 94:4, May 04:7, Mar 09:8; *CPT Changes: An Insider's View* 2004

(Do not report 43259 in conjunction with 76975)

⊙ **43260** Endoscopic retrograde cholangiopancreatography (ERCP); diagnostic, with or without collection of specimen(s) by brushing or washing (separate procedure)
→ *CPT Assistant* Spring 94:5, Oct 04:13, May 08:14, Aug 08:12, Jan 12:12

(For radiological supervision and interpretation, see 74328, 74329, 74330)

Endoscopic Retrograde Cholangiopancreatography (ERCP)
43260

Examination of the hepatobiliary system (pancreatic ducts, hepatic ducts, common bile ducts, duodenal papilla [ampulla of Vater] and gallbladder [if present]) is performed through a side-viewing flexible fiberoptic endoscope.

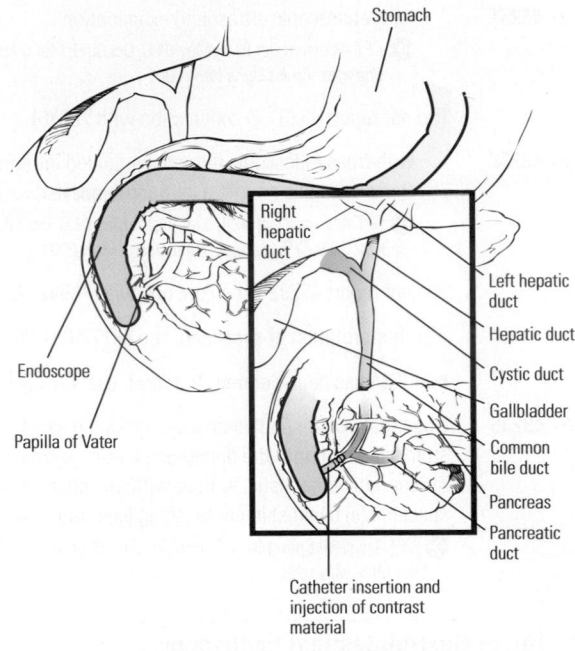

Stomach · Right hepatic duct · Left hepatic duct · Hepatic duct · Cystic duct · Gallbladder · Common bile duct · Pancreas · Pancreatic duct · Endoscope · Papilla of Vater · Catheter insertion and injection of contrast material

⊙ **43261** with biopsy, single or multiple
→ *CPT Assistant* Spring 94:5, Aug 08:12, Jun 11:13

(For radiological supervision and interpretation, see 74328, 74329, 74330)

⊙ **43262** with sphincterotomy/papillotomy
→ *CPT Assistant* Spring 94:5, Oct 04:13, Jul 09:10

(For radiological supervision and interpretation, see 74328, 74329, 74330)

⊙ **43263** with pressure measurement of sphincter of Oddi (pancreatic duct or common bile duct)
→ *CPT Assistant* Spring 94:5, Oct 04:13

(For radiological supervision and interpretation, see 74328, 74329, 74330)

⊙ **43264** with endoscopic retrograde removal of calculus/calculi from biliary and/or pancreatic ducts
→ *CPT Assistant* Spring 94:5; *CPT Changes: An Insider's View* 2002

(When done with sphincterotomy, also use 43262)

(For radiological supervision and interpretation, see 74328, 74329, 74330)

⊙ **43265** with endoscopic retrograde destruction, lithotripsy of calculus/calculi, any method
→ *CPT Assistant* Spring 94:5; *CPT Changes: An Insider's View* 2002

(When done with sphincterotomy, also use 43262)

(For radiological supervision and interpretation, see 74328, 74329, 74330)

⊙ **43267**   with endoscopic retrograde insertion of nasobiliary or nasopancreatic drainage tube

➔ *CPT Assistant* Spring 94:6

(When done with sphincterotomy, also use 43262)

(For radiological supervision and interpretation, see 74328, 74329, 74330)

⊙ **43268**   with endoscopic retrograde insertion of tube or stent into bile or pancreatic duct

➔ *CPT Assistant* Spring 94:6, Sep 04:13, Oct 04:12, Jan 12:11

(When done with sphincterotomy, also use 43262)

(For radiological supervision and interpretation, see 74328, 74329, 74330)

⊙ **43269**   with endoscopic retrograde removal of foreign body and/or change of tube or stent

➔ *CPT Assistant* Spring 94:6, Jan 12:12

(When done with sphincterotomy, also use 43262)

(For radiological supervision and interpretation, see 74328, 74329, 74330)

⊙ **43271**   with endoscopic retrograde balloon dilation of ampulla, biliary and/or pancreatic duct(s)

➔ *CPT Assistant* Spring 94:6

(When done with sphincterotomy, also use 43262)

(For radiological supervision and interpretation, see 74328, 74329, 74330)

⊙ **43272**   with ablation of tumor(s), polyp(s), or other lesion(s) not amenable to removal by hot biopsy forceps, bipolar cautery or snare technique

(For radiological supervision and interpretation, see 74328, 74329, 74330)

⊙+ **43273**   Endoscopic cannulation of papilla with direct visualization of common bile duct(s) and/or pancreatic duct(s) (List separately in addition to code(s) for primary procedure)

➔ *CPT Changes: An Insider's View* 2009

(Use 43273 in conjunction with 43260-43265, 43267-43272)

Laparoscopy

Surgical laparoscopy always includes diagnostic laparoscopy. To report a diagnostic laparoscopy (peritoneoscopy) (separate procedure), use 49320.

43279   Laparoscopy, surgical, esophagomyotomy (Heller type), with fundoplasty, when performed

➔ *CPT Assistant* Feb 12:3; *CPT Changes: An Insider's View* 2009

(For open approach, see 43330, 43331)

(Do not report 43279 in conjunction with 43280)

43280   Laparoscopy, surgical, esophagogastric fundoplasty (eg, Nissen, Toupet procedures)

➔ *CPT Assistant* Nov 99:22, Mar 00:8, Dec 02:2, Jun 11:8, Feb 12:3; *CPT Changes: An Insider's View* 2000

(Do not report 43280 in conjunction with 43279)

(For open approach, see 43327, 43328)

Laparoscopic Fundoplasty
43280

With the esophagus and fundus held aside, sutures are placed in both crus diaphragmatis muscles below the esophagus to bring them together to close the hiatal hernia, and the anterior and posterior walls of the fundus are wrapped and stitched around the esophagus to complete the laparoscopic fundoplasty.

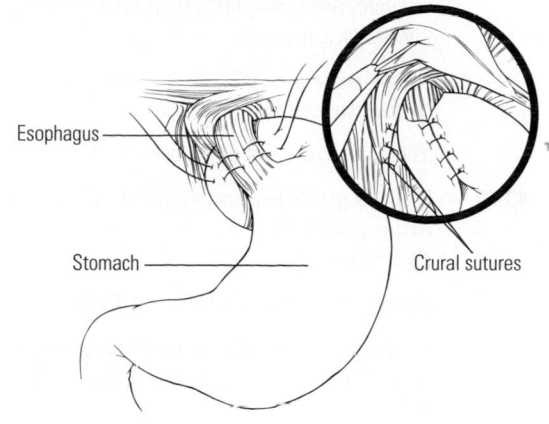

Esophagus

Stomach

Crural sutures

43281   Laparoscopy, surgical, repair of paraesophageal hernia, includes fundoplasty, when performed; without implantation of mesh

➔ *CPT Assistant* Jun 11:9, Feb 12:3; *CPT Changes: An Insider's View* 2010

43282   with implantation of mesh

➔ *CPT Assistant* Jun 11:9, Feb 12:3; *CPT Changes: An Insider's View* 2010

(To report transabdominal paraesophageal hiatal hernia repair, see 43332, 43333. To report transthoracic diaphragmatic hernia repair, see 43334, 43335)

(Do not report 43281, 43282 in conjunction with 43280, 43450, 43453, 43456, 43458, 49568)

+ **43283**   Laparoscopy, surgical, esophageal lengthening procedure (eg, Collis gastroplasty or wedge gastroplasty) (List separately in addition to code for primary procedure)

➔ *CPT Assistant* Jun 11:9, Feb 12:3; *CPT Changes: An Insider's View* 2011

(Use 43283 in conjunction with 43280, 43281, 43282)

43289   Unlisted laparoscopy procedure, esophagus

➔ *CPT Assistant* Nov 99:22, Mar 00:8; *CPT Changes: An Insider's View* 2000

Repair

43300   Esophagoplasty (plastic repair or reconstruction), cervical approach; without repair of tracheoesophageal fistula

43305   with repair of tracheoesophageal fistula

Digestive

43310 Esophagoplasty (plastic repair or reconstruction), thoracic approach; without repair of tracheoesophageal fistula

43312   with repair of tracheoesophageal fistula

43313 Esophagoplasty for congenital defect (plastic repair or reconstruction), thoracic approach; without repair of congenital tracheoesophageal fistula
➜ *CPT Changes: An Insider's View* 2002

43314   with repair of congenital tracheoesophageal fistula
➜ *CPT Changes: An Insider's View* 2002

(Do not report modifier 63 in conjunction with 43313, 43314)

43320 Esophagogastrostomy (cardioplasty), with or without vagotomy and pyloroplasty, transabdominal or transthoracic approach

(43324 has been deleted. To report esophagogastric fundoplasty, see 43327, 43328)

(For laparoscopic procedure, use 43280)

43325 Esophagogastric fundoplasty; with fundic patch (Thal-Nissen procedure)
➜ *CPT Assistant* Winter 90:6

(For cricopharyngeal myotomy, use 43030)

(43326 has been deleted. To report esophagogastric fundoplasty with gastroplasty, see 43327, 43328, 43332-43338)

43327 Esophagogastric fundoplasty partial or complete; laparotomy
➜ *CPT Assistant* Jun 11:8, Feb 12:3; *CPT Changes: An Insider's View* 2011

43328   thoracotomy
➜ *CPT Assistant* Jun 11:8, Feb 12:3; *CPT Changes: An Insider's View* 2011

43330 Esophagomyotomy (Heller type); abdominal approach
➜ *CPT Assistant* Nov 99:22; *CPT Changes: An Insider's View* 2000

(For laparoscopic esophagomyotomy procedure, use 43279)

43331   thoracic approach
➜ *CPT Assistant* Nov 99:22; *CPT Changes: An Insider's View* 2000

(For thoracoscopic esophagomyotomy, use 32665)

43332 Repair, paraesophageal hiatal hernia (including fundoplication), via laparotomy, except neonatal; without implantation of mesh or other prosthesis
➜ *CPT Assistant* Feb 12:3; *CPT Changes: An Insider's View* 2011

43333   with implantation of mesh or other prosthesis
➜ *CPT Assistant* Feb 12:3; *CPT Changes: An Insider's View* 2011

(For neonatal diaphragmatic hernia repair, use 39503)

43334 Repair, paraesophageal hiatal hernia (including fundoplication), via thoracotomy, except neonatal; without implantation of mesh or other prosthesis
➜ *CPT Assistant* Feb 12:3; *CPT Changes: An Insider's View* 2011

Nissen Fundoplasty
43327, 43328

The lower esophagus is accessed through an upper abdominal or lower thoracic incision. The fundus of the stomach is mobilized and wrapped around the lower esophageal sphincter, and the wrap is sutured into place.

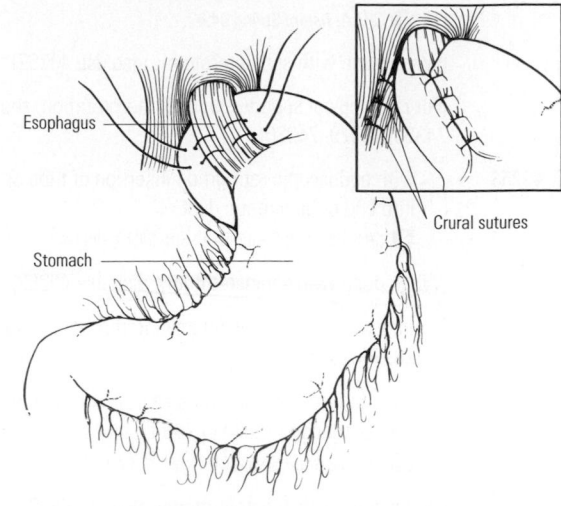

43335   with implantation of mesh or other prosthesis
➜ *CPT Assistant* Feb 12:3; *CPT Changes: An Insider's View* 2011

(For neonatal diaphragmatic hernia repair, use 39503)

43336 Repair, paraesophageal hiatal hernia, (including fundoplication), via thoracoabdominal incision, except neonatal; without implantation of mesh or other prosthesis
➜ *CPT Assistant* Feb 12:3; *CPT Changes: An Insider's View* 2011

43337   with implantation of mesh or other prosthesis
➜ *CPT Assistant* Feb 12:3; *CPT Changes: An Insider's View* 2011

(For neonatal diaphragmatic hernia repair, use 39503)

+ 43338 Esophageal lengthening procedure (eg, Collis gastroplasty or wedge gastroplasty) (List separately in addition to code for primary procedure)
➜ *CPT Assistant* Jun 11:10, Feb 12:3; *CPT Changes: An Insider's View* 2011

(Use 43338 in conjunction with 43280, 43327-43337)

43340 Esophagojejunostomy (without total gastrectomy); abdominal approach

43341   thoracic approach

43350 Esophagostomy, fistulization of esophagus, external; abdominal approach

43351   thoracic approach

43352   cervical approach

43360 Gastrointestinal reconstruction for previous esophagectomy, for obstructing esophageal lesion or fistula, or for previous esophageal exclusion; with stomach, with or without pyloroplasty

---

43361   with colon interposition or small intestine reconstruction, including intestine mobilization, preparation, and anastomosis(es)
→ *CPT Changes: An Insider's View* 2002

43400   Ligation, direct, esophageal varices

43401   Transection of esophagus with repair, for esophageal varices

43405   Ligation or stapling at gastroesophageal junction for pre-existing esophageal perforation

43410   Suture of esophageal wound or injury; cervical approach
→ *CPT Assistant* Jun 96:7

43415   transthoracic or transabdominal approach

43420   Closure of esophagostomy or fistula; cervical approach

43425   transthoracic or transabdominal approach

(To report transabdominal paraesophageal hiatal hernia repair, see 43332, 43333. To report transthoracic diaphragmatic hernia repair, see 43334, 43335)

Manipulation

(For associated esophagogram, use 74220)

43450   Dilation of esophagus, by unguided sound or bougie, single or multiple passes
→ *CPT Assistant* Spring 94:1, Jan 97:10, Apr 98:14, Jun 98:10

(For radiological supervision and interpretation, use 74360)

⊙ **43453**   Dilation of esophagus, over guide wire
→ *CPT Assistant* Spring 94:1, Jan 97:10, Dec 97:11

(For dilation with direct visualization, use 43220)

(For dilation of esophagus, by balloon or dilator, see 43220, 43458, and 74360)

(For radiological supervision and interpretation, use 74360)

⊙ **43456**   Dilation of esophagus, by balloon or dilator, retrograde
→ *CPT Assistant* Spring 94:3, Jan 97:10, May 05:3

(For radiological supervision and interpretation, use 74360)

⊙ **43458**   Dilation of esophagus with balloon (30 mm diameter or larger) for achalasia
→ *CPT Assistant* Spring 94:3, Jan 97:10, May 05:3

(For dilation with balloon less than 30 mm diameter, use 43220)

(For radiological supervision and interpretation, use 74360)

43460   Esophagogastric tamponade, with balloon (Sengstaken type)
→ *CPT Changes: An Insider's View* 2009

(For removal of esophageal foreign body by balloon catheter, see 43215, 43247, 74235)

Other Procedures

43496   Free jejunum transfer with microvascular anastomosis
→ *CPT Assistant* Nov 96:8, Apr 97:4, Jun 97:10, Nov 97:17, Nov 98:16

(Do not report code 69990 in addition to code 43496)

43499   Unlisted procedure, esophagus
→ *CPT Assistant* May 07:10, Oct 10:12, Dec 10:12, May 11:9, Dec 11:19

Stomach

Incision

43500   Gastrotomy; with exploration or foreign body removal

43501   with suture repair of bleeding ulcer

43502   with suture repair of pre-existing esophagogastric laceration (eg, Mallory-Weiss)

43510   with esophageal dilation and insertion of permanent intraluminal tube (eg, Celestin or Mousseaux-Barbin)

43520   Pyloromyotomy, cutting of pyloric muscle (Fredet-Ramstedt type operation)

(Do not report modifier 63 in conjunction with 43520)

Excision

(43600 has been deleted)

43605   Biopsy of stomach, by laparotomy
→ *CPT Changes: An Insider's View* 2011

43610   Excision, local; ulcer or benign tumor of stomach

43611   malignant tumor of stomach

43620   Gastrectomy, total; with esophagoenterostomy

43621   with Roux-en-Y reconstruction

43622   with formation of intestinal pouch, any type

43631   Gastrectomy, partial, distal; with gastroduodenostomy

43632   with gastrojejunostomy

43633   with Roux-en-Y reconstruction

43634   with formation of intestinal pouch

+ **43635**   Vagotomy when performed with partial distal gastrectomy (List separately in addition to code[s] for primary procedure)
→ *CPT Assistant* Nov 97:17

(Use 43635 in conjunction with 43631, 43632, 43633, 43634)

43640   Vagotomy including pyloroplasty, with or without gastrostomy; truncal or selective

(For pyloroplasty, use 43800)

(For vagotomy, see 64752-64760)

43641   parietal cell (highly selective)

►(For upper gastrointestinal endoscopy, see 43235-43259)◄

Digestive

Laparoscopy

Surgical laparoscopy always includes diagnostic laparoscopy. To report a diagnostic laparoscopy (peritoneoscopy) (separate procedure), use 49320.

(For upper gastrointestinal endoscopy including esophagus, stomach, and either the duodenum and/or jejunum, see 43235-43259)

43644 Laparoscopy, surgical, gastric restrictive procedure; with gastric bypass and Roux-en-Y gastroenterostomy (roux limb 150 cm or less)

➲ *CPT Assistant* May 05:3; *CPT Changes: An Insider's View* 2005

(Do not report 43644 in conjunction with 43846, 49320)

(Esophagogastroduodenoscopy [EGD] performed for a separate condition should be reported with modifier 59)

(For greater than 150 cm, use 43645)

(For open procedure, use 43846)

43645 with gastric bypass and small intestine reconstruction to limit absorption

➲ *CPT Assistant* May 05:3; *CPT Changes: An Insider's View* 2005

(Do not report 43645 in conjunction with 49320, 43847)

43647 Laparoscopy, surgical; implantation or replacement of gastric neurostimulator electrodes, antrum

➲ *CPT Assistant* Mar 07:4; *CPT Changes: An Insider's View* 2007

43648 revision or removal of gastric neurostimulator electrodes, antrum

➲ *CPT Assistant* Mar 07:4; *CPT Changes: An Insider's View* 2007

(For open approach, see 43881, 43882)

(For insertion of gastric neurostimulator pulse generator, use 64590)

(For revision or removal of gastric neurostimulator pulse generator, use 64595)

(For electronic analysis and programming of gastric neurostimulator pulse generator, see 95980-95982)

(For laparoscopic implantation, revision, or removal of gastric neurostimulator electrodes, lesser curvature [morbid obesity], use 43659)

►(For laparoscopic implantation, revision, replacement, or removal of vagus nerve blocking neurostimulator electrode array and/or pulse generator at the esophagogastric junction, see 0312T-0317T)◄

43651 Laparoscopy, surgical; transection of vagus nerves, truncal

➲ *CPT Assistant* Nov 99:22, Mar 00:8; *CPT Changes: An Insider's View* 2000

43652 transection of vagus nerves, selective or highly selective

➲ *CPT Assistant* Nov 99:22, Mar 00:8; *CPT Changes: An Insider's View* 2000

43653 gastrostomy, without construction of gastric tube (eg, Stamm procedure) (separate procedure)

➲ *CPT Assistant* Nov 99:22, Mar 00:8; *CPT Changes: An Insider's View* 2000

43659 Unlisted laparoscopy procedure, stomach

➲ *CPT Assistant* Nov 99:22, Mar 00:8, Apr 06:19, Jun 06:16, Dec 07:12, Jun 11:8, Dec 11:19; *CPT Changes: An Insider's View* 2000

Introduction

43752 Naso- or oro-gastric tube placement, requiring physician's skill and fluoroscopic guidance (includes fluoroscopy, image documentation and report)

➲ *CPT Assistant* Jan 02:11, Apr 03:7, Oct 03:2, Jul 06:4, Feb 07:10, Jul 07:1, Aug 08:7, Sep 11:4; *CPT Changes: An Insider's View* 2001, 2004

(Do not report 43752 in conjunction with critical care codes 99291-99292, neonatal critical care codes 99468, 99469, pediatric critical care codes 99471, 99472 or low birth weight intensive care service codes 99478, 99479)

(For percutaneous placement of gastrostomy tube, use 49440)

(For enteric tube placement, see 44500, 74340)

Gastric Intubation
43753

A large-bore gastric lavage tube is inserted orally through the esophagus into the stomach for expedient lavage and evacuation of stomach contents (eg, poisonings, hemorrhage).

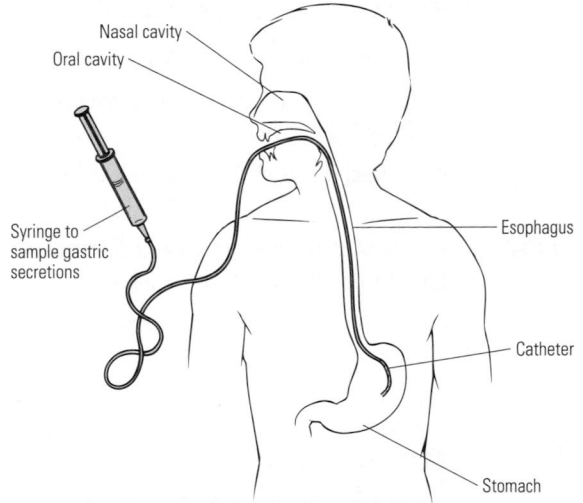

43753 Gastric intubation and aspiration(s) therapeutic, necessitating physician's skill (eg, for gastrointestinal hemorrhage), including lavage if performed

➲ *CPT Assistant* Sep 11:3; *CPT Changes: An Insider's View* 2011

43754 Gastric intubation and aspiration, diagnostic; single specimen (eg, acid analysis)

➲ *CPT Assistant* Dec 10:10, Sep 11:3; *CPT Changes: An Insider's View* 2011

43755 collection of multiple fractional specimens with gastric stimulation, single or double lumen tube (gastric secretory study) (eg, histamine, insulin, pentagastrin, calcium, secretin), includes drug administration

➔ *CPT Assistant* Dec 10:10, Sep 11:3; *CPT Changes: An Insider's View* 2011

(For gastric acid analysis, use 82930)

(For naso- or oro-gastric tube placement by physician with fluoroscopic guidance, use 43752)

(Report the drug[s] or substance[s] administered. The fluid used to administer the drug[s] is not separately reported)

43756 Duodenal intubation and aspiration, diagnostic, includes image guidance; single specimen (eg, bile study for crystals or afferent loop culture)

➔ *CPT Assistant* Dec 10:10, Sep 11:3; *CPT Changes: An Insider's View* 2011

43757 collection of multiple fractional specimens with pancreatic or gallbladder stimulation, single or double lumen tube, includes drug administration

➔ *CPT Assistant* Dec 10:10, Sep 11:3; *CPT Changes: An Insider's View* 2011

(For appropriate chemical analysis procedures, see 89049-89240)

(Report the substances[s] or drug[s] administered. The fluid used to administer the drug[s] is not separately reported)

43760 Change of gastrostomy tube, percutaneous, without imaging or endoscopic guidance

➔ *CPT Assistant* Apr 08:11, Aug 08:7, Sep 10:9; *CPT Changes: An Insider's View* 2008

(To report fluoroscopically guided replacement of gastrostomy tube, use 49450)

(For endoscopic placement of gastrostomy tube, use 43246)

43761 Repositioning of a naso- or oro-gastric feeding tube, through the duodenum for enteric nutrition

➔ *CPT Assistant* Oct 96:9, Nov 99:22, Jun 08:8, Aug 08:7; *CPT Changes: An Insider's View* 2000, 2008, 2010

(Do not report 43761 in conjunction with 44500, 49446)

(If imaging guidance is performed, use 76000)

(For endoscopic conversion of a gastrostomy tube to jejunostomy tube, use 44373)

(For placement of a long gastrointestinal tube into the duodenum, use 44500)

Bariatric Surgery

Bariatric surgical procedures may involve the stomach, duodenum, jejunum, and/or the ileum.

Laparoscopy

Surgical laparoscopy always includes diagnostic laparoscopy. To report a diagnostic laparoscopy (separate procedure), use 49320.

Typical postoperative follow-up care (see Surgery Guidelines, CPT Surgical Package Definition) after gastric restriction using the adjustable gastric restrictive device includes subsequent restrictive device adjustment(s) through the postoperative period for the typical patient. Adjustment consists of changing the gastric restrictive device component diameter by injection or aspiration of fluid through the subcutaneous port component.

43770 Laparoscopy, surgical, gastric restrictive procedure; placement of adjustable gastric restrictive device (eg, gastric band and subcutaneous port components)

➔ *CPT Assistant* Dec 10:13; *CPT Changes: An Insider's View* 2006, 2008

(For individual component placement, report 43770 with modifier 52)

43771 revision of adjustable gastric restrictive device component only

➔ *CPT Changes: An Insider's View* 2006, 2008

43772 removal of adjustable gastric restrictive device component only

➔ *CPT Changes: An Insider's View* 2006, 2008

43773 removal and replacement of adjustable gastric restrictive device component only

➔ *CPT Changes: An Insider's View* 2006, 2008

(Do not report 43773 in conjunction with 43772)

43774 removal of adjustable gastric restrictive device and subcutaneous port components

➔ *CPT Changes: An Insider's View* 2006, 2008

(For removal and replacement of both gastric band and subcutaneous port components, use 43659)

43775 longitudinal gastrectomy (ie, sleeve gastrectomy)

➔ *CPT Changes: An Insider's View* 2010

(For open gastric restrictive procedure, without gastric bypass, for morbid obesity, other than vertical-banded gastroplasty, use 43843)

▶(For laparoscopic implantation, revision, replacement, removal or reprogramming of vagus nerve blocking neurostimulator electrode array and/or pulse generator at the esophagogastric junction, see 0312T-0317T)◀

Other Procedures

43800   Pyloroplasty

(For pyloroplasty and vagotomy, use 43640)

43810   Gastroduodenostomy

43820   Gastrojejunostomy; without vagotomy

43825   with vagotomy, any type

43830   Gastrostomy, open; without construction of gastric tube (eg, Stamm procedure) (separate procedure)
→ *CPT Assistant* Nov 99:22; *CPT Changes: An Insider's View* 2000

43831   neonatal, for feeding
→ *CPT Assistant* Nov 99:22; *CPT Changes: An Insider's View* 2000

(For change of gastrostomy tube, use 43760)

(Do not report modifier 63 in conjunction with 43831)

43832   with construction of gastric tube (eg, Janeway procedure)
→ *CPT Assistant* Nov 99:22; *CPT Changes: An Insider's View* 2000

(For percutaneous endoscopic gastrostomy, use 43246)

43840   Gastrorrhaphy, suture of perforated duodenal or gastric ulcer, wound, or injury

43842   Gastric restrictive procedure, without gastric bypass, for morbid obesity; vertical-banded gastroplasty
→ *CPT Assistant* May 98:5

43843   other than vertical-banded gastroplasty
→ *CPT Assistant* May 98:5

(For laparoscopic longitudinal gastrectomy [ie, sleeve gastrectomy], use 43775)

43845   Gastric restrictive procedure with partial gastrectomy, pylorus-preserving duodenoileostomy and ileoileostomy (50 to 100 cm common channel) to limit absorption (biliopancreatic diversion with duodenal switch)
→ *CPT Assistant* May 05:3; *CPT Changes: An Insider's View* 2005

(Do not report 43845 in conjunction with 43633, 43847, 44130, 49000)

43846   Gastric restrictive procedure, with gastric bypass for morbid obesity; with short limb (150 cm or less) Roux-en-Y gastroenterostomy
→ *CPT Assistant* May 98:5, May 05:3; *CPT Changes: An Insider's View* 2005

(For greater than 150 cm, use 43847)

(For laparoscopic procedure, use 43644)

43847   with small intestine reconstruction to limit absorption
→ *CPT Assistant* May 98:5, May 02:7; *CPT Changes: An Insider's View* 2002

43848   Revision, open, of gastric restrictive procedure for morbid obesity, other than adjustable gastric restrictive device (separate procedure)
→ *CPT Assistant* May 98:5, Apr 06:1; *CPT Changes: An Insider's View* 2006, 2008

Gastric Bypass for Morbid Obesity
43846

The stomach is partitioned with a staple line on the lesser curvature (no band, no gastric transection). A short limb of small bowel (less than 100 cm) is divided and anastomosed to the small upper stomach pouch.

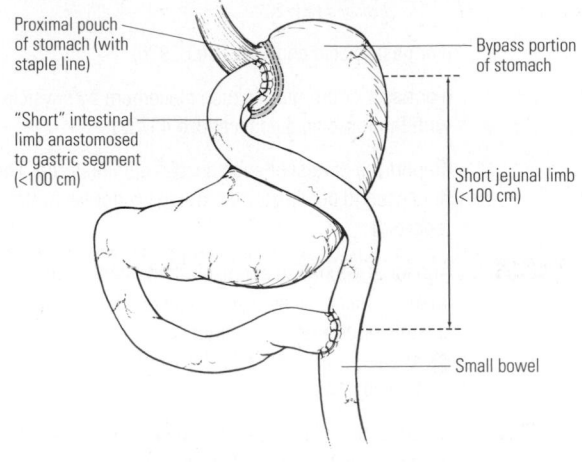

Proximal pouch of stomach (with staple line)

"Short" intestinal limb anastomosed to gastric segment (<100 cm)

Bypass portion of stomach

Short jejunal limb (<100 cm)

Small bowel

(For laparoscopic adjustable gastric restrictive procedures, see 43770-43774)

(For gastric restrictive port procedures, see 43886-43888)

43850   Revision of gastroduodenal anastomosis (gastroduodenostomy) with reconstruction; without vagotomy

43855   with vagotomy

43860   Revision of gastrojejunal anastomosis (gastrojejunostomy) with reconstruction, with or without partial gastrectomy or intestine resection; without vagotomy
→ *CPT Changes: An Insider's View* 2002

43865   with vagotomy

43870   Closure of gastrostomy, surgical

43880   Closure of gastrocolic fistula

43881   Implantation or replacement of gastric neurostimulator electrodes, antrum, open
→ *CPT Assistant* Mar 07:4; *CPT Changes: An Insider's View* 2007

43882   Revision or removal of gastric neurostimulator electrodes, antrum, open
→ *CPT Assistant* Mar 07:4; *CPT Changes: An Insider's View* 2007

(For laparoscopic approach, see 43647, 43648)

(For insertion of gastric neurostimulator pulse generator, use 64590)

(For revision or removal of gastric neurostimulator pulse generator, use 64595)

(For electronic analysis and programming of gastric neurostimulator pulse generator, see 95980-95982)

Digestive

(For open implantation, revision, or removal of gastric neurostimulator electrodes, lesser curvature [morbid obesity], use 43999)

►(For laparoscopic implantation, revision, replacement, removal or reprogramming of vagus nerve blocking neurostimulator electrode array and/or pulse generator at the esophagogastric junction, see 0312T-0317T)◄

►(For open implantation, revision, or removal of gastric lesser curvature or vagal trunk (EGJ) neurostimulator electrodes, [morbid obesity], use 43999)◄

43886   Gastric restrictive procedure, open; revision of subcutaneous port component only
➔ *CPT Changes: An Insider's View* 2006

43887   removal of subcutaneous port component only
➔ *CPT Changes: An Insider's View* 2006

43888   removal and replacement of subcutaneous port component only
➔ *CPT Changes: An Insider's View* 2006

(Do not report 43888 in conjunction with 43774, 43887)

(For laparoscopic removal of both gastric restrictive device and subcutaneous port components, use 43774)

(For removal and replacement of both gastric restrictive device and subcutaneous port components, use 43659)

43999   Unlisted procedure, stomach
➔ *CPT Assistant* Mar 10:10, Jun 11:13

Intestines (Except Rectum)

Incision

44005   Enterolysis (freeing of intestinal adhesion) (separate procedure)
➔ *CPT Assistant* Winter 90:6, Nov 97:17, Nov 99:23, Jan 00:11, Apr 00:10; *CPT Changes: An Insider's View* 2000

(Do not report 44005 in addition to 45136)

(For laparoscopic approach, use 44180)

44010   Duodenotomy, for exploration, biopsy(s), or foreign body removal

+ 44015   Tube or needle catheter jejunostomy for enteral alimentation, intraoperative, any method (List separately in addition to primary procedure)
➔ *CPT Assistant* Mar 02:10, Jul 10:10

44020   Enterotomy, small intestine, other than duodenum; for exploration, biopsy(s), or foreign body removal
➔ *CPT Changes: An Insider's View* 2002

44021   for decompression (eg, Baker tube)

44025   Colotomy, for exploration, biopsy(s), or foreign body removal

(For exteriorization of intestine (Mikulicz resection with crushing of spur), see 44602-44605)

44050   Reduction of volvulus, intussusception, internal hernia, by laparotomy

44055   Correction of malrotation by lysis of duodenal bands and/or reduction of midgut volvulus (eg, Ladd procedure)

(Do not report modifier 63 in conjunction with 44055)

Excision

Intestinal allotransplantation involves three distinct components of physician work:

1. ***Cadaver donor enterectomy,*** which includes harvesting the intestine graft and cold preservation of the graft (perfusing with cold preservation solution and cold maintenance) (use 44132). ***Living donor enterectomy,*** which includes harvesting the intestine graft, cold preservation of the graft (perfusing with cold preservation solution and cold maintenance), and care of the donor (use 44133).

2. ***Backbench work:***

   Standard preparation of an intestine allograft prior to transplantation includes mobilization and fashioning of the superior mesenteric artery and vein (see 44715).

   Additional reconstruction of an intestine allograft prior to transplantation may include venous and/or arterial anastomosis(es) (see 44720-44721).

3. ***Recipient intestinal allotransplantation with or without recipient enterectomy,*** which includes transplantation of allograft and care of the recipient (see 44135, 44136).

44100   Biopsy of intestine by capsule, tube, peroral (1 or more specimens)

44110   Excision of 1 or more lesions of small or large intestine not requiring anastomosis, exteriorization, or fistulization; single enterotomy
➔ *CPT Changes: An Insider's View* 2002

44111   multiple enterotomies

44120   Enterectomy, resection of small intestine; single resection and anastomosis
➔ *CPT Assistant* Mar 04:3, Aug 08:7

(Do not report 44120 in addition to 45136)

+ 44121   each additional resection and anastomosis (List separately in addition to code for primary procedure)

(Use 44121 in conjunction with 44120)

44125   with enterostomy

44126   Enterectomy, resection of small intestine for congenital atresia, single resection and anastomosis of proximal segment of intestine; without tapering

➔ *CPT Changes: An Insider's View* 2002

44127   with tapering

➔ *CPT Changes: An Insider's View* 2002

Enterectomy, Resection for Congenital Atresia
44127

+ 44128   each additional resection and anastomosis (List separately in addition to code for primary procedure)

➔ *CPT Changes: An Insider's View* 2002

(Use 44128 in conjunction with 44126, 44127)

(Do not report modifier 63 in conjunction with 44126, 44127, 44128)

44130   Enteroenterostomy, anastomosis of intestine, with or without cutaneous enterostomy (separate procedure)

44132   Donor enterectomy (including cold preservation), open; from cadaver donor

➔ *CPT Changes: An Insider's View* 2001, 2005

44133   partial, from living donor

➔ *CPT Changes: An Insider's View* 2001

(For backbench intestinal graft preparation or reconstruction, see 44715, 44720, 44721)

44135   Intestinal allotransplantation; from cadaver donor

➔ *CPT Changes: An Insider's View* 2001

44136   from living donor

➔ *CPT Changes: An Insider's View* 2001

44137   Removal of transplanted intestinal allograft, complete

➔ *CPT Changes: An Insider's View* 2005

(For partial removal of transplant allograft, see 44120, 44121, 44140)

+ 44139   Mobilization (take-down) of splenic flexure performed in conjunction with partial colectomy (List separately in addition to primary procedure)

(Use 44139 in conjunction with 44140-44147)

44140   Colectomy, partial; with anastomosis

➔ *CPT Assistant* Fall 92:23, Aug 08:7, Nov 08:7, Sep 10:7

(For laparoscopic procedure, use 44204)

Colectomy, Partial
44140

A segment of the colon is resected and an anastomosis is performed between the remaining ends of the colon.

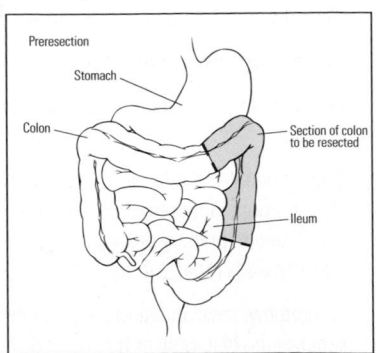

44141   with skin level cecostomy or colostomy

➔ *CPT Assistant* Fall 92:24, Nov 08:7

44143   with end colostomy and closure of distal segment (Hartmann type procedure)

➔ *CPT Assistant* Fall 92:24, Nov 08:7

(For laparoscopic procedure, use 44206)

44144   with resection, with colostomy or ileostomy and creation of mucofistula
> *CPT Assistant* Fall 92:24, Nov 08:7

44145   with coloproctostomy (low pelvic anastomosis)
> *CPT Assistant* Fall 92:24

(For laparoscopic procedure, use 44207)

44146   with coloproctostomy (low pelvic anastomosis), with colostomy
> *CPT Assistant* Fall 92:24, Nov 08:7

(For laparoscopic procedure, use 44208)

44147   abdominal and transanal approach
> *CPT Assistant* Fall 92:24, Nov 08:7

44150   Colectomy, total, abdominal, without proctectomy; with ileostomy or ileoproctostomy

(For laparoscopic procedure, use 44210)

44151   with continent ileostomy

44155   Colectomy, total, abdominal, with proctectomy; with ileostomy

(For laparoscopic procedure, use 44212)

44156   with continent ileostomy

44157   with ileoanal anastomosis, includes loop ileostomy, and rectal mucosectomy, when performed
> *CPT Changes: An Insider's View* 2007

44158   with ileoanal anastomosis, creation of ileal reservoir (S or J), includes loop ileostomy, and rectal mucosectomy, when performed
> *CPT Changes: An Insider's View* 2007

(For laparoscopic procedure, use 44211)

44160   Colectomy, partial, with removal of terminal ileum with ileocolostomy
> *CPT Changes: An Insider's View* 2002

(For laparoscopic procedure, use 44205)

Laparoscopy

Surgical laparoscopy always includes diagnostic laparoscopy. To report a diagnostic laparoscopy (peritoneoscopy) (separate procedure), use 49320.

Incision

44180   Laparoscopy, surgical, enterolysis (freeing of intestinal adhesion) (separate procedure)
> *CPT Changes: An Insider's View* 2006

(For laparoscopy with salpingolysis, ovariolysis, use 58660)

Colectomy With Removal of Terminal Ileum and Ileocolostomy
44160

A segment of the colon and terminal ileum is removed and an anastomosis is performed between the remaining ileum and colon.

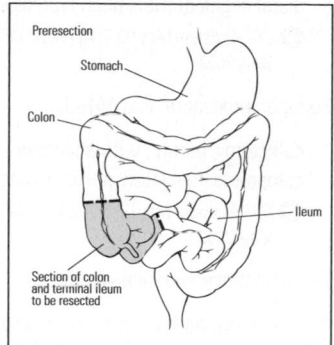

Enterostomy—External Fistulization of Intestines

44186   Laparoscopy, surgical; jejunostomy (eg, for decompression or feeding)
> *CPT Changes: An Insider's View* 2006

44187   ileostomy or jejunostomy, non-tube
> *CPT Changes: An Insider's View* 2006

(For open procedure, use 44310)

44188   Laparoscopy, surgical, colostomy or skin level cecostomy
> *CPT Changes: An Insider's View* 2006

(For open procedure, use 44320)

(Do not report 44188 in conjunction with 44970)

Excision

44202   Laparoscopy, surgical; enterectomy, resection of small intestine, single resection and anastomosis
> *CPT Assistant* Nov 99:23, Mar 00:9, May 03:2, Apr 06:1; *CPT Changes: An Insider's View* 2000, 2002, 2006

Digestive

+ 44203 each additional small intestine resection and anastomosis (List separately in addition to code for primary procedure)

➔ *CPT Assistant* May 03:2; *CPT Changes: An Insider's View* 2002

(Use 44203 in conjunction with 44202)

(For open procedure, see 44120, 44121)

44204 colectomy, partial, with anastomosis

➔ *CPT Assistant* May 03:3, Apr 06:1, 19; *CPT Changes: An Insider's View* 2002

(For open procedure, use 44140)

44205 colectomy, partial, with removal of terminal ileum with ileocolostomy

➔ *CPT Assistant* May 03:3, Apr 06:1; *CPT Changes: An Insider's View* 2002

(For open procedure, use 44160)

44206 colectomy, partial, with end colostomy and closure of distal segment (Hartmann type procedure)

➔ *CPT Assistant* May 03:3, Apr 06:1; *CPT Changes: An Insider's View* 2003

(For open procedure, use 44143)

44207 colectomy, partial, with anastomosis, with coloproctostomy (low pelvic anastomosis)

➔ *CPT Assistant* May 03:3, Apr 06:1; *CPT Changes: An Insider's View* 2003

(For open procedure, use 44145)

44208 colectomy, partial, with anastomosis, with coloproctostomy (low pelvic anastomosis) with colostomy

➔ *CPT Assistant* May 03:3, Apr 06:1; *CPT Changes: An Insider's View* 2003

(For open procedure, use 44146)

44210 colectomy, total, abdominal, without proctectomy, with ileostomy or ileoproctostomy

➔ *CPT Assistant* May 03:3; *CPT Changes: An Insider's View* 2003

(For open procedure, use 44150)

44211 colectomy, total, abdominal, with proctectomy, with ileoanal anastomosis, creation of ileal reservoir (S or J), with loop ileostomy, includes rectal mucosectomy, when performed

➔ *CPT Assistant* May 03:3; *CPT Changes: An Insider's View* 2003, 2007

(For open procedure, see 44157, 44158)

44212 colectomy, total, abdominal, with proctectomy, with ileostomy

➔ *CPT Assistant* May 03:3; *CPT Changes: An Insider's View* 2003

(For open procedure, use 44155)

+ 44213 Laparoscopy, surgical, mobilization (take-down) of splenic flexure performed in conjunction with partial colectomy (List separately in addition to primary procedure)

➔ *CPT Changes: An Insider's View* 2006

(Use 44213 in conjunction with 44204-44208)

(For open procedure, use 44139)

Repair

44227 Laparoscopy, surgical, closure of enterostomy, large or small intestine, with resection and anastomosis

➔ *CPT Changes: An Insider's View* 2006

(For open procedure, see 44625, 44626)

Other Procedures

44238 Unlisted laparoscopy procedure, intestine (except rectum)

➔ *CPT Assistant* May 03:4; *CPT Changes: An Insider's View* 2003

Enterostomy—External Fistulization of Intestines

44300 Placement, enterostomy or cecostomy, tube open (eg, for feeding or decompression) (separate procedure)

➔ *CPT Assistant* Mar 02:10, Aug 08:7; *CPT Changes: An Insider's View* 2008

(For percutaneous placement of duodenostomy, jejunostomy, gastro-jejunostomy or cecostomy [or other colonic] tube including fluoroscopic imaging guidance, see 49441-49442)

44310 Ileostomy or jejunostomy, non-tube

➔ *CPT Assistant* Mar 02:10, Apr 06:1; *CPT Changes: An Insider's View* 2006

(For laparoscopic procedure, use 44187)

(Do not report 44310 in conjunction with 44144, 44150-44151, 44155, 44156, 45113, 45119, 45136)

44312 Revision of ileostomy; simple (release of superficial scar) (separate procedure)

➔ *CPT Assistant* Spring 93:35

44314 complicated (reconstruction in-depth) (separate procedure)

44316 Continent ileostomy (Kock procedure) (separate procedure)

(For fiberoptic evaluation, use 44385)

44320 Colostomy or skin level cecostomy;

➔ *CPT Changes: An Insider's View* 2006

(For laparoscopic procedure, use 44188)

(Do not report 44320 in conjunction with 44141, 44144, 44146, 44605, 45110, 45119, 45126, 45563, 45805, 45825, 50810, 51597, 57307, or 58240)

44322   with multiple biopsies (eg, for congenital megacolon) (separate procedure)

→ *CPT Changes: An Insider's View* 2002

44340   Revision of colostomy; simple (release of superficial scar) (separate procedure)

44345   complicated (reconstruction in-depth) (separate procedure)

44346   with repair of paracolostomy hernia (separate procedure)

Endoscopy, Small Intestine and Stomal

Surgical endoscopy always includes diagnostic endoscopy.

▸(For upper gastrointestinal endoscopy, see 43235-43258)◂

⊙ 44360   Small intestinal endoscopy, enteroscopy beyond second portion of duodenum, not including ileum; diagnostic, with or without collection of specimen(s) by brushing or washing (separate procedure)

→ *CPT Assistant* Spring 94:7, Mar 11:10

⊙ 44361   with biopsy, single or multiple

⊙ 44363   with removal of foreign body

⊙ 44364   with removal of tumor(s), polyp(s), or other lesion(s) by snare technique

⊙ 44365   with removal of tumor(s), polyp(s), or other lesion(s) by hot biopsy forceps or bipolar cautery

⊙ 44366   with control of bleeding (eg, injection, bipolar cautery, unipolar cautery, laser, heater probe, stapler, plasma coagulator)

→ *CPT Assistant* Jun 10:4; *CPT Changes: An Insider's View* 2002

⊙ 44369   with ablation of tumor(s), polyp(s), or other lesion(s) not amenable to removal by hot biopsy forceps, bipolar cautery or snare technique

⊙ 44370   with transendoscopic stent placement (includes predilation)

→ *CPT Assistant* Nov 01:7; *CPT Changes: An Insider's View* 2001

⊙ 44372   with placement of percutaneous jejunostomy tube

→ *CPT Assistant* Spring 94:7

⊙ 44373   with conversion of percutaneous gastrostomy tube to percutaneous jejunostomy tube

→ *CPT Assistant* Spring 94:7

(For fiberoptic jejunostomy through stoma, use 43235)

⊙ 44376   Small intestinal endoscopy, enteroscopy beyond second portion of duodenum, including ileum; diagnostic, with or without collection of specimen(s) by brushing or washing (separate procedure)

→ *CPT Assistant* Spring 94:7, Mar 11:10

⊙ 44377   with biopsy, single or multiple

→ *CPT Assistant* Spring 94:7

⊙ 44378   with control of bleeding (eg, injection, bipolar cautery, unipolar cautery, laser, heater probe, stapler, plasma coagulator)

→ *CPT Assistant* Spring 94:7, Jun 10:4, Apr 12:17; *CPT Changes: An Insider's View* 2002

⊙ 44379   with transendoscopic stent placement (includes predilation)

→ *CPT Assistant* Nov 01:7; *CPT Changes: An Insider's View* 2001

⊙ 44380   Ileoscopy, through stoma; diagnostic, with or without collection of specimen(s) by brushing or washing (separate procedure)

⊙ 44382   with biopsy, single or multiple

⊙ 44383   with transendoscopic stent placement (includes predilation)

→ *CPT Assistant* Nov 01:7; *CPT Changes: An Insider's View* 2001

⊙ 44385   Endoscopic evaluation of small intestinal (abdominal or pelvic) pouch; diagnostic, with or without collection of specimen(s) by brushing or washing (separate procedure)

⊙ 44386   with biopsy, single or multiple

⊙ 44388   Colonoscopy through stoma; diagnostic, with or without collection of specimen(s) by brushing or washing (separate procedure)

→ *CPT Assistant* Nov 07:8

⊙ 44389   with biopsy, single or multiple

⊙ 44390   with removal of foreign body

⊙ 44391   with control of bleeding (eg, injection, bipolar cautery, unipolar cautery, laser, heater probe, stapler, plasma coagulator)

→ *CPT Assistant* Jun 10:4; *CPT Changes: An Insider's View* 2002

⊙ 44392   with removal of tumor(s), polyp(s), or other lesion(s) by hot biopsy forceps or bipolar cautery

⊙ 44393   with ablation of tumor(s), polyp(s), or other lesion(s) not amenable to removal by hot biopsy forceps, bipolar cautery or snare technique

⊙ 44394   with removal of tumor(s), polyp(s), or other lesion(s) by snare technique

(For colonoscopy per rectum, see 45330-45385)

⊙ 44397   with transendoscopic stent placement (includes predilation)

→ *CPT Assistant* Nov 01:7; *CPT Changes: An Insider's View* 2001

Introduction

⊙⊘ 44500   Introduction of long gastrointestinal tube (eg, Miller-Abbott) (separate procedure)

(For radiological supervision and interpretation, use 74340)

(For naso- or oro-gastric tube placement, use 43752)

Repair

44602 Suture of small intestine (enterorrhaphy) for perforated ulcer, diverticulum, wound, injury or rupture; single perforation

44603   multiple perforations

44604 Suture of large intestine (colorrhaphy) for perforated ulcer, diverticulum, wound, injury or rupture (single or multiple perforations); without colostomy

44605   with colostomy

44615 Intestinal stricturoplasty (enterotomy and enterorrhaphy) with or without dilation, for intestinal obstruction

44620 Closure of enterostomy, large or small Intestine;
➡ *CPT Assistant* Nov 97:17, May 02:7

44625   with resection and anastomosis other than colorectal
➡ *CPT Assistant* Nov 97:17

44626   with resection and colorectal anastomosis (eg, closure of Hartmann type procedure)
➡ *CPT Assistant* Nov 97:17

(For laparoscopic procedure, use 44227)

44640 Closure of intestinal cutaneous fistula

44650 Closure of enteroenteric or enterocolic fistula

44660 Closure of enterovesical fistula; without intestinal or bladder resection

44661   with intestine and/or bladder resection
➡ *CPT Changes: An Insider's View* 2002

(For closure of renocolic fistula, see 50525, 50526)

(For closure of gastrocolic fistula, use 43880)

(For closure of rectovesical fistula, see 45800, 45805)

44680 Intestinal plication (separate procedure)

Other Procedures

44700 Exclusion of small intestine from pelvis by mesh or other prosthesis, or native tissue (eg, bladder or omentum)
➡ *CPT Assistant* Nov 97:18; *CPT Changes: An Insider's View* 2002

(For therapeutic radiation clinical treatment, see **Radiation Oncology** section)

+ 44701 Intraoperative colonic lavage (List separately in addition to code for primary procedure)
➡ *CPT Changes: An Insider's View* 2003

(Use 44701 in conjunction with 44140, 44145, 44150, or 44604 as appropriate)

(Do not report 44701 in conjunction with 44300, 44950-44960)

● 44705 Preparation of fecal microbiota for instillation, including assessment of donor specimen
➡ *CPT Changes: An Insider's View* 2013

►(Do not report 44705 in conjunction with 74283)◄

►(For fecal instillation by oro-nasogastric tube or enema, use 44799)◄

44715 Backbench standard preparation of cadaver or living donor intestine allograft prior to transplantation, including mobilization and fashioning of the superior mesenteric artery and vein
➡ *CPT Changes: An Insider's View* 2005

44720 Backbench reconstruction of cadaver or living donor intestine allograft prior to transplantation; venous anastomosis, each
➡ *CPT Changes: An Insider's View* 2005

44721   arterial anastomosis, each
➡ *CPT Assistant* Apr 05:10-11; *CPT Changes: An Insider's View* 2005

44799 Unlisted procedure, intestine
➡ *CPT Assistant* Dec 00:14, May 08:15, Nov 08:11, Mar 10:10, Jul 10:10, Mar 11:10, May 11:9

(For unlisted laparoscopic procedure, intestine except rectum, use 44238)

Meckel's Diverticulum and the Mesentery

Excision

44800 Excision of Meckel's diverticulum (diverticulectomy) or omphalomesenteric duct

44820 Excision of lesion of mesentery (separate procedure)

(With intestine resection, see 44120 or 44140 et seq)

Suture

44850 Suture of mesentery (separate procedure)

(For reduction and repair of internal hernia, use 44050)

Other Procedures

44899 Unlisted procedure, Meckel's diverticulum and the mesentery

Appendix

Incision

44900 Incision and drainage of appendiceal abscess; open
➡ *CPT Assistant* Nov 97:18

⊙ 44901   percutaneous
➡ *CPT Assistant* Nov 97:18, Mar 98:8

(For radiological supervision and interpretation, use 75989)

Excision

44950   Appendectomy;
→ *CPT Assistant* February 92:22, Sep 96:4, Aug 02:2, Nov 08:7

(Incidental appendectomy during intra-abdominal surgery does not usually warrant a separate identification. If necessary to report, add modifier 52)

+ 44955   when done for indicated purpose at time of other major procedure (not as separate procedure) (List separately in addition to code for primary procedure)
→ *CPT Assistant* Fall 92:22, Sep 96:4, Apr 97:3, Nov 08:7, Jan 12:13

44960   for ruptured appendix with abscess or generalized peritonitis
→ *CPT Assistant* Fall 92:22, Nov 08:7

Laparoscopy

Surgical laparoscopy always includes diagnostic laparoscopy. To report a diagnostic laparoscopy (peritoneoscopy) (separate procedure), use 49320.

44970   Laparoscopy, surgical, appendectomy
→ *CPT Assistant* Nov 99:23, Mar 00:9, Apr 06:1, 20; *CPT Changes: An Insider's View* 2000

44979   Unlisted laparoscopy procedure, appendix
→ *CPT Assistant* Nov 99:23, Mar 00:9, Jan 12:13; *CPT Changes: An Insider's View* 2000

Rectum

Incision

45000   Transrectal drainage of pelvic abscess

45005   Incision and drainage of submucosal abscess, rectum

45020   Incision and drainage of deep supralevator, pelvirectal, or retrorectal abscess

(See also 46050, 46060)

Excision

45100   Biopsy of anorectal wall, anal approach (eg, congenital megacolon)

(For endoscopic biopsy, use 45305)

45108   Anorectal myomectomy

45110   Proctectomy; complete, combined abdominoperineal, with colostomy

(For laparoscopic procedure, use 45395)

45111   partial resection of rectum, transabdominal approach

45112   Proctectomy, combined abdominoperineal, pull-through procedure (eg, colo-anal anastomosis)
→ *CPT Assistant* Nov 97:18

(For colo-anal anastomosis with colonic reservoir or pouch, use 45119)

45113   Proctectomy, partial, with rectal mucosectomy, ileoanal anastomosis, creation of ileal reservoir (S or J), with or without loop ileostomy

45114   Proctectomy, partial, with anastomosis; abdominal and transsacral approach

45116   transsacral approach only (Kraske type)

45119   Proctectomy, combined abdominoperineal pull-through procedure (eg, colo-anal anastomosis), with creation of colonic reservoir (eg, J-pouch), with diverting enterostomy when performed
→ *CPT Assistant* Nov 97:18, Apr 06:1; *CPT Changes: An Insider's View* 2006

(For laparoscopic procedure, use 45397)

45120   Proctectomy, complete (for congenital megacolon), abdominal and perineal approach; with pull-through procedure and anastomosis (eg, Swenson, Duhamel, or Soave type operation)

45121   with subtotal or total colectomy, with multiple biopsies

45123   Proctectomy, partial, without anastomosis, perineal approach

45126   Pelvic exenteration for colorectal malignancy, with proctectomy (with or without colostomy), with removal of bladder and ureteral transplantations, and/or hysterectomy, or cervicectomy, with or without removal of tube(s), with or without removal of ovary(s), or any combination thereof
→ *CPT Assistant* Nov 98:16

45130   Excision of rectal procidentia, with anastomosis; perineal approach

45135   abdominal and perineal approach

45136   Excision of ileoanal reservoir with ileostomy
→ *CPT Changes: An Insider's View* 2002

(Do not report 45136 in addition to 44005, 44120, 44310)

45150   Division of stricture of rectum

45160   Excision of rectal tumor by proctotomy, transsacral or transcoccygeal approach

(45170 has been deleted. To report excision of rectal tumor, transanal approach, see 45171, 45172)

45171   Excision of rectal tumor, transanal approach; not including muscularis propria (ie, partial thickness)
→ *CPT Assistant* Jun 10:3; *CPT Changes: An Insider's View* 2010

45172   including muscularis propria (ie, full thickness)

➔ *CPT Assistant* Jun 10:3; *CPT Changes: An Insider's View* 2010

(For destruction of rectal tumor, transanal approach, use 45190)

(For transanal endoscopic microsurgical [ie, TEMS] excision of rectal tumor, including muscularis propria [ie, full thickness], use 0184T)

Rectal Tumor Excision
45171-45172

A rectal tumor is excised via transanal approach.

Destruction

45190   Destruction of rectal tumor (eg, electrodesiccation, electrosurgery, laser ablation, laser resection, cryosurgery) transanal approach

➔ *CPT Assistant* Jun 10:3; *CPT Changes: An Insider's View* 2002

(For excision of rectal tumor, transanal approach, see 45171, 45172)

(For transanal endoscopic microsurgical [ie, TEMS] excision of rectal tumor, including muscularis propria [ie, full thickness], use 0184T)

Endoscopy

Definitions

Proctosigmoidoscopy is the examination of the rectum and sigmoid colon.

Sigmoidoscopy is the examination of the entire rectum, sigmoid colon and may include examination of a portion of the descending colon.

Colonoscopy is the examination of the entire colon, from the rectum to the cecum, and may include the examination of the terminal ileum.

When performing an endoscopy on a patient who is scheduled and prepared for a total colonoscopy, if the physician is unable to advance the colonoscope beyond the splenic flexure, due to unforeseen circumstances, report the colonoscopy code with modifier 53 and appropriate documentation.

Surgical endoscopy always includes diagnostic endoscopy.

For computed tomographic colonography, see 74261-74263.

45300   Proctosigmoidoscopy, rigid; diagnostic, with or without collection of specimen(s) by brushing or washing (separate procedure)

➔ *CPT Assistant* Spring 94:8, Oct 97:6, Apr 06:1

⊙ **45303**   with dilation (eg, balloon, guide wire, bougie)

➔ *CPT Assistant* Spring 94:8, Oct 97:6, Apr 06:1; *CPT Changes: An Insider's View* 2002

(For radiological supervision and interpretation, use 74360)

⊙ **45305**   with biopsy, single or multiple

➔ *CPT Assistant* Spring 94:8, Oct 97:6, Apr 06:1

⊙ **45307**   with removal of foreign body

➔ *CPT Assistant* Spring 94:8, Oct 97:6, Apr 06:1

⊙ **45308**   with removal of single tumor, polyp, or other lesion by hot biopsy forceps or bipolar cautery

➔ *CPT Assistant* Spring 94:8, Oct 97:6, Apr 06:1

⊙ **45309**   with removal of single tumor, polyp, or other lesion by snare technique

➔ *CPT Assistant* Spring 94:8, Oct 97:6, Apr 06:1

⊙ **45315**   with removal of multiple tumors, polyps, or other lesions by hot biopsy forceps, bipolar cautery or snare technique

➔ *CPT Assistant* Spring 94:8, Oct 97:6, Apr 06:1

⊙ **45317**   with control of bleeding (eg, injection, bipolar cautery, unipolar cautery, laser, heater probe, stapler, plasma coagulator)

➔ *CPT Assistant* Spring 94:8, Oct 97:6, Apr 06:1; *CPT Changes: An Insider's View* 2002

⊙ **45320**   with ablation of tumor(s), polyp(s), or other lesion(s) not amenable to removal by hot biopsy forceps, bipolar cautery or snare technique (eg, laser)

➔ *CPT Assistant* Spring 94:8, Oct 97:6, Apr 06:1

⊙ **45321**   with decompression of volvulus

➔ *CPT Assistant* Spring 94:8, Oct 97:6, Apr 06:1

⊙ **45327**   with transendoscopic stent placement (includes predilation)

➔ *CPT Assistant* Nov 01:7, Apr 06:1; *CPT Changes: An Insider's View* 2001

—— Coding Tip ——

Definition of Sigmoidoscopy

Sigmoidoscopy is the examination of the entire rectum, sigmoid colon and may include examination of a portion of the descending colon.

CPT Coding Guidelines, Endoscopy

45330 Sigmoidoscopy, flexible; diagnostic, with or without collection of specimen(s) by brushing or washing (separate procedure)

➔ *CPT Assistant* Spring 94:9, May 05:3, May 07:10, Nov 07:8

45331 with biopsy, single or multiple

➔ *CPT Assistant* Spring 94:9, Sep 96:6, Jan 07:28

⊙ **45332** with removal of foreign body

➔ *CPT Assistant* Winter 90:3, Spring 94:9

⊙ **45333** with removal of tumor(s), polyp(s), or other lesion(s) by hot biopsy forceps or bipolar cautery

➔ *CPT Assistant* Winter 90:3, Spring 94:9

⊙ **45334** with control of bleeding (eg, injection, bipolar cautery, unipolar cautery, laser, heater probe, stapler, plasma coagulator)

➔ *CPT Assistant* Spring 94:9, Sep 96:6, Jan 07:28, Jun 10:5; *CPT Changes: An Insider's View* 2002

⊙ **45335** with directed submucosal injection(s), any substance

➔ *CPT Assistant* Mar 03:22, Jun 10:5; *CPT Changes: An Insider's View* 2003

⊙ **45337** with decompression of volvulus, any method

➔ *CPT Assistant* Spring 94:9

⊙ **45338** with removal of tumor(s), polyp(s), or other lesion(s) by snare technique

➔ *CPT Assistant* Spring 94:9

⊙ **45339** with ablation of tumor(s), polyp(s), or other lesion(s) not amenable to removal by hot biopsy forceps, bipolar cautery or snare technique

➔ *CPT Assistant* Spring 94:9

⊙ **45340** with dilation by balloon, 1 or more strictures

➔ *CPT Changes: An Insider's View* 2003

(Do not report 45340 in conjunction with 45345)

⊙ **45341** with endoscopic ultrasound examination

➔ *CPT Assistant* Oct 01:4, May 05:3; *CPT Changes: An Insider's View* 2001

⊙ **45342** with transendoscopic ultrasound guided intramural or transmural fine needle aspiration/biopsy(s)

➔ *CPT Assistant* Oct 01:4, May 05:3; *CPT Changes: An Insider's View* 2001

(Do not report 45341, 45342 in conjunction with 76942, 76975)

(For interpretation of specimen, see 88172-88173)

(For transrectal ultrasound utilizing rigid probe device, use 76872)

⊙ **45345** with transendoscopic stent placement (includes predilation)

➔ *CPT Assistant* Nov 01:7; *CPT Changes: An Insider's View* 2001

—— Coding Tip ——

Definition of Colonoscopy

Colonoscopy is the examination of the entire colon, from the rectum to the cecum, and may include the examination of the terminal ileum. When performing an endoscopy on a patient who is scheduled and prepared for a total colonoscopy, if the physician is unable to advance the colonoscope beyond the splenic flexure, due to unforeseen circumstances, report the colonoscopy code with modifier 53 and appropriate documentation.

CPT Coding Guidelines, Endoscopy

⊙ **45355** Colonoscopy, rigid or flexible, transabdominal via colotomy, single or multiple

(For fiberoptic colonoscopy beyond 25cm to splenic flexure, see 45330-45345)

⊙ **45378** Colonoscopy, flexible, proximal to splenic flexure; diagnostic, with or without collection of specimen(s) by brushing or washing, with or without colon decompression (separate procedure)

➔ *CPT Assistant* Spring 94:9, Aug 99:3, Jan 02:12, Jan 04:4, May 05:3, Dec 10:3, Apr 11:12

Colonoscopy
45378

A colonoscope is inserted in the anus and moved through the colon past the splenic flexure in order to visualize the lumen of the rectum and colon.

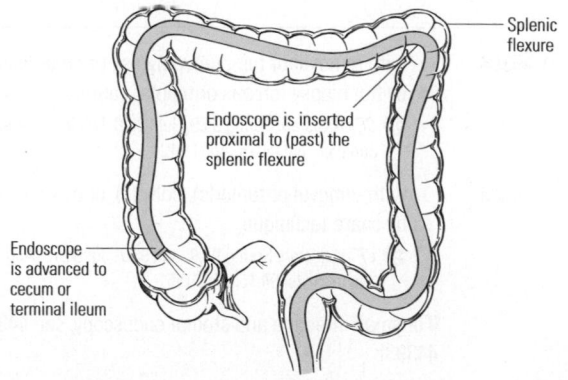

Splenic flexure

Endoscope is inserted proximal to (past) the splenic flexure

Endoscope is advanced to cecum or terminal ileum

⊙ **45379** with removal of foreign body

➔ *CPT Assistant* Spring 94:9, Aug 99:3

⊙ **45380** with biopsy, single or multiple

➔ *CPT Assistant* Spring 94:9, Jan 96:7, Feb 99:11, Aug 99:3, Jan 04:7, Jul 04:15

⊙ **45381** with directed submucosal injection(s), any substance

➔ *CPT Assistant* Mar 03:22, Jan 04:7, Jun 10:5; *CPT Changes: An Insider's View* 2003

⊙ **45382**   with control of bleeding (eg, injection, bipolar cautery, unipolar cautery, laser, heater probe, stapler, plasma coagulator)

➜ *CPT Assistant* Spring 94:9, Aug 99:3, Jun 10:5; *CPT Changes: An Insider's View* 2002

⊙ **45383**   with ablation of tumor(s), polyp(s), or other lesion(s) not amenable to removal by hot biopsy forceps, bipolar cautery or snare technique

➜ *CPT Assistant* Spring 94:9, Aug 99:3, Jan 04:4, Dec 10:3

Colonoscopy With Lesion Ablation or Removal
45383, 45385

Insertion and advancement of a colonoscope through the colon and past the splenic flexure for ablation (45383) or removal (45385) of tumors, polyps, or other lesions

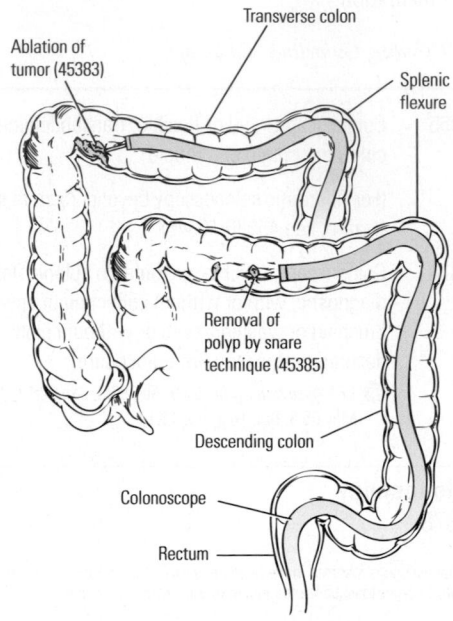

⊙ **45384**   with removal of tumor(s), polyp(s), or other lesion(s) by hot biopsy forceps or bipolar cautery

➜ *CPT Assistant* Spring 94:9, Jul 98:10, Feb 99:11, Aug 99:3, Jan 04:6, Jul 04:15, Apr 11:12

⊙ **45385**   with removal of tumor(s), polyp(s), or other lesion(s) by snare technique

➜ *CPT Assistant* Spring 94:9, Jan 96:7, Jul 98:10, Aug 99:3, Jan 04:5, Jul 04:15, Jun 10:5

(For small intestine and stomal endoscopy, see 44360-44393)

⊙ **45386**   with dilation by balloon, 1 or more strictures

➜ *CPT Changes: An Insider's View* 2003

(Do not report 45386 in conjunction with 45387)

⊙ **45387**   with transendoscopic stent placement (includes predilation)

➜ *CPT Assistant* Nov 01:7; *CPT Changes: An Insider's View* 2001

⊙ **45391**   with endoscopic ultrasound examination

➜ *CPT Assistant* May 05:3; *CPT Changes: An Insider's View* 2005

(Do not report 45391 in conjunction with 45330, 45341, 45342, 45378, 76872)

⊙ **45392**   with transendoscopic ultrasound guided intramural or transmural fine needle aspiration/biopsy(s)

➜ *CPT Assistant* May 05:3; *CPT Changes: An Insider's View* 2005

(Do not report 45392 in conjunction with 45330, 45341, 45342, 45378, 76872)

Laparoscopy

Surgical laparoscopy always includes diagnostic laparoscopy. To report a diagnostic laparoscopy (peritoneoscopy) (separate procedure), use 49320.

Excision

45395   Laparoscopy, surgical; proctectomy, complete, combined abdominoperineal, with colostomy

➜ *CPT Changes: An Insider's View* 2006

(For open procedure, use 45110)

45397   proctectomy, combined abdominoperineal pull-through procedure (eg, colo-anal anastomosis), with creation of colonic reservoir (eg, J-pouch), with diverting enterostomy, when performed

➜ *CPT Changes: An Insider's View* 2006

(For open procedure, use 45119)

Repair

45400   Laparoscopy, surgical; proctopexy (for prolapse)

➜ *CPT Changes: An Insider's View* 2006

(For open procedure, use 45540, 45541)

45402   proctopexy (for prolapse), with sigmoid resection

➜ *CPT Changes: An Insider's View* 2006

(For open procedure, use 45550)

45499   Unlisted laparoscopy procedure, rectum

➜ *CPT Changes: An Insider's View* 2006

Repair

45500   Proctoplasty; for stenosis

45505   for prolapse of mucous membrane

45520   Perirectal injection of sclerosing solution for prolapse

➜ *CPT Assistant* Jul 01:11, Aug 01:10

45540   Proctopexy (eg, for prolapse); abdominal approach

➜ *CPT Changes: An Insider's View* 2006

(For laparoscopic procedure, use 45400)

45541   perineal approach

45550   with sigmoid resection, abdominal approach

➜ *CPT Changes: An Insider's View* 2006

(For laparoscopic procedure, use 45402)

Digestive

45560	Repair of rectocele (separate procedure)

(For repair of rectocele with posterior colporrhaphy, use 57250)

45562	Exploration, repair, and presacral drainage for rectal injury;
45563	with colostomy
45800	Closure of rectovesical fistula;
45805	with colostomy
45820	Closure of rectourethral fistula;
45825	with colostomy

(For rectovaginal fistula closure, see 57300-57308)

Manipulation

45900	Reduction of procidentia (separate procedure) under anesthesia
45905	Dilation of anal sphincter (separate procedure) under anesthesia other than local
45910	Dilation of rectal stricture (separate procedure) under anesthesia other than local
45915	Removal of fecal impaction or foreign body (separate procedure) under anesthesia

➔ *CPT Changes: An Insider's View* 2003

Other Procedures

Surgical diagnostic anorectal exam (45990) includes the following elements: external perineal exam, digital rectal exam, pelvic exam (when performed), diagnostic anoscopy, and diagnostic rigid proctoscopy.

45990	Anorectal exam, surgical, requiring anesthesia (general, spinal, or epidural), diagnostic

➔ *CPT Changes: An Insider's View* 2006

(Do not report 45990 in conjunction with 45300-45327, 46600, 57410, 99170)

45999	Unlisted procedure, rectum

(For unlisted laparoscopic procedure, rectum, use 45499)

Anus

For incision of thrombosed external hemorrhoid, use 46083. For ligation of internal hemorrhoid(s), see 46221, 46945, 46946. For excision of internal and/or external hemorrhoid(s), see 46250-46262, 46320. For injection of hemorrhoid(s), use 46500. For destruction of internal hemorrhoid(s) by thermal energy, use 46930. For destruction of hemorrhoid(s) by cryosurgery, use 46999. For hemorrhoidopexy, use 46947.

Incision

(For subcutaneous fistulotomy, use 46270)

46020	Placement of seton

➔ *CPT Changes: An Insider's View* 2002

(Do not report 46020 in addition to 46060, 46280, 46600, 0249T)

Placement of Seton
46020

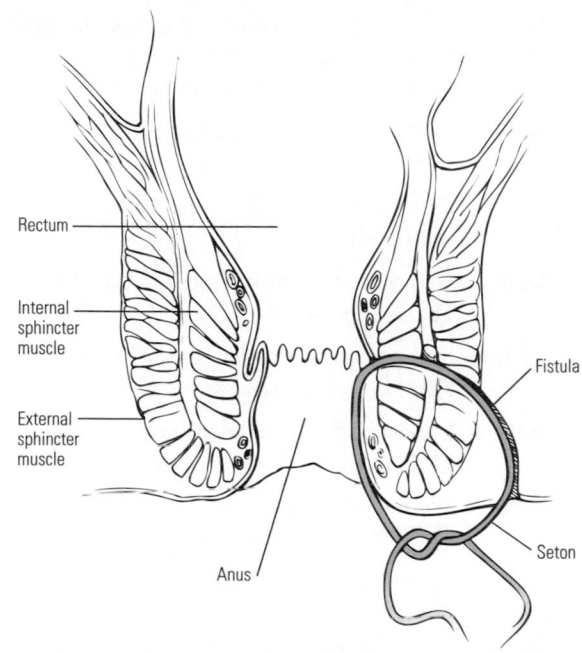

46030	Removal of anal seton, other marker
46040	Incision and drainage of ischiorectal and/or perirectal abscess (separate procedure)
46045	Incision and drainage of intramural, intramuscular, or submucosal abscess, transanal, under anesthesia
46050	Incision and drainage, perianal abscess, superficial

(See also 45020, 46060)

46060	Incision and drainage of ischiorectal or intramural abscess, with fistulectomy or fistulotomy, submuscular, with or without placement of seton

(Do not report 46060 in addition to 46020)

(See also 45020)

46070	Incision, anal septum (infant)

(For anoplasty, see 46700-46705)

(Do not report modifier 63 in conjunction with 46070)

46080	Sphincterotomy, anal, division of sphincter (separate procedure)
46083	Incision of thrombosed hemorrhoid, external

➔ *CPT Assistant* Jun 97:10

Excision

46200 Fissurectomy, including sphincterotomy, when performed
➲ *CPT Changes: An Insider's View* 2010

(46210, 46211 have been deleted. To report, use 46999)

46220 Code is out of numerical sequence. See 46200-46288

46221 Hemorrhoidectomy, internal, by rubber band ligation(s)
➲ *CPT Assistant* Oct 97:8; *CPT Changes: An Insider's View* 2010

(For ligation, hemorrhoidal vascular bundle(s), including ultrasound guidance, use 0249T)

 # 46945 Hemorrhoidectomy, internal, by ligation other than rubber band; single hemorrhoid column/group
➲ *CPT Changes: An Insider's View* 2010

 # 46946 2 or more hemorrhoid columns/groups
➲ *CPT Changes: An Insider's View* 2010

(Do not report 46221, 46945, and 46946 in conjunction with 0249T)

 # 46220 Excision of single external papilla or tag, anus
➲ *CPT Changes: An Insider's View* 2010

46230 Excision of multiple external papillae or tags, anus
➲ *CPT Changes: An Insider's View* 2010

 # 46320 Excision of thrombosed hemorrhoid, external
➲ *CPT Changes: An Insider's View* 2010

46250 Hemorrhoidectomy, external, 2 or more columns/groups
➲ *CPT Changes: An Insider's View* 2010

(For hemorrhoidectomy, external, single column/group, use 46999)

46255 Hemorrhoidectomy, internal and external, single column/group;
➲ *CPT Changes: An Insider's View* 2010

46257 with fissurectomy

46258 with fistulectomy, including fissurectomy, when performed
➲ *CPT Changes: An Insider's View* 2010

46260 Hemorrhoidectomy, internal and external, 2 or more columns/groups;
➲ *CPT Changes: An Insider's View* 2010

46261 with fissurectomy

46262 with fistulectomy, including fissurectomy, when performed
➲ *CPT Assistant* May 05:3; *CPT Changes: An Insider's View* 2010

(Do not report 46250-46262 in conjunction with 0249T)

46270 Surgical treatment of anal fistula (fistulectomy/ fistulotomy); subcutaneous

46275 intersphincteric
➲ *CPT Changes: An Insider's View* 2010

Hemorrhoidectomy of Internal Prolapsed Hemorrhoid Columns
46250-46262

Hemorrhoidectomy of Internal Prolapsed Hemorrhoid Columns 46250-46262

Internal prolapsed hemorrhoid columns

Anal column is considered to be an internal hemorrhoid with 3 major areas in the anal canal: right posterior (1 o'clock), right anterior (5 o'clock), and left lateral (9 o'clock) positions of the anus

46280 transsphincteric, suprasphincteric, extrasphincteric or multiple, including placement of seton, when performed
➲ *CPT Changes: An Insider's View* 2010

(Do not report 46280 in conjunction with 46020)

46285 second stage

46288 Closure of anal fistula with rectal advancement flap

46320 Code is out of numerical sequence. See 46200-46288

Introduction

46500 Injection of sclerosing solution, hemorrhoids
➲ *CPT Assistant* May 05:3

46505 Chemodenervation of internal anal sphincter
➲ *CPT Changes: An Insider's View* 2006

(For chemodenervation of other muscles, see 64612-64614. For destruction of nerve by neurolytic agent, see 64630, 64640)

(Report the specific service in conjunction with the specific substance(s) or drug(s) provided)

Endoscopy

Surgical endoscopy always includes diagnostic endoscopy.

46600   Anoscopy; diagnostic, with or without collection of specimen(s) by brushing or washing (separate procedure)
> *CPT Assistant* Spring 94:9, Oct 97:6, Apr 06:1, Jun 10:3, Aug 11:9

(Do not report 46600 in conjunction with 46020, 0249T)

(For diagnostic high resolution anoscopy [HRA], use 0226T)

46604   with dilation (eg, balloon, guide wire, bougie)
> *CPT Assistant* Spring 94:9, Oct 97:6; *CPT Changes: An Insider's View* 2002

46606   with biopsy, single or multiple
> *CPT Assistant* Spring 94:9, Oct 97:6

(For high resolution anoscopy [HRA] with biopsy, use 0227T)

46608   with removal of foreign body
> *CPT Assistant* Spring 94:9, Oct 97:6

46610   with removal of single tumor, polyp, or other lesion by hot biopsy forceps or bipolar cautery
> *CPT Assistant* Spring 94:10, Oct 97:6

46611   with removal of single tumor, polyp, or other lesion by snare technique
> *CPT Assistant* Spring 94:10, Oct 97:6

46612   with removal of multiple tumors, polyps, or other lesions by hot biopsy forceps, bipolar cautery or snare technique
> *CPT Assistant* Spring 94:10, Oct 97:6

46614   with control of bleeding (eg, injection, bipolar cautery, unipolar cautery, laser, heater probe, stapler, plasma coagulator)
> *CPT Assistant* Spring 94:10, Oct 97:6; *CPT Changes: An Insider's View* 2002

46615   with ablation of tumor(s), polyp(s), or other lesion(s) not amenable to removal by hot biopsy forceps, bipolar cautery or snare technique
> *CPT Assistant* Spring 94:10, Oct 97:6

(For delivery of thermal energy to the muscle of the anal canal, use 0288T)

Repair

46700   Anoplasty, plastic operation for stricture; adult

46705   infant

(Do not report modifier 63 in conjunction with 46705)

(For simple incision of anal septum, use 46070)

46706   Repair of anal fistula with fibrin glue
> *CPT Changes: An Insider's View* 2003

46707   Repair of anorectal fistula with plug (eg, porcine small intestine submucosa [SIS])
> *CPT Assistant* Jan 12:10; *CPT Changes: An Insider's View* 2010

46710   Repair of ileoanal pouch fistula/sinus (eg, perineal or vaginal), pouch advancement; transperineal approach
> *CPT Changes: An Insider's View* 2006

46712   combined transperineal and transabdominal approach
> *CPT Changes: An Insider's View* 2006

46715   Repair of low imperforate anus; with anoperineal fistula (cut-back procedure)

46716   with transposition of anoperineal or anovestibular fistula

(Do not report modifier 63 in conjunction with 46715, 46716)

46730   Repair of high imperforate anus without fistula; perineal or sacroperineal approach

46735   combined transabdominal and sacroperineal approaches

(Do not report modifier 63 in conjunction with 46730, 46735)

46740   Repair of high imperforate anus with rectourethral or rectovaginal fistula; perineal or sacroperineal approach

46742   combined transabdominal and sacroperineal approaches

(Do not report modifier 63 in conjunction with 46740, 46742)

46744   Repair of cloacal anomaly by anorectovaginoplasty and urethroplasty, sacroperineal approach

(Do not report modifier 63 in conjunction with 46744)

46746   Repair of cloacal anomaly by anorectovaginoplasty and urethroplasty, combined abdominal and sacroperineal approach;

46748   with vaginal lengthening by intestinal graft or pedicle flaps

46750   Sphincteroplasty, anal, for incontinence or prolapse; adult

46751   child

46753   Graft (Thiersch operation) for rectal incontinence and/or prolapse

46754   Removal of Thiersch wire or suture, anal canal

46760   Sphincteroplasty, anal, for incontinence, adult; muscle transplant

46761   levator muscle imbrication (Park posterior anal repair)

46762   implantation artificial sphincter

 # 46947   Hemorrhoidopexy (eg, for prolapsing internal hemorrhoids) by stapling
> *CPT Assistant* May 05:3, 14; *CPT Changes: An Insider's View* 2005

▲=Revised code   ●=New code   ▶◀=Contains new or revised text   ⊘=Modifier 51 exempt

Digestive

Destruction

46900 Destruction of lesion(s), anus (eg, condyloma, papilloma, molluscum contagiosum, herpetic vesicle), simple; chemical

46910 electrodesiccation

46916 cryosurgery

46917 laser surgery

46922 surgical excision

46924 Destruction of lesion(s), anus (eg, condyloma, papilloma, molluscum contagiosum, herpetic vesicle), extensive (eg, laser surgery, electrosurgery, cryosurgery, chemosurgery)
→ CPT Changes: An Insider's View 2002

46930 Destruction of internal hemorrhoid(s) by thermal energy (eg, infrared coagulation, cautery, radiofrequency)
→ CPT Changes: An Insider's View 2009

(46934-46936 have been deleted)

(46937, 46938 have been deleted. To report, use 45190)

46940 Curettage or cautery of anal fissure, including dilation of anal sphincter (separate procedure); initial
→ CPT Changes: An Insider's View 2002

46942 subsequent

46945 Code is out of numerical sequence. See 46200-46288

46946 Code is out of numerical sequence. See 46200-46288

46947 Code is out of numerical sequence. See 46700-46947

Other Procedures

46999 Unlisted procedure, anus
→ CPT Assistant Oct 97:8

Liver

Incision

⊙ **47000** Biopsy of liver, needle; percutaneous
→ CPT Assistant Fall 93:12; CPT Changes: An Insider's View 2012

(If imaging guidance is performed, see 76942, 77002, 77012, 77021)

+ **47001** when done for indicated purpose at time of other major procedure (List separately in addition to code for primary procedure)
→ CPT Assistant Jun 07:10

(If imaging guidance is performed, see 76942, 77002)

(For fine needle aspiration in conjunction with 47000, 47001, see 10021, 10022)

(For evaluation of fine needle aspirate in conjunction with 47000, 47001, see 88172, 88173)

47010 Hepatotomy; for open drainage of abscess or cyst, 1 or 2 stages
→ CPT Assistant Nov 97:18

⊙ **47011** for percutaneous drainage of abscess or cyst, 1 or 2 stages
→ CPT Assistant Nov 97:18, Mar 98:8

(For radiological supervision and interpretation, use 75989)

47015 Laparotomy, with aspiration and/or injection of hepatic parasitic (eg, amoebic or echinococcal) cyst(s) or abscess(es)

Excision

47100 Biopsy of liver, wedge

47120 Hepatectomy, resection of liver; partial lobectomy
→ CPT Assistant May 98:10

47122 trisegmentectomy

47125 total left lobectomy

47130 total right lobectomy

Liver Transplantation

Liver allotransplantation involves three distinct components of physician work:

1. *Cadaver donor hepatectomy,* which includes harvesting the graft and cold preservation of the graft (perfusing with cold preservation solution and cold maintenance) (use 47133). *Living donor hepatectomy,* which includes harvesting the graft, cold preservation of the graft (perfusing with cold preservation solution and cold maintenance), and care of the donor (see 47140-47142).

2. *Backbench work:*

   Standard preparation of the whole liver graft will include one of the following:

   Preparation of whole liver graft (including cholecystectomy, if necessary, and dissection and removal of surrounding soft tissues to prepare vena cava, portal vein, hepatic artery, and common bile duct for implantation) (use 47143).

   Preparation as described for whole liver graft, plus trisegment split into two partial grafts (use 47144).

   Preparation as described for whole liver graft, plus lobe split into two partial grafts (use 47145).

   Additional reconstruction of the liver graft may include venous and/or arterial anastomosis(es) (see 47146, 47147).

3. *Recipient liver allotransplantation,* which includes recipient hepatectomy (partial or whole), transplantation of the allograft (partial or whole), and care of the recipient (see 47135, 47136).

47133 Donor hepatectomy (including cold preservation), from cadaver donor
→ CPT Changes: An Insider's View 2005

47135   Liver allotransplantation; orthotopic, partial or whole, from cadaver or living donor, any age
> *CPT Assistant* Dec 11:16

47136   heterotopic, partial or whole, from cadaver or living donor, any age
> *CPT Assistant* Dec 11:16

47140   Donor hepatectomy (including cold preservation), from living donor; left lateral segment only (segments II and III)
> *CPT Assistant* Aug 11:9; *CPT Changes: An Insider's View* 2004, 2005

47141   total left lobectomy (segments II, III and IV)
> *CPT Changes: An Insider's View* 2004

47142   total right lobectomy (segments V, VI, VII and VIII)
> *CPT Changes: An Insider's View* 2004

47143   Backbench standard preparation of cadaver donor whole liver graft prior to allotransplantation, including cholecystectomy, if necessary, and dissection and removal of surrounding soft tissues to prepare the vena cava, portal vein, hepatic artery, and common bile duct for implantation; without trisegment or lobe split
> *CPT Assistant* Apr 05:10, 12; *CPT Changes: An Insider's View* 2005

47144   with trisegment split of whole liver graft into 2 partial liver grafts (ie, left lateral segment [segments II and III] and right trisegment [segments I and IV through VIII])
> *CPT Changes: An Insider's View* 2005, 2009

47145   with lobe split of whole liver graft into 2 partial liver grafts (ie, left lobe [segments II, III, and IV] and right lobe [segments I and V through VIII])
> *CPT Changes: An Insider's View* 2005

47146   Backbench reconstruction of cadaver or living donor liver graft prior to allotransplantation; venous anastomosis, each
> *CPT Changes: An Insider's View* 2005

47147   arterial anastomosis, each
> *CPT Changes: An Insider's View* 2005

(Do not report 47143-47147 in conjunction with 47120-47125, 47600, 47610)

Repair

47300   Marsupialization of cyst or abscess of liver

47350   Management of liver hemorrhage; simple suture of liver wound or injury

47360   complex suture of liver wound or injury, with or without hepatic artery ligation

47361   exploration of hepatic wound, extensive debridement, coagulation and/or suture, with or without packing of liver

47362   re-exploration of hepatic wound for removal of packing

Laparoscopy

Surgical laparoscopy always includes diagnostic laparoscopy. To report a diagnostic laparoscopy (peritoneoscopy) (separate procedure), use 49320.

47370   Laparoscopy, surgical, ablation of 1 or more liver tumor(s); radiofrequency
> *CPT Assistant* Oct 02:2; *CPT Changes: An Insider's View* 2002

(For imaging guidance, use 76940)

47371   cryosurgical
> *CPT Changes: An Insider's View* 2002

(For imaging guidance, use 76940)

47379   Unlisted laparoscopic procedure, liver
> *CPT Assistant* Aug 06:10, Dec 07:12; *CPT Changes: An Insider's View* 2001

Other Procedures

47380   Ablation, open, of 1 or more liver tumor(s); radiofrequency
> *CPT Assistant* Oct 02:1; *CPT Changes: An Insider's View* 2002
> *Clinical Examples in Radiology* Summer 08:3

(For imaging guidance, use 76940)

47381   cryosurgical
> *CPT Changes: An Insider's View* 2002

(For imaging guidance, use 76940)

⊙ **47382**   Ablation, 1 or more liver tumor(s), percutaneous, radiofrequency
> *CPT Assistant* Oct 02:1; *CPT Changes: An Insider's View* 2002, 2010
> *Clinical Examples in Radiology* Spring 08:1, 2, Summer 08:3

(For imaging guidance and monitoring, see 76940, 77013, 77022)

47399   Unlisted procedure, liver

Biliary Tract

Incision

47400   Hepaticotomy or hepaticostomy with exploration, drainage, or removal of calculus

47420   Choledochotomy or choledochostomy with exploration, drainage, or removal of calculus, with or without cholecystotomy; without transduodenal sphincterotomy or sphincteroplasty

47425   with transduodenal sphincterotomy or sphincteroplasty

47460   Transduodenal sphincterotomy or sphincteroplasty, with or without transduodenal extraction of calculus (separate procedure)

47480 Cholecystotomy or cholecystostomy, open, with exploration, drainage, or removal of calculus (separate procedure)

➲ *CPT Assistant* Apr 11:12; *CPT Changes: An Insider's View* 2011

➲ *Clinical Examples in Radiology* Summer 11:3

(For percutaneous cholecystostomy, use 47490)

Introduction

47490 Cholecystostomy, percutaneous, complete procedure, including imaging guidance, catheter placement, cholecystogram when performed, and radiological supervision and interpretation

➲ *CPT Assistant* Apr 11:12; *CPT Changes: An Insider's View* 2011

➲ *Clinical Examples in Radiology* Summer 11:1-3, Winter 11:10

(Do not report 47490 in conjunction with 47505, 74305, 75989, 76942, 77002, 77012, 77021)

47500 Injection procedure for percutaneous transhepatic cholangiography

(For radiological supervision and interpretation, use 74320)

47505 Injection procedure for cholangiography through an existing catheter (eg, percutaneous transhepatic or T-tube)

➲ *CPT Assistant* Apr 11:12

➲ *Clinical Examples in Radiology* Summer 10:11, Summer 11:3

(For radiological supervision and interpretation, use 74305)

47510 Introduction of percutaneous transhepatic catheter for biliary drainage

(For radiological supervision and interpretation, use 75980)

47511 Introduction of percutaneous transhepatic stent for internal and external biliary drainage

(For radiological supervision and interpretation, use 75982)

⊙ **47525** Change of percutaneous biliary drainage catheter

➲ *CPT Changes: An Insider's View* 2010

➲ *Clinical Examples in Radiology* Summer 10:11

(For radiological supervision and interpretation, use 75984)

47530 Revision and/or reinsertion of transhepatic tube

(For radiological supervision and interpretation, use 75984)

Endoscopy

Surgical endoscopy always includes diagnostic endoscopy.

✚ **47550** Biliary endoscopy, intraoperative (choledochoscopy) (List separately in addition to code for primary procedure)

47552 Biliary endoscopy, percutaneous via T-tube or other tract; diagnostic, with or without collection of specimen(s) by brushing and/or washing (separate procedure)

47553 with biopsy, single or multiple

47554 with removal of calculus/calculi

➲ *CPT Changes: An Insider's View* 2002

47555 with dilation of biliary duct stricture(s) without stent

47556 with dilation of biliary duct stricture(s) with stent

(For ERCP, see 43260-43272, 74363)

(If imaging guidance is performed, see 74363, 75982)

Laparoscopy

Surgical laparoscopy always includes diagnostic laparoscopy. To report a diagnostic laparoscopy (peritoneoscopy) (separate procedure), use 49320.

47560 Laparoscopy, surgical; with guided transhepatic cholangiography, without biopsy

➲ *CPT Assistant* Nov 99:23, Mar 00:9; *CPT Changes: An Insider's View* 2000

47561 with guided transhepatic cholangiography with biopsy

➲ *CPT Assistant* Nov 99:23, Mar 00:9; *CPT Changes: An Insider's View* 2000

47562 cholecystectomy

➲ *CPT Assistant* Nov 99:23, Mar 00:9, Sep 03:3, Dec 07:12; *CPT Changes: An Insider's View* 2000

Laparoscopic Cholecystectomy
47562

The gallbladder is dissected and removed from the liver bed under laparoscopic guidance.

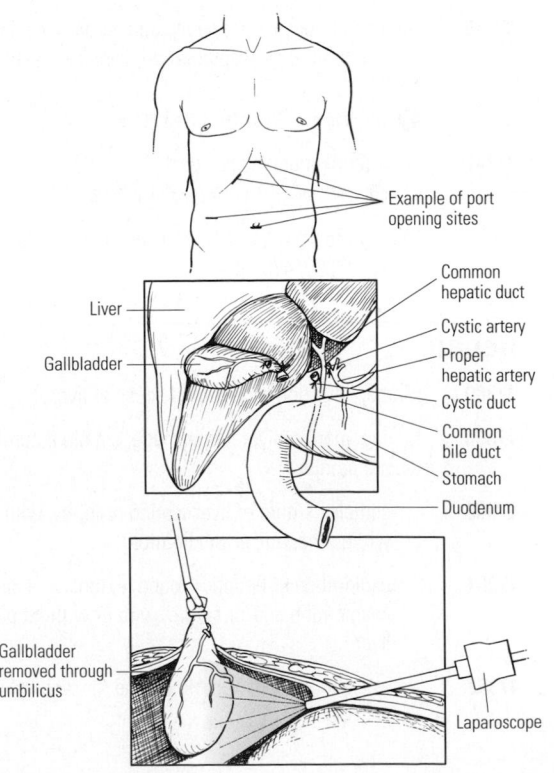

Example of port opening sites

Common hepatic duct

Cystic artery

Proper hepatic artery

Cystic duct

Common bile duct

Stomach

Duodenum

Liver

Gallbladder

Gallbladder removed through umbilicus

Laparoscope

47563   cholecystectomy with cholangiography
→ *CPT Assistant* Nov 99:23, Mar 00:9, Dec 00:14, Dec 07:12; *CPT Changes: An Insider's View* 2000

47564   cholecystectomy with exploration of common duct
→ *CPT Assistant* Nov 99:23, Mar 00:9; *CPT Changes: An Insider's View* 2000

47570   cholecystoenterostomy
→ *CPT Assistant* Nov 99:23, Mar 00:9; *CPT Changes: An Insider's View* 2000

47579   Unlisted laparoscopy procedure, biliary tract
→ *CPT Assistant* Nov 99:23, Mar 00:9; *CPT Changes: An Insider's View* 2000

Excision

47600   Cholecystectomy;
→ *CPT Assistant* Fall 92:19, Nov 99:24; *CPT Changes: An Insider's View* 2000

47605   with cholangiography
→ *CPT Assistant* Nov 99:24, Apr 02:19; *CPT Changes: An Insider's View* 2000

(For laparoscopic approach, see 47562-47564)

47610   Cholecystectomy with exploration of common duct;
→ *CPT Assistant* Apr 02:19

(For cholecystectomy with exploration of common duct with biliary endoscopy, use 47610 with 47550)

47612   with choledochoenterostomy

47620   with transduodenal sphincterotomy or sphincteroplasty, with or without cholangiography

47630   Biliary duct stone extraction, percutaneous via T-tube tract, basket, or snare (eg, Burhenne technique)
→ *CPT Assistant* Jun 98:10

(For radiological supervision and interpretation, use 74327)

47700   Exploration for congenital atresia of bile ducts, without repair, with or without liver biopsy, with or without cholangiography

(Do not report modifier 63 in conjunction with 47700)

47701   Portoenterostomy (eg, Kasai procedure)

(Do not report modifier 63 in conjunction with 47701)

47711   Excision of bile duct tumor, with or without primary repair of bile duct; extrahepatic

47712   intrahepatic

(For anastomosis, see 47760-47800)

47715   Excision of choledochal cyst

Repair

47720   Cholecystoenterostomy; direct
→ *CPT Assistant* Nov 99:24; *CPT Changes: An Insider's View* 2000

(For laparoscopic approach, use 47570)

47721   with gastroenterostomy

47740   Roux-en-Y

47741   Roux-en-Y with gastroenterostomy

47760   Anastomosis, of extrahepatic biliary ducts and gastrointestinal tract

47765   Anastomosis, of intrahepatic ducts and gastrointestinal tract

47780   Anastomosis, Roux-en-Y, of extrahepatic biliary ducts and gastrointestinal tract

47785   Anastomosis, Roux-en-Y, of intrahepatic biliary ducts and gastrointestinal tract

47800   Reconstruction, plastic, of extrahepatic biliary ducts with end-to-end anastomosis

47801   Placement of choledochal stent
→ *CPT Assistant* Dec 10:13

47802   U-tube hepaticoenterostomy

47900   Suture of extrahepatic biliary duct for pre-existing injury (separate procedure)

Other Procedures

47999   Unlisted procedure, biliary tract
→ *CPT Assistant* May 11:9

Pancreas

(For peroral pancreatic endoscopic procedures, see 43260-43272)

Incision

48000   Placement of drains, peripancreatic, for acute pancreatitis;

48001   with cholecystostomy, gastrostomy, and jejunostomy

48020   Removal of pancreatic calculus
→ *CPT Assistant* Spring 91:7

Excision

48100   Biopsy of pancreas, open (eg, fine needle aspiration, needle core biopsy, wedge biopsy)
→ *CPT Changes: An Insider's View* 2002

48102   Biopsy of pancreas, percutaneous needle

(For radiological supervision and interpretation, see 76942, 77002, 77012, 77021)

(For fine needle aspiration, use 10022)

(For evaluation of fine needle aspirate, see 88172, 88173)

48105   Resection or debridement of pancreas and peripancreatic tissue for acute necrotizing pancreatitis
→ *CPT Changes: An Insider's View* 2007

48120   Excision of lesion of pancreas (eg, cyst, adenoma)

48140 Pancreatectomy, distal subtotal, with or without splenectomy; without pancreaticojejunostomy

48145 with pancreaticojejunostomy

48146 Pancreatectomy, distal, near-total with preservation of duodenum (Child-type procedure)

48148 Excision of ampulla of Vater

48150 Pancreatectomy, proximal subtotal with total duodenectomy, partial gastrectomy, choledochoenterostomy and gastrojejunostomy (Whipple-type procedure); with pancreatojejunostomy

48152 without pancreatojejunostomy

48153 Pancreatectomy, proximal subtotal with near-total duodenectomy, choledochoenterostomy and duodenojejunostomy (pylorus-sparing, Whipple-type procedure); with pancreatojejunostomy

48154 without pancreatojejunostomy

48155 Pancreatectomy, total

48160 Pancreatectomy, total or subtotal, with autologous transplantation of pancreas or pancreatic islet cells
➔ *CPT Changes: An Insider's View* 2002

Introduction

✛ 48400 Injection procedure for intraoperative pancreatography (List separately in addition to code for primary procedure)
➔ *CPT Assistant* Dec 07:12

(For radiological supervision and interpretation, see 74300-74305)

Repair

48500 Marsupialization of pancreatic cyst
➔ *CPT Changes: An Insider's View* 2002

48510 External drainage, pseudocyst of pancreas; open
➔ *CPT Assistant* Nov 97:18

⊙ 48511 percutaneous
➔ *CPT Assistant* Nov 97:18, Mar 98:8

(For radiological supervision and interpretation, use 75989)

48520 Internal anastomosis of pancreatic cyst to gastrointestinal tract; direct

48540 Roux-en-Y

48545 Pancreatorrhaphy for injury
➔ *CPT Changes: An Insider's View* 2002

48547 Duodenal exclusion with gastrojejunostomy for pancreatic injury
➔ *CPT Changes: An Insider's View* 2002

48548 Pancreaticojejunostomy, side-to-side anastomosis (Puestow-type operation)
➔ *CPT Changes: An Insider's View* 2007

Pancreas Transplantation

Pancreas allotransplantation involves three distinct components of physician work:

1. ***Cadaver donor pancreatectomy,*** which includes harvesting the pancreas graft, with or without duodenal segment, and cold preservation of the graft (perfusing with cold preservation solution and cold maintenance) (use 48550).

2. ***Backbench work:***

   Standard preparation of a cadaver donor pancreas allograft prior to transplantation includes dissection of the allograft from surrounding soft tissues, splenectomy, duodenotomy, ligation of bile duct, ligation of mesenteric vessels, and Y-graft arterial anastomoses from the iliac artery to the superior mesenteric artery and to the splenic artery (use 48551).

   Additional reconstruction of a cadaver donor pancreas allograft prior to transplantation may include venous anastomosis(es) (use 48552).

3. ***Recipient pancreas allotransplantation,*** which includes transplantation of allograft, and care of the recipient (use 48554).

48550 Donor pancreatectomy (including cold preservation), with or without duodenal segment for transplantation
➔ *CPT Assistant* Apr 05:10, 12; *CPT Changes: An Insider's View* 2005

48551 Backbench standard preparation of cadaver donor pancreas allograft prior to transplantation, including dissection of allograft from surrounding soft tissues, splenectomy, duodenotomy, ligation of bile duct, ligation of mesenteric vessels, and Y-graft arterial anastomoses from iliac artery to superior mesenteric artery and to splenic artery
➔ *CPT Changes: An Insider's View* 2005

48552 Backbench reconstruction of cadaver donor pancreas allograft prior to transplantation, venous anastomosis, each
➔ *CPT Changes: An Insider's View* 2005

(Do not report 48551 and 48552 in conjunction with 35531, 35563, 35685, 38100-38102, 44010, 44820, 44850, 47460, 47505-47525, 47550-47556, 48100-48120, 48545)

48554 Transplantation of pancreatic allograft

48556 Removal of transplanted pancreatic allograft

Other Procedures

48999 Unlisted procedure, pancreas
➔ *CPT Assistant* Dec 07:12, May 11:9

Abdomen, Peritoneum, and Omentum

Incision

49000 Exploratory laparotomy, exploratory celiotomy with or without biopsy(s) (separate procedure)
➔ *CPT Assistant* Fall 92:23, Mar 01:10, Nov 08:7

(To report wound exploration due to penetrating trauma without laparotomy, use 20102)

49002 Reopening of recent laparotomy
➔ *CPT Assistant* Fall 92:23, Nov 08:7

(To report re-exploration of hepatic wound for removal of packing, use 47362)

49010 Exploration, retroperitoneal area with or without biopsy(s) (separate procedure)

(To report wound exploration due to penetrating trauma without laparotomy, use 20102)

49020 Drainage of peritoneal abscess or localized peritonitis, exclusive of appendiceal abscess; open

(For appendiceal abscess, use 44900)

⊙ **49021**   percutaneous

(For radiological supervision and interpretation, use 75989)

49040 Drainage of subdiaphragmatic or subphrenic abscess; open
➔ *CPT Assistant* Nov 97:18

⊙ **49041**   percutaneous
➔ *CPT Assistant* Nov 97:18, Mar 98:8

(For radiological supervision and interpretation, use 75989)

49060 Drainage of retroperitoneal abscess; open
➔ *CPT Assistant* Nov 97:18, Nov 99:24, Jul 01:11, Aug 01:10; *CPT Changes: An Insider's View* 2000

⊙ **49061**   percutaneous
➔ *CPT Assistant* Nov 97:18, Mar 98:8, Nov 99:24, Jul 01:11, Aug 01:10; *CPT Changes: An Insider's View* 2000

(For laparoscopic drainage, use 49323)

(For radiological supervision and interpretation, use 75989)

49062 Drainage of extraperitoneal lymphocele to peritoneal cavity, open
➔ *CPT Assistant* Nov 97:19, Jul 01:11, Aug 01:10

(49080, 49081 have been deleted. To report, see 49082-49084)

49082 Abdominal paracentesis (diagnostic or therapeutic); without imaging guidance
➔ *CPT Changes: An Insider's View* 2012
➔ *Clinical Examples in Radiology* Fall 11:11, Spring 12:10, Winter 12:9

49083 with imaging guidance
➔ *CPT Changes: An Insider's View* 2012
➔ *Clinical Examples in Radiology* Fall 11:11, Spring 12:10, Winter 12:9

(Do not report 49083 in conjunction with 76942, 77002, 77012, 77021)

49084 Peritoneal lavage, including imaging guidance, when performed
➔ *CPT Changes: An Insider's View* 2012
➔ *Clinical Examples in Radiology* Fall 11:11, Winter 12:9

(Do not report 49084 in conjunction with 76942, 77002, 77012, 77021)

Excision, Destruction

(For lysis of intestinal adhesions, use 44005)

49180 Biopsy, abdominal or retroperitoneal mass, percutaneous needle
➔ *CPT Assistant* Fall 93:11
➔ *Clinical Examples in Radiology* Fall 10:7

(If imaging guidance is performed, see 76942, 77002, 77012, 77021)

(For fine needle aspiration, use 10021 or 10022)

(For evaluation of fine needle aspirate, see 88172, 88173)

49203 Excision or destruction, open, intra-abdominal tumors, cysts or endometriomas, 1 or more peritoneal, mesenteric, or retroperitoneal primary or secondary tumors; largest tumor 5 cm diameter or less
➔ *CPT Assistant* Aug 08:7, Dec 10:16; *CPT Changes: An Insider's View* 2008

49204   largest tumor 5.1-10.0 cm diameter
➔ *CPT Assistant* Aug 08:7, Dec 10:16; *CPT Changes: An Insider's View* 2008

49205   largest tumor greater than 10.0 cm diameter
➔ *CPT Assistant* Aug 08:7, Dec 10:16; *CPT Changes: An Insider's View* 2008

(Do not report 49203-49205 in conjunction with 38770, 38780, 49000, 49010, 49215, 50010, 50205, 50225, 50236, 50250, 50290, 58900-58960)

(For partial or total nephrectomy, use 50220 or 50240 in conjunction with 49203-49205)

(For colectomy, use 44140 in conjunction with 49203-49205)

(For small bowel resection, use 44120 in conjunction with 49203-49205)

(For vena caval resection with reconstruction, use 49203-49205 in conjunction with 37799)

(For resection of recurrent ovarian, tubal, primary peritoneal, or uterine malignancy, see 58957, 58958)

(For cryoablation of renal tumors, see 50250, 50593)

49215 Excision of presacral or sacrococcygeal tumor

(Do not report modifier 63 in conjunction with 49215)

Digestive

49220 Staging laparotomy for Hodgkins disease or lymphoma (includes splenectomy, needle or open biopsies of both liver lobes, possibly also removal of abdominal nodes, abdominal node and/or bone marrow biopsies, ovarian repositioning)

➔ *CPT Changes: An Insider's View* 2002

49250 Umbilectomy, omphalectomy, excision of umbilicus (separate procedure)

49255 Omentectomy, epiploectomy, resection of omentum (separate procedure)

➔ *CPT Assistant* Nov 99:24; *CPT Changes: An Insider's View* 2000

Laparoscopy

Surgical laparoscopy always includes diagnostic laparoscopy. To report a diagnostic laparoscopy (peritoneoscopy), (separate procedure), use 49320.

For laparoscopic fulguration or excision of lesions of the ovary, pelvic viscera, or peritoneal surface use 58662.

49320 Laparoscopy, abdomen, peritoneum, and omentum, diagnostic, with or without collection of specimen(s) by brushing or washing (separate procedure)

➔ *CPT Assistant* Nov 99:24, Mar 00:9, Apr 06:19, Mar 07:4, Nov 07:1, Dec 08:7, Jun 10:7; *CPT Changes: An Insider's View* 2000, 2001

Laparoscopy
49320

The physician inserts a fiberoptic laparoscope to observe the necessary organs in these procedures.

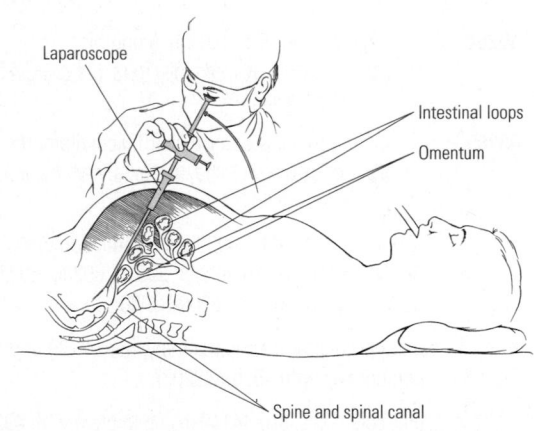

Laparoscope

Intestinal loops

Omentum

Spine and spinal canal

49321 Laparoscopy, surgical; with biopsy (single or multiple)

➔ *CPT Assistant* Nov 99:24, Mar 00:9; *CPT Changes: An Insider's View* 2000, 2001

49322 with aspiration of cavity or cyst (eg, ovarian cyst) (single or multiple)

➔ *CPT Assistant* Nov 99:24, Mar 00:9; *CPT Changes: An Insider's View* 2000

49323 with drainage of lymphocele to peritoneal cavity

➔ *CPT Assistant* Nov 99:24, Mar 00:9, May 00:4, Jul 01:11, Aug 01:10; *CPT Changes: An Insider's View* 2000

(For percutaneous or open drainage, see 49060, 49061)

49324 with insertion of tunneled intraperitoneal catheter

➔ *CPT Changes: An Insider's View* 2007, 2011

(For subcutaneous extension of intraperitoneal catheter with remote chest exit site, use 49435 in conjunction with 49324)

(For open insertion of tunneled intraperitoneal catheter, use 49421)

49325 with revision of previously placed intraperitoneal cannula or catheter, with removal of intraluminal obstructive material if performed

➔ *CPT Changes: An Insider's View* 2007

+ 49326 with omentopexy (omental tacking procedure) (List separately in addition to code for primary procedure)

➔ *CPT Changes: An Insider's View* 2007

(Use 49326 in conjunction with 49324, 49325)

+ 49327 with placement of interstitial device(s) for radiation therapy guidance (eg, fiducial markers, dosimeter), intra-abdominal, intrapelvic, and/or retroperitoneum, including imaging guidance, if performed, single or multiple (List separately in addition to code for primary procedure)

➔ *CPT Changes: An Insider's View* 2011

(Use 49327 in conjunction with laparoscopic abdominal, pelvic, or retroperitoneal procedure[s] performed concurrently)

(For placement of interstitial device[s] for intra-abdominal, intrapelvic, and/or retroperitoneal radiation therapy guidance concurrent with open procedure, use 49412)

(For percutaneous placement of interstitial device[s] for intra-abdominal, intrapelvic, and/or retroperitoneal radiation therapy guidance, use 49411)

49329 Unlisted laparoscopy procedure, abdomen, peritoneum and omentum

➔ *CPT Assistant* Nov 99:24, Mar 00:9, Feb 06:16, Dec 11:16; *CPT Changes: An Insider's View* 2000

Introduction, Revision, Removal

49400 Injection of air or contrast into peritoneal cavity (separate procedure)

➔ *CPT Assistant* Dec 10:13

➔ *Clinical Examples in Radiology* Fall 07:1, 2

(For radiological supervision and interpretation, use 74190)

49402 Removal of peritoneal foreign body from peritoneal cavity

➔ *CPT Changes: An Insider's View* 2007

(For lysis of intestinal adhesions, use 44005)

⊙ 49411 Placement of interstitial device(s) for radiation therapy guidance (eg, fiducial markers, dosimeter), percutaneous, intra-abdominal, intra-pelvic (except prostate), and/or retroperitoneum, single or multiple

➔ *CPT Assistant* Feb 10:7; *CPT Changes: An Insider's View* 2010

(Report supply of device separately)

(For imaging guidance, see 76942, 77002, 77012, 77021)

(For percutaneous placement of interstitial device[s] for intra-thoracic radiation therapy guidance, use 32553)

+ 49412   Placement of interstitial device(s) for radiation therapy guidance (eg, fiducial markers, dosimeter), open, intra-abdominal, intrapelvic, and/or retroperitoneum, including image guidance, if performed, single or multiple (List separately in addition to code for primary procedure)
➜ *CPT Changes: An Insider's View* 2011

(Use 49412 in conjunction with open abdominal, pelvic, or retroperitoneal procedure[s] performed concurrently)

(For placement of interstitial device[s] for intra-abdominal, intrapelvic, and/or retroperitoneal radiation therapy guidance concurrent with laparoscopic procedure, use 49327)

(For percutaneous placement of interstitial device[s] for intra-abdominal, intrapelvic, and/or retroperitoneal radiation therapy guidance, use 49411)

⊙ 49418   Insertion of tunneled intraperitoneal catheter (eg, dialysis, intraperitoneal chemotherapy instillation, management of ascites), complete procedure, including imaging guidance, catheter placement, contrast injection when performed, and radiological supervision and interpretation, percutaneous
➜ *CPT Changes: An Insider's View* 2011

49419   Insertion of tunneled intraperitoneal catheter, with subcutaneous port (ie, totally implantable)
➜ *CPT Changes: An Insider's View* 2003, 2011

(For removal, use 49422)

(49420 has been deleted. To report open placement of a tunneled intraperitoneal catheter for dialysis, use 49421. To report open or percutaneous peritoneal drainage or lavage, see 49020, 49021, 49040, 49041, 49082-49084, as appropriate. To report percutaneous insertion of a tunneled intraperitoneal catheter without subcutaneous port, use 49418)

49421   Insertion of tunneled intraperitoneal catheter for dialysis, open
➜ *CPT Assistant* Fall 93:2, Jul 06:19; *CPT Changes: An Insider's View* 2011

(For laparoscopic insertion of tunneled intraperitoneal catheter, use 49324)

(For subcutaneous extension of intraperitoneal catheter with remote chest exit site, use 49435 in conjunction with 49421)

49422   Removal of tunneled intraperitoneal catheter
➜ *CPT Changes: An Insider's View* 2011

(For removal of a non-tunneled catheter, use appropriate E/M code)

49423   Exchange of previously placed abscess or cyst drainage catheter under radiological guidance (separate procedure)
➜ *CPT Assistant* Nov 97:19, Mar 98:8

(For radiological supervision and interpretation, use 75984)

49424   Contrast injection for assessment of abscess or cyst via previously placed drainage catheter or tube (separate procedure)
➜ *CPT Assistant* Nov 97:19, Mar 98:8, Nov 03:14; *CPT Changes: An Insider's View* 2002
➜ *Clinical Examples in Radiology* Fall 09:9

(For radiological supervision and interpretation, use 76080)

49425   Insertion of peritoneal-venous shunt

49426   Revision of peritoneal-venous shunt

(For shunt patency test, use 78291)

49427   Injection procedure (eg, contrast media) for evaluation of previously placed peritoneal-venous shunt

(For radiological supervision and interpretation, see 75809, 78291)

49428   Ligation of peritoneal-venous shunt

49429   Removal of peritoneal-venous shunt

+ 49435   Insertion of subcutaneous extension to intraperitoneal cannula or catheter with remote chest exit site (List separately in addition to code for primary procedure)
➜ *CPT Changes: An Insider's View* 2007

(Use 49435 in conjunction with 49324, 49421)

49436   Delayed creation of exit site from embedded subcutaneous segment of intraperitoneal cannula or catheter
➜ *CPT Changes: An Insider's View* 2007

Initial Placement

Do not additionally report 43752 for placement of a nasogastric (NG) or orogastric (OG) tube to insufflate the stomach prior to percutaneous gastrointestinal tube placement. NG or OG tube placement is considered part of the procedure in this family of codes.

⊙ 49440   Insertion of gastrostomy tube, percutaneous, under fluoroscopic guidance including contrast injection(s), image documentation and report
➜ *CPT Assistant* Jan 08:8, Jun 08:8, Aug 08:7, Sep 10:9; *CPT Changes: An Insider's View* 2008

(For conversion to a gastro-jejunostomy tube at the time of initial gastrostomy tube placement, use 49440 in conjunction with 49446)

⊙ 49441   Insertion of duodenostomy or jejunostomy tube, percutaneous, under fluoroscopic guidance including contrast injection(s), image documentation and report
➜ *CPT Assistant* Jan 08:8, Jun 08:8, Aug 08:7; *CPT Changes: An Insider's View* 2008

(For conversion of gastrostomy tube to gastro-jejunostomy tube, use 49446)

⊙ **49442** Insertion of cecostomy or other colonic tube, percutaneous, under fluoroscopic guidance including contrast injection(s), image documentation and report

➥ *CPT Assistant* Jan 08:8, Jun 08:8, Aug 08:7; *CPT Changes: An Insider's View* 2008

Conversion

⊙ **49446** Conversion of gastrostomy tube to gastro-jejunostomy tube, percutaneous, under fluoroscopic guidance including contrast injection(s), image documentation and report

➥ *CPT Changes: An Insider's View* 2008

(For conversion to a gastro-jejunostomy tube at the time of initial gastrostomy tube placement, use 49446 in conjunction with 49440)

Replacement

If an existing gastrostomy, duodenostomy, jejunostomy, gastro-jejunostomy, or cecostomy (or other colonic) tube is removed and a new tube is placed via a separate percutaneous access site, the placement of the new tube is not considered a replacement and would be reported using the appropriate initial placement codes 49440-49442.

49450 Replacement of gastrostomy or cecostomy (or other colonic) tube, percutaneous, under fluoroscopic guidance including contrast injection(s), image documentation and report

➥ *CPT Assistant* Sep 10:9; *CPT Changes: An Insider's View* 2008

(To report a percutaneous change of a gastrostomy tube without imaging or endoscopic guidance, use 43760)

49451 Replacement of duodenostomy or jejunostomy tube, percutaneous, under fluoroscopic guidance including contrast injection(s), image documentation and report

➥ *CPT Assistant* Jan 08:8, Jun 08:8, Aug 08:7, Jul 10:10; *CPT Changes: An Insider's View* 2008

49452 Replacement of gastro-jejunostomy tube, percutaneous, under fluoroscopic guidance including contrast injection(s), image documentation and report

➥ *CPT Assistant* Mar 10:10; *CPT Changes: An Insider's View* 2008

Mechanical Removal of Obstructive Material

49460 Mechanical removal of obstructive material from gastrostomy, duodenostomy, jejunostomy, gastro-jejunostomy, or cecostomy (or other colonic) tube, any method, under fluoroscopic guidance including contrast injection(s), if performed, image documentation and report

➥ *CPT Changes: An Insider's View* 2008

(Do not report 49460 in conjunction with 49450-49452, 49465)

Other

49465 Contrast injection(s) for radiological evaluation of existing gastrostomy, duodenostomy, jejunostomy, gastro-jejunostomy, or cecostomy (or other colonic) tube, from a percutaneous approach including image documentation and report

➥ *CPT Changes: An Insider's View* 2008

(Do not report 49465 in conjunction with 49450-49460)

Repair

Hernioplasty, Herniorrhaphy, Herniotomy

The hernia repair codes in this section are categorized primarily by the type of hernia (inguinal, femoral, incisional, etc).

Some types of hernias are further categorized as "initial" or "recurrent" based on whether or not the hernia has required previous repair(s).

Additional variables accounted for by some of the codes include patient age and clinical presentation (reducible vs. incarcerated or strangulated).

With the exception of the incisional hernia repairs (see 49560-49566) the use of mesh or other prostheses is not separately reported.

The excision/repair of strangulated organs or structures such as testicle(s), intestine, ovaries are reported by using the appropriate code for the excision/repair (eg, 44120, 54520, and 58940) in addition to the appropriate code for the repair of the strangulated hernia.

(For reduction and repair of intra-abdominal hernia, use 44050)

(For debridement of abdominal wall, see 11042, 11043)

(Codes 49491-49651 are unilateral procedures. To report bilateral procedure, report modifier 50 with the appropriate procedure code)

49491 Repair, initial inguinal hernia, preterm infant (younger than 37 weeks gestation at birth), performed from birth up to 50 weeks postconception age, with or without hydrocelectomy; reducible

➥ *CPT Assistant* Mar 04:2, Jun 08:3; *CPT Changes: An Insider's View* 2002

49492 incarcerated or strangulated

➥ *CPT Assistant* Mar 04:2, Jun 08:3; *CPT Changes: An Insider's View* 2002

(Do not report modifier 63 in conjunction with 49491, 49492)

(Postconception age equals gestational age at birth plus age of infant in weeks at the time of the hernia repair. Initial inguinal hernia repairs that are performed on preterm infants who are older than 50 weeks postconception age and younger than age 6 months at the time of surgery, should be reported using codes 49495, 49496)

49495 Repair, initial inguinal hernia, full term infant younger than age 6 months, or preterm infant older than 50 weeks postconception age and younger than age 6 months at the time of surgery, with or without hydrocelectomy; reducible

➔ *CPT Assistant* Winter 93:6, Winter 94:13, Jan 04:27, Mar 04:10, May 04:14, Nov 07:9, Jun 08:3; *CPT Changes: An Insider's View* 2002

49496   incarcerated or strangulated

➔ *CPT Assistant* Winter 93:6, Winter 94:13, Jan 04:27, Mar 04:10, May 04:14, Jun 08:3

(Do not report modifier 63 in conjunction with 49495, 49496)

(Postconception age equals gestational age at birth plus age in weeks at the time of the hernia repair. Initial inguinal hernia repairs that are performed on preterm infants who are younger than or up to 50 weeks postconception age but younger than 6 months of age since birth, should be reported using codes 49491, 49492. Inguinal hernia repairs on infants age 6 months to younger than 5 years should be reported using codes 49500-49501)

49500 Repair initial inguinal hernia, age 6 months to younger than 5 years, with or without hydrocelectomy; reducible

➔ *CPT Assistant* Winter 94:13, Jan 04:27, Mar 04:10, Nov 07:9, Jun 08:3; *CPT Changes: An Insider's View* 2002

49501   incarcerated or strangulated

➔ *CPT Assistant* Winter 94:13, Jan 04:27, Mar 04:12, Jun 08:3; *CPT Changes: An Insider's View* 2002

49505 Repair initial inguinal hernia, age 5 years or older; reducible

➔ *CPT Assistant* Winter 94:13, Sep 00:10, Jan 04:27, Mar 04:12, Jun 08:3

49507   incarcerated or strangulated

➔ *CPT Assistant* Winter 94:13, Jan 04:27, Mar 04:10, Jun 08:3

(For inguinal hernia repair, with simple orchiectomy, see 49505 or 49507 and 54520)

(For inguinal hernia repair, with excision of hydrocele or spermatocele, see 49505 or 49507 and 54840 or 55040)

49520 Repair recurrent inguinal hernia, any age; reducible

➔ *CPT Assistant* Winter 94:13, Sep 03:3, Jan 04:27, Mar 04:3, Jun 08:3

49521   incarcerated or strangulated

➔ *CPT Assistant* Winter 94:13, Jan 04:27, Mar 04:10, Jun 08:3

49525 Repair inguinal hernia, sliding, any age

➔ *CPT Assistant* Winter 94:14, Jan 04:27, Mar 04:10, Nov 07:9, Jun 08:3

(For incarcerated or strangulated inguinal hernia repair, see 49496, 49501, 49507, 49521)

49540 Repair lumbar hernia

➔ *CPT Assistant* Winter 94:14, Jun 08:3

49550 Repair initial femoral hernia, any age; reducible

➔ *CPT Assistant* Winter 94:14, Jun 08:3

49553   incarcerated or strangulated

➔ *CPT Assistant* Winter 94:14, Jun 08:3

49555 Repair recurrent femoral hernia; reducible

➔ *CPT Assistant* Winter 94:14, Jun 08:3

49557   incarcerated or strangulated

➔ *CPT Assistant* Winter 94:14, Jun 08:3

49560 Repair initial incisional or ventral hernia; reducible

➔ *CPT Assistant* Winter 93:6, Winter 94:14, Nov 97:19, Jun 08:3, Jan 12:10

49561   incarcerated or strangulated

➔ *CPT Assistant* Winter 94:14, Jun 08:3, Jan 12:10

49565 Repair recurrent incisional or ventral hernia; reducible

➔ *CPT Assistant* Winter 94:14, Nov 97:19, Jun 08:3, Jan 12:10

49566   incarcerated or strangulated

➔ *CPT Assistant* Winter 94:14, Jun 08:3, Jan 12:10

─── *Coding Tip* ───

Restrictions for Reporting Insertion of Mesh and Other Prostheses with Hernia Repairs

With the exception of the incisional hernia repairs (see 49560-49566) the use of mesh or other prostheses is not separately reported.

CPT Coding Guidelines, Hernioplasty, Herniorrhaphy, Herniotomy

+ 49568 Implantation of mesh or other prosthesis for open incisional or ventral hernia repair or mesh for closure of debridement for necrotizing soft tissue infection (List separately in addition to code for the incisional or ventral hernia repair)

➔ *CPT Assistant* Winter 94:14, Nov 97:19, Sep 01:11, Nov 05:15, Nov 07:9, Jun 08:3, Jan 12:10; *CPT Changes: An Insider's View* 2008, 2009

(Use 49568 in conjunction with 11004-11006, 49560-49566)

49570 Repair epigastric hernia (eg, preperitoneal fat); reducible (separate procedure)

➔ *CPT Assistant* Winter 94:15, Jun 08:3

49572   incarcerated or strangulated

➔ *CPT Assistant* Winter 94:15, Jun 08:3

49580 Repair umbilical hernia, younger than age 5 years; reducible

➔ *CPT Assistant* Winter 94:15, Jun 08:3

49582   incarcerated or strangulated

➔ *CPT Assistant* Winter 94:15, Jun 08:3

49585 Repair umbilical hernia, age 5 years or older; reducible

➔ *CPT Assistant* Winter 94:15

49587   incarcerated or strangulated

➔ *CPT Assistant* Winter 94:15

49590 Repair spigelian hernia
➔ *CPT Assistant* Winter 94:15

49600 Repair of small omphalocele, with primary closure
➔ *CPT Assistant* Winter 94:15

(Do not report modifier 63 in conjunction with 49600)

49605 Repair of large omphalocele or gastroschisis; with or without prosthesis
➔ *CPT Assistant* Winter 94:15

49606 with removal of prosthesis, final reduction and closure, in operating room
➔ *CPT Assistant* Winter 94:15

(Do not report modifier 63 in conjunction with 49605, 49606)

49610 Repair of omphalocele (Gross type operation); first stage
➔ *CPT Assistant* Winter 94:15

49611 second stage
➔ *CPT Assistant* Winter 94:15

(Do not report modifier 63 in conjunction with 49610, 49611)

(For diaphragmatic or hiatal hernia repair, see 39503, 43332)

(For surgical repair of omentum, use 49999)

Laparoscopy

Surgical laparoscopy always includes diagnostic laparoscopy. To report a diagnostic laparoscopy (peritoneoscopy) (separate procedure), use 49320.

49650 Laparoscopy, surgical; repair initial inguinal hernia
➔ *CPT Assistant* Nov 99:24, Mar 00:9; *CPT Changes: An Insider's View* 2000

49651 repair recurrent inguinal hernia
➔ *CPT Assistant* Nov 99:24, Mar 00:9; *CPT Changes: An Insider's View* 2000

49652 Laparoscopy, surgical, repair, ventral, umbilical, spigelian or epigastric hernia (includes mesh insertion, when performed); reducible
➔ *CPT Changes: An Insider's View* 2009

(Do not report 49652 in conjunction with 44180, 49568)

49653 incarcerated or strangulated
➔ *CPT Changes: An Insider's View* 2009

(Do not report 49653 in conjunction with 44180, 49568)

49654 Laparoscopy, surgical, repair, incisional hernia (includes mesh insertion, when performed); reducible
➔ *CPT Changes: An Insider's View* 2009

(Do not report 49654 in conjunction with 44180, 49568)

49655 incarcerated or strangulated
➔ *CPT Changes: An Insider's View* 2009

(Do not report 49655 in conjunction with 44180, 49568)

49656 Laparoscopy, surgical, repair, recurrent incisional hernia (includes mesh insertion, when performed); reducible
➔ *CPT Changes: An Insider's View* 2009

(Do not report 49656 in conjunction with 44180, 49568)

49657 incarcerated or strangulated
➔ *CPT Changes: An Insider's View* 2009

(Do not report 49657 in conjunction with 44180, 49568)

49659 Unlisted laparoscopy procedure, hernioplasty, herniorrhaphy, herniotomy
➔ *CPT Assistant* Nov 99:25, Mar 00:9, Sep 01:11, Nov 05:15, Feb 06:16, Jan 09:7; *CPT Changes: An Insider's View* 2000

Suture

49900 Suture, secondary, of abdominal wall for evisceration or dehiscence
➔ *CPT Assistant* Sep 10:7

(For suture of ruptured diaphragm, see 39540, 39541)

(For debridement of abdominal wall, see 11042, 11043)

Other Procedures

49904 Omental flap, extra-abdominal (eg, for reconstruction of sternal and chest wall defects)
➔ *CPT Changes: An Insider's View* 2003

(Code 49904 includes harvest and transfer. If a second surgeon harvests the omental flap, then the 2 surgeons should code 49904 as co-surgeons, using modifier 62)

+ 49905 Omental flap, intra-abdominal (List separately in addition to code for primary procedure)
➔ *CPT Assistant* Nov 00:11; *CPT Changes: An Insider's View* 2003

(Do not report 49905 in conjunction with 44700)

49906 Free omental flap with microvascular anastomosis
➔ *CPT Assistant* Nov 96:8, Apr 97:8, Nov 98:16

(Do not report code 69990 in addition to 49906)

49999 Unlisted procedure, abdomen, peritoneum and omentum
➔ *CPT Assistant* Jul 06:19, Sep 07:10, Nov 07:9, Aug 08:7, Apr 10:10, Dec 10:13, Jun 11:13
➔ *Clinical Examples in Radiology* Fall 07:1, 2

Surgery

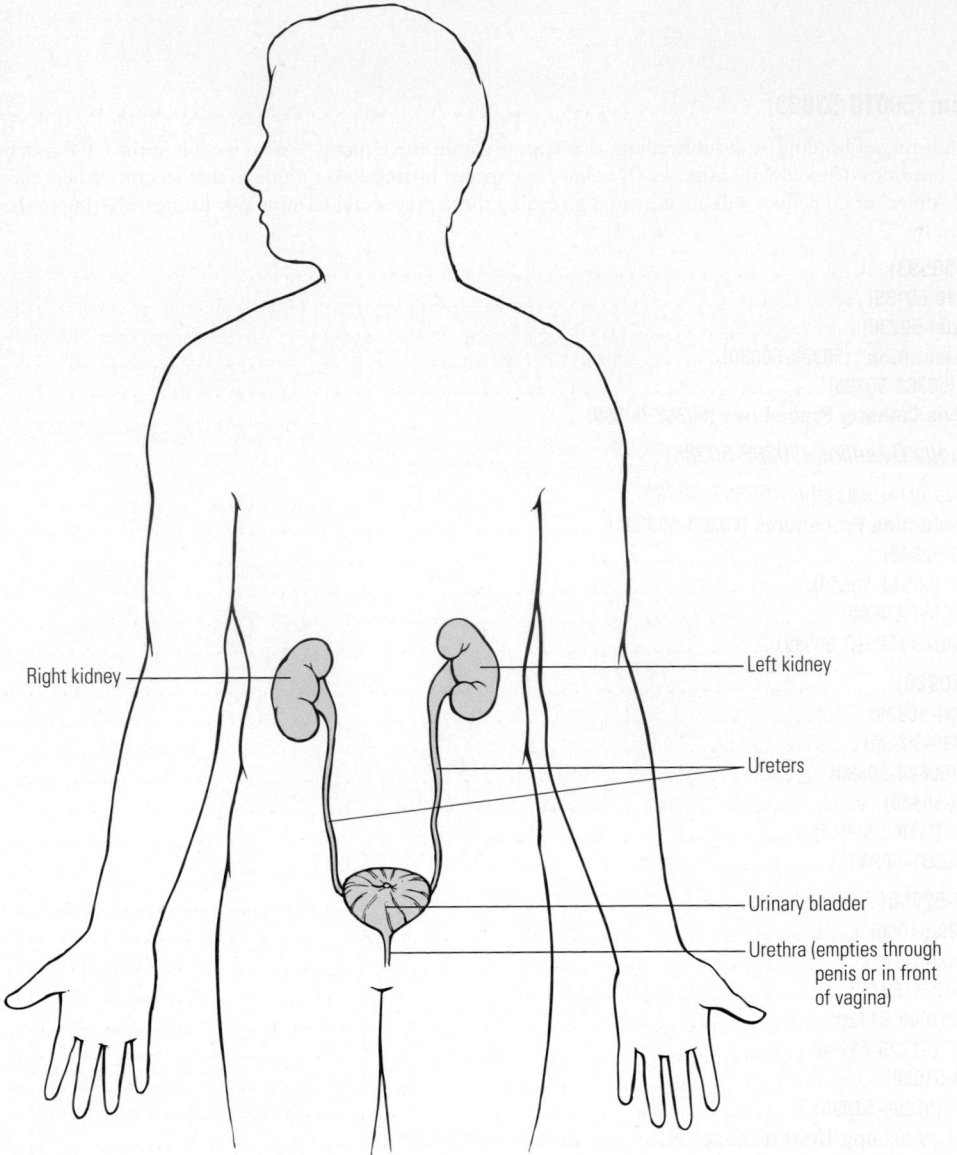

Right kidney

Left kidney

Ureters

Urinary bladder

Urethra (empties through
penis or in front
of vagina)

Urinary System

(For provision of chemotherapeutic agents, report both the specific service in addition to code(s) for the specific substance(s) or drug(s) provided)

Kidney

Incision

(For retroperitoneal exploration, abscess, tumor, or cyst, see 49010, 49060, 49203-49205)

50010   Renal exploration, not necessitating other specific procedures

(For laparoscopic ablation of renal mass lesion(s), use 50542)

50020   Drainage of perirenal or renal abscess; open
⟹ *CPT Assistant* Nov 97:19, Oct 01:8

Drainage of Renal Abscess
50020

An incision is made to the abscess cavity and the site is irrigated and drained.

⊙ 50021   percutaneous
⟹ *CPT Assistant* Nov 97:19, Mar 98:8, Oct 01:8

(For radiological supervision and interpretation, use 75989)

50040   Nephrostomy, nephrotomy with drainage
⟹ *CPT Assistant* Spring 93:35, Oct 01:8

50045   Nephrotomy, with exploration
⟹ *CPT Assistant* Oct 01:8

(For renal endoscopy performed in conjunction with this procedure, see 50570-50580)

50060   Nephrolithotomy; removal of calculus
⟹ *CPT Assistant* Oct 01:8

Nephrolithotomy With Calculus Removal
50060-50075

A kidney stone (calculus) is removed by an incision in the kidney. Use 50070 if complicated by a congenital kidney abnormality.

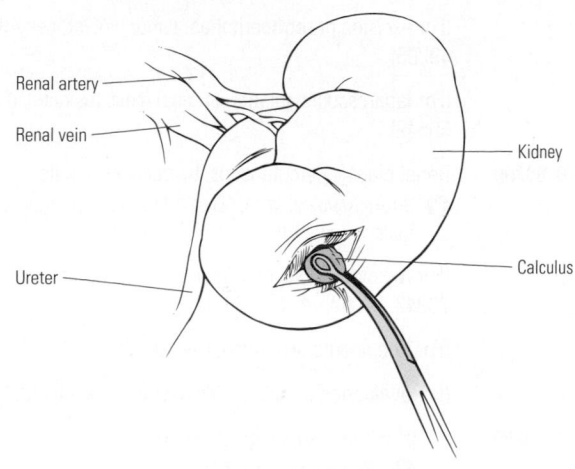

50065   secondary surgical operation for calculus
⟹ *CPT Assistant* Oct 01:8

50070   complicated by congenital kidney abnormality
⟹ *CPT Assistant* Oct 01:8

50075   removal of large staghorn calculus filling renal pelvis and calyces (including anatrophic pyelolithotomy)
⟹ *CPT Assistant* Oct 01:8

50080   Percutaneous nephrostolithotomy or pyelostolithotomy, with or without dilation, endoscopy, lithotripsy, stenting, or basket extraction; up to 2 cm
⟹ *CPT Assistant* Oct 01:8, Dec 08:7, Jun 09:10

50081   over 2 cm
⟹ *CPT Assistant* Oct 01:8, Dec 08:7, Jun 09:10

(For establishment of nephrostomy without nephrostolithotomy, see 50040, 50395, 52334)

(For fluoroscopic guidance, see 76000, 76001)

50100   Transection or repositioning of aberrant renal vessels (separate procedure)
⟹ *CPT Assistant* Oct 01:8

50120   Pyelotomy; with exploration
⟹ *CPT Assistant* Oct 01:8

(For renal endoscopy performed in conjunction with this procedure, see 50570-50580)

50125   with drainage, pyelostomy
⟹ *CPT Assistant* Oct 01:8

50130   with removal of calculus (pyelolithotomy, pelviolithotomy, including coagulum pyelolithotomy)
⟹ *CPT Assistant* Oct 01:8

▲=Revised code   ●=New code   ▶◀=Contains new or revised text   ⊘=Modifier 51 exempt

Urinary

50135   complicated (eg, secondary operation, congenital kidney abnormality)
➔ *CPT Assistant* Oct 01:8

(For supply of anticarcinogenic agents, use 99070 in addition to code for primary procedure)

Excision

(For excision of retroperitoneal tumor or cyst, see 49203-49205)

(For laparoscopic ablation of renal mass lesion(s), use 50542)

⊙ **50200**   Renal biopsy; percutaneous, by trocar or needle
➔ *CPT Assistant* Fall 93:13, Oct 01:8, Feb 10:7; *CPT Changes: An Insider's View* 2010

(For radiological supervision and interpretation, see 76942, 77002, 77012, 77021)

(For fine needle aspiration, use 10022)

(For evaluation of fine needle aspirate, see 88172, 88173)

50205   by surgical exposure of kidney
➔ *CPT Assistant* Oct 01:8

50220   Nephrectomy, including partial ureterectomy, any open approach including rib resection;
➔ *CPT Assistant* Oct 01:8, Nov 02:3, Aug 08:7; *CPT Changes: An Insider's View* 2002

50225   complicated because of previous surgery on same kidney
➔ *CPT Assistant* Oct 01:8, Nov 02:3

50230   radical, with regional lymphadenectomy and/or vena caval thrombectomy
➔ *CPT Assistant* Oct 01:8, Nov 02:3

(When vena caval resection with reconstruction is necessary, use 37799)

50234   Nephrectomy with total ureterectomy and bladder cuff; through same incision
➔ *CPT Assistant* Oct 01:8, Nov 02:3

50236   through separate incision
➔ *CPT Assistant* Oct 01:8, Nov 02:3

50240   Nephrectomy, partial
➔ *CPT Assistant* Oct 01:8, Nov 02:3, Jan 03:20, Apr 05:10, 12, Aug 08:7

(For laparoscopic partial nephrectomy, use 50543)

50250   Ablation, open, 1 or more renal mass lesion(s), cryosurgical, including intraoperative ultrasound guidance and monitoring, if performed
➔ *CPT Assistant* May 06:17; *CPT Changes: An Insider's View* 2006, 2011

(For laparoscopic ablation of renal mass lesions, use 50542)

(For percutaneous ablation of renal tumors, see 50592, 50593)

50280   Excision or unroofing of cyst(s) of kidney
➔ *CPT Assistant* Nov 99:25, Oct 01:8; *CPT Changes: An Insider's View* 2000

(For laparoscopic ablation of renal cysts, use 50541)

50290   Excision of perinephric cyst
➔ *CPT Assistant* Oct 01:8

Renal Transplantation

Renal *auto*transplantation includes reimplantation of the autograft as the primary procedure, along with secondary extra-corporeal procedure(s) (eg, partial nephrectomy, nephrolithotomy) reported with modifier 51 (see 50380 and applicable secondary procedure(s)).

Renal *allo*transplantation involves three distinct components of physician work:

1. *Cadaver donor nephrectomy, unilateral or bilateral,* which includes harvesting the graft(s) and cold preservation of the graft(s) (perfusing with cold preservation solution and cold maintenance) (use 50300). *Living donor nephrectomy,* which includes harvesting the graft, cold preservation of the graft (perfusing with cold preservation solution and cold maintenance), and care of the donor (see 50320, 50547).

2. *Backbench work:*

   Standard preparation of a cadaver donor renal allograft prior to transplantation including dissection and removal of perinephric fat, diaphragmatic and retroperitoneal attachments; excision of adrenal gland; and preparation of ureter(s), renal vein(s), and renal artery(s), ligating branches, as necessary (use 50323).

   Standard preparation of a living donor renal allograft (open or laparoscopic) prior to transplantation including dissection and removal of perinephric fat and preparation of ureter(s), renal vein(s), and renal artery(s), ligating branches, as necessary (use 50325).

   Additional reconstruction of a cadaver or living donor renal allograft prior to transplantation may include venous, arterial, and/or ureteral anastomosis(es) necessary for implantation (see 50327-50329).

3. *Recipient renal allotransplantation,* which includes transplantation of the allograft (with or without recipient nephrectomy) and care of the recipient (see 50360, 50365).

   (For dialysis, see 90935-90999)

   (For laparoscopic donor nephrectomy, use 50547)

   (For laparoscopic drainage of lymphocele to peritoneal cavity, use 49323)

50300　Donor nephrectomy (including cold preservation); from cadaver donor, unilateral or bilateral

> ➔ *CPT Assistant* Nov 99:25, Apr 05:10-12; *CPT Changes: An Insider's View* 2000, 2005

50320　　open, from living donor

> ➔ *CPT Assistant* Nov 99:25, May 00:4; *CPT Changes: An Insider's View* 2000, 2005

50323　Backbench standard preparation of cadaver donor renal allograft prior to transplantation, including dissection and removal of perinephric fat, diaphragmatic and retroperitoneal attachments, excision of adrenal gland, and preparation of ureter(s), renal vein(s), and renal artery(s), ligating branches, as necessary

> ➔ *CPT Assistant* Apr 05:10-11; *CPT Changes: An Insider's View* 2005

(Do not report 50323 in conjunction with 60540, 60545)

50325　Backbench standard preparation of living donor renal allograft (open or laparoscopic) prior to transplantation, including dissection and removal of perinephric fat and preparation of ureter(s), renal vein(s), and renal artery(s), ligating branches, as necessary

> ➔ *CPT Changes: An Insider's View* 2005

50327　Backbench reconstruction of cadaver or living donor renal allograft prior to transplantation; venous anastomosis, each

> ➔ *CPT Changes: An Insider's View* 2005

50328　　arterial anastomosis, each

> ➔ *CPT Changes: An Insider's View* 2005

50329　　ureteral anastomosis, each

> ➔ *CPT Changes: An Insider's View* 2005

50340　Recipient nephrectomy (separate procedure)

(For bilateral procedure, report 50340 with modifier 50)

50360　Renal allotransplantation, implantation of graft; without recipient nephrectomy

> ➔ *CPT Changes: An Insider's View* 2005

50365　　with recipient nephrectomy

> ➔ *CPT Assistant* Apr 05:10-11

(For bilateral procedure, report 50365 with modifier 50)

50370　Removal of transplanted renal allograft

50380　Renal autotransplantation, reimplantation of kidney

> ➔ *CPT Assistant* Apr 05:10, 12

(For renal autotransplantation extra-corporeal [bench] surgery, use autotransplantation as the primary procedure and report secondary procedure[s] [eg, partial nephrectomy, nephrolithotomy] with modifier 51)

Introduction

Renal Pelvis Catheter Procedures

Internally Dwelling

⊙ **50382**　Removal (via snare/capture) and replacement of internally dwelling ureteral stent via percutaneous approach, including radiological supervision and interpretation

> ➔ *CPT Assistant* Sep 06:1, 16, Oct 08:8, Dec 09:4; *CPT Changes: An Insider's View* 2006
>
> ➔ *Clinical Examples in Radiology* Winter 06:15, Spring 08:5

(For bilateral procedure, use modifier 50)

(For removal and replacement of an internally dwelling ureteral stent via a transurethral approach, use 50385)

⊙ **50384**　Removal (via snare/capture) of internally dwelling ureteral stent via percutaneous approach, including radiological supervision and interpretation

> ➔ *CPT Assistant* Sep 06:2, 16, Oct 08:8; *CPT Changes: An Insider's View* 2006
>
> ➔ *Clinical Examples in Radiology* Winter 06:16, Spring 08:5

(For bilateral procedure, use modifier 50)

(Do not report 50382, 50384 in conjunction with 50395)

(For removal of an internally dwelling ureteral stent via a transurethral approach, use 50386)

⊙ **50385**　Removal (via snare/capture) and replacement of internally dwelling ureteral stent via transurethral approach, without use of cystoscopy, including radiological supervision and interpretation

> ➔ *CPT Assistant* Oct 08:8, Dec 09:4; *CPT Changes: An Insider's View* 2008
>
> ➔ *Clinical Examples in Radiology* Spring 08:5

⊙ **50386**　Removal (via snare/capture) of internally dwelling ureteral stent via transurethral approach, without use of cystoscopy, including radiological supervision and interpretation

> ➔ *CPT Assistant* Oct 08:8; *CPT Changes: An Insider's View* 2008
>
> ➔ *Clinical Examples in Radiology* Spring 08:4

Externally Accessible

⊙ **50387**　Removal and replacement of externally accessible transnephric ureteral stent (eg, external/internal stent) requiring fluoroscopic guidance, including radiological supervision and interpretation

> ➔ *CPT Assistant* Sep 06:2, 4, 16, Dec 09:4, Mar 12:3; *CPT Changes: An Insider's View* 2006
>
> ➔ *Clinical Examples in Radiology* Winter 06:16, Spring 08:5

(For bilateral procedure, use modifier 50)

(For removal and replacement of externally accessible ureteral stent via ureterostomy or ilieal conduit, use 50688)

Urinary

(For removal without replacement of an externally accessible ureteral stent not requiring fluoroscopic guidance, see Evaluation and Management services codes)

50389   Removal of nephrostomy tube, requiring fluoroscopic guidance (eg, with concurrent indwelling ureteral stent)

➔ *CPT Assistant* Sep 06:1, 2, 4; *CPT Changes: An Insider's View* 2006

➔ *Clinical Examples in Radiology* Winter 06:16

(Removal of nephrostomy tube not requiring fluoroscopic guidance is considered inherent to E/M services. Report the appropriate level of E/M service provided)

Other Introduction Procedures

50390   Aspiration and/or injection of renal cyst or pelvis by needle, percutaneous

➔ *CPT Assistant* Fall 93:14, Dec 97:7, Oct 01:8, Oct 05:18, Oct 08:8

(For radiological supervision and interpretation, see 74425, 74470, 76942, 77002, 77012, 77021)

(For evaluation of fine needle aspirate, see 88172, 88173)

50391   Instillation(s) of therapeutic agent into renal pelvis and/or ureter through established nephrostomy, pyelostomy or ureterostomy tube (eg, anticarcinogenic or antifungal agent)

➔ *CPT Assistant* Oct 05:18; *CPT Changes: An Insider's View* 2005

50392   Introduction of intracatheter or catheter into renal pelvis for drainage and/or injection, percutaneous

➔ *CPT Assistant* Dec 97:7, Oct 01:8, Oct 05:18, Oct 08:8

(For radiological supervision and interpretation, see 74475, 76942, 77012)

Introduction of Catheter Into Renal Pelvis
50392

The physician inserts a catheter into the renal pelvis in order to drain urine and/or give an injection.

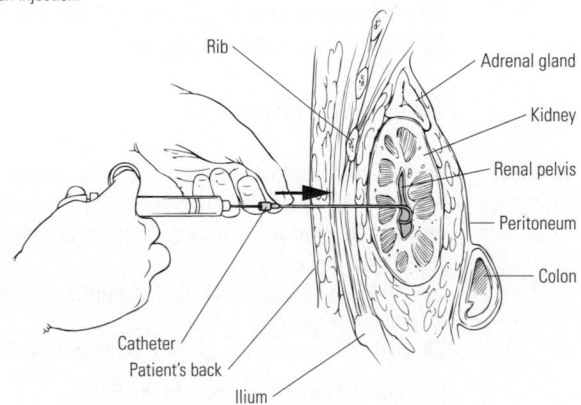

50393   Introduction of ureteral catheter or stent into ureter through renal pelvis for drainage and/or injection, percutaneous

➔ *CPT Assistant* Fall 93:14, Oct 01:8, Oct 05:18, Dec 09:4, Mar 12:10

➔ *Clinical Examples in Radiology* Summer 06:1-3

(For radiological supervision and interpretation, see 74480, 76942, 77002, 77012)

50394   Injection procedure for pyelography (as nephrostogram, pyelostogram, antegrade pyeloureterograms) through nephrostomy or pyelostomy tube, or indwelling ureteral catheter

➔ *CPT Assistant* Fall 93:15, Dec 97:7, Oct 01:8, Oct 05:18

➔ *Clinical Examples in Radiology* Summer 06:1-3

(For radiological supervision and interpretation, use 74425)

50395   Introduction of guide into renal pelvis and/or ureter with dilation to establish nephrostomy tract, percutaneous

➔ *CPT Assistant* Oct 01:8, Oct 05:18, Sep 06:1, Dec 08:7, Jan 09:7

(For radiological supervision and interpretation, see 74475, 74480, 74485)

(For nephrostolithotomy, see 50080, 50081)

(For retrograde percutaneous nephrostomy, use 52334)

(For endoscopic surgery, see 50551-50561)

50396   Manometric studies through nephrostomy or pyelostomy tube, or indwelling ureteral catheter

➔ *CPT Assistant* Fall 93:16, Dec 97:7, Oct 01:8

(For radiological supervision and interpretation, see 74425, 74475, 74480)

50398   Change of nephrostomy or pyelostomy tube

➔ *CPT Assistant* Oct 01:8, Mar 12:10

(For radiological supervision and interpretation, use 75984)

Repair

50400   Pyeloplasty (Foley Y-pyeloplasty), plastic operation on renal pelvis, with or without plastic operation on ureter, nephropexy, nephrostomy, pyelostomy, or ureteral splinting; simple

➔ *CPT Assistant* Nov 99:25, May 00:4, Oct 01:8; *CPT Changes: An Insider's View* 2000

50405   complicated (congenital kidney abnormality, secondary pyeloplasty, solitary kidney, calycoplasty)

➔ *CPT Assistant* Nov 99:25, May 00:4, Oct 01:8; *CPT Changes: An Insider's View* 2000

(For laparoscopic approach, use 50544)

50500   Nephrorrhaphy, suture of kidney wound or injury

50520   Closure of nephrocutaneous or pyelocutaneous fistula

50525   Closure of nephrovisceral fistula (eg, renocolic), including visceral repair; abdominal approach

50526   thoracic approach

50540   Symphysiotomy for horseshoe kidney with or without pyeloplasty and/or other plastic procedure, unilateral or bilateral (1 operation)

Laparoscopy

Surgical laparoscopy always includes diagnostic laparoscopy. To report a diagnostic laparoscopy (peritoneoscopy) (separate procedure), use 49320.

50541   Laparoscopy, surgical; ablation of renal cysts

> ↪ *CPT Assistant* Nov 99:25, May 00:4, Oct 01:8, Nov 02:3, Jan 03:20; *CPT Changes: An Insider's View* 2000

50542   ablation of renal mass lesion(s), including intraoperative ultrasound guidance and monitoring, when performed

> ↪ *CPT Assistant* Nov 02:3, Jan 03:21, Aug 04:12; *CPT Changes: An Insider's View* 2003, 2011

(For open procedure, use 50250)

(For percutaneous ablation of renal tumors, see 50592, 50593)

50543   partial nephrectomy

> ↪ *CPT Assistant* Nov 02:3, Jan 03:21; *CPT Changes: An Insider's View* 2003

(For open procedure, use 50240)

50544   pyeloplasty

> ↪ *CPT Assistant* Nov 99:25, May 00:4, Oct 01:8; *CPT Changes: An Insider's View* 2000

50545   radical nephrectomy (includes removal of Gerota's fascia and surrounding fatty tissue, removal of regional lymph nodes, and adrenalectomy)

> ↪ *CPT Assistant* Oct 01:8; *CPT Changes: An Insider's View* 2001

(For open procedure, use 50230)

Laparoscopic Radical Nephrectomy
50545

Radical nephrectomy (includes removal of Gerota's fascia and surrounding fatty tissue, removal of regional lymph nodes, and adrenalectomy)

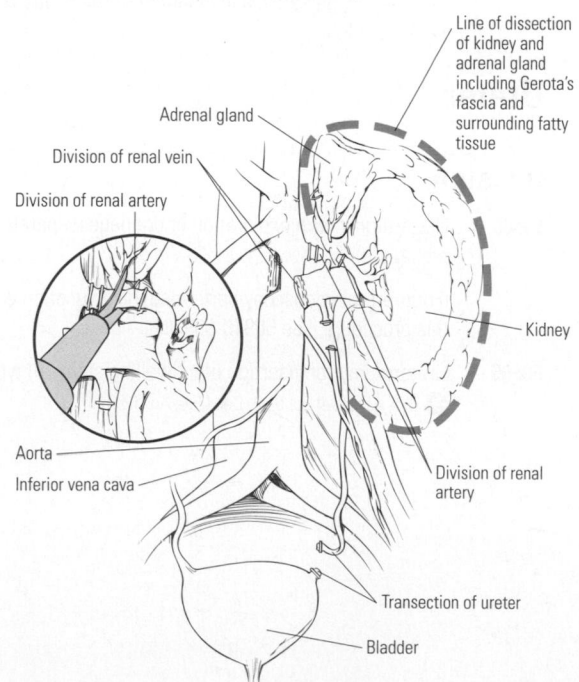

50546   nephrectomy, including partial ureterectomy

> ↪ *CPT Assistant* Nov 99:25, May 00:4, Oct 01:8; *CPT Changes: An Insider's View* 2000, 2001

Laparoscopic Nephrectomy
50546

A kidney is dissected and removed under laparoscopic guidance.

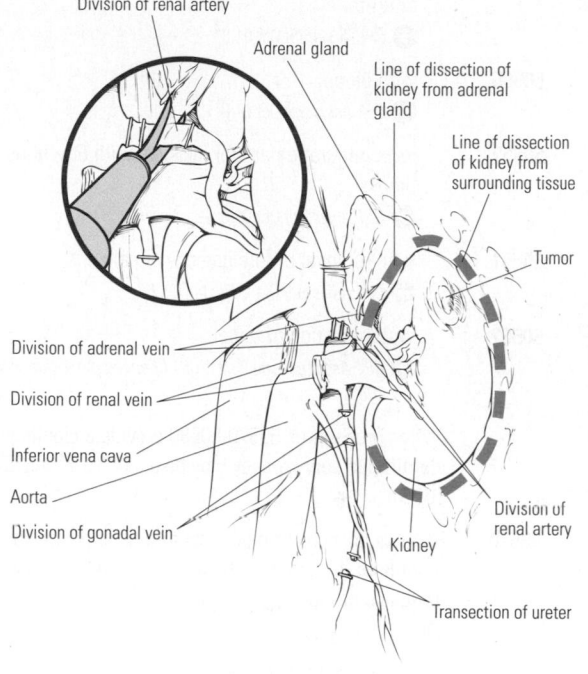

50547   donor nephrectomy (including cold preservation), from living donor

> ↪ *CPT Assistant* Nov 99:25, May 00:4, Oct 01:8; *CPT Changes: An Insider's View* 2000, 2006

(For open procedure, use 50320)

(For backbench renal allograft standard preparation prior to transplantation, use 50325)

(For backbench renal allograft reconstruction prior to transplantation, see 50327-50329)

50548   nephrectomy with total ureterectomy

> ↪ *CPT Assistant* Nov 99:25, May 00:4, Oct 01:8; *CPT Changes: An Insider's View* 2000, 2001

(For open procedure, see 50234, 50236)

50549   Unlisted laparoscopy procedure, renal

> ↪ *CPT Assistant* Nov 99:25, Mar 00:9, May 00:4, Feb 06:16; *CPT Changes: An Insider's View* 2000

(For laparoscopic drainage of lymphocele to peritoneal cavity, use 49323)

Endoscopy

(For supplies and materials, use 99070)

50551 Renal endoscopy through established nephrostomy or pyelostomy, with or without irrigation, instillation, or ureteropyelography, exclusive of radiologic service;
➲ *CPT Assistant* Oct 01:8, Jan 03:21

50553 with ureteral catheterization, with or without dilation of ureter
➲ *CPT Assistant* Oct 01:8

50555 with biopsy
➲ *CPT Assistant* Oct 01:8

50557 with fulguration and/or incision, with or without biopsy
➲ *CPT Assistant* Oct 01:8

50561 with removal of foreign body or calculus
➲ *CPT Assistant* Oct 01:8, Jan 03:21

50562 with resection of tumor
➲ *CPT Assistant* Jan 03:21; *CPT Changes: An Insider's View* 2003

(When procedures 50570-50580 provide a significant identifiable service, they may be added to 50045 and 50120)

50570 Renal endoscopy through nephrotomy or pyelotomy, with or without irrigation, instillation, or ureteropyelography, exclusive of radiologic service;
➲ *CPT Assistant* Oct 01:8

(For nephrotomy, use 50045)

(For pyelotomy, use 50120)

50572 with ureteral catheterization, with or without dilation of ureter
➲ *CPT Assistant* Oct 01:8

50574 with biopsy
➲ *CPT Assistant* Oct 01:8

50575 with endopyelotomy (includes cystoscopy, ureteroscopy, dilation of ureter and ureteral pelvic junction, incision of ureteral pelvic junction and insertion of endopyelotomy stent)
➲ *CPT Assistant* Oct 01:8, Aug 02:11

50576 with fulguration and/or incision, with or without biopsy
➲ *CPT Assistant* Oct 01:8

50580 with removal of foreign body or calculus
➲ *CPT Assistant* Oct 01:8

Other Procedures

50590 Lithotripsy, extracorporeal shock wave
➲ *CPT Assistant* Jul 01:11, Aug 01:10, Oct 01:8, Jul 03:16, Aug 03:14

Lithotripsy
50590

The physician breaks up a kidney stone (calculus) by directing shock waves through a liquid surrounding the patient.

Kidney stone (calculus)
Radiologic monitors for guidance
Medium
Shock waves are concentrated on stone
Electrode
Patient, transverse section

⊙ **50592** Ablation, 1 or more renal tumor(s), percutaneous, unilateral, radiofrequency
➲ *CPT Changes: An Insider's View* 2006
➲ *Clinical Examples in Radiology* Winter 06:16

(50592 is a unilateral procedure. For bilateral procedure, report 50592 with modifier 50)

(For imaging guidance and monitoring, see 76940, 77013, 77022)

⊙ **50593** Ablation, renal tumor(s), unilateral, percutaneous, cryotherapy
➲ *CPT Changes: An Insider's View* 2008

(50593 is a unilateral procedure. For bilateral procedure, report 50593 with modifier 50)

(For imaging guidance and monitoring, see codes 76940, 77013, 77022)

Ureter

Incision

50600 Ureterotomy with exploration or drainage (separate procedure)

(For ureteral endoscopy performed in conjunction with this procedure, see 50970-50980)

50605 Ureterotomy for insertion of indwelling stent, all types
➲ *CPT Assistant* Oct 01:8, Dec 09:4, Apr 12:18

Indwelling Ureteral Stent
50605

The physician makes an incision in the ureter (ureterotomy) and inserts a stent. For placement using cystourethroscopic technique, use 52332.

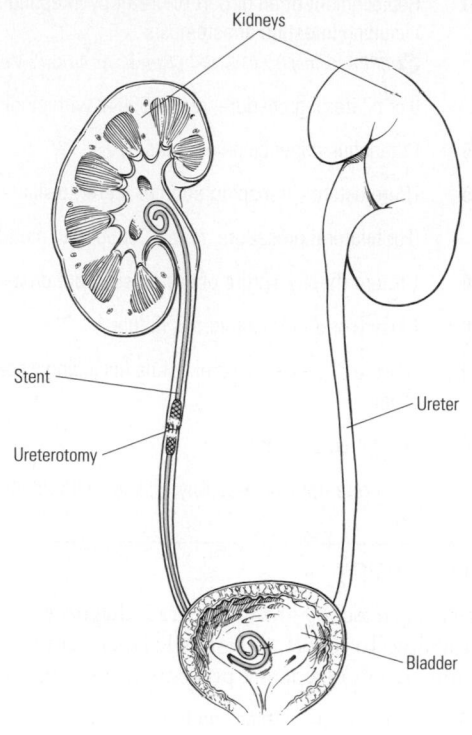

Kidneys

Stent

Ureterotomy

Ureter

Bladder

50610   Ureterolithotomy; upper one-third of ureter
> *CPT Assistant* Nov 99:26, Oct 01:8; *CPT Changes: An Insider's View* 2000

50620   middle one-third of ureter
> *CPT Assistant* Nov 99:26, Oct 01:8; *CPT Changes: An Insider's View* 2000

50630   lower one-third of ureter
> *CPT Assistant* Nov 99:26, Oct 01:8; *CPT Changes: An Insider's View* 2000

(For laparoscopic approach, use 50945)

(For transvesical ureterolithotomy, use 51060)

(For cystotomy with stone basket extraction of ureteral calculus, use 51065)

(For endoscopic extraction or manipulation of ureteral calculus, see 50080, 50081, 50561, 50961, 50980, 52320-52330, 52352, 52353)

Excision

(For ureterocele, see 51535, 52300)

50650   Ureterectomy, with bladder cuff (separate procedure)

50660   Ureterectomy, total, ectopic ureter, combination abdominal, vaginal and/or perineal approach

Introduction

50684   Injection procedure for ureterography or ureteropyelography through ureterostomy or indwelling ureteral catheter

(For radiological supervision and interpretation, use 74425)

50686   Manometric studies through ureterostomy or indwelling ureteral catheter

50688   Change of ureterostomy tube or externally accessible ureteral stent via ileal conduit
> *CPT Changes: An Insider's View* 2006
> *Clinical Examples in Radiology* Winter 06:20

(If imaging guidance is performed, use 75984)

50690   Injection procedure for visualization of ileal conduit and/or ureteropyelography, exclusive of radiologic service

(For radiological supervision and interpretation, use 74425)

Repair

50700   Ureteroplasty, plastic operation on ureter (eg, stricture)

50715   Ureterolysis, with or without repositioning of ureter for retroperitoneal fibrosis

(For bilateral procedure, report 50715 with modifier 50)

50722   Ureterolysis for ovarian vein syndrome

50725   Ureterolysis for retrocaval ureter, with reanastomosis of upper urinary tract or vena cava

50727   Revision of urinary-cutaneous anastomosis (any type urostomy);

50728   with repair of fascial defect and hernia

50740   Ureteropyelostomy, anastomosis of ureter and renal pelvis
> *CPT Assistant* Oct 01:8

50750   Ureterocalycostomy, anastomosis of ureter to renal calyx
> *CPT Assistant* Oct 01:8

50760   Ureteroureterostomy
> *CPT Assistant* Oct 01:8

50770   Transureteroureterostomy, anastomosis of ureter to contralateral ureter

(Codes 50780-50785 include minor procedures to prevent vesicoureteral reflux)

50780   Ureteroneocystostomy; anastomosis of single ureter to bladder
> *CPT Assistant* Oct 01:8

(For bilateral procedure, report 50780 with modifier 50)

(When combined with cystourethroplasty or vesical neck revision, use 51820)

50782   anastomosis of duplicated ureter to bladder
> *CPT Assistant* Oct 01:8

Urinary

Urinary

50783   with extensive ureteral tailoring
> *CPT Assistant* Oct 01:8

50785   with vesico-psoas hitch or bladder flap
> *CPT Assistant* Oct 01:8

(For bilateral procedure, report 50785 with modifier 50)

50800   Ureteroenterostomy, direct anastomosis of ureter to intestine
> *CPT Assistant* Oct 01:8

(For bilateral procedure, report 50800 with modifier 50)

50810   Ureterosigmoidostomy, with creation of sigmoid bladder and establishment of abdominal or perineal colostomy, including intestine anastomosis
> *CPT Assistant* Oct 01:8; *CPT Changes: An Insider's View* 2002

50815   Ureterocolon conduit, including intestine anastomosis
> *CPT Assistant* Oct 01:8

(For bilateral procedure, report 50815 with modifier 50)

50820   Ureteroileal conduit (ileal bladder), including intestine anastomosis (Bricker operation)
> *CPT Assistant* Oct 01:8; *CPT Changes: An Insider's View* 2002

(For bilateral procedure, report 50820 with modifier 50)

(For combination of 50800-50820 with cystectomy, see 51580-51595)

Ureteroileal Conduit
50820

The ureters are connected to a segment of intestine to divert urine flow through an opening in the skin.

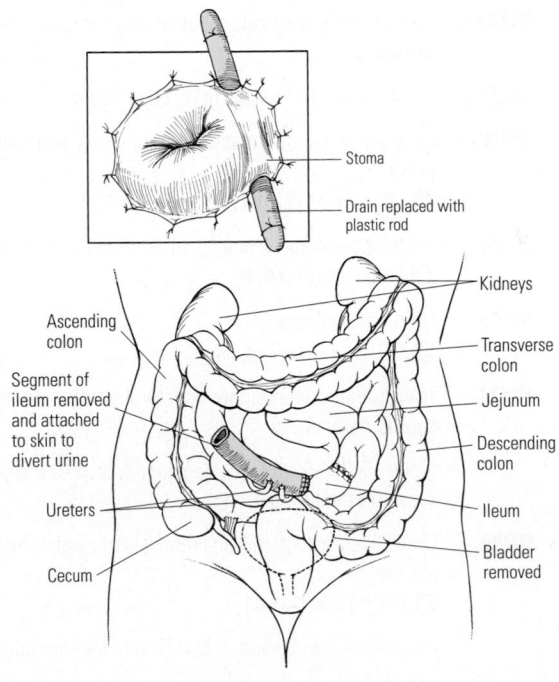

50825   Continent diversion, including intestine anastomosis using any segment of small and/or large intestine (Kock pouch or Camey enterocystoplasty)
> *CPT Assistant* Oct 01:8; *CPT Changes: An Insider's View* 2002

50830   Urinary undiversion (eg, taking down of ureteroileal conduit, ureterosigmoidostomy or ureteroenterostomy with ureteroureterostomy or ureteroneocystostomy)
> *CPT Assistant* Oct 01:8

50840   Replacement of all or part of ureter by intestine segment, including intestine anastomosis
> *CPT Assistant* Oct 01:8; *CPT Changes: An Insider's View* 2002

(For bilateral procedure, report 50840 with modifier 50)

50845   Cutaneous appendico-vesicostomy

50860   Ureterostomy, transplantation of ureter to skin

(For bilateral procedure, report 50860 with modifier 50)

50900   Ureterorrhaphy, suture of ureter (separate procedure)

50920   Closure of ureterocutaneous fistula

50930   Closure of ureterovisceral fistula (including visceral repair)

50940   Deligation of ureter

(For ureteroplasty, ureterolysis, see 50700-50860)

Laparoscopy

Surgical laparoscopy always includes diagnostic laparoscopy. To report a diagnostic laparoscopy (peritoneoscopy) (separate procedure), use 49320.

50945   Laparoscopy, surgical; ureterolithotomy
> *CPT Assistant* Nov 99:26, May 00:4, Oct 01:8, Sep 06:13; *CPT Changes: An Insider's View* 2000

50947   ureteroneocystostomy with cystoscopy and ureteral stent placement
> *CPT Assistant* Oct 01:8; *CPT Changes: An Insider's View* 2001

Laparoscopic Ureteroneocystostomy
50947

Ureteroneocystostomy with cystoscopy and ureteral stent placement

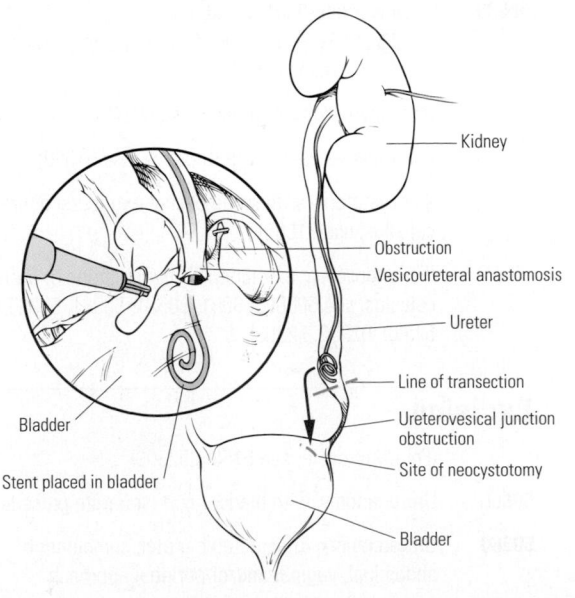

50948   ureteroneocystostomy without cystoscopy and ureteral stent placement

> *CPT Assistant* Oct 01:8; *CPT Changes: An Insider's View* 2001

(For open ureteroneocystostomy, see 50780-50785)

50949   Unlisted laparoscopy procedure, ureter

> *CPT Assistant* Oct 01:8; *CPT Changes: An Insider's View* 2001

Endoscopy

50951   Ureteral endoscopy through established ureterostomy, with or without irrigation, instillation, or ureteropyelography, exclusive of radiologic service;

> *CPT Assistant* Oct 01:8

50953   with ureteral catheterization, with or without dilation of ureter

> *CPT Assistant* Oct 01:8

50955   with biopsy

> *CPT Assistant* Oct 01:8

50957   with fulguration and/or incision, with or without biopsy

> *CPT Assistant* Oct 01:8

50961   with removal of foreign body or calculus

> *CPT Assistant* Oct 01:8, Mar 07:10, Apr 07:12

(When procedures 50970-50980 provide a significant identifiable service, they may be added to 50600)

50970   Ureteral endoscopy through ureterotomy, with or without irrigation, instillation, or ureteropyelography, exclusive of radiologic service;

> *CPT Assistant* Oct 01:8

(For ureterotomy, use 50600)

50972   with ureteral catheterization, with or without dilation of ureter

> *CPT Assistant* Oct 01:8

50974   with biopsy

> *CPT Assistant* Oct 01:8

50976   with fulguration and/or incision, with or without biopsy

> *CPT Assistant* Oct 01:8

50980   with removal of foreign body or calculus

> *CPT Assistant* Oct 01:8

Bladder

Incision

51020   Cystotomy or cystostomy; with fulguration and/or insertion of radioactive material

51030   with cryosurgical destruction of intravesical lesion

51040   Cystostomy, cystotomy with drainage

51045   Cystotomy, with insertion of ureteral catheter or stent (separate procedure)

51050   Cystolithotomy, cystotomy with removal of calculus, without vesical neck resection

51060   Transvesical ureterolithotomy

51065   Cystotomy, with calculus basket extraction and/or ultrasonic or electrohydraulic fragmentation of ureteral calculus

> *CPT Changes: An Insider's View* 2002

51080   Drainage of perivesical or prevesical space abscess

Removal

51100   Aspiration of bladder; by needle

> *CPT Assistant* Jun 08:11; *CPT Changes: An Insider's View* 2008

51101   by trocar or intracatheter

> *CPT Assistant* Jun 08:11; *CPT Changes: An Insider's View* 2008

51102   with insertion of suprapubic catheter

> *CPT Assistant* Jun 08:11; *CPT Changes: An Insider's View* 2008

(For imaging guidance, see 76942, 77002, 77012)

Excision

51500   Excision of urachal cyst or sinus, with or without umbilical hernia repair

51520   Cystotomy; for simple excision of vesical neck (separate procedure)

51525   for excision of bladder diverticulum, single or multiple (separate procedure)

51530   for excision of bladder tumor

(For transurethral resection, see 52234-52240, 52305)

51535   Cystotomy for excision, incision, or repair of ureterocele

(For bilateral procedure, report 51535 with modifier 50)

(For transurethral excision, use 52300)

51550   Cystectomy, partial; simple

51555   complicated (eg, postradiation, previous surgery, difficult location)

51565   Cystectomy, partial, with reimplantation of ureter(s) into bladder (ureteroneocystostomy)

51570   Cystectomy, complete; (separate procedure)

> *CPT Assistant* Spring 93:35

51575   with bilateral pelvic lymphadenectomy, including external iliac, hypogastric, and obturator nodes

> *CPT Assistant* Spring 93:35

51580   Cystectomy, complete, with ureterosigmoidostomy or ureterocutaneous transplantations;

51585   with bilateral pelvic lymphadenectomy, including external iliac, hypogastric, and obturator nodes

51590   Cystectomy, complete, with ureteroileal conduit or sigmoid bladder, including intestine anastomosis;

> *CPT Changes: An Insider's View* 2002

▲=Revised code   ●=New code   ►◄=Contains new or revised text   ⊘=Modifier 51 exempt

Urinary

Urinary

51595 with bilateral pelvic lymphadenectomy, including external iliac, hypogastric, and obturator nodes

51596 Cystectomy, complete, with continent diversion, any open technique, using any segment of small and/or large intestine to construct neobladder

➔ *CPT Changes: An Insider's View* 2002

51597 Pelvic exenteration, complete, for vesical, prostatic or urethral malignancy, with removal of bladder and ureteral transplantations, with or without hysterectomy and/or abdominoperineal resection of rectum and colon and colostomy, or any combination thereof

(For pelvic exenteration for gynecologic malignancy, use 58240)

Introduction

51600 Injection procedure for cystography or voiding urethrocystography

(For radiological supervision and interpretation, see 74430, 74455)

51605 Injection procedure and placement of chain for contrast and/or chain urethrocystography

(For radiological supervision and interpretation, use 74430)

51610 Injection procedure for retrograde urethrocystography

(For radiological supervision and interpretation, use 74450)

51700 Bladder irrigation, simple, lavage and/or instillation

(Codes 51701-51702 are reported only when performed independently. Do not report 51701-51702 when catheter insertion is an inclusive component of another procedure.)

51701 Insertion of non-indwelling bladder catheter (eg, straight catheterization for residual urine)

➔ *CPT Assistant* Jul 06:4, Jan 07:31, Jul 07:1; *CPT Changes: An Insider's View* 2003

51702 Insertion of temporary indwelling bladder catheter; simple (eg, Foley)

➔ *CPT Assistant* Oct 03:10, Jul 06:4, Jan 07:31, Jul 07:1; *CPT Changes: An Insider's View* 2003

➔ *Clinical Examples in Radiology* Spring 12:1

51703 complicated (eg, altered anatomy, fractured catheter/balloon)

➔ *CPT Assistant* Jan 07:31; *CPT Changes: An Insider's View* 2003

51705 Change of cystostomy tube; simple

➔ *CPT Assistant* Dec 07:13

51710 complicated

➔ *CPT Assistant* Dec 07:13

(If imaging guidance is performed, use 75984)

51715 Endoscopic injection of implant material into the submucosal tissues of the urethra and/or bladder neck

51720 Bladder instillation of anticarcinogenic agent (including retention time)

➔ *CPT Assistant* Nov 02:11; *CPT Changes: An Insider's View* 2007

Urodynamics

▶The following section (51725-51798) lists procedures that may be used separately or in many and varied combinations.◀

When multiple procedures are performed in the same investigative session, modifier 51 should be employed.

▶All procedures in this section imply that these services are performed by, or are under the direct supervision of, a physician or other qualified health care professional and that all instruments, equipment, fluids, gases, probes, catheters, technician's fees, medications, gloves, trays, tubing, and other sterile supplies be provided by that individual. When the individual only interprets the results and/or operates the equipment, a professional component, modifier 26, should be used to identify these services.◀

51725 Simple cystometrogram (CMG) (eg, spinal manometer)

➔ *CPT Assistant* Sep 02:6, Feb 10:7

51726 Complex cystometrogram (ie, calibrated electronic equipment);

➔ *CPT Assistant* Sep 02:6, Feb 10:7; *CPT Changes: An Insider's View* 2010

51727 with urethral pressure profile studies (ie, urethral closure pressure profile), any technique

➔ *CPT Assistant* Feb 10:7; *CPT Changes: An Insider's View* 2010

51728 with voiding pressure studies (ie, bladder voiding pressure), any technique

➔ *CPT Assistant* Feb 10:7; *CPT Changes: An Insider's View* 2010

51729 with voiding pressure studies (ie, bladder voiding pressure) and urethral pressure profile studies (ie, urethral closure pressure profile), any technique

➔ *CPT Assistant* Feb 10:7; *CPT Changes: An Insider's View* 2010

#+ 51797 Voiding pressure studies, intra-abdominal (ie, rectal, gastric, intraperitoneal) (List separately in addition to code for primary procedure)

➔ *CPT Assistant* Dec 01:7, Sep 02:6, Oct 09:7, Feb 10:7; *CPT Changes: An Insider's View* 2008, 2010

(Use 51797 in conjunction with 51728, 51729)

51736 Simple uroflowmetry (UFR) (eg, stop-watch flow rate, mechanical uroflowmeter)

➔ *CPT Assistant* Sep 02:6, Feb 10:7

51741 Complex uroflowmetry (eg, calibrated electronic equipment)

➔ *CPT Assistant* Sep 02:6, Feb 10:7

(51772 has been deleted. To report urethral pressure profile studies, see 51727, 51729)

51784   Electromyography studies (EMG) of anal or urethral sphincter, other than needle, any technique
⮕ *CPT Assistant* Sep 02:6, Feb 10:7

51785   Needle electromyography studies (EMG) of anal or urethral sphincter, any technique
⮕ *CPT Assistant* Apr 02:6, Sep 02:6, Jul 04:13, Feb 10:7

51792   Stimulus evoked response (eg, measurement of bulbocavernosus reflex latency time)
⮕ *CPT Assistant* Apr 02:6, Sep 02:6, Feb 10:7

(51795 has been deleted. To report bladder voiding pressure studies, see 51728, 51729)

51797   Code is out of numerical sequence. See 51725-51798

51798   Measurement of post-voiding residual urine and/or bladder capacity by ultrasound, non-imaging
⮕ *CPT Assistant* Dec 05:3, Feb 10:7; *CPT Changes: An Insider's View* 2003

Measurement of Postvoiding
51798

Bladder

Ultrasound scanner

Repair

51800   Cystoplasty or cystourethroplasty, plastic operation on bladder and/or vesical neck (anterior Y-plasty, vesical fundus resection), any procedure, with or without wedge resection of posterior vesical neck

51820   Cystourethroplasty with unilateral or bilateral ureteroneocystostomy

51840   Anterior vesicourethropexy, or urethropexy (eg, Marshall-Marchetti-Krantz, Burch); simple
⮕ *CPT Assistant* Jan 97:1, Nov 97:19, Apr 98:15, Jun 02:7, May 06:17, Jun 10:6

51841   complicated (eg, secondary repair)
⮕ *CPT Assistant* Jan 97:1, Jun 02:7, Jun 10:6

(For urethropexy (Pereyra type), use 57289)

51845   Abdomino-vaginal vesical neck suspension, with or without endoscopic control (eg, Stamey, Raz, modified Pereyra)
⮕ *CPT Assistant* Jan 97:3

51860   Cystorrhaphy, suture of bladder wound, injury or rupture; simple

51865   complicated

51880   Closure of cystostomy (separate procedure)

51900   Closure of vesicovaginal fistula, abdominal approach

(For vaginal approach, see 57320-57330)

51920   Closure of vesicouterine fistula;

51925   with hysterectomy

(For closure of vesicoenteric fistula, see 44660, 44661)

(For closure of rectovesical fistula, see 45800-45805)

51940   Closure, exstrophy of bladder
⮕ *CPT Changes: An Insider's View* 2002

(See also 54390)

51960   Enterocystoplasty, including intestinal anastomosis
⮕ *CPT Changes: An Insider's View* 2002

51980   Cutaneous vesicostomy

Laparoscopy

Surgical laparoscopy always includes diagnostic laparoscopy. To report a diagnostic laparoscopy (peritoneoscopy) (separate procedure), use 49320.

51990   Laparoscopy, surgical; urethral suspension for stress incontinence
⮕ *CPT Assistant* Nov 99:26, May 00:4, Jun 10:6, Mar 12:10; *CPT Changes: An Insider's View* 2000

51992   sling operation for stress incontinence (eg, fascia or synthetic)
⮕ *CPT Assistant* Nov 99:26, May 00:4, Mar 12:10; *CPT Changes: An Insider's View* 2000

(For open sling operation for stress incontinence, use 57288)

(For reversal or removal of sling operation for stress incontinence, use 57287)

Laparoscopic Sling Suspension Urinary Incontinence
51990

Nonabsorbable sutures are placed laparoscopically into the endopelvic fascia at the bladder neck region on each side and secured to the ipsilateral pectineal ligament. The sutures are tied using extra vaginal-urethral knots so as to create a hammock type suspension of the bladder neck, without urethral occlusion.

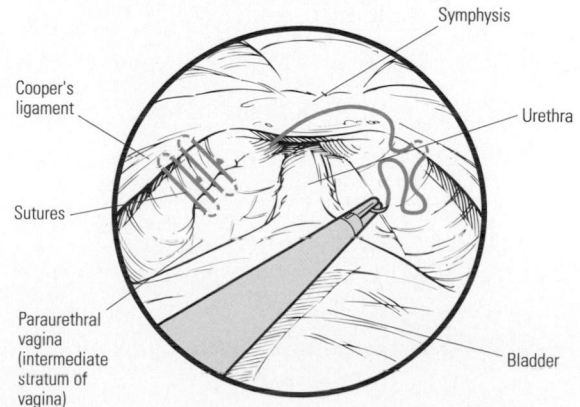

Symphysis

Cooper's ligament

Urethra

Sutures

Paraurethral vagina (intermediate stratum of vagina)

Bladder

51999   Unlisted laparoscopy procedure, bladder

➔ *CPT Changes: An Insider's View* 2006

Endoscopy—Cystoscopy, Urethroscopy, Cystourethroscopy

Endoscopic descriptions are listed so that the main procedure can be identified without having to list all the minor related functions performed at the same time. For example: meatotomy, urethral calibration and/or dilation, urethroscopy, and cystoscopy prior to a transurethral resection of prostate; ureteral catheterization following extraction of ureteral calculus; internal urethrotomy and bladder neck fulguration when performing a cystourethroscopy for the female urethral syndrome. When the secondary procedure requires significant additional time and effort, it may be identified by the addition of modifier 22.

For example: urethrotomy performed for a documented pre-existing stricture or bladder neck contracture.

52000   Cystourethroscopy (separate procedure)

➔ *CPT Assistant* Oct 00:7, May 01:5, Sep 04:11, Oct 05:23, Nov 07:9

52001   Cystourethroscopy with irrigation and evacuation of multiple obstructing clots

➔ *CPT Changes: An Insider's View* 2002, 2003

(Do not report 52001 in conjunction with 52000)

— *Coding Tip* —

Restrictions for Reporting Temporary Catheter Insertion and Removal with Cystourethroscopy

The insertion and removal of a temporary ureteral catheter (52005) during diagnostic or therapeutic cystourethroscopic with ureteroscopy and/or pyeloscopy is included in 52320-52355 and should not be reported separately.

CPT Coding Guidelines, Urinary System, Bladder Transurethral Surgery, Ureter and Pelvis

---

52005   Cystourethroscopy, with ureteral catheterization, with or without irrigation, instillation, or ureteropyelography, exclusive of radiologic service;

➔ *CPT Assistant* Sep 00:11, Jan 01:13, May 01:5, Oct 01:8, Dec 10:15

Cystourethroscopy With Ureteral Catheterization
52005

A cystourethroscope is passed through the urethra and bladder in order to view the urinary collecting system.

52007   with brush biopsy of ureter and/or renal pelvis

➔ *CPT Assistant* May 01:5, Oct 01:8

52010   Cystourethroscopy, with ejaculatory duct catheterization, with or without irrigation, instillation, or duct radiography, exclusive of radiologic service

➔ *CPT Assistant* May 01:5

(For radiological supervision and interpretation, use 74440)

Transurethral Surgery

Urethra and Bladder

52204   Cystourethroscopy, with biopsy(s)

➔ *CPT Assistant* May 01:5, Sep 01:1, Sep 03:16, Aug 09:6; *CPT Changes: An Insider's View* 2007

52214   Cystourethroscopy, with fulguration (including cryosurgery or laser surgery) of trigone, bladder neck, prostatic fossa, urethra, or periurethral glands

➔ *CPT Assistant* May 01:5, Sep 01:1, Aug 09:6

(For transurethral fulguration of prostate tissue performed within the postoperative period of 52601 or 52630 performed by the same physician, append modifier 78)

(For transurethral fulguration of prostate tissue performed within the postoperative period of a related procedure performed by the same physician, append modifier 78)

(For transurethral fulguration of prostate for postoperative bleeding performed by the same physician, append modifier 78)

Urinary

52224   Cystourethroscopy, with fulguration (including cryosurgery or laser surgery) or treatment of MINOR (less than 0.5 cm) lesion(s) with or without biopsy
> *CPT Assistant* May 01:5, Sep 01:1, Dec 07:7, Jun 09:10, Aug 09:6

52234   Cystourethroscopy, with fulguration (including cryosurgery or laser surgery) and/or resection of; SMALL bladder tumor(s) (0.5 up to 2.0 cm)
> *CPT Assistant* May 01:5, Sep 01:1, Oct 02:12, Jan 03:21, Jun 09:10, Aug 09:6; *CPT Changes: An Insider's View* 2005

52235   MEDIUM bladder tumor(s) (2.0 to 5.0 cm)
> *CPT Assistant* May 01:5, Sep 01:1, Oct 02:12, Jan 03:21, Jun 09:10, Aug 09:6

52240   LARGE bladder tumor(s)
> *CPT Assistant* May 01:5, Sep 01:1, Jun 09:10, Aug 09:6

52250   Cystourethroscopy with insertion of radioactive substance, with or without biopsy or fulguration
> *CPT Assistant* May 01:5, Sep 01:1

52260   Cystourethroscopy, with dilation of bladder for interstitial cystitis; general or conduction (spinal) anesthesia
> *CPT Assistant* May 01:5, Sep 01:1, Oct 05:23

52265   local anesthesia
> *CPT Assistant* May 01:5, Sep 01:1

52270   Cystourethroscopy, with internal urethrotomy; female
> *CPT Assistant* May 01:5, Sep 01:1

52275   male
> *CPT Assistant* May 01:5, Sep 01:1

52276   Cystourethroscopy with direct vision internal urethrotomy
> *CPT Assistant* May 01:5, Sep 01:1, May 09:8, Feb 10:7

52277   Cystourethroscopy, with resection of external sphincter (sphincterotomy)
> *CPT Assistant* May 01:5, Sep 01:1

52281   Cystourethroscopy, with calibration and/or dilation of urethral stricture or stenosis, with or without meatotomy, with or without injection procedure for cystography, male or female
> *CPT Assistant* Nov 97:20, May 01:5, Sep 01:1, Jun 07:10

52282   Cystourethroscopy, with insertion of permanent urethral stent
> *CPT Assistant* Nov 97:20, May 01:5, Sep 01:1, Feb 10:7; *CPT Changes: An Insider's View* 2010

(For placement of temporary prostatic urethral stent, use 53855)

52283   Cystourethroscopy, with steroid injection into stricture
> *CPT Assistant* May 01:5, Sep 01:1

52285   Cystourethroscopy for treatment of the female urethral syndrome with any or all of the following: urethral meatotomy, urethral dilation, internal urethrotomy, lysis of urethrovaginal septal fibrosis, lateral incisions of the bladder neck, and fulguration of polyp(s) of urethra, bladder neck, and/or trigone
> *CPT Assistant* May 01:5, Sep 01:1

● **52287**   Cystourethroscopy, with injection(s) for chemodenervation of the bladder
> *CPT Changes: An Insider's View* 2013

►(The supply of the chemodenervation agent is reported separately)◄

52290   Cystourethroscopy; with ureteral meatotomy, unilateral or bilateral
> *CPT Assistant* May 01:5, Sep 01:1

52300   with resection or fulguration of orthotopic ureterocele(s), unilateral or bilateral
> *CPT Assistant* May 01:5, Sep 01:1

52301   with resection or fulguration of ectopic ureterocele(s), unilateral or bilateral
> *CPT Assistant* May 01:5, Sep 01:1

52305   with incision or resection of orifice of bladder diverticulum, single or multiple
> *CPT Assistant* May 01:5, Sep 01:1

--- *Coding Tip* ---

Instructions for Reporting Stent Removal

To report cystourethroscopic removal of a self-retaining, indwelling ureteral stent, see 52310, 52315, and append modifier 58, if appropriate.

CPT Coding Guidelines, Urinary System, Bladder Transurethral Surgery, Ureter and Pelvis

52310   Cystourethroscopy, with removal of foreign body, calculus, or ureteral stent from urethra or bladder (separate procedure); simple
> *CPT Assistant* May 01:5, Sep 01:1

52315   complicated
> *CPT Assistant* May 01:5, Sep 01:1

52317   Litholapaxy: crushing or fragmentation of calculus by any means in bladder and removal of fragments; simple or small (less than 2.5 cm)
> *CPT Assistant* May 01:5, Sep 01:1, Feb 12:11

52318   complicated or large (over 2.5 cm)
> *CPT Assistant* May 01:5, Sep 01:1, Feb 12:11

Ureter and Pelvis

Therapeutic cystourethroscopy always includes diagnostic cystourethroscopy. To report a diagnostic cystourethroscopy, use 52000. Therapeutic cystourethroscopy with ureteroscopy and/or pyeloscopy always includes diagnostic cystourethroscopy with ureteroscopy and/or pyeloscopy. To report a diagnostic cystourethroscopy with ureteroscopy and/or pyeloscopy, use 52351.

Do not report 52000 in conjunction with 52320-52343.

Do not report 52351 in conjunction with 52344-52346, 52352-52355.

The insertion and removal of a temporary ureteral catheter (52005) during diagnostic or therapeutic cystourethroscopic with ureteroscopy and/or pyeloscopy is included in 52320-52355 and should not be reported separately.

To report insertion of a self-retaining, indwelling stent performed during diagnostic or therapeutic cystourethroscopy with ureteroscopy and/or pyeloscopy, report 52332, in addition to primary procedure(s) performed (52320-52355), and append modifier 51. 52332 is used to report a unilateral procedure unless otherwise specified.

For bilateral insertion of self-retaining, indwelling ureteral stents, use code 52332, and append modifier 50.

To report cystourethroscopic removal of a self-retaining, indwelling ureteral stent, see 52310, 52315, and append modifier 58, if appropriate.

52320 Cystourethroscopy (including ureteral catheterization); with removal of ureteral calculus
> *CPT Assistant* Mar 96:1, May 96:11, Jan 01:13, May 01:5, Sep 01:1, Oct 01:8

52325 with fragmentation of ureteral calculus (eg, ultrasonic or electro-hydraulic technique)
> *CPT Assistant* Mar 96:1, May 96:11, May 01:5, Sep 01:1, Oct 01:8, Dec 07:13

52327 with subureteric injection of implant material
> *CPT Assistant* Mar 96:1, May 96:11, May 01:5, Sep 01:1, Oct 01:8

52330 with manipulation, without removal of ureteral calculus
> *CPT Assistant* Mar 96:1, May 96:11, Sep 00:11, May 01:5, Sep 01:1, Oct 01:8

52332 Cystourethroscopy, with insertion of indwelling ureteral stent (eg, Gibbons or double-J type)
> *CPT Assistant* Mar 96:1, May 96:11, Nov 96:8, Jan 01:13, May 01:5, Sep 01:1, Oct 01:8, Oct 05:18, Dec 09:4, 12

52334 Cystourethroscopy with insertion of ureteral guide wire through kidney to establish a percutaneous nephrostomy, retrograde
> *CPT Assistant* Mar 96:11, May 96:11, May 01:5, Sep 01:1, Oct 01:8

(For percutaneous nephrostolithotomy, see 50080, 50081; for establishment of nephrostomy tract only, use 50395)

(For cystourethroscopy, with ureteroscopy and/or pyeloscopy, see 52351-52355)

(For cystourethroscopy with incision, fulguration, or resection of congenital posterior urethral valves or obstructive hypertrophic mucosal folds, use 52400)

52341 Cystourethroscopy; with treatment of ureteral stricture (eg, balloon dilation, laser, electrocautery, and incision)
> *CPT Assistant* Nov 96:9, Apr 01:4, May 01:5, Sep 01:1, Oct 01:8; *CPT Changes: An Insider's View* 2001

52342 with treatment of ureteropelvic junction stricture (eg, balloon dilation, laser, electrocautery, and incision)
> *CPT Assistant* Apr 01:4, May 01:5, Sep 01:1, Oct 01:8, Aug 02:11; *CPT Changes: An Insider's View* 2001

52343 with treatment of intra-renal stricture (eg, balloon dilation, laser, electrocautery, and incision)
> *CPT Assistant* Apr 01:4, May 01:5, Sep 01:1, Oct 01:8; *CPT Changes: An Insider's View* 2001

52344 Cystourethroscopy with ureteroscopy; with treatment of ureteral stricture (eg, balloon dilation, laser, electrocautery, and incision)
> *CPT Assistant* Apr 01:4, May 01:5, Sep 01:1, Oct 01:8; *CPT Changes: An Insider's View* 2001

52345 with treatment of ureteropelvic junction stricture (eg, balloon dilation, laser, electrocautery, and incision)
> *CPT Assistant* Apr 01:4, May 01:5, Sep 01:1, Oct 01:8; *CPT Changes: An Insider's View* 2001

52346 with treatment of intra-renal stricture (eg, balloon dilation, laser, electrocautery, and incision)
> *CPT Assistant* Apr 01:4, May 01:5, Sep 01:1, Oct 01:8; *CPT Changes: An Insider's View* 2001

(For transurethral resection or incision of ejaculatory ducts, use 52402)

52351 Cystourethroscopy, with ureteroscopy and/or pyeloscopy; diagnostic
> *CPT Assistant* Apr 01:4, May 01:5, Sep 01:1, Oct 01:8; *CPT Changes: An Insider's View* 2001

(For radiological supervision and interpretation, use 74485)

(Do not report 52351 in conjunction with 52341-52346, 52352-52355)

52352 with removal or manipulation of calculus (ureteral catheterization is included)
> *CPT Assistant* Apr 01:4, May 01:5, Sep 01:1, Oct 01:8, Jun 07:10, Feb 10:13; *CPT Changes: An Insider's View* 2001

52353 with lithotripsy (ureteral catheterization is included)
> *CPT Assistant* Apr 01:4, May 01:5, Sep 01:1, Oct 01:8, Dec 07:13, Apr 09:8; *CPT Changes: An Insider's View* 2001

52354 with biopsy and/or fulguration of ureteral or renal pelvic lesion
> *CPT Assistant* Apr 01:4, May 01:5, Sep 01:1, Oct 01:8; *CPT Changes: An Insider's View* 2001, 2003

52355 with resection of ureteral or renal pelvic tumor
> *CPT Assistant* Apr 01:4, May 01:5, Sep 01:1, Oct 01:8, Jan 03:21; *CPT Changes: An Insider's View* 2001, 2003

Vesical Neck and Prostate

52400 Cystourethroscopy with incision, fulguration, or resection of congenital posterior urethral valves, or congenital obstructive hypertrophic mucosal folds
> *CPT Assistant* Apr 01:4; *CPT Changes: An Insider's View* 2001

52402 Cystourethroscopy with transurethral resection or incision of ejaculatory ducts
> *CPT Changes: An Insider's View* 2005

52450 Transurethral incision of prostate
➔ *CPT Assistant* Apr 01:4, Jul 05:15

52500 Transurethral resection of bladder neck (separate procedure)
➔ *CPT Assistant* Apr 01:4, Jan 04:27, Jul 05:15, May 09:8

52601 Transurethral electrosurgical resection of prostate, including control of postoperative bleeding, complete (vasectomy, meatotomy, cystourethroscopy, urethral calibration and/or dilation, and internal urethrotomy are included)
➔ *CPT Assistant* Nov 97:20, Apr 01:4, Jun 03:6, Oct 11:10

(For other approaches, see 55801-55845)

Transurethral Resection of Prostate, Complete
52601

The physician removes the prostate gland using an electrocautery knife.

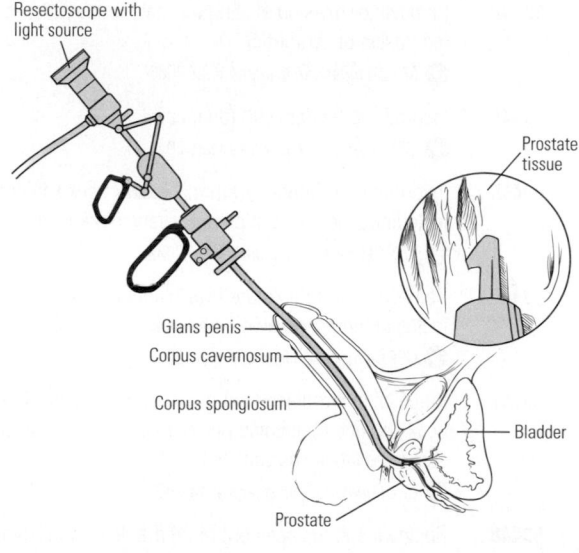

(52606 has been deleted. For transurethral fulguration of prostate, use 52214)

(52612, 52614, 52620 have been deleted. For first stage transurethral partial resection of prostate, use 52601. For second stage partial resection of prostate, use 52601 with modifier 58. For transurethral resection of residual or regrowth of obstructive prostate tissue, use 52630)

52630 Transurethral resection; residual or regrowth of obstructive prostate tissue including control of postoperative bleeding, complete (vasectomy, meatotomy, cystourethroscopy, urethral calibration and/or dilation, and internal urethrotomy are included)
➔ *CPT Assistant* Apr 01:4; *CPT Changes: An Insider's View* 2009

(For resection of residual prostate tissue performed within the postoperative period of a related procedure performed by the same physician, append modifier 78)

52640 of postoperative bladder neck contracture
➔ *CPT Assistant* Apr 01:4

52647 Laser coagulation of prostate, including control of postoperative bleeding, complete (vasectomy, meatotomy, cystourethroscopy, urethral calibration and/or dilation, and internal urethrotomy are included if performed)
➔ *CPT Assistant* Nov 97:20, Mar 98:11, Apr 01:4, Nov 06:21; *CPT Changes: An Insider's View* 2006

52648 Laser vaporization of prostate, including control of postoperative bleeding, complete (vasectomy, meatotomy, cystourethroscopy, urethral calibration and/or dilation, internal urethrotomy and transurethral resection of prostate are included if performed)
➔ *CPT Assistant* Mar 98:11, Apr 01:5, Jul 05:15, Nov 06:21; *CPT Changes: An Insider's View* 2006

Contact Laser Vaporization of Prostate
52648

A laser is used to vaporize the prostate.

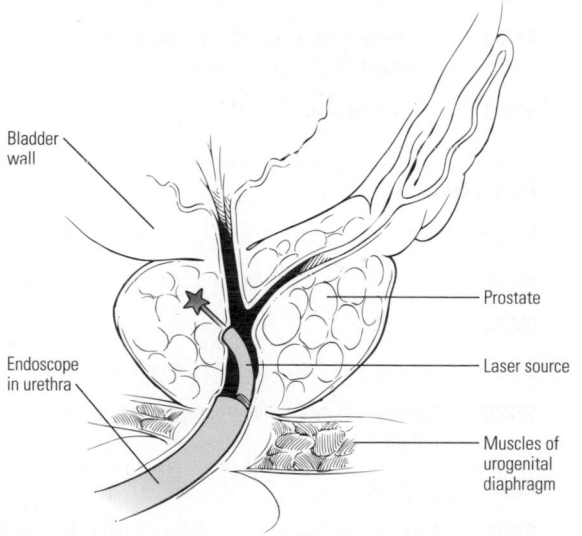

52649 Laser enucleation of the prostate with morcellation, including control of postoperative bleeding, complete (vasectomy, meatotomy, cystourethroscopy, urethral calibration and/or dilation, internal urethrotomy and transurethral resection of prostate are included if performed)
➔ *CPT Changes: An Insider's View* 2008

(Do not report 52649 in conjunction with 52000, 52276, 52281, 52601, 52647, 52648, 53020, 55250)

52700 Transurethral drainage of prostatic abscess
➔ *CPT Assistant* Apr 01:4

(For litholapaxy, use 52317, 52318)

Urethra

(For endoscopy, see cystoscopy, urethroscopy, cystourethroscopy, 52000-52700)

(For injection procedure for urethrocystography, see 51600-51610)

Incision

53000 Urethrotomy or urethrostomy, external (separate procedure); pendulous urethra

53010   perineal urethra, external

53020 Meatotomy, cutting of meatus (separate procedure); except infant

53025   infant

(Do not report modifier 63 in conjunction with 53025)

53040 Drainage of deep periurethral abscess

(For subcutaneous abscess, see 10060, 10061)

53060 Drainage of Skene's gland abscess or cyst

53080 Drainage of perineal urinary extravasation; uncomplicated (separate procedure)

53085   complicated

Excision

53200 Biopsy of urethra

53210 Urethrectomy, total, including cystostomy; female

53215   male

53220 Excision or fulguration of carcinoma of urethra

53230 Excision of urethral diverticulum (separate procedure); female

53235   male

53240 Marsupialization of urethral diverticulum, male or female

53250 Excision of bulbourethral gland (Cowper's gland)

53260 Excision or fulguration; urethral polyp(s), distal urethra

(For endoscopic approach, see 52214, 52224)

53265   urethral caruncle

53270   Skene's glands

53275   urethral prolapse

Repair

(For hypospadias, see 54300-54352)

53400 Urethroplasty; first stage, for fistula, diverticulum, or stricture (eg, Johannsen type)

53405   second stage (formation of urethra), including urinary diversion

53410 Urethroplasty, 1-stage reconstruction of male anterior urethra

53415 Urethroplasty, transpubic or perineal, 1-stage, for reconstruction or repair of prostatic or membranous urethra

53420 Urethroplasty, 2-stage reconstruction or repair of prostatic or membranous urethra; first stage

53425   second stage

53430 Urethroplasty, reconstruction of female urethra

53431 Urethroplasty with tubularization of posterior urethra and/or lower bladder for incontinence (eg, Tenago, Leadbetter procedure)

➥ CPT Changes: An Insider's View 2002

53440 Sling operation for correction of male urinary incontinence (eg, fascia or synthetic)

➥ CPT Changes: An Insider's View 2003

53442 Removal or revision of sling for male urinary incontinence (eg, fascia or synthetic)

➥ CPT Changes: An Insider's View 2003

53444 Insertion of tandem cuff (dual cuff)

➥ CPT Changes: An Insider's View 2002

53445 Insertion of inflatable urethral/bladder neck sphincter, including placement of pump, reservoir, and cuff

➥ CPT Changes: An Insider's View 2002

53446 Removal of inflatable urethral/bladder neck sphincter, including pump, reservoir, and cuff

➥ CPT Changes: An Insider's View 2002

53447 Removal and replacement of inflatable urethral/bladder neck sphincter including pump, reservoir, and cuff at the same operative session

➥ CPT Changes: An Insider's View 2002

53448 Removal and replacement of inflatable urethral/bladder neck sphincter including pump, reservoir, and cuff through an infected field at the same operative session including irrigation and debridement of infected tissue

➥ CPT Changes: An Insider's View 2002

(Do not report 11042, 11043 in addition to 53448)

53449 Repair of inflatable urethral/bladder neck sphincter, including pump, reservoir, and cuff

➥ CPT Changes: An Insider's View 2002

53450 Urethromeatoplasty, with mucosal advancement

(For meatotomy, see 53020, 53025)

53460 Urethromeatoplasty, with partial excision of distal urethral segment (Richardson type procedure)

53500 Urethrolysis, transvaginal, secondary, open, including cystourethroscopy (eg, postsurgical obstruction, scarring)

➥ CPT Assistant Sep 04:11; CPT Changes: An Insider's View 2004

(For urethrolysis by retropubic approach, use 53899)

(Do not report 53500 in conjunction with 52000)

| 53502 | Urethrorrhaphy, suture of urethral wound or injury, female |

53502 Urethrorrhaphy, suture of urethral wound or injury, female

53505 Urethrorrhaphy, suture of urethral wound or injury; penile

53510   perineal

53515   prostatomembranous

53520 Closure of urethrostomy or urethrocutaneous fistula, male (separate procedure)

(For closure of urethrovaginal fistula, use 57310)

(For closure of urethrorectal fistula, see 45820, 45825)

Manipulation

(For radiological supervision and interpretation, use 74485)

53600 Dilation of urethral stricture by passage of sound or urethral dilator, male; initial

53601   subsequent

53605 Dilation of urethral stricture or vesical neck by passage of sound or urethral dilator, male, general or conduction (spinal) anesthesia

(For dilation of urethral stricture, male, performed under local anesthesia, see 53600, 53601, 53620, 53621)

53620 Dilation of urethral stricture by passage of filiform and follower, male; initial

53621   subsequent

53660 Dilation of female urethra including suppository and/or instillation; initial

53661   subsequent

53665 Dilation of female urethra, general or conduction (spinal) anesthesia

(For urethral catheterization, see 51701-51703)

(For dilation of urethra performed under local anesthesia, female, see 53660, 53661)

Other Procedures

(For 2 or 3 glass urinalysis, use 81020)

53850 Transurethral destruction of prostate tissue; by microwave thermotherapy
➔ *CPT Assistant* Nov 97:20, Apr 01:6, Feb 10:7

53852   by radiofrequency thermotherapy
➔ *CPT Assistant* Nov 97:20, Apr 01:6

(53853 has been deleted. To report, use 55899)

53855 Insertion of a temporary prostatic urethral stent, including urethral measurement
➔ *CPT Assistant* Feb 10:7; *CPT Changes: An Insider's View* 2010

(For insertion of permanent urethral stent, use 52282)

Temporary Prostatic Urethral Stent Insertion
53855

A temporary prostatic urethral stent is inserted.

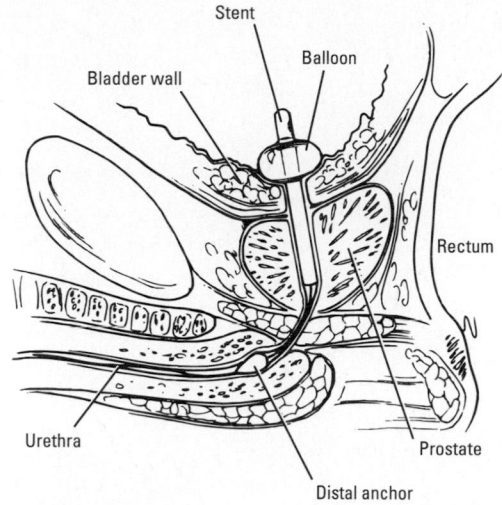

53860 Transurethral radiofrequency micro-remodeling of the female bladder neck and proximal urethra for stress urinary incontinence
➔ *CPT Changes: An Insider's View* 2011

53899 Unlisted procedure, urinary system
➔ *CPT Assistant* Aug 04:12, Sep 04:11, Oct 05:18, 23-24, Feb 06:14, May 10:10
➔ *Clinical Examples in Radiology* Summer 06:1-3

Notes

⊙=Moderate sedation ✚=Add-on code ✗=FDA approval pending #=Resequenced code ○=Recycled/reinstated code ➜➜=See p xiii for details

Surgery

Deferent duct

Urinary bladder and cavity

Corpus cavernosa

Corpus spongiosum

Penis

Glans penis

Prepuce

Seminal vesicle

Ejaculatory duct

Prostate gland

Spermatic cord and deferent duct

Epididymus

Testes

Scrotum

Male Genital

Male Genital System

Penis

Incision

(For abdominal perineal gangrene debridement, see 11004-11006)

54000 Slitting of prepuce, dorsal or lateral (separate procedure); newborn

(Do not report modifier 63 in conjunction with 54000)

54001 except newborn

54015 Incision and drainage of penis, deep

(For skin and subcutaneous abscess, see 10060-10160)

Destruction

54050 Destruction of lesion(s), penis (eg, condyloma, papilloma, molluscum contagiosum, herpetic vesicle), simple; chemical

54055 electrodesiccation

54056 cryosurgery

54057 laser surgery

54060 surgical excision

54065 Destruction of lesion(s), penis (eg, condyloma, papilloma, molluscum contagiosum, herpetic vesicle), extensive (eg, laser surgery, electrosurgery, cryosurgery, chemosurgery)
➜ *CPT Changes: An Insider's View* 2002

(For destruction or excision of other lesions, see **Integumentary System**)

Excision

54100 Biopsy of penis; (separate procedure)
➜ *CPT Assistant* Nov 99:26; *CPT Changes: An Insider's View* 2000

54105 deep structures

54110 Excision of penile plaque (Peyronie disease);

54111 with graft to 5 cm in length
➜ *CPT Assistant* Aug 99:5

54112 with graft greater than 5 cm in length

54115 Removal foreign body from deep penile tissue (eg, plastic implant)

54120 Amputation of penis; partial

54125 complete

54130 Amputation of penis, radical; with bilateral inguinofemoral lymphadenectomy

54135 in continuity with bilateral pelvic lymphadenectomy, including external iliac, hypogastric and obturator nodes

(For lymphadenectomy [separate procedure], see 38760-38770)

54150 Circumcision, using clamp or other device with regional dorsal penile or ring block
➜ *CPT Assistant* Sep 96:11, May 98:11, Apr 03:27, Aug 03:6, May 07:10, Jul 07:5; *CPT Changes: An Insider's View* 2007

(Do not report modifier 63 in conjunction with 54150)

(Report 54150 with modifier 52 when performed without dorsal penile or ring block)

54160 Circumcision, surgical excision other than clamp, device, or dorsal slit; neonate (28 days of age or less)
➜ *CPT Assistant* Sep 96:11, May 98:11, May 07:10, Jul 07:5; *CPT Changes: An Insider's View* 2007

(Do not report modifier 63 in conjunction with 54160)

54161 older than 28 days of age
➜ *CPT Assistant* Sep 96:11, Dec 96:10, May 98:11, Jul 07:5; *CPT Changes: An Insider's View* 2007

54162 Lysis or excision of penile post-circumcision adhesions
➜ *CPT Changes: An Insider's View* 2002

54163 Repair incomplete circumcision
➜ *CPT Changes: An Insider's View* 2002

54164 Frenulotomy of penis
➜ *CPT Changes: An Insider's View* 2002

(Do not report 54164 with circumcision codes 54150-54161, 54162, 54163)

Introduction

54200 Injection procedure for Peyronie disease;

54205 with surgical exposure of plaque

54220 Irrigation of corpora cavernosa for priapism

54230 Injection procedure for corpora cavernosography

(For radiological supervision and interpretation, use 74445)

54231 Dynamic cavernosometry, including intracavernosal injection of vasoactive drugs (eg, papaverine, phentolamine)

54235 Injection of corpora cavernosa with pharmacologic agent(s) (eg, papaverine, phentolamine)
➜ *CPT Assistant* Sep 96:10

54240 Penile plethysmography

54250 Nocturnal penile tumescence and/or rigidity test

Repair

(For other urethroplasties, see 53400-53430)

(For penile revascularization, use 37788)

54300 Plastic operation of penis for straightening of chordee (eg, hypospadias), with or without mobilization of urethra

Male Genital

54304 Plastic operation on penis for correction of chordee or for first stage hypospadias repair with or without transplantation of prepuce and/or skin flaps

54308 Urethroplasty for second stage hypospadias repair (including urinary diversion); less than 3 cm

54312   greater than 3 cm

54316 Urethroplasty for second stage hypospadias repair (including urinary diversion) with free skin graft obtained from site other than genitalia

54318 Urethroplasty for third stage hypospadias repair to release penis from scrotum (eg, third stage Cecil repair)

54322 1-stage distal hypospadias repair (with or without chordee or circumcision); with simple meatal advancement (eg, Magpi, V-flap)

54324   with urethroplasty by local skin flaps (eg, flip-flap, prepucial flap)

54326   with urethroplasty by local skin flaps and mobilization of urethra

54328   with extensive dissection to correct chordee and urethroplasty with local skin flaps, skin graft patch, and/or island flap

➔ *CPT Assistant* Oct 04:15

(For urethroplasty and straightening of chordee, use 54308)

54332 1-stage proximal penile or penoscrotal hypospadias repair requiring extensive dissection to correct chordee and urethroplasty by use of skin graft tube and/or island flap

➔ *CPT Assistant* Mar 04:11, Sep 04:12

54336 1-stage perineal hypospadias repair requiring extensive dissection to correct chordee and urethroplasty by use of skin graft tube and/or island flap

➔ *CPT Assistant* Oct 04:15

54340 Repair of hypospadias complications (ie, fistula, stricture, diverticula); by closure, incision, or excision, simple

54344   requiring mobilization of skin flaps and urethroplasty with flap or patch graft

54348   requiring extensive dissection and urethroplasty with flap, patch or tubed graft (includes urinary diversion)

54352 Repair of hypospadias cripple requiring extensive dissection and excision of previously constructed structures including re-release of chordee and reconstruction of urethra and penis by use of local skin as grafts and island flaps and skin brought in as flaps or grafts

54360 Plastic operation on penis to correct angulation

54380 Plastic operation on penis for epispadias distal to external sphincter;

54385   with incontinence

54390   with exstrophy of bladder

54400 Insertion of penile prosthesis; non-inflatable (semi-rigid)

54401   inflatable (self-contained)

(For removal or replacement of penile prosthesis, see 54415, 54416)

54405 Insertion of multi-component, inflatable penile prosthesis, including placement of pump, cylinders, and reservoir

➔ *CPT Changes: An Insider's View* 2002

(For reduced services, report 54405 with modifier 52)

54406 Removal of all components of a multi-component, inflatable penile prosthesis without replacement of prosthesis

➔ *CPT Changes: An Insider's View* 2002

(For reduced services, report 54406 with modifier 52)

54408 Repair of component(s) of a multi-component, inflatable penile prosthesis

➔ *CPT Changes: An Insider's View* 2002

54410 Removal and replacement of all component(s) of a multi-component, inflatable penile prosthesis at the same operative session

➔ *CPT Changes: An Insider's View* 2002

54411 Removal and replacement of all components of a multi-component inflatable penile prosthesis through an infected field at the same operative session, including irrigation and debridement of infected tissue

➔ *CPT Changes: An Insider's View* 2002

(For reduced services, report 54411 with modifier 52)

(Do not report 11042, 11043 in addition to 54411)

54415 Removal of non-inflatable (semi-rigid) or inflatable (self-contained) penile prosthesis, without replacement of prosthesis

➔ *CPT Changes: An Insider's View* 2002

54416 Removal and replacement of non-inflatable (semi-rigid) or inflatable (self-contained) penile prosthesis at the same operative session

➔ *CPT Changes: An Insider's View* 2002

54417 Removal and replacement of non-inflatable (semi-rigid) or inflatable (self-contained) penile prosthesis through an infected field at the same operative session, including irrigation and debridement of infected tissue

➔ *CPT Changes: An Insider's View* 2002

(Do not report 11042, 11043 in addition to 54417)

54420 Corpora cavernosa-saphenous vein shunt (priapism operation), unilateral or bilateral

54430 Corpora cavernosa-corpus spongiosum shunt (priapism operation), unilateral or bilateral

54435 Corpora cavernosa-glans penis fistulization (eg, biopsy needle, Winter procedure, rongeur, or punch) for priapism

54440 Plastic operation of penis for injury

Manipulation

54450   Foreskin manipulation including lysis of preputial adhesions and stretching

Testis

Excision

(For abdominal perineal gangrene debridement, see 11004-11006)

54500   Biopsy of testis, needle (separate procedure)

(For fine needle aspiration, see 10021, 10022)

(For evaluation of fine needle aspirate, see 88172, 88173)

54505   Biopsy of testis, incisional (separate procedure)
> *CPT Assistant* Oct 01:8

(For bilateral procedure, report 54505 with modifier 50)

(When combined with vasogram, seminal vesiculogram, or epididymogram, use 55300)

54512   Excision of extraparenchymal lesion of testis
> *CPT Assistant* Oct 01:8, Aug 05:13; *CPT Changes: An Insider's View* 2001

54520   Orchiectomy, simple (including subcapsular), with or without testicular prosthesis, scrotal or inguinal approach
> *CPT Assistant* Winter 94:13, Oct 01:8, Mar 04:3

(For bilateral procedure, report 54520 with modifier 50)

54522   Orchiectomy, partial
> *CPT Assistant* Oct 01:8; *CPT Changes: An Insider's View* 2001

54530   Orchiectomy, radical, for tumor; inguinal approach
> *CPT Assistant* Oct 01:8

54535   with abdominal exploration
> *CPT Assistant* Oct 01:8

(For orchiectomy with repair of hernia, see 49505 or 49507 and 54520)

(For radical retroperitoneal lymphadenectomy, use 38780)

Exploration

54550   Exploration for undescended testis (inguinal or scrotal area)
> *CPT Assistant* Oct 01:8

(For bilateral procedure, report 54550 with modifier 50)

54560   Exploration for undescended testis with abdominal exploration
> *CPT Assistant* Oct 01:8

(For bilateral procedure, report 54560 with modifier 50)

Repair

54600   Reduction of torsion of testis, surgical, with or without fixation of contralateral testis
> *CPT Assistant* Aug 05:13

54620   Fixation of contralateral testis (separate procedure)

54640   Orchiopexy, inguinal approach, with or without hernia repair
> *CPT Assistant* Oct 01:8, Jan 04:27, Mar 04:10, Jun 08:4

(For bilateral procedure, report 54640 with modifier 50)

(For inguinal hernia repair performed in conjunction with inguinal orchiopexy, see 49495-49525)

54650   Orchiopexy, abdominal approach, for intra-abdominal testis (eg, Fowler-Stephens)
> *CPT Assistant* Nov 99:26, May 00:4, Oct 01:8; *CPT Changes: An Insider's View* 2000

(For laparoscopic approach, use 54692)

54660   Insertion of testicular prosthesis (separate procedure)
> *CPT Assistant* Oct 01:8

(For bilateral procedure, report 54660 with modifier 50)

54670   Suture or repair of testicular injury
> *CPT Assistant* Oct 01:8

54680   Transplantation of testis(es) to thigh (because of scrotal destruction)
> *CPT Assistant* Oct 01:8

Laparoscopy

Surgical laparoscopy always includes diagnostic laparoscopy. To report a diagnostic laparoscopy (peritoneoscopy) (separate procedure), use 49320.

54690   Laparoscopy, surgical; orchiectomy
> *CPT Assistant* Nov 99:26, Mar 00:5, Oct 01:8; *CPT Changes: An Insider's View* 2000

54692   orchiopexy for intra-abdominal testis
> *CPT Assistant* Nov 99:27, May 00:4, Oct 01:8; *CPT Changes: An Insider's View* 2000

Laparoscopic Orchiopexy
54692

Surgical fixation of an undescended testis in the scrotum under laparoscopic guidance

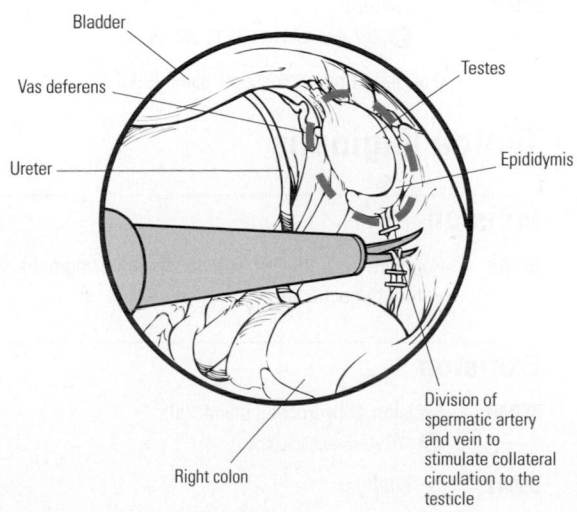

Bladder | Testes | Vas deferens | Ureter | Epididymis | Right colon | Division of spermatic artery and vein to stimulate collateral circulation to the testicle

Male Genital

54699 Unlisted laparoscopy procedure, testis

➔ *CPT Assistant* Nov 99:27, Mar 00:9; *CPT Changes: An Insider's View* 2000

Epididymis

Incision

54700 Incision and drainage of epididymis, testis and/or scrotal space (eg, abscess or hematoma)

➔ *CPT Assistant* Oct 01:8

(For debridement of necrotizing soft tissue infection of external genitalia, see 11004-11006)

Excision

54800 Biopsy of epididymis, needle

➔ *CPT Assistant* Oct 01:8

(For fine needle aspiration, see 10021, 10022)

(For evaluation of fine needle aspirate, see 88172, 88173)

54830 Excision of local lesion of epididymis

➔ *CPT Assistant* Oct 01:8

54840 Excision of spermatocele, with or without epididymectomy

➔ *CPT Assistant* Oct 01:8

54860 Epididymectomy; unilateral

54861 bilateral

Exploration

54865 Exploration of epididymis, with or without biopsy

➔ *CPT Changes: An Insider's View* 2007

Repair

54900 Epididymovasostomy, anastomosis of epididymis to vas deferens; unilateral

➔ *CPT Assistant* Nov 98:16, Jun 04:11

54901 bilateral

➔ *CPT Assistant* Nov 98:16, Jun 04:11

(For operating microscope, use 69990)

Tunica Vaginalis

Incision

55000 Puncture aspiration of hydrocele, tunica vaginalis, with or without injection of medication

Excision

55040 Excision of hydrocele; unilateral

➔ *CPT Assistant* Jun 08:4

55041 bilateral

(With hernia repair, see 49495-49501)

Repair

55060 Repair of tunica vaginalis hydrocele (Bottle type)

Scrotum

Incision

55100 Drainage of scrotal wall abscess

(See also 54700)

(For debridement of necrotizing soft tissue infection of external genitalia, see 11004-11006)

55110 Scrotal exploration

55120 Removal of foreign body in scrotum

Excision

(For excision of local lesion of skin of scrotum, see **Integumentary System**)

55150 Resection of scrotum

Repair

55175 Scrotoplasty; simple

55180 complicated

Vas Deferens

Incision

55200 Vasotomy, cannulization with or without incision of vas, unilateral or bilateral (separate procedure)

Excision

55250 Vasectomy, unilateral or bilateral (separate procedure), including postoperative semen examination(s)

➔ *CPT Assistant* Jun 98:10, Jul 98:10

Introduction

55300 Vasotomy for vasograms, seminal vesiculograms, or epididymograms, unilateral or bilateral

(For radiological supervision and interpretation, use 74440)

(When combined with biopsy of testis, see 54505 and use modifier 51)

Repair

55400 Vasovasostomy, vasovasorrhaphy

➔ *CPT Assistant* Nov 98:16, Oct 01:8, Jun 04:11

(For bilateral procedure, report 55400 with modifier 50)

(For operating microscope, use 69990)

Male Genital

Suture

55450   Ligation (percutaneous) of vas deferens, unilateral or bilateral (separate procedure)

Spermatic Cord

Excision

55500   Excision of hydrocele of spermatic cord, unilateral (separate procedure)
> *CPT Assistant* Oct 01:8

55520   Excision of lesion of spermatic cord (separate procedure)
> *CPT Assistant* Sep 00:10, Oct 01:8

55530   Excision of varicocele or ligation of spermatic veins for varicocele; (separate procedure)
> *CPT Assistant* Oct 01:8

55535   abdominal approach
> *CPT Assistant* Oct 01:8

55540   with hernia repair
> *CPT Assistant* Oct 01:8

Laparoscopy

Surgical laparoscopy always includes diagnostic laparoscopy. To report a diagnostic laparoscopy (peritoneoscopy) (separate procedure), use 49320.

55550   Laparoscopy, surgical, with ligation of spermatic veins for varicocele
> *CPT Assistant* Nov 99:27, Mar 00:9, Oct 01:8; *CPT Changes: An Insider's View* 2000

55559   Unlisted laparoscopy procedure, spermatic cord
> *CPT Assistant* Nov 99:27, Mar 00:9; *CPT Changes: An Insider's View* 2000

Seminal Vesicles

Incision

55600   Vesiculotomy;
(For bilateral procedure, report 55600 with modifier 50)

55605   complicated

Excision

55650   Vesiculectomy, any approach
(For bilateral procedure, report 55650 with modifier 50)

55680   Excision of Mullerian duct cyst
(For injection procedure, see 52010, 55300)

Prostate

Incision

55700   Biopsy, prostate; needle or punch, single or multiple, any approach
> *CPT Assistant* May 96:3, Nov 10:5

(If imaging guidance is performed, use 76942)

(For fine needle aspiration, see 10021, 10022)

(For evaluation of fine needle aspirate, see 88172, 88173)

(For transperineal stereotactic template guided saturation prostate biopsies, use 55706)

55705   incisional, any approach

55706   Biopsies, prostate, needle, transperineal, stereotactic template guided saturation sampling, including imaging guidance
> *CPT Assistant* Nov 10:5; *CPT Changes: An Insider's View* 2009

(Do not report 55706 in conjunction with 55700)

55720   Prostatotomy, external drainage of prostatic abscess, any approach; simple

55725   complicated

(For transurethral drainage, use 52700)

Excision

(For transurethral removal of prostate, see 52601-52640)

(For transurethral destruction of prostate, see 53850-53852)

(For limited pelvic lymphadenectomy for staging [separate procedure], use 38562)

(For independent node dissection, see 38770-38780)

55801   Prostatectomy, perineal, subtotal (including control of postoperative bleeding, vasectomy, meatotomy, urethral calibration and/or dilation, and internal urethrotomy)
> *CPT Assistant* Jun 03:6-7

55810   Prostatectomy, perineal radical;
> *CPT Assistant* Jun 03:7

55812   with lymph node biopsy(s) (limited pelvic lymphadenectomy)

55815   with bilateral pelvic lymphadenectomy, including external iliac, hypogastric and obturator nodes

(If 55815 is carried out on separate days, use 38770 with modifier 50 and 55810)

55821   Prostatectomy (including control of postoperative bleeding, vasectomy, meatotomy, urethral calibration and/or dilation, and internal urethrotomy); suprapubic, subtotal, 1 or 2 stages
> *CPT Assistant* Jun 03:6

55831   retropubic, subtotal
> *CPT Assistant* Jun 03:7

Male Genital

Male Genital

55840 Prostatectomy, retropubic radical, with or without nerve sparing;
➔ *CPT Assistant* Jun 03:8

55842 with lymph node biopsy(s) (limited pelvic lymphadenectomy)
➔ *CPT Assistant* Jun 03:8

55845 with bilateral pelvic lymphadenectomy, including external iliac, hypogastric, and obturator nodes
➔ *CPT Assistant* Jun 03:8

(If 55845 is carried out on separate days, use 38770 with modifier 50 and 55840)

(For laparoscopic retropubic radical prostatectomy, use 55866)

55860 Exposure of prostate, any approach, for insertion of radioactive substance;

(For application of interstitial radioelement, see 77776-77778)

55862 with lymph node biopsy(s) (limited pelvic lymphadenectomy)

55865 with bilateral pelvic lymphadenectomy, including external iliac, hypogastric and obturator nodes

Laparoscopy

Surgical laparoscopy always includes diagnostic laparoscopy. To report a diagnostic laparoscopy (peritoneoscopy) (separate procedure), use 49320.

55866 Laparoscopy, surgical prostatectomy, retropubic radical, including nerve sparing, includes robotic assistance, when performed
➔ *CPT Assistant* Jun 03:8, Mar 12:10; *CPT Changes: An Insider's View* 2003, 2011

(For open procedure, use 55840)

Other Procedures

(For artificial insemination, see 58321, 58322)

55870 Electroejaculation

55873 Cryosurgical ablation of the prostate (includes ultrasonic guidance and monitoring)
➔ *CPT Assistant* Apr 01:4, Sep 02:9, Jun 03:8, Feb 10:7; *CPT Changes: An Insider's View* 2001, 2010

55875 Transperineal placement of needles or catheters into prostate for interstitial radioelement application, with or without cystoscopy
➔ *CPT Assistant* May 07:1, Apr 09:3; *CPT Changes: An Insider's View* 2007

(For placement of needles or catheters into pelvic organs and/or genitalia [except prostate] for interstitial radioelement application, use 55920)

(For interstitial radioelement application, see 77776-77787)

(For ultrasonic guidance for interstitial radioelement application, use 76965)

55876 Placement of interstitial device(s) for radiation therapy guidance (eg, fiducial markers, dosimeter), prostate (via needle, any approach), single or multiple
➔ *CPT Assistant* May 07:1, Oct 07:1, Feb 10:7, 12; *CPT Changes: An Insider's View* 2007, 2010, 2011

(Report supply of device separately)

(For imaging guidance, see 76942, 77002, 77012, 77021)

55899 Unlisted procedure, male genital system
➔ *CPT Assistant* Jun 03:8, May 07:11
➔ *Clinical Examples in Radiology* Spring 06:8-9

Reproductive System Procedures

55920 Placement of needles or catheters into pelvic organs and/or genitalia (except prostate) for subsequent interstitial radioelement application
➔ *CPT Assistant* Apr 09:10; *CPT Changes: An Insider's View* 2008

(For placement of needles or catheters into prostate, use 55875)

(For insertion of uterine tandems and/or vaginal ovoids for clinical brachytherapy, use 57155)

(For insertion of Heyman capsules for clinical brachytherapy, use 58346)

Intersex Surgery

55970 Intersex surgery; male to female

55980 female to male

Surgery

Female Genital System (56405-58999) 303

The following is a listing of headings and subheadings that appear within the Female Genital System section of the CPT codebook. The subheadings or subsections denoted with asterisks (*) below have special instructions unique to that section. Where these are indicated, special "notes" or guidelines will be presented preceding those procedural terminology listings, referring to that subsection specifically.

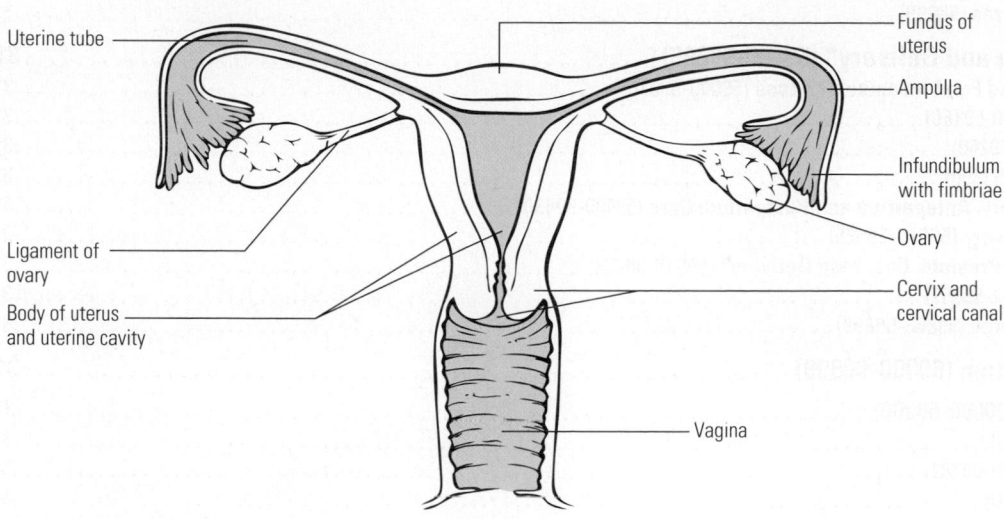

Female Genital

Female Genital System

(For pelvic laparotomy, use 49000)

(For excision or destruction of endometriomas, open method, see 49203-49205, 58957, 58958)

(For paracentesis, see 49082, 49083, 49084)

(For secondary closure of abdominal wall evisceration or disruption, use 49900)

(For fulguration or excision of lesions, laparoscopic approach, use 58662)

(For chemotherapy, see 96401-96549)

Vulva, Perineum, and Introitus

Definitions

The following definitions apply to the vulvectomy codes (56620-56640):

A *simple* procedure is the removal of skin and superficial subcutaneous tissues.

A *radical* procedure is the removal of skin and deep subcutaneous tissue.

A *partial* procedure is the removal of less than 80% of the vulvar area.

A *complete* procedure is the removal of greater than 80% of the vulvar area.

Incision

(For incision and drainage of sebaceous cyst, furuncle, or abscess, see 10040, 10060, 10061)

56405 Incision and drainage of vulva or perineal abscess

56420 Incision and drainage of Bartholin's gland abscess

(For incision and drainage of Skene's gland abscess or cyst, use 53060)

56440 Marsupialization of Bartholin's gland cyst

56441 Lysis of labial adhesions
→ *CPT Assistant* Winter 90:7

56442 Hymenotomy, simple incision
→ *CPT Changes: An Insider's View* 2007

Destruction

56501 Destruction of lesion(s), vulva; simple (eg, laser surgery, electrosurgery, cryosurgery, chemosurgery)
→ *CPT Changes: An Insider's View* 2002

56515 extensive (eg, laser surgery, electrosurgery, cryosurgery, chemosurgery)
→ *CPT Changes: An Insider's View* 2002

(For destruction of Skene's gland cyst or abscess, use 53270)

(For cautery destruction of urethral caruncle, use 53265)

Excision

56605 Biopsy of vulva or perineum (separate procedure); 1 lesion
→ *CPT Assistant* Sep 00:9, Jun 08:6

+ 56606 each separate additional lesion (List separately in addition to code for primary procedure)

(Use 56606 in conjunction with 56605)

(For excision of local lesion, see 11420-11426, 11620-11626)

56620 Vulvectomy simple; partial

56625 complete

(For skin graft, see 15002 et seq)

56630 Vulvectomy, radical, partial;

(For skin graft, if used, see 15004-15005, 15120, 15121, 15240, 15241)

56631 with unilateral inguinofemoral lymphadenectomy

56632 with bilateral inguinofemoral lymphadenectomy

56633 Vulvectomy, radical, complete;

56634 with unilateral inguinofemoral lymphadenectomy

56637 with bilateral inguinofemoral lymphadenectomy

56640 Vulvectomy, radical, complete, with inguinofemoral, iliac, and pelvic lymphadenectomy

(For bilateral procedure, report 56640 with modifier 50)

(For lymphadenectomy, see 38760-38780)

56700 Partial hymenectomy or revision of hymenal ring

56740 Excision of Bartholin's gland or cyst

(For excision of Skene's gland, use 53270)

(For excision of urethral caruncle, use 53265)

(For excision or fulguration of urethral carcinoma, use 53220)

(For excision or marsupialization of urethral diverticulum, see 53230, 53240)

Repair

(For repair of urethra for mucosal prolapse, use 53275)

56800 Plastic repair of introitus

56805 Clitoroplasty for intersex state

56810 Perineoplasty, repair of perineum, nonobstetrical (separate procedure)

(See also 56800)

(For repair of wounds to genitalia, see 12001-12007, 12041-12047, 13131-13133)

▲ =Revised code   ● =New code   ▶ ◀ =Contains new or revised text   ⊘ =Modifier 51 exempt

(For repair of recent injury of vagina and perineum, nonobstetrical, use 57210)

(For anal sphincteroplasty, see 46750, 46751)

(For episiorrhaphy, episioperineorrhaphy for recent injury of vulva and/or perineum, nonobstetrical, use 57210)

Endoscopy

56820 Colposcopy of the vulva;

➔ *CPT Assistant* Feb 03:5; *CPT Changes: An Insider's View* 2003

56821 with biopsy(s)

➔ *CPT Assistant* Feb 03:5, Jun 03:11; *CPT Changes: An Insider's View* 2003

(For colposcopic examinations/procedures involving the vagina, see 57420, 57421; cervix, see 57452-57461)

Vagina

Incision

57000 Colpotomy; with exploration

➔ *CPT Assistant* Nov 07:1

57010 with drainage of pelvic abscess

57020 Colpocentesis (separate procedure)

57022 Incision and drainage of vaginal hematoma; obstetrical/postpartum

➔ *CPT Changes: An Insider's View* 2001, 2002

57023 non-obstetrical (eg, post-trauma, spontaneous bleeding)

➔ *CPT Changes: An Insider's View* 2001

Destruction

57061 Destruction of vaginal lesion(s); simple (eg, laser surgery, electrosurgery, cryosurgery, chemosurgery)

➔ *CPT Assistant* Apr 96:11; *CPT Changes: An Insider's View* 2002

57065 extensive (eg, laser surgery, electrosurgery, cryosurgery, chemosurgery)

➔ *CPT Assistant* Apr 96:11; *CPT Changes: An Insider's View* 2002

Excision

57100 Biopsy of vaginal mucosa; simple (separate procedure)

57105 extensive, requiring suture (including cysts)

57106 Vaginectomy, partial removal of vaginal wall;

➔ *CPT Assistant* Nov 98:17, Oct 99:5

Vaginectomy, Partial Removal of Vaginal Wall
57106

A specific portion of the upper or lower vaginal wall is excised.

57107 with removal of paravaginal tissue (radical vaginectomy)

➔ *CPT Assistant* Nov 98:17, Oct 99:5

57109 with removal of paravaginal tissue (radical vaginectomy) with bilateral total pelvic lymphadenectomy and para-aortic lymph node sampling (biopsy)

➔ *CPT Assistant* Nov 98:17, Oct 99:5

57110 Vaginectomy, complete removal of vaginal wall;

➔ *CPT Assistant* Nov 98:17, Oct 99:5

57111 with removal of paravaginal tissue (radical vaginectomy)

➔ *CPT Assistant* Nov 98:17, Oct 99:5

Vaginectomy, Complete Removal of Vaginal Wall (Radical Vaginectomy)
57111

Removal of all of the vaginal wall and removal of paravaginal tissue (the highly vascular supporting connective tissue next to the vagina)

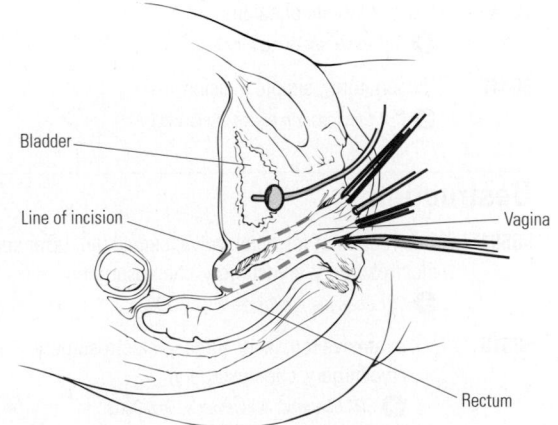

57112　　with removal of paravaginal tissue (radical vaginectomy) with bilateral total pelvic lymphadenectomy and para-aortic lymph node sampling (biopsy)

➔ *CPT Assistant* Nov 98:17, Oct 99:5

57120　　Colpocleisis (Le Fort type)

57130　　Excision of vaginal septum

57135　　Excision of vaginal cyst or tumor

Introduction

57150　　Irrigation of vagina and/or application of medicament for treatment of bacterial, parasitic, or fungoid disease

⊙ **57155**　　Insertion of uterine tandem and/or vaginal ovoids for clinical brachytherapy

➔ *CPT Assistant* Feb 02:8, Apr 09:3; *CPT Changes: An Insider's View* 2002, 2011

(For placement of needles or catheters into pelvic organs and/or genitalia [except prostate] for interstitial radioelement application, use 55920)

(For insertion of radioelement sources or ribbons, see 77761-77763, 77785-77787)

57156　　Insertion of a vaginal radiation afterloading apparatus for clinical brachytherapy

➔ *CPT Changes: An Insider's View* 2011

57160　　Fitting and insertion of pessary or other intravaginal support device

➔ *CPT Assistant* Nov 96:9, Oct 98:11, Jun 00:11, May 10:10

57170　　Diaphragm or cervical cap fitting with instructions

57180　　Introduction of any hemostatic agent or pack for spontaneous or traumatic nonobstetrical vaginal hemorrhage (separate procedure)

➔ *CPT Assistant* Nov 07:1

Repair

(For urethral suspension, Marshall-Marchetti-Krantz type, abdominal approach, see 51840, 51841)

(For laparoscopic suspension, use 51990)

57200　　Colporrhaphy, suture of injury of vagina (nonobstetrical)

57210　　Colpoperineorrhaphy, suture of injury of vagina and/or perineum (nonobstetrical)

57220　　Plastic operation on urethral sphincter, vaginal approach (eg, Kelly urethral plication)

➔ *CPT Assistant* Winter 90:7

57230　　Plastic repair of urethrocele

➔ *CPT Assistant* Winter 90:7

57240　　Anterior colporrhaphy, repair of cystocele with or without repair of urethrocele

➔ *CPT Assistant* Winter 90:7, Jan 97:3, Jun 02:5, Jun 10:6

57250　　Posterior colporrhaphy, repair of rectocele with or without perineorrhaphy

➔ *CPT Assistant* Winter 90:7, Jun 02:4, May 11:9

(For repair of rectocele [separate procedure] without posterior colporrhaphy, use 45560)

57260　　Combined anteroposterior colporrhaphy;

➔ *CPT Assistant* Jun 02:5, Jun 10:6

57265　　　with enterocele repair

➔ *CPT Assistant* Jun 02:6, Jun 10:6

+ 57267　　Insertion of mesh or other prosthesis for repair of pelvic floor defect, each site (anterior, posterior compartment), vaginal approach (List separately in addition to code for primary procedure)

➔ *CPT Assistant* Jul 05:16, May 11:9, Jan 12:10; *CPT Changes: An Insider's View* 2005

(Use 57267 in conjunction with 45560, 57240-57265, 57285)

57268　　Repair of enterocele, vaginal approach (separate procedure)

➔ *CPT Assistant* Jun 02:6

57270　　Repair of enterocele, abdominal approach (separate procedure)

➔ *CPT Assistant* Jun 02:6

57280　　Colpopexy, abdominal approach

➔ *CPT Assistant* Jan 97:3, Jun 02:6

57282　　Colpopexy, vaginal; extra-peritoneal approach (sacrospinous, iliococcygeus)

➔ *CPT Assistant* Jan 97:3, Jun 02:6; *CPT Changes: An Insider's View* 2005

57283　　　intra-peritoneal approach (uterosacral, levator myorrhaphy)

➔ *CPT Assistant* May 11:9; *CPT Changes: An Insider's View* 2005

(Do not report 57283 in conjunction with 57556, 58263, 58270, 58280, 58292, 58294)

57284　　Paravaginal defect repair (including repair of cystocele, if performed); open abdominal approach

➔ *CPT Assistant* Jan 97:1, Jun 02:7, Jul 05:16, Jun 10:6; *CPT Changes: An Insider's View* 2008

(Do not report 57284 in conjunction with 51840, 51841, 51990, 57240, 57260, 57265, 58152, 58267)

57285　　　vaginal approach

➔ *CPT Assistant* Jun 10:6; *CPT Changes: An Insider's View* 2008

(Do not report 57285 in conjunction with 51990, 57240, 57260, 57265, 58267)

57287　　Removal or revision of sling for stress incontinence (eg, fascia or synthetic)

➔ *CPT Assistant* Jun 02:7, Nov 07:9; *CPT Changes: An Insider's View* 2001

57288 Sling operation for stress incontinence (eg, fascia or synthetic)

> *CPT Assistant* Nov 99:28, May 00:4, Oct 00:7, Apr 02:18, Jun 02:7; *CPT Changes: An Insider's View* 2000

(For laparoscopic approach, use 51992)

57289 Pereyra procedure, including anterior colporrhaphy

> *CPT Assistant* Jan 97:3, Jun 02:7

57291 Construction of artificial vagina; without graft

57292 with graft

57295 Revision (including removal) of prosthetic vaginal graft; vaginal approach

> *CPT Changes: An Insider's View* 2006

57296 open abdominal approach

> *CPT Changes: An Insider's View* 2007

(For laparoscopic approach, use 57426)

57300 Closure of rectovaginal fistula; vaginal or transanal approach

> *CPT Assistant* Nov 97:21

57305 abdominal approach

> *CPT Assistant* Nov 97:21

57307 abdominal approach, with concomitant colostomy

> *CPT Assistant* Nov 97:21

57308 transperineal approach, with perineal body reconstruction, with or without levator plication

> *CPT Assistant* Nov 97:21

57310 Closure of urethrovaginal fistula;

57311 with bulbocavernosus transplant

57320 Closure of vesicovaginal fistula; vaginal approach

(For concomitant cystostomy, see 51020-51040, 51101, 51102)

57330 transvesical and vaginal approach

(For abdominal approach, use 51900)

57335 Vaginoplasty for intersex state

Manipulation

57400 Dilation of vagina under anesthesia (other than local)

> *CPT Changes: An Insider's View* 2009

57410 Pelvic examination under anesthesia (other than local)

> *CPT Assistant* Spring 93:34, Apr 06:1, Nov 07:1; *CPT Changes: An Insider's View* 2009

57415 Removal of impacted vaginal foreign body (separate procedure) under anesthesia (other than local)

> *CPT Changes: An Insider's View* 2009

(For removal without anesthesia of an impacted vaginal foreign body, use the appropriate E/M code)

Endoscopy/Laparoscopy

57420 Colposcopy of the entire vagina, with cervix if present;

> *CPT Assistant* Feb 03:5; *CPT Changes: An Insider's View* 2003

57421 with biopsy(s) of vagina/cervix

> *CPT Assistant* Feb 03:5, Jun 03:11, Jun 06:16; *CPT Changes: An Insider's View* 2003, 2006

(For colposcopic visualization of cervix and adjacent upper vagina, use 57452)

(When reporting colposcopies of multiple sites, use modifier 51 as appropriate. For colposcopic examinations/procedures involving the vulva, see 56820, 56021; cervix, see 57452-57461)

(For endometrial sampling [biopsy] performed in conjunction with colposcopy, use 58110)

57423 Paravaginal defect repair (including repair of cystocele, if performed), laparoscopic approach

> *CPT Assistant* Jun 10:6; *CPT Changes: An Insider's View* 2008

(Do not report 57423 in conjunction with 49320, 51840, 51841, 51990, 57240, 57260, 58152, 58267)

57425 Laparoscopy, surgical, colpopexy (suspension of vaginal apex)

> *CPT Changes: An Insider's View* 2004

57426 Revision (including removal) of prosthetic vaginal graft, laparoscopic approach

> *CPT Changes: An Insider's View* 2010

(For vaginal approach, see 57295. For open abdominal approach, see 57296)

Laparoscopic Revision of Prosthetic Vaginal Graft
57426

Location of prosthetic vaginal graft.

Sacral promontory

Prosthetic graft

Sutures

Bladder

Rectum

Rectovaginal septum

Vagina

Cervix Uteri

(For cervicography, use Category III code 0003T)

Endoscopy

(For colposcopic examinations/procedures involving the vulva, see 56820, 56821; vagina, see 57420, 57421)

57452　Colposcopy of the cervix including upper/adjacent vagina;

➡ *CPT Assistant* Apr 00:5, Feb 03:5, Jun 03:10; *CPT Changes: An Insider's View* 2003

(Do not report 57452 in addition to 57454-57461)

57454　　with biopsy(s) of the cervix and endocervical curettage

➡ *CPT Assistant* Apr 00:5, Feb 03:5, Jun 03:10, Aug 11:9; *CPT Changes: An Insider's View* 2003

57455　　with biopsy(s) of the cervix

➡ *CPT Assistant* Apr 00:5, Feb 03:5, Jun 03:10; *CPT Changes: An Insider's View* 2003

57456　　with endocervical curettage

➡ *CPT Assistant* Apr 00:5, Jan 03:23, Feb 03:5, Jun 03:10; *CPT Changes: An Insider's View* 2003

57460　　with loop electrode biopsy(s) of the cervix

➡ *CPT Assistant* Apr 00:5, Jan 03:23, Feb 03:5, Jun 03:10, Jul 05:15; *CPT Changes: An Insider's View* 2003

57461　　with loop electrode conization of the cervix

➡ *CPT Assistant* Jan 03:23, Feb 03:5, Jun 03:10, Dec 06:15; *CPT Changes: An Insider's View* 2003

(Do not report 57461 in addition to 57456)

(For endometrial sampling [biopsy] performed in conjunction with colposcopy, use 58110)

Excision

(For radical surgical procedures, see 58200-58240)

57500　Biopsy of cervix, single or multiple, or local excision of lesion, with or without fulguration (separate procedure)

➡ *CPT Changes: An Insider's View* 2008

57505　Endocervical curettage (not done as part of a dilation and curettage)

➡ *CPT Assistant* Jul 05:15

57510　Cautery of cervix; electro or thermal

➡ *CPT Changes: An Insider's View* 2002

57511　　cryocautery, initial or repeat

57513　　laser ablation

57520　Conization of cervix, with or without fulguration, with or without dilation and curettage, with or without repair; cold knife or laser

➡ *CPT Assistant* Apr 00:5

(See also 58120)

57522　　loop electrode excision

➡ *CPT Assistant* Apr 00:5, Mar 03:22, Jul 03:15

57530　Trachelectomy (cervicectomy), amputation of cervix (separate procedure)

57531　Radical trachelectomy, with bilateral total pelvic lymphadenectomy and para-aortic lymph node sampling biopsy, with or without removal of tube(s), with or without removal of ovary(s)

➡ *CPT Assistant* Nov 97:21

(For radical abdominal hysterectomy, use 58210)

57540　Excision of cervical stump, abdominal approach;

57545　　with pelvic floor repair

57550　Excision of cervical stump, vaginal approach;

57555　　with anterior and/or posterior repair

57556　　with repair of enterocele

(For insertion of intrauterine device, use 58300)

(For insertion of any hemostatic agent or pack for control of spontaneous non-obstetrical hemorrhage, see 57180)

57558　Dilation and curettage of cervical stump

➡ *CPT Changes: An Insider's View* 2007

Repair

57700　Cerclage of uterine cervix, nonobstetrical

57720　Trachelorrhaphy, plastic repair of uterine cervix, vaginal approach

Manipulation

57800　Dilation of cervical canal, instrumental (separate procedure)

Corpus Uteri

Excision

58100　Endometrial sampling (biopsy) with or without endocervical sampling (biopsy), without cervical dilation, any method (separate procedure)

(For endocervical curettage only, use 57505)

(For endometrial sampling [biopsy] performed in conjunction with colposcopy [57420, 57421, 57452-57461], use 58110)

+ 58110　Endometrial sampling (biopsy) performed in conjunction with colposcopy (List separately in addition to code for primary procedure)

➡ *CPT Assistant* Jun 06:17; *CPT Changes: An Insider's View* 2006

(Use 58110 in conjunction with 57420, 57421, 57452-57461)

58120　Dilation and curettage, diagnostic and/or therapeutic (nonobstetrical)

➡ *CPT Assistant* Fall 95:16, Nov 97:21, May 03:19

(For postpartum hemorrhage, use 59160)

Female Genital

58140 Myomectomy, excision of fibroid tumor(s) of uterus, 1 to 4 intramural myoma(s) with total weight of 250 g or less and/or removal of surface myomas; abdominal approach

➡ *CPT Assistant* Feb 03:15, Jun 03:5; *CPT Changes: An Insider's View* 2002, 2003

58145   vaginal approach

58146 Myomectomy, excision of fibroid tumor(s) of uterus, 5 or more intramural myomas and/or intramural myomas with total weight greater than 250 g, abdominal approach

➡ *CPT Assistant* Feb 03:15, Jun 03:5; *CPT Changes: An Insider's View* 2003

(Do not report 58146 in addition to 58140-58145, 58150-58240)

Hysterectomy Procedures

58150 Total abdominal hysterectomy (corpus and cervix), with or without removal of tube(s), with or without removal of ovary(s);

➡ *CPT Assistant* Dec 96:10, Apr 97:3, Nov 97:21, Sep 00:9, Aug 01:11

58152   with colpo-urethrocystopexy (eg, Marshall-Marchetti-Krantz, Burch)

➡ *CPT Assistant* Jan 97:1, Nov 97:22, Jun 10:6

(For urethrocystopexy without hysterectomy, see 51840, 51841)

58180 Supracervical abdominal hysterectomy (subtotal hysterectomy), with or without removal of tube(s), with or without removal of ovary(s)

58200 Total abdominal hysterectomy, including partial vaginectomy, with para-aortic and pelvic lymph node sampling, with or without removal of tube(s), with or without removal of ovary(s)

58210 Radical abdominal hysterectomy, with bilateral total pelvic lymphadenectomy and para-aortic lymph node sampling (biopsy), with or without removal of tube(s), with or without removal of ovary(s)

➡ *CPT Assistant* Fall 92:21, May 12:14

(For radical hysterectomy with ovarian transposition, use also 58825)

58240 Pelvic exenteration for gynecologic malignancy, with total abdominal hysterectomy or cervicectomy, with or without removal of tube(s), with or without removal of ovary(s), with removal of bladder and ureteral transplantations, and/or abdominoperineal resection of rectum and colon and colostomy, or any combination thereof

(For pelvic exenteration for lower urinary tract or male genital malignancy, use 51597)

58260 Vaginal hysterectomy, for uterus 250 g or less;

➡ *CPT Assistant* May 11:9; *CPT Changes: An Insider's View* 2003

58262   with removal of tube(s), and/or ovary(s)

58263   with removal of tube(s), and/or ovary(s), with repair of enterocele

58267   with colpo-urethrocystopexy (Marshall-Marchetti-Krantz type, Pereyra type) with or without endoscopic control

➡ *CPT Assistant* Jun 10:6

58270   with repair of enterocele

(For repair of enterocele with removal of tubes and/or ovaries, use 58263)

58275 Vaginal hysterectomy, with total or partial vaginectomy;

➡ *CPT Changes: An Insider's View* 2002

58280   with repair of enterocele

58285 Vaginal hysterectomy, radical (Schauta type operation)

➡ *CPT Assistant* Nov 07:1

58290 Vaginal hysterectomy, for uterus greater than 250 g;

➡ *CPT Changes: An Insider's View* 2003

58291   with removal of tube(s) and/or ovary(s)

➡ *CPT Changes: An Insider's View* 2003

58292   with removal of tube(s) and/or ovary(s), with repair of enterocele

➡ *CPT Changes: An Insider's View* 2003

58293   with colpo-urethrocystopexy (Marshall-Marchetti-Krantz type, Pereyra type) with or without endoscopic control

➡ *CPT Changes: An Insider's View* 2003

58294   with repair of enterocele

➡ *CPT Changes: An Insider's View* 2003

Introduction

(To report insertion of non-biodegradable drug delivery implant for contraception, use 11981. To report removal of implantable contraceptive capsules with subsequent insertion of non-biodegradable drug delivery implant, use 11976 and 11981)

58300 Insertion of intrauterine device (IUD)

➡ *CPT Assistant* Apr 98:14

58301 Removal of intrauterine device (IUD)

➡ *CPT Assistant* Apr 98:14

58321 Artificial insemination; intra-cervical

58322   intra-uterine

58323 Sperm washing for artificial insemination

➡ *CPT Assistant* Jan 98:6

58340 Catheterization and introduction of saline or contrast material for saline infusion sonohysterography (SIS) or hysterosalpingography

➡ *CPT Assistant* Nov 97:22, Jul 99:8, Mar 09:11; *CPT Changes: An Insider's View* 2004

(For radiological supervision and interpretation of saline infusion sonohysterography, use 76831)

(For radiological supervision and interpretation of hysterosalpingography, use 74740)

58345   Transcervical introduction of fallopian tube catheter for diagnosis and/or re-establishing patency (any method), with or without hysterosalpingography

→ *CPT Assistant* Nov 97:22, Mar 09:11

(For radiological supervision and interpretation, use 74742)

58346   Insertion of Heyman capsules for clinical brachytherapy

→ *CPT Assistant* Feb 02:8, Apr 09:3; *CPT Changes: An Insider's View* 2002

(For placement of needles or catheters into pelvic organs and/or genitalia [except prostate] for interstitial radioelement application, use 55920)

(For insertion of radioelement sources or ribbons, see 77761-77763, 77785-77787)

58350   Chromotubation of oviduct, including materials

→ *CPT Assistant* May 02:19, Dec 08:7

►(To report the supply of any materials, use 99070)◄

58353   Endometrial ablation, thermal, without hysteroscopic guidance

→ *CPT Assistant* Mar 02:11, Apr 02:19; *CPT Changes: An Insider's View* 2001

(For hysteroscopic procedure, use 58563)

58356   Endometrial cryoablation with ultrasonic guidance, including endometrial curettage, when performed

→ *CPT Changes: An Insider's View* 2005

(Do not report 58356 in conjunction with 58100, 58120, 58340, 76700, 76856)

Repair

58400   Uterine suspension, with or without shortening of round ligaments, with or without shortening of sacrouterine ligaments; (separate procedure)

58410   with presacral sympathectomy

→ *CPT Assistant* Mar 07:9

(For anastomosis of tubes to uterus, use 58752)

58520   Hysterorrhaphy, repair of ruptured uterus (nonobstetrical)

58540   Hysteroplasty, repair of uterine anomaly (Strassman type)

(For closure of vesicouterine fistula, use 51920)

Laparoscopy/Hysteroscopy

Surgical laparoscopy always includes diagnostic laparoscopy. To report a diagnostic laparoscopy (peritoneoscopy) (separate procedure), use 49320. To report a diagnostic hysteroscopy (separate procedure), use 58555.

58541   Laparoscopy, surgical, supracervical hysterectomy, for uterus 250 g or less;

→ *CPT Assistant* Nov 07:1; *CPT Changes: An Insider's View* 2007

58542   with removal of tube(s) and/or ovary(s)

→ *CPT Assistant* Nov 07:1; *CPT Changes: An Insider's View* 2007

(Do not report 58541, 58542 in conjunction with 49320, 57000, 57180, 57410, 58140-58146, 58545, 58546, 58561, 58661, 58670, 58671)

58543   Laparoscopy, surgical, supracervical hysterectomy, for uterus greater than 250 g;

→ *CPT Assistant* Nov 07:1; *CPT Changes: An Insider's View* 2007

58544   with removal of tube(s) and/or ovary(s)

→ *CPT Assistant* Nov 07:1; *CPT Changes: An Insider's View* 2007

(Do not report 58543-58544 in conjunction with 49320, 57000, 57180, 57410, 58140-58146, 58545, 58546, 58561, 58661, 58670, 58671)

58545   Laparoscopy, surgical, myomectomy, excision; 1 to 4 intramural myomas with total weight of 250 g or less and/or removal of surface myomas

→ *CPT Assistant* Jun 03:5, 12; *CPT Changes: An Insider's View* 2003

58546   5 or more intramural myomas and/or intramural myomas with total weight greater than 250 g

→ *CPT Assistant* Jun 03:12, Jan 04:26; *CPT Changes: An Insider's View* 2003

58548   Laparoscopy, surgical, with radical hysterectomy, with bilateral total pelvic lymphadenectomy and para-aortic lymph node sampling (biopsy), with removal of tube(s) and ovary(s), if performed

→ *CPT Assistant* Nov 07:1; *CPT Changes: An Insider's View* 2007

(Do not report 58548 in conjunction with 38570-38572, 58210, 58285, 58550-58554)

58550   Laparoscopy, surgical, with vaginal hysterectomy, for uterus 250 g or less;

→ *CPT Assistant* Nov 99:28, Mar 00:9; *CPT Changes: An Insider's View* 2000, 2003

58552   with removal of tube(s) and/or ovary(s)

→ *CPT Assistant* Nov 07:1; *CPT Changes: An Insider's View* 2003

(Do not report 58550-58552 in conjunction with 49320, 57000, 57180, 57410, 58140-58146, 58545, 58546, 58561, 58661, 58670, 58671)

58553   Laparoscopy, surgical, with vaginal hysterectomy, for uterus greater than 250 g;

→ *CPT Changes: An Insider's View* 2003

58554   with removal of tube(s) and/or ovary(s)

→ *CPT Changes: An Insider's View* 2003

(Do not report 58553-58554 in conjunction with 49320, 57000, 57180, 57410, 58140-58146, 58545, 58546, 58561, 58661, 58670, 58671)

58555   Hysteroscopy, diagnostic (separate procedure)

→ *CPT Assistant* Nov 99:28, Mar 00:10; *CPT Changes: An Insider's View* 2000

58558   Hysteroscopy, surgical; with sampling (biopsy) of endometrium and/or polypectomy, with or without D & C

→ *CPT Assistant* Nov 99:28, Mar 00:10, Sep 02:10, Jan 03:7, May 03:19; *CPT Changes: An Insider's View* 2000

Female Genital

58559   with lysis of intrauterine adhesions (any method)
> *CPT Assistant* Nov 99:28, Mar 00:10; *CPT Changes: An Insider's View* 2000

58560   with division or resection of intrauterine septum (any method)
> *CPT Assistant* Nov 99:28, Mar 00:10; *CPT Changes: An Insider's View* 2000

58561   with removal of leiomyomata
> *CPT Assistant* Nov 99:28, Mar 00:10, Jan 03:7; *CPT Changes: An Insider's View* 2000

58562   with removal of impacted foreign body
> *CPT Assistant* Nov 99:28, Mar 00:10; *CPT Changes: An Insider's View* 2000

58563   with endometrial ablation (eg, endometrial resection, electrosurgical ablation, thermoablation)
> *CPT Assistant* Nov 99:28, Mar 00:10, Mar 02:11, Apr 02:19, Jan 03:7, Feb 12:11; *CPT Changes: An Insider's View* 2000, 2002

Hysteroscopy
58563

58565   with bilateral fallopian tube cannulation to induce occlusion by placement of permanent implants
> *CPT Assistant* Jan 11:9, Feb 12:11; *CPT Changes: An Insider's View* 2005

(Do not report 58565 in conjunction with 58555 or 57800)

(For unilateral procedure, use modifier 52)

58570   Laparoscopy, surgical, with total hysterectomy, for uterus 250 g or less;
> *CPT Changes: An Insider's View* 2008

58571   with removal of tube(s) and/or ovary(s)
> *CPT Assistant* May 12:14; *CPT Changes: An Insider's View* 2008

58572   Laparoscopy, surgical, with total hysterectomy, for uterus greater than 250 g;
> *CPT Changes: An Insider's View* 2008

58573   with removal of tube(s) and/or ovary(s)
> *CPT Assistant* May 12:14; *CPT Changes: An Insider's View* 2008

(Do not report 58570-58573 in conjunction with 49320, 57000, 57180, 57410, 58140-58146, 58150, 58545, 58546, 58561, 58661, 58670, 58671)

58578   Unlisted laparoscopy procedure, uterus
> *CPT Assistant* Nov 99:28, Mar 00:10, Mar 07:9; *CPT Changes: An Insider's View* 2000

58579   Unlisted hysteroscopy procedure, uterus
> *CPT Assistant* Nov 99:28, Mar 00:10; *CPT Changes: An Insider's View* 2000

Oviduct/Ovary

Incision

58600   Ligation or transection of fallopian tube(s), abdominal or vaginal approach, unilateral or bilateral
> *CPT Assistant* Nov 99:28; *CPT Changes: An Insider's View* 2000

58605   Ligation or transection of fallopian tube(s), abdominal or vaginal approach, postpartum, unilateral or bilateral, during same hospitalization (separate procedure)
> *CPT Assistant* Nov 99:28; *CPT Changes: An Insider's View* 2000

(For laparoscopic procedures, use 58670, 58671)

+ 58611   Ligation or transection of fallopian tube(s) when done at the time of cesarean delivery or intra-abdominal surgery (not a separate procedure) (List separately in addition to code for primary procedure)
> *CPT Changes: An Insider's View* 2002

58615   Occlusion of fallopian tube(s) by device (eg, band, clip, Falope ring) vaginal or suprapubic approach
> *CPT Assistant* Nov 99:28; *CPT Changes: An Insider's View* 2000

(For laparoscopic approach, use 58671)

(For lysis of adnexal adhesions, use 58740)

Laparoscopy

Surgical laparoscopy always includes diagnostic laparoscopy. To report a diagnostic laparoscopy (peritoneoscopy) (separate procedure), use 49320.

58660   Laparoscopy, surgical; with lysis of adhesions (salpingolysis, ovariolysis) (separate procedure)
> *CPT Assistant* Nov 99:28, Mar 00:10, Mar 03:22, Dec 11:16; *CPT Changes: An Insider's View* 2000

58661   with removal of adnexal structures (partial or total oophorectomy and/or salpingectomy)
➔ *CPT Assistant* Nov 99:28, Mar 00:10, Jan 02:11, Nov 07:1, May 10:10; *CPT Changes: An Insider's View* 2000

58662   with fulguration or excision of lesions of the ovary, pelvic viscera, or peritoneal surface by any method
➔ *CPT Assistant* Nov 99:28, Mar 00:10, *CPT Changes: An Insider's View* 2000

58670   with fulguration of oviducts (with or without transection)
➔ *CPT Assistant* Nov 99:29, Mar 00:10, Nov 07:2; *CPT Changes: An Insider's View* 2000

58671   with occlusion of oviducts by device (eg, band, clip, or Falope ring)
➔ *CPT Assistant* Nov 99:29, Mar 00:10; *CPT Changes: An Insider's View* 2000

58672   with fimbrioplasty
➔ *CPT Assistant* Nov 99:29, Mar 00:10; *CPT Changes: An Insider's View* 2000

58673   with salpingostomy (salpingoneostomy)
➔ *CPT Assistant* Nov 99:29, Mar 00:10, May 02:19; *CPT Changes: An Insider's View* 2000

(Codes 58672 and 58673 are used to report unilateral procedures. For bilateral procedure, use modifier 50)

58679   Unlisted laparoscopy procedure, oviduct, ovary
➔ *CPT Assistant* Nov 99:29, Mar 00:10; *CPT Changes: An Insider's View* 2000

(For laparoscopic aspiration of ovarian cyst, use 49322)

(For laparoscopic biopsy of the ovary or fallopian tube, use 49321)

Excision

58700   Salpingectomy, complete or partial, unilateral or bilateral (separate procedure)

58720   Salpingo-oophorectomy, complete or partial, unilateral or bilateral (separate procedure)
➔ *CPT Assistant* Sep 00:9, Jul 06:19

Repair

58740   Lysis of adhesions (salpingolysis, ovariolysis)
➔ *CPT Assistant* Sep 96:9, Nov 99:29; *CPT Changes: An Insider's View* 2000

(For laparoscopic approach, use 58660)

(For excision or destruction of endometriomas, open method, see 49203-49205, 58957, 58958)

(For fulguration or excision of lesions, laparoscopic approach, use 58662)

58750   Tubotubal anastomosis

58752   Tubouterine implantation

58760   Fimbrioplasty
➔ *CPT Assistant* Nov 99:29; *CPT Changes: An Insider's View* 2000

(For laparoscopic approach, use 58672)

58770   Salpingostomy (salpingoneostomy)
➔ *CPT Assistant* Nov 99:29; *CPT Changes: An Insider's View* 2000

(For laparoscopic approach, use 58673)

Ovary

Incision

58800   Drainage of ovarian cyst(s), unilateral or bilateral (separate procedure); vaginal approach

58805   abdominal approach

58820   Drainage of ovarian abscess; vaginal approach, open
➔ *CPT Assistant* Nov 97:22

58822   abdominal approach
➔ *CPT Assistant* Nov 97:22

⊙ **58823**   Drainage of pelvic abscess, transvaginal or transrectal approach, percutaneous (eg, ovarian, pericolic)
➔ *CPT Assistant* Nov 97:22, Mar 98:8

(For radiological supervision and interpretation, use 75989)

58825   Transposition, ovary(s)

Excision

58900   Biopsy of ovary, unilateral or bilateral (separate procedure)
➔ *CPT Assistant* Nov 99:29; *CPT Changes: An Insider's View* 2000

(For laparoscopic biopsy of the ovary or fallopian tube, use 49321)

58920   Wedge resection or bisection of ovary, unilateral or bilateral

58925   Ovarian cystectomy, unilateral or bilateral

58940   Oophorectomy, partial or total, unilateral or bilateral;
➔ *CPT Assistant* Mar 04:3

(For oophorectomy with concomitant debulking for ovarian malignancy, use 58952)

58943   for ovarian, tubal or primary peritoneal malignancy, with para-aortic and pelvic lymph node biopsies, peritoneal washings, peritoneal biopsies, diaphragmatic assessments, with or without salpingectomy(s), with or without omentectomy
➔ *CPT Assistant* Oct 10:16, Dec 10:16; *CPT Changes: An Insider's View* 2001

58950   Resection (initial) of ovarian, tubal or primary peritoneal malignancy with bilateral salpingo-oophorectomy and omentectomy;
➔ *CPT Assistant* Oct 10:16, Dec 10:16; *CPT Changes: An Insider's View* 2001, 2007

58951   with total abdominal hysterectomy, pelvic and limited para-aortic lymphadenectomy

⮕ *CPT Assistant* Aug 01:11, Oct 10:16, Dec 10:16

58952   with radical dissection for debulking (ie, radical excision or destruction, intra-abdominal or retroperitoneal tumors)

⮕ *CPT Assistant* Dec 96:10, Aug 01:11, Oct 10:16, Dec 10:16; *CPT Changes: An Insider's View* 2001

(For resection of recurrent ovarian, tubal, primary peritoneal, or uterine malignancy, see 58957, 58958)

58953   Bilateral salpingo-oophorectomy with omentectomy, total abdominal hysterectomy and radical dissection for debulking;

⮕ *CPT Assistant* Feb 02:8, Oct 10:16, Dec 10:16; *CPT Changes: An Insider's View* 2002

58954   with pelvic lymphadenectomy and limited para-aortic lymphadenectomy

⮕ *CPT Assistant* Feb 02:9, Oct 10:16, Dec 10:16; *CPT Changes: An Insider's View* 2002

58956   Bilateral salpingo-oophorectomy with total omentectomy, total abdominal hysterectomy for malignancy

⮕ *CPT Changes: An Insider's View* 2005

(Do not report 58956 in conjunction with 49255, 58150, 58180, 58262, 58263, 58550, 58661, 58700, 58720, 58900, 58925, 58940, 58957, 58958)

58957   Resection (tumor debulking) of recurrent ovarian, tubal, primary peritoneal, uterine malignancy (intra-abdominal, retroperitoneal tumors), with omentectomy, if performed;

⮕ *CPT Changes: An Insider's View* 2007

58958   with pelvic lymphadenectomy and limited para-aortic lymphadenectomy

⮕ *CPT Changes: An Insider's View* 2007

(Do not report 58957, 58958 in conjunction with 38770, 38780, 44005, 49000, 49203-49215, 49255, 58900-58960)

58960   Laparotomy, for staging or restaging of ovarian, tubal, or primary peritoneal malignancy (second look), with or without omentectomy, peritoneal washing, biopsy of abdominal and pelvic peritoneum, diaphragmatic assessment with pelvic and limited para-aortic lymphadenectomy

⮕ *CPT Changes: An Insider's View* 2001

(Do not report 58960 in conjunction with 58957, 58958)

In Vitro Fertilization

58970   Follicle puncture for oocyte retrieval, any method

(For radiological supervision and interpretation, use 76948)

58974   Embryo transfer, intrauterine

58976   Gamete, zygote, or embryo intrafallopian transfer, any method

⮕ *CPT Assistant* Nov 99:29; *CPT Changes: An Insider's View* 2000

(For laparoscopic adnexal procedures, see 58660-58673)

Other Procedures

58999   Unlisted procedure, female genital system (nonobstetrical)

⮕ *CPT Assistant* Apr 09:9, 10

Maternity Care and Delivery

The services normally provided in uncomplicated maternity cases include antepartum care, delivery, and postpartum care.

Antepartum care includes the initial and subsequent history, physical examinations, recording of weight, blood pressures, fetal heart tones, routine chemical urinalysis, and monthly visits up to 28 weeks gestation, biweekly visits to 36 weeks gestation, and weekly visits until delivery. Any other visits or services within this time period should be coded separately.

Postpartum care only services (59430) include office or other outpatient visits following vaginal or cesarean section delivery.

▶Delivery services include admission to the hospital, the admission history and physical examination, management of uncomplicated labor, vaginal delivery (with or without episiotomy, with or without forceps), or cesarean delivery. When reporting delivery only services (59409, 59514, 59612, 59620), report inpatient postdelivery management and discharge services using Evaluation and Management Services codes (99217-99239). Delivery and postpartum services (59410, 59515, 59614, 59622) include delivery services and all inpatient and outpatient postpartum services. Medical complications of pregnancy (eg, cardiac problems, neurological problems, diabetes, hypertension, toxemia, hyperemesis, preterm labor, premature rupture of membranes, trauma) and medical problems complicating labor and delivery management may require additional resources and may be reported separately.◀

For surgical complications of pregnancy (eg, appendectomy, hernia, ovarian cyst, Bartholin cyst), see services in the **Surgery** section.

▶If all or part of the antepartum and/or postpartum patient care is provided except delivery due to termination of pregnancy by abortion or referral to another physician or other qualified health care professional for delivery, see the antepartum and postpartum care codes 59425, 59426, and 59430.◀

(For circumcision of newborn, see 54150, 54160)

Antepartum and Fetal Invasive Services

(For fetal intrauterine transfusion, use 36460)

(For unlisted fetal invasive procedure, use 59897)

59000   Amniocentesis; diagnostic
➔ *CPT Assistant* Apr 97:2, Feb 02:7, Aug 02:2, May 04:2; *CPT Changes: An Insider's View* 2002

(For radiological supervision and interpretation, use 76946)

59001   therapeutic amniotic fluid reduction (includes ultrasound guidance)
➔ *CPT Assistant* Feb 02:7, Aug 02:2; *CPT Changes: An Insider's View* 2002

Amniocentesis, Therapeutic Amniotic Fluid Reduction
59001

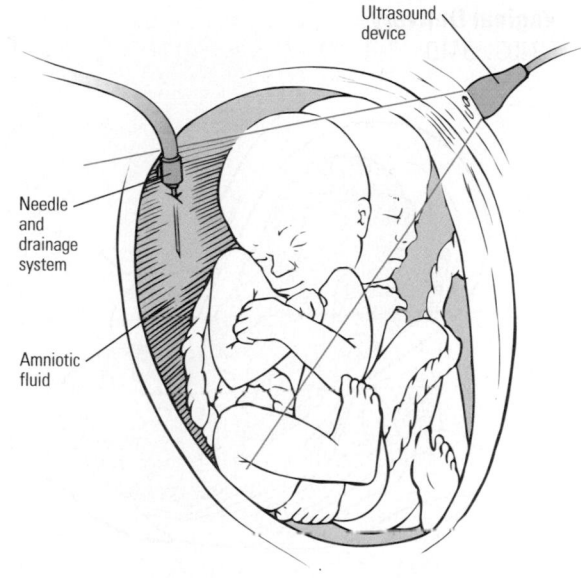

Ultrasound device

Needle and drainage system

Amniotic fluid

59012   Cordocentesis (intrauterine), any method
➔ *CPT Assistant* Aug 02:2

(For radiological supervision and interpretation, use 76941)

59015   Chorionic villus sampling, any method
➔ *CPT Assistant* Apr 97:2, Aug 02:2

(For radiological supervision and interpretation, use 76945)

59020   Fetal contraction stress test
➔ *CPT Assistant* Apr 97:2, Aug 02:2

59025   Fetal non-stress test
➔ *CPT Assistant* Apr 97:2, May 98:10, Oct 04:10, Dec 08:8

59030   Fetal scalp blood sampling
➔ *CPT Assistant* Aug 02:3

(For repeat fetal scalp blood sampling, use 59030 and see modifiers 76 and 77)

59050   Fetal monitoring during labor by consulting physician (ie, non-attending physician) with written report; supervision and interpretation
➔ *CPT Assistant* Nov 97:22

59051   interpretation only
➔ *CPT Assistant* Nov 97:22

59070   Transabdominal amnioinfusion, including ultrasound guidance
➔ *CPT Assistant* May 04:2, Jun 04:11; *CPT Changes: An Insider's View* 2004

59072   Fetal umbilical cord occlusion, including ultrasound guidance
➔ *CPT Assistant* May 04:2, Jun 04:11; *CPT Changes: An Insider's View* 2004

59074   Fetal fluid drainage (eg, vesicocentesis, thoracocentesis, paracentesis), including ultrasound guidance
➔ *CPT Assistant* May 04:2, 4, Jun 04:11, Dec 04:19; *CPT Changes: An Insider's View* 2004

59076   Fetal shunt placement, including ultrasound guidance
➔ *CPT Assistant* May 04:2, 4, Jun 04:11, Dec 04:19; *CPT Changes: An Insider's View* 2004

Excision

59100   Hysterotomy, abdominal (eg, for hydatidiform mole, abortion)

(When tubal ligation is performed at the same time as hysterotomy, use 58611 in addition to 59100)

59120   Surgical treatment of ectopic pregnancy; tubal or ovarian, requiring salpingectomy and/or oophorectomy, abdominal or vaginal approach

59121   tubal or ovarian, without salpingectomy and/or oophorectomy

59130   abdominal pregnancy

59135   interstitial, uterine pregnancy requiring total hysterectomy

59136   interstitial, uterine pregnancy with partial resection of uterus

59140   cervical, with evacuation

Female Genital

Female Genital

59150   Laparoscopic treatment of ectopic pregnancy; without salpingectomy and/or oophorectomy
➔ *CPT Assistant* Sep 96:9

Laparoscopic Treatment of Ectopic Pregnancy
59150

The site of gestation is located with a laparoscope, and a small incision is made above the site. The ectopic pregnancy is then removed.

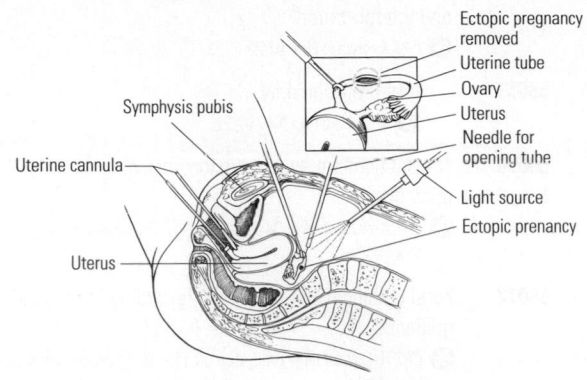

59151   with salpingectomy and/or oophorectomy

59160   Curettage, postpartum
➔ *CPT Assistant* Nov 97:22, Sep 02:11

Introduction

(For intrauterine fetal transfusion, use 36460)

(For introduction of hypertonic solution and/or prostaglandins to initiate labor, see 59850-59857)

59200   Insertion of cervical dilator (eg, laminaria, prostaglandin) (separate procedure)
➔ *CPT Assistant* Fall 93:9, Apr 97:3, Jul 05:15

Repair

(For tracheloplasty, use 57700)

▲ **59300**   Episiotomy or vaginal repair, by other than attending
➔ *CPT Changes: An Insider's View* 2013

59320   Cerclage of cervix, during pregnancy; vaginal
➔ *CPT Assistant* Aug 02:2, Nov 06:21, Feb 07:10

59325   abdominal
➔ *CPT Assistant* Aug 02:2, Nov 06:21, Feb 07:10

59350   Hysterorrhaphy of ruptured uterus
➔ *CPT Assistant* Aug 02:2

Vaginal Delivery, Antepartum and Postpartum Care

—— *Coding Tip* ——

Instructions for Reporting Antepartum and Postpartum Care

The services normally provided in uncomplicated maternity cases include antepartum care, delivery, and postpartum care.

CPT Coding Guidelines, Maternity Care and Delivery

59400   Routine obstetric care including antepartum care, vaginal delivery (with or without episiotomy, and/or forceps) and postpartum care
➔ *CPT Assistant* Feb 96:1, Mar 96:11, Feb 97:11, Apr 97:3, Apr 98:15, Jun 98:10, Aug 02:3, Feb 03:15

Vaginal Delivery
59400-59410

59409   Vaginal delivery only (with or without episiotomy and/or forceps);
➔ *CPT Assistant* Feb 96:1, Mar 96:11, Jul 96:11, Sep 96:4, Feb 97:11, Apr 97:1, Aug 02:3, Dec 07:13, Jun 09:10

59410   including postpartum care

59412   External cephalic version, with or without tocolysis
➔ *CPT Assistant* Fall 94:21, Feb 96:1, Aug 02:2-3

(Use 59412 in addition to code[s] for delivery)

59414   Delivery of placenta (separate procedure)
➔ *CPT Assistant* Jun 96:10, Jun 98:10, Aug 02:3

(For antepartum care only, see 59425, 59426 or appropriate E/M code[s])

(For 1-3 antepartum care visits, see appropriate E/M code[s])

59425   Antepartum care only; 4-6 visits
➔ *CPT Assistant* Fall 94:21, Apr 97:11, Aug 02:3

59426   7 or more visits
➔ *CPT Assistant* Fall 94:21, Apr 97:11, Aug 02:3

59430   Postpartum care only (separate procedure)
➔ *CPT Assistant* Jun 96:10, Aug 02:3

Cesarean Delivery

(For standby attendance for infant, use 99360)

(For low cervical cesarean section, see 59510, 59515, 59525)

—— *Coding Tip* ——

Instructions for Reporting Cesarean Delivery

Patients who have had a previous cesarean delivery and now present with the expectation of a vaginal delivery are coded using codes 59610-59622. If the patient has a successful vaginal delivery after a previous cesarean delivery (VBAC), use codes 59610-59614. If the attempt is unsuccessful and another cesarean delivery is carried out, use codes 59618-59622. To report elective cesarean deliveries use code 59510, 59514 or 59515.

CPT Coding Guidelines, Maternity Care and Delivery, Delivery After Previous Cesarean Delivery

Cesarean Delivery
59510-59515

Vertical incision

Transverse incision

59510   Routine obstetric care including antepartum care, cesarean delivery, and postpartum care
➔ *CPT Assistant* Jul 96:11, Sep 96:4, Oct 96:10, Feb 97:11, Apr 97:2, Aug 02:3

59514   Cesarean delivery only;
➔ *CPT Assistant* Oct 96:10, Feb 97:11

59515   including postpartum care

(For classic cesarean section, see 59510, 59515, 59525)

+ 59525   Subtotal or total hysterectomy after cesarean delivery (List separately in addition to code for primary procedure)

(Use 59525 in conjunction with 59510, 59514, 59515, 59618, 59620, 59622)

(For extraperitoneal cesarean section, or cesarean section with subtotal or total hysterectomy, see 59510, 59515, 59525)

Delivery After Previous Cesarean Delivery

Patients who have had a previous cesarean delivery and now present with the expectation of a vaginal delivery are coded using codes 59610-59622. If the patient has a successful vaginal delivery after a previous cesarean delivery (VBAC), use codes 59610-59614. If the attempt is unsuccessful and another cesarean delivery is carried out, use codes 59618-59622. To report elective cesarean deliveries use code 59510, 59514 or 59515.

59610   Routine obstetric care including antepartum care, vaginal delivery (with or without episiotomy, and/or forceps) and postpartum care, after previous cesarean delivery
➔ *CPT Assistant* Feb 96:2, Apr 97:3, Aug 02:3

59612   Vaginal delivery only, after previous cesarean delivery (with or without episiotomy and/or forceps);
➔ *CPT Assistant* Feb 96:2, Aug 02:3

59614   including postpartum care
➔ *CPT Assistant* Feb 96:2

59618   Routine obstetric care including antepartum care, cesarean delivery, and postpartum care, following attempted vaginal delivery after previous cesarean delivery
➔ *CPT Assistant* Feb 96:2, Aug 02:4

59620   Cesarean delivery only, following attempted vaginal delivery after previous cesarean delivery;
➔ *CPT Assistant* Feb 96:2

59622   including postpartum care
➔ *CPT Assistant* Feb 96:2

Abortion

(For medical treatment of spontaneous complete abortion, any trimester, use E/M codes 99201-99233)

(For surgical treatment of spontaneous abortion, use 59812)

59812   Treatment of incomplete abortion, any trimester, completed surgically
➔ *CPT Assistant* Fall 93:9, Fall 95:16

Female Genital

59820   Treatment of missed abortion, completed surgically; first trimester
   → *CPT Assistant* Fall 93:9, Fall 95:16, Feb 99:10

59821   second trimester
   → *CPT Assistant* Fall 93:9, Fall 95:16

59830   Treatment of septic abortion, completed surgically
   → *CPT Assistant* Fall 93:9

59840   Induced abortion, by dilation and curettage
   → *CPT Assistant* Fall 93:9, Sep 03:16

59841   Induced abortion, by dilation and evacuation
   → *CPT Assistant* Fall 93:9

59850   Induced abortion, by 1 or more intra-amniotic injections (amniocentesis-injections), including hospital admission and visits, delivery of fetus and secundines;
   → *CPT Assistant* Fall 93:10

59851   with dilation and curettage and/or evacuation
   → *CPT Assistant* Fall 93:10

59852   with hysterotomy (failed intra-amniotic injection)
   → *CPT Assistant* Fall 93:10

   (For insertion of cervical dilator, use 59200)

59855   Induced abortion, by 1 or more vaginal suppositories (eg, prostaglandin) with or without cervical dilation (eg, laminaria), including hospital admission and visits, delivery of fetus and secundines;

59856   with dilation and curettage and/or evacuation

59857   with hysterotomy (failed medical evacuation)

Other Procedures

59866   Multifetal pregnancy reduction(s) (MPR)

59870   Uterine evacuation and curettage for hydatidiform mole
   → *CPT Assistant* Feb 99:10

59871   Removal of cerclage suture under anesthesia (other than local)
   → *CPT Assistant* Nov 97:22, Nov 06:21, Feb 07:10

59897   Unlisted fetal invasive procedure, including ultrasound guidance, when performed
   → *CPT Assistant* May 04:5; *CPT Changes: An Insider's View* 2004, 2010

59898   Unlisted laparoscopy procedure, maternity care and delivery
   → *CPT Assistant* Nov 99:29, Mar 00:10; *CPT Changes: An Insider's View* 2000

59899   Unlisted procedure, maternity care and delivery
   → *CPT Assistant* Jun 97:10, May 04:2

Endocrine System

(For pituitary and pineal surgery, see Nervous System)

Thyroid Gland

Incision

60000   Incision and drainage of thyroglossal duct cyst, infected
   → *CPT Changes: An Insider's View* 2002

Excision

60100   Biopsy thyroid, percutaneous core needle
   → *CPT Assistant* Jun 97:5, Jun 07:10

   (If imaging guidance is performed, see 76942, 77002, 77012, 77021)

   (For fine needle aspiration, use 10021 or 10022)

   (For evaluation of fine needle aspirate, see 88172, 88173)

60200   Excision of cyst or adenoma of thyroid, or transection of isthmus
   → *CPT Assistant* Aug 11:10

60210   Partial thyroid lobectomy, unilateral; with or without isthmusectomy
   → *CPT Assistant* Winter 94:7, Aug 11:9

60212   with contralateral subtotal lobectomy, including isthmusectomy

60220   Total thyroid lobectomy, unilateral; with or without isthmusectomy
   → *CPT Assistant* Oct 10:13, Dec 10:13, Aug 11:10

Thyroid Lobectomy
60220

The thyroid is exposed via a transverse cervical incision. The superior and inferior thyroid vessels serving the lobe are ligated, the isthmus is severed, and the entire thyroid lobe is resected.

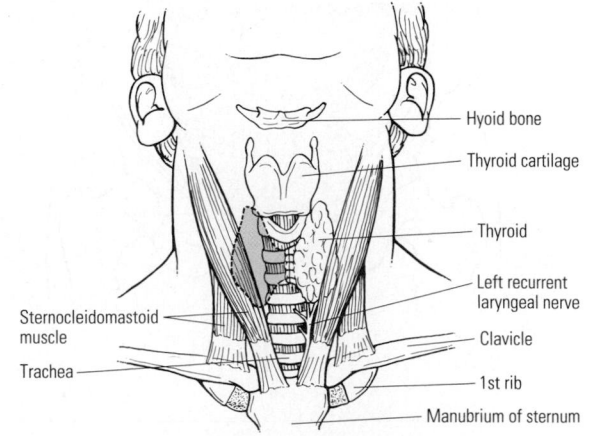

Labels: Hyoid bone; Thyroid cartilage; Thyroid; Left recurrent laryngeal nerve; Clavicle; 1st rib; Manubrium of sternum; Sternocleidomastoid muscle; Trachea

Female Genital

60225   with contralateral subtotal lobectomy, including isthmusectomy

60240   Thyroidectomy, total or complete

(For thyroidectomy, subtotal or partial, use 60271)

60252   Thyroidectomy, total or subtotal for malignancy; with limited neck dissection

➔ *CPT Assistant* Nov 00:10

60254   with radical neck dissection

➔ *CPT Assistant* Nov 00:10

60260   Thyroidectomy, removal of all remaining thyroid tissue following previous removal of a portion of thyroid

➔ *CPT Assistant* Oct 10:13, Dec 10:13

(For bilateral procedure, report 60260 with modifier 50)

60270   Thyroidectomy, including substernal thyroid; sternal split or transthoracic approach

➔ *CPT Changes: An Insider's View* 2002

60271   cervical approach

60280   Excision of thyroglossal duct cyst or sinus;

60281   recurrent

(For thyroid ultrasonography, use 76536)

Removal

60300   Aspiration and/or injection, thyroid cyst

➔ *CPT Changes: An Insider's View* 2008

(For fine needle aspiration, see 10021, 10022)

(If imaging guidance is performed, see 76942, 77012)

Parathyroid, Thymus, Adrenal Glands, Pancreas, and Carotid Body

Excision

(For pituitary and pineal surgery, see **Nervous System**)

60500   Parathyroidectomy or exploration of parathyroid(s);

60502   re-exploration

60505   with mediastinal exploration, sternal split or transthoracic approach

+ 60512   Parathyroid autotransplantation (List separately in addition to code for primary procedure)

➔ *CPT Assistant* Aug 11:9

(Use 60512 in conjunction with 60500, 60502, 60505, 60212, 60225, 60240, 60252, 60254, 60260, 60270, 60271)

Posterior View of the Pharynx
60512

Epiglottis

Thyroid cartilage

Thyroid gland

Parathyroid glands

Trachea

Esophagus

60520   Thymectomy, partial or total; transcervical approach (separate procedure)

60521   sternal split or transthoracic approach, without radical mediastinal dissection (separate procedure)

➔ *CPT Assistant* Dec 07:12

60522   sternal split or transthoracic approach, with radical mediastinal dissection (separate procedure)

(For thoracoscopic [VATS] thymectomy, see 32673)

60540   Adrenalectomy, partial or complete, or exploration of adrenal gland with or without biopsy, transabdominal, lumbar or dorsal (separate procedure);

➔ *CPT Assistant* Nov 98:17

60545   with excision of adjacent retroperitoneal tumor

➔ *CPT Assistant* Nov 98:17

(Do not report 60540, 60545 in conjunction with 50323)

(For bilateral procedure, report 60540 with modifier 50)

(For excision of remote or disseminated pheochromocytoma, see 49203-49205)

(For laparoscopic approach, use 60650)

Female Genital

60600   Excision of carotid body tumor; without excision of
            carotid artery

60605   with excision of carotid artery

Laparoscopy

Surgical laparoscopy always includes diagnostic
laparoscopy. To report a diagnostic laparoscopy
(peritoneoscopy) (separate procedure), use 49320.

60650   Laparoscopy, surgical, with adrenalectomy, partial or
            complete, or exploration of adrenal gland with or without
            biopsy, transabdominal, lumbar or dorsal

   ➔ *CPT Assistant* Nov 99:30, Mar 00:10, Nov 01:8; *CPT Changes: An
      Insider's View* 2000

Laparoscopic Adrenalectomy
60650

An adrenal gland is dissected and removed under laparoscopic guidance. Multiple small
blood vessels from the vena cava and the aorta do not follow standard anatomic
pattern, requiring intricate dissection.

Left

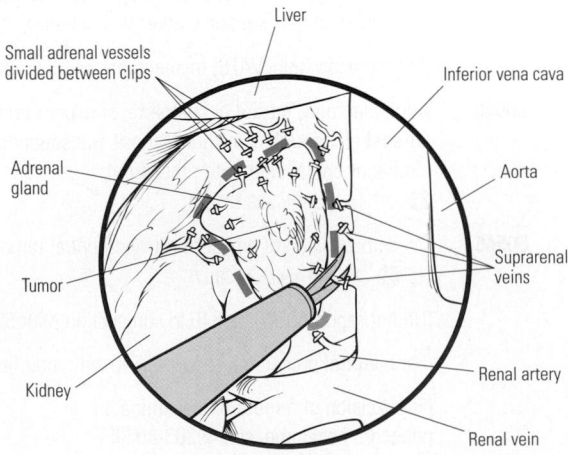

Right

60659   Unlisted laparoscopy procedure, endocrine system

   ➔ *CPT Assistant* Nov 99:30, Mar 00:10; *CPT Changes: An Insider's
      View* 2000

Other Procedures

60699   Unlisted procedure, endocrine system

   ➔ *CPT Assistant* Feb 06:16, Dec 07:12

⊙=Moderate sedation   ✚=Add-on code   ✐=FDA approval pending   #=Resequenced code   ○=Recycled/reinstated code   ➔➔=See p xiii for details

Female Genital

Surgery

Brain
Cerebellum
Spinal cord
Brachial plexus
Musculocutaneous n.
Radial nerve
Intercostal nerves (with ribs)
Subcostal nerve (12th thoracic)
Median nerve
Iliohypogastric nerve
Ilioinguinal nerve
Deep branch of radial nerve
Lat. femoral cutaneous nerve
Genitofemoral nerve
Superficial branch of radial nerve
Obturator nerve
Ulnar nerve
Lumbar plexus
Sacral plexus
Femoral nerve
Pudendal nerve
Sciatic nerve
Muscular branches of femoral nerve
Saphenous nerve
Tibial nerve
Common peroneal nerve
Deep peroneal nerve
Superficial peroneal nerve

Nervous

Nervous

Nervous System

Skull, Meninges, and Brain

(For injection procedure for cerebral angiography, see 36100-36218)

(For injection procedure for ventriculography, see 61026, 61120)

(For injection procedure for pneumoencephalography, use 61055)

Injection, Drainage, or Aspiration

61000 Subdural tap through fontanelle, or suture, infant, unilateral or bilateral; initial

61001 subsequent taps

61020 Ventricular puncture through previous burr hole, fontanelle, suture, or implanted ventricular catheter/reservoir; without injection

61026 with injection of medication or other substance for diagnosis or treatment
➔ *CPT Changes: An Insider's View* 2002

61050 Cisternal or lateral cervical (C1-C2) puncture; without injection (separate procedure)

61055 with injection of medication or other substance for diagnosis or treatment (eg, C1-C2)
➔ *CPT Changes: An Insider's View* 2002

(For radiological supervision and interpretation, see **Radiology**)

61070 Puncture of shunt tubing or reservoir for aspiration or injection procedure

(For radiological supervision and interpretation, use 75809)

Twist Drill, Burr Hole(s), or Trephine

61105 Twist drill hole for subdural or ventricular puncture

⊘ **61107** Twist drill hole(s) for subdural, intracerebral, or ventricular puncture; for implanting ventricular catheter, pressure recording device, or other intracerebral monitoring device
➔ *CPT Changes: An Insider's View* 2007

(For intracranial neuroendoscopic ventricular catheter placement, use 62160)

61108 for evacuation and/or drainage of subdural hematoma

61120 Burr hole(s) for ventricular puncture (including injection of gas, contrast media, dye, or radioactive material)

61140 Burr hole(s) or trephine; with biopsy of brain or intracranial lesion

61150 with drainage of brain abscess or cyst

61151 with subsequent tapping (aspiration) of intracranial abscess or cyst

61154 Burr hole(s) with evacuation and/or drainage of hematoma, extradural or subdural

(For bilateral procedure, report 61154 with modifier 50)

61156 Burr hole(s); with aspiration of hematoma or cyst, intracerebral

61210 for implanting ventricular catheter, reservoir, EEG electrode(s), pressure recording device, or other cerebral monitoring device (separate procedure)
➔ *CPT Changes: An Insider's View* 2007, 2008

(For intracranial neuroendoscopic ventricular catheter placement, use 62160)

61215 Insertion of subcutaneous reservoir, pump or continuous infusion system for connection to ventricular catheter
➔ *CPT Assistant* Spring 93:13

(For refilling and maintenance of an implantable infusion pump for spinal or brain drug therapy, use 95990)

(For chemotherapy, use 96450)

61250 Burr hole(s) or trephine, supratentorial, exploratory, not followed by other surgery

(For bilateral procedure, report 61250 with modifier 50)

61253 Burr hole(s) or trephine, infratentorial, unilateral or bilateral
➔ *CPT Assistant* Sep 02:10

(If burr hole[s] or trephine are followed by craniotomy at same operative session, use 61304-61321; do not use 61250 or 61253)

Craniectomy or Craniotomy

61304 Craniectomy or craniotomy, exploratory; supratentorial

61305 infratentorial (posterior fossa)

61312 Craniectomy or craniotomy for evacuation of hematoma, supratentorial; extradural or subdural

61313 intracerebral

61314 Craniectomy or craniotomy for evacuation of hematoma, infratentorial; extradural or subdural

61315 intracerebellar

➕ **61316** Incision and subcutaneous placement of cranial bone graft (List separately in addition to code for primary procedure)
➔ *CPT Changes: An Insider's View* 2003

(Use 61316 in conjunction with 61304, 61312, 61313, 61322, 61323, 61340, 61570, 61571, 61680-61705)

61320 Craniectomy or craniotomy, drainage of intracranial abscess; supratentorial

61321 infratentorial

61322 Craniectomy or craniotomy, decompressive, with or without duraplasty, for treatment of intracranial hypertension, without evacuation of associated intraparenchymal hematoma; without lobectomy
➔ *CPT Changes: An Insider's View* 2003

(Do not report 61313 in addition to 61322)

(For subtemporal decompression, use 61340)

61323 with lobectomy
   → *CPT Changes: An Insider's View* 2003

(Do not report 61313 in addition to 61323)

(For subtemporal decompression, use 61340)

61330 Decompression of orbit only, transcranial approach

(For bilateral procedure, report 61330 with modifier 50)

61332 Exploration of orbit (transcranial approach); with biopsy

61333 with removal of lesion

61334 with removal of foreign body

61340 Subtemporal cranial decompression (pseudotumor cerebri, slit ventricle syndrome)
   → *CPT Changes: An Insider's View* 2003

(For bilateral procedure, report 61340 with modifier 50)

(For decompressive craniotomy or craniectomy for intracranial hypertension, without hematoma evacuation, see 61322, 61323)

61343 Craniectomy, suboccipital with cervical laminectomy for decompression of medulla and spinal cord, with or without dural graft (eg, Arnold-Chiari malformation)

61345 Other cranial decompression, posterior fossa

(For orbital decompression by lateral wall approach, Kroenlein type, use 67445)

61440 Craniotomy for section of tentorium cerebelli (separate procedure)

61450 Craniectomy, subtemporal, for section, compression, or decompression of sensory root of gasserian ganglion

61458 Craniectomy, suboccipital; for exploration or decompression of cranial nerves

61460 for section of 1 or more cranial nerves

61470 for medullary tractotomy

61480 for mesencephalic tractotomy or pedunculotomy

61490 Craniotomy for lobotomy, including cingulotomy

(For bilateral procedure, report 61490 with modifier 50)

61500 Craniectomy; with excision of tumor or other bone lesion of skull

61501 for osteomyelitis

61510 Craniectomy, trephination, bone flap craniotomy; for excision of brain tumor, supratentorial, except meningioma

61512 for excision of meningioma, supratentorial

61514 for excision of brain abscess, supratentorial

61516 for excision or fenestration of cyst, supratentorial

(For excision of pituitary tumor or craniopharyngioma, see 61545, 61546, 61548)

+ 61517 Implantation of brain intracavitary chemotherapy agent (List separately in addition to code for primary procedure)
   → *CPT Changes: An Insider's View* 2003

(Use 61517 only in conjunction with 61510 or 61518)

(Do not report 61517 for brachytherapy insertion. For intracavitary insertion of radioelement sources or ribbons, see 77785-77787)

61518 Craniectomy for excision of brain tumor, infratentorial or posterior fossa; except meningioma, cerebellopontine angle tumor, or midline tumor at base of skull

61519 meningioma

61520 cerebellopontine angle tumor

61521 midline tumor at base of skull

61522 Craniectomy, infratentorial or posterior fossa; for excision of brain abscess

61524 for excision or fenestration of cyst

61526 Craniectomy, bone flap craniotomy, transtemporal (mastoid) for excision of cerebellopontine angle tumor;
   → *CPT Assistant* Summer 91:8

61530 combined with middle/posterior fossa craniotomy/craniectomy

61531 Subdural implantation of strip electrodes through 1 or more burr or trephine hole(s) for long-term seizure monitoring

(For stereotactic implantation of electrodes, use 61760)

(For craniotomy for excision of intracranial arteriovenous malformation, see 61680-61692)

61533 Craniotomy with elevation of bone flap; for subdural implantation of an electrode array, for long-term seizure monitoring

(For continuous EEG monitoring, see 95950-95954)

61534 for excision of epileptogenic focus without electrocorticography during surgery

61535 for removal of epidural or subdural electrode array, without excision of cerebral tissue (separate procedure)

61536 for excision of cerebral epileptogenic focus, with electrocorticography during surgery (includes removal of electrode array)

61537 for lobectomy, temporal lobe, without electrocorticography during surgery
   → *CPT Changes: An Insider's View* 2004

61538 for lobectomy, temporal lobe, with electrocorticography during surgery
   → *CPT Changes: An Insider's View* 2004

61539 for lobectomy, other than temporal lobe, partial or total, with electrocorticography during surgery
   → *CPT Changes: An Insider's View* 2004

61540 for lobectomy, other than temporal lobe, partial or total, without electrocorticography during surgery
   → *CPT Changes: An Insider's View* 2004

Nervous

61541   for transection of corpus callosum

61542   for total hemispherectomy

61543   for partial or subtotal (functional) hemispherectomy
> *CPT Changes: An Insider's View* 2004

61544   for excision or coagulation of choroid plexus

61545   for excision of craniopharyngioma

(For craniotomy for selective amygdalohippocampectomy, use 61566)

(For craniotomy for multiple subpial transections during surgery, use 61567)

61546 Craniotomy for hypophysectomy or excision of pituitary tumor, intracranial approach

61548 Hypophysectomy or excision of pituitary tumor, transnasal or transseptal approach, nonstereotactic
> *CPT Assistant* Nov 98:17, Jul 11:13

(Do not report code 69990 in addition to code 61548)

61550 Craniectomy for craniosynostosis; single cranial suture
> *CPT Assistant* Feb 12:11

61552   multiple cranial sutures
> *CPT Assistant* Feb 12:11

(For cranial reconstruction for orbital hypertelorism, see 21260-21263)

(For reconstruction, see 21172-21180)

61556 Craniotomy for craniosynostosis; frontal or parietal bone flap
> *CPT Assistant* Feb 12:11

61557   bifrontal bone flap
> *CPT Assistant* Feb 12:11

61558 Extensive craniectomy for multiple cranial suture craniosynostosis (eg, cloverleaf skull); not requiring bone grafts
> *CPT Assistant* Feb 12:11

61559   recontouring with multiple osteotomies and bone autografts (eg, barrel-stave procedure) (includes obtaining grafts)
> *CPT Assistant* Feb 12:11

(For reconstruction, see 21172-21180)

61563 Excision, intra and extracranial, benign tumor of cranial bone (eg, fibrous dysplasia); without optic nerve decompression

61564   with optic nerve decompression

(For reconstruction, see 21181-21183)

61566 Craniotomy with elevation of bone flap; for selective amygdalohippocampectomy
> *CPT Changes: An Insider's View* 2004

61567   for multiple subpial transections, with electrocorticography during surgery
> *CPT Changes: An Insider's View* 2004

61570 Craniectomy or craniotomy; with excision of foreign body from brain

61571   with treatment of penetrating wound of brain

(For sequestrectomy for osteomyelitis, use 61501)

61575 Transoral approach to skull base, brain stem or upper spinal cord for biopsy, decompression or excision of lesion;

61576   requiring splitting of tongue and/or mandible (including tracheostomy)

(For arthrodesis, use 22548)

Surgery of Skull Base

The surgical management of lesions involving the skull base (base of anterior, middle, and posterior cranial fossae) often requires the skills of several surgeons of different surgical specialties working together or in tandem during the operative session. These operations are usually not staged because of the need for definitive closure of dura, subcutaneous tissues, and skin to avoid serious infections such as osteomyelitis and/or meningitis.

The procedures are categorized according to

(1) *approach procedure* necessary to obtain adequate exposure to the lesion (pathologic entity), (2) *definitive procedure(s)* necessary to biopsy, excise or otherwise treat the lesion, and (3) *repair/reconstruction* of the defect present following the definitive procedure(s).

The *approach procedure* is described according to anatomical area involved, ie, anterior cranial fossa, middle cranial fossa, posterior cranial fossa, and brain stem or upper spinal cord.

The *definitive procedure(s)* describes the repair, biopsy, resection, or excision of various lesions of the skull base and, when appropriate, primary closure of the dura, mucous membranes, and skin.

The *repair/reconstruction procedure(s)* is reported separately if extensive dural grafting, cranioplasty, local or regional myocutaneous pedicle flaps, or extensive skin grafts are required.

For primary closure, see the appropriate codes (ie, 15732, 15756-15758).

When one surgeon performs the approach procedure, another surgeon performs the definitive procedure, and another surgeon performs the repair/reconstruction procedure, each surgeon reports only the code for the specific procedure performed.

If one surgeon performs more than one procedure (ie, approach procedure and definitive procedure), then both codes are reported, adding modifier 51 to the secondary, additional procedure(s).

Approach Procedures

Anterior Cranial Fossa

61580   Craniofacial approach to anterior cranial fossa; extradural, including lateral rhinotomy, ethmoidectomy, sphenoidectomy, without maxillectomy or orbital exenteration
➔ *CPT Assistant* Winter 93:17, Spring 94:11

61581   extradural, including lateral rhinotomy, orbital exenteration, ethmoidectomy, sphenoidectomy and/or maxillectomy
➔ *CPT Assistant* Winter 93:17, Spring 94:11

61582   extradural, including unilateral or bifrontal craniotomy, elevation of frontal lobe(s), osteotomy of base of anterior cranial fossa
➔ *CPT Assistant* Winter 93:17, Spring 94:11

61583   intradural, including unilateral or bifrontal craniotomy, elevation or resection of frontal lobe, osteotomy of base of anterior cranial fossa
➔ *CPT Assistant* Winter 93:17, Spring 94:11

61584   Orbitocranial approach to anterior cranial fossa, extradural, including supraorbital ridge osteotomy and elevation of frontal and/or temporal lobe(s); without orbital exenteration
➔ *CPT Assistant* Winter 93:18

61585   with orbital exenteration
➔ *CPT Assistant* Winter 93:18

61586   Bicoronal, transzygomatic and/or LeFort I osteotomy approach to anterior cranial fossa with or without internal fixation, without bone graft
➔ *CPT Assistant* Winter 93:18, Nov 96:12

Middle Cranial Fossa

61590   Infratemporal pre-auricular approach to middle cranial fossa (parapharyngeal space, infratemporal and midline skull base, nasopharynx), with or without disarticulation of the mandible, including parotidectomy, craniotomy, decompression and/or mobilization of the facial nerve and/or petrous carotid artery
➔ *CPT Assistant* Winter 93:18

61591   Infratemporal post-auricular approach to middle cranial fossa (internal auditory meatus, petrous apex, tentorium, cavernous sinus, parasellar area, infratemporal fossa) including mastoidectomy, resection of sigmoid sinus, with or without decompression and/or mobilization of contents of auditory canal or petrous carotid artery
➔ *CPT Assistant* Winter 93:18

61592   Orbitocranial zygomatic approach to middle cranial fossa (cavernous sinus and carotid artery, clivus, basilar artery or petrous apex) including osteotomy of zygoma, craniotomy, extra- or intradural elevation of temporal lobe
➔ *CPT Assistant* Winter 93:18

Posterior Cranial Fossa

61595   Transtemporal approach to posterior cranial fossa, jugular foramen or midline skull base, including mastoidectomy, decompression of sigmoid sinus and/or facial nerve, with or without mobilization
➔ *CPT Assistant* Winter 93:18

61596   Transcochlear approach to posterior cranial fossa, jugular foramen or midline skull base, including labyrinthectomy, decompression, with or without mobilization of facial nerve and/or petrous carotid artery
➔ *CPT Assistant* Winter 93:18

61597   Transcondylar (far lateral) approach to posterior cranial fossa, jugular foramen or midline skull base, including occipital condylectomy, mastoidectomy, resection of C1-C3 vertebral body(s), decompression of vertebral artery, with or without mobilization
➔ *CPT Assistant* Winter 93:18

61598   Transpetrosal approach to posterior cranial fossa, clivus or foramen magnum, including ligation of superior petrosal sinus and/or sigmoid sinus
➔ *CPT Assistant* Winter 93:18

Definitive Procedures

Base of Anterior Cranial Fossa

61600   Resection or excision of neoplastic, vascular or infectious lesion of base of anterior cranial fossa; extradural
➔ *CPT Assistant* Winter 93:19, Spring 94:12, Nov 96:12

61601   intradural, including dural repair, with or without graft
➔ *CPT Assistant* Winter 93:19, Spring 94:12

Base of Middle Cranial Fossa

61605   Resection or excision of neoplastic, vascular or infectious lesion of infratemporal fossa, parapharyngeal space, petrous apex; extradural
➔ *CPT Assistant* Winter 93:19

61606   intradural, including dural repair, with or without graft
➔ *CPT Assistant* Winter 93:20

61607   Resection or excision of neoplastic, vascular or infectious lesion of parasellar area, cavernous sinus, clivus or midline skull base; extradural
➔ *CPT Assistant* Winter 93:20

61608   intradural, including dural repair, with or without graft
➔ *CPT Assistant* Winter 93:20

Codes 61609-61612 are reported in addition to code(s) for primary procedure(s) 61605-61608. Report only one transection or ligation of carotid artery code per operative session.

+ 61609   Transection or ligation, carotid artery in cavernous sinus; without repair (List separately in addition to code for primary procedure)
➔ *CPT Assistant* Winter 93:20

+ 61610 with repair by anastomosis or graft (List separately in addition to code for primary procedure)

➔ *CPT Assistant* Winter 93:20

+ 61611 Transection or ligation, carotid artery in petrous canal; without repair (List separately in addition to code for primary procedure)

➔ *CPT Assistant* Winter 93:20

+ 61612 with repair by anastomosis or graft (List separately in addition to code for primary procedure)

➔ *CPT Assistant* Winter 93:20

61613 Obliteration of carotid aneurysm, arteriovenous malformation, or carotid-cavernous fistula by dissection within cavernous sinus

➔ *CPT Assistant* Winter 93:20

Base of Posterior Cranial Fossa

61615 Resection or excision of neoplastic, vascular or infectious lesion of base of posterior cranial fossa, jugular foramen, foramen magnum, or C1-C3 vertebral bodies; extradural

➔ *CPT Assistant* Winter 93:20

61616 intradural, including dural repair, with or without graft

Repair and/or Reconstruction of Surgical Defects of Skull Base

61618 Secondary repair of dura for cerebrospinal fluid leak, anterior, middle or posterior cranial fossa following surgery of the skull base; by free tissue graft (eg, pericranium, fascia, tensor fascia lata, adipose tissue, homologous or synthetic grafts)

➔ *CPT Assistant* Winter 93:20, Spring 94:19, Mar 00:11

61619 by local or regionalized vascularized pedicle flap or myocutaneous flap (including galea, temporalis, frontalis or occipitalis muscle)

➔ *CPT Assistant* Winter 93:20, Spring 94:19, Mar 00:11

Endovascular Therapy

61623 Endovascular temporary balloon arterial occlusion, head or neck (extracranial/intracranial) including selective catheterization of vessel to be occluded, positioning and inflation of occlusion balloon, concomitant neurological monitoring, and radiologic supervision and interpretation of all angiography required for balloon occlusion and to exclude vascular injury post occlusion

➔ *CPT Changes: An Insider's View* 2003

(If selective catheterization and angiography of arteries other than artery to be occluded is performed, use appropriate catheterization and radiologic supervision and interpretation codes)

(If complete diagnostic angiography of the artery to be occluded is performed immediately prior to temporary occlusion, use appropriate radiologic supervision and interpretation codes only)

61624 Transcatheter permanent occlusion or embolization (eg, for tumor destruction, to achieve hemostasis, to occlude a vascular malformation), percutaneous, any method; central nervous system (intracranial, spinal cord)

➔ *CPT Assistant* Jun 99:10, Nov 06:8; *CPT Changes: An Insider's View* 2003

➔ *Clinical Examples in Radiology* Summer 07:2

(See also 37204)

(For radiological supervision and interpretation, use 75894)

61626 non-central nervous system, head or neck (extracranial, brachiocephalic branch)

(See also 37204)

(For radiological supervision and interpretation, use 75894)

61630 Balloon angioplasty, intracranial (eg, atherosclerotic stenosis), percutaneous

➔ *CPT Changes: An Insider's View* 2006

➔ *Clinical Examples in Radiology* Winter 06:16

61635 Transcatheter placement of intravascular stent(s), intracranial (eg, atherosclerotic stenosis), including balloon angioplasty, if performed

➔ *CPT Changes: An Insider's View* 2006

➔ *Clinical Examples in Radiology* Winter 06:16

(61630 and 61635 include all selective vascular catheterization of the target vascular family, all diagnostic imaging for arteriography of the target vascular family, and all related radiological supervision and interpretation. When diagnostic arteriogram [including imaging and selective catheterization] confirms the need for angioplasty or stent placement, 61630 and 61635 are inclusive of these services. If angioplasty or stenting are not indicated, then the appropriate codes for selective catheterization and imaging should be reported in lieu of 61630 and 61635)

61640 Balloon dilatation of intracranial vasospasm, percutaneous; initial vessel

➔ *CPT Changes: An Insider's View* 2006

➔ *Clinical Examples in Radiology* Winter 06:16

+ 61641 each additional vessel in same vascular family (List separately in addition to code for primary procedure)

➔ *CPT Changes: An Insider's View* 2006

➔ *Clinical Examples in Radiology* Winter 06:16

+ 61642 each additional vessel in different vascular family (List separately in addition to code for primary procedure)

➔ *CPT Changes: An Insider's View* 2006

➔ *Clinical Examples in Radiology* Winter 06:16

(Use 61641 and 61642 in conjunction with 61640)

(61640, 61641, 61642 include all selective vascular catheterization of the target vessel, contrast injection[s], vessel measurement, roadmapping, postdilatation angiography, and fluoroscopic guidance for the balloon dilatation)

Surgery for Aneurysm, Arteriovenous Malformation, or Vascular Disease

Includes craniotomy when appropriate for procedure.

61680   Surgery of intracranial arteriovenous malformation; supratentorial, simple

61682   supratentorial, complex

61684   infratentorial, simple

61686   infratentorial, complex

61690   dural, simple

61692   dural, complex

61697   Surgery of complex intracranial aneurysm, intracranial approach; carotid circulation
> *CPT Changes: An Insider's View* 2001

61698   vertebrobasilar circulation
> *CPT Changes: An Insider's View* 2001

(61697, 61698 involve aneurysms that are larger than 15 mm or with calcification of the aneurysm neck, or with incorporation of normal vessels into the aneurysm neck, or a procedure requiring temporary vessel occlusion, trapping or cardiopulmonary bypass to successfully treat the aneurysm)

61700   Surgery of simple intracranial aneurysm, intracranial approach; carotid circulation
> *CPT Assistant* Jun 99:11, Jul 99:10; *CPT Changes: An Insider's View* 2001

61702   vertebrobasilar circulation
> *CPT Changes: An Insider's View* 2001

61703   Surgery of intracranial aneurysm, cervical approach by application of occluding clamp to cervical carotid artery (Selverstone-Crutchfield type)

(For cervical approach for direct ligation of carotid artery, see 37600-37606)

61705   Surgery of aneurysm, vascular malformation or carotid-cavernous fistula; by intracranial and cervical occlusion of carotid artery

61708   by intracranial electrothrombosis

(For ligation or gradual occlusion of internal/common carotid artery, see 37605, 37606)

61710   by intra-arterial embolization, injection procedure, or balloon catheter

61711   Anastomosis, arterial, extracranial-intracranial (eg, middle cerebral/cortical) arteries

(For carotid or vertebral thromboendarterectomy, use 35301)

(Use 69990 when the surgical microscope is employed for the microsurgical procedure. Do not use 69990 for visualization with magnifying loupes or corrected vision)

Intracranial Aneurysm, Intracranial Approach
61700

Placement of ligating clip across the neck of an intracranial aneurysm

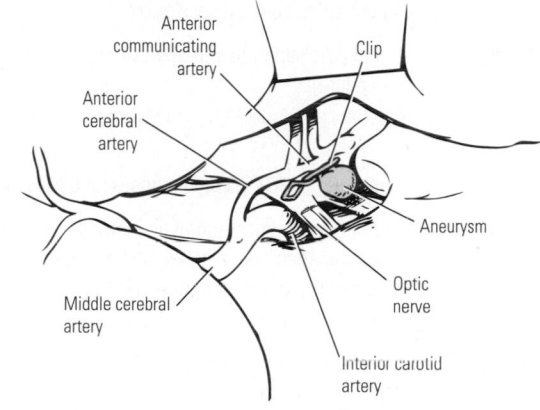

Stereotaxis

61720   Creation of lesion by stereotactic method, including burr hole(s) and localizing and recording techniques, single or multiple stages; globus pallidus or thalamus
> *CPT Assistant* Jul 11:12

61735   subcortical structure(s) other than globus pallidus or thalamus
> *CPT Assistant* Jul 11:12

61750   Stereotactic biopsy, aspiration, or excision, including burr hole(s), for intracranial lesion;
> *CPT Assistant* Nov 99:30; *CPT Changes: An Insider's View* 2000

61751   with computed tomography and/or magnetic resonance guidance
> *CPT Assistant* Jun 96:10, Nov 99:30, Dec 04:20, Jul 11:12; *CPT Changes: An Insider's View* 2000, 2003

(For radiological supervision and interpretation of computerized tomography, see 70450, 70460, or 70470 as appropriate)

(For radiological supervision and interpretation of magnetic resonance imaging, see 70551, 70552, or 70553 as appropriate)

61760 Stereotactic implantation of depth electrodes into the cerebrum for long-term seizure monitoring

→ *CPT Assistant* Jul 11:12

61770 Stereotactic localization, including burr hole(s), with insertion of catheter(s) or probe(s) for placement of radiation source

→ *CPT Assistant* Jul 11:12; *CPT Changes: An Insider's View* 2001

+ 61781 Stereotactic computer-assisted (navigational) procedure; cranial, intradural (List separately in addition to code for primary procedure)

→ *CPT Assistant* Jul 11:12; *CPT Changes: An Insider's View* 2011

(Do not report 61781 in conjunction with 61720-61791, 61796-61799, 61863-61868, 62201, 77371-77373, 77432)

+ 61782 cranial, extradural (List separately in addition to code for primary procedure)

→ *CPT Assistant* Jul 11:12; *CPT Changes: An Insider's View* 2011

▶(Do not report 61781, 61782 by the same individual during the same surgical session)◀

+ 61783 spinal (List separately in addition to code for primary procedure)

→ *CPT Assistant* Jul 11:12; *CPT Changes: An Insider's View* 2011

(Do not report 61783 in conjunction with 63620, 63621)

61790 Creation of lesion by stereotactic method, percutaneous, by neurolytic agent (eg, alcohol, thermal, electrical, radiofrequency); gasserian ganglion

→ *CPT Assistant* Jul 11:12

61791 trigeminal medullary tract

→ *CPT Assistant* Jul 11:12

(61793 has been deleted. To report, see 61796-61800, 63620-63621)

Stereotactic Radiosurgery (Cranial)

▶Cranial stereotactic radiosurgery is a distinct procedure that utilizes externally generated ionizing radiation to inactivate or eradicate defined target(s) in the head without the need to make an incision. The target is defined by and the treatment is delivered using high-resolution stereotactic imaging. Stereotactic radiosurgery codes and headframe application procedures are reported by the neurosurgeon. The radiation oncologist reports the appropriate code(s) for clinical treatment planning, physics and dosimetry, treatment delivery, and management from the **Radiation Oncology** section (77261-77790). Any necessary planning, dosimetry, targeting, positioning, or blocking by the neurosurgeon is included in the stereotactic radiation surgery services. The same individual should not report stereotactic radiosurgery services with radiation treatment management codes (77427-77435).◀

Cranial stereotactic radiosurgery is typically performed in a single planning and treatment session, using a rigidly attached stereotactic guiding device, other immobilization technology and/or a stereotactic image-guidance system, but can be performed with more than one planning session and in a limited number of treatment sessions, up to a maximum of five sessions. Do not report stereotactic radiosurgery more than once per lesion per course of treatment when the treatment requires more than one session.

Codes 61796 and 61797 involve stereotactic radiosurgery for simple cranial lesions. Simple cranial lesions are lesions less than 3.5 cm in maximum dimension that do not meet the definition of a complex lesion provided below. Report code 61796 when all lesions are simple.

Codes 61798 and 61799 involve stereotactic radiosurgery for complex cranial lesions and procedures that create therapeutic lesions (eg, thalamotomy or pallidotomy). All lesions 3.5 cm in maximum dimension or greater are complex. When performing therapeutic lesion creation procedures, report code 61798 only once regardless of the number of lesions created. Schwannomas, arterio-venous malformations, pituitary tumors, glomus tumors, pineal region tumors and cavernous sinus/parasellar/petroclival tumors are complex. Any lesion that is adjacent (5mm or less) to the optic nerve/optic chasm/optic tract or within the brainstem is complex. If treating multiple lesions, and any single lesion treated is complex, use 61798.

Do not report codes 61796-61800 in conjunction with code 20660.

Codes 61796-61799 include computer-assisted planning. Do not report codes 61796-61799 in conjunction with 61781-61783.

(For intensity modulated beam delivery plan and treatment, see 77301, 77418. For stereotactic body radiation therapy, see 77373, 77435)

(61795 has been deleted. To report, see 61781, 61782, 61783)

61796 Stereotactic radiosurgery (particle beam, gamma ray, or linear accelerator); 1 simple cranial lesion

→ *CPT Assistant* Jul 11:12, Apr 12:11; *CPT Changes: An Insider's View* 2009

(Do not report 61796 more than once per course of treatment)

(Do not report 61796 in conjunction with 61798)

+ 61797 each additional cranial lesion, simple (List separately in addition to code for primary procedure)

→ *CPT Assistant* Jul 11:12, Apr 12:11; *CPT Changes: An Insider's View* 2009

(Use 61797 in conjunction with 61796, 61798)

(For each course of treatment, 61797 and 61799 may be reported no more than once per lesion. Do not report any combination of 61797 and 61799 more than 4 times for entire course of treatment regardless of number of lesions treated)

Nervous

61798   1 complex cranial lesion

➔ *CPT Assistant* Jul 11:12, Apr 12:11; *CPT Changes: An Insider's View* 2009

(Do not report 61798 more than once per course of treatment)

(Do not report 61798 in conjunction with 61796)

+ 61799   each additional cranial lesion, complex (List separately in addition to code for primary procedure)

➔ *CPT Assistant* Jul 11:12, Apr 12:11; *CPT Changes: An Insider's View* 2009

(Use 61799 in conjunction with 61798)

(For each course of treatment, 61797 and 61799 may be reported no more than once per lesion. Do not report any combination of 61797 and 61799 more than 4 times for entire course of treatment regardless of number of lesions treated)

+ 61800   Application of stereotactic headframe for stereotactic radiosurgery (List separately in addition to code for primary procedure)

➔ *CPT Assistant* Apr 12:11; *CPT Changes: An Insider's View* 2009

(Use 61800 in conjunction with 61796, 61798)

Neurostimulators (Intracranial)

Codes 61850-61888 apply to both simple and complex neurostimulators. For initial or subsequent electronic analysis and programming of neurostimulator pulse generators, see codes 95970-95975.

►Microelectrode recording, when performed by the operating surgeon in association with implantation of neurostimulator electrode arrays, is an inclusive service and should not be reported separately. If another individual participates in neurophysiological mapping during a deep brain stimulator implantation procedure, this service may be reported by the second individual with codes 95961-95962.◄

61850   Twist drill or burr hole(s) for implantation of neurostimulator electrodes, cortical

➔ *CPT Assistant* Sep 99:5, Nov 99:30; *CPT Changes: An Insider's View* 2000

61860   Craniectomy or craniotomy for implantation of neurostimulator electrodes, cerebral, cortical

➔ *CPT Assistant* Sep 99:5, Nov 99:30; *CPT Changes: An Insider's View* 2000

61863   Twist drill, burr hole, craniotomy, or craniectomy with stereotactic implantation of neurostimulator electrode array in subcortical site (eg, thalamus, globus pallidus, subthalamic nucleus, periventricular, periaqueductal gray), without use of intraoperative microelectrode recording; first array

➔ *CPT Assistant* Sep 99:5, Oct 10:10, Jul 11:12; *CPT Changes: An Insider's View* 2004

+ 61864   each additional array (List separately in addition to primary procedure)

➔ *CPT Assistant* Sep 99:5, Jul 11:12; *CPT Changes: An Insider's View* 2004

(Use 61864 in conjunction with 61863)

61867   Twist drill, burr hole, craniotomy, or craniectomy with stereotactic implantation of neurostimulator electrode array in subcortical site (eg, thalamus, globus pallidus, subthalamic nucleus, periventricular, periaqueductal gray), with use of intraoperative microelectrode recording; first array

➔ *CPT Assistant* Jul 11:12; *CPT Changes: An Insider's View* 2004

+ 61868   each additional array (List separately in addition to primary procedure)

➔ *CPT Assistant* Jul 11:12; *CPT Changes: An Insider's View* 2004

(Use 61868 in conjunction with 61867)

Placement of Cranial Neurostimulator
61867-61868, 61885

Placement of subcortical (eg, thalamic) neurostimulator electrode via burr hole (61867-61868) with connection of the electrode to an implanted programmable pulse generator (61885) in the infraclavicular area

Cranium

Brain

Multi-contact (eg, quadripolar) (61867-61868)

Pulse generator (61885)

61870   Craniectomy for implantation of neurostimulator electrodes, cerebellar; cortical

61875   subcortical

61880   Revision or removal of intracranial neurostimulator electrodes

61885   Insertion or replacement of cranial neurostimulator pulse generator or receiver, direct or inductive coupling; with connection to a single electrode array

➔ *CPT Assistant* Sep 99:5, Nov 99:30, Jun 00:3, Apr 01:8, Sep 03:3, Dec 10:14, Feb 11:5, Sep 11:8; *CPT Changes: An Insider's View* 2000, 2005

Nervous

61886 with connection to 2 or more electrode arrays
➔ *CPT Assistant* Nov 99:30, Jun 00:3, Apr 01:8, Feb 11:5, Sep 11:8; *CPT Changes: An Insider's View* 2000

(For percutaneous placement of cranial nerve [eg, vagus, trigeminal] neurostimulator electrode(s), use 64553)

(For revision or removal of cranial nerve [eg, vagus, trigeminal] neurostimulator electrode array, use 64569)

61888 Revision or removal of cranial neurostimulator pulse generator or receiver
➔ *CPT Assistant* Sep 11:8

(Do not report 61888 in conjunction with 61885 or 61886 for the same pulse generator)

Repair

62000 Elevation of depressed skull fracture; simple, extradural

62005 compound or comminuted, extradural

62010 with repair of dura and/or debridement of brain

62100 Craniotomy for repair of dural/cerebrospinal fluid leak, including surgery for rhinorrhea/otorrhea
➔ *CPT Changes: An Insider's View* 2002

(For repair of spinal dural/CSF leak, see 63707, 63709)

62115 Reduction of craniomegalic skull (eg, treated hydrocephalus); not requiring bone grafts or cranioplasty

62116 with simple cranioplasty

62117 requiring craniotomy and reconstruction with or without bone graft (includes obtaining grafts)

62120 Repair of encephalocele, skull vault, including cranioplasty

62121 Craniotomy for repair of encephalocele, skull base

62140 Cranioplasty for skull defect; up to 5 cm diameter

62141 larger than 5 cm diameter

62142 Removal of bone flap or prosthetic plate of skull

62143 Replacement of bone flap or prosthetic plate of skull

62145 Cranioplasty for skull defect with reparative brain surgery

62146 Cranioplasty with autograft (includes obtaining bone grafts); up to 5 cm diameter

62147 larger than 5 cm diameter

✚ 62148 Incision and retrieval of subcutaneous cranial bone graft for cranioplasty (List separately in addition to code for primary procedure)
➔ *CPT Changes: An Insider's View* 2003

(Use 62148 in conjunction with 62140-62147)

Neuroendoscopy

Surgical endoscopy always includes diagnostic endoscopy.

✚ 62160 Neuroendoscopy, intracranial, for placement or replacement of ventricular catheter and attachment to shunt system or external drainage (List separately in addition to code for primary procedure)
➔ *CPT Assistant* Jun 07:11; *CPT Changes: An Insider's View* 2003

(Use 62160 only in conjunction with 61107, 61210, 62220-62230, 62258)

62161 Neuroendoscopy, intracranial; with dissection of adhesions, fenestration of septum pellucidum or intraventricular cysts (including placement, replacement, or removal of ventricular catheter)
➔ *CPT Changes: An Insider's View* 2003

62162 with fenestration or excision of colloid cyst, including placement of external ventricular catheter for drainage
➔ *CPT Changes: An Insider's View* 2003

62163 with retrieval of foreign body
➔ *CPT Changes: An Insider's View* 2003

62164 with excision of brain tumor, including placement of external ventricular catheter for drainage
➔ *CPT Changes: An Insider's View* 2003

62165 with excision of pituitary tumor, transnasal or trans-sphenoidal approach
➔ *CPT Changes: An Insider's View* 2003

Cerebrospinal Fluid (CSF) Shunt

62180 Ventriculocisternostomy (Torkildsen type operation)

62190 Creation of shunt; subarachnoid/subdural-atrial, -jugular, -auricular

62192 subarachnoid/subdural-peritoneal, -pleural, other terminus

62194 Replacement or irrigation, subarachnoid/subdural catheter
➔ *CPT Assistant* Dec 11:6

62200 Ventriculocisternostomy, third ventricle;

62201 stereotactic, neuroendoscopic method
➔ *CPT Assistant* Aug 07:15, Jul 11:12; *CPT Changes: An Insider's View* 2003

(For intracranial neuroendoscopic procedures, see 62161-62165)

62220 Creation of shunt; ventriculo-atrial, -jugular, -auricular

(For intracranial neuroendoscopic ventricular catheter placement, use 62160)

62223 ventriculo-peritoneal, -pleural, other terminus

(For intracranial neuroendoscopic ventricular catheter placement, use 62160)

Nervous

Cerebrospinal Fluid (CSF) Shunt (Ventricular Peritoneal)
62223

A ventriculostomy is performed to drain CSF into the peritoneal cavity.

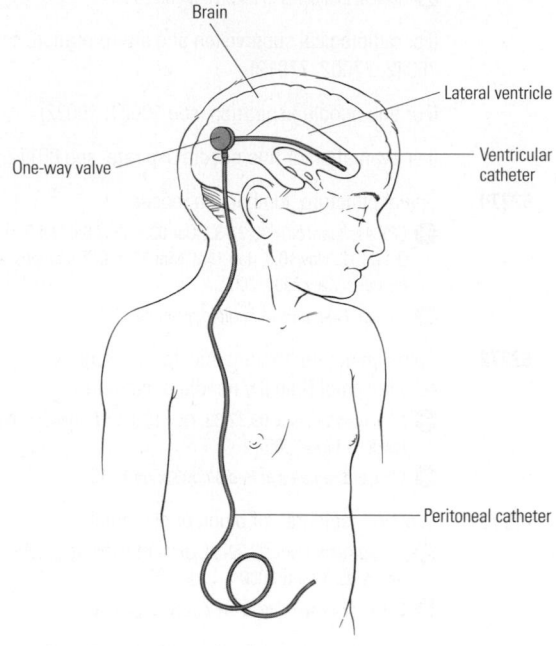

62225   Replacement or irrigation, ventricular catheter
> *CPT Assistant* Dec 11:6

(For intracranial neuroendoscopic ventricular catheter placement, use 62160)

62230   Replacement or revision of cerebrospinal fluid shunt, obstructed valve, or distal catheter in shunt system
> *CPT Assistant* Dec 11:6; *CPT Changes: An Insider's View* 2002

(For intracranial neuroendoscopic ventricular catheter placement, use 62160)

62252   Reprogramming of programmable cerebrospinal shunt
> *CPT Changes: An Insider's View* 2001, 2002

62256   Removal of complete cerebrospinal fluid shunt system; without replacement
> *CPT Changes: An Insider's View* 2002

62258   with replacement by similar or other shunt at same operation
> *CPT Assistant* Dec 11:6

(For percutaneous irrigation or aspiration of shunt reservoir, use 61070)

(For reprogramming of programmable CSF shunt, use 62252)

(For intracranial neuroendoscopic ventricular catheter placement, use 62160)

Spine and Spinal Cord

(For application of caliper or tongs, use 20660)

(For treatment of fracture or dislocation of spine, see 22305-22327)

Injection, Drainage, or Aspiration

Injection of contrast during fluoroscopic guidance and localization is an inclusive component of 62263, 62264, 62267, 62270-62273, 62280-62282, 62310-62319. Fluoroscopic guidance and localization is reported with 77003, unless a formal contrast study (myelography, epidurography, or arthrography) is performed, in which case the use of fluoroscopy is included in the supervision and interpretation codes.

For radiologic supervision and interpretation of epidurography, use 72275. Code 72275 is only to be used when an epidurogram is performed, images documented, and a formal radiologic report is issued.

Code 62263 describes a catheter-based treatment involving targeted injection of various substances (eg, hypertonic saline, steroid, anesthetic) via an indwelling epidural catheter. Code 62263 includes percutaneous insertion and removal of an epidural catheter (remaining in place over a several-day period), for the administration of multiple injections of a neurolytic agent(s) performed during serial treatment sessions (ie, spanning two or more treatment days). If required, adhesions or scarring may also be lysed by mechanical means. Code 62263 is **not** reported for each adhesiolysis treatment, but should be reported **once** to describe the entire series of injections/infusions spanning two or more treatment days.

Code 62264 describes multiple adhesiolysis treatment sessions performed on the same day. Adhesions or scarring may be lysed by injections of neurolytic agent(s). If required, adhesions or scarring may also be lysed mechanically using a percutaneously-deployed catheter.

Codes 62263 and 62264 include the procedure of injections of contrast for epidurography (72275) and fluoroscopic guidance and localization (77003) during initial or subsequent sessions.

Fluoroscopy (for localization) may be used in the placement of injections reported with 62310-62319, but is not required. If used, fluoroscopy should be reported with 77003. For epidurography, use 72275.

The placement and use of a catheter to administer one or more epidural or subarachnoid injections on a single calendar day should be reported in the same manner as if a needle had been used, ie, as a single injection using either 62310 or 62311. Such injections should not be reported with 62318 or 62319.

Nervous

Threading a catheter into the epidural space, injecting substances at one or more levels and then removing the catheter should be treated as a single injection (62310, 62311). If the catheter is left in place to deliver substance(s) over a prolonged period (ie, more than a single calendar day) either continuously or via intermittent bolus, use 62318, 62319 as appropriate.

When reporting 62310-62319, code choice is based on the region at which the needle or catheter entered the body (eg, lumbar). Codes 62310-62319 should be reported only once, when the substance injected spreads or catheter tip insertion moves into another spinal region (eg, 62311 is reported only once for injection or catheter insertion at L3-4 with spread of the substance or placement of the catheter tip to the thoracic region).

Percutaneous spinal procedures are done with indirect visualization (eg, image guidance or endoscopic approaches) and without direct visualization (including through a microscope). Endoscopic assistance during an open procedure with direct visualization is reported using excision codes (eg, 63020-63035).

(Report 01996 for daily hospital management of continuous epidural or subarachnoid drug administration performed in conjunction with 62318-62319)

62263 Percutaneous lysis of epidural adhesions using solution injection (eg, hypertonic saline, enzyme) or mechanical means (eg, catheter) including radiologic localization (includes contrast when administered), multiple adhesiolysis sessions; 2 or more days
➜ *CPT Assistant* Nov 99:33, Dec 99:11, Mar 02:11, Dec 02:10, Nov 05:14, Jul 08:9, Oct 09:12, Nov 10:3, Jan 11:8, Jun 12:12; *CPT Changes: An Insider's View* 2000, 2003
➜ *Clinical Examples in Radiology* Spring 11:10

(62263 includes codes 72275 and 77003)

62264 1 day
➜ *CPT Assistant* Nov 05:14, Jul 08:9, Oct 09:12, Nov 10:3, Jan 11:8, Jun 12:12; *CPT Changes: An Insider's View* 2003
➜ *Clinical Examples in Radiology* Spring 11:10

(Do not report 62264 with 62263)

(62264 includes codes 72275 and 77003)

62267 Percutaneous aspiration within the nucleus pulposus, intervertebral disc, or paravertebral tissue for diagnostic purposes
➜ *CPT Assistant* Nov 10:3, Jan 11:8, Jul 12:3; *CPT Changes: An Insider's View* 2009
➜ *Clinical Examples in Radiology* Fall 10:8, Spring 11:10

(For imaging, use 77003)

(Do not report 62267 in conjunction with 10022, 20225, 62287, 62290, 62291)

62268 Percutaneous aspiration, spinal cord cyst or syrinx

(For radiological supervision and interpretation, see 76942, 77002, 77012)

62269 Biopsy of spinal cord, percutaneous needle
➜ *Clinical Examples in Radiology* Fall 10:7

(For radiological supervision and interpretation, see 76942, 77002, 77012)

(For fine needle aspiration, see 10021, 10022)

(For evaluation of fine needle aspirate, see 88172, 88173)

62270 Spinal puncture, lumbar, diagnostic
➜ *CPT Assistant* Nov 99:32-33, Oct 03:2, Jul 06:4, Jul 07:1, Oct 09:12, Nov 10:3, Jan 11:8, Mar 12:3; *CPT Changes: An Insider's View* 2000, 2002
➜ *Clinical Examples in Radiology* Spring 11:9

62272 Spinal puncture, therapeutic, for drainage of cerebrospinal fluid (by needle or catheter)
➜ *CPT Assistant* Nov 99:32-33, Nov 10:3; *CPT Changes: An Insider's View* 2000
➜ *Clinical Examples in Radiology* Spring 11:10

62273 Injection, epidural, of blood or clot patch
➜ *CPT Assistant* Nov 99:32-34, Oct 09:12, Nov 10:3; *CPT Changes: An Insider's View* 2000
➜ *Clinical Examples in Radiology* Spring 11:10

(For injection of diagnostic or therapeutic substance(s), see 62310, 62311, 62318, 62319)

62280 Injection/infusion of neurolytic substance (eg, alcohol, phenol, iced saline solutions), with or without other therapeutic substance; subarachnoid
➜ *CPT Assistant* Nov 99:32-34, Jan 00:2, Jul 08:9, Oct 09:12, Feb 10:11, Nov 10:3, Jan 11:8, Jun 12:12; *CPT Changes: An Insider's View* 2000
➜ *Clinical Examples in Radiology* Spring 11:10

62281 epidural, cervical or thoracic
➜ *CPT Assistant* Apr 96:11, Nov 99:32-34, Jan 00:2, Jul 08:9, Oct 09:12, Feb 10:11, May 10:10, Nov 10:3, Jan 11:8, Jun 12:12; *CPT Changes: An Insider's View* 2000
➜ *Clinical Examples in Radiology* Spring 11:10

62282 epidural, lumbar, sacral (caudal)
➜ *CPT Assistant* Apr 96:11, Nov 99:32-34, Jan 00:2, Jul 08:9, Oct 09:12, Feb 10:11, Nov 10:3, Jan 11:8, Jun 12:12; *CPT Changes: An Insider's View* 2000
➜ *Clinical Examples in Radiology* Spring 11:10

62284 Injection procedure for myelography and/or computed tomography, spinal (other than C1-C2 and posterior fossa)
➜ *CPT Assistant* Fall 93:13, Sep 04:13; *CPT Changes: An Insider's View* 2003, 2008
➜ *Clinical Examples in Radiology* Fall 06:5-6, 11-12, Spring 11:9

(For injection procedure at C1-C2, use 61055)

(For radiological supervision and interpretation, see **Radiology**)

62287   Decompression procedure, percutaneous, of nucleus pulposus of intervertebral disc, any method utilizing needle based technique to remove disc material under fluoroscopic imaging or other form of indirect visualization, with the use of an endoscope, with discography and/or epidural injection(s) at the treated level(s), when performed, single or multiple levels, lumbar

➔ *CPT Assistant* Nov 99:34, Mar 02:11, Oct 10:9, Jul 12:3; *CPT Changes: An Insider's View* 2000, 2009, 2012

(This includes endoscopic approach)

(Do not report 62287 in conjunction with 62267, 62290, 62311, 77003, 77012, 72295, when performed at same level)

(For non-needle based technique for percutaneous decompression of nucleus pulposus of intervertebral disc, see 0274T, 0275T)

62290   Injection procedure for discography, each level; lumbar

➔ *CPT Assistant* Nov 99:35, Apr 03:27, Mar 11:7, Jul 12:3; *CPT Changes: An Insider's View* 2000

➔ *Clinical Examples in Radiology* Fall 10:10

62291   cervical or thoracic

➔ *CPT Assistant* Nov 99:35, Mar 11:7; *CPT Changes: An Insider's View* 2000

➔ *Clinical Examples in Radiology* Fall 10:10

(For radiological supervision and interpretation, see 72285, 72295)

62292   Injection procedure for chemonucleolysis, including discography, intervertebral disc, single or multiple levels, lumbar

➔ *CPT Assistant* Oct 99:10

62294   Injection procedure, arterial, for occlusion of arteriovenous malformation, spinal

62310   Injection(s), of diagnostic or therapeutic substance(s) (including anesthetic, antispasmodic, opioid, steroid, other solution), not including neurolytic substances, including needle or catheter placement, includes contrast for localization when performed, epidural or subarachnoid; cervical or thoracic

➔ *CPT Assistant* Nov 99:32-35, Jan 00:2, Dec 00:15, Sep 04:5, Jul 08:9, Nov 08:11, Oct 09:12, Feb 10:12, May 10:10, Nov 10:3, Jan 11:8, Jul 12:4, 5; *CPT Changes: An Insider's View* 2000, 2012

➔ *Clinical Examples in Radiology* Spring 11:10

62311   lumbar or sacral (caudal)

➔ *CPT Assistant* Nov 99:32-35, Jan 00:1, Dec 00:15, Sep 04:5, Jul 08:9, Nov 08:11, Oct 09:12, Nov 10:3, Jan 11:8, Jul 12:3-5; *CPT Changes: An Insider's View* 2000, 2012

➔ *Clinical Examples in Radiology* Winter 10:14, Spring 11:10

62318   Injection(s), including indwelling catheter placement, continuous infusion or intermittent bolus, of diagnostic or therapeutic substance(s) (including anesthetic, antispasmodic, opioid, steroid, other solution), not including neurolytic substances, includes contrast for localization when performed, epidural or subarachnoid; cervical or thoracic

➔ *CPT Assistant* Nov 99:32-35, Jan 00:2, Dec 00:15, Oct 01:9, Jul 08:9, Nov 08:11, Oct 09:12, Nov 10:3, Jan 11:8, Jul 12:4, 5; *CPT Changes: An Insider's View* 2000, 2012

➔ *Clinical Examples in Radiology* Spring 11:10

62319   lumbar or sacral (caudal)

➔ *CPT Assistant* Nov 99:32-35, Jan 00:2, Dec 00:15, Oct 01:9, Jul 08:9, Nov 08:11, Oct 09:12, Nov 10:3, Jan 11:8, Jul 12:4, 5; *CPT Changes: An Insider's View* 2000, 2012

➔ *Clinical Examples in Radiology* Spring 11:10

(For transforaminal epidural injection, see 64479-64484)

(Report 01996 for daily hospital management of continuous epidural or subarachnoid drug administration performed in conjunction with 62318-62319)

Catheter Implantation

(For percutaneous placement of intrathecal or epidural catheter, see codes 62270-62273, 62280-62284, 62310-62319)

62350   Implantation, revision or repositioning of tunneled intrathecal or epidural catheter, for long-term medication administration via an external pump or implantable reservoir/infusion pump; without laminectomy

➔ *CPT Assistant* Nov 99:36; *CPT Changes: An Insider's View* 2000, 2001

62351   with laminectomy

➔ *CPT Assistant* Nov 99:36; *CPT Changes: An Insider's View* 2000

(For refilling and maintenance of an implantable infusion pump for spinal or brain drug therapy, see 95990, 95991)

62355   Removal of previously implanted intrathecal or epidural catheter

Reservoir/Pump Implantation

62360   Implantation or replacement of device for intrathecal or epidural drug infusion; subcutaneous reservoir

62361   nonprogrammable pump

Nervous

62362   programmable pump, including preparation of pump, with or without programming

> *CPT Assistant* Mar 97:11

Intrathecal or Epidural Drug Infusion Pump Implantation
62362

The reservoir is placed in the subcutaneous tissues and attached to a previously placed catheter for intrathecal or epidural drug infusion.

Catheter

Implanted infusion pump

62365   Removal of subcutaneous reservoir or pump, previously implanted for intrathecal or epidural infusion

62367   Electronic analysis of programmable, implanted pump for intrathecal or epidural drug infusion (includes evaluation of reservoir status, alarm status, drug prescription status); without reprogramming or refill

> *CPT Assistant* Jul 12:5, 6; *CPT Changes: An Insider's View* 2012

62368   with reprogramming

> *CPT Assistant* Nov 02:10, Jul 06:1, Jul 12:5, 6

(For refilling and maintenance of an implantable infusion pump for spinal or brain drug therapy, see 95990-95991)

62369   with reprogramming and refill

> *CPT Assistant* Jul 12:5, 6; *CPT Changes: An Insider's View* 2012

▲ **62370**   with reprogramming and refill (requiring skill of a physician or other qualified health care professional)

> *CPT Assistant* Jul 12:5, 6; *CPT Changes: An Insider's View* 2012, 2013

(Do not report 62367-62370 in conjunction with 95990, 95991. For refilling and maintenance of a reservoir or an implantable infusion pump for spinal or brain drug delivery without reprogramming, see 95990, 95991)

Posterior Extradural Laminotomy or Laminectomy for Exploration/ Decompression of Neural Elements or Excision of Herniated Intervertebral Discs

Endoscopically assisted laminotomy (hemilaminectomy) requires open and direct visualization. When visualization is only endoscopic and/or image guidance, the procedure is percutaneous and reported using 0274T, 0275T.

(When 63001-63048 are followed by arthrodesis, see 22590-22614)

63001   Laminectomy with exploration and/or decompression of spinal cord and/or cauda equina, without facetectomy, foraminotomy or discectomy (eg, spinal stenosis), 1 or 2 vertebral segments; cervical

> *CPT Assistant* Jan 01:12, Jun 07:1, Jul 11:13, Jul 12:3

63003   thoracic

> *CPT Assistant* Jan 01:12, Jul 12:3

63005   lumbar, except for spondylolisthesis

> *CPT Assistant* Jan 01:12, Jul 12:3

Lumbar Laminectomy
63005

With the patient prone and under general anesthesia, the laminae and underlying ligamentum flavum are removed.

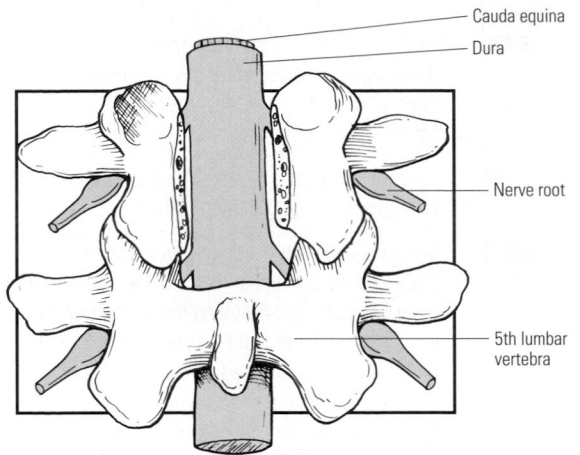

Cauda equina

Dura

Nerve root

5th lumbar vertebra

63011   sacral

> *CPT Assistant* Jan 01:12

63012   Laminectomy with removal of abnormal facets and/or pars inter-articularis with decompression of cauda equina and nerve roots for spondylolisthesis, lumbar (Gill type procedure)

> *CPT Assistant* Jan 01:12

63015   Laminectomy with exploration and/or decompression of spinal cord and/or cauda equina, without facetectomy, foraminotomy or discectomy (eg, spinal stenosis), more than 2 vertebral segments; cervical

> *CPT Assistant* Jan 01:12

Nervous

63016   thoracic
    ➔ *CPT Assistant* Jan 01:12

63017   lumbar
    ➔ *CPT Assistant* Jan 01:12

63020   Laminotomy (hemilaminectomy), with decompression of nerve root(s), including partial facetectomy, foraminotomy and/or excision of herniated intervertebral disc; 1 interspace, cervical
    ➔ *CPT Assistant* Nov 99:36, Jan 01:12, Jul 12:4; *CPT Changes: An Insider's View* 2000, 2009, 2012

(For bilateral procedure, report 63020 with modifier 50)

63030   1 interspace, lumbar
    ➔ *CPT Assistant* Mar 96:7, Nov 99:36, Jan 01:12, Feb 01:10, Sep 02:10, Oct 04:12, Oct 08:10, Oct 09:9, Nov 10:3, Mar 11:7, Jul 11:13, Jul 12:3, 4; *CPT Changes: An Insider's View* 2000, 2009, 2012

(For bilateral procedure, report 63030 with modifier 50)

+ 63035   each additional interspace, cervical or lumbar (List separately in addition to code for primary procedure)
    ➔ *CPT Assistant* Fall 91:8, Mar 96:7, Nov 99:36, Jan 01:12, Feb 01:10, Jul 12:4; *CPT Changes: An Insider's View* 2000, 2009, 2012

(Use 63035 in conjunction with 63020-63030)

(For bilateral procedure, report 63035 with modifier 50)

(For percutaneous endoscopic approach, see 0274T, 0275T)

63040   Laminotomy (hemilaminectomy), with decompression of nerve root(s), including partial facetectomy, foraminotomy and/or excision of herniated intervertebral disc, reexploration, single interspace; cervical
    ➔ *CPT Assistant* Jan 99:11, Jan 01:12; *CPT Changes: An Insider's View* 2001

(For bilateral procedure, report 63040 with modifier 50)

63042   lumbar
    ➔ *CPT Assistant* Jan 99:11, Jan 01:12, Oct 08:10, Oct 09:9, Jul 11:13

(For bilateral procedure, report 63042 with modifier 50)

+ 63043   each additional cervical interspace (List separately in addition to code for primary procedure)
    ➔ *CPT Changes: An Insider's View* 2001

(Use 63043 in conjunction with 63040)

(For bilateral procedure, report 63043 with modifier 50)

+ 63044   each additional lumbar interspace (List separately in addition to code for primary procedure)
    ➔ *CPT Changes: An Insider's View* 2001

(Use 63044 in conjunction with 63042)

(For bilateral procedure, report 63044 with modifier 50)

63045   Laminectomy, facetectomy and foraminotomy (unilateral or bilateral with decompression of spinal cord, cauda equina and/or nerve root[s], [eg, spinal or lateral recess stenosis]), single vertebral segment; cervical
    ➔ *CPT Assistant* Jan 01:12

63046   thoracic
    ➔ *CPT Assistant* Jan 99:11, Jan 01:12

63047   lumbar
    ➔ *CPT Assistant* Jan 99:11, Jan 01:12, Feb 01:10, Nov 02:11, Apr 08:11, Jul 08:7, Oct 08:10, Oct 09:9, Nov 10:4, Jul 11:13

+ 63048   each additional segment, cervical, thoracic, or lumbar (List separately in addition to code for primary procedure)
    ➔ *CPT Assistant* Fall 91:8, Jan 99:11, Jan 01:12

(Use 63048 in conjunction with 63045-63047)

63050   Laminoplasty, cervical, with decompression of the spinal cord, 2 or more vertebral segments;
    ➔ *CPT Changes: An Insider's View* 2005

63051   with reconstruction of the posterior bony elements (including the application of bridging bone graft and non-segmental fixation devices [eg, wire, suture, mini-plates], when performed]
    ➔ *CPT Assistant* Jul 11:13; *CPT Changes: An Insider's View* 2005

(Do not report 63050 or 63051 in conjunction with 22600, 22614, 22840-22842, 63001, 63015, 63045, 63048, 63295 for the same vertebral segment(s))

Transpedicular or Costovertebral Approach for Posterolateral Extradural Exploration/Decompression

63055   Transpedicular approach with decompression of spinal cord, equina and/or nerve root(s) (eg, herniated intervertebral disc), single segment; thoracic
    ➔ *CPT Assistant* Nov 99:36; *CPT Changes: An Insider's View* 2000

63056   lumbar (including transfacet, or lateral extraforaminal approach) (eg, far lateral herniated intervertebral disc)
    ➔ *CPT Assistant* Nov 99:36, Oct 09:9, Nov 11:10, Jul 12:3; *CPT Changes: An Insider's View* 2000

+ 63057   each additional segment, thoracic or lumbar (List separately in addition to code for primary procedure)
    ➔ *CPT Assistant* Nov 99:36; *CPT Changes: An Insider's View* 2000

(Use 63057 in conjunction with 63055, 63056)

63064   Costovertebral approach with decompression of spinal cord or nerve root(s) (eg, herniated intervertebral disc), thoracic; single segment
    ➔ *CPT Assistant* Fall 92:19

+ 63066   each additional segment (List separately in addition to code for primary procedure)

(Use 63066 in conjunction with 63064)

(For excision of thoracic intraspinal lesions by laminectomy, see 63266, 63271, 63276, 63281, 63286)

Nervous

Anterior or Anterolateral Approach for Extradural Exploration/Decompression

For the following codes, when two surgeons work together as primary surgeons performing distinct part(s) of spinal cord exploration/decompression operation, each surgeon should report his/her distinct operative work by appending modifier 62 to the procedure code (and any associated add-on codes for that procedure code as long as both surgeons continue to work together as primary surgeons). In this situation, modifier 62 may be appended to the definitive procedure code(s) 63075, 63077, 63081, 63085, 63087, 63090 and, as appropriate, to associated additional interspace add-on code(s) 63076, 63078 or additional segment add-on code(s) 63082, 63086, 63088, 63091 as long as both surgeons continue to work together as primary surgeons.

63075   Discectomy, anterior, with decompression of spinal cord and/or nerve root(s), including osteophytectomy; cervical, single interspace

➔ *CPT Assistant* Nov 98:18, Jan 01:12, Feb 02:4; *CPT Changes: An Insider's View* 2002

▶(Do not report 63075 in conjunction with 22554, even if performed by separate individuals. To report anterior cervical discectomy and interbody fusion at the same level during the same session, use 22551)◀

+ 63076   cervical, each additional interspace (List separately in addition to code for primary procedure)

➔ *CPT Assistant* Nov 98:18, Jan 01:12, Feb 02:4; *CPT Changes: An Insider's View* 2002

▶(Do not report 63076 in conjunction with 22554, even if performed by separate individuals. To report anterior cervical discectomy and interbody fusion at the same level during the same session, use 22552)◀

(Use 63076 in conjunction with 63075)

63077   thoracic, single interspace

➔ *CPT Assistant* Nov 98:18, Jan 01:12, Feb 02:4; *CPT Changes: An Insider's View* 2002

+ 63078   thoracic, each additional interspace (List separately in addition to code for primary procedure)

➔ *CPT Assistant* Nov 98:18, Jan 01:12, Feb 02:4; *CPT Changes: An Insider's View* 2002

(Use 63078 in conjunction with 63077)

(Do not report code 69990 in addition to codes 63075-63078)

63081   Vertebral corpectomy (vertebral body resection), partial or complete, anterior approach with decompression of spinal cord and/or nerve root(s); cervical, single segment

➔ *CPT Assistant* Spring 93:37, Feb 02:4; *CPT Changes: An Insider's View* 2002

+ 63082   cervical, each additional segment (List separately in addition to code for primary procedure)

➔ *CPT Assistant* Spring 93:37, Feb 02:4; *CPT Changes: An Insider's View* 2002

(Use 63082 in conjunction with 63081)

(For transoral approach, see 61575, 61576)

63085   Vertebral corpectomy (vertebral body resection), partial or complete, transthoracic approach with decompression of spinal cord and/or nerve root(s); thoracic, single segment

➔ *CPT Assistant* Spring 93:37, Feb 02:4; *CPT Changes: An Insider's View* 2002

+ 63086   thoracic, each additional segment (List separately in addition to code for primary procedure)

➔ *CPT Assistant* Spring 93:37, Feb 02:4; *CPT Changes: An Insider's View* 2002

(Use 63086 in conjunction with 63085)

63087   Vertebral corpectomy (vertebral body resection), partial or complete, combined thoracolumbar approach with decompression of spinal cord, cauda equina or nerve root(s), lower thoracic or lumbar; single segment

➔ *CPT Assistant* Spring 93:37, Feb 02:4; *CPT Changes: An Insider's View* 2002

+ 63088   each additional segment (List separately in addition to code for primary procedure)

➔ *CPT Assistant* Spring 93:37, Feb 02:4; *CPT Changes: An Insider's View* 2002

(Use 63088 in conjunction with 63087)

63090   Vertebral corpectomy (vertebral body resection), partial or complete, transperitoneal or retroperitoneal approach with decompression of spinal cord, cauda equina or nerve root(s), lower thoracic, lumbar, or sacral; single segment

➔ *CPT Assistant* Spring 93:37, Mar 96:6, Feb 02:4; *CPT Changes: An Insider's View* 2002

+ 63091   each additional segment (List separately in addition to code for primary procedure)

➔ *CPT Assistant* Spring 93:37, Mar 96:6, Feb 02:4; *CPT Changes: An Insider's View* 2002

(Use 63091 in conjunction with 63090)

(Procedures 63081-63091 include discectomy above and/or below vertebral segment)

(If followed by arthrodesis, see 22548-22812)

(For reconstruction of spine, use appropriate vertebral corpectomy codes 63081-63091, bone graft codes 20930-20938, arthrodesis codes 22548-22812, and spinal instrumentation codes 22840-22855)

Lateral Extracavitary Approach for Extradural Exploration/Decompression

63101   Vertebral corpectomy (vertebral body resection), partial or complete, lateral extracavitary approach with decompression of spinal cord and/or nerve root(s) (eg, for tumor or retropulsed bone fragments); thoracic, single segment

➔ *CPT Changes: An Insider's View* 2004

63102   lumbar, single segment

➔ *CPT Changes: An Insider's View* 2004

+ 63103   thoracic or lumbar, each additional segment (List separately in addition to code for primary procedure)

➔ *CPT Changes: An Insider's View* 2004

(Use 63103 in conjunction with 63101 and 63102)

Nervous

Incision

63170 Laminectomy with myelotomy (eg, Bischof or DREZ type), cervical, thoracic, or thoracolumbar

63172 Laminectomy with drainage of intramedullary cyst/syrinx; to subarachnoid space

63173 to peritoneal or pleural space
➔ *CPT Changes: An Insider's View* 2004

63180 Laminectomy and section of dentate ligaments, with or without dural graft, cervical; 1 or 2 segments

63182 more than 2 segments

63185 Laminectomy with rhizotomy; 1 or 2 segments

63190 more than 2 segments

63191 Laminectomy with section of spinal accessory nerve

(For bilateral procedure, report 63191 with modifier 50)

(For resection of sternocleidomastoid muscle, use 21720)

63194 Laminectomy with cordotomy, with section of 1 spinothalamic tract, 1 stage; cervical

63195 thoracic

63196 Laminectomy with cordotomy, with section of both spinothalamic tracts, 1 stage; cervical

63197 thoracic

63198 Laminectomy with cordotomy with section of both spinothalamic tracts, 2 stages within 14 days; cervical

63199 thoracic

63200 Laminectomy, with release of tethered spinal cord, lumbar

Excision by Laminectomy of Lesion Other Than Herniated Disc

63250 Laminectomy for excision or occlusion of arteriovenous malformation of spinal cord; cervical

63251 thoracic

63252 thoracolumbar

63265 Laminectomy for excision or evacuation of intraspinal lesion other than neoplasm, extradural; cervical

63266 thoracic

63267 lumbar

63268 sacral

63270 Laminectomy for excision of intraspinal lesion other than neoplasm, intradural; cervical

63271 thoracic

63272 lumbar

63273 sacral

63275 Laminectomy for biopsy/excision of intraspinal neoplasm; extradural, cervical

63276 extradural, thoracic

63277 extradural, lumbar

63278 extradural, sacral

63280 intradural, extramedullary, cervical

63281 intradural, extramedullary, thoracic

63282 intradural, extramedullary, lumbar

63283 intradural, sacral

63285 intradural, intramedullary, cervical

63286 intradural, intramedullary, thoracic

63287 intradural, intramedullary, thoracolumbar

63290 combined extradural-intradural lesion, any level

(For drainage of intramedullary cyst/syrinx, use 63172, 63173)

+ 63295 Osteoplastic reconstruction of dorsal spinal elements, following primary intraspinal procedure (List separately in addition to code for primary procedure)
➔ *CPT Changes: An Insider's View* 2005

(Use 63295 in conjunction with 63172, 63173, 63185, 63190, 63200-63290)

(Do not report 63295 in conjunction with 22590-22614, 22840-22844, 63050, 63051 for the same vertebral segment[s])

Excision, Anterior or Anterolateral Approach, Intraspinal Lesion

For the following codes, when two surgeons work together as primary surgeons performing distinct part(s) of an anterior approach for an intraspinal excision, each surgeon should report his/her distinct operative work by appending modifier 62 to the single definitive procedure code. In this situation, modifier 62 may be appended to the definitive procedure code(s) 63300-63307 and, as appropriate, to the associated additional segment add-on code 63308 as long as both surgeons continue to work together as primary surgeons.

(For arthrodesis, see 22548-22585)

(For reconstruction of spine, see 20930-20938)

63300 Vertebral corpectomy (vertebral body resection), partial or complete, for excision of intraspinal lesion, single segment; extradural, cervical
➔ *CPT Assistant* Feb 02:4

63301 extradural, thoracic by transthoracic approach
➔ *CPT Assistant* Feb 02:4

63302 extradural, thoracic by thoracolumbar approach
➔ *CPT Assistant* Feb 02:4

63303 extradural, lumbar or sacral by transperitoneal or retroperitoneal approach
➔ *CPT Assistant* Feb 02:4

Nervous

63304 intradural, cervical
→ *CPT Assistant* Feb 02:4

63305 intradural, thoracic by transthoracic approach
→ *CPT Assistant* Feb 02:4

63306 intradural, thoracic by thoracolumbar approach
→ *CPT Assistant* Feb 02:4

63307 intradural, lumbar or sacral by transperitoneal or retroperitoneal approach
→ *CPT Assistant* Feb 02:4

+ 63308 each additional segment (List separately in addition to codes for single segment)
→ *CPT Assistant* Feb 02:4

(Use 63308 in conjunction with 63300-63307)

Stereotaxis

63600 Creation of lesion of spinal cord by stereotactic method, percutaneous, any modality (including stimulation and/or recording)

63610 Stereotactic stimulation of spinal cord, percutaneous, separate procedure not followed by other surgery

63615 Stereotactic biopsy, aspiration, or excision of lesion, spinal cord

Stereotactic Radiosurgery (Spinal)

►Spinal stereotactic radiosurgery is a distinct procedure that utilizes externally generated ionizing radiation to inactivate or eradicate defined target(s) in the spine without the need to make an incision. The target is defined by and the treatment is delivered using high-resolution stereotactic imaging. These codes are reported by the surgeon. The radiation oncologist reports the appropriate code(s) for clinical treatment planning, physics and dosimetry, treatment delivery and management from the **Radiation Oncology** section (77261-77790). Any necessary planning, dosimetry, targeting, positioning, or blocking by the neurosurgeon is included in the stereotactic radiation surgery services. The same individual should not report stereotactic radiosurgery services with radiation treatment management codes (77427-77432).◄

Spinal stereotactic radiosurgery is typically performed in a single planning and treatment session using a stereotactic image-guidance system, but can be performed with a planning session and in a limited number of treatment sessions, up to a maximum of five sessions. Do not report stereotactic radiosurgery more than once per lesion per course of treatment when the treatment requires greater than one session.

Stereotactic spinal surgery is only used when the tumor being treated affects spinal neural tissue or abuts the dura mater. Arteriovenous malformations must be subdural. For other radiation services of the spine, see **Radiation Oncology** services.

Codes 63620, 63621 include computer-assisted planning. Do not report 63620, 63621 in conjunction with 61781-61783.

(For intensity modulated beam delivery plan and treatment, see 77301, 77418. For stereotactic body radiation therapy, see 77373, 77435)

63620 Stereotactic radiosurgery (particle beam, gamma ray, or linear accelerator); 1 spinal lesion
→ *CPT Assistant* Oct 10:3, Jul 11:12; *CPT Changes: An Insider's View* 2009

(Do not report 63620 more than once per course of treatment)

+ 63621 each additional spinal lesion (List separately in addition to code for primary procedure)
→ *CPT Assistant* Oct 10:3, Jul 11:12; *CPT Changes: An Insider's View* 2009

(Report 63621 in conjunction with 63620)

(For each course of treatment, 63621 may be reported no more than once per lesion. Do not report 63621 more than 2 times for entire course of treatment regardless of number of lesions treated)

Neurostimulators (Spinal)

Codes 63650-63688 apply to both simple and complex neurostimulators. For initial or subsequent electronic analysis and programming of neurostimulator pulse generators, see codes 95970-95975.

Codes 63650, 63655, and 63661-63664 describe the operative placement, revision, replacement, or removal of the spinal neurostimulator system components to provide spinal electrical stimulation. A neurostimulator system includes an implanted neurostimulator, external controller, extension, and collection of contacts. Multiple contacts or electrodes (4 or more) provide the actual electrical stimulation in the epidural space.

For percutaneously placed neurostimulator systems (63650, 63661, 63663), the contacts are on a catheter-like lead. An array defines the collection of contacts that are on one catheter.

For systems placed via an open surgical exposure (63655, 63662, 63664), the contacts are on a plate or paddle-shaped surface.

Do not report 63661 or 63663 when removing or replacing a temporary percutaneously placed array for an external generator.

63650 Percutaneous implantation of neurostimulator electrode array, epidural
→ *CPT Assistant* Jun 98:3-4, Nov 98:18, Mar 99:11, Apr 99:10, Sep 99:3, Dec 08:8, Feb 10:9, Aug 10:8, Oct 10:14, Dec 10:14, Apr 11:10; *CPT Changes: An Insider's View* 2010

Percutaneous Implantation of Neurostimulator Electrodes
63650

Single catheter electrode array is inserted percutaneously into the epidural space. A simple or complex receiver is subcutaneously implanted.

Dura mater and spinal cord
Single catheter with 8 contacts
Thoracic vertebra
Single catheter
Subcutaneous complex receiver
External antenna on top of skin
External transmitter
Epidural fat
Spinal cord
Catheter in epidural space
Dura

63655   Laminectomy for implantation of neurostimulator electrodes, plate/paddle, epidural

→ *CPT Assistant* Jun 98:3-4, Nov 98:18, Sep 99:3-4, Dec 08:8, Aug 10:8, Dec 10:14, Apr 11:10

Placement of Neurostimulator Electrodes Through Laminectomy
63655

The electrode plate or paddle is placed in the epidural space via open exposure through large laminotomy or small laminectomy. The simple or complex receiver is subcutaneously implanted.

Dura mater and spinal cord
Electrode plate/paddle with 4 contacts
Lead with 16 contacts
Thoracic vertebra
Small laminectomy
Dual array plate/paddle with 16 contacts in epidural space
Subcutaneous complex receiver
External antenna on top of skin
External transmitter
Epidural fat
Dura
Spinal cord
Epidural space with lamitrode in place
Anterior longitudinal ligament
Posterior longitudinal ligament

(63660 has been deleted. To report, see 63661-63664)

63661   Removal of spinal neurostimulator electrode percutaneous array(s), including fluoroscopy, when performed

→ *CPT Assistant* Feb 10:9, Aug 10:8, Jan 11:8, Apr 11:10; *CPT Changes: An Insider's View* 2010

→ *Clinical Examples in Radiology* Spring 11:10

63662   Removal of spinal neurostimulator electrode plate/paddle(s) placed via laminotomy or laminectomy, including fluoroscopy, when performed

→ *CPT Assistant* Feb 10:9, Aug 10:8, Apr 11:10; *CPT Changes: An Insider's View* 2010

→ *Clinical Examples in Radiology* Spring 11:10

63663   Revision including replacement, when performed, of spinal neurostimulator electrode percutaneous array(s), including fluoroscopy, when performed

→ *CPT Assistant* Feb 10:9, Aug 10:8, Apr 11:10; *CPT Changes: An Insider's View* 2010

→ *Clinical Examples in Radiology* Spring 11:10

(Do not report 63663 in conjunction with 63661, 63662 for the same spinal level)

63664   Revision including replacement, when performed, of spinal neurostimulator electrode plate/paddle(s) placed via laminotomy or laminectomy, including fluoroscopy, when performed

→ *CPT Assistant* Feb 10:9, Aug 10:8, Apr 11:10; *CPT Changes: An Insider's View* 2010

→ *Clinical Examples in Radiology* Spring 11:10

(Do not report 63664 in conjunction with 63661, 63662 for the same spinal level)

63685   Insertion or replacement of spinal neurostimulator pulse generator or receiver, direct or inductive coupling

→ *CPT Assistant* Jun 98:3-4, Sep 99:5, Feb 10:9, Oct 10:14, Dec 10:14, Apr 11:10; *CPT Changes: An Insider's View* 2005

(Do not report 63685 in conjunction with 63688 for the same pulse generator or receiver)

63688   Revision or removal of implanted spinal neurostimulator pulse generator or receiver

→ *CPT Assistant* Jun 98:3-4, Sep 99:5, Feb 10:9, Apr 11:11

(For electronic analysis of implanted neurostimulator pulse generator system, see 95970-95975)

Repair

63700   Repair of meningocele; less than 5 cm diameter

63702   larger than 5 cm diameter

(Do not use modifier 63 in conjunction with 63700, 63702)

63704   Repair of myelomeningocele; less than 5 cm diameter

63706   larger than 5 cm diameter

(Do not use modifier 63 in conjunction with 63704, 63706)

(For complex skin closure, see **Integumentary System**)

63707 Repair of dural/cerebrospinal fluid leak, not requiring laminectomy

➔ *CPT Changes: An Insider's View* 2002

63709 Repair of dural/cerebrospinal fluid leak or pseudomeningocele, with laminectomy

➔ *CPT Changes: An Insider's View* 2002

63710 Dural graft, spinal

(For laminectomy and section of dentate ligaments, with or without dural graft, cervical, see 63180, 63182)

Shunt, Spinal CSF

63740 Creation of shunt, lumbar, subarachnoid-peritoneal, -pleural, or other; including laminectomy

➔ *CPT Assistant* Winter 90:8

63741 percutaneous, not requiring laminectomy

➔ *CPT Assistant* Winter 90:8

63744 Replacement, irrigation or revision of lumbosubarachnoid shunt

63746 Removal of entire lumbosubarachnoid shunt system without replacement

(For insertion of subarachnoid catheter with reservoir and/or pump for intermittent or continuous infusion of drug including laminectomy, see 62351 and 62360, 62361 or 62362)

(For insertion or replacement of subarachnoid or epidural catheter, with reservoir and/or pump for drug infusion without laminectomy, see 62350 and 62360, 62361 or 62362)

Extracranial Nerves, Peripheral Nerves, and Autonomic Nervous System

(For intracranial surgery on cranial nerves, see 61450, 61460, 61790)

Introduction/Injection of Anesthetic Agent (Nerve Block), Diagnostic or Therapeutic

(For destruction by neurolytic agent or chemodenervation, see 62280-62282, 64600-64681)

(For epidural or subarachnoid injection, see 62310-62319)

(64479-64495 are unilateral procedures. For bilateral procedures, use modifier 50)

Somatic Nerves

64400 Injection, anesthetic agent; trigeminal nerve, any division or branch

➔ *CPT Assistant* Jul 98:10, May 99:8, Nov 99:36, Apr 05:13, Feb 10:9; *CPT Changes: An Insider's View* 2000

64402 facial nerve

➔ *CPT Assistant* Jul 98:10, Apr 05:13

64405 greater occipital nerve

➔ *CPT Assistant* Jul 98:10, Apr 05:13

64408 vagus nerve

➔ *CPT Assistant* Jul 98:10, Apr 05:13

64410 phrenic nerve

➔ *CPT Assistant* Jul 98:10, Apr 05:13

64412 spinal accessory nerve

➔ *CPT Assistant* Jul 98:10, Apr 05:13, Aug 07:15

64413 cervical plexus

➔ *CPT Assistant* Jul 98:10, Apr 05:13

64415 brachial plexus, single

➔ *CPT Assistant* Fall 92:17, Jul 98:10, May 99:8, Oct 01:9, Feb 04:7, Apr 05:13, Nov 06:23; *CPT Changes: An Insider's View* 2003

64416 brachial plexus, continuous infusion by catheter (including catheter placement)

➔ *CPT Assistant* Feb 04:7, Apr 05:13; *CPT Changes: An Insider's View* 2003, 2009

(Do not report 64416 in conjunction with 01996)

64417 axillary nerve

➔ *CPT Assistant* Jul 98:10, Apr 05:13

64418 suprascapular nerve

➔ *CPT Assistant* Jul 98:10, Apr 05:13, Aug 07:15

64420 intercostal nerve, single

➔ *CPT Assistant* Jul 98:10, Apr 05:13, Aug 10:12, Nov 10:9

64421 intercostal nerves, multiple, regional block

➔ *CPT Assistant* Jul 98:10, Apr 05:13, Aug 10:12, Nov 10:9

64425 ilioinguinal, iliohypogastric nerves

➔ *CPT Assistant* Jul 98:10, Apr 05:13

64430 pudendal nerve

➔ *CPT Assistant* Jul 98:10, Apr 05:13

64435 paracervical (uterine) nerve

➔ *CPT Assistant* Jul 98:10, Mar 03:22, Jul 03:15, Apr 05:13, Feb 12:11

64445 sciatic nerve, single

➔ *CPT Assistant* Jul 98:10, May 99:8, Feb 04:8, Apr 05:13, Dec 11:8; *CPT Changes: An Insider's View* 2003

64446 sciatic nerve, continuous infusion by catheter (including catheter placement)

➔ *CPT Assistant* Feb 04:9, Apr 05:13; *CPT Changes: An Insider's View* 2003, 2009

(Do not report 64446 in conjunction with 01996)

64447 femoral nerve, single

➔ *CPT Assistant* Feb 04:9, Apr 05:13; *CPT Changes: An Insider's View* 2003

(Do not report 64447 in conjunction with 01996)

64448   femoral nerve, continuous infusion by catheter (including catheter placement)

➔ *CPT Assistant* Feb 04:10, Apr 05:13; *CPT Changes: An Insider's View* 2003, 2009

(Do not report 64448 in conjunction with 01996)

64449   lumbar plexus, posterior approach, continuous infusion by catheter (including catheter placement)

➔ *CPT Assistant* Apr 05:13; *CPT Changes: An Insider's View* 2004, 2009

(Do not report 64449 in conjunction with 01996)

64450   other peripheral nerve or branch

➔ *CPT Assistant* Jul 98:10, Nov 99:37, Dec 99:7, Oct 01:9, Aug 03:6, Apr 05:13, Jan 09:6; *CPT Changes: An Insider's View* 2000

64455   Injection(s), anesthetic agent and/or steroid, plantar common digital nerve(s) (eg, Morton's neuroma)

➔ *CPT Changes: An Insider's View* 2009

(Do not report 64455 in conjunction with 64632)

(Imaging guidance [fluoroscopy or CT] and any injection of contrast are inclusive components of 64479-64484. Imaging guidance and localization are required for the performance of 64479-64484)

(64470-64476 have been deleted. To report, see 64490-64495)

64479   Injection(s), anesthetic agent and/or steroid, transforaminal epidural, with imaging guidance (fluoroscopy or CT); cervical or thoracic, single level

➔ *CPT Assistant* Nov 99:33, 37, Feb 00:4, Jul 08:9, Nov 08:11, Feb 10:9, Jan 11:8, Feb 11:4, Jul 11:16, Jul 12:5; *CPT Changes: An Insider's View* 2000, 2011

➔ *Clinical Examples in Radiology* Summer 08:9, Spring 11:10

(For transforaminal epidural injection under ultrasound guidance, use 0228T)

+ 64480   cervical or thoracic, each additional level (List separately in addition to code for primary procedure)

➔ *CPT Assistant* Nov 99:33, 37, Feb 00:4, Feb 05:14, Jul 08:9, Feb 10:9, Jan 11:8, Feb 11:4, Jul 11:16, Jul 12:5; *CPT Changes: An Insider's View* 2000, 2011

➔ *Clinical Examples in Radiology* Summer 08:9, Spring 11:10

(Use 64480 in conjunction with 64479)

(For transforaminal epidural injection under ultrasound guidance, use 0229T)

(For transforaminal epidural injection at the T12-L1 level, use 64479)

64483   lumbar or sacral, single level

➔ *CPT Assistant* Nov 99:33, 37, Feb 00:4, Jul 08:9, Feb 10:9, Jan 11:8, Feb 11:4, Jul 11:16, May 12:14, Jul 12:5; *CPT Changes: An Insider's View* 2000, 2011

➔ *Clinical Examples in Radiology* Spring 11:10

(For transforaminal epidural injection under ultrasound guidance, use 0230T)

+ 64484   lumbar or sacral, each additional level (List separately in addition to code for primary procedure)

➔ *CPT Assistant* Nov 99:33, 37, Feb 00:4, Feb 05:14, Jul 08:9, Nov 08:11, Feb 10:9, Feb 11:4, Jul 11:16, Jul 12:5; *CPT Changes: An Insider's View* 2000, 2011

➔ *Clinical Examples in Radiology* Spring 11:10

(Use 64484 in conjunction with 64483)

(For transforaminal epidural injection under ultrasound guidance, use 0231T)

(64479-64484 are unilateral procedures. For bilateral procedures, use modifier 50)

Paravertebral Spinal Nerves and Branches

(Image guidance [fluoroscopy or CT] and any injection of contrast are inclusive components of 64490-64495. Imaging guidance and localization are required for the performance of paravertebral facet joint injections described by codes 64490-64495. If imaging is not used, report 20552-20553. If ultrasound guidance is used, report 0213T-0218T)

(For bilateral paravertebral facet injection procedures, use modifier 50)

(For paravertebral facet injection of the T12-L1 joint, or nerves innervating that joint, use 64490)

64490   Injection(s), diagnostic or therapeutic agent, paravertebral facet (zygapophyseal) joint (or nerves innervating that joint) with image guidance (fluoroscopy or CT), cervical or thoracic; single level

➔ *CPT Assistant* Feb 10:9, Aug 10:12, Dec 10:13, Jan 11:8, Feb 11:4, Jun 12:10; *CPT Changes: An Insider's View* 2010

➔ *Clinical Examples in Radiology* Winter 10:15, Spring 11:10

+ 64491   second level (List separately in addition to code for primary procedure)

➔ *CPT Assistant* Aug 10:12, Jun 12:10; *CPT Changes: An Insider's View* 2010

➔ *Clinical Examples in Radiology* Winter 10:15

+ 64492   third and any additional level(s) (List separately in addition to code for primary procedure)

➔ *CPT Assistant* Feb 10:9, Aug 10:12, Jan 11:8, Feb 11:4, Jun 12:10; *CPT Changes: An Insider's View* 2010

➔ *Clinical Examples in Radiology* Winter 10:14, Spring 11:10

(Do not report 64492 more than once per day)

(Use 64491, 64492 in conjunction with 64490)

Nervous

64493 Injection(s), diagnostic or therapeutic agent, paravertebral facet (zygapophyseal) joint (or nerves innervating that joint) with image guidance (fluoroscopy or CT), lumbar or sacral; single level
➔ *CPT Assistant* Feb 10:9, Aug 10:12, Jan 11:8, Feb 11:4, Jun 12:10; *CPT Changes: An Insider's View* 2010
➔ *Clinical Examples in Radiology* Winter 10:14, Spring 11:10

+ 64494 second level (List separately in addition to code for primary procedure)
➔ *CPT Assistant* Feb 10:9, Aug 10:12, Jan 11:8, Feb 11:4, Jun 12:10; *CPT Changes: An Insider's View* 2010
➔ *Clinical Examples in Radiology* Winter 10:14, Spring 11:10

+ 64495 third and any additional level(s) (List separately in addition to code for primary procedure)
➔ *CPT Assistant* Feb 10:9, Aug 10:12, Jan 11:8, Feb 11:4, Jun 12:10; *CPT Changes: An Insider's View* 2010
➔ *Clinical Examples in Radiology* Winter 10:14, Spring 11:10

(Do not report 64495 more than once per day)

(Use 64494, 64495 in conjunction with 64493)

Autonomic Nerves

64505 Injection, anesthetic agent; sphenopalatine ganglion
➔ *CPT Assistant* Jul 98:10, Apr 05:13

64508 carotid sinus (separate procedure)
➔ *CPT Assistant* Jul 98:10, Apr 05:13

64510 stellate ganglion (cervical sympathetic)
➔ *CPT Assistant* Jul 98:10, Apr 05:13

64517 superior hypogastric plexus
➔ *CPT Assistant* Oct 04:11, Apr 05:13; *CPT Changes: An Insider's View* 2004

64520 lumbar or thoracic (paravertebral sympathetic)
➔ *CPT Assistant* Jul 98:10, Apr 05:13, Dec 10:14

64530 celiac plexus, with or without radiologic monitoring
➔ *CPT Assistant* Jul 98:10, Apr 05:13

Neurostimulators (Peripheral Nerve)

Codes 64553-64595 apply to both simple and complex neurostimulators. For initial or subsequent electronic analysis and programming of neurostimulator pulse generators, see codes 95970-95975. An electrode array is a catheter or other device with more than one contact. The function of each contact may be capable of being adjusted during programming services.

(For implantation of trial or permanent electrode arrays or pulse generators for peripheral subcutaneous field stimulation, see 0282T-0284T)

64550 Application of surface (transcutaneous) neurostimulator
➔ *CPT Assistant* Jan 02:11, Apr 02:18

64553 Percutaneous implantation of neurostimulator electrode array; cranial nerve
➔ *CPT Assistant* Nov 99:38, Apr 01:9; *CPT Changes: An Insider's View* 2000, 2012

(For open placement of cranial nerve [eg, vagus, trigeminal] neurostimulator pulse generator or receiver, see 61885, 61886, as appropriate)

64555 peripheral nerve (excludes sacral nerve)
➔ *CPT Changes: An Insider's View* 2002, 2012

(Do not report 64555 in conjunction with 64566)

(64560 has been deleted)

▲ **64561** sacral nerve (transforaminal placement) including image guidance, if performed
➔ *CPT Changes: An Insider's View* 2002, 2012, 2013

64565 neuromuscular
➔ *CPT Assistant* Jul 00:11, Dec 08:8; *CPT Changes: An Insider's View* 2012

64566 Posterior tibial neurostimulation, percutaneous needle electrode, single treatment, includes programming
➔ *CPT Assistant* Feb 11:5, Sep 11:8; *CPT Changes: An Insider's View* 2011

(Do not report 64566 in conjunction with 64555, 95970-95972)

64568 Incision for implantation of cranial nerve (eg, vagus nerve) neurostimulator electrode array and pulse generator
➔ *CPT Assistant* Feb 11:5, Sep 11:8, 10, 12; *CPT Changes: An Insider's View* 2011

(Do not report 64568 in conjunction with 61885, 61886, 64570)

64569 Revision or replacement of cranial nerve (eg, vagus nerve) neurostimulator electrode array, including connection to existing pulse generator
➔ *CPT Assistant* Feb 11:5, Sep 11:8; *CPT Changes: An Insider's View* 2011

(Do not report 64569 in conjunction with 64570 or 61888)

(For replacement of pulse generator, use 61885)

64570 Removal of cranial nerve (eg, vagus nerve) neurostimulator electrode array and pulse generator
➔ *CPT Assistant* Feb 11:5, Sep 11:10; *CPT Changes: An Insider's View* 2011

(Do not report 64570 in conjunction with 61888)

▶(For laparoscopic implantation, revision, replacement, or removal of vagus nerve blocking neurostimulator electrode array and/or pulse generator at the esophagogastric junction, see 0312T-0317T)◀

⊙=Moderate sedation +=Add-on code ✗=FDA approval pending #=Resequenced code ○=Recycled/reinstated code ➔➔=See p xiii for details

Implantation Neurostimulator Electrodes, Cranial Nerve (Vagus Nerve Stimulation)
64568-64570

Implantation of a cranial nerve (eg, vagus nerve) neurostimulator electrode with connection of the electrode to an implanted programmable pulse generator in the infraclavicular area (64568). Revision or replacement of the cranial nerve electrode (64569). Replacement of the cranial nerve pulse generator (61885).

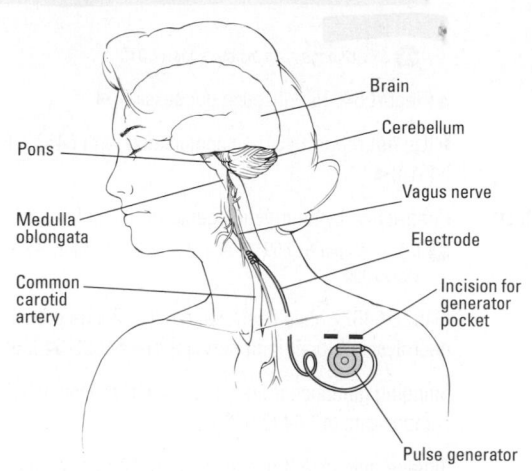

(64573 has been deleted)

64575   Incision for implantation of neurostimulator electrode array; peripheral nerve (excludes sacral nerve)
→ *CPT Changes: An Insider's View* 2002, 2011, 2012

(64577 has been deleted)

64580   neuromuscular
→ *CPT Changes: An Insider's View* 2012

64581   sacral nerve (transforaminal placement)
→ *CPT Changes: An Insider's View* 2002, 2012

Incisional Implantation of Sacral Nerve Neurostimulator
64581

Posterior View

64585   Revision or removal of peripheral neurostimulator electrode array
→ *CPT Changes: An Insider's View* 2012

64590   Insertion or replacement of peripheral or gastric neurostimulator pulse generator or receiver, direct or inductive coupling
→ *CPT Assistant* Sep 99:4, Apr 01:8, Mar 07:4, Apr 07:7, Sep 11:9; *CPT Changes: An Insider's View* 2002, 2005, 2007

(Do not report 64590 in conjunction with 64595)

64595   Revision or removal of peripheral or gastric neurostimulator pulse generator or receiver
→ *CPT Assistant* Sep 99:3, Mar 07:4, Jan 08:8; *CPT Changes: An Insider's View* 2007

►Destruction by Neurolytic Agent (eg, Chemical, Thermal, Electrical or Radiofrequency), Chemodenervation◄

►Codes 64600-64681 include the injection of other therapeutic agents (eg, corticosteroids). Do not report diagnostic/therapeutic injections separately. Do not report a code labeled as destruction when using therapies that are not destructive of the target nerve (eg, pulsed radiofrequency), use 64999. For codes labeled as chemodenervation, the supply of the chemodenervation agent is reported separately.◄

►(For chemodenervation of internal anal sphincter, use 46505)◄

►(For chemodenervation of the bladder, use 52287)◄

►(For chemodenervation for strabismus involving the extraocular muscles, use 67345)◄

►(For chemodenervation guided by needle electromyography or muscle electrical stimulation, see 95873, 95874)◄

Somatic Nerves

64600   Destruction by neurolytic agent, trigeminal nerve; supraorbital, infraorbital, mental, or inferior alveolar branch
→ *CPT Assistant* Aug 05:13, Feb 10:9

64605   second and third division branches at foramen ovale
→ *CPT Assistant* Aug 05:13, Feb 10:9

64610   second and third division branches at foramen ovale under radiologic monitoring
→ *CPT Assistant* Aug 05:13, Feb 10:9

64611   Chemodenervation of parotid and submandibular salivary glands, bilateral
→ *CPT Assistant* Feb 11:10; *CPT Changes: An Insider's View* 2011

(Report 64611 with modifier 52 if fewer than four salivary glands are injected)

▲ **64612** Chemodenervation of muscle(s); muscle(s) innervated by facial nerve, unilateral (eg, for blepharospasm, hemifacial spasm)

Botox injector

→ *CPT Assistant* Oct 98:10, Apr 01:2, Aug 05:13, Sep 06:5, Dec 08:9, Jan 09:8, Feb 10:9, 13, Dec 11:19; *CPT Changes: An Insider's View* 2000, 2001, 2013

►(To report a bilateral procedure, use modifier 50)◄

Chemodenervation of Extremity
64614

Flexor digitorum superficialis m. (cut)

Botulinum injection

Flexor digitorum profundus m.

Flexor carpi ulnaris m.

Cramped hand

Cramping relieved

64613 neck muscle(s) (eg, for spasmodic torticollis, spasmodic dysphonia)

→ *CPT Assistant* Sep 00:10, Apr 01:2, Aug 05:13, Sep 06:5, Dec 08:9, Jan 09:8, Feb 10:9, Jun 10:8; *CPT Changes: An Insider's View* 2001, 2006

►(Report 64613 only once per session)◄

►(Do not report 64613 with modifier 50)◄

▲ **64614** extremity and/or trunk muscle(s) (eg, for dystonia, cerebral palsy, multiple sclerosis)

→ *CPT Assistant* Apr 01:2, Feb 05:14, Aug 05:13, Sep 06:5, Dec 08:9, Feb 10:9, Sep 10:10; *CPT Changes: An Insider's View* 2001, 2013

►(Report 64614 only once per session)◄

● **64615** muscle(s) innervated by facial, trigeminal, cervical spinal and accessory nerves, bilateral (eg, for chronic migraine)

→ *CPT Changes: An Insider's View* 2013

►(Report 64615 only once per session)◄

►(Do not report 64615 in conjunction with 64612, 64613, 64614)◄

64620 Destruction by neurolytic agent, intercostal nerve

→ *CPT Assistant* Nov 99:38, Aug 05:13; *CPT Changes: An Insider's View* 2000

(64622-64627 have been deleted. For image guided neurolysis of facet joint nerve[s], see 64633-64636)

(Imaging guidance [fluoroscopy or CT] are inclusive components of 64333-64636)

(Image guidance [fluoroscopy or CT] and any injection of contrast are inclusive components of 64633-64636. Image guidance and localization are required for the performance of paravertebral facet joint nerve destruction by neurolytic agent described by 64633-64636. If CT or fluoroscopic imaging is not used, report 64999)

(For paravertebral facet destruction by neurolysis of the T12-L1 joint, or nerves innervating that joint, use 64633)

\# **64633** Destruction by neurolytic agent, paravertebral facet joint nerve(s), with imaging guidance (fluoroscopy or CT); cervical or thoracic, single facet joint

→ *CPT Assistant* Jun 12:10, Jul 12:6; *CPT Changes: An Insider's View* 2012

(For bilateral procedure, report 64633 with modifier 50)

\#+ **64634** cervical or thoracic, each additional facet joint (List separately in addition to code for primary procedure)

→ *CPT Assistant* Jun 12:10, Jul 12:6; *CPT Changes: An Insider's View* 2012

(Use 64634 in conjunction with 64633)

(For bilateral procedure, report 64634 with modifier 50)

\# **64635** lumbar or sacral, single facet joint

→ *CPT Assistant* Jun 12:10, Jul 12:6, 14; *CPT Changes: An Insider's View* 2012

(For bilateral procedure, report 64635 with modifier 50)

\#+ **64636** lumbar or sacral, each additional facet joint (List separately in addition to code for primary procedure)

→ *CPT Assistant* Jun 12:10, Jul 12:6, 14; *CPT Changes: An Insider's View* 2012

(Use 64636 in conjunction with 64635)

Nervous

(For bilateral procedure, report 64636 with modifier 50)

(Do not report 64633-64636 in conjunction with 77003, 77012)

64630   Destruction by neurolytic agent; pudendal nerve
    ➲ *CPT Assistant* Aug 05:13, Feb 10:9; *CPT Changes: An Insider's View* 2001

64632   plantar common digital nerve
    ➲ *CPT Assistant* Jan 09:6; *CPT Changes: An Insider's View* 2009

(Do not report 64632 in conjunction with 64455)

64633   Code is out of numerical sequence. See 64600-64640

64634   Code is out of numerical sequence. See 64600-64640

64635   Code is out of numerical sequence. See 64600-64640

64636   Code is out of numerical sequence. See 64600-64640

64640   other peripheral nerve or branch
    ➲ *CPT Assistant* Aug 05:13, Dec 09:11, Feb 10:9, Jun 12:15

Sympathetic Nerves

64650   Chemodenervation of eccrine glands; both axillae
    ➲ *CPT Assistant* Jun 08:9, Feb 10:11; *CPT Changes: An Insider's View* 2006

64653   other area(s) (eg, scalp, face, neck), per day
    ➲ *CPT Assistant* Jun 08:9; *CPT Changes: An Insider's View* 2006

(Report the specific service in conjunction with code(s) for the specific substance(s) or drug(s) provided)

(For chemodenervation of extremities (eg, hands or feet), use 64999)

▶(For chemodenervation of bladder, use 52287)◀

64680   Destruction by neurolytic agent, with or without radiologic monitoring; celiac plexus
    ➲ *CPT Assistant* Feb 99:10, Aug 05:13, Jun 08:9; *CPT Changes: An Insider's View* 2004

64681   superior hypogastric plexus
    ➲ *CPT Assistant* Aug 05:13, Dec 07:13; *CPT Changes: An Insider's View* 2004

Neuroplasty (Exploration, Neurolysis or Nerve Decompression)

Neuroplasty is the surgical decompression or freeing of intact nerve from scar tissue, including external neurolysis and/or transposition to repair or restore the nerve.

(For percutaneous neurolysis, see 62263, 62264, 62280-62282)

(For internal neurolysis requiring use of operating microscope, use 64727)

(For facial nerve decompression, use 69720)

(For neuroplasty with nerve wrapping, see 64702-64727, 64999)

64702   Neuroplasty; digital, 1 or both, same digit
    ➲ *CPT Assistant* Jun 01:11

64704   nerve of hand or foot
    ➲ *CPT Assistant* Jun 01:11

64708   Neuroplasty, major peripheral nerve, arm or leg, open; other than specified
    ➲ *CPT Assistant* Jun 01:11, Jun 12:12; *CPT Changes: An Insider's View* 2011

64712   sciatic nerve
    ➲ *CPT Assistant* Jun 01:11, Jun 12:12; *CPT Changes: An Insider's View* 2011

64713   brachial plexus
    ➲ *CPT Assistant* Jun 01:11, Jun 12:12; *CPT Changes: An Insider's View* 2011

64714   lumbar plexus
    ➲ *CPT Assistant* Jun 97:11, Sep 98:16, Jun 01:11, Jun 12:12; *CPT Changes: An Insider's View* 2011

64716   Neuroplasty and/or transposition; cranial nerve (specify)
    ➲ *CPT Assistant* Jun 01:11

64718   ulnar nerve at elbow
    ➲ *CPT Assistant* Jun 01:11, Mar 09:10

64719   ulnar nerve at wrist
    ➲ *CPT Assistant* Jun 01:11, Mar 09:10

64721   median nerve at carpal tunnel
    ➲ *CPT Assistant* Fall 92:17, Sep 97:10, Jun 01:11, Nov 06:23, Aug 09:11, Jun 12:15

(For arthroscopic procedure, use 29848)

64722   Decompression; unspecified nerve(s) (specify)
    ➲ *CPT Assistant* Sep 98:16, May 99:11, Jun 01:11, Oct 04:12

64726   plantar digital nerve
    ➲ *CPT Assistant* Jun 01:11

+ 64727 Internal neurolysis, requiring use of operating microscope (List separately in addition to code for neuroplasty) (Neuroplasty includes external neurolysis)
    ➲ *CPT Assistant* Nov 98:19, Jun 01:11, Jun 12:13

(Do not report code 69990 in addition to code 64727)

Transection or Avulsion

(For stereotactic lesion of gasserian ganglion, use 61790)

64732   Transection or avulsion of; supraorbital nerve
    ➲ *CPT Assistant* Nov 99:39; *CPT Changes: An Insider's View* 2000

64734   infraorbital nerve

64736   mental nerve

64738   inferior alveolar nerve by osteotomy

64740   lingual nerve

64742   facial nerve, differential or complete

64744   greater occipital nerve

64746   phrenic nerve

(For section of recurrent laryngeal nerve, use 31595)

Nervous

64752 vagus nerve (vagotomy), transthoracic

64755 vagus nerves limited to proximal stomach (selective proximal vagotomy, proximal gastric vagotomy, parietal cell vagotomy, supra- or highly selective vagotomy)

➔ *CPT Assistant* Nov 99:39; *CPT Changes: An Insider's View* 2000, 2002

(For laparoscopic approach, use 43652)

64760 vagus nerve (vagotomy), abdominal

➔ *CPT Assistant* Nov 99:39; *CPT Changes: An Insider's View* 2000

(For laparoscopic approach, use 43651)

64761 pudendal nerve

(For bilateral procedure, report 64761 with modifier 50)

64763 Transection or avulsion of obturator nerve, extrapelvic, with or without adductor tenotomy

(For bilateral procedure, report 64763 with modifier 50)

64766 Transection or avulsion of obturator nerve, intrapelvic, with or without adductor tenotomy

(For bilateral procedure, report 64766 with modifier 50)

64771 Transection or avulsion of other cranial nerve, extradural

64772 Transection or avulsion of other spinal nerve, extradural

(For excision of tender scar, skin and subcutaneous tissue, with or without tiny neuroma, see 11400-11446, 13100-13153)

Excision

Somatic Nerves

(For Morton neurectomy, use 28080)

64774 Excision of neuroma; cutaneous nerve, surgically identifiable

64776 digital nerve, 1 or both, same digit

+ 64778 digital nerve, each additional digit (List separately in addition to code for primary procedure)

(Use 64778 in conjunction with 64776)

64782 hand or foot, except digital nerve

+ 64783 hand or foot, each additional nerve, except same digit (List separately in addition to code for primary procedure)

(Use 64783 in conjunction with 64782)

64784 major peripheral nerve, except sciatic

64786 sciatic nerve

+ 64787 Implantation of nerve end into bone or muscle (List separately in addition to neuroma excision)

(Use 64787 in conjunction with 64774-64786)

64788 Excision of neurofibroma or neurolemmoma; cutaneous nerve

64790 major peripheral nerve

64792 extensive (including malignant type)

64795 Biopsy of nerve

Sympathetic Nerves

64802 Sympathectomy, cervical

(For bilateral procedure, report 64802 with modifier 50)

64804 Sympathectomy, cervicothoracic

(For bilateral procedure, report 64804 with modifier 50)

64809 Sympathectomy, thoracolumbar

(For bilateral procedure, report 64809 with modifier 50)

64818 Sympathectomy, lumbar

(For bilateral procedure, report 64818 with modifier 50)

64820 Sympathectomy; digital arteries, each digit

➔ *CPT Assistant* Jan 04:27; *CPT Changes: An Insider's View* 2002

(Do not report 69990 in addition to code 64820)

64821 radial artery

➔ *CPT Changes: An Insider's View* 2002

(Do not report 69990 in addition to code 64821)

64822 ulnar artery

➔ *CPT Changes: An Insider's View* 2002

(Do not report 69990 in addition to code 64822)

64823 superficial palmar arch

➔ *CPT Changes: An Insider's View* 2002

(Do not report 69990 in addition to code 64823)

Neurorrhaphy

64831 Suture of digital nerve, hand or foot; 1 nerve

➔ *CPT Assistant* Apr 00:5

+ 64832 each additional digital nerve (List separately in addition to code for primary procedure)

➔ *CPT Assistant* Apr 00:5

(Use 64832 in conjunction with 64831)

64834 Suture of 1 nerve; hand or foot, common sensory nerve

➔ *CPT Changes: An Insider's View* 2008

64835 median motor thenar

➔ *CPT Changes: An Insider's View* 2008

64836 ulnar motor

➔ *CPT Changes: An Insider's View* 2008

+ 64837 Suture of each additional nerve, hand or foot (List separately in addition to code for primary procedure)

(Use 64837 in conjunction with 64834-64836)

64840 Suture of posterior tibial nerve

64856 Suture of major peripheral nerve, arm or leg, except sciatic; including transposition

64857   without transposition

64858 Suture of sciatic nerve

+ 64859 Suture of each additional major peripheral nerve (List separately in addition to code for primary procedure)

(Use 64859 in conjunction with 64856, 64857)

64861 Suture of; brachial plexus

64862   lumbar plexus

64864 Suture of facial nerve; extracranial

64865   infratemporal, with or without grafting

64866 Anastomosis; facial-spinal accessory

64868   facial-hypoglossal

64870   facial-phrenic

+ 64872 Suture of nerve; requiring secondary or delayed suture (List separately in addition to code for primary neurorrhaphy)

(Use 64872 in conjunction with 64831-64865)

+ 64874   requiring extensive mobilization, or transposition of nerve (List separately in addition to code for nerve suture)

(Use 64874 in conjunction with 64831-64865)

+ 64876   requiring shortening of bone of extremity (List separately in addition to code for nerve suture)

(Use 64876 in conjunction with 64831-64865)

Neurorrhaphy With Nerve Graft, Vein Graft, or Conduit

64885 Nerve graft (includes obtaining graft), head or neck; up to 4 cm in length
  → *CPT Assistant* Nov 00:11

64886   more than 4 cm length
  → *CPT Assistant* Nov 00:11

64890 Nerve graft (includes obtaining graft), single strand, hand or foot; up to 4 cm length

64891   more than 4 cm length

64892 Nerve graft (includes obtaining graft), single strand, arm or leg; up to 4 cm length

64893   more than 4 cm length

64895 Nerve graft (includes obtaining graft), multiple strands (cable), hand or foot; up to 4 cm length
  → *CPT Assistant* Nov 00:11

64896   more than 4 cm length
  → *CPT Assistant* Nov 00:11

64897 Nerve graft (includes obtaining graft), multiple strands (cable), arm or leg; up to 4 cm length
  → *CPT Assistant* Nov 00:11

64898   more than 4 cm length
  → *CPT Assistant* Nov 00:11

+ 64901 Nerve graft, each additional nerve; single strand (List separately in addition to code for primary procedure)
  → *CPT Assistant* Nov 00:11

(Use 64901 in conjunction with 64885-64893)

+ 64902   multiple strands (cable) (List separately in addition to code for primary procedure)
  → *CPT Assistant* Nov 00:11

(Use 64902 in conjunction with 64885, 64886, 64895-64898)

64905 Nerve pedicle transfer; first stage

64907   second stage

64910 Nerve repair; with synthetic conduit or vein allograft (eg, nerve tube), each nerve
  → *CPT Assistant* Nov 07:4; *CPT Changes: An Insider's View* 2007

64911   with autogenous vein graft (includes harvest of vein graft), each nerve
  → *CPT Assistant* Nov 07:4; *CPT Changes: An Insider's View* 2007

(Do not report 69990 in addition to 64910, 64911)

Other Procedures

64999 Unlisted procedure, nervous system
  → *CPT Assistant* Apr 96:11, Sep 98:16, Oct 98:10, Jan 00:10, Aug 00:7, Sep 00:10, Feb 02:10, Nov 03:5, Oct 04:11, Apr 05:13, Aug 05:13, Sep 05:9, Sep 07:10, Nov 07:4, Dec 07:8, Jul 08:9, Sep 08:11, Aug 09:8, Dec 09:11, Jun 10:8, Sep 10:10, Nov 10:4, Apr 11:12, Jul 11:12, 16-17, Sep 11:12, Jan 12:14, Feb 12:11, May 12:14

Notes

⊙=Moderate sedation ✚=Add-on code ✗=FDA approval pending #=Resequenced code ○=Recycled/reinstated code ➔➔=See p xiii for details

Surgery

Eye anatomy

Eye and Ocular Adnexa

(For diagnostic and treatment ophthalmological services, see **Medicine, Ophthalmology,** and 92002 et seq)

(Do not report code 69990 in addition to codes 65091-68850)

Eyeball

Removal of Eye

65091   Evisceration of ocular contents; without implant

65093   with implant

65101   Enucleation of eye; without implant

65103   with implant, muscles not attached to implant

65105   with implant, muscles attached to implant

(For conjunctivoplasty after enucleation, see 68320 et seq)

65110   Exenteration of orbit (does not include skin graft), removal of orbital contents; only

65112   with therapeutic removal of bone

65114   with muscle or myocutaneous flap

(For skin graft to orbit (split skin), see 15120, 15121; free, full thickness, see 15260, 15261)

(For eyelid repair involving more than skin, see 67930 et seq)

Secondary Implant(s) Procedures

An ocular implant is an implant inside muscular cone; an orbital implant is an implant outside muscular cone.

65125   Modification of ocular implant with placement or replacement of pegs (eg, drilling receptacle for prosthesis appendage) (separate procedure)

65130   Insertion of ocular implant secondary; after evisceration, in scleral shell

65135   after enucleation, muscles not attached to implant

65140   after enucleation, muscles attached to implant

65150   Reinsertion of ocular implant, with or without conjunctival graft

65155   with use of foreign material for reinforcement and/or attachment of muscles to implant

65175   Removal of ocular implant

(For orbital implant (implant outside muscle cone) insertion, use 67550; removal, use 67560)

Removal of Foreign Body

(For removal of implanted material: ocular implant, use 65175; anterior segment implant, use 65920; posterior segment implant, use 67120; orbital implant, use 67560)

(For diagnostic x-ray for foreign body, use 70030)

(For diagnostic echography for foreign body, use 76529)

(For removal of foreign body from orbit: frontal approach, use 67413; lateral approach, use 67430; transcranial approach, use 61334)

(For removal of foreign body from eyelid, embedded, use 67938)

(For removal of foreign body from lacrimal system, use 68530)

65205   Removal of foreign body, external eye; conjunctival superficial
> *CPT Assistant* Mar 05:17

65210   conjunctival embedded (includes concretions), subconjunctival, or scleral nonperforating

65220   corneal, without slit lamp

65222   corneal, with slit lamp

(For repair of corneal laceration with foreign body, use 65275)

65235   Removal of foreign body, intraocular; from anterior chamber of eye or lens
> *CPT Changes: An Insider's View* 2002

(For removal of implanted material from anterior segment, use 65920)

65260   from posterior segment, magnetic extraction, anterior or posterior route

65265   from posterior segment, nonmagnetic extraction

(For removal of implanted material from posterior segment, use 67120)

Repair of Laceration

(For fracture of orbit, see 21385 et seq)

(For repair of wound of eyelid, skin, linear, simple, see 12011-12018; intermediate, layered closure, see 12051-12057; linear, complex, see 13150-13160; other, see 67930, 67935)

(For repair of wound of lacrimal system, use 68700)

(For repair of operative wound, use 66250)

65270   Repair of laceration; conjunctiva, with or without nonperforating laceration sclera, direct closure

65272   conjunctiva, by mobilization and rearrangement, without hospitalization

65273   conjunctiva, by mobilization and rearrangement, with hospitalization

Eye/Occular Adnexa

65275   cornea, nonperforating, with or without removal foreign body

65280   cornea and/or sclera, perforating, not involving uveal tissue

65285   cornea and/or sclera, perforating, with reposition or resection of uveal tissue

(65280 and 65285 are not used for repair of a surgical wound)

65286   application of tissue glue, wounds of cornea and/or sclera

➔ *CPT Assistant* May 99:11, Apr 09:5

(Repair of laceration includes use of conjunctival flap and restoration of anterior chamber, by air or saline injection when indicated)

(For repair of iris or ciliary body, use 66680)

65290   Repair of wound, extraocular muscle, tendon and/or Tenon's capsule

Anterior Segment

Cornea

Excision

65400   Excision of lesion, cornea (keratectomy, lamellar, partial), except pterygium

65410   Biopsy of cornea

65420   Excision or transposition of pterygium; without graft
➔ *CPT Assistant* Dec 07:13

65426   with graft

Removal or Destruction

65430   Scraping of cornea, diagnostic, for smear and/or culture

65435   Removal of corneal epithelium; with or without chemocauterization (abrasion, curettage)

65436   with application of chelating agent (eg, EDTA)

65450   Destruction of lesion of cornea by cryotherapy, photocoagulation or thermocauterization

Cryotherapy of Lesion on Cornea
65450

A freezing probe is applied directly to the corneal defect to destroy it.

- Cryoprobe
- Frozen area
- Anterior chamber
- Lens
- Cornea
- Ciliary body
- Conjunctiva

65600   Multiple punctures of anterior cornea (eg, for corneal erosion, tattoo)

Keratoplasty

Corneal transplant includes use of fresh or preserved grafts. The preparation of donor material is included for penetrating or anterior lamellar keratoplasty, but reported separately for endothelial keratoplasty. Do not report 65710-65757 in conjunction with 92025.

(Keratoplasty excludes refractive keratoplasty procedures, 65760, 65765, and 65767)

65710   Keratoplasty (corneal transplant); anterior lamellar
➔ *CPT Assistant* Oct 02:8, Apr 09:5, Dec 09:13; *CPT Changes: An Insider's View* 2009

65730   penetrating (except in aphakia or pseudophakia)
➔ *CPT Assistant* Oct 02:8, Feb 06:1, Apr 09:5, Dec 09:13; *CPT Changes: An Insider's View* 2009

65750   penetrating (in aphakia)
➔ *CPT Assistant* Oct 02:8, Apr 09:5, Dec 09:13

65755   penetrating (in pseudophakia)
➔ *CPT Assistant* Winter 90:8, Oct 02:9, Apr 09:5, Dec 09:13

65756   endothelial
➔ *CPT Changes: An Insider's View* 2009

+ 65757   Backbench preparation of corneal endothelial allograft prior to transplantation (List separately in addition to code for primary procedure)
➔ *CPT Changes: An Insider's View* 2009

(Use 65757 in conjunction with 65756)

Other Procedures

Do not report 65760-65771 in conjunction with 92025.

65760   Keratomileusis
➔ *CPT Assistant* Oct 02:9

65765   Keratophakia
➔ *CPT Assistant* Oct 02:10

65767   Epikeratoplasty
    ↪ *CPT Assistant* Winter 90:8, Oct 02:10

65770   Keratoprosthesis
    ↪ *CPT Assistant* Oct 02:10

65771   Radial keratotomy
    ↪ *CPT Assistant* Winter 90:8, Oct 02:10

65772   Corneal relaxing incision for correction of surgically
    induced astigmatism
    ↪ *CPT Assistant* Oct 02:10, 12

65775   Corneal wedge resection for correction of surgically
    induced astigmatism
    ↪ *CPT Assistant* Oct 02:10, 12

(For fitting of contact lens for treatment of disease, see
92071, 92072)

(For unlisted procedures on cornea, use 66999)

65778   Placement of amniotic membrane on the ocular surface
    for wound healing; self-retaining
    ↪ *CPT Changes: An Insider's View* 2011

65779   single layer, sutured
      ↪ *CPT Changes: An Insider's View* 2011

(Do not report 65778, 65779 in conjunction with 65430,
65435, 65780)

(For placement of amniotic membrane using tissue glue,
use 66999)

65780   Ocular surface reconstruction; amniotic membrane
    transplantation, multiple layers
    ↪ *CPT Assistant* May 04:10, Jun 09:9; *CPT Changes: An Insider's
    View* 2004, 2011

(For placement of amniotic membrane without
reconstruction using self-retaining or single layer suture
technique, see 65778, 65779)

65781   limbal stem cell allograft (eg, cadaveric or living
      donor)
      ↪ *CPT Assistant* May 04:10; *CPT Changes: An Insider's View*
      2004

65782   limbal conjunctival autograft (includes obtaining
      graft)
      ↪ *CPT Assistant* Feb 04:11, May 04:10, Feb 05:15-16; *CPT
      Changes: An Insider's View* 2004

(For harvesting conjunctival allograft, living donor, use
68371)

Anterior Chamber

Incision

▲ **65800**   Paracentesis of anterior chamber of eye (separate
    procedure); with removal of aqueous
    ↪ *CPT Changes: An Insider's View* 2013

▶(65805 has been deleted. To report, use 65800)◀

65810   with removal of vitreous and/or discission of anterior
      hyaloid membrane, with or without air injection

65815   with removal of blood, with or without irrigation and/
      or air injection

(For injection, see 66020-66030)

(For removal of blood clot, use 65930)

65820   Goniotomy
    ↪ *CPT Assistant* Sep 05:12

(Do not report modifier 63 in conjunction with 65820)

(For use of ophthalmic endoscope with 65820, use 66990)

65850   Trabeculotomy ab externo

65855   Trabeculoplasty by laser surgery, 1 or more sessions
    (defined treatment series)
    ↪ *CPT Assistant* Mar 98:7, Mar 03:23

(If re-treatment is necessary after several months
because of disease progression, a new treatment or
treatment series should be reported with a modifier, if
necessary, to indicate lesser or greater complexity)

(For trabeculectomy, use 66170)

65860   Severing adhesions of anterior segment, laser technique
    (separate procedure)

65865   Severing adhesions of anterior segment of eye, incisional
    technique (with or without injection of air or liquid)
    (separate procedure); goniosynechiae

(For trabeculoplasty by laser surgery, use 65855)

65870   anterior synechiae, except goniosynechiae

65875   posterior synechiae
      ↪ *CPT Assistant* Sep 05:12

(For use of ophthalmic endoscope with 65875, use 66990)

65880   corneovitreal adhesions

(For laser surgery, use 66821)

Removal

65900   Removal of epithelial downgrowth, anterior chamber of
    eye
    ↪ *CPT Changes: An Insider's View* 2002

65920   Removal of implanted material, anterior segment of eye
    ↪ *CPT Assistant* Sep 05:12; *CPT Changes: An Insider's View* 2002

(For use of ophthalmic endoscope with 65920, use 66990)

65930   Removal of blood clot, anterior segment of eye
    ↪ *CPT Changes: An Insider's View* 2002

Introduction

66020   Injection, anterior chamber of eye (separate procedure);
    air or liquid
    ↪ *CPT Changes: An Insider's View* 2002

66030   medication

(For unlisted procedures on anterior segment, use 66999)

Eye/Occular Adnexa

Anterior Sclera

Excision

(For removal of intraocular foreign body, use 65235)

(For operations on posterior sclera, use 67250, 67255)

66130 Excision of lesion, sclera

66150 Fistulization of sclera for glaucoma; trephination with iridectomy

66155 thermocauterization with iridectomy

66160 sclerectomy with punch or scissors, with iridectomy

66165 iridencleisis or iridotasis

66170 trabeculectomy ab externo in absence of previous surgery
➔ *CPT Assistant* Jul 03:4, Nov 03:10

(For trabeculotomy ab externo, use 65850)

(For repair of operative wound, use 66250)

66172 trabeculectomy ab externo with scarring from previous ocular surgery or trauma (includes injection of antifibrotic agents)
➔ *CPT Assistant* Jul 03:4, Nov 03:10

66174 Transluminal dilation of aqueous outflow canal; without retention of device or stent
➔ *CPT Changes: An Insider's View* 2011

66175 with retention of device or stent
➔ *CPT Changes: An Insider's View* 2011

Aqueous Shunt

66180 Aqueous shunt to extraocular reservoir (eg, Molteno, Schocket, Denver-Krupin)
➔ *CPT Assistant* Winter 90:8, Aug 03:9, Sep 03:2, Jun 12:15

66185 Revision of aqueous shunt to extraocular reservoir
➔ *CPT Assistant* Winter 90:8

(For removal of implanted shunt, use 67120)

Repair or Revision

(For scleral procedures in retinal surgery, see 67101 et seq)

66220 Repair of scleral staphyloma; without graft

66225 with graft

(For scleral reinforcement, see 67250, 67255)

66250 Revision or repair of operative wound of anterior segment, any type, early or late, major or minor procedure
➔ *CPT Assistant* Oct 10:15, Dec 10:15

(For unlisted procedures on anterior sclera, use 66999)

Iris, Ciliary Body

Incision

66500 Iridotomy by stab incision (separate procedure); except transfixion

66505 with transfixion as for iris bombe

(For iridotomy by photocoagulation, use 66761)

Excision

66600 Iridectomy, with corneoscleral or corneal section; for removal of lesion

66605 with cyclectomy

66625 peripheral for glaucoma (separate procedure)

66630 sector for glaucoma (separate procedure)

66635 optical (separate procedure)

(For coreoplasty by photocoagulation, use 66762)

Repair

66680 Repair of iris, ciliary body (as for iridodialysis)

(For reposition or resection of uveal tissue with perforating wound of cornea or sclera, use 65285)

66682 Suture of iris, ciliary body (separate procedure) with retrieval of suture through small incision (eg, McCannel suture)

Destruction

66700 Ciliary body destruction; diathermy

66710 cyclophotocoagulation, transscleral
➔ *CPT Assistant* Mar 05:20, Sep 05:5; *CPT Changes: An Insider's View* 2005

66711 cyclophotocoagulation, endoscopic
➔ *CPT Assistant* Mar 05:20, Sep 05:5, 12; *CPT Changes: An Insider's View* 2005

(Do not report 66711 in conjunction with 66990)

⊙ **66720** cryotherapy

66740 cyclodialysis

66761 Iridotomy/iridectomy by laser surgery (eg, for glaucoma) (per session)
➔ *CPT Assistant* Mar 98:7; *CPT Changes: An Insider's View* 2011

66762 Iridoplasty by photocoagulation (1 or more sessions) (eg, for improvement of vision, for widening of anterior chamber angle)
➔ *CPT Assistant* Mar 98:7

66770   Destruction of cyst or lesion iris or ciliary body (nonexcisional procedure)

(For excision lesion iris, ciliary body, see 66600, 66605; for removal of epithelial downgrowth, use 65900)

(For unlisted procedures on iris, ciliary body, use 66999)

Lens

Incision

66820   Discission of secondary membranous cataract (opacified posterior lens capsule and/or anterior hyaloid); stab incision technique (Ziegler or Wheeler knife)

66821   laser surgery (eg, YAG laser) (1 or more stages)

66825   Repositioning of intraocular lens prosthesis, requiring an incision (separate procedure)

Removal

Lateral canthotomy, iridectomy, iridotomy, anterior capsulotomy, posterior capsulotomy, the use of viscoelastic agents, enzymatic zonulysis, use of other pharmacologic agents, and subconjunctival or sub-tenon injections are included as part of the code for the extraction of lens.

66830   Removal of secondary membranous cataract (opacified posterior lens capsule and/or anterior hyaloid) with corneo-scleral section, with or without iridectomy (iridocapsulotomy, iridocapsulectomy)

66840   Removal of lens material; aspiration technique, 1 or more stages
→ *CPT Assistant* Fall 92:4, Jan 09:7, Apr 09:9, Sep 09:5

66850   phacofragmentation technique (mechanical or ultrasonic) (eg, phacoemulsification), with aspiration
→ *CPT Assistant* Fall 92:6, Jan 09:7, Apr 09:9, Sep 09:5

66852   pars plana approach, with or without vitrectomy
→ *CPT Assistant* Fall 92:8, Jan 09:7, Apr 09:9, Sep 09:5

66920   intracapsular
→ *CPT Assistant* Fall 92:8, Sep 09:5

66930   intracapsular, for dislocated lens
→ *CPT Assistant* Fall 92:8, Sep 09:5

66940   extracapsular (other than 66840, 66850, 66852)
→ *CPT Assistant* Fall 92:4, Jan 09:7, Apr 09:9, Sep 09:5

(For removal of intralenticular foreign body without lens extraction, use 65235)

(For repair of operative wound, use 66250)

Intraocular Lens Procedures

66982   Extracapsular cataract removal with insertion of intraocular lens prosthesis (1-stage procedure), manual or mechanical technique (eg, irrigation and aspiration or phacoemulsification), complex, requiring devices or techniques not generally used in routine cataract surgery (eg, iris expansion device, suture support for intraocular lens, or primary posterior capsulorrhexis) or performed on patients in the amblyogenic developmental stage
→ *CPT Assistant* Feb 01:7, Nov 03:10, Sep 09:5; *CPT Changes: An Insider's View* 2001, 2002

►(For insertion of ocular telescope prosthesis including removal of crystalline lens, use 0308T)◄

66983   Intracapsular cataract extraction with insertion of intraocular lens prosthesis (1 stage procedure)
→ *CPT Assistant* Fall 92:5, 8, Nov 03:10, Sep 09:5

►(Do not report 66983 in conjunction with 0308T)◄

66984   Extracapsular cataract removal with insertion of intraocular lens prosthesis (1 stage procedure), manual or mechanical technique (eg, irrigation and aspiration or phacoemulsification)
→ *CPT Assistant* Fall 92:5, 8, Feb 01:7, Nov 03:10, Mar 05:11, Sep 09:5

(For complex extracapsular cataract removal, use 66982)

►(For insertion of ocular telescope prosthesis including removal of crystalline lens, use 0308T)◄

66985   Insertion of intraocular lens prosthesis (secondary implant), not associated with concurrent cataract removal
→ *CPT Assistant* Sep 05:12, Sep 09:5, Dec 11:16

(To code implant at time of concurrent cataract surgery, see 66982, 66983, 66984)

►(To report supply of intraocular lens prosthesis, use 99070)◄

(For ultrasonic determination of intraocular lens power, use 76519)

(For removal of implanted material from anterior segment, use 65920)

(For secondary fixation (separate procedure), use 66682)

(For use of ophthalmic endoscope with 66985, use 66990)

66986   Exchange of intraocular lens
→ *CPT Assistant* Sep 05:12

(For use of ophthalmic endoscope with 66986, use 66990)

Other Procedures

+ **66990**   Use of ophthalmic endoscope (List separately in addition to code for primary procedure)
→ *CPT Assistant* Sep 05:12, Oct 08:3; *CPT Changes: An Insider's View* 2003

(66990 may be used only with codes 65820, 65875, 65920, 66985, 66986, 67036, 67039, 67040, 67041, 67042, 67043, 67112, 67113)

66999   Unlisted procedure, anterior segment of eye

▲=Revised code   ●=New code   ► ◄=Contains new or revised text   ⊘=Modifier 51 exempt

Posterior Segment

Vitreous

67005   Removal of vitreous, anterior approach (open sky technique or limbal incision); partial removal
   ➔ *CPT Assistant* Fall 92:4

67010   subtotal removal with mechanical vitrectomy
   ➔ *CPT Assistant* Fall 92:4

   (For removal of vitreous by paracentesis of anterior chamber, use 65810)

   (For removal of corneovitreal adhesions, use 65880)

67015   Aspiration or release of vitreous, subretinal or choroidal fluid, pars plana approach (posterior sclerotomy)

67025   Injection of vitreous substitute, pars plana or limbal approach (fluid-gas exchange), with or without aspiration (separate procedure)

67027   Implantation of intravitreal drug delivery system (eg, ganciclovir implant), includes concomitant removal of vitreous
   ➔ *CPT Assistant* Nov 97:23, Nov 98:1

Intravitreal Drug Delivery System
67027

A drug delivery system that releases medication into the vitreous is implanted into the vitreous by pars plana incision.

(For removal, use 67121)

67028   Intravitreal injection of a pharmacologic agent (separate procedure)
   ➔ *CPT Assistant* Winter 90:9

67030   Discission of vitreous strands (without removal), pars plana approach

67031   Severing of vitreous strands, vitreous face adhesions, sheets, membranes or opacities, laser surgery (1 or more stages)

67036   Vitrectomy, mechanical, pars plana approach;
   ➔ *CPT Assistant* Fall 92:6, Oct 08:3

   (For application of intraocular epiretinal radiation with 67036, use 0190T)

67039   with focal endolaser photocoagulation
   ➔ *CPT Assistant* Winter 90:9, Sep 05:12

67040   with endolaser panretinal photocoagulation
   ➔ *CPT Assistant* Winter 90:9, Sep 05:12, Jul 07:12

67041   with removal of preretinal cellular membrane (eg, macular pucker)
   ➔ *CPT Changes: An Insider's View* 2008

67042   with removal of internal limiting membrane of retina (eg, for repair of macular hole, diabetic macular edema), includes, if performed, intraocular tamponade (ie, air, gas or silicone oil)
   ➔ *CPT Changes: An Insider's View* 2008

67043   with removal of subretinal membrane (eg, choroidal neovascularization), includes, if performed, intraocular tamponade (ie, air, gas or silicone oil) and laser photocoagulation
   ➔ *CPT Changes: An Insider's View* 2008

   (For use of ophthalmic endoscope with 67036, 67039, 67040-67043, use 66990)

   (For associated lensectomy, use 66850)

   (For use of vitrectomy in retinal detachment surgery, see 67108, 67113)

   (For associated removal of foreign body, see 65260, 65265)

   (For unlisted procedures on vitreous, use 67299)

Retina or Choroid

Repair

(If diathermy, cryotherapy and/or photocoagulation are combined, report under principal modality used)

67101   Repair of retinal detachment, 1 or more sessions; cryotherapy or diathermy, with or without drainage of subretinal fluid
   ➔ *CPT Assistant* Mar 98:7

67105   photocoagulation, with or without drainage of subretinal fluid
   ➔ *CPT Assistant* Mar 98:7

67107   Repair of retinal detachment; scleral buckling (such as lamellar scleral dissection, imbrication or encircling procedure), with or without implant, with or without cryotherapy, photocoagulation, and drainage of subretinal fluid

Repair of Retinal Detachment
67107

The retinal tear is treated externally by placing a hot or cold probe over the sclera and then depressing it. The burn seals the choroid to the retina at the site of the tear. The healing scar is supported by the encircling band, which buckles the eye.

Clove hitch suture securing ends of buckle

Silicone sponge

Encircling silicone exoplant

67108   with vitrectomy, any method, with or without air or gas tamponade, focal endolaser photocoagulation, cryotherapy, drainage of subretinal fluid, scleral buckling, and/or removal of lens by same technique
➔ *CPT Assistant* Winter 90:9, Mar 12:9

67110   by injection of air or other gas (eg, pneumatic retinopexy)
➔ *CPT Assistant* Winter 90:9

67112   by scleral buckling or vitrectomy, on patient having previous ipsilateral retinal detachment repair(s) using scleral buckling or vitrectomy techniques

(For aspiration or drainage of subretinal or subchoroidal fluid, use 67015)

(For use of ophthalmic endoscope with 67112, use 66990)

67113   Repair of complex retinal detachment (eg, proliferative vitreoretinopathy, stage C-1 or greater, diabetic traction retinal detachment, retinopathy of prematurity, retinal tear of greater than 90 degrees), with vitrectomy and membrane peeling, may include air, gas, or silicone oil tamponade, cryotherapy, endolaser photocoagulation, drainage of subretinal fluid, scleral buckling, and/or removal of lens
➔ *CPT Changes: An Insider's View* 2008

(To report vitrectomy, pars plana approach, other than in retinal detachment surgery, see 67036-67043)

(For use of ophthalmic endoscope with 67113, use 66990)

67115   Release of encircling material (posterior segment)

67120   Removal of implanted material, posterior segment; extraocular

67121   intraocular
➔ *CPT Assistant* Nov 97:23, Nov 98:19

(For removal from anterior segment, use 65920)

(For removal of foreign body, see 65260, 65265)

Prophylaxis

Codes 67141, 67145 include treatment at one or more sessions that may occur at different encounters. These codes should be reported once during a defined treatment period.

Repetitive services. The services listed below are often performed in multiple sessions or groups of sessions. The methods of reporting vary.

The following descriptors are intended to include all sessions in a defined treatment period.

67141   Prophylaxis of retinal detachment (eg, retinal break, lattice degeneration) without drainage, 1 or more sessions; cryotherapy, diathermy
➔ *CPT Assistant* Mar 98:7, Oct 08:3

67145   photocoagulation (laser or xenon arc)
➔ *CPT Assistant* Fall 92:4, Mar 98:7

Destruction

Codes 67208, 67210, 67218, 67220, 67227, 67228, 67229 include treatment at one or more sessions that may occur at different encounters. These codes should be reported once during a defined treatment period.

67208   Destruction of localized lesion of retina (eg, macular edema, tumors), 1 or more sessions; cryotherapy, diathermy
➔ *CPT Assistant* Mar 98:7, Nov 98:19, Oct 08:3

67210   photocoagulation
➔ *CPT Assistant* Mar 98:7, Nov 98:19, Oct 08:3, Jan 12:3

67218   radiation by implantation of source (includes removal of source)
➔ *CPT Assistant* Mar 98:7, Oct 08:3

67220   Destruction of localized lesion of choroid (eg, choroidal neovascularization); photocoagulation (eg, laser), 1 or more sessions
➔ *CPT Assistant* Nov 98:19, Nov 99:39, Feb 01:8, Oct 08:3, Jan 12:3; *CPT Changes: An Insider's View* 2000, 2001

67221   photodynamic therapy (includes intravenous infusion)
➔ *CPT Assistant* Feb 01:8, Sep 01:10, Jun 02:10; *CPT Changes: An Insider's View* 2001

+ 67225   photodynamic therapy, second eye, at single session (List separately in addition to code for primary eye treatment)
➔ *CPT Assistant* Jun 02:10; *CPT Changes: An Insider's View* 2002

(Use 67225 in conjunction with 67221)

Eye/Occular Adnexa

67227 Destruction of extensive or progressive retinopathy (eg, diabetic retinopathy), 1 or more sessions, cryotherapy, diathermy

> *CPT Assistant* Mar 98:7, Oct 08:3; *CPT Changes: An Insider's View* 2008

67228 Treatment of extensive or progressive retinopathy, 1 or more sessions; (eg, diabetic retinopathy), photocoagulation

> *CPT Assistant* Mar 98:7, Oct 08:3; *CPT Changes: An Insider's View* 2008

67229 preterm infant (less than 37 weeks gestation at birth), performed from birth up to 1 year of age (eg, retinopathy of prematurity), photocoagulation or cryotherapy

> *CPT Changes: An Insider's View* 2008

(For bilateral procedure, use modifier 50)

(For unlisted procedures on retina, use 67299)

Posterior Sclera

Repair

(For excision lesion sclera, use 66130)

67250 Scleral reinforcement (separate procedure); without graft

67255 with graft

> *CPT Assistant* Jun 12:15

(For repair scleral staphyloma, see 66220, 66225)

Other Procedures

67299 Unlisted procedure, posterior segment

Ocular Adnexa

Extraocular Muscles of Right Eye

Extraocular Muscles

67311 Strabismus surgery, recession or resection procedure; 1 horizontal muscle

> *CPT Assistant* Summer 93:20, Mar 97:5, Nov 98:19, Sep 02:10

Strabismus Surgery—Horizontal Muscles
67311-67312

In Figure A, the medial or lateral rectus muscle is made weaker by recession (retroplacement of the muscle attachment). In Figure B, it is made stronger by resection (removal of a segment). Use 67311 for one horizontal muscle and 67312 for two muscles of the same eye.

67312 2 horizontal muscles

> *CPT Assistant* Summer 93:20, Mar 97:5

67314 1 vertical muscle (excluding superior oblique)

> *CPT Assistant* Summer 93:20, Mar 97:5

67316   2 or more vertical muscles (excluding superior oblique)

➔ *CPT Assistant* Summer 93:20, Mar 97:5

(For adjustable sutures, use 67335 in addition to codes 67311-67334 for primary procedure reflecting number of muscles operated on)

Strabismus Surgery—Vertical Muscles
67314-67316

Either the superior or inferior rectus muscle is strengthened or weakened. Use 67316 for two muscles of the same eye.

Inferior (or superior) rectus muscle

67318   Strabismus surgery, any procedure, superior oblique muscle

➔ *CPT Assistant* Summer 93:20, Mar 97:5, Nov 98:19

+ 67320   Transposition procedure (eg, for paretic extraocular muscle), any extraocular muscle (specify) (List separately in addition to code for primary procedure)

➔ *CPT Assistant* Summer 93:20, Mar 97:5

(Use 67320 in conjunction with 67311-67318)

Transposition Procedure
67320

The extraocular muscles are transposed.

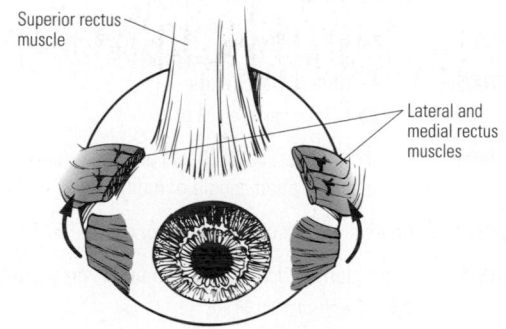

Superior rectus muscle

Lateral and medial rectus muscles

+ 67331   Strabismus surgery on patient with previous eye surgery or injury that did not involve the extraocular muscles (List separately in addition to code for primary procedure)

➔ *CPT Assistant* Summer 93:20, Mar 97:5

(Use 67331 in conjunction with 67311-67318)

+ 67332   Strabismus surgery on patient with scarring of extraocular muscles (eg, prior ocular injury, strabismus or retinal detachment surgery) or restrictive myopathy (eg, dysthyroid ophthalmopathy) (List separately in addition to code for primary procedure)

➔ *CPT Assistant* Summer 93:20, Mar 97:5

(Use 67332 in conjunction with 67311-67318)

+ 67334   Strabismus surgery by posterior fixation suture technique, with or without muscle recession (List separately in addition to code for primary procedure)

➔ *CPT Assistant* Summer 93:20, Mar 97:5

(Use 67334 in conjunction with 67311-67318)

+ 67335   Placement of adjustable suture(s) during strabismus surgery, including postoperative adjustment(s) of suture(s) (List separately in addition to code for specific strabismus surgery)

➔ *CPT Assistant* Summer 93:20, Mar 97:5

(Use 67335 in conjunction with 67311-67334)

Strabismus Surgery—Adjustable Sutures
67335

Sutures are tied in such a way as to allow the tension on the muscle to be adjusted after the anesthetic is not affecting the position of the globe.

Superior rectus muscle

Adjustable suture

+ 67340   Strabismus surgery involving exploration and/or repair of detached extraocular muscle(s) (List separately in addition to code for primary procedure)

➔ *CPT Assistant* Summer 93:20, Mar 97:5

(Use 67340 in conjunction with 67311-67334)

67343   Release of extensive scar tissue without detaching extraocular muscle (separate procedure)

➔ *CPT Assistant* Summer 93:20, Mar 97:5

(Use 67343 in conjunction with 67311-67340, when such procedures are performed other than on the affected muscle)

67345   Chemodenervation of extraocular muscle

➔ *CPT Assistant* Summer 93:20, Mar 97:5, Apr 00:2, Feb 10:13

(For chemodenervation for blepharospasm and other neurological disorders, see 64612 and 64613)

Eye/Occular Adnexa

67346   Biopsy of extraocular muscle
> *CPT Changes: An Insider's View* 2007

(For repair of wound, extraocular muscle, tendon or Tenon's capsule, use 65290)

Other Procedures

67399   Unlisted procedure, ocular muscle

Orbit

Exploration, Excision, Decompression

67400   Orbitotomy without bone flap (frontal or transconjunctival approach); for exploration, with or without biopsy

67405   with drainage only

67412   with removal of lesion

67413   with removal of foreign body

67414   with removal of bone for decompression
> *CPT Assistant* Jul 99:10

67415   Fine needle aspiration of orbital contents

(For exenteration, enucleation, and repair, see 65101 et seq; for optic nerve decompression, use 67570)

67420   Orbitotomy with bone flap or window, lateral approach (eg, Kroenlein); with removal of lesion

67430   with removal of foreign body

67440   with drainage

67445   with removal of bone for decompression

(For optic nerve sheath decompression, use 67570)

67450   for exploration, with or without biopsy

(For orbitotomy, transcranial approach, see 61330-61334)

(For orbital implant, see 67550, 67560)

(For removal of eyeball or for repair after removal, see 65091-65175)

Other Procedures

67500   Retrobulbar injection; medication (separate procedure, does not include supply of medication)

67505   alcohol

67515   Injection of medication or other substance into Tenon's capsule
> *CPT Changes: An Insider's View* 2002

(For subconjunctival injection, use 68200)

67550   Orbital implant (implant outside muscle cone); insertion

67560   removal or revision

(For ocular implant (implant inside muscle cone), see 65093-65105, 65130-65175)

(For treatment of fractures of malar area, orbit, see 21355 et seq)

67570   Optic nerve decompression (eg, incision or fenestration of optic nerve sheath)

67599   Unlisted procedure, orbit

Eyelids

Incision

67700   Blepharotomy, drainage of abscess, eyelid

67710   Severing of tarsorrhaphy

67715   Canthotomy (separate procedure)

(For canthoplasty, use 67950)

(For division of symblepharon, use 68340)

#▲ **67810**   Incisional biopsy of eyelid skin including lid margin
> *CPT Assistant* Dec 04:19; *CPT Changes: An Insider's View* 2013

►(For biopsy of skin of the eyelid, see 11100, 11101, 11310-11313)◄

Excision, Destruction

Codes for removal of lesion include more than skin (ie, involving lid margin, tarsus, and/or palpebral conjunctiva).

(For removal of lesion, involving mainly skin of eyelid, see 11310-11313; 11440-11446, 11640-11646; 17000-17004)

(For repair of wounds, blepharoplasty, grafts, reconstructive surgery, see 67930-67975)

67800   Excision of chalazion; single
> *CPT Assistant* Sep 99:10

67801   multiple, same lid

67805   multiple, different lids
> *CPT Assistant* Sep 99:10

67808   under general anesthesia and/or requiring hospitalization, single or multiple

67810   Code is out of numerical sequence. See 67700-67810

67820   Correction of trichiasis; epilation, by forceps only
> *CPT Assistant* Jul 98:10

Trichiasis
67820-67825

When the eyelashes are ingrown or misdirected (trichiasis), the physician uses a biomicroscope and forceps to remove the offending eyelashes. Report 67825 when cryosurgery or electrosurgery is used to destroy the follicles.

Forceps

Ingrown or misdirected eyelashes

67825   epilation by other than forceps (eg, by electrosurgery, cryotherapy, laser surgery)
➔ *CPT Assistant* Jul 98:10

67830   incision of lid margin

67835   incision of lid margin, with free mucous membrane graft

67840   Excision of lesion of eyelid (except chalazion) without closure or with simple direct closure

(For excision and repair of eyelid by reconstructive surgery, see 67961, 67966)

67850   Destruction of lesion of lid margin (up to 1 cm)

(For Mohs micrographic surgery, see 17311-17315)

(For initiation or follow-up care of topical chemotherapy (eg, 5-FU or similar agents), see appropriate office visits)

Tarsorrhaphy

67875   Temporary closure of eyelids by suture (eg, Frost suture)
➔ *CPT Assistant* Winter 90:9

67880   Construction of intermarginal adhesions, median tarsorrhaphy, or canthorrhaphy;

67882   with transposition of tarsal plate

(For severing of tarsorrhaphy, use 67710)

(For canthoplasty, reconstruction canthus, use 67950)

(For canthotomy, use 67715)

Repair (Brow Ptosis, Blepharoptosis, Lid Retraction, Ectropion, Entropion)

67900   Repair of brow ptosis (supraciliary, mid-forehead or coronal approach)

(For forehead rhytidectomy, use 15824)

67901   Repair of blepharoptosis; frontalis muscle technique with suture or other material (eg, banked fascia)
➔ *CPT Assistant* Sep 00:7, Oct 06:11; *CPT Changes: An Insider's View* 2006

67902   frontalis muscle technique with autologous fascial sling (includes obtaining fascia)
➔ *CPT Assistant* Sep 00:7, Oct 06:11; *CPT Changes: An Insider's View* 2006

67903   (tarso) levator resection or advancement, internal approach
➔ *CPT Assistant* Sep 00:7, Oct 06:11

67904   (tarso) levator resection or advancement, external approach
➔ *CPT Assistant* Sep 00:7, Oct 06:11, Aug 11:8

67906   superior rectus technique with fascial sling (includes obtaining fascia)
➔ *CPT Assistant* Sep 00:7, Oct 06:11

67908   conjunctivo-tarso-Muller's muscle-levator resection (eg, Fasanella-Servat type)
➔ *CPT Assistant* Sep 00:7, Oct 06:11

67909   Reduction of overcorrection of ptosis

67911   Correction of lid retraction

(For obtaining autogenous graft materials, see 20920, 20922 or 20926)

(For correction of trichiasis by mucous membrane graft, use 67835)

67912   Correction of lagophthalmos, with implantation of upper eyelid lid load (eg, gold weight)
➔ *CPT Assistant* May 04:12, Aug 04:10, Oct 06:11; *CPT Changes: An Insider's View* 2004

67914   Repair of ectropion; suture

67915   thermocauterization

67916   excision tarsal wedge
➔ *CPT Assistant* Feb 04:11, May 04:12, Feb 05:16, Oct 06:11; *CPT Changes: An Insider's View* 2004

67917   extensive (eg, tarsal strip operations)
➔ *CPT Assistant* Feb 04:11, May 04:12, Oct 06:11; *CPT Changes: An Insider's View* 2004

(For correction of everted punctum, use 68705)

67921   Repair of entropion; suture

67922   thermocauterization

67923   excision tarsal wedge
➔ *CPT Assistant* May 04:12, Oct 06:11; *CPT Changes: An Insider's View* 2004

67924   extensive (eg, tarsal strip or capsulopalpebral fascia repairs operation)
➔ *CPT Assistant* May 04:12, Oct 06:11; *CPT Changes: An Insider's View* 2004

(For repair of cicatricial ectropion or entropion requiring scar excision or skin graft, see also 67961 et seq)

Eye/Occular Adnexa

Reconstruction

Codes for blepharoplasty involve more than skin (ie, involving lid margin, tarsus, and/or palpebral conjunctiva).

67930 Suture of recent wound, eyelid, involving lid margin, tarsus, and/or palpebral conjunctiva direct closure; partial thickness

67935 full thickness

67938 Removal of embedded foreign body, eyelid

(For repair of skin of eyelid, see 12011-12018; 12051-12057; 13150-13153)

(For tarsorrhaphy, canthorrhaphy, see 67880, 67882)

(For repair of blepharoptosis and lid retraction, see 67901-67911)

(For blepharoplasty for entropion, ectropion, see 67916, 67917, 67923, 67924)

(For correction of blepharochalasis (blepharorhytidectomy), see 15820-15823)

(For repair of skin of eyelid, adjacent tissue transfer, see 14060, 14061; preparation for graft, use 15004; free graft, see 15120, 15121, 15260, 15261)

(For excision of lesion of eyelid, use 67800 et seq)

(For repair of lacrimal canaliculi, use 68700)

67950 Canthoplasty (reconstruction of canthus)

67961 Excision and repair of eyelid, involving lid margin, tarsus, conjunctiva, canthus, or full thickness, may include preparation for skin graft or pedicle flap with adjacent tissue transfer or rearrangement; up to one-fourth of lid margin

67966 over one-fourth of lid margin

(For canthoplasty, use 67950)

(For free skin grafts, see 15120, 15121, 15260, 15261)

(For tubed pedicle flap preparation, use 15576; for delay, use 15630; for attachment, use 15650)

67971 Reconstruction of eyelid, full thickness by transfer of tarsoconjunctival flap from opposing eyelid; up to two-thirds of eyelid, 1 stage or first stage

67973 total eyelid, lower, 1 stage or first stage

67974 total eyelid, upper, 1 stage or first stage

67975 second stage

Other Procedures

67999 Unlisted procedure, eyelids

Conjunctiva

(For removal of foreign body, see 65205 et seq)

Incision and Drainage

68020 Incision of conjunctiva, drainage of cyst

68040 Expression of conjunctival follicles (eg, for trachoma)

Excision and/or Destruction

68100 Biopsy of conjunctiva

68110 Excision of lesion, conjunctiva; up to 1 cm

68115 over 1 cm

68130 with adjacent sclera

68135 Destruction of lesion, conjunctiva

Injection

(For injection into Tenon's capsule or retrobulbar injection, see 67500-67515)

68200 Subconjunctival injection
➔ *CPT Assistant* Aug 03:15

Conjunctivoplasty

(For wound repair, see 65270-65273)

68320 Conjunctivoplasty; with conjunctival graft or extensive rearrangement
➔ *CPT Assistant* Feb 04:11

68325 with buccal mucous membrane graft (includes obtaining graft)

68326 Conjunctivoplasty, reconstruction cul-de-sac; with conjunctival graft or extensive rearrangement

68328 with buccal mucous membrane graft (includes obtaining graft)

68330 Repair of symblepharon; conjunctivoplasty, without graft

68335 with free graft conjunctiva or buccal mucous membrane (includes obtaining graft)

68340 division of symblepharon, with or without insertion of conformer or contact lens

Other Procedures

68360 Conjunctival flap; bridge or partial (separate procedure)

68362 total (such as Gunderson thin flap or purse string flap)

(For conjunctival flap for perforating injury, see 65280, 65285)

(For repair of operative wound, use 66250)

(For removal of conjunctival foreign body, see 65205, 65210)

68371 Harvesting conjunctival allograft, living donor
> *CPT Assistant* May 04:10; *CPT Changes: An Insider's View* 2004

68399 Unlisted procedure, conjunctiva

Lacrimal System

Incision

68400 Incision, drainage of lacrimal gland

68420 Incision, drainage of lacrimal sac (dacryocystotomy or dacryocystostomy)

68440 Snip incision of lacrimal punctum

Excision

68500 Excision of lacrimal gland (dacryoadenectomy), except for tumor; total

68505   partial

68510 Biopsy of lacrimal gland

68520 Excision of lacrimal sac (dacryocystectomy)

68525 Biopsy of lacrimal sac

68530 Removal of foreign body or dacryolith, lacrimal passages

68540 Excision of lacrimal gland tumor; frontal approach

68550   involving osteotomy

Repair

68700 Plastic repair of canaliculi

68705 Correction of everted punctum, cautery

68720 Dacryocystorhinostomy (fistulization of lacrimal sac to nasal cavity)
> *CPT Assistant* Sep 01:10, Jul 03:15, Aug 03:14, Aug 09:11

68745 Conjunctivorhinostomy (fistulization of conjunctiva to nasal cavity); without tube

68750   with insertion of tube or stent

68760 Closure of the lacrimal punctum; by thermocauterization, ligation, or laser surgery

68761   by plug, each
> *CPT Assistant* Jun 96:10, Jan 07:28

Closure of Lacrimal Punctum by Plug
68761

The physician inserts a lacrimal duct implant into a lacrimal punctum.

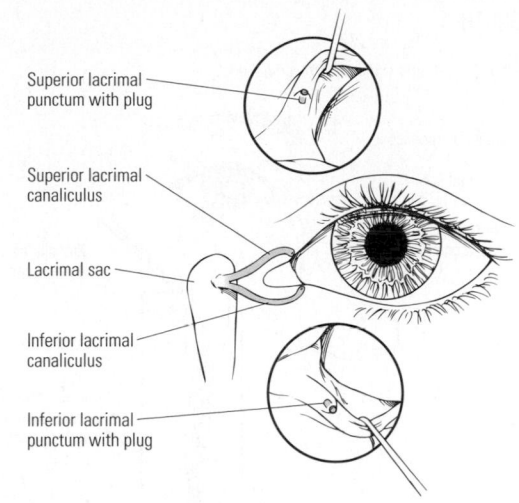

68770 Closure of lacrimal fistula (separate procedure)

Probing and/or Related Procedures

68801 Dilation of lacrimal punctum, with or without irrigation

(To report a bilateral procedure, use 68801 with modifier 50)

68810 Probing of nasolacrimal duct, with or without irrigation;
> *CPT Assistant* Nov 02:11, Oct 08:3

(For bilateral procedure, report 68810 with modifier 50)

68811   requiring general anesthesia
> *CPT Assistant* Nov 02:11, Oct 08:3

(For bilateral procedure, report 68811 with modifier 50)

68815   with insertion of tube or stent
> *CPT Assistant* Nov 02:11, Oct 08:3, Aug 09:11, Nov 10:9

(See also 92018)

(For bilateral procedure, report 68815 with modifier 50)

Eye/Occular Adnexa

68816   with transluminal balloon catheter dilation

> CPT Changes: An Insider's View 2008

Probing of Nasolacrimal Duct
68816

A balloon catheter is in the nasolacrimal duct.

Superior canaliculus

Lacrimal sac

Narrowing of
nasolacrimal duct

Cannula inserted into
superior canaliculus

Guidewire

Balloon catheter inserted
retrograde expanding
nasolacrimal duct

(Do not report 68816 in conjunction with 68810, 68811,
68815)

(For bilateral procedure, report 68816 with modifier 50)

68840   Probing of lacrimal canaliculi, with or without irrigation

68850   Injection of contrast medium for dacryocystography

> CPT Assistant Feb 01:9

(For radiological supervision and interpretation, see
70170, 78660)

Other Procedures

68899   Unlisted procedure, lacrimal system

Surgery

The following is a listing of headings and subheadings that appear within the Auditory System and Operating Microscope sections of the CPT codebook. The subheadings or subsections denoted with asterisks (*) below have special instructions unique to that section. Where these are indicated, special "notes" or guidelines will be presented preceding those procedural terminology listings, referring to that subsection specifically.

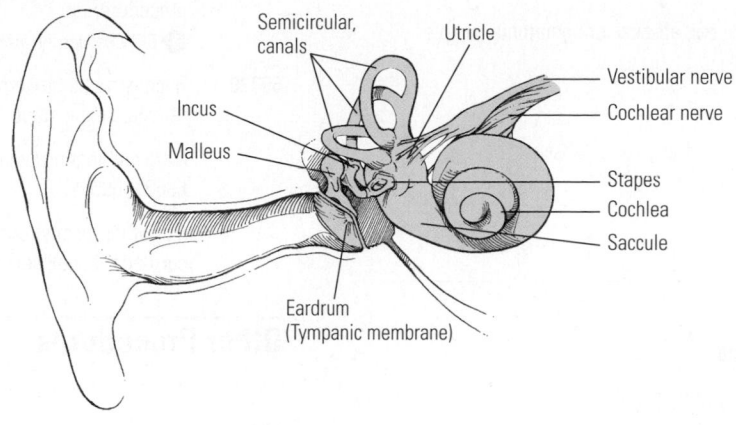

Auditory System

(For diagnostic services (eg, audiometry, vestibular tests), see 92502 et seq)

External Ear

Incision

69000   Drainage external ear, abscess or hematoma; simple
> *CPT Assistant* Oct 97:11, Oct 99:10

69005   complicated

69020   Drainage external auditory canal, abscess
> *CPT Assistant* Oct 97:11

69090   Ear piercing

Excision

69100   Biopsy external ear

69105   Biopsy external auditory canal

69110   Excision external ear; partial, simple repair

69120   complete amputation

(For reconstruction of ear, see 15120 et seq)

69140   Excision exostosis(es), external auditory canal

69145   Excision soft tissue lesion, external auditory canal

69150   Radical excision external auditory canal lesion; without neck dissection

69155   with neck dissection

(For resection of temporal bone, use 69535)

(For skin grafting, see 15004-15261)

Removal

69200   Removal foreign body from external auditory canal; without general anesthesia

69205   with general anesthesia

69210   Removal impacted cerumen (separate procedure), 1 or both ears
> *CPT Assistant* Apr 03:9, Jul 05:14

69220   Debridement, mastoidectomy cavity, simple (eg, routine cleaning)

(For bilateral procedure, report 69220 with modifier 50)

69222   Debridement, mastoidectomy cavity, complex (eg, with anesthesia or more than routine cleaning)

(For bilateral procedure, report 69222 with modifier 50)

Repair

(For suture of wound or injury of external ear, see 12011-14302)

⊙ **69300**   Otoplasty, protruding ear, with or without size reduction

(For bilateral procedure, report 69300 with modifier 50)

69310   Reconstruction of external auditory canal (meatoplasty) (eg, for stenosis due to injury, infection) (separate procedure)
> *CPT Changes: An Insider's View* 2002

69320   Reconstruction external auditory canal for congenital atresia, single stage

(For combination with middle ear reconstruction, see 69631, 69641)

(For other reconstructive procedures with grafts (eg, skin, cartilage, bone), see 13150-15760, 21230-21235)

Other Procedures

(For otoscopy under general anesthesia, use 92502)

69399   Unlisted procedure, external ear

Middle Ear

Introduction

69400   Eustachian tube inflation, transnasal; with catheterization

69401   without catheterization

69405   Eustachian tube catheterization, transtympanic

Incision

69420   Myringotomy including aspiration and/or eustachian tube inflation
> *CPT Assistant* May 11:8

69421   Myringotomy including aspiration and/or eustachian tube inflation requiring general anesthesia
> *CPT Assistant* May 11:8

69424   Ventilating tube removal requiring general anesthesia
> *CPT Assistant* Mar 05:17, Jun 10:11, Nov 10:9; *CPT Changes: An Insider's View* 2003

(For bilateral procedure, report 69424 with modifier 50)

(Do not report code 69424 in conjunction with 69205, 69210, 69420, 69421, 69433-69676, 69710-69745, 69801-69930)

69433   Tympanostomy (requiring insertion of ventilating tube), local or topical anesthesia
> *CPT Assistant* May 11:8

(For bilateral procedure, report 69433 with modifier 50)

Tympanostomy
69433-69436

A ventilating tube is inserted into the opening of the tympanum.

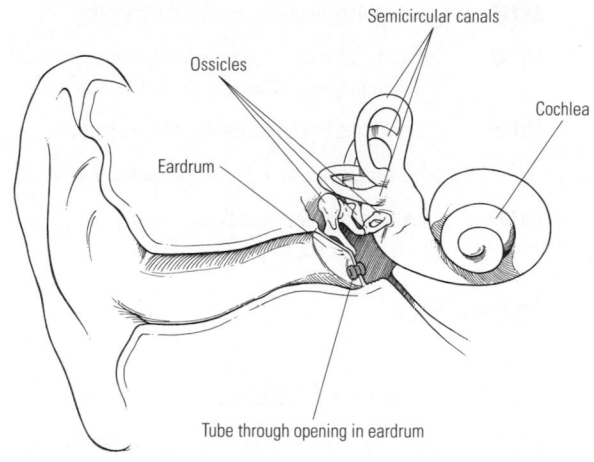

69436   Tympanostomy (requiring insertion of ventilating tube), general anesthesia
> *CPT Assistant* May 11:8, May 12:14

(For bilateral procedure, report 69436 with modifier 50)

69440   Middle ear exploration through postauricular or ear canal incision

(For atticotomy, see 69601 et seq)

69450   Tympanolysis, transcanal

Excision

69501   Transmastoid antrotomy (simple mastoidectomy)

69502   Mastoidectomy; complete

69505   modified radical

69511   radical

(For skin graft, see 15004 et seq)

(For mastoidectomy cavity debridement, see 69220, 69222)

69530   Petrous apicectomy including radical mastoidectomy

69535   Resection temporal bone, external approach

(For middle fossa approach, see 69950-69970)

69540   Excision aural polyp

69550   Excision aural glomus tumor; transcanal

69552   transmastoid

69554   extended (extratemporal)

Repair

69601   Revision mastoidectomy; resulting in complete mastoidectomy

69602   resulting in modified radical mastoidectomy

69603   resulting in radical mastoidectomy

69604   resulting in tympanoplasty

(For planned secondary tympanoplasty after mastoidectomy, see 69631, 69632)

69605   with apicectomy

(For skin graft, see 15120, 15121, 15260, 15261)

69610   Tympanic membrane repair, with or without site preparation of perforation for closure, with or without patch
> *CPT Assistant* Mar 01:10, Mar 03:21, Aug 08:4

69620   Myringoplasty (surgery confined to drumhead and donor area)
> *CPT Assistant* Mar 01:10, Aug 08:4

69631   Tympanoplasty without mastoidectomy (including canalplasty, atticotomy and/or middle ear surgery), initial or revision; without ossicular chain reconstruction
> *CPT Assistant* Jul 98:11, Mar 01:10, Mar 07:9, Aug 08:4

69632   with ossicular chain reconstruction (eg, postfenestration)

69633   with ossicular chain reconstruction and synthetic prosthesis (eg, partial ossicular replacement prosthesis [PORP], total ossicular replacement prosthesis [TORP])

69635   Tympanoplasty with antrotomy or mastoidotomy (including canalplasty, atticotomy, middle ear surgery, and/or tympanic membrane repair); without ossicular chain reconstruction

69636   with ossicular chain reconstruction

Tympanoplasty
69635-69646

A graft is used to repair the tympanic membrane perforation.

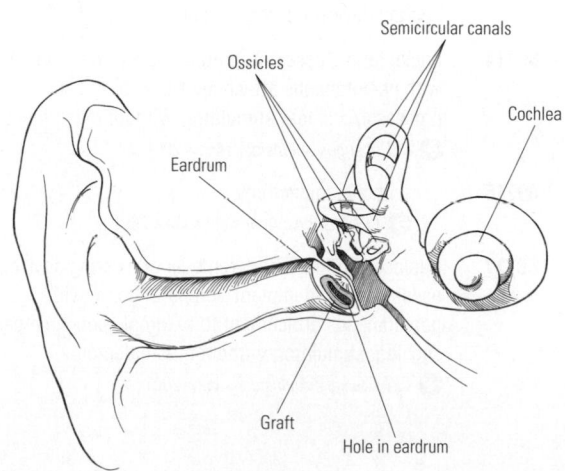

Auditory

69637   with ossicular chain reconstruction and synthetic prosthesis (eg, partial ossicular replacement prosthesis [PORP], total ossicular replacement prosthesis [TORP])

69641   Tympanoplasty with mastoidectomy (including canalplasty, middle ear surgery, tympanic membrane repair); without ossicular chain reconstruction

69642   with ossicular chain reconstruction

69643   with intact or reconstructed wall, without ossicular chain reconstruction

69644   with intact or reconstructed canal wall, with ossicular chain reconstruction

69645   radical or complete, without ossicular chain reconstruction

69646   radical or complete, with ossicular chain reconstruction

69650   Stapes mobilization

69660   Stapedectomy or stapedotomy with reestablishment of ossicular continuity, with or without use of foreign material;

69661   with footplate drill out

69662   Revision of stapedectomy or stapedotomy

69666   Repair oval window fistula

69667   Repair round window fistula

69670   Mastoid obliteration (separate procedure)

69676   Tympanic neurectomy

(For bilateral procedure, report 69676 with modifier 50)

Other Procedures

69700   Closure postauricular fistula, mastoid (separate procedure)

69710   Implantation or replacement of electromagnetic bone conduction hearing device in temporal bone

(Replacement procedure includes removal of old device)

69711   Removal or repair of electromagnetic bone conduction hearing device in temporal bone

69714   Implantation, osseointegrated implant, temporal bone, with percutaneous attachment to external speech processor/cochlear stimulator; without mastoidectomy
  ➔ *CPT Changes: An Insider's View* 2001

69715   with mastoidectomy
  ➔ *CPT Changes: An Insider's View* 2001

69717   Replacement (including removal of existing device), osseointegrated implant, temporal bone, with percutaneous attachment to external speech processor/cochlear stimulator; without mastoidectomy
  ➔ *CPT Changes: An Insider's View* 2001

69718   with mastoidectomy
  ➔ *CPT Changes: An Insider's View* 2001

69720   Decompression facial nerve, intratemporal; lateral to geniculate ganglion

69725   including medial to geniculate ganglion

69740   Suture facial nerve, intratemporal, with or without graft or decompression; lateral to geniculate ganglion

69745   including medial to geniculate ganglion

(For extracranial suture of facial nerve, use 64864)

69799   Unlisted procedure, middle ear
  ➔ *CPT Assistant* Oct 99:10

Inner Ear

Incision and/or Destruction

69801   Labyrinthotomy, with perfusion of vestibuloactive drug(s); transcanal
  ➔ *CPT Assistant* Nov 96:12, May 11:8; *CPT Changes: An Insider's View* 2011

(Do not report 69801 more than once per day)

(Do not report 69801 in conjunction with 69420, 69421, 69433, 69436 when performed on the same ear)

(69802 has been deleted)

69805   Endolymphatic sac operation; without shunt

69806   with shunt
  ➔ *CPT Assistant* Nov 96:12

69820   Fenestration semicircular canal

69840   Revision fenestration operation

Excision

69905   Labyrinthectomy; transcanal

69910   with mastoidectomy

69915   Vestibular nerve section, translabyrinthine approach

(For transcranial approach, use 69950)

Introduction

69930   Cochlear device implantation, with or without mastoidectomy

Cochlear Device Implantation
69930

An internal coil is attached to the temporal bone and the ground wire attached to the internal coil is connected to the temporalis muscle.

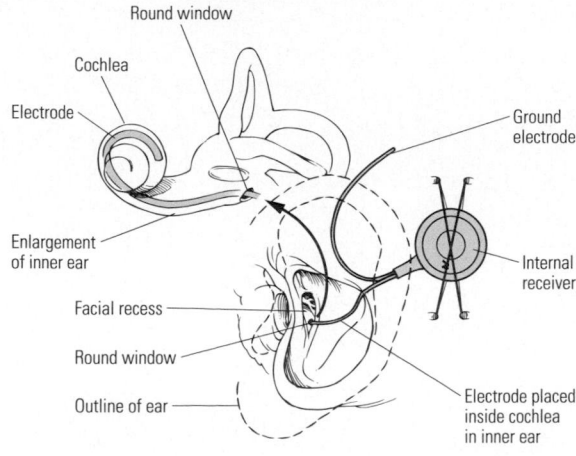

Round window
Cochlea
Electrode
Ground electrode
Enlargement of inner ear
Internal receiver
Facial recess
Round window
Outline of ear
Electrode placed inside cochlea in inner ear

Other Procedures

69949   Unlisted procedure, inner ear

Temporal Bone, Middle Fossa Approach

(For external approach, use 69535)

69950   Vestibular nerve section, transcranial approach

69955   Total facial nerve decompression and/or repair (may include graft)

69960   Decompression internal auditory canal

69970   Removal of tumor, temporal bone

Other Procedures

69979   Unlisted procedure, temporal bone, middle fossa approach

   ➔ *CPT Assistant* Jan 07:30

Operating Microscope

▶The surgical microscope is employed when the surgical services are performed using the techniques of microsurgery. Code 69990 should be reported (without modifier 51 appended) in addition to the code for the primary procedure performed. Do not use 69990 for visualization with magnifying loupes or corrected vision. Do not report 69990 in addition to procedures where use of the operating microscope is an inclusive component (15756-15758, 15842, 19364, 19368, 20955-20962, 20969-20973, 22551, 22552, 22856-22861, 26551-26554, 26556, 31526, 31531, 31536, 31541, 31545, 31546, 31561, 31571, 43116, 43496, 49906, 61548, 63075-63078, 64727, 64820-64823, 65091-68850, 0184T, 0226T, 0227T, 0308T).◀

+ 69990   Microsurgical techniques, requiring use of operating microscope (List separately in addition to code for primary procedure)

   ➔ *CPT Assistant* Nov 98:20, Apr 99:11, Jun 99:11, Jul 99:10, Oct 99:10, Oct 00:3, Oct 02:8, Jan 04:28, Mar 05:11, Jul 05:14, Aug 05:1, Nov 07:4, Sep 08:10, Mar 09:10, Dec 11:14, Mar 12:9, Jun 12:17; *CPT Changes: An Insider's View* 2002

Operating Microscope
69990

A surgical operating microscope is used to obtain good visualization of the fine structures in the operating field. The lens system may be operated by hand or foot controls to adjust to working distance, with interchangeable oculars providing magnification as needed.

Eye piece
Lens

Auditory

Notes

⊙=Moderate sedation   ✚=Add-on code   ✗=FDA approval pending   #=Resequenced code   ○=Recycled/reinstated code   ➋➋=See p xiii for details

Radiology Guidelines
(Including Nuclear Medicine and Diagnostic Ultrasound)

Radiology

The following is a listing of headings and subheadings that appear within the Radiology section of the CPT codebook. The subheadings or subsections denoted with asterisks (*) below have special instructions unique to that section. Where these are indicated, special "notes" or guidelines will be presented preceding those procedural terminology listings, referring to that subsection specifically.

Radiology

Radiology Guidelines (Including Nuclear Medicine and Diagnostic Ultrasound)

►Guidelines to direct general reporting of services are presented in the **Introduction.** Some of the commonalities are repeated here for the convenience of those referring to this section on **Radiology (Including Nuclear Medicine and Diagnostic Ultrasound).** Other definitions and items unique to Radiology are also listed.◄

Subject Listings

►Subject listings apply when radiological services are performed by or under the responsible supervision of a physician or other qualified health care professional.◄

Separate Procedures

Some of the procedures or services listed in the CPT codebook that are commonly carried out as an integral component of a total service or procedure have been identified by the inclusion of the term "separate procedure." The codes designated as "separate procedure" should not be reported in addition to the code for the total procedure or service of which it is considered an integral component.

However, when a procedure or service that is designated as a "separate procedure" is carried out independently or considered to be unrelated or distinct from other procedures/services provided at that time, it may be reported by itself, or in addition to other procedures/services by appending modifier 59 to the specific "separate procedure" code to indicate that the procedure is not considered to be a component of another procedure, but is a distinct, independent procedure. This may represent a different session or patient encounter, different procedure or surgery, different site or organ system, separate incision/excision, separate lesion, separate injury, or area of injury in extensive injuries.

Unlisted Service or Procedure

A service or procedure may be provided that is not listed in this edition of the CPT codebook. When reporting such a service, the appropriate "Unlisted Procedure" code may be used to indicate the service, identifying it by "Special Report" as discussed below. The "Unlisted Procedures" and accompanying codes for **Radiology (Including Nuclear Medicine and Diagnostic Ultrasound)** are as follows:

76496	Unlisted fluoroscopic procedure (eg, diagnostic, interventional)
76497	Unlisted computed tomography procedure (eg, diagnostic, interventional)
76498	Unlisted magnetic resonance procedure (eg, diagnostic, interventional)
76499	Unlisted diagnostic radiographic procedure
76999	Unlisted ultrasound procedure (eg, diagnostic, interventional)
77299	Unlisted procedure, therapeutic radiology clinical treatment planning
77399	Unlisted procedure, medical radiation physics, dosimetry and treatment devices, and special services
77499	Unlisted procedure, therapeutic radiology treatment management
77799	Unlisted procedure, clinical brachytherapy
78099	Unlisted endocrine procedure, diagnostic nuclear medicine
78199	Unlisted hematopoietic, reticuloendothelial and lymphatic procedure, diagnostic nuclear medicine
78299	Unlisted gastrointestinal procedure, diagnostic nuclear medicine
78399	Unlisted musculoskeletal procedure, diagnostic nuclear medicine
78499	Unlisted cardiovascular procedure, diagnostic nuclear medicine
78599	Unlisted respiratory procedure, diagnostic nuclear medicine

⊙=Moderate sedation ✚=Add-on code ✗=FDA approval pending #=Resequenced code ○=Recycled/reinstated code ➤➤=See p xiii for details

78699	Unlisted nervous system procedure, diagnostic nuclear medicine
78799	Unlisted genitourinary procedure, diagnostic nuclear medicine
78999	Unlisted miscellaneous procedure, diagnostic nuclear medicine
79999	Radiopharmaceutical therapy, unlisted procedure

Special Report

A service that is rarely provided, unusual, variable, or new may require a special report. Pertinent information should include an adequate definition or description of the nature, extent, and need for the procedure; and the time, effort, and equipment necessary to provide the service.

Supervision and Interpretation

▶Imaging may be required during the performance of certain procedures or certain imaging procedures may require surgical procedures to access the imaged area. Many services include image guidance, which is not separately reportable and is so stated in the descriptor or guidelines. When imaging is not included in a surgical procedure or procedure from the **Medicine** section, image guidance codes or codes labeled "radiological supervision and interpretation" may be reported for the portion of the service that requires imaging. Both services require image documentation and radiological supervision, interpretation, and report services require a separate interpretation.◀

(The Radiological Supervision and Interpretation codes are not applicable to the Radiation Oncology subsection.)

Administration of Contrast Material(s)

The phrase "with contrast" used in the codes for procedures performed using contrast for imaging enhancement represents contrast material administered intravascularly, intra-articularly, or intrathecally.

For intra-articular injection, use the appropriate joint injection code. If radiographic arthrography is performed, also use the arthrography supervision and interpretation code for the appropriate joint (which includes fluoroscopy). If computed tomography (CT) or magnetic resonance (MR) arthrography are performed without radiographic arthrography, use the appropriate joint injection code, the appropriate CT or MR code ("with contrast" or "without followed by contrast"), and the appropriate imaging guidance code for needle placement for contrast injection.

For spine examinations using computed tomography, magnetic resonance imaging, magnetic resonance angiography, "with contrast" includes intrathecal or intravascular injection. For intrathecal injection, use also 61055 or 62284.

Injection of intravascular contrast material is part of the "with contrast" CT, computed tomographic angiography (CTA), magnetic resonance imaging (MRI), and magnetic resonance angiography (MRA) procedures.

Oral and/or rectal contrast administration alone does not qualify as a study "with contrast."

Written Report(s)

▶A written report signed by the interpreting individual should be considered an integral part of a radiologic procedure or interpretation.◀

Radiology

Radiology

Diagnostic Radiology (Diagnostic Imaging)

Head and Neck

70010 Myelography, posterior fossa, radiological supervision and interpretation
> CPT Assistant Mar 05:11, Dec 07:16

70015 Cisternography, positive contrast, radiological supervision and interpretation

70030 Radiologic examination, eye, for detection of foreign body

70100 Radiologic examination, mandible; partial, less than 4 views

70110   complete, minimum of 4 views

70120 Radiologic examination, mastoids; less than 3 views per side

70130   complete, minimum of 3 views per side

70134 Radiologic examination, internal auditory meati, complete

70140 Radiologic examination, facial bones; less than 3 views

70150   complete, minimum of 3 views

70160 Radiologic examination, nasal bones, complete, minimum of 3 views

70170 Dacryocystography, nasolacrimal duct, radiological supervision and interpretation

70190 Radiologic examination; optic foramina

70200   orbits, complete, minimum of 4 views

70210 Radiologic examination, sinuses, paranasal, less than 3 views

70220 Radiologic examination, sinuses, paranasal, complete, minimum of 3 views

70240 Radiologic examination, sella turcica

70250 Radiologic examination, skull; less than 4 views
> CPT Changes: An Insider's View 2004

70260   complete, minimum of 4 views
> CPT Changes: An Insider's View 2004

70300 Radiologic examination, teeth; single view

70310   partial examination, less than full mouth

70320   complete, full mouth

70328 Radiologic examination, temporomandibular joint, open and closed mouth; unilateral

70330   bilateral
> CPT Assistant May 11:10

70332 Temporomandibular joint arthrography, radiological supervision and interpretation
> CPT Assistant Feb 07:11

(Do not report 70332 in conjunction with 77002)

70336 Magnetic resonance (eg, proton) imaging, temporomandibular joint(s)
> CPT Assistant Jul 99:11, Jul 01:7; CPT Changes: An Insider's View 2001

70350 Cephalogram, orthodontic

70355 Orthopantogram (eg, panoramic x-ray)
> CPT Changes: An Insider's View 2012
> Clinical Examples in Radiology Fall 11:11

70360 Radiologic examination; neck, soft tissue

70370   pharynx or larynx, including fluoroscopy and/or magnification technique

70371 Complex dynamic pharyngeal and speech evaluation by cine or video recording
> CPT Assistant Dec 04:17

70373 Laryngography, contrast, radiological supervision and interpretation

70380 Radiologic examination, salivary gland for calculus

70390 Sialography, radiological supervision and interpretation
> Clinical Examples in Radiology Fall 09:9

70450 Computed tomography, head or brain; without contrast material
> CPT Assistant Apr 96:11; CPT Changes: An Insider's View 2003
> Clinical Examples in Radiology Winter 08:6

70460   with contrast material(s)
> CPT Assistant Apr 96:11
> Clinical Examples in Radiology Winter 10:11

70470   without contrast material, followed by contrast material(s) and further sections
> CPT Assistant Apr 96:11

(To report 3D rendering, see 76376, 76377)

70480 Computed tomography, orbit, sella, or posterior fossa or outer, middle, or inner ear; without contrast material
> CPT Changes: An Insider's View 2003

70481   with contrast material(s)
> CPT Assistant Apr 08:11

70482   without contrast material, followed by contrast material(s) and further sections

(To report 3D rendering, see 76376, 76377)

70486 Computed tomography, maxillofacial area; without contrast material
> CPT Assistant Mar 02:11; CPT Changes: An Insider's View 2003
> Clinical Examples in Radiology Spring 07:4, Winter 07:4-5, Fall 09:9

70487   with contrast material(s)

70488   without contrast material, followed by contrast material(s) and further sections

(To report 3D rendering, see 76376, 76377)

70490   Computed tomography, soft tissue neck; without contrast material
> *CPT Changes: An Insider's View* 2003

70491   with contrast material(s)

70492   without contrast material followed by contrast material(s) and further sections

(To report 3D rendering, see 76376, 76377)

(For cervical spine, see 72125, 72126)

70496   Computed tomographic angiography, head, with contrast material(s), including noncontrast images, if performed, and image postprocessing
> *CPT Assistant* Jul 01:4, Dec 05:7, Jan 07:31; *CPT Changes: An Insider's View* 2001, 2008

70498   Computed tomographic angiography, neck, with contrast material(s), including noncontrast images, if performed, and image postprocessing
> *CPT Assistant* Jul 01:4, Dec 05:7, Jan 07:31; *CPT Changes: An Insider's View* 2001, 2008
> *Clinical Examples in Radiology* Winter 09:2

70540   Magnetic resonance (eg, proton) imaging, orbit, face, and/or neck; without contrast material(s)
> *CPT Assistant* Jul 01:6, Mar 07:7, Sep 10:10; *CPT Changes: An Insider's View* 2001, 2007
> *Clinical Examples in Radiology* Spring 05:3, Summer 07:7

(For head or neck magnetic resonance angiography studies, see 70544-70546, 70547-70549)

70542   with contrast material(s)
> *CPT Assistant* Jul 01:6, Sep 10:10; *CPT Changes: An Insider's View* 2001
> *Clinical Examples in Radiology* Spring 05:3, Summer 07:7

70543   without contrast material(s), followed by contrast material(s) and further sequences
> *CPT Assistant* Jul 01:6, Sep 10:10; *CPT Changes: An Insider's View* 2001
> *Clinical Examples in Radiology* Spring 05:2-3, Summer 07:7, Winter 07:7, 11

(Report 70540-70543 once per imaging session)

70544   Magnetic resonance angiography, head; without contrast material(s)
> *CPT Assistant* Sep 01:5, Dec 05:7, Jan 07:31; *CPT Changes: An Insider's View* 2001

70545   with contrast material(s)
> *CPT Assistant* Jul 01:5, Dec 05:7; *CPT Changes: An Insider's View* 2001

70546   without contrast material(s), followed by contrast material(s) and further sequences
> *CPT Assistant* Jul 01:5, Dec 05:7, Jan 07:31; *CPT Changes: An Insider's View* 2001

70547   Magnetic resonance angiography, neck; without contrast material(s)
> *CPT Assistant* Sep 01:5, Dec 05:7, Jan 07:31; *CPT Changes: An Insider's View* 2001
> *Clinical Examples in Radiology* Winter 09:2

70548   with contrast material(s)
> *CPT Assistant* Sep 01:6, Dec 05:7, Jan 07:31; *CPT Changes: An Insider's View* 2001
> *Clinical Examples in Radiology* Winter 09:2

70549   without contrast material(s), followed by contrast material(s) and further sequences
> *CPT Assistant* Sep 01:6, Dec 05:7, Jan 07:31; *CPT Changes: An Insider's View* 2001
> *Clinical Examples in Radiology* Winter 09:2

70551   Magnetic resonance (eg, proton) imaging, brain (including brain stem); without contrast material
> *CPT Assistant* May 98:10, Mar 05:20, Feb 07:6

70552   with contrast material(s)
> *CPT Assistant* Jul 01:6, Mar 05:20, Feb 07:6

70553   without contrast material, followed by contrast material(s) and further sequences
> *CPT Assistant* Nov 97:24, Jul 01:6, Mar 05:20, Feb 07:6
> *Clinical Examples in Radiology* Spring 05:2, Spring 06:4-5

(For magnetic spectroscopy, use 76390)

Functional MRI involves identification and mapping of stimulation of brain function. When neurofunctional tests are administered by a technologist or other non-physician or non-psychologist, use 70554. When neurofunctional tests are entirely administered by a physician or psychologist, use 70555.

70554   Magnetic resonance imaging, brain, functional MRI; including test selection and administration of repetitive body part movement and/or visual stimulation, not requiring physician or psychologist administration
> *CPT Assistant* Feb 07:6, Mar 07:7, Aug 08:13; *CPT Changes: An Insider's View* 2007

(Do not report 70554 in conjunction with 96020)

70555   requiring physician or psychologist administration of entire neurofunctional testing
> *CPT Assistant* Feb 07:6, Mar 07:7; *CPT Changes: An Insider's View* 2007

(Do not report 70555 unless 96020 is performed)

(Do not report 70554, 70555 in conjunction with 70551-70553 unless a separate diagnostic MRI is performed)

70557   Magnetic resonance (eg, proton) imaging, brain (including brain stem and skull base), during open intracranial procedure (eg, to assess for residual tumor or residual vascular malformation); without contrast material
> *CPT Changes: An Insider's View* 2004

70558   with contrast material(s)
> *CPT Changes: An Insider's View* 2004

Radiology

70559 without contrast material(s), followed by contrast material(s) and further sequences

➔ *CPT Changes: An Insider's View* 2004

(For stereotactic biopsy of intracranial lesion with magnetic resonance guidance, use 61751. Codes 70557, 70558, or 70559 may be reported only if a separate report is generated. Report only 1 of the above codes once per operative session. Do not use these codes in conjunction with 61751, 77021, 77022)

Chest

(For fluoroscopic or ultrasonic guidance for needle placement procedures (eg, biopsy, aspiration, injection, localization device) of the thorax, see 76942, 77002)

71010 Radiologic examination, chest; single view, frontal

➔ *CPT Assistant* Aug 00:1, Feb 07:10, Jul 07:1, 6

➔ *Clinical Examples in Radiology* Summer 09:11, Fall 09:10

71015 stereo, frontal

➔ *CPT Assistant* Feb 07:10, Jul 07:1

71020 Radiologic examination, chest, 2 views, frontal and lateral;

➔ *CPT Assistant* Sep 03:3, Mar 05:11, Feb 07:10, Jul 07:1, 6, Dec 09:14, Sep 10:6

71021 with apical lordotic procedure

71022 with oblique projections

➔ *CPT Assistant* Jul 07:6

71023 with fluoroscopy

➔ *CPT Assistant* Aug 03:14, Dec 08:7

71030 Radiologic examination, chest, complete, minimum of 4 views;

➔ *CPT Assistant* Jul 07:6, Dec 09:14

(For concurrent computer-aided detection [CAD] performed in addition to codes 71010, 71020, 71021, 71022, and 71030, use 0174T. Do not report 71010, 71020, 71021, 71022, and 71030 in conjunction with 0175T for CAD performed remotely from the primary interpretation)

71034 with fluoroscopy

➔ *CPT Assistant* Aug 03:14, Dec 08:7

(For separate chest fluoroscopy, use 76000)

71035 Radiologic examination, chest, special views (eg, lateral decubitus, Bucky studies)

▶(71040, 71060 have been deleted. To report, use 76499)◀

(71090 has been deleted. To report pacemaker or pacing cardioverter-defibrillator lead insertion, replacement, or revision procedures with fluoroscopic guidance, see 33206-33249. To report fluoroscopic guidance for diagnostic lead evaluation without lead insertion, replacement, or revision procedures, use 76000)

71100 Radiologic examination, ribs, unilateral; 2 views

71101 including posteroanterior chest, minimum of 3 views

71110 Radiologic examination, ribs, bilateral; 3 views

71111 including posteroanterior chest, minimum of 4 views

71120 Radiologic examination; sternum, minimum of 2 views

71130 sternoclavicular joint or joints, minimum of 3 views

71250 Computed tomography, thorax; without contrast material

➔ *CPT Assistant* Jul 07:13, Aug 11:10; *CPT Changes: An Insider's View* 2003

➔ *Clinical Examples in Radiology* Fall 08:7

71260 with contrast material(s)

➔ *CPT Assistant* Jul 01:4, Jun 09:9

➔ *Clinical Examples in Radiology* Summer 05:4, Fall 08:7, 11, 12

71270 without contrast material, followed by contrast material(s) and further sections

➔ *CPT Assistant* Jun 01:10, Jul 07:13

➔ *Clinical Examples in Radiology* Fall 08:7

(For cardiac computed tomography of the heart, see 75571-75574)

(To report 3D rendering, see 76376, 76377)

71275 Computed tomographic angiography, chest (noncoronary), with contrast material(s), including noncontrast images, if performed, and image postprocessing

➔ *CPT Assistant* Jul 01:4, Jun 05:11, Dec 05:7, Jan 07:31, Mar 07:7, Jun 09:9, Aug 11:10; *CPT Changes: An Insider's View* 2001, 2007, 2008

➔ *Clinical Examples in Radiology* Spring 05:7, Fall 08:11, 12, Spring 09:11, Fall 09:10, Winter 10:2

(For coronary artery computed tomographic angiography including calcification score and/or cardiac morphology, use 75574)

71550 Magnetic resonance (eg, proton) imaging, chest (eg, for evaluation of hilar and mediastinal lymphadenopathy); without contrast material(s)

➔ *CPT Assistant* Jul 01:7, Apr 10:10, Sep 10:10; *CPT Changes: An Insider's View* 2001

71551 with contrast material(s)

➔ *CPT Assistant* Jul 01:7, Sep 10:10; *CPT Changes: An Insider's View* 2001

71552 without contrast material(s), followed by contrast material(s) and further sequences

➔ *CPT Assistant* Jul 01:7, Apr 10:10, Sep 10:10; *CPT Changes: An Insider's View* 2001

(For breast MRI, see 77058, 77059)

71555 Magnetic resonance angiography, chest (excluding myocardium), with or without contrast material(s)

➔ *CPT Assistant* Fall 95:2, Dec 05:7, Jan 07:31

Spine and Pelvis

72010 Radiologic examination, spine, entire, survey study, anteroposterior and lateral

➔ *CPT Assistant* May 02:18, Jan 07:29

➔ *Clinical Examples in Radiology* Fall 09:10

72020 Radiologic examination, spine, single view, specify level

▲ **72040**   Radiologic examination, spine, cervical; 3 views or less

➔ *CPT Assistant* Sep 01:7; *CPT Changes: An Insider's View* 2001, 2013

➔ *Clinical Examples in Radiology* Fall 09:10, Summer 11:8, Fall 11:9

▲ **72050**   4 or 5 views

➔ *CPT Changes: An Insider's View* 2013

➔ *Clinical Examples in Radiology* Summer 11:8, Fall 11:9

▲ **72052**   6 or more views

➔ *CPT Changes: An Insider's View* 2013

➔ *Clinical Examples in Radiology* Summer 11:8, Fall 11:9

72069   Radiologic examination, spine, thoracolumbar, standing (scoliosis)

➔ *CPT Assistant* Winter 90:9

➔ *Clinical Examples in Radiology* Fall 11:9

72070   Radiologic examination, spine; thoracic, 2 views

➔ *CPT Assistant* Sep 01:7; *CPT Changes: An Insider's View* 2001

➔ *Clinical Examples in Radiology* Fall 11:9

72072   thoracic, 3 views

➔ *CPT Assistant* Sep 01:7; *CPT Changes: An Insider's View* 2001

➔ *Clinical Examples in Radiology* Fall 11:9

72074   thoracic, minimum of 4 views

➔ *CPT Assistant* Sep 01:7; *CPT Changes: An Insider's View* 2001

➔ *Clinical Examples in Radiology* Fall 11:9

72080   thoracolumbar, 2 views

➔ *CPT Assistant* Sep 01:7; *CPT Changes: An Insider's View* 2001

➔ *Clinical Examples in Radiology* Fall 11:9

72090   scoliosis study, including supine and erect studies

➔ *Clinical Examples in Radiology* Fall 11:9

72100   Radiologic examination, spine, lumbosacral; 2 or 3 views

➔ *CPT Assistant* Sep 01:7; *CPT Changes: An Insider's View* 2001

➔ *Clinical Examples in Radiology* Fall 11:9, 10

72110   minimum of 4 views

➔ *CPT Assistant* Sep 01:7; *CPT Changes: An Insider's View* 2001

➔ *Clinical Examples in Radiology* Fall 11:9, 10

72114   complete, including bending views, minimum of 6 views

➔ *CPT Changes: An Insider's View* 2012

72120   bending views only, 2 or 3 views

➔ *CPT Changes: An Insider's View* 2012

➔ *Clinical Examples in Radiology* Fall 11:9, 10

(Contrast material in CT of spine is either by intrathecal or intravenous injection. For intrathecal injection, use also 61055 or 62284. IV injection of contrast material is part of the CT procedure)

72125   Computed tomography, cervical spine; without contrast material

➔ *CPT Changes: An Insider's View* 2003

72126   with contrast material

72127   without contrast material, followed by contrast material(s) and further sections

(For intrathecal injection procedure, see 61055, 62284)

72128   Computed tomography, thoracic spine; without contrast material

➔ *CPT Changes: An Insider's View* 2003

72129   with contrast material

(For intrathecal injection procedure, see 61055, 62284)

72130   without contrast material, followed by contrast material(s) and further sections

(For intrathecal injection procedure, see 61055, 62284)

72131   Computed tomography, lumbar spine; without contrast material

➔ *CPT Changes: An Insider's View* 2003

➔ *Clinical Examples in Radiology* Summer 07:11, Spring 12:10

72132   with contrast material

➔ *CPT Assistant* Fall 93:13

➔ *Clinical Examples in Radiology* Fall 06:5-6, 11-12

72133   without contrast material, followed by contrast material(s) and further sections

(For intrathecal injection procedure, see 61055, 62284)

(To report 3D rendering, see 76376, 76377)

72141   Magnetic resonance (eg, proton) imaging, spinal canal and contents, cervical; without contrast material

➔ *CPT Assistant* Apr 10:10

72142   with contrast material(s)

➔ *CPT Assistant* Apr 10:10

(For cervical spinal canal imaging without contrast material followed by contrast material, use 72156)

72146   Magnetic resonance (eg, proton) imaging, spinal canal and contents, thoracic; without contrast material

➔ *CPT Assistant* May 99:10, Apr 10:10

72147   with contrast material(s)

➔ *CPT Assistant* May 99:10, Apr 10:10

(For thoracic spinal canal imaging without contrast material followed by contrast material, use 72157)

72148   Magnetic resonance (eg, proton) imaging, spinal canal and contents, lumbar; without contrast material

➔ *CPT Assistant* Nov 05:15

➔ *Clinical Examples in Radiology* Spring 06:6, 11

72149   with contrast material(s)

(For lumbar spinal canal imaging without contrast material followed by contrast material, use 72158)

72156   Magnetic resonance (eg, proton) imaging, spinal canal and contents, without contrast material, followed by contrast material(s) and further sequences; cervical

72157   thoracic

72158   lumbar

Radiology

72159 Magnetic resonance angiography, spinal canal and contents, with or without contrast material(s)
➔ *CPT Assistant* Dec 05:7, Jan 07:31

72170 Radiologic examination, pelvis; 1 or 2 views
➔ *CPT Assistant* Sep 01:7, Mar 03:23; *CPT Changes: An Insider's View* 2001
➔ *Clinical Examples in Radiology* Spring 05:12

72190   complete, minimum of 3 views

(For pelvimetry, use 74710)

(For a combined computed tomography [CT] or computed tomographic angiography abdomen and pelvis study, see 74174, 74176-74178)

72191 Computed tomographic angiography, pelvis, with contrast material(s), including noncontrast images, if performed, and image postprocessing
➔ *CPT Assistant* Jul 01:4, 6, Dec 05:7, Jan 07:31; *CPT Changes: An Insider's View* 2001, 2008
➔ *Clinical Examples in Radiology* Summer 08:8, Fall 09:10, Fall 11:9

(Do not report 72191 in conjunction with 73706 or 75635. For CTA aorto-iliofemoral runoff, use 75635)

(Do not report 72191 in conjunction with 74175. For a combined computed tomographic angiography abdomen and pelvis study, use 74174)

72192 Computed tomography, pelvis; without contrast material
➔ *CPT Assistant* Mar 05:1, 4, Mar 07:10, Apr 10:9, Nov 11:6; *CPT Changes: An Insider's View* 2003
➔ *Clinical Examples in Radiology* Winter 06:11, Spring 07:3, 11, Summer 07:11, Fall 09:9, Fall 11:8, Winter 11:8-10

72193   with contrast material(s)
➔ *CPT Assistant* Mar 05:1, 4, Mar 07:10, Apr 10:9, Nov 11:6
➔ *Clinical Examples in Radiology* Winter 05:1, 7, Spring 07:3, 11, Fall 11:8, Winter 11:8-10

72194   without contrast material, followed by contrast material(s) and further sections
➔ *CPT Assistant* Mar 05:1, 4, Mar 07:10, Apr 10:9, Nov 11:6
➔ *Clinical Examples in Radiology* Spring 07:3, 11, Fall 11:8, Winter 11:8-10

(For a combined CT abdomen and pelvis study, see 74176-74178)

(To report 3D rendering, see 76376, 76377)

(For computed tomographic colonography, diagnostic, see 74261-74262. For computed tomographic colonography, screening, use 74263)

(Do not report 72192-72194 in conjunction with 74261-74263)

72195 Magnetic resonance (eg, proton) imaging, pelvis; without contrast material(s)
➔ *CPT Assistant* Jul 01:7, Jun 06:17; *CPT Changes: An Insider's View* 2001
➔ *Clinical Examples in Radiology* Spring 06:8-9, Fall 06:7-8, Summer 07:4, 5

72196   with contrast material(s)
➔ *CPT Assistant* Jul 01:7, Jun 06:17; *CPT Changes: An Insider's View* 2001
➔ *Clinical Examples in Radiology* Spring 06:8-9, Fall 06:7-8

72197   without contrast material(s), followed by contrast material(s) and further sequences
➔ *CPT Assistant* Jul 01:7; *CPT Changes: An Insider's View* 2001
➔ *Clinical Examples in Radiology* Spring 06:8-9, Fall 06:2-3, 7-8

72198 Magnetic resonance angiography, pelvis, with or without contrast material(s)
➔ *CPT Assistant* Dec 05:7, Jan 07:31

72200 Radiologic examination, sacroiliac joints; less than 3 views

72202   3 or more views

72220 Radiologic examination, sacrum and coccyx, minimum of 2 views

72240 Myelography, cervical, radiological supervision and interpretation
➔ *CPT Assistant* Fall 93:13
➔ *Clinical Examples in Radiology* Fall 06:5-6, 11-12

(For complete cervical myelography, see 61055, 62284, 72240)

72255 Myelography, thoracic, radiological supervision and interpretation

(For complete thoracic myelography, see 61055, 62284, 72255)

72265 Myelography, lumbosacral, radiological supervision and interpretation
➔ *CPT Assistant* Fall 93:13, Aug 00:7

(For complete lumbosacral myelography, see 61055, 62284, 72265)

72270 Myelography, 2 or more regions (eg, lumbar/thoracic, cervical/thoracic, lumbar/cervical, lumbar/thoracic/cervical), radiological supervision and interpretation
➔ *CPT Changes: An Insider's View* 2004

(For complete myelography of entire spinal canal, see 61055, 62284, 72270)

72275 Epidurography, radiological supervision and interpretation
➔ *CPT Assistant* Nov 99:40, Jan 00:2, Aug 00:7, Jul 08:9, Oct 09:12, Feb 10:12, May 10:10, Jun 12:12, Jul 12:5; *CPT Changes: An Insider's View* 2000

(72275 includes 77003)

(For injection procedure, see 62280-62282, 62310-62319, 64479-64484)

(Use 72275 only when an epidurogram is performed, images documented, and a formal radiologic report is issued)

▶(Do not report 72275 in conjunction with 22586, 0195T, 0196T, 0309T)◄

Epidurography
72275

Epidural space
surrounding
spinal cord

Subarachnoid
space

Spinal cord

Catheter

Epidural
space

72285 Discography, cervical or thoracic, radiological supervision
and interpretation

➜ *CPT Assistant* Nov 99:35, 40, Mar 11:7; *CPT Changes: An
Insider's View* 2000

➜ *Clinical Examples in Radiology* Fall 10:10

72291 Radiological supervision and interpretation, percutaneous
vertebroplasty, vertebral augmentation, or sacral
augmentation (sacroplasty), including cavity creation, per
vertebral body or sacrum; under fluoroscopic guidance

➜ *CPT Assistant* Mar 07:7; *CPT Changes: An Insider's View* 2007,
2010

72292 under CT guidance

➜ *CPT Assistant* Mar 07:7; *CPT Changes: An Insider's View*
2007, 2010

(For procedure, see 22520-22525, 0200T, 0201T)

72295 Discography, lumbar, radiological supervision and
interpretation

➜ *CPT Assistant* Apr 03:27, Mar 11:7, Jul 12:3

➜ *Clinical Examples in Radiology* Fall 10:10

Upper Extremities

(For stress views, any joint, use 77071)

73000 Radiologic examination; clavicle, complete

73010 scapula, complete

73020 Radiologic examination, shoulder; 1 view

73030 complete, minimum of 2 views

73040 Radiologic examination, shoulder, arthrography,
radiological supervision and interpretation

➜ *CPT Assistant* Jul 01:7, Feb 07:11

➜ *Clinical Examples in Radiology* Spring 05:6, Spring 09:6, 7

(Do not report 77002 in conjunction with 73040)

73050 Radiologic examination; acromioclavicular joints,
bilateral, with or without weighted distraction

73060 humerus, minimum of 2 views

73070 Radiologic examination, elbow; 2 views

➜ *CPT Assistant* Winter 90:9, Sep 01:8; *CPT Changes: An Insider's
View* 2001

73080 complete, minimum of 3 views

73085 Radiologic examination, elbow, arthrography, radiological
supervision and interpretation

➜ *CPT Assistant* Feb 07:11

➜ *Clinical Examples in Radiology* Spring 05:6

(Do not report 77002 in conjunction with 73085)

73090 Radiologic examination; forearm, 2 views

➜ *CPT Assistant* Sep 01:8, Apr 02:14; *CPT Changes: An Insider's
View* 2001

73092 upper extremity, infant, minimum of 2 views

73100 Radiologic examination, wrist; 2 views

➜ *CPT Assistant* Winter 90:9, Sep 01:8; *CPT Changes: An Insider's
View* 2001

73110 complete, minimum of 3 views

➜ *CPT Assistant* Mar 97:10, Nov 06:22

73115 Radiologic examination, wrist, arthrography, radiological
supervision and interpretation

➜ *CPT Assistant* Feb 07:11

➜ *Clinical Examples in Radiology* Spring 05:6

(Do not report 77002 in conjunction with 73115)

73120 Radiologic examination, hand; 2 views

➜ *CPT Assistant* Winter 90:9

73130 minimum of 3 views

➜ *Clinical Examples in Radiology* Winter 05:9, Spring 11:8

73140 Radiologic examination, finger(s), minimum of 2 views

➜ *CPT Assistant* Jan 07:29

➜ *Clinical Examples in Radiology* Spring 11:8

73200 Computed tomography, upper extremity; without contrast
material

➜ *CPT Assistant* Jul 11:17; *CPT Changes: An Insider's View* 2003

Radiology

73201 with contrast material(s)
➔ *CPT Assistant* Jul 11:17
➔ *Clinical Examples in Radiology* Spring 09:6, 7

73202 without contrast material, followed by contrast material(s) and further sections

(To report 3D rendering, see 76376, 76377)

73206 Computed tomographic angiography, upper extremity, with contrast material(s), including noncontrast images, if performed, and image postprocessing
➔ *CPT Assistant* Jul 01:5, Dec 05:7, Jan 07:31; *CPT Changes: An Insider's View* 2001, 2008

73218 Magnetic resonance (eg, proton) imaging, upper extremity, other than joint; without contrast material(s)
➔ *CPT Assistant* Jul 01:7, Sep 10:10, Feb 11:9; *CPT Changes: An Insider's View* 2001

73219 with contrast material(s)
➔ *CPT Assistant* Jul 01:7, Sep 10:10; *CPT Changes: An Insider's View* 2001

73220 without contrast material(s), followed by contrast material(s) and further sequences
➔ *CPT Assistant* Jul 01:7, Sep 10:10; *CPT Changes: An Insider's View* 2001

73221 Magnetic resonance (eg, proton) imaging, any joint of upper extremity; without contrast material(s)
➔ *CPT Assistant* Jul 01:7, Sep 10:10, Feb 11:9; *CPT Changes: An Insider's View* 2001

73222 with contrast material(s)
➔ *CPT Assistant* Jul 01:7, Sep 10:10; *CPT Changes: An Insider's View* 2001
➔ *Clinical Examples in Radiology* Spring 05:5

73223 without contrast material(s), followed by contrast material(s) and further sequences
➔ *CPT Assistant* Jul 01:7, Sep 10:10; *CPT Changes: An Insider's View* 2001
➔ *Clinical Examples in Radiology* Spring 09:6

73225 Magnetic resonance angiography, upper extremity, with or without contrast material(s)
➔ *CPT Assistant* Dec 05:7, Jan 07:31

Lower Extremities

(For stress views, any joint, use 77071)

73500 Radiologic examination, hip, unilateral; 1 view
➔ *Clinical Examples in Radiology* Spring 05:12

73510 complete, minimum of 2 views
➔ *CPT Assistant* Spring 92:9, May 99:10, Apr 02:19, Mar 03:23
➔ *Clinical Examples in Radiology* Spring 05:12

73520 Radiologic examination, hips, bilateral, minimum of 2 views of each hip, including anteroposterior view of pelvis
➔ *CPT Assistant* Apr 02:19
➔ *Clinical Examples in Radiology* Spring 05:12

73525 Radiologic examination, hip, arthrography, radiological supervision and interpretation
➔ *CPT Assistant* Feb 07:11, Jun 12:14
➔ *Clinical Examples in Radiology* Spring 05:6

(Do not report 73525 in conjunction with 77002)

73530 Radiologic examination, hip, during operative procedure

73540 Radiologic examination, pelvis and hips, infant or child, minimum of 2 views

(73542 has been deleted, for arthrography use 27096)

73550 Radiologic examination, femur, 2 views
➔ *CPT Assistant* Sep 01:8; *CPT Changes: An Insider's View* 2001

73560 Radiologic examination, knee; 1 or 2 views

73562 3 views
➔ *CPT Assistant* Apr 02:15
➔ *Clinical Examples in Radiology* Fall 06:4

73564 complete, 4 or more views
➔ *CPT Assistant* Jun 98:11, Nov 98:21
➔ *Clinical Examples in Radiology* Fall 06:4

73565 both knees, standing, anteroposterior
➔ *CPT Assistant* Winter 90:9
➔ *Clinical Examples in Radiology* Fall 06:4

73580 Radiologic examination, knee, arthrography, radiological supervision and interpretation
➔ *CPT Assistant* Feb 07:11
➔ *Clinical Examples in Radiology* Spring 05:6

(Do not report 73580 in conjunction with 77002)

73590 Radiologic examination; tibia and fibula, 2 views
➔ *CPT Assistant* Sep 01:8; *CPT Changes: An Insider's View* 2001

73592 lower extremity, infant, minimum of 2 views

73600 Radiologic examination, ankle; 2 views
➔ *CPT Assistant* Sep 01:8, Apr 02:15, Mar 03:9; *CPT Changes: An Insider's View* 2001

73610 complete, minimum of 3 views
➔ *CPT Assistant* Apr 02:15, Mar 03:9

73615 Radiologic examination, ankle, arthrography, radiological supervision and interpretation
➔ *CPT Assistant* Feb 07:11

(Do not report 73615 in conjunction with 77002)

73620 Radiologic examination, foot; 2 views
➔ *CPT Assistant* Sep 01:8, Apr 02:15, Mar 03:9; *CPT Changes: An Insider's View* 2001

73630 complete, minimum of 3 views
➔ *Clinical Examples in Radiology* Summer 07:12

73650 Radiologic examination; calcaneus, minimum of 2 views

73660 toe(s), minimum of 2 views

73700 Computed tomography, lower extremity; without contrast material
➔ *CPT Assistant* Mar 07:10, Jul 11:17; *CPT Changes: An Insider's View* 2003
➔ *Clinical Examples in Radiology* Fall 08:10, Fall 10:6

73701   with contrast material(s)
> *CPT Assistant* Mar 07:10, Jul 11:17
> *Clinical Examples in Radiology* Summer 10:10

73702   without contrast material, followed by contrast
material(s) and further sections
> *CPT Assistant* Mar 07:10, Jul 11:17

(To report 3D rendering, see 76376, 76377)

73706   Computed tomographic angiography, lower extremity,
with contrast material(s), including noncontrast images, if
performed, and image postprocessing
> *CPT Assistant* Jul 01:5-6, Dec 05:7, Jan 07:31, Apr 08:11,
Apr 11:13; *CPT Changes: An Insider's View* 2001, 2008
> *Clinical Examples in Radiology* Summer 08:8

(For CTA aorto-iliofemoral runoff, use 75635)

73718   Magnetic resonance (eg, proton) imaging, lower
extremity other than joint; without contrast material(s)
> *CPT Assistant* Jul 01:3; *CPT Changes: An Insider's View* 2001
> *Clinical Examples in Radiology* Spring 07:7-9, 12, Summer 07:4, 5

73719   with contrast material(s)
> *CPT Assistant* Jul 01:3; *CPT Changes: An Insider's View*
2001
> *Clinical Examples in Radiology* Spring 07:7-9, 12,
Summer 07:4, 5

73720   without contrast material(s), followed by contrast
material(s) and further sequences
> *CPT Assistant* Jul 01:3; *CPT Changes: An Insider's View*
2001
> *Clinical Examples in Radiology* Spring 07:7-9, 12,
Summer 07:4, 5

73721   Magnetic resonance (eg, proton) imaging, any joint of
lower extremity; without contrast material
> *CPT Assistant* Jul 01:3, Jun 06:17; *CPT Changes: An Insider's
View* 2001
> *Clinical Examples in Radiology* Spring 07:7-9, 12, Summer 07:4, 5

73722   with contrast material(s)
> *CPT Assistant* Jul 01:3, Jun 06:17; *CPT Changes: An Insider's
View* 2001
> *Clinical Examples in Radiology* Spring 07:7-9, 12,
Summer 07:4, 5

73723   without contrast material(s), followed by contrast
material(s) and further sequences
> *CPT Assistant* Jul 01:3; *CPT Changes: An Insider's View*
2001
> *Clinical Examples in Radiology* Spring 07:7-9, 12,
Summer 07:4, 5

73725   Magnetic resonance angiography, lower extremity, with
or without contrast material(s)
> *CPT Assistant* Dec 05:7, Jan 07:31
> *Clinical Examples in Radiology* Spring 06:1-3

Abdomen

74000   Radiologic examination, abdomen; single anteroposterior
view
> *CPT Assistant* Nov 98:21
> *Clinical Examples in Radiology* Spring 07:4, Summer 09:11

74010   anteroposterior and additional oblique and cone
views
> *CPT Assistant* Jan 07:29
> *Clinical Examples in Radiology* Spring 07:4, 8, Summer 11:11

74020   complete, including decubitus and/or erect views

74022   complete acute abdomen series, including supine,
erect, and/or decubitus views, single view chest
> *CPT Changes: An Insider's View* 2003

74150   Computed tomography, abdomen; without contrast
material
> *CPT Assistant* Oct 02:12, Mar 05:1, 4, Apr 10:9, Nov 11:6; *CPT
Changes: An Insider's View* 2003
> *Clinical Examples in Radiology* Spring 07:3, 11, Fall 08:7,
Fall 09:9, Fall 11:8, Winter 11:8, 9

74160   with contrast material(s)
> *CPT Assistant* Mar 05:1, 4, Apr 10:9, Nov 11:6
> *Clinical Examples in Radiology* Spring 07:3, 11, Fall 08:7,
Summer 10:10, Fall 11:8, Winter 11:8, 9

74170   without contrast material, followed by contrast
material(s) and further sections
> *CPT Assistant* Mar 05:4, Apr 10:9, Nov 11:6
> *Clinical Examples in Radiology* Winter 05:1, 7-8, 12,
Spring 07:3, 11, Fall 08:7, Fall 11:8, Winter 11:8, 9

(For a combined CT abdomen and pelvis study, see
74176-74178)

(To report 3D rendering, see 76376, 76377)

(For computed tomographic colonography, diagnostic, see
74261-74262. For computed tomographic colonography,
screening, use 74263)

(Do not report 74150-74170 in conjunction with 74261-
74263)

74174   Computed tomographic angiography, abdomen and
pelvis, with contrast material(s), including noncontrast
images, if performed, and image postprocessing
> *CPT Changes: An Insider's View* 2012
> *Clinical Examples in Radiology* Fall 11:8

(Do not report 74174 in conjunction with 72191, 73706,
74175, 75635, 76376, 76377)

(For CTA aorto-iliofemoral runoff, use 75635)

74175   Computed tomographic angiography, abdomen, with
contrast material(s), including noncontrast images, if
performed, and image postprocessing
> *CPT Assistant* Jul 01:6, Dec 05:7, Jan 07:31, Apr 11:13; *CPT
Changes: An Insider's View* 2001, 2008
> *Clinical Examples in Radiology* Summer 08:8, Fall 09:10, Fall 11:8

(Do not report 74175 in conjunction with 73706 or 75635.
For CTA aorto-iliofemoral runoff, use 75635)

(Do not report 74175 in conjunction with 72191. For a
combined computed tomographic angiography abdomen
and pelvis study, use 74174)

Radiology

For combinations of CT of the abdomen with CT of the pelvis performed at the same session, use the following table. Do not report more than one CT of the abdomen or CT of the pelvis for any session.

Stand Alone Code	74150 CT Abdomen WO Contrast	74160 CT Abdomen W Contrast	74170 CT Abdomen WO/W Contrast
72192 CT Pelvis WO Contrast	74176	74178	74178
72193 CT Pelvis W Contrast	74178	74177	74178
72194 CT Pelvis WO/W Contrast	74178	74178	74178

74176 Computed tomography, abdomen and pelvis; without contrast material

➔ *CPT Assistant* Nov 11:6; *CPT Changes: An Insider's View* 2011

➔ *Clinical Examples in Radiology* Fall 11:8, Winter 11:9

74177 with contrast material(s)

➔ *CPT Assistant* Nov 11:6; *CPT Changes: An Insider's View* 2011

➔ *Clinical Examples in Radiology* Fall 11:8, Winter 11:9

74178 without contrast material in one or both body regions, followed by contrast material(s) and further sections in one or both body regions

➔ *CPT Assistant* Nov 11:6; *CPT Changes: An Insider's View* 2011

➔ *Clinical Examples in Radiology* Fall 11:8, Winter 11:8

(Do not report 74176-74178 in conjunction with 72192-72194, 74150-74170)

(Report 74176, 74177, or 74178 only once per CT abdomen and pelvis examination)

74181 Magnetic resonance (eg, proton) imaging, abdomen; without contrast material(s)

➔ *CPT Assistant* Jul 01:3, Nov 07:9, May 09:9, Jul 09:10; *CPT Changes: An Insider's View* 2001

➔ *Clinical Examples in Radiology* Fall 07:3, Spring 09:4

74182 with contrast material(s)

➔ *CPT Assistant* Jul 01:3, May 09:9, Jul 09:10; *CPT Changes: An Insider's View* 2001

74183 without contrast material(s), followed by with contrast material(s) and further sequences

➔ *CPT Assistant* Jul 01:3, May 09:9, Jul 09:10; *CPT Changes: An Insider's View* 2001

74185 Magnetic resonance angiography, abdomen, with or without contrast material(s)

➔ *CPT Assistant* Dec 05:7, Jan 07:31

➔ *Clinical Examples in Radiology* Spring 06:1-3

74190 Peritoneogram (eg, after injection of air or contrast), radiological supervision and interpretation

➔ *CPT Assistant* Dec 10:13

➔ *Clinical Examples in Radiology* Fall 07:1, 2

(For procedure, use 49400)

(For computed tomography, see 72192 or 74150)

Gastrointestinal Tract

(For percutaneous placement of gastrostomy tube, use 43246)

74210 Radiologic examination; pharynx and/or cervical esophagus

74220 esophagus

74230 Swallowing function, with cineradiography/ videoradiography

➔ *CPT Assistant* Dec 04:17; *CPT Changes: An Insider's View* 2002

➔ *Clinical Examples in Radiology* Summer 06:4-5

74235 Removal of foreign body(s), esophageal, with use of balloon catheter, radiological supervision and interpretation

(For procedure, see 43215, 43247)

74240 Radiologic examination, gastrointestinal tract, upper; with or without delayed films, without KUB

74241 with or without delayed films, with KUB

74245 with small intestine, includes multiple serial films

➔ *CPT Changes: An Insider's View* 2002

74246 Radiological examination, gastrointestinal tract, upper, air contrast, with specific high density barium, effervescent agent, with or without glucagon; with or without delayed films, without KUB

74247 with or without delayed films, with KUB

74249 with small intestine follow-through

➔ *CPT Changes: An Insider's View* 2002

74250 Radiologic examination, small intestine, includes multiple serial films;

➔ *CPT Changes: An Insider's View* 2002

74251 via enteroclysis tube

74260 Duodenography, hypotonic

74261 Computed tomographic (CT) colonography, diagnostic, including image postprocessing; without contrast material

➔ *CPT Assistant* Apr 10:9; *CPT Changes: An Insider's View* 2010

➔ *Clinical Examples in Radiology* Winter 10:6

74262 with contrast material(s) including non-contrast images, if performed

➔ *CPT Assistant* Apr 10:9; *CPT Changes: An Insider's View* 2010

➔ *Clinical Examples in Radiology* Winter 10:4-6

(Do not report 74261, 74262 in conjunction with 72192-72194, 74150-74170, 74263, 76376, 76377)

74263 Computed tomographic (CT) colonography, screening, including image postprocessing

➔ *CPT Assistant* Apr 10:9; *CPT Changes: An Insider's View* 2010

➔ *Clinical Examples in Radiology* Winter 10:6

(Do not report 74263 in conjunction with 72192-72194, 74150-74170, 74261, 74262, 76376, 76377)

74270   Radiologic examination, colon; contrast (eg, barium) enema, with or without KUB

→ *CPT Assistant* May 03:19; *CPT Changes: An Insider's View* 2009

74280   air contrast with specific high density barium, with or without glucagon

74283   Therapeutic enema, contrast or air, for reduction of intussusception or other intraluminal obstruction (eg, meconium ileus)

→ *CPT Assistant* Nov 97:24

74290   Cholecystography, oral contrast;

74291   additional or repeat examination or multiple day examination

74300   Cholangiography and/or pancreatography; intraoperative, radiological supervision and interpretation

→ *CPT Assistant* Nov 99:41, Dec 00:14; *CPT Changes: An Insider's View* 2000

+ 74301   additional set intraoperative, radiological supervision and interpretation (List separately in addition to code for primary procedure)

(Use 74301 in conjunction with 74300)

74305   through existing catheter, radiological supervision and interpretation

→ *CPT Assistant* Nov 99:41, Apr 11:12; *CPT Changes: An Insider's View* 2000, 2002

→ *Clinical Examples in Radiology* Summer 10:11, Summer 11:3

(For procedure, see 47505, 48400, 47560-47561, 47563)

(For biliary duct stone extraction, percutaneous, see 47630, 74327)

74320   Cholangiography, percutaneous, transhepatic, radiological supervision and interpretation

→ *CPT Assistant* Feb 07:11, Nov 10:3, Jan 11:8

74327   Postoperative biliary duct calculus removal, percutaneous via T-tube tract, basket, or snare (eg, Burhenne technique), radiological supervision and interpretation

→ *CPT Changes: An Insider's View* 2002

(For procedure, use 47630)

74328   Endoscopic catheterization of the biliary ductal system, radiological supervision and interpretation

(For procedure, see 43260-43272 as appropriate)

74329   Endoscopic catheterization of the pancreatic ductal system, radiological supervision and interpretation

(For procedure, see 43260-43272 as appropriate)

74330   Combined endoscopic catheterization of the biliary and pancreatic ductal systems, radiological supervision and interpretation

(For procedure, see 43260-43272 as appropriate)

74340   Introduction of long gastrointestinal tube (eg, Miller-Abbott), including multiple fluoroscopies and films, radiological supervision and interpretation

(For tube placement, use 44500)

74355   Percutaneous placement of enteroclysis tube, radiological supervision and interpretation

→ *CPT Assistant* Feb 07:11, Nov 10:3, Jan 11:8

74360   Intraluminal dilation of strictures and/or obstructions (eg, esophagus), radiological supervision and interpretation

→ *CPT Assistant* Spring 94:3, Oct 08:6

74363   Percutaneous transhepatic dilation of biliary duct stricture with or without placement of stent, radiological supervision and interpretation

→ *CPT Changes: An Insider's View* 2002

(For procedure, see 47510, 47511, 47555, 47556)

Urinary Tract

74400   Urography (pyelography), intravenous, with or without KUB, with or without tomography

74410   Urography, infusion, drip technique and/or bolus technique;

74415   with nephrotomography

74420   Urography, retrograde, with or without KUB

→ *CPT Assistant* Sep 00:11, Dec 10:15

74425   Urography, antegrade (pyelostogram, nephrostogram, loopogram), radiological supervision and interpretation

→ *CPT Assistant* Fall 93:14, Dec 97:7, Oct 05:18

→ *Clinical Examples in Radiology* Summer 06:1-3

74430   Cystography, minimum of 3 views, radiological supervision and interpretation

74440   Vasography, vesiculography, or epididymography, radiological supervision and interpretation

74445   Corpora cavernosography, radiological supervision and interpretation

→ *CPT Assistant* Feb 07:11, Nov 10:3, Jan 11:8

74450   Urethrocystography, retrograde, radiological supervision and interpretation

74455   Urethrocystography, voiding, radiological supervision and interpretation

74470   Radiologic examination, renal cyst study, translumbar, contrast visualization, radiological supervision and interpretation

→ *CPT Assistant* Oct 05:18, Feb 07:11, Nov 10:3, Jan 11:8

74475   Introduction of intracatheter or catheter into renal pelvis for drainage and/or injection, percutaneous, radiological supervision and interpretation

→ *CPT Assistant* Dec 97:7, Oct 05:18, Feb 07:11, Nov 10:3, Jan 11:8

74480   Introduction of ureteral catheter or stent into ureter through renal pelvis for drainage and/or injection, percutaneous, radiological supervision and interpretation

→ *CPT Assistant* Fall 93:14, Oct 05:18

→ *Clinical Examples in Radiology* Summer 06:1-3, Summer 08:12

(For transurethral surgery [ureter and pelvis], see 52320-52355)

74485 Dilation of nephrostomy, ureters, or urethra, radiological supervision and interpretation

→ *CPT Assistant* Oct 05:18, Dec 08:7, Jan 09:7

→ *Clinical Examples in Radiology* Summer 06:1-3

(For dilation of ureter without radiologic guidance, use 52341, 52344)

(For change of nephrostomy or pyelostomy tube, use 50398)

Gynecological and Obstetrical

(For abdomen and pelvis, see 72170-72190, 74000-74170)

74710 Pelvimetry, with or without placental localization

74740 Hysterosalpingography, radiological supervision and interpretation

→ *CPT Assistant* Nov 97:24, Jul 99:8, Mar 09:11

(For introduction of saline or contrast for hysterosalpingography, see 58340)

74742 Transcervical catheterization of fallopian tube, radiological supervision and interpretation

(For procedure, use 58345)

74775 Perineogram (eg, vaginogram, for sex determination or extent of anomalies)

Heart

Cardiac magnetic imaging differs from traditional magnetic resonance imaging (MRI) in its ability to provide a physiologic evaluation of cardiac function. Traditional MRI relies on static images to obtain clinical diagnoses based upon anatomic information. Improvement in spatial and temporal resolution has expanded the application from an anatomic test and includes physiologic evaluation of cardiac function. Flow and velocity assessment for valves and intracardiac shunts is performed in addition to a function and morphologic evaluation. Use 75559 with 75565 to report flow with pharmacologic wall motion stress evaluation without contrast. Use 75563 with 75565 to report flow with pharmacologic perfusion stress with contrast.

Cardiac MRI for velocity flow mapping can be reported in conjunction with 75557, 75559, 75561, or 75563.

►Listed procedures may be performed independently or in the course of overall medical care. If the individual providing these services is also responsible for diagnostic workup and/or follow-up care of the patient, also see appropriate sections. Only one procedure in the series 75557-75563 is appropriately reported per session. Only one add-on code for flow velocity can be reported per session.◄

Cardiac MRI studies may be performed at rest and/or during pharmacologic stress. Therefore, the appropriate stress testing code from the 93015-93018 series should be reported in addition to 75559 or 75563.

Cardiac computed tomography (CT) and coronary computed tomographic angiography (CTA) include the axial source images of the pre-contrast, arterial phase sequence, and venous phase sequence (if performed), as well as the two-dimensional and three-dimensional reformatted images resulting from the study, including cine review. Contrast enhanced cardiac CT and coronary CTA codes 75571-75574 include any quantitative assessment when performed as part of the same encounter. Report only one computed tomography heart service per encounter.

(For separate injection procedures for vascular radiology, see **Surgery** section, 36000 36299)

(For cardiac catheterization procedures, see 93451-93572)

(75552-75556 have been deleted. To report, see 75557, 75559, 75561, 75563, 75565)

75557 Cardiac magnetic resonance imaging for morphology and function without contrast material;

→ *CPT Assistant* Jul 10:7; *CPT Changes: An Insider's View* 2008

→ *Clinical Examples in Radiology* Spring 09:2

75559 with stress imaging

→ *CPT Changes: An Insider's View* 2008

→ *Clinical Examples in Radiology* Spring 09:2

75561 Cardiac magnetic resonance imaging for morphology and function without contrast material(s), followed by contrast material(s) and further sequences;

→ *CPT Assistant* Jul 10:7; *CPT Changes: An Insider's View* 2008

→ *Clinical Examples in Radiology* Spring 09:2

75563 with stress imaging

→ *CPT Assistant* Jul 10:7; *CPT Changes: An Insider's View* 2008

→ *Clinical Examples in Radiology* Spring 09:2

(75558, 75560, 75562, 75564 have been deleted. To report flow velocity, use 75565)

+ **75565** Cardiac magnetic resonance imaging for velocity flow mapping (List separately in addition to code for primary procedure)

→ *CPT Assistant* Jul 10:7; *CPT Changes: An Insider's View* 2010

(Use 75565 in conjunction with 75557, 75559, 75561, 75563)

(Do not report 75557, 75559, 75561, 75563, 75565 in conjunction with 76376, 76377)

75571 Computed tomography, heart, without contrast material, with quantitative evaluation of coronary calcium

→ *CPT Assistant* Jul 10:7; *CPT Changes: An Insider's View* 2010

→ *Clinical Examples in Radiology* Winter 10:2, 3

75572 Computed tomography, heart, with contrast material, for evaluation of cardiac structure and morphology (including 3D image postprocessing, assessment of cardiac function, and evaluation of venous structures, if performed)

→ *CPT Assistant* Jul 10:7; *CPT Changes: An Insider's View* 2010

→ *Clinical Examples in Radiology* Winter 10:2, 3

Radiology

75573 Computed tomography, heart, with contrast material, for evaluation of cardiac structure and morphology in the setting of congenital heart disease (including 3D image postprocessing, assessment of LV cardiac function, RV structure and function and evaluation of venous structures, if performed)

➔ *CPT Assistant* Jul 10:7; *CPT Changes: An Insider's View* 2010

➔ *Clinical Examples in Radiology* Winter 10:2, 3

75574 Computed tomographic angiography, heart, coronary arteries and bypass grafts (when present), with contrast material, including 3D image postprocessing (including evaluation of cardiac structure and morphology, assessment of cardiac function, and evaluation of venous structures, if performed)

➔ *CPT Assistant* Jul 10:7; *CPT Changes: An Insider's View* 2010

➔ *Clinical Examples in Radiology* Winter 10:1-3

Vascular Procedures

Aorta and Arteries

Selective vascular catheterizations should be coded to include introduction and all lesser order selective catheterizations used in the approach (eg, the description for a selective right middle cerebral artery catheterization includes the introduction and placement catheterization of the right common and internal carotid arteries).

Additional second and/or third order arterial catheterizations within the same family of arteries supplied by a single first order artery should be expressed by 36218 or 36248. Additional first order or higher catheterizations in vascular families supplied by a first order vessel different from a previously selected and coded family should be separately coded using the conventions described above.

The lower extremity endovascular revascularization codes describing services performed for occlusive disease (37220-37235) include catheterization (36200, 36140, 36245-36248) in the work described by the codes. Catheterization codes are not additionally reported for diagnostic lower extremity angiography when performed through the same access site as the therapy (37220-37235) performed in the same session. However, catheterization for the diagnostic lower extremity angiogram may be reported separately if a different arterial puncture site is necessary.

For angiography performed in conjunction with therapeutic transcatheter radiological supervision and interpretation services, see the **Radiology Transcatheter Procedures** guidelines.

Diagnostic angiography (radiological supervision and interpretation) codes should NOT be used with interventional procedures for:

1. Contrast injections, angiography, roadmapping, and/or fluoroscopic guidance for the intervention,

2. Vessel measurement, and

3. Post-angioplasty/stent/atherectomy angiography, as this work is captured in the radiological supervision and interpretation code(s). In those therapeutic codes that include radiological supervision and interpretation, this work is captured in the therapeutic code.

Diagnostic angiography performed at the time of an interventional procedure is separately reportable if:

1. No prior catheter-based angiographic study is available and a full diagnostic study is performed, and the decision to intervene is based on the diagnostic study, OR

2. A prior study is available, but as documented in the medical record:

    a. The patient's condition with respect to the clinical indication has changed since the prior study, OR

    b. There is inadequate visualization of the anatomy and/or pathology, OR

    c. There is a clinical change during the procedure that requires new evaluation outside the target area of intervention.

Diagnostic angiography performed at a separate sessions from an interventional procedure is separately reported.

If diagnostic angiography is necessary, is performed at the same session as the interventional procedure and meets the above criteria, modifier 59 must be appended to the diagnostic radiological supervision and interpretation code(s) to denote that diagnostic work has been done following these guidelines.

Diagnostic angiography performed at the time of an interventional procedure is NOT separately reportable if it is specifically included in the interventional code descriptor.

    (For intravenous procedure, see 36000, 36005-36015, and for intra-arterial procedure, see 36100-36248)

    (For radiological supervision and interpretation, see 75600-75893)

75600 Aortography, thoracic, without serialography, radiological supervision and interpretation

    ▶(For supravalvular aortography performed at the time of cardiac catheterization, use 93567, which includes imaging supervision, interpretation, and report)◀

75605 Aortography, thoracic, by serialography, radiological supervision and interpretation

➔ *CPT Assistant* Spring 94:29, Dec 98:9

    ▶(For supravalvular aortography performed at the time of cardiac catheterization, use 93567, which includes imaging supervision, interpretation, and report)◀

Radiology

Aortography
75600-75630

A radiographic contrast study is performed on the abdominal or thoracic aorta.

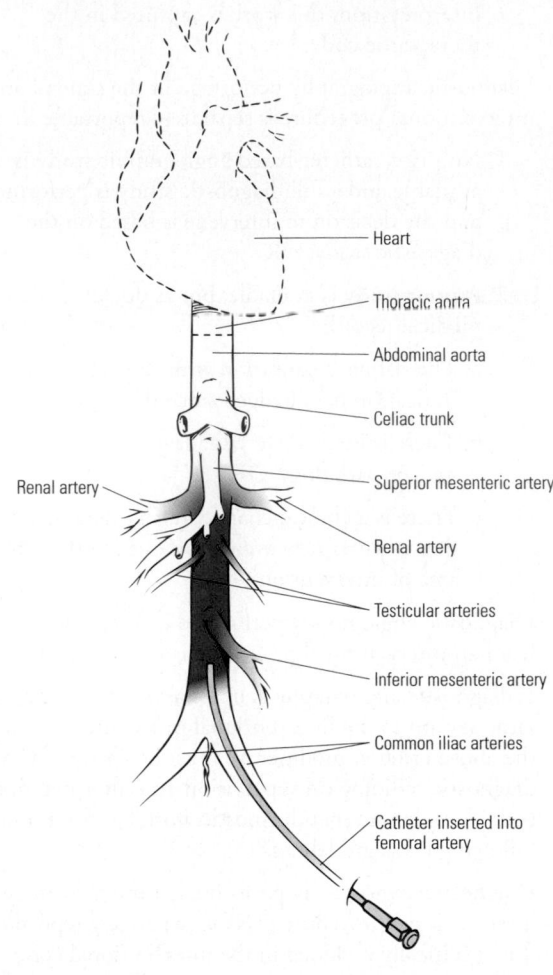

- Heart
- Thoracic aorta
- Abdominal aorta
- Celiac trunk
- Superior mesenteric artery
- Renal artery
- Renal artery
- Testicular arteries
- Inferior mesenteric artery
- Common iliac arteries
- Catheter inserted into femoral artery

75625 Aortography, abdominal, by serialography, radiological supervision and interpretation

➡ *CPT Assistant* Fall 93:16, Jan 01:14, Dec 07:14, Apr 08:11, Dec 09:13

➡ *Clinical Examples in Radiology* Winter 08:1, 2, 4, 5, 9

75630 Aortography, abdominal plus bilateral iliofemoral lower extremity, catheter, by serialography, radiological supervision and interpretation

➡ *CPT Assistant* Fall 93:16, Jan 01:14, Apr 08:11, Dec 09:13

75635 Computed tomographic angiography, abdominal aorta and bilateral iliofemoral lower extremity runoff, with contrast material(s), including noncontrast images, if performed, and image postprocessing

➡ *CPT Assistant* Jul 01:4-5, Dec 05:7, Jan 07:31, Apr 11:13; *CPT Changes: An Insider's View* 2001, 2008

➡ *Clinical Examples in Radiology* Spring 06:1-3, Summer 08:7, 8, Summer 10:10

(Do not report 75635 in conjunction with 72191, 73706, 74175 or 74174)

►(75650 has been deleted. To report, see 36221-36226)◄

75658 Angiography, brachial, retrograde, radiological supervision and interpretation

►(75660 has been deleted. To report, use 36227)◄

►(75662 has been deleted. To report, use 36227 and append modifier 50)◄

►(75665 has been deleted. To report, see 36223, 36224)◄

►(75671 has been deleted. To report, see 36223 and 36224 and append modifier 50 as appropriate)◄

►(75676 has been deleted. To report, see 36222-36224)◄

►(75680 has been deleted. To report, see 36222-36224 and append modifier 50 as appropriate)◄

►(75685 has been deleted. To report, see 36225, 36226)◄

75705 Angiography, spinal, selective, radiological supervision and interpretation

75710 Angiography, extremity, unilateral, radiological supervision and interpretation

➡ *CPT Assistant* Apr 99:11, Jan 01:14

➡ *Clinical Examples in Radiology* Spring 11:1, Winter 11:1, Spring 12:4

75716 Angiography, extremity, bilateral, radiological supervision and interpretation

➡ *CPT Assistant* Fall 93:16, Jan 01:14, Dec 07:14, Apr 08:11, Dec 09:13

➡ *Clinical Examples in Radiology* Winter 08:1, 2, 4, 5, 9

(75722 has been deleted. To report, see 36251, 36253)

(75724 has been deleted. To report, see 36252, 36254)

75726 Angiography, visceral, selective or supraselective (with or without flush aortogram), radiological supervision and interpretation

➡ *Clinical Examples in Radiology* Summer 08:1, 2, 3

(For selective angiography, each additional visceral vessel studied after basic examination, use 75774)

75731 Angiography, adrenal, unilateral, selective, radiological supervision and interpretation

75733 Angiography, adrenal, bilateral, selective, radiological supervision and interpretation

75736 Angiography, pelvic, selective or supraselective, radiological supervision and interpretation

➡ *Clinical Examples in Radiology* Spring 05:14, Winter 08:4, 5

75741 Angiography, pulmonary, unilateral, selective, radiological supervision and interpretation

➡ *CPT Assistant* Mar 12:10

75743 Angiography, pulmonary, bilateral, selective, radiological supervision and interpretation

➡ *CPT Assistant* Spring 94:29, Apr 98:7

Radiology

75746   Angiography, pulmonary, by nonselective catheter or venous injection, radiological supervision and interpretation

►(For pulmonary angiography by nonselective catheter or venous injection performed at the time of cardiac catheterization, use 93568, which includes imaging supervision, interpretation, and report)◄

75756   Angiography, internal mammary, radiological supervision and interpretation

►(For internal mammary angiography performed at the time of cardiac catheterization, see 93455, 93457, 93459, 93461, 93564, which include imaging supervision, interpretation, and report)◄

+ 75774   Angiography, selective, each additional vessel studied after basic examination, radiological supervision and interpretation (List separately in addition to code for primary procedure)

➔ *CPT Assistant* Fall 93:17, Spring 94:29, Apr 11:13
➔ *Clinical Examples in Radiology* Summer 08:1, 2, 3, Winter 08:1, 2, 4, 5

(Use 75774 in addition to code for specific initial vessel studied)

►(Do not report 75774 as part of diagnostic angiography of the extracranial and intracranial cervicocerebral vessels. It may be appropriate to report 75774 for diagnostic angiography of upper extremities and other vascular beds performed in the same session)◄

(For angiography, see 36147, 75600-75756, 75791)

(For catheterizations, see codes 36215-36248)

►(For cardiac catheterization procedures, see 93452-93462, 93531-93533, 93563-93568)◄

(75790 has been deleted. To report, see 36147, 75791)

75791   Angiography, arteriovenous shunt (eg, dialysis patient fistula/graft), complete evaluation of dialysis access, including fluoroscopy, image documentation and report (includes injections of contrast and all necessary imaging from the arterial anastomosis and adjacent artery through entire venous outflow including the inferior or superior vena cava), radiological supervision and interpretation

➔ *CPT Assistant* Dec 11:16; *CPT Changes: An Insider's View* 2010
➔ *Clinical Examples in Radiology* Winter 10:8

(Do not report 75791 in conjunction with 36147, 36148)

(For introduction of catheter, if necessary, see 36140, 36215-36217, 36245-36247)

(Use 75791 only if radiological evaluation is performed through an already existing access into the shunt or from an access that is not a direct puncture of the shunt)

(For radiological evaluation with needle/catheter introduction, AV dialysis shunt, complete procedure, use 36147)

Veins and Lymphatics

For venography performed in conjunction with therapeutic transcatheter radiological supervision and interpretation services, see the **Radiology Transcatheter Procedures** guidelines.

Diagnostic venography (radiological supervision and interpretation) codes should NOT be used with interventional procedures for:

1. Contrast injections, venography, roadmapping, and/or fluoroscopic guidance for the intervention,

2. Vessel measurement, and

3. Post-angioplasty/stent venography, as this work is captured in the radiological supervision and intrepretation code(s).

Diagnostic venography performed at the time of an interventional procedure is separately reportable if:

1. No prior catheter-based venographic study is available and a full diagnostic study is performed, and decision to intervene is based on the diagnostic study, OR

2. A prior study is available, but as documented in the medical record:

   a. The patient's condition with respect to the clinical indication has changed since the prior study, OR

   b. There is inadequate visualization of the anatomy and/or pathology, OR

   c. There is a clinical change during the procedure that requires new evaluation outside the target area of intervention.

Diagnostic venography performed at a separate setting from an interventional procedure is separately reported.

Diagnostic venography performed at the time of an interventional procedure is NOT separately reportable if it is specifically included in the interventional code descriptor.

(For injection procedure for venous system, see 36000-36015, 36400-36510)

(For injection procedure for lymphatic system, use 38790)

75801   Lymphangiography, extremity only, unilateral, radiological supervision and interpretation

75803   Lymphangiography, extremity only, bilateral, radiological supervision and interpretation

75805   Lymphangiography, pelvic/abdominal, unilateral, radiological supervision and interpretation

75807   Lymphangiography, pelvic/abdominal, bilateral, radiological supervision and interpretation

75809   Shuntogram for investigation of previously placed indwelling nonvascular shunt (eg, LeVeen shunt, ventriculoperitoneal shunt, indwelling infusion pump), radiological supervision and interpretation

➔ *CPT Assistant* Feb 07:11, Jul 08:13, Aug 08:13, Sep 08:10, Nov 10:3, Jan 11:8; *CPT Changes: An Insider's View* 2001

Radiology

(For procedure, see 49427 or 61070)

75810 Splenoportography, radiological supervision and interpretation

➔ *CPT Assistant* Feb 07:11, Nov 10:3, Jan 11:8

75820 Venography, extremity, unilateral, radiological supervision and interpretation

➔ *CPT Assistant* Oct 97:10, May 08:14

➔ *Clinical Examples in Radiology* Summer 06:8-9, Spring 08:12

Venography
75820-75822

A radiographic contrast study is performed on the veins of the lower extremities.

Inferior vena cava
Common iliac
Percutaneous catheter
Deep femoral vein
Femoral vein
Great saphenous vein
Popliteal vein
Anterior tibial vein
Small saphenous vein
Posterior tibial vein
Peroneal vein
Venous arch on dorsum of foot

75822 Venography, extremity, bilateral, radiological supervision and interpretation

75825 Venography, caval, inferior, with serialography, radiological supervision and interpretation

➔ *Clinical Examples in Radiology* Winter 05:5-6, Winter 12:3

75827 Venography, caval, superior, with serialography, radiological supervision and interpretation

➔ *CPT Assistant* Apr 98:12

➔ *Clinical Examples in Radiology* Winter 12:3

75831 Venography, renal, unilateral, selective, radiological supervision and interpretation

➔ *CPT Assistant* Sep 98:7

➔ *Clinical Examples in Radiology* Winter 12:3

75833 Venography, renal, bilateral, selective, radiological supervision and interpretation

➔ *CPT Assistant* Sep 98:7

➔ *Clinical Examples in Radiology* Winter 12:3

75840 Venography, adrenal, unilateral, selective, radiological supervision and interpretation

75842 Venography, adrenal, bilateral, selective, radiological supervision and interpretation

75860 Venography, venous sinus (eg, petrosal and inferior sagittal) or jugular, catheter, radiological supervision and interpretation

➔ *CPT Changes: An Insider's View* 2004

75870 Venography, superior sagittal sinus, radiological supervision and interpretation

75872 Venography, epidural, radiological supervision and interpretation

75880 Venography, orbital, radiological supervision and interpretation

75885 Percutaneous transhepatic portography with hemodynamic evaluation, radiological supervision and interpretation

➔ *CPT Assistant* Oct 96:4, Mar 02:10, Dec 03:2, Feb 07:11, Nov 10:3, Jan 11:8

75887 Percutaneous transhepatic portography without hemodynamic evaluation, radiological supervision and interpretation

➔ *CPT Assistant* Mar 02:10, Dec 03:2, Feb 07:11, Jan 11:8

75889 Hepatic venography, wedged or free, with hemodynamic evaluation, radiological supervision and interpretation

75891 Hepatic venography, wedged or free, without hemodynamic evaluation, radiological supervision and interpretation

75893 Venous sampling through catheter, with or without angiography (eg, for parathyroid hormone, renin), radiological supervision and interpretation

(For procedure, use 36500)

Transcatheter Procedures

Therapeutic transcatheter radiological supervision and interpretation code(s) include the following services associated with that intervention:

1. Contrast injections, angiography/venography, roadmapping, and fluoroscopic guidance for the intervention,

2. Vessel measurement, and

3. Completion angiography/venography (except for those uses permitted by 75898).

Unless specifically included in the code descriptor, diagnostic angiography/venography performed at the time of transcatheter therapeutic radiological and interpretation service(s) is separately reportable (eg, no prior catheter-based diagnostic angiography/venography study of the target vessel is available, prior diagnostic study is inadequate, patient's condition with respect to the clinical indication has changed since the prior study or during the intervention). See 75600-75893.

Codes 75956 and 75957 include all angiography of the thoracic aorta and its branches for diagnostic imaging prior to deployment of the primary endovascular devices (including all routine components of modular devices), fluoroscopic guidance in the delivery of the endovascular components, and intraprocedural arterial angiography (eg, confirm position, detect endoleak, evaluate runoff).

Code 75958 includes the analogous services for placement of each proximal thoracic endovascular extension. Code 75959 includes the analogous services for placement of a distal thoracic endovascular extension(s) placed during a procedure after the primary repair.

75894   Transcatheter therapy, embolization, any method, radiological supervision and interpretation

➔ *CPT Assistant* Sep 98:7, Feb 08:5, Apr 12:5

➔ *Clinical Examples in Radiology* Summer 07:2, Winter 07:1-3, Summer 08:1, 2, 3, Winter 08:4, 5, Fall 11:3

(For uterine fibroid embolization [uterine artery embolization performed to treat uterine fibroids], use 37210)

(For obstetrical and gynecologic embolization procedures other than uterine fibroid embolization [eg, embolization to treat obstetrical or postpartum hemorrhage], use 37204)

▲ **75896**   Transcatheter therapy, infusion, other than for thrombolysis, radiological supervision and interpretation

➔ *CPT Assistant* May 01:4; *CPT Changes: An Insider's View* 2013

➔ *Clinical Examples in Radiology* Spring 08:7, 8, Winter 12:3

▶(For radiological supervision and interpretation for thrombolysis other than coronary, see 37211-37214)◀

▶(Do not report 75896 in conjunction with 37211-37214)◀

(For infusion for coronary disease, see 92975, 92977)

▲ **75898**   Angiography through existing catheter for follow-up study for transcatheter therapy, embolization or infusion, other than for thrombolysis

➔ *CPT Assistant* Dec 07:11, Nov 11:11; *CPT Changes: An Insider's View* 2002, 2013

➔ *Clinical Examples in Radiology* Summer 07:2, Summer 08:1, 2, 3, Winter 08:4, 5

▶(For thrombolysis infusion management other than coronary, see 37211-37214)◀

▶(Do not report 75898 in conjunction with 37211-37214)◀

▶(75900 has been deleted. For exchange of a previously placed intravascular catheter during thrombolytic therapy with contrast monitoring, radiological supervision and interpretation, see 37211-37214)◀

75901   Mechanical removal of pericatheter obstructive material (eg, fibrin sheath) from central venous device via separate venous access, radiologic supervision and interpretation

➔ *CPT Assistant* Jul 03:13, Dec 04:12; *CPT Changes: An Insider's View* 2003

(For procedure, use 36595)

(For venous catheterization, see 36010-36012)

75902   Mechanical removal of intraluminal (intracatheter) obstructive material from central venous device through device lumen, radiologic supervision and interpretation

➔ *CPT Assistant* Jul 03:13, Dec 04:12; *CPT Changes: An Insider's View* 2003

(For procedure, use 36596)

(For venous catheterization, see 36010-36012)

(75940 has been deleted. To report, use 37191)

75945   Intravascular ultrasound (non-coronary vessel), radiological supervision and interpretation; initial vessel

➔ *Clinical Examples in Radiology* Winter 12:3

+ **75946**   each additional non-coronary vessel (List separately in addition to code for primary procedure)

➔ *Clinical Examples in Radiology* Winter 12:3

(Use 75946 in conjunction with 75945)

(For catheterizations, see codes 36215-36248)

(For transcatheter therapies, see codes 37200-37208, 61624, 61626)

(For procedure, see 37250, 37251)

75952   Endovascular repair of infrarenal abdominal aortic aneurysm or dissection, radiological supervision and interpretation

➔ *CPT Assistant* Apr 12:3; *CPT Changes: An Insider's View* 2001

(For implantation of endovascular grafts, see 34800-34805)

(For radiologic supervision and interpretation of endovascular repair of abdominal aortic aneurysm involving visceral vessels, see Category III codes 0080T, 0081T)

75953   Placement of proximal or distal extension prosthesis for endovascular repair of infrarenal aortic or iliac artery aneurysm, pseudoaneurysm, or dissection, radiological supervision and interpretation

➔ *CPT Assistant* Feb 03:3; *CPT Changes: An Insider's View* 2001, 2003

(For implantation of endovascular extension prostheses, see 34825, 34826)

75954   Endovascular repair of iliac artery aneurysm, pseudoaneurysm, arteriovenous malformation, or trauma, using ilio-iliac tube endoprosthesis, radiological supervision and interpretation

➔ *CPT Assistant* Feb 03:3; *CPT Changes: An Insider's View* 2003, 2011

Radiology

(For implantation of endovascular graft, see 34900)

(For endovascular repair of iliac artery bifurcation [eg, aneurysm, pseudoaneurysm, arteriovenous malformation, trauma] using bifurcated endoprosthesis, radiological supervision and interpretation, use 0255T)

75956 Endovascular repair of descending thoracic aorta (eg, aneurysm, pseudoaneurysm, dissection, penetrating ulcer, intramural hematoma, or traumatic disruption); involving coverage of left subclavian artery origin, initial endoprosthesis plus descending thoracic aortic extension(s), if required, to level of celiac artery origin, radiological supervision and interpretation

➔ *CPT Changes: An Insider's View* 2006

➔ *Clinical Examples in Radiology* Winter 06:17

(For implantation of endovascular graft, use 33880)

75957 not involving coverage of left subclavian artery origin, initial endoprosthesis plus descending thoracic aortic extension(s), if required, to level of celiac artery origin, radiological supervision and interpretation

➔ *CPT Changes: An Insider's View* 2006

➔ *Clinical Examples in Radiology* Winter 06:17

(For implantation of endovascular graft, use 33881)

75958 Placement of proximal extension prosthesis for endovascular repair of descending thoracic aorta (eg, aneurysm, pseudoaneurysm, dissection, penetrating ulcer, intramural hematoma, or traumatic disruption), radiological supervision and interpretation

➔ *CPT Changes: An Insider's View* 2006

➔ *Clinical Examples in Radiology* Winter 06:17

(Report 75958 for each proximal extension)

(For implantation of proximal endovascular extension, see 33883, 33884)

75959 Placement of distal extension prosthesis(s) (delayed) after endovascular repair of descending thoracic aorta, as needed, to level of celiac origin, radiological supervision and interpretation

➔ *CPT Changes: An Insider's View* 2006

➔ *Clinical Examples in Radiology* Winter 06:17

(Do not report 75959 in conjunction with 75956, 75957)

(Report 75959 once, regardless of number of modules deployed)

(For implantation of distal endovascular extension, use 33886)

75960 Transcatheter introduction of intravascular stent(s) (except coronary, carotid, vertebral, iliac, and lower extremity artery), percutaneous and/or open, radiological supervision and interpretation, each vessel

➔ *CPT Assistant* Fall 93:18, Oct 96:2, May 01:4, Dec 03:2, Jul 11:5, Apr 12:5; *CPT Changes: An Insider's View* 2005, 2011

(For stent placement, including radiological supervision and interpretation, in iliac, femoral, popliteal, and tibial/peroneal arteries, see 37221, 37223, 37226, 37227, 37230, 37231, 37234, 37235)

(For procedure, see 37205-37208)

(For radiologic supervision and interpretation for transcatheter placement of extracranial vertebral or intrathoracic carotid artery stent(s), see Category III codes 0075T, 0076T)

▶(75961 has been deleted. To report, use 37197)◀

(For removal of a vena cava filter, use 37193)

75962 Transluminal balloon angioplasty, peripheral artery other than renal, or other visceral artery, iliac or lower extremity, radiological supervision and interpretation

➔ *CPT Assistant* Fall 93:18, May 01:4, Jul 11:5, Apr 12:6; *CPT Changes: An Insider's View* 2011, 2012

➔ *Clinical Examples in Radiology* Spring 07:1-3, Winter 08:1, 2, 4, 5, Winter 10:9

(For radiological supervision and interpretation for transluminal balloon angioplasty in iliac, femoral, popliteal, and tibial/peroneal arteries, see 37220-37235)

(For procedure, see 35458, 35475)

+ 75964 Transluminal balloon angioplasty, each additional peripheral artery other than renal or other visceral artery, iliac or lower extremity, radiological supervision and interpretation (List separately in addition to code for primary procedure)

➔ *CPT Assistant* Dec 07:10, Jul 11:5; *CPT Changes: An Insider's View* 2011, 2012

(Use 75964 in conjunction with 75962)

75966 Transluminal balloon angioplasty, renal or other visceral artery, radiological supervision and interpretation

➔ *Clinical Examples in Radiology* Fall 11:3

+ 75968 Transluminal balloon angioplasty, each additional visceral artery, radiological supervision and interpretation (List separately in addition to code for primary procedure)

(Use 75968 in conjunction with 75966)

▶(For percutaneous transluminal coronary angioplasty, see 92920-92944)◀

75970 Transcatheter biopsy, radiological supervision and interpretation

(For injection procedure only for transcatheter therapy or biopsy, see 36100-36299)

(For transcatheter renal and ureteral biopsy, use 52007)

(For percutaneous needle biopsy of pancreas, use 48102; of retroperitoneal lymph node or mass, use 49180)

75978 Transluminal balloon angioplasty, venous (eg, subclavian stenosis), radiological supervision and interpretation

➔ *CPT Assistant* Oct 96:4, Feb 97:2, May 01:4, Dec 03:2, Dec 11:16, Apr 12:6

➔ *Clinical Examples in Radiology* Spring 05:8-10, Spring 07:1-3, Winter 10:7-9, Spring 12:6

75980 Percutaneous transhepatic biliary drainage with contrast monitoring, radiological supervision and interpretation

➔ *CPT Assistant* Feb 07:11, Nov 10:3, Jan 11:8

75982   Percutaneous placement of drainage catheter for combined internal and external biliary drainage or of a drainage stent for internal biliary drainage in patients with an inoperable mechanical biliary obstruction, radiological supervision and interpretation
➔ *CPT Assistant* Feb 07:11, Nov 10:3, Jan 11:8

75984   Change of percutaneous tube or drainage catheter with contrast monitoring (eg, genitourinary system, abscess), radiological supervision and interpretation
➔ *CPT Assistant* Nov 97:24; *CPT Changes: An Insider's View* 2008
➔ *Clinical Examples in Radiology* Summer 10:11

(For percutaneous replacement of gastrostomy, duodenostomy, jejunostomy, gastro-jejunostomy, or cecostomy [or other colonic] tube including fluoroscopic imaging guidance, see 49450-49452)

(For change of nephrostomy or pyelostomy tube only, use 50398)

(For introduction procedure only for percutaneous biliary drainage, see 47510, 47511)

(For percutaneous cholecystostomy, use 47490)

(For change of percutaneous biliary drainage catheter only, use 47525)

(For percutaneous nephrostolithotomy or pyelostolithotomy, see 50080, 50081)

(For removal and/or replacement of an internally dwelling ureteral stent via a transurethral approach, see 50385-50386)

75989   Radiological guidance (ie, fluoroscopy, ultrasound, or computed tomography), for percutaneous drainage (eg, abscess, specimen collection), with placement of catheter, radiological supervision and interpretation
➔ *CPT Assistant* Nov 97:24, Mar 98:8, Feb 07:11, Nov 10:3, Apr 11:12; *CPT Changes: An Insider's View* 2001, 2002
➔ *Clinical Examples in Radiology* Summer 10:3, Summer 11:3, Winter 11:10

▶(Do not report 75989 in conjunction with 32554, 32555, 32556, 32557, 47490)◀

Transluminal Atherectomy

(75992 has been deleted. To report, see 37225, 37227, 37229, 37231, 0238T)

(75993 has been deleted. To report, see 37233, 37235, 0238T)

(75994 has been deleted. To report, use 0234T)

(75995 has been deleted. To report, use 0235T)

(75996 has been deleted. To report, use 0235T)

Other Procedures

(For computed tomography cerebral perfusion analysis, see Category III code 0042T)

(For arthrography of shoulder, use 73040; elbow, use 73085; wrist, use 73115; hip, use 73525; knee, use 73580; ankle, use 73615)

▲ **76000**   Fluoroscopy (separate procedure), up to 1 hour physician or other qualified health care professional time, other than 71023 or 71034 (eg, cardiac fluoroscopy)
➔ *CPT Assistant* Apr 96:11, Nov 99:32, Dec 00:14, Apr 03:7, Jul 03:16, Aug 03:14, Jul 08:9, Aug 08:7, Dec 08:7, 9, Aug 10:8, Oct 10:14, Nov 10:3, Dec 10:14, Jul 11:5, Nov 11:11; *CPT Changes: An Insider's View* 2000, 2013

▲ **76001**   Fluoroscopy, physician or other qualified health care professional time more than 1 hour, assisting a nonradiologic physician or other qualified health care professional (eg, nephrostolithotomy, ERCP, bronchoscopy, transbronchial biopsy)
➔ *CPT Assistant* Nov 10:3, Nov 11:11; *CPT Changes: An Insider's View* 2013

76010   Radiologic examination from nose to rectum for foreign body, single view, child
➔ *CPT Assistant* Feb 10:12; *CPT Changes: An Insider's View* 2001
➔ *Clinical Examples in Radiology* Summer 09:11

76080   Radiologic examination, abscess, fistula or sinus tract study, radiological supervision and interpretation
➔ *CPT Assistant* Nov 97:24, Mar 98:8, Nov 03:14, Dec 06:10, Jan 09:8
➔ *Clinical Examples in Radiology* Fall 09:9

(For contrast injection[s] and radiological assessment of gastrostomy, duodenostomy, jejunostomy, gastro-jejunostomy, or cecostomy [or other colonic] tube including fluoroscopic imaging guidance, use 49465)

76098   Radiological examination, surgical specimen
➔ *Clinical Examples in Radiology* Fall 10:1

76100   Radiologic examination, single plane body section (eg, tomography), other than with urography

76101   Radiologic examination, complex motion (ie, hypercycloidal) body section (eg, mastoid polytomography), other than with urography; unilateral

76102   bilateral

(Do not report 76101, 76102 more than once per day)

(For panoramic X-ray, use 70355)

(For nephrotomography, use 74415)

76120   Cineradiography/videoradiography, except where specifically included
➔ *CPT Assistant* Sep 00:4, Apr 04:15, Apr 11:13; *CPT Changes: An Insider's View* 2002

+ **76125**   Cineradiography/videoradiography to complement routine examination (List separately in addition to code for primary procedure)
➔ *CPT Assistant* Oct 97:1, Sep 00:4; *CPT Changes: An Insider's View* 2002

Radiology

76140 Consultation on X-ray examination made elsewhere, written report

➲ *CPT Assistant* Summer 91:13, Oct 97:1

(76150 has been deleted)

(76350 has been deleted)

(2D reformatting is no longer separately reported. To report 3D rendering, see 76376, 76377)

▲ **76376** 3D rendering with interpretation and reporting of computed tomography, magnetic resonance imaging, ultrasound, or other tomographic modality with image postprocessing under concurrent supervision; not requiring image postprocessing on an independent workstation

➲ *CPT Assistant* Dec 05:1, 7, Jan 07:31, Jul 08:3, May 09:9, Jun 09:9, Jul 09:10, Apr 10:5, Jul 10:7; *CPT Changes: An Insider's View* 2006, 2013

➲ *Clinical Examples in Radiology* Spring 06:8-9, Fall 06:9-10, Winter 06:17, Winter 07:4-5, Summer 08:8, Fall 08:12, Spring 09:4, Summer 09:14, Fall 09:9, Spring 10:2, Summer 10:10, Fall 10:6, Winter 10:6

(Use 76376 in conjunction with code[s] for base imaging procedure[s])

►(Do not report 76376 in conjunction with 31627, 70496, 70498, 70544-70549, 71275, 71555, 72159, 72191, 72198, 73206, 73225, 73706, 73725, 74174, 74175, 74185, 74261-74263, 75557, 75559, 75561, 75563, 75565, 75571-75574, 75635, 76377, 78012-78999, 0159T)◄

▲ **76377** requiring image postprocessing on an independent workstation

➲ *CPT Assistant* Dec 05:1, Jan 07:31, Jul 08:3, May 09:9, Jun 09:9, Jul 09:10, Dec 09:13, Feb 10:6, Apr 10:5, 9, Jul 10:7; *CPT Changes: An Insider's View* 2006, 2013

➲ *Clinical Examples in Radiology* Spring 06:8-9, Fall 06:9-10, Winter 06:17, Summer 07:1, 2, Winter 07:4-5, Summer 08:8, Fall 08:12, Spring 09:5, Summer 09:14, Fall 09:9, Spring 10:2, Summer 10:10, Fall 10:6, Winter 10:6

(Use 76377 in conjunction with code[s] for base imaging procedure[s])

►(Do not report 76377 in conjunction with 70496, 70498, 70544-70549, 71275, 71555, 72159, 72191, 72198, 73206, 73225, 73706, 73725, 74174, 74175, 74185, 74261-74263, 75557, 75559, 75561, 75563, 75565, 75571-75574, 75635, 76376, 78012-78999, 0159T)◄

(To report computer-aided detection, including computer algorithm analysis of MRI data for lesion detection/characterization, pharmacokinetic analysis, breast MRI, use Category III code 0159T)

►(76376, 76377 require concurrent supervision of image postprocessing 3D manipulation of volumetric data set and image rendering)◄

76380 Computed tomography, limited or localized follow-up study

➲ *CPT Assistant* Jul 07:13; *CPT Changes: An Insider's View* 2002, 2003

76390 Magnetic resonance spectroscopy

➲ *CPT Assistant* Nov 97:25

(For magnetic resonance imaging, use appropriate MRI body site code)

76496 Unlisted fluoroscopic procedure (eg, diagnostic, interventional)

➲ *CPT Changes: An Insider's View* 2003

➲ *Clinical Examples in Radiology* Fall 07:3

76497 Unlisted computed tomography procedure (eg, diagnostic, interventional)

➲ *CPT Assistant* Jun 05:11; *CPT Changes: An Insider's View* 2003

➲ *Clinical Examples in Radiology* Spring 05:1, 7

76498 Unlisted magnetic resonance procedure (eg, diagnostic, interventional)

➲ *CPT Assistant* Dec 11:17; *CPT Changes: An Insider's View* 2003

➲ *Clinical Examples in Radiology* Fall 08:11, Spring 09:11

76499 Unlisted diagnostic radiographic procedure

➲ *CPT Assistant* Jul 99:10, Sep 00:4, Apr 04:15, Nov 06:22, Mar 08:15, Dec 11:17; *CPT Changes: An Insider's View* 2003

➲ *Clinical Examples in Radiology* Spring 11:8

Diagnostic Ultrasound

All diagnostic ultrasound examinations require permanently recorded images with measurements, when such measurements are clinically indicated. For those codes whose sole diagnostic goal is a biometric measure (ie, 76514, 76516, and 76519), permanently recorded images are not required. A final, written report should be issued for inclusion in the patient's medical record. The prescription form for the intraocular lens satisfies the written report requirement for 76519. For those anatomic regions that have "complete" and "limited" ultrasound codes, note the elements that comprise a "complete" exam. The report should contain a description of these elements or the reason that an element could not be visualized (eg, obscured by bowel gas, surgically absent).

If less than the required elements for a "complete" exam are reported (eg, limited number of organs or limited portion of region evaluated), the "limited" code for that anatomic region should be used once per patient exam session. A "limited" exam of an anatomic region should not be reported for the same exam session as a "complete" exam of that same region.

Evaluation of vascular structures using both color and spectral Doppler is separately reportable. To report, see **Noninvasive Vascular Diagnostic Studies** (93880-93990). However, color Doppler alone, when performed for anatomic structure identification in conjunction with a real-time ultrasound examination, is not reported separately.

Ultrasound guidance procedures also require permanently recorded images of the site to be localized, as well as a documented description of the localization process, either separately or within the report of the procedure for which the guidance is utilized.

Use of ultrasound, without thorough evaluation of organ(s) or anatomic region, image documentation, and final, written report, is not separately reportable.

Definitions

A-mode implies a one-dimensional ultrasonic measurement procedure.

M-mode implies a one-dimensional ultrasonic measurement procedure with movement of the trace to record amplitude and velocity of moving echo-producing structures.

B-scan implies a two-dimensional ultrasonic scanning procedure with a two-dimensional display.

Real-time scan implies a two-dimensional ultrasonic scanning procedure with display of both two-dimensional structure and motion with time.

(To report diagnostic vascular ultrasound studies, see 93880-93990)

(For focused ultrasound ablation treatment of uterine leiomyomata, see Category III codes 0071T, 0072T)

Head and Neck

76506 Echoencephalography, real time with image documentation (gray scale) (for determination of ventricular size, delineation of cerebral contents, and detection of fluid masses or other intracranial abnormalities), including A-mode encephalography as secondary component where indicated
➔ *CPT Assistant* Mar 07:7; *CPT Changes: An Insider's View* 2007, 2008

76510 Ophthalmic ultrasound, diagnostic; B-scan and quantitative A-scan performed during the same patient encounter
➔ *CPT Assistant* Dec 05:3; *CPT Changes: An Insider's View* 2005

76511 quantitative A-scan only
➔ *CPT Assistant* Winter 93:12, Oct 96:9, Nov 99:42, Jul 04:12, Dec 05:3; *CPT Changes: An Insider's View* 2005

76512 B-scan (with or without superimposed non-quantitative A-scan)
➔ *CPT Assistant* Winter 93:12, Oct 96:9, Dec 05:3; *CPT Changes: An Insider's View* 2005

76513 anterior segment ultrasound, immersion (water bath) B-scan or high resolution biomicroscopy
➔ *CPT Assistant* Winter 93:12, Nov 99:42, Nov 09:9; *CPT Changes: An Insider's View* 2000

(For scanning computerized ophthalmic diagnostic imaging of the anterior and posterior segments using technology other than ultrasound, see 92132, 92133, 92134)

76514 corneal pachymetry, unilateral or bilateral (determination of corneal thickness)
➔ *CPT Assistant* Jul 04:12, 15, Feb 05:13, Jun 05:11, Dec 05:3; *CPT Changes: An Insider's View* 2004

76516 Ophthalmic biometry by ultrasound echography, A-scan;
➔ *CPT Assistant* Oct 03:10, Dec 05:3

76519 with intraocular lens power calculation
➔ *CPT Assistant* Winter 93:12, Oct 03:10, Dec 05:3, Sep 09:5

(For partial coherence interferometry, use 92136)

76529 Ophthalmic ultrasonic foreign body localization
➔ *CPT Assistant* Winter 93:12

76536 Ultrasound, soft tissues of head and neck (eg, thyroid, parathyroid, parotid), real time with image documentation
➔ *CPT Assistant* Mar 07:7, May 09:7; *CPT Changes: An Insider's View* 2002, 2007

Chest

76604 Ultrasound, chest (includes mediastinum), real time with image documentation
➔ *CPT Changes: An Insider's View* 2002, 2007

76645 Ultrasound, breast(s) (unilateral or bilateral), real time with image documentation
➔ *CPT Changes: An Insider's View* 2002, 2007
➔ *Clinical Examples in Radiology* Fall 05:8, Fall 08:2, 3, 9

▶(Do not report 76645 in conjunction with 0301T)◀

Abdomen and Retroperitoneum

A complete ultrasound examination of the abdomen (76700) consists of real time scans of the liver, gall bladder, common bile duct, pancreas, spleen, kidneys, and the upper abdominal aorta and inferior vena cava including any demonstrated abdominal abnormality.

A complete ultrasound examination of the retroperitoneum (76770) consists of real time scans of the kidneys, abdominal aorta, common iliac artery origins, and inferior vena cava, including any demonstrated retroperitoneal abnormality. Alternatively, if clinical history suggests urinary tract pathology, complete evaluation of the kidneys and urinary bladder also comprises a complete retroperitoneal ultrasound.

Use of ultrasound, without thorough evaluation of organ(s) or anatomic region, image documentation and final, written report, is not separately reportable.

76700 Ultrasound, abdominal, real time with image documentation; complete
➔ *CPT Assistant* Fall 93:13, Oct 01:3, Dec 05:3, Mar 07:7; *CPT Changes: An Insider's View* 2002, 2007
➔ *Clinical Examples in Radiology* Winter 05:9, 11, Fall 07:4, Spring 08:10

76705 limited (eg, single organ, quadrant, follow-up)
➔ *CPT Assistant* Fall 93:13, Oct 01:3, Apr 03:27, Dec 05:3, Feb 09:22, May 09:7, Mar 12:10
➔ *Clinical Examples in Radiology* Winter 05:9, 11, Fall 07:4, Summer 11:11, Spring 12:10, Winter 12:10

76770 Ultrasound, retroperitoneal (eg, renal, aorta, nodes), real time with image documentation; complete
➔ *CPT Assistant* May 99:10, Jun 99:10; *CPT Changes: An Insider's View* 2002, 2007
➔ *Clinical Examples in Radiology* Winter 05:9, 11, Fall 07:4, Winter 08:12, Summer 09:12

Radiology

76775   limited
> *CPT Assistant* May 99:10, Jun 99:10, Dec 05:3, Feb 09:22
> *Clinical Examples in Radiology* Winter 05:9, 11, Spring 07:5-6, Fall 07:4, Winter 07:8-10, Summer 09:12

76776   Ultrasound, transplanted kidney, real time and duplex Doppler with image documentation
> *CPT Assistant* Mar 07:7; *CPT Changes: An Insider's View* 2007

(For ultrasound of transplanted kidney without duplex Doppler, use 76775)

(For ultrasound and duplex Doppler of a transplanted kidney, do not report 76776 in conjunction with 93975, 93976)

Spinal Canal

76800   Ultrasound, spinal canal and contents
> *CPT Assistant* Apr 98:15; *CPT Changes: An Insider's View* 2002

Pelvis

Obstetrical

Codes 76801 and 76802 include determination of the number of gestational sacs and fetuses, gestational sac/fetal measurements appropriate for gestation (younger than 14 weeks 0 days), survey of visible fetal and placental anatomic structure, qualitative assessment of amniotic fluid volume/gestational sac shape and examination of the maternal uterus and adnexa.

Codes 76805 and 76810 include determination of number of fetuses and amniotic/chorionic sacs, measurements appropriate for gestational age (older than or equal to 14 weeks 0 days), survey of intracranial/spinal/abdominal anatomy, 4 chambered heart, umbilical cord insertion site, placenta location and amniotic fluid assessment and, when visible, examination of maternal adnexa.

Codes 76811 and 76812 include all elements of codes 76805 and 76810 plus detailed anatomic evaluation of the fetal brain/ventricles, face, heart/outflow tracts and chest anatomy, abdominal organ specific anatomy, number/length/architecture of limbs and detailed evaluation of the umbilical cord and placenta and other fetal anatomy as clinically indicated.

Report should document the results of the evaluation of each element described above or the reason for non-visualization.

Code 76815 represents a focused "quick look" exam limited to the assessment of one or more of the elements listed in code 76815.

Code 76816 describes an examination designed to reassess fetal size and interval growth or reevaluate one or more anatomic abnormalities of a fetus previously demonstrated on ultrasound, and should be coded once for each fetus requiring reevaluation using modifier 59 for each fetus after the first.

Code 76817 describes a transvaginal obstetric ultrasound performed separately or in addition to one of the transabdominal examinations described above. For transvaginal examinations performed for non-obstetrical purposes, use code 76830.

76801   Ultrasound, pregnant uterus, real time with image documentation, fetal and maternal evaluation, first trimester (< 14 weeks 0 days), transabdominal approach; single or first gestation
> *CPT Assistant* Mar 03:7, Nov 05:15; *CPT Changes: An Insider's View* 2003
> *Clinical Examples in Radiology* Winter 07:6-7, Summer 10:8

(To report first trimester fetal nuchal translucency measurement, use 76813)

+ 76802   each additional gestation (List separately in addition to code for primary procedure)
> *CPT Assistant* Mar 03:7, Nov 05:15; *CPT Changes: An Insider's View* 2003
> *Clinical Examples in Radiology* Winter 07:6-7, Summer 11:10

(Use 76802 in conjunction with 76801)

(To report first trimester fetal nuchal translucency measurement, use 76814)

76805   Ultrasound, pregnant uterus, real time with image documentation, fetal and maternal evaluation, after first trimester (> or = 14 weeks 0 days), transabdominal approach; single or first gestation
> *CPT Assistant* Apr 97:2, Nov 97:25, Oct 01:3, Aug 02:2, Mar 03:7; *CPT Changes: An Insider's View* 2002, 2003
> *Clinical Examples in Radiology* Winter 05:3-4

+ 76810   each additional gestation (List separately in addition to code for primary procedure)
> *CPT Assistant* Apr 97:2, Oct 01:3, Aug 02:2, Mar 03:7; *CPT Changes: An Insider's View* 2003
> *Clinical Examples in Radiology* Winter 05:4, Summer 11:10

(Use 76810 in conjunction with 76805)

76811   Ultrasound, pregnant uterus, real time with image documentation, fetal and maternal evaluation plus detailed fetal anatomic examination, transabdominal approach; single or first gestation
> *CPT Assistant* Mar 03:7; *CPT Changes: An Insider's View* 2003
> *Clinical Examples in Radiology* Winter 05:4

+ 76812   each additional gestation (List separately in addition to code for primary procedure)
> *CPT Assistant* Mar 03:7; *CPT Changes: An Insider's View* 2003
> *Clinical Examples in Radiology* Summer 11:10

(Use 76812 in conjunction with 76811)

76813   Ultrasound, pregnant uterus, real time with image documentation, first trimester fetal nuchal translucency measurement, transabdominal or transvaginal approach; single or first gestation
> *CPT Assistant* Mar 07:7; *CPT Changes: An Insider's View* 2007
> *Clinical Examples in Radiology* Winter 07:6

+ 76814   each additional gestation (List separately in addition to code for primary procedure)
> CPT Assistant Mar 07:7; CPT Changes: An Insider's View 2007
> Clinical Examples in Radiology Winter 07:6, Summer 11:10

(Use 76814 in conjunction with 76813)

76815   Ultrasound, pregnant uterus, real time with image documentation, limited (eg, fetal heart beat, placental location, fetal position and/or qualitative amniotic fluid volume), 1 or more fetuses
> CPT Assistant Apr 97:2, Nov 97:25, Oct 01:3, Dec 01:6, Aug 02:2, Mar 03:7, Nov 03:14, May 10:9; CPT Changes: An Insider's View 2003
> Clinical Examples in Radiology Winter 07:6-7, Summer 10:8, 9

(Use 76815 only once per exam and not per element)

(To report first trimester fetal nuchal translucency measurement, see 76813, 76814)

76816   Ultrasound, pregnant uterus, real time with image documentation, follow-up (eg, re-evaluation of fetal size by measuring standard growth parameters and amniotic fluid volume, re-evaluation of organ system(s) suspected or confirmed to be abnormal on a previous scan), transabdominal approach, per fetus
> CPT Assistant Apr 97:2, Oct 01:3, Aug 02:2, Mar 03:7, May 10:9, Nov 11:10; CPT Changes: An Insider's View 2003
> Clinical Examples in Radiology Summer 10:9

(Report 76816 with modifier 59 for each additional fetus examined in a multiple pregnancy)

76817   Ultrasound, pregnant uterus, real time with image documentation, transvaginal
> CPT Assistant Mar 03:7, Nov 11:10; CPT Changes: An Insider's View 2003
> Clinical Examples in Radiology Summer 10:8, Summer 11:10

(For non-obstetrical transvaginal ultrasound, use 76830)

(If transvaginal examination is done in addition to transabdominal obstetrical ultrasound exam, use 76817 in addition to appropriate transabdominal exam code)

76818   Fetal biophysical profile; with non-stress testing
> CPT Assistant Apr 97:2, May 98:10, Sep 01:4, Oct 01:3, Dec 01:6, Nov 04:10; CPT Changes: An Insider's View 2001

76819   without non-stress testing
> CPT Assistant Sep 01:8, Dec 01:6; CPT Changes: An Insider's View 2001, 2002

(Fetal biophysical profile assessments for the second and any additional fetuses, should be reported separately by code 76818 or 76819 with the modifier 59 appended)

(For amniotic fluid index without non-stress test, use 76815)

76820   Doppler velocimetry, fetal; umbilical artery
> CPT Assistant Dec 05:3; CPT Changes: An Insider's View 2005

76821   middle cerebral artery
> CPT Assistant Dec 05:3; CPT Changes: An Insider's View 2005

76825   Echocardiography, fetal, cardiovascular system, real time with image documentation (2D), with or without M-mode recording;
> CPT Assistant Apr 97:2, Aug 02:2

76826   follow-up or repeat study
> CPT Assistant Apr 97:2, Aug 02:2

76827   Doppler echocardiography, fetal, pulsed wave and/or continuous wave with spectral display; complete
> CPT Assistant Apr 97:2, Aug 02:2, Dec 05:3; CPT Changes: An Insider's View 2005

76828   follow-up or repeat study
> CPT Assistant Apr 97:2, Aug 02:2, Dec 05:3

(To report the use of color mapping, use 93325)

Nonobstetrical

Code 76856 includes the complete evaluation of the female pelvic anatomy. Elements of this examination include a description and measurements of the uterus and adnexal structures, measurement of the endometrium, measurement of the bladder (when applicable), and a description of any pelvic pathology (eg, ovarian cysts, uterine leiomyomata, free pelvic fluid).

Code 76856 is also applicable to a complete evaluation of the male pelvis. Elements of the examination include evaluation and measurement (when applicable) of the urinary bladder, evaluation of the prostate and seminal vesicles to the extent that they are visualized transabdominally, and any pelvic pathology (eg, bladder tumor, enlarged prostate, free pelvic fluid, pelvic abscess).

Code 76857 represents a focused examination limited to the assessment of one or more elements listed in code 76856 and/or the reevaluation of one or more pelvic abnormalities previously demonstrated on ultrasound. Code 76857, rather than 76770, should be utilized if the urinary bladder alone (ie, not including the kidneys) is imaged, whereas code 51798 should be utilized if a bladder volume or post-void residual measurement is obtained without imaging the bladder.

Use of ultrasound, without thorough evaluation of organ(s) or anatomic region, image documentation, and final, written report, is not separately reportable.

76830   Ultrasound, transvaginal
> CPT Assistant Aug 96:10, Jul 99:8, Aug 02:2, Mar 03:7, Dec 05:3, Feb 09:22, Nov 11:10; CPT Changes: An Insider's View 2002
> Clinical Examples in Radiology 2004_Inaugural 04:6-7, Spring 08:9, Summer 10:8, 9

(For obstetrical transvaginal ultrasound, use 76817)

(If transvaginal examination is done in addition to transabdominal non-obstetrical ultrasound exam, use 76830 in addition to appropriate transabdominal exam code)

76831 Saline infusion sonohysterography (SIS), including color flow Doppler, when performed

→ *CPT Assistant* Nov 97:25, Jul 99:8, Dec 05:3, Mar 09:11; *CPT Changes: An Insider's View* 2004

(For introduction of saline for saline infusion sonohysterography, use 58340)

76856 Ultrasound, pelvic (nonobstetric), real time with image documentation; complete

→ *CPT Assistant* Oct 01:3, Dec 05:3, Jan 06:47, Mar 07:7, Feb 09:22; *CPT Changes: An Insider's View* 2002, 2007

→ *Clinical Examples in Radiology* 2004_Inaugural 04:6-7, Spring 08:9, Summer 10:8

76857 limited or follow-up (eg, for follicles)

→ *CPT Assistant* Jun 97:10, Oct 01:3, Dec 05:3, Sep 07:10, May 09:7

→ *Clinical Examples in Radiology* Spring 08:9, Summer 10:8

Genitalia

76870 Ultrasound, scrotum and contents

→ *CPT Assistant* May 05:3; *CPT Changes: An Insider's View* 2002

76872 Ultrasound, transrectal;

→ *CPT Assistant* May 96:3, Nov 99:42; *CPT Changes: An Insider's View* 2000, 2004

(Do not report 76872 in conjunction with 0249T)

76873 prostate volume study for brachytherapy treatment planning (separate procedure)

→ *CPT Assistant* Nov 99:42; *CPT Changes: An Insider's View* 2000

Extremities

A complete ultrasound examination of an extremity (76881) consists of real time scans of a specific joint that includes examination of the muscles, tendons, joint, other soft tissue structures, and any identifiable abnormality.

Code 76882 refers to an examination of an extremity that would be performed primarily for evaluation of muscles, tendons, joints, and/or soft tissues. This is a limited examination of the extremity where a specific anatomic structure such as a tendon or muscle is assessed. In addition, the code would be used to evaluate a soft-tissue mass that may be present in an extremity where knowledge of its cystic or solid characteristics is needed.

For spectral and color Doppler evaluation of the extremities, use 93925, 93926, 93930, 93931, 93970, or 93971 as appropriate.

(76880 has been deleted. To report ultrasound examination of an extremity, see 76881, 76882)

76881 Ultrasound, extremity, nonvascular, real-time with image documentation; complete

→ *CPT Changes: An Insider's View* 2011

→ *Clinical Examples in Radiology* Winter 11:7, 11

76882 limited, anatomic specific

→ *CPT Changes: An Insider's View* 2011

→ *Clinical Examples in Radiology* Summer 11:11, Winter 11:7

▲ **76885** Ultrasound, infant hips, real time with imaging documentation; dynamic (requiring physician or other qualified health care professional manipulation)

→ *CPT Assistant* Nov 97:25; *CPT Changes: An Insider's View* 2002, 2013

▲ **76886** limited, static (not requiring physician or other qualified health care professional manipulation)

→ *CPT Assistant* Nov 97:25; *CPT Changes: An Insider's View* 2002, 2013

Ultrasonic Guidance Procedures

76930 Ultrasonic guidance for pericardiocentesis, imaging supervision and interpretation

→ *CPT Changes: An Insider's View* 2001

76932 Ultrasonic guidance for endomyocardial biopsy, imaging supervision and interpretation

→ *CPT Changes: An Insider's View* 2001

76936 Ultrasound guided compression repair of arterial pseudoaneurysm or arteriovenous fistulae (includes diagnostic ultrasound evaluation, compression of lesion and imaging)

+ **76937** Ultrasound guidance for vascular access requiring ultrasound evaluation of potential access sites, documentation of selected vessel patency, concurrent realtime ultrasound visualization of vascular needle entry, with permanent recording and reporting (List separately in addition to code for primary procedure)

→ *CPT Assistant* Dec 04:13, Jan 09:7, Jul 10:6, Nov 10:3, Jan 11:8, Apr 12:6; *CPT Changes: An Insider's View* 2004

→ *Clinical Examples in Radiology* 2004_Inaugural 04:1-2, Winter 05:5-6, Summer 06:8-9, Spring 08:7, 8, Fall 08:5, 6, Spring 09:10, Winter 09:8, 9, Summer 10:1, 3, 4, Spring 12:4, Winter 12:3

(Do not report 76937 in conjunction with 37191, 37192, 37193, 37760, 37761, 76942)

(If extremity venous non-invasive vascular diagnostic study is performed separate from venous access guidance, use 93965, 93970 or 93971)

76940 Ultrasound guidance for, and monitoring of, parenchymal tissue ablation

→ *CPT Assistant* Oct 02:2, Mar 07:7; *CPT Changes: An Insider's View* 2004, 2007

→ *Clinical Examples in Radiology* Spring 08:1, 2

(Do not report 76940 in conjunction with 50250, 50542, 76942, 76998)

(For ablation, see 32998, 47370-47382, 50592, 50593)

76941 Ultrasonic guidance for intrauterine fetal transfusion or cordocentesis, imaging supervision and interpretation

→ *CPT Changes: An Insider's View* 2001

(For procedure, see 36460, 59012)

76942   Ultrasonic guidance for needle placement (eg, biopsy, aspiration, injection, localization device), imaging supervision and interpretation

➔ *CPT Assistant* Fall 93:12, Fall 94:2, May 96:3, Jun 97:5, Oct 01:2, May 04:7, Dec 04:12, Apr 05:15-16, Aug 08:7, Mar 09:8, Feb 10:6, Mar 10:9, Jul 10:6, Feb 11:4, Mar 11:9, Apr 11:12; *CPT Changes: An Insider's View* 2001

➔ *Clinical Examples in Radiology* Summer 05:1, 2, 6, Fall 05:1, Summer 08:5, 6, Fall 08:2, 3, Fall 09:8, Winter 09:9, Summer 10:1, 3, 4, Fall 10:3, Summer 11:3

▶(Do not report 76942 in conjunction with 27096, 32554, 32555, 32556, 32557, 37760, 37761, 43232, 43237, 43242, 45341, 45342, 64479-64484, 64490-64495, 76975, 0213T-0218T, 0228T-0231T, 0232T, 0249T, 0301T)◀

(For injection(s) of platelet rich plasma, use 0232T)

76945   Ultrasonic guidance for chorionic villus sampling, imaging supervision and interpretation

➔ *CPT Changes: An Insider's View* 2001

(For procedure, use 59015)

76946   Ultrasonic guidance for amniocentesis, imaging supervision and interpretation

➔ *CPT Changes: An Insider's View* 2001

76948   Ultrasonic guidance for aspiration of ova, imaging supervision and interpretation

➔ *CPT Changes: An Insider's View* 2001

76950   Ultrasonic guidance for placement of radiation therapy fields

➔ *CPT Changes: An Insider's View* 2001

(For placement of interstitial device[s] for radiation therapy guidance, see 31627, 32553, 49411, 55876)

76965   Ultrasonic guidance for interstitial radioelement application

Other Procedures

76970   Ultrasound study follow-up (specify)

76975   Gastrointestinal endoscopic ultrasound, supervision and interpretation

➔ *CPT Assistant* Spring 94:5, May 04:7, Mar 09:8; *CPT Changes: An Insider's View* 2001

(Do not report 76975 in conjunction with 43231, 43232, 43237, 43238, 43242, 43259, 45341, 45342, or 76942)

76977   Ultrasound bone density measurement and interpretation, peripheral site(s), any method

➔ *CPT Assistant* Nov 98:21

76998   Ultrasonic guidance, intraoperative

➔ *CPT Assistant* Mar 07:7, Jul 10:6; *CPT Changes: An Insider's View* 2007

➔ *Clinical Examples in Radiology* Winter 12:11

▶(Do not report 76998 in conjunction with 36475-36479, 37760, 37761, 47370-47382, 0249T, 0301T)◀

(For ultrasound guidance for open and laparoscopic radiofrequency tissue ablation, use 76940)

76999   Unlisted ultrasound procedure (eg, diagnostic, interventional)

➔ *CPT Changes: An Insider's View* 2003

Radiologic Guidance

Fluoroscopic Guidance

(Do not report guidance codes 77001, 77002, 77003 for services in which fluoroscopic guidance is included in the descriptor)

+ 77001   Fluoroscopic guidance for central venous access device placement, replacement (catheter only or complete), or removal (includes fluoroscopic guidance for vascular access and catheter manipulation, any necessary contrast injections through access site or catheter with related venography radiologic supervision and interpretation, and radiographic documentation of final catheter position) (List separately in addition to code for primary procedure)

➔ *CPT Assistant* Mar 07:7, Jul 08:9, Nov 10:3, Jan 11:8; *CPT Changes: An Insider's View* 2007

➔ *Clinical Examples in Radiology* Spring 08:7, 8, Fall 08:5, 6, Winter 09:8, 9, Summer 10:11

(Do not use 77001 in conjunction with 77002)

(If formal extremity venography is performed from separate venous access and separately interpreted, use 36005 and 75820, 75822, 75825, or 75827)

77002   Fluoroscopic guidance for needle placement (eg, biopsy, aspiration, injection, localization device)

➔ *CPT Assistant* Feb 07:11, Mar 07:7, May 07:1, Jun 07:10, Jul 08:9, Aug 08:7, Dec 08:9, Dec 09:12, Feb 10:6, Nov 10:3, Jan 11:8, Apr 11:12, Feb 12:11, Apr 12:19, Jun 12:14; *CPT Changes: An Insider's View* 2007

➔ *Clinical Examples in Radiology* Summer 08:5, 6, Spring 09:6, 7, Fall 09:7, Winter 09:9, Fall 10:10, Summer 11:3

(See appropriate surgical code for procedure and anatomic location)

(77002 includes all radiographic arthrography with the exception of supervision and interpretation for CT and MR arthrography)

▶(Do not report 77002 in conjunction with 32554, 32555, 32556, 32557, 70332, 73040, 73085, 73115, 73525, 73580, 73615, 0232T)◀

(For injection(s) of platelet rich plasma, use 0232T)

(77002 is included in the organ/anatomic specific radiological supervision and interpretation procedures 49440, 74320, 74355, 74445, 74470, 74475, 75809, 75810, 75885, 75887, 75980, 75982, 75989)

Radiology

77003 Fluoroscopic guidance and localization of needle or catheter tip for spine or paraspinous diagnostic or therapeutic injection procedures (epidural or subarachnoid)

➜ *CPT Assistant* Mar 07:7, Jul 08:9, Feb 10:12, May 10:10, Aug 10:8, Oct 10:14, Nov 10:3, Dec 10:14, Jan 11:8, Feb 11:4, Mar 11:7, Jul 11:17, Jun 12:12, Jul 12:3, 5, 6; *CPT Changes: An Insider's View* 2007, 2010, 2011, 2012

➜ *Clinical Examples in Radiology* Summer 08:9, 13, Winter 09:9, Spring 11:9

(Injection of contrast during fluoroscopic guidance and localization [77003] is included in 22526, 22527, 27096, 62263, 62264, 62267, 62270-62282, 62310-62319)

(Fluoroscopic guidance for subarachnoid puncture for diagnostic radiographic myelography is included in supervision and interpretation codes 72240-72270)

(For epidural or subarachnoid needle or catheter placement and injection, see 62270-62282, 62310-62319)

(For sacroiliac joint arthrography, see 27096)

(For paravertebral facet joint injection, see 64490-64495. For paravertebral facet joint nerve destruction by neurolysis, see 64633-64636. For transforaminal epidural needle placement and injection, see 64479-64484)

▶(Do not report 77002, 77003 in conjunction with 22586, 27096, 64479–64484, 64490-64495, 64633-64636, 0195T, 0196T, 0309T)◀

(For percutaneous or endoscopic lysis of epidural adhesions, 62263, 62264 include fluoroscopic guidance and localization)

Computed Tomography Guidance

77011 Computed tomography guidance for stereotactic localization

➜ *CPT Assistant* Mar 07:7; *CPT Changes: An Insider's View* 2007

77012 Computed tomography guidance for needle placement (eg, biopsy, aspiration, injection, localization device), radiological supervision and interpretation

➜ *CPT Assistant* Mar 07:7, May 07:1, Jun 07:10, Aug 08:7, Feb 10:6, Feb 11:4, Apr 11:12, Jul 12:3, 6; *CPT Changes: An Insider's View* 2007

➜ *Clinical Examples in Radiology* Summer 08:5, 6, Fall 08:3, Fall 09:6, Fall 10:3, Summer 11:3

▶(Do not report 77011, 77012 in conjunction with 22586, 0195T, 0196T, 0309T)◀

▶(Do not report 77012 in conjunction with 27096, 32554, 32555, 32556, 32557, 64479-64484, 64490-64495, 64633-64636, 0232T)◀

(For injection(s) of platelet rich plasma, use 0232T)

77013 Computed tomography guidance for, and monitoring of, parenchymal tissue ablation

➜ *CPT Assistant* Mar 07:7; *CPT Changes: An Insider's View* 2007

(Do not report 77013 in conjunction with 20982)

(For percutaneous radiofrequency ablation, see 32998, 47382, 50592, 50593)

77014 Computed tomography guidance for placement of radiation therapy fields

➜ *CPT Assistant* Mar 07:7; *CPT Changes: An Insider's View* 2007

➜ *Clinical Examples in Radiology* Summer 09:2, 4, Spring 12:10

(For placement of interstitial device[s] for radiation therapy guidance, see 31627, 32553, 49411, 55876)

Magnetic Resonance Guidance

77021 Magnetic resonance guidance for needle placement (eg, for biopsy, needle aspiration, injection, or placement of localization device) radiological supervision and interpretation

➜ *CPT Assistant* Mar 07:7, May 07:1, Jun 07:10, Aug 08:7, Feb 10:6, Apr 11:12; *CPT Changes: An Insider's View* 2007

➜ *Clinical Examples in Radiology* Summer 08:5, 6, 13, Fall 08:3, Fall 10:3, Summer 11:3

(For procedure, see appropriate organ or site)

▶(Do not report 77021 in conjunction with 32554, 32555, 32556, 32557, 0232T)◀

(For injection(s) of platelet rich plasma, use 0232T)

77022 Magnetic resonance guidance for, and monitoring of, parenchymal tissue ablation

➜ *CPT Assistant* Mar 07:7; *CPT Changes: An Insider's View* 2007

(For percutaneous radiofrequency ablation, see 32998, 47382, 50592, 50593)

(For focused ultrasound ablation treatment of uterine leiomyomata, see Category III codes 0071T, 0072T)

Other Radiologic Guidance

77031 Stereotactic localization guidance for breast biopsy or needle placement (eg, for wire localization or for injection), each lesion, radiological supervision and interpretation

➜ *CPT Assistant* Mar 07:7, May 10:9; *CPT Changes: An Insider's View* 2007

➜ *Clinical Examples in Radiology* Fall 08:3, Fall 10:1

(For procedure, see 10022, 19000-19103, 19290, 19291)

(For injection for sentinel node localization without lymphoscintigraphy, use 38792)

77032 Mammographic guidance for needle placement, breast (eg, for wire localization or for injection), each lesion, radiological supervision and interpretation

➜ *CPT Assistant* Mar 07:7; *CPT Changes: An Insider's View* 2007

➜ *Clinical Examples in Radiology* Fall 08:3, 4, Fall 10:3

(For procedure, see 10022, 19000, 19102, 19103, 19290, 19291)

(For injection for sentinel node localization without lymphoscintigraphy, use 38792)

Radiology

Breast, Mammography

(For mammographic guidance for needle placement of breast lesion, use 77032)

+▲ 77051   Computer-aided detection (computer algorithm analysis of digital image data for lesion detection) with further review for interpretation, with or without digitization of film radiographic images; diagnostic mammography (List separately in addition to code for primary procedure)

➔ *CPT Assistant* Mar 07:7, Apr 07:1; *CPT Changes: An Insider's View* 2007, 2013

➔ *Clinical Examples in Radiology* Winter 09:7

(Use 77051 in conjunction with 77055, 77056)

+▲ 77052   screening mammography (List separately in addition to code for primary procedure)

➔ *CPT Assistant* Mar 07:7, Apr 07:1; *CPT Changes: An Insider's View* 2007, 2013

➔ *Clinical Examples in Radiology* Winter 09:6, 7, 8

(Use 77052 in conjunction with 77057)

77053   Mammary ductogram or galactogram, single duct, radiological supervision and interpretation

➔ *CPT Assistant* Mar 07:7; *CPT Changes: An Insider's View* 2007

(For mammary ductogram or galactogram injection, use 19030)

77054   Mammary ductogram or galactogram, multiple ducts, radiological supervision and interpretation

➔ *CPT Assistant* Mar 07:7; *CPT Changes: An Insider's View* 2007

77055   Mammography; unilateral

➔ *CPT Assistant* Mar 07:7; *CPT Changes: An Insider's View* 2007

➔ *Clinical Examples in Radiology* Fall 08:2, 4, Winter 09:7, Fall 10:3

77056   bilateral

➔ *CPT Assistant* Mar 07:7; *CPT Changes: An Insider's View* 2007

➔ *Clinical Examples in Radiology* Winter 09:7

(Use 77055, 77056 in conjunction with 77051 for computer-aided detection applied to a diagnostic mammogram)

77057   Screening mammography, bilateral (2-view film study of each breast)

➔ *CPT Assistant* Mar 07:7; *CPT Changes: An Insider's View* 2007

➔ *Clinical Examples in Radiology* Winter 09:6, 7

(Use 77057 in conjunction with 77052 for computer-aided detection applied to a screening mammogram)

(For electrical impedance breast scan, use 76499)

77058   Magnetic resonance imaging, breast, without and/or with contrast material(s); unilateral

➔ *CPT Assistant* Mar 07:7; *CPT Changes: An Insider's View* 2007

77059   bilateral

➔ *CPT Assistant* Mar 07:7, Jul 07:6; *CPT Changes: An Insider's View* 2007

Screening Mammography
77057

Mammogram

Medial lateral oblique view

Cranial caudal view

Bone/Joint Studies

▲ 77071   Manual application of stress performed by physician or other qualified health care professional for joint radiography, including contralateral joint if indicated

➔ *CPT Assistant* Mar 07:7; *CPT Changes: An Insider's View* 2007, 2013

(For radiographic interpretation of stressed images, see appropriate anatomic site and number of views)

77072   Bone age studies

➔ *CPT Assistant* Mar 07:7; *CPT Changes: An Insider's View* 2007

77073   Bone length studies (orthoroentgenogram, scanogram)

➔ *CPT Assistant* Mar 07:7; *CPT Changes: An Insider's View* 2007

➔ *Clinical Examples in Radiology* Summer 07:12, Fall 08:10, Fall 10:6

77074   Radiologic examination, osseous survey; limited (eg, for metastases)

➔ *CPT Assistant* Mar 07:7; *CPT Changes: An Insider's View* 2007

Radiology

77075   complete (axial and appendicular skeleton)
> *CPT Assistant* Mar 07:7; *CPT Changes: An Insider's View* 2007

77076   Radiologic examination, osseous survey, infant
> *CPT Assistant* Mar 07:7; *CPT Changes: An Insider's View* 2007

77077   Joint survey, single view, 2 or more joints (specify)
> *CPT Assistant* Mar 07:7; *CPT Changes: An Insider's View* 2007

77078   Computed tomography, bone mineral density study, 1 or more sites; axial skeleton (eg, hips, pelvis, spine)
> *CPT Assistant* Mar 07:7; *CPT Changes: An Insider's View* 2007

(77079 has been deleted)

77080   Dual-energy X-ray absorptiometry (DXA), bone density study, 1 or more sites; axial skeleton (eg, hips, pelvis, spine)
> *CPT Assistant* Mar 07:7; *CPT Changes: An Insider's View* 2007
> *Clinical Examples in Radiology* Fall 07:11, Summer 10:6

77081   appendicular skeleton (peripheral) (eg, radius, wrist, heel)
> *CPT Assistant* Mar 07:7; *CPT Changes: An Insider's View* 2007

77082   vertebral fracture assessment
> *CPT Assistant* Mar 07:7; *CPT Changes: An Insider's View* 2007
> *Clinical Examples in Radiology* Summer 10:6

(For dual energy x-ray absorptiometry [DXA] body composition study, use 76499)

(77083 has been deleted)

77084   Magnetic resonance (eg, proton) imaging, bone marrow blood supply
> *CPT Assistant* Mar 07:7; *CPT Changes: An Insider's View* 2007

Radiation Oncology

Listings for Radiation Oncology provide for teletherapy and brachytherapy to include initial consultation, clinical treatment planning, simulation, medical radiation physics, dosimetry, treatment devices, special services, and clinical treatment management procedures. They include normal follow-up care during course of treatment and for three months following its completion.

When a service or procedure is provided that is not listed in this edition of the CPT codebook it should be identified by a Special Report (see page 375) and one of the following unlisted procedure codes:

77299 Unlisted procedure, therapeutic radiology clinical treatment planning

77399 Unlisted procedure, medical radiation physics, dosimetry and treatment devices, and special services

77499 Unlisted procedure, therapeutic radiology treatment management

77799 Unlisted procedure, clinical brachytherapy

For treatment by injectable or ingestible isotopes, see subsection Nuclear Medicine.

Consultation: Clinical Management

Preliminary consultation, evaluation of patient prior to decision to treat, or full medical care (in addition to treatment management) when provided by the therapeutic radiologist may be identified by the appropriate procedure codes from **Evaluation and Management, Medicine,** or **Surgery** sections.

Clinical Treatment Planning (External and Internal Sources)

The clinical treatment planning process is a complex service including interpretation of special testing, tumor localization, treatment volume determination, treatment time/dosage determination, choice of treatment modality, determination of number and size of treatment ports, selection of appropriate treatment devices, and other procedures.

Definitions

Simple planning requires a single treatment area of interest encompassed in a single port or simple parallel opposed ports with simple or no blocking.

Intermediate planning requires 3 or more converging ports, 2 separate treatment areas, multiple blocks, or special time dose constraints.

Complex planning requires highly complex blocking, custom shielding blocks, tangential ports, special wedges or compensators, three or more separate treatment areas, rotational or special beam considerations, combination of therapeutic modalities.

77261   Therapeutic radiology treatment planning; simple
> *CPT Assistant* Fall 91:12, 15, Oct 97:2, Oct 10:3
> *Clinical Examples in Radiology* Summer 09:4

77262   intermediate
> *CPT Assistant* Fall 91:12, 15, Oct 97:2, Apr 09:3, Nov 09:6, Oct 10:3
> *Clinical Examples in Radiology* Summer 09:4

77263   complex
> *CPT Assistant* Fall 91:15, Oct 97:2, Apr 09:3, Nov 09:6, Oct 10:3
> *Clinical Examples in Radiology* Summer 09:2, 4

Definitions

Simple simulation of a single treatment area with either a single port or parallel opposed ports. Simple or no blocking.

Intermediate simulation of three or more converging ports, two separate treatment areas, multiple blocks.

Complex simulation of tangential portals, three or more treatment areas, rotation or arc therapy, complex blocking, custom shielding blocks, brachytherapy source verification, hyperthermia probe verification, any use of contrast materials.

Three-dimensional (3D) computer-generated 3D reconstruction of tumor volume and surrounding critical normal tissue structures from direct CT scans and/or MRI data in preparation for non-coplanar or coplanar therapy. The simulation uses documented 3D beam's eye view volume-dose displays of multiple or moving beams. Documentation with 3D volume reconstruction and dose distribution is required.

Simulation may be carried out on a dedicated simulator, a radiation therapy treatment unit, or diagnostic X-ray machine.

77280   Therapeutic radiology simulation-aided field setting; simple
> *CPT Assistant* Fall 91:15, Oct 97:2, Nov 97:26, Apr 09:10, Nov 09:6, Oct 10:3
> *Clinical Examples in Radiology* Summer 08:12, Summer 09:2, 4, 5

77285   intermediate
> *CPT Assistant* Fall 91:15, Oct 97:3, Nov 09:6, Oct 10:3
> *Clinical Examples in Radiology* Summer 08:12, Summer 09:4

77290   complex
> *CPT Assistant* Fall 91:12, 15, Oct 97:3, Apr 09:3, 10, Nov 09:6, Oct 10:3
> *Clinical Examples in Radiology* Summer 08:12, Summer 09:4

77295   3-dimensional
> *CPT Assistant* Fall 91:15, Oct 97:3, Nov 97:26, May 05:7, Oct 07:1, Nov 09:3, Oct 10:3
> *Clinical Examples in Radiology* Summer 08:12, Summer 09:2, 5

77299   Unlisted procedure, therapeutic radiology clinical treatment planning
> *CPT Assistant* Oct 10:3

Medical Radiation Physics, Dosimetry, Treatment Devices, and Special Services

77300   Basic radiation dosimetry calculation, central axis depth dose calculation, TDF, NSD, gap calculation, off axis factor, tissue inhomogeneity factors, calculation of non-ionizing radiation surface and depth dose, as required during course of treatment, only when prescribed by the treating physician
> *CPT Assistant* Fall 91:14, Oct 97:3, Dec 08:9, Nov 09:3, Oct 10:3; *CPT Changes: An Insider's View* 2002
> *Clinical Examples in Radiology* Summer 08:12, Summer 09:2, 5, 6

77301   Intensity modulated radiotherapy plan, including dose-volume histograms for target and critical structure partial tolerance specifications
> *CPT Assistant* Mar 05:1, 6, May 05:7, Oct 07:1, Nov 09:3, Oct 10:3; *CPT Changes: An Insider's View* 2002

(Dose plan is optimized using inverse or forward planning technique for modulated beam delivery [eg, binary, dynamic MLC] to create highly conformal dose distribution. Computer plan distribution must be verified for positional accuracy based on dosimetric verification of the intensity map with verification of treatment set-up and interpretation of verification methodology)

77305   Teletherapy, isodose plan (whether hand or computer calculated); simple (1 or 2 parallel opposed unmodified ports directed to a single area of interest)
> *CPT Assistant* Fall 91:15, Oct 97:3, Oct 10:3
> *Clinical Examples in Radiology* Summer 09:5

77310   intermediate (3 or more treatment ports directed to a single area of interest)
> *CPT Assistant* Fall 91:15, Oct 97:3, Oct 10:3
> *Clinical Examples in Radiology* Summer 09:5, 6

77315   complex (mantle or inverted Y, tangential ports, the use of wedges, compensators, complex blocking, rotational beam, or special beam considerations)
> *CPT Assistant* Fall 91:15, Oct 97:3, Oct 10:3
> *Clinical Examples in Radiology* Summer 09:5, 6

(Only 1 teletherapy isodose plan may be reported for a given course of therapy to a specific treatment area)

77321   Special teletherapy port plan, particles, hemibody, total body
> *CPT Assistant* Fall 91:14, Oct 97:4, Oct 10:3
> *Clinical Examples in Radiology* Summer 09:5, 6

77326   Brachytherapy isodose plan; simple (calculation made from single plane, 1 to 4 sources/ribbon application, remote afterloading brachytherapy, 1 to 8 sources)
> *CPT Assistant* Winter 91:17, Apr 09:3, Oct 10:3; *CPT Changes: An Insider's View* 2003

(For definition of source/ribbon, see page 407)

77327   intermediate (multiplane dosage calculations, application involving 5 to 10 sources/ribbons, remote afterloading brachytherapy, 9 to 12 sources)
> *CPT Assistant* Winter 91:17, Apr 09:3, Oct 10:3

77328   complex (multiplane isodose plan, volume implant calculations, over 10 sources/ribbons used, special spatial reconstruction, remote afterloading brachytherapy, over 12 sources)
> *CPT Assistant* Winter 91:17, Apr 09:3, Oct 10:3

77331   Special dosimetry (eg, TLD, microdosimetry) (specify), only when prescribed by the treating physician
> *CPT Assistant* Fall 91:13, Oct 97:4
> *Clinical Examples in Radiology* Summer 09:5, 6

77332   Treatment devices, design and construction; simple (simple block, simple bolus)
> *CPT Assistant* Oct 97:4, Oct 10:3
> *Clinical Examples in Radiology* Summer 07:10, Summer 08:12, Summer 09:6

77333   intermediate (multiple blocks, stents, bite blocks, special bolus)
> *CPT Assistant* Oct 97:3, Oct 10:3
> *Clinical Examples in Radiology* Summer 07:10, Summer 08:12, Summer 09:6

77334   complex (irregular blocks, special shields, compensators, wedges, molds or casts)
> *CPT Assistant* Fall 91:14, Oct 97:4, Dec 08:9, Nov 09:3, Oct 10:3, Dec 10:15
> *Clinical Examples in Radiology* Summer 07:9, 10, Summer 08:12, Summer 09:2, 6

Radiology

77336 Continuing medical physics consultation, including assessment of treatment parameters, quality assurance of dose delivery, and review of patient treatment documentation in support of the radiation oncologist, reported per week of therapy

➔ *CPT Assistant* Fall 91:15, Oct 97:4, Nov 98:21, Oct 10:3

➔ *Clinical Examples in Radiology* Summer 08:12, Summer 09:2, 6

77338 Multi-leaf collimator (MLC) device(s) for intensity modulated radiation therapy (IMRT), design and construction per IMRT plan

➔ *CPT Assistant* Oct 10:3, Dec 10:15; *CPT Changes: An Insider's View* 2010

(Do not report 77338 more than once per IMRT plan)

(For immobilization in IMRT treatment, see 77332-77334)

(Do not report 77338 in conjunction with 0073T, compensator based IMRT)

77370 Special medical radiation physics consultation

➔ *CPT Assistant* Fall 91:14, Oct 97:4, May 09:8, Oct 10:3

➔ *Clinical Examples in Radiology* Summer 08:12, Summer 09:6, 9

Stereotactic Radiation Treatment Delivery

⊙ **77371** Radiation treatment delivery, stereotactic radiosurgery (SRS), complete course of treatment of cranial lesion(s) consisting of 1 session; multi-source Cobalt 60 based

➔ *CPT Assistant* Mar 07:7, Oct 07:1, Oct 10:3, Jul 11:12; *CPT Changes: An Insider's View* 2007, 2008, 2010

➔ *Clinical Examples in Radiology* Summer 09:7

77372 linear accelerator based

➔ *CPT Assistant* Mar 07:7, Oct 07:1, Oct 10:3, Jul 11:12; *CPT Changes: An Insider's View* 2007, 2008

➔ *Clinical Examples in Radiology* Summer 09:7

(For radiation treatment management, use 77432)

77373 Stereotactic body radiation therapy, treatment delivery, per fraction to 1 or more lesions, including image guidance, entire course not to exceed 5 fractions

➔ *CPT Assistant* Mar 07:7, Oct 07:1, Oct 10:3, Jul 11:12; *CPT Changes: An Insider's View* 2007

➔ *Clinical Examples in Radiology* Summer 09:7

(Do not report 77373 in conjunction with 77401-77416, 77418)

(For single fraction cranial lesion[s], see 77371, 77372)

Other Procedures

77399 Unlisted procedure, medical radiation physics, dosimetry and treatment devices, and special services

➔ *CPT Assistant* Nov 98:21, Oct 10:3

Radiation Treatment Delivery

(Radiation treatment delivery [77401-77416] recognizes the technical component and the various energy levels)

(For intra-fraction localization and tracking of target, use 0197T)

77401 Radiation treatment delivery, superficial and/or ortho voltage

➔ *CPT Assistant* Apr 03:14, Aug 03:10, Oct 07:1, Oct 10:3

➔ *Clinical Examples in Radiology* Summer 08:12, Summer 09:7

77402 Radiation treatment delivery, single treatment area, single port or parallel opposed ports, simple blocks or no blocks; up to 5 MeV

➔ *CPT Assistant* Apr 03:14, Aug 03:10, Oct 07:1, Oct 10:3

➔ *Clinical Examples in Radiology* Spring 07:7-9, 12, Summer 08:12, Summer 09:7

77403 6-10 MeV

➔ *CPT Assistant* Apr 03:14, Oct 10:3

➔ *Clinical Examples in Radiology* Spring 07:7-9, 12, Summer 08:12, Summer 09:7

77404 11-19 MeV

➔ *CPT Assistant* Apr 03:14, Oct 10:3

➔ *Clinical Examples in Radiology* Spring 07:7-9, 12, Summer 08:12, Summer 09:7

77406 20 MeV or greater

➔ *CPT Assistant* Apr 03:14, Aug 03:10, Oct 07:1, Oct 10:3

➔ *Clinical Examples in Radiology* Spring 07:7-9, 12, Summer 08:12, Summer 09:7

77407 Radiation treatment delivery, 2 separate treatment areas, 3 or more ports on a single treatment area, use of multiple blocks; up to 5 MeV

➔ *CPT Assistant* Apr 03:14, Aug 03:10, Oct 07:1

➔ *Clinical Examples in Radiology* Spring 07:7-9, 12, Summer 08:12, Summer 09:7

77408 6-10 MeV

➔ *CPT Assistant* Apr 03:14

➔ *Clinical Examples in Radiology* Spring 07:7-9, 12, Summer 08:12, Summer 09:7

77409 11-19 MeV

➔ *CPT Assistant* Apr 03:14

➔ *Clinical Examples in Radiology* Spring 07:7, Summer 08:12, Summer 09:7

77411 20 MeV or greater

➔ *CPT Assistant* Apr 03:14, Aug 03:10, Oct 07:1

➔ *Clinical Examples in Radiology* Spring 07:7-9, 12, Summer 08:12, Summer 09:7

77412 Radiation treatment delivery, 3 or more separate treatment areas, custom blocking, tangential ports, wedges, rotational beam, compensators, electron beam; up to 5 MeV

➔ *CPT Assistant* Apr 03:14, Aug 03:10, Oct 07:1; *CPT Changes: An Insider's View* 2006

➔ *Clinical Examples in Radiology* Winter 06:20, Spring 07:7-9, 12, Summer 08:12, Summer 09:7

77413 6-10 MeV

➔ *CPT Assistant* Fall 91:14, Apr 03:14

➔ *Clinical Examples in Radiology* Spring 07:7-9, 12, Summer 08:12, Summer 09:2, 7

77414 11-19 MeV

➔ *CPT Assistant* Apr 03:14

➔ *Clinical Examples in Radiology* Spring 07:7-9, 12, Summer 08:12, Summer 09:7

77416   20 MeV or greater
→ *CPT Assistant* Aug 03:10, Oct 07:1
→ *Clinical Examples in Radiology* Spring 07:7-9, 12, Summer 08:12, Summer 09:7

77417   Therapeutic radiology port film(s)
→ *CPT Assistant* Fall 91:14, Dec 97:11, Feb 06:14, Oct 07:1
→ *Clinical Examples in Radiology* Summer 09:2, 7

77418   Intensity modulated treatment delivery, single or multiple fields/arcs, via narrow spatially and temporally modulated beams, binary, dynamic MLC, per treatment session
→ *CPT Assistant* Mar 05:1, 6, May 05:7, Mar 10:9; *CPT Changes: An Insider's View* 2002, 2005
→ *Clinical Examples in Radiology* Summer 07:9, Summer 09:7, Spring 12:10

(For intensity modulated treatment planning, use 77301)

(For compensator-based beam modulation treatment delivery, use Category III code 0073T)

77421   Stereoscopic X-ray guidance for localization of target volume for the delivery of radiation therapy
→ *CPT Assistant* Oct 07:1; *CPT Changes: An Insider's View* 2006
→ *Clinical Examples in Radiology* Winter 06:18, Fall 08:10, Summer 09:7, Spring 12:11

(Do not report 77421 in conjunction with 77432, 77435)

(Do not report 77421 more than once per treatment delivery session)

(For placement of interstitial device[s] for radiation therapy guidance, see 31627, 32553, 49411, 55876)

77424   Intraoperative radiation treatment delivery, x-ray, single treatment session
→ *CPT Changes: An Insider's View* 2012
→ *Clinical Examples in Radiology* Fall 11:11

77425   Intraoperative radiation treatment delivery, electrons, single treatment session
→ *CPT Changes: An Insider's View* 2012
→ *Clinical Examples in Radiology* Fall 11:11

Neutron Beam Treatment Delivery

77422   High energy neutron radiation treatment delivery; single treatment area using a single port or parallel-opposed ports with no blocks or simple blocking
→ *CPT Changes: An Insider's View* 2006
→ *Clinical Examples in Radiology* Winter 06:18

77423   1 or more isocenter(s) with coplanar or non-coplanar geometry with blocking and/or wedge, and/or compensator(s)
→ *CPT Changes: An Insider's View* 2006
→ *Clinical Examples in Radiology* Winter 06:18

77424   Code is out of numerical sequence. See 77401-77425

77425   Code is out of numerical sequence. See 77401-77425

Radiation Treatment Management

Radiation treatment management is reported in units of five fractions or treatment sessions, regardless of the actual time period in which the services are furnished. The services need not be furnished on consecutive days. Multiple fractions representing two or more treatment sessions furnished on the same day may be counted separately as long as there has been a distinct break in therapy sessions, and the fractions are of the character usually furnished on different days. Code 77427 is also reported if there are three or four fractions beyond a multiple of five at the end of a course of treatment; one or two fractions beyond a multiple of five at the end of a course of treatment are not reported separately.

Radiation treatment management requires **and includes** a minimum of one examination of the patient by the physician for medical evaluation and management (eg, assessment of the patient's response to treatment, coordination of care and treatment, review of imaging and/or lab test results with documentation) for each reporting of the radiation treatment management service. Code 77469 represents only the intraoperative session management and does not include medical evaluation and management outside of that session. The professional services furnished during treatment management typically include:

■ Review of port films;

■ Review of dosimetry, dose delivery, and treatment parameters;

■ Review of patient treatment set-up.

77427   Radiation treatment management, 5 treatments
→ *CPT Assistant* Nov 99:42, Feb 00:7, Oct 07:1, Nov 09:6; *CPT Changes: An Insider's View* 2000
→ *Clinical Examples in Radiology* Summer 08:12, Summer 09:2, 7, 8

77431   Radiation therapy management with complete course of therapy consisting of 1 or 2 fractions only
→ *CPT Assistant* Winter 90:10, Oct 97:4, Nov 09:6
→ *Clinical Examples in Radiology* Summer 08:12, Summer 09:7, 8

(77431 is not to be used to fill in the last week of a long course of therapy)

77432   Stereotactic radiation treatment management of cranial lesion(s) (complete course of treatment consisting of 1 session)
→ *CPT Assistant* Oct 97:4, Nov 09:6, Jul 11:12; *CPT Changes: An Insider's View* 2008
→ *Clinical Examples in Radiology* Summer 09:7, 8

(The same physician should not report both stereotactic radiosurgery services [61796-61800] and radiation treatment management [77432 or 77435] for cranial lesions)

(For stereotactic body radiation therapy treatment, use 77435)

77435 Stereotactic body radiation therapy, treatment management, per treatment course, to 1 or more lesions, including image guidance, entire course not to exceed 5 fractions

> *CPT Assistant* Mar 07:7, Oct 07:1, Nov 09:6; *CPT Changes: An Insider's View* 2007

> *Clinical Examples in Radiology* Summer 09:7, 8

(Do not report 77435 in conjunction with 77427-77432)

►(The same physician should not report both stereotactic radiosurgery services [32701, 63620, 63621] and radiation treatment management [77435])◄

77469 Intraoperative radiation treatment management

> *CPT Changes: An Insider's View* 2012

> *Clinical Examples in Radiology* Summer 09:7, Fall 11:11

77470 Special treatment procedure (eg, total body irradiation, hemibody radiation, per oral or endocavitary irradiation)

> *CPT Assistant* Winter 91:22, Oct 97:1, Apr 09:3; *CPT Changes: An Insider's View* 2001, 2012

> *Clinical Examples in Radiology* Summer 08:12, Summer 09:7, 8, Spring 12:11

(77470 assumes that the procedure is performed 1 or more times during the course of therapy, in addition to daily or weekly patient management)

(For intraoperative radiation treatment delivery and management, see 77424, 77425, 77469)

77499 Unlisted procedure, therapeutic radiology treatment management

> *CPT Assistant* Nov 99:42, Feb 00:7, Nov 09:6; *CPT Changes: An Insider's View* 2000

> *Clinical Examples in Radiology* Summer 09:7, 8

Proton Beam Treatment Delivery

Definitions

Simple proton treatment delivery to a single treatment area utilizing a single non-tangential/oblique port, custom block with compensation (77522) and without compensation (77520).

Intermediate proton treatment delivery to one or more treatment areas utilizing two or more ports or one or more tangential/oblique ports, with custom blocks and compensators.

Complex proton treatment delivery to one or more treatment areas utilizing two or more ports per treatment area with matching or patching fields and/or multiple isocenters, with custom blocks and compensators.

77520 Proton treatment delivery; simple, without compensation

> *CPT Assistant* Nov 99:43; *CPT Changes: An Insider's View* 2000, 2001

77522 simple, with compensation

> *CPT Changes: An Insider's View* 2001

77523 intermediate

> *CPT Assistant* Nov 99:43; *CPT Changes: An Insider's View* 2000, 2001

77525 complex

> *CPT Changes: An Insider's View* 2001

Hyperthermia

Hyperthermia treatments as listed in this section include external (superficial and deep), interstitial, and intracavitary.

Radiation therapy when given concurrently is listed separately.

Hyperthermia is used only as an adjunct to radiation therapy or chemotherapy. It may be induced by a variety of sources (eg, microwave, ultrasound, low energy radio-frequency conduction, or by probes).

The listed treatments include management during the course of therapy and follow-up care for three months after completion.

Preliminary consultation is not included (see **Evaluation and Management** 99241-99255).

Physics planning and interstitial insertion of temperature sensors, and use of external or interstitial heat generating sources are included.

The following descriptors are included in the treatment schedule:

⊙ **77600** Hyperthermia, externally generated; superficial (ie, heating to a depth of 4 cm or less)

> *CPT Assistant* Winter 91:22

⊙ **77605** deep (ie, heating to depths greater than 4 cm)

> *CPT Assistant* Winter 91:22

►(For focused microwave thermotherapy of the breast, use 0301T)◄

⊙ **77610** Hyperthermia generated by interstitial probe(s); 5 or fewer interstitial applicators

> *CPT Assistant* Winter 91:22

⊙ **77615** more than 5 interstitial applicators

> *CPT Assistant* Winter 91:22

Clinical Intracavitary Hyperthermia

77620 Hyperthermia generated by intracavitary probe(s)

> *CPT Assistant* Winter 91:22

Clinical Brachytherapy

Clinical brachytherapy requires the use of either natural or man-made radioelements applied into or around a treatment field of interest. The supervision of radioelements and dose interpretation are performed solely by the therapeutic radiologist.

Services 77750-77799 include admission to the hospital and daily visits.

For insertion of ovoids and tandems, use 57155.

For insertion of Heyman capsules, use 58346.

Definitions

(Sources refer to intracavitary placement or permanent interstitial placement; ribbons refer to temporary interstitial placement)

A simple application has one to four sources/ribbons.

An intermediate application has five to 10 sources/ribbons.

A complex application has greater than 10 sources/ribbons.

    (For high dose rate electronic brachytherapy, per fraction, use Category III code 0182T)

77750   Infusion or instillation of radioelement solution (includes 3-month follow-up care)

    ⮕ *CPT Assistant* Sep 05:1; *CPT Changes: An Insider's View* 2005

    (For administration of radiolabeled monoclonal antibodies, use 79403)

    (For non-antibody radiopharmaceutical therapy by intravenous administration only, not including 3-month follow-up care, use 79101)

77761   Intracavitary radiation source application; simple

    ⮕ *CPT Assistant* Winter 91:23, Jan 96:7, Mar 99:3, Feb 02:7, Sep 05:1; *CPT Changes: An Insider's View* 2001

77762   intermediate

    ⮕ *CPT Assistant* Winter 91:23, Feb 02:7, Sep 05:1

77763   complex

    ⮕ *CPT Assistant* Winter 91:23, Mar 99:3, Feb 02:7, Sep 05:1

    (Do not report 77761-77763 in conjunction with Category III code 0182T)

77776   Interstitial radiation source application; simple

    ⮕ *CPT Assistant* Winter 91:23, Sep 05:1, Aug 08:7; *CPT Changes: An Insider's View* 2001

77777   intermediate

    ⮕ *CPT Assistant* Winter 91:23, Sep 05:1, May 07:1, Aug 08:7

77778   complex

    ⮕ *CPT Assistant* Winter 91:23, Apr 04:6, Sep 05:1, May 07:1

    (Do not report 77776-77778 in conjunction with Category III code 0182T)

    (77781 has been deleted. To report, see 77785, 77786)

    (77782-77784 have been deleted. To report, see 77785-77787)

77785   Remote afterloading high dose rate radionuclide brachytherapy; 1 channel

    ⮕ *CPT Changes: An Insider's View* 2009

77786   2-12 channels

    ⮕ *CPT Changes: An Insider's View* 2009

77787   over 12 channels

    ⮕ *CPT Changes: An Insider's View* 2009

    (Do not report 77785-77787 in conjunction with Category III code 0182T)

77789   Surface application of radiation source

    ⮕ *CPT Assistant* Sep 05:1; *CPT Changes: An Insider's View* 2001

    (Do not report 77789 in conjunction with Category III code 0182T)

77790   Supervision, handling, loading of radiation source

    ⮕ *CPT Assistant* Sep 05:1; *CPT Changes: An Insider's View* 2001

77799   Unlisted procedure, clinical brachytherapy

    ⮕ *CPT Assistant* Sep 05:1

Nuclear Medicine

▶Listed procedures may be performed independently or in the course of overall medical care. If the individual providing these services is also responsible for diagnostic workup and/or follow-up care of patient, see appropriate sections also.◀

Radioimmunoassay tests are found in the **Clinical Pathology** section (codes 82000-84999). These codes can be appropriately used by any specialist performing such tests in a laboratory licensed and/or certified for radioimmunoassays. The reporting of these tests is not confined to clinical pathology laboratories alone.

▶The services listed do not include the radiopharmaceutical or drug. To separately report supply of diagnostic and therapeutic radiopharmaceuticals and drugs, use the appropriate supply code(s), in addition to the procedure code.◀

Diagnostic

Endocrine System

    ▶(78000-78011 have been deleted. To report, see 78012-78014)◀

● **78012**   Thyroid uptake, single or multiple quantitative measurement(s) (including stimulation, suppression, or discharge, when performed)

    ⮕ *CPT Changes: An Insider's View* 2013

● **78013**   Thyroid imaging (including vascular flow, when performed);

    ⮕ *CPT Changes: An Insider's View* 2013

● **78014**   with single or multiple uptake(s) quantitative measurement(s) (including stimulation, suppression, or discharge, when performed)

    ⮕ *CPT Changes: An Insider's View* 2013

78015   Thyroid carcinoma metastases imaging; limited area (eg, neck and chest only)

    ⮕ *CPT Assistant* Nov 98:21, Jan 07:31

78016   with additional studies (eg, urinary recovery)

    ⮕ *CPT Assistant* Jan 07:31

78018   whole body

    ⮕ *CPT Assistant* Apr 99:4, Jan 07:31

    ⮕ *Clinical Examples in Radiology* Fall 09:3-5

＋ **78020**   Thyroid carcinoma metastases uptake (List separately in addition to code for primary procedure)

    ⮕ *CPT Assistant* Nov 98:21, Apr 99:4, Jan 07:31

    ⮕ *Clinical Examples in Radiology* Fall 09:3-5

    (Use 78020 in conjunction with 78018 only)

▲ **78070**   Parathyroid planar imaging (including subtraction, when performed);

    ⮕ *CPT Assistant* Jan 07:31; *CPT Changes: An Insider's View* 2013

    ⮕ *Clinical Examples in Radiology* Summer 11:4, 5

Radiology

● **78071**   with tomographic (SPECT)
→ *CPT Changes: An Insider's View* 2013

● **78072**   with tomographic (SPECT), and concurrently acquired computed tomography (CT) for anatomical localization
→ *CPT Changes: An Insider's View* 2013

78075   Adrenal imaging, cortex and/or medulla
→ *CPT Assistant* Jan 07:31, Feb 12:9

78099   Unlisted endocrine procedure, diagnostic nuclear medicine
→ *CPT Assistant* Dec 05:7, Jan 07:31

(For chemical analysis, see **Chemistry** section)

Hematopoietic, Reticuloendothelial and Lymphatic System

78102   Bone marrow imaging; limited area
→ *CPT Assistant* Dec 05:7, Feb 12:9

78103   multiple areas

78104   whole body

78110   Plasma volume, radiopharmaceutical volume-dilution technique (separate procedure); single sampling

78111   multiple samplings

78120   Red cell volume determination (separate procedure); single sampling

78121   multiple samplings

78122   Whole blood volume determination, including separate measurement of plasma volume and red cell volume (radiopharmaceutical volume-dilution technique)

78130   Red cell survival study;

78135   differential organ/tissue kinetics (eg, splenic and/or hepatic sequestration)

78140   Labeled red cell sequestration, differential organ/tissue (eg, splenic and/or hepatic)

78185   Spleen imaging only, with or without vascular flow

(If combined with liver study, use procedures 78215 and 78216)

78190   Kinetics, study of platelet survival, with or without differential organ/tissue localization

78191   Platelet survival study

78195   Lymphatics and lymph nodes imaging
→ *CPT Assistant* Nov 98:22, Jul 99:6, Nov 99:43, Dec 99:8, Sep 08:5, Feb 12:9; *CPT Changes: An Insider's View* 2000, 2002

(For sentinel node identification without scintigraphy imaging, use 38792)

(For sentinel node excision, see 38500-38542)

78199   Unlisted hematopoietic, reticuloendothelial and lymphatic procedure, diagnostic nuclear medicine
→ *CPT Assistant* Dec 05:7

(For chemical analysis, see **Chemistry** section)

Gastrointestinal System

78201   Liver imaging; static only
→ *CPT Assistant* Dec 05:7, Feb 12:9

78202   with vascular flow
→ *CPT Assistant* Feb 12:9

(For spleen imaging only, use 78185)

78205   Liver imaging (SPECT);
→ *CPT Assistant* Nov 98:22

78206   with vascular flow
→ *CPT Assistant* Nov 98:22

78215   Liver and spleen imaging; static only

78216   with vascular flow

(78220 has been deleted)

(78223 has been deleted. To report hepatobiliary system imaging, see 78226, 78227)

78226   Hepatobiliary system imaging, including gallbladder when present;
→ *CPT Changes: An Insider's View* 2012
→ *Clinical Examples in Radiology* Winter 12:6

78227   with pharmacologic intervention, including quantitative measurement(s) when performed
→ *CPT Changes: An Insider's View* 2012
→ *Clinical Examples in Radiology* Winter 12:5

78230   Salivary gland imaging;

78231   with serial images

78232   Salivary gland function study

78258   Esophageal motility

78261   Gastric mucosa imaging

78262   Gastroesophageal reflux study

78264   Gastric emptying study

78267   Urea breath test, C-14 (isotopic); acquisition for analysis
→ *CPT Assistant* Nov 99:43; *CPT Changes: An Insider's View* 2000, 2005
→ *Clinical Examples in Radiology* Fall 07:9

78268   analysis
→ *CPT Assistant* Nov 99:43; *CPT Changes: An Insider's View* 2000
→ *Clinical Examples in Radiology* Fall 07:9

78270   Vitamin B-12 absorption study (eg, Schilling test); without intrinsic factor

78271   with intrinsic factor

78272   Vitamin B-12 absorption studies combined, with and without intrinsic factor

78278   Acute gastrointestinal blood loss imaging

78282   Gastrointestinal protein loss

78290   Intestine imaging (eg, ectopic gastric mucosa, Meckel's localization, volvulus)
→ *CPT Changes: An Insider's View* 2002

78291 Peritoneal-venous shunt patency test (eg, for LeVeen, Denver shunt)
➔ *CPT Assistant* Feb 12:9

(For injection procedure, use 49427)

78299 Unlisted gastrointestinal procedure, diagnostic nuclear medicine
➔ *CPT Assistant* Dec 05:7

Musculoskeletal System

Bone and joint imaging can be used in the diagnosis of a variety of inflammatory processes (eg, osteomyelitis), as well as for localization of primary and/or metastatic neoplasms.

78300 Bone and/or joint imaging; limited area
➔ *CPT Assistant* Mar 97:11, Dec 05:7, Feb 12:9
➔ *Clinical Examples in Radiology* Winter 09:5, Spring 10:9

78305   multiple areas
➔ *CPT Assistant* Mar 97:11
➔ *Clinical Examples in Radiology* Winter 09:5, Spring 10:9

78306   whole body
➔ *CPT Assistant* Mar 97:11, Jan 02:10, Jun 03:11, Feb 12:10
➔ *Clinical Examples in Radiology* Summer 06:7, 12, Winter 09:3, 4, 5, Spring 10:9

78315   3 phase study
➔ *CPT Assistant* Jan 02:10
➔ *Clinical Examples in Radiology* Summer 06:7, 12, Winter 09:4, 5, Spring 10:9

78320   tomographic (SPECT)
➔ *CPT Assistant* Mar 97:11, Jun 03:11, Jan 08:9
➔ *Clinical Examples in Radiology* Winter 09:4, 5, Spring 10:9

78350 Bone density (bone mineral content) study, 1 or more sites; single photon absorptiometry
➔ *CPT Assistant* Nov 97:26

78351   dual photon absorptiometry, 1 or more sites
➔ *CPT Assistant* Nov 97:26, Feb 12:9

78399 Unlisted musculoskeletal procedure, diagnostic nuclear medicine
➔ *CPT Assistant* Dec 05:7

Cardiovascular System

Myocardial perfusion and cardiac blood pool imaging studies may be performed at rest and/or during stress. When performed during exercise and/or pharmacologic stress, the appropriate stress testing code from the 93015-93018 series should be reported in addition to 78451-78454, 78472-78492.

78414 Determination of central c-v hemodynamics (non-imaging) (eg, ejection fraction with probe technique) with or without pharmacologic intervention or exercise, single or multiple determinations
➔ *CPT Assistant* Dec 05:7, May 10:6, Feb 12:9

78428 Cardiac shunt detection
➔ *CPT Assistant* May 10:6

78445 Non-cardiac vascular flow imaging (ie, angiography, venography)
➔ *CPT Assistant* May 10:6
➔ *Clinical Examples in Radiology* Spring 10:9

78451 Myocardial perfusion imaging, tomographic (SPECT) (including attenuation correction, qualitative or quantitative wall motion, ejection fraction by first pass or gated technique, additional quantification, when performed); single study, at rest or stress (exercise or pharmacologic)
➔ *CPT Assistant* May 10:5, Feb 11:9, Feb 12:10; *CPT Changes: An Insider's View* 2010
➔ *Clinical Examples in Radiology* Spring 10:9, Winter 10:11

78452   multiple studies, at rest and/or stress (exercise or pharmacologic) and/or redistribution and/or rest reinjection
➔ *CPT Assistant* May 10:5, Feb 11:9, Feb 12:9; *CPT Changes: An Insider's View* 2010
➔ *Clinical Examples in Radiology* Spring 10:9, Winter 10:10, 11

78453 Myocardial perfusion imaging, planar (including qualitative or quantitative wall motion, ejection fraction by first pass or gated technique, additional quantification, when performed); single study, at rest or stress (exercise or pharmacologic)
➔ *CPT Assistant* May 10:5; *CPT Changes: An Insider's View* 2010
➔ *Clinical Examples in Radiology* Winter 10:11

78454   multiple studies, at rest and/or stress (exercise or pharmacologic) and/or redistribution and/or rest reinjection
➔ *CPT Assistant* May 10:5; *CPT Changes: An Insider's View* 2010
➔ *Clinical Examples in Radiology* Winter 10:11

78456 Acute venous thrombosis imaging, peptide
➔ *CPT Assistant* Nov 99:43, May 10:6; *CPT Changes: An Insider's View* 2000

78457 Venous thrombosis imaging, venogram; unilateral
➔ *CPT Assistant* Nov 99:43; *CPT Changes: An Insider's View* 2000

78458   bilateral
➔ *CPT Assistant* Nov 99:43, May 10:6; *CPT Changes: An Insider's View* 2000

78459 Myocardial imaging, positron emission tomography (PET), metabolic evaluation
➔ *CPT Assistant* Jun 96:5, Nov 97:26, May 10:6
➔ *Clinical Examples in Radiology* Summer 10:11

(For myocardial perfusion study, see 78491-78492)

(78460-78465 have been deleted. To report, see 78451-78454)

78466 Myocardial imaging, infarct avid, planar; qualitative or quantitative
➔ *CPT Assistant* May 10:6

78468   with ejection fraction by first pass technique
➔ *CPT Assistant* May 10:6

78469   tomographic SPECT with or without quantification
➔ *CPT Assistant* May 10:6

78472 Cardiac blood pool imaging, gated equilibrium; planar, single study at rest or stress (exercise and/or pharmacologic), wall motion study plus ejection fraction, with or without additional quantitative processing

➜ *CPT Assistant* Nov 98:22, Nov 99:44, May 10:6; *CPT Changes: An Insider's View* 2000

(For assessment of right ventricular ejection fraction by first pass technique, use 78496)

78473 multiple studies, wall motion study plus ejection fraction, at rest and stress (exercise and/or pharmacologic), with or without additional quantification

➜ *CPT Assistant* May 10:6

(Do not report 78472, 78473 in conjunction with 78451-78454, 78481, 78483, 78494)

(78478, 78480 have been deleted. To report, see 78451-78454)

78481 Cardiac blood pool imaging (planar), first pass technique; single study, at rest or with stress (exercise and/or pharmacologic), wall motion study plus ejection fraction, with or without quantification

➜ *CPT Assistant* May 10:6

78483 multiple studies, at rest and with stress (exercise and/or pharmacologic), wall motion study plus ejection fraction, with or without quantification

➜ *CPT Assistant* May 10:6

(For cerebral blood flow study, use 78610)

(Do not report 78481-78483 in conjunction with 78451-78454)

78491 Myocardial imaging, positron emission tomography (PET), perfusion; single study at rest or stress

➜ *CPT Assistant* Nov 97:27, May 10:6

➜ *Clinical Examples in Radiology* Summer 10:11

78492 multiple studies at rest and/or stress

➜ *CPT Assistant* Nov 97:27, May 10:6

➜ *Clinical Examples in Radiology* Summer 10:11

78494 Cardiac blood pool imaging, gated equilibrium, SPECT, at rest, wall motion study plus ejection fraction, with or without quantitative processing

➜ *CPT Assistant* Nov 98:22, Jun 99:3, May 10:6

+ 78496 Cardiac blood pool imaging, gated equilibrium, single study, at rest, with right ventricular ejection fraction by first pass technique (List separately in addition to code for primary procedure)

➜ *CPT Assistant* Nov 98:22, Jun 99:3, 11, May 10:6, Feb 12:9

(Use 78496 in conjunction with 78472)

78499 Unlisted cardiovascular procedure, diagnostic nuclear medicine

➜ *CPT Assistant* Dec 05:7, May 10:6

➜ *Clinical Examples in Radiology* Summer 08:12

Respiratory System

78579 Pulmonary ventilation imaging (eg, aerosol or gas)

➜ *CPT Assistant* Feb 12:9; *CPT Changes: An Insider's View* 2012

➜ *Clinical Examples in Radiology* Fall 11:5

78580 Pulmonary perfusion imaging (eg, particulate)

➜ *CPT Assistant* Mar 99:4, Dec 05:7, May 10:6; *CPT Changes: An Insider's View* 2012

78582 Pulmonary ventilation (eg, aerosol or gas) and perfusion imaging

➜ *CPT Changes: An Insider's View* 2012

➜ *Clinical Examples in Radiology* Fall 11:4, 5

78597 Quantitative differential pulmonary perfusion, including imaging when performed

➜ *CPT Changes: An Insider's View* 2012

➜ *Clinical Examples in Radiology* Fall 11:5, 6

78598 Quantitative differential pulmonary perfusion and ventilation (eg, aerosol or gas), including imaging when performed

➜ *CPT Assistant* Feb 12:9; *CPT Changes: An Insider's View* 2012

➜ *Clinical Examples in Radiology* Fall 11:5

(Report 78579, 78580, 78582-78598 only once per imaging session)

(Do not report 78580, 78582-78598 in conjunction with 78451-78454)

(78584-78596 have been deleted. To report, see 78579, 78582-78598)

78599 Unlisted respiratory procedure, diagnostic nuclear medicine

➜ *CPT Assistant* Dec 05:7

Nervous System

78600 Brain imaging, less than 4 static views;

➜ *CPT Assistant* Dec 05:7, Feb 12:9; *CPT Changes: An Insider's View* 2008

78601 with vascular flow

➜ *CPT Changes: An Insider's View* 2008

78605 Brain imaging, minimum 4 static views;

➜ *CPT Changes: An Insider's View* 2008

78606 with vascular flow

➜ *CPT Changes: An Insider's View* 2008

78607 Brain imaging, tomographic (SPECT)

➜ *CPT Changes: An Insider's View* 2008

➜ *Clinical Examples in Radiology* Spring 12:9

78608 Brain imaging, positron emission tomography (PET); metabolic evaluation

➜ *Clinical Examples in Radiology* Spring 10:1, 2

78609 perfusion evaluation

78610 Brain imaging, vascular flow only

78630 Cerebrospinal fluid flow, imaging (not including introduction of material); cisternography

(For injection procedure, see 61000-61070, 62270-62319)

78635   ventriculography

(For injection procedure, see 61000-61070, 62270-62294)

78645   shunt evaluation

(For injection procedure, see 61000-61070, 62270-62294)

78647   tomographic (SPECT)

78650   Cerebrospinal fluid leakage detection and localization
➔ *CPT Changes: An Insider's View* 2002

(For injection procedure, see 61000-61070, 62270-62294)

78660   Radiopharmaceutical dacryocystography
➔ *CPT Assistant* Feb 12:9

78699   Unlisted nervous system procedure, diagnostic nuclear medicine
➔ *CPT Assistant* Dec 05:7

Genitourinary System

78700   Kidney imaging morphology;
➔ *CPT Assistant* Dec 05:7, Mar 07:7, Feb 12:9; *CPT Changes: An Insider's View* 2007
➔ *Clinical Examples in Radiology* Fall 09:2

78701   with vascular flow
➔ *Clinical Examples in Radiology* Fall 09:2

78707   with vascular flow and function, single study without pharmacological intervention
➔ *CPT Assistant* Nov 97:27, Mar 07:7; *CPT Changes: An Insider's View* 2007

78708   with vascular flow and function, single study, with pharmacological intervention (eg, angiotensin converting enzyme inhibitor and/or diuretic)
➔ *CPT Assistant* Nov 97:27, Mar 07:7; *CPT Changes: An Insider's View* 2007
➔ *Clinical Examples in Radiology* Fall 09:2

78709   with vascular flow and function, multiple studies, with and without pharmacological intervention (eg, angiotensin converting enzyme inhibitor and/or diuretic)
➔ *CPT Assistant* Nov 97:27, Mar 07:7; *CPT Changes: An Insider's View* 2007
➔ *Clinical Examples in Radiology* Fall 09:2

(For introduction of radioactive substance in association with renal endoscopy, see 77776-77778)

78710   tomographic (SPECT)
➔ *CPT Assistant* Nov 97:27, Mar 07:7; *CPT Changes: An Insider's View* 2007

78725   Kidney function study, non-imaging radioisotopic study
➔ *CPT Assistant* Nov 98:22
➔ *Clinical Examples in Radiology* Fall 09:2

+ 78730   Urinary bladder residual study (List separately in addition to code for primary procedure)
➔ *CPT Assistant* Mar 07:7; *CPT Changes: An Insider's View* 2007
➔ *Clinical Examples in Radiology* Spring 12:2

(Use 78730 in conjunction with 78740)

(For measurement of postvoid residual urine and/or bladder capacity by ultrasound, nonimaging, use 51798)

(For ultrasound imaging of the bladder only, with measurement of postvoid residual urine when performed, use 76857)

78740   Ureteral reflux study (radiopharmaceutical voiding cystogram)
➔ *Clinical Examples in Radiology* Spring 12:1

(Use 78740 in conjunction with 78730 for urinary bladder residual study)

(For catheterization, see 51701, 51702, 51703)

78761   Testicular imaging with vascular flow
➔ *CPT Assistant* Mar 07:7, Feb 12:9; *CPT Changes: An Insider's View* 2007

78799   Unlisted genitourinary procedure, diagnostic nuclear medicine
➔ *CPT Assistant* Dec 05:7

(For chemical analysis, see **Chemistry** section)

Other Procedures

(For specific organ, see appropriate heading)

(For radiophosphorus tumor identification, ocular, see 78800)

78800   Radiopharmaceutical localization of tumor or distribution of radiopharmaceutical agent(s); limited area
➔ *CPT Assistant* Dec 05:7, Dec 11:17, Feb 12:9; *CPT Changes: An Insider's View* 2004
➔ *Clinical Examples in Radiology* Summer 06:6, 10-11, Spring 10:4, 8, Fall 10:11

(For specific organ, see appropriate heading)

78801   multiple areas
➔ *CPT Assistant* Dec 11:17, Feb 12:9

78802   whole body, single day imaging
➔ *CPT Assistant* Jun 03:11, Feb 12:9; *CPT Changes: An Insider's View* 2004
➔ *Clinical Examples in Radiology* Summer 06:6, 10-11

78803   tomographic (SPECT)
➔ *CPT Assistant* Jun 03:11, Feb 12:9
➔ *Clinical Examples in Radiology* Summer 06:6, 10-11

78804   whole body, requiring 2 or more days imaging
➔ *CPT Assistant* Feb 12:9; *CPT Changes: An Insider's View* 2004

78805   Radiopharmaceutical localization of inflammatory process; limited area
➔ *CPT Assistant* Nov 99:44, Feb 12:9; *CPT Changes: An Insider's View* 2001

78806   whole body
➔ *CPT Assistant* Nov 99:44, Jun 03:11, Feb 12:9; *CPT Changes: An Insider's View* 2000

78807   tomographic (SPECT)
➔ *CPT Assistant* Jun 03:11, Feb 12:9

Radiology

(For imaging bone infectious or inflammatory disease with a bone imaging radiopharmaceutical, see 78300, 78305, 78306)

78808   Injection procedure for radiopharmaceutical localization by non-imaging probe study, intravenous (eg, parathyroid adenoma)

➔ *CPT Assistant* Feb 12:9; *CPT Changes: An Insider's View* 2009

(For sentinel lymph node identification, use 38792)

(For PET of brain, see 78608, 78609)

(For PET myocardial imaging, see 78459, 78491, 78492)

78811   Positron emission tomography (PET) imaging; limited area (eg, chest, head/neck)

➔ *CPT Assistant* Dec 05:7, Feb 12:9; *CPT Changes: An Insider's View* 2005, 2008

➔ *Clinical Examples in Radiology* Spring 05:13, 15, Spring 10:2, 7

78812   skull base to mid-thigh

➔ *CPT Assistant* Dec 05:7, Feb 12:9; *CPT Changes: An Insider's View* 2005, 2008

➔ *Clinical Examples in Radiology* Spring 05:13, 15, Spring 10:1, 2

78813   whole body

➔ *CPT Assistant* Dec 05:7, Feb 12:9; *CPT Changes: An Insider's View* 2005, 2008

➔ *Clinical Examples in Radiology* Spring 05:13, 15, Spring 10:2

78814   Positron emission tomography (PET) with concurrently acquired computed tomography (CT) for attenuation correction and anatomical localization imaging; limited area (eg, chest, head/neck)

➔ *CPT Assistant* Feb 05:13, Jun 05:10, Dec 05:7, Feb 12:9; *CPT Changes: An Insider's View* 2005, 2008

➔ *Clinical Examples in Radiology* Spring 05:13, 15, Spring 10:2, 4

78815   skull base to mid-thigh

➔ *CPT Assistant* Feb 05:13, Jun 05:10, Dec 05:7, Feb 12:9; *CPT Changes: An Insider's View* 2005, 2008

➔ *Clinical Examples in Radiology* Spring 05:13, 15, Spring 10:2, 4

78816   whole body

➔ *CPT Assistant* Feb 05:13, Jun 05:10, Dec 05:7, Feb 12:9; *CPT Changes: An Insider's View* 2005, 2008

➔ *Clinical Examples in Radiology* Spring 05:13, 15, Spring 10:2

(Report 78811-78816 only once per imaging session)

(Computed tomography [CT] performed for other than attenuation correction and anatomical localization is reported using the appropriate site specific CT code with modifier 59)

(78890, 78891 have been deleted)

78999   Unlisted miscellaneous procedure, diagnostic nuclear medicine

➔ *CPT Assistant* Dec 05:7, Feb 12:9

➔ *Clinical Examples in Radiology* Summer 08:12, Spring 10:2, 11

Therapeutic

The oral and intravenous administration codes in this section are inclusive of the mode of administration. For intra-arterial, intra-cavitary, and intra-articular

administration, also use the appropriate injection and/or procedure codes, as well as imaging guidance and radiological supervision and interpretation codes, when appropriate.

79005   Radiopharmaceutical therapy, by oral administration

➔ *CPT Assistant* Sep 05:1, Feb 12:9; *CPT Changes: An Insider's View* 2005

➔ *Clinical Examples in Radiology* Spring 05:14, Fall 09:5, Winter 12:8

(For monoclonal antibody therapy, use 79403)

79101   Radiopharmaceutical therapy, by intravenous administration

➔ *CPT Assistant* Sep 05:1, Feb 12:9; *CPT Changes: An Insider's View* 2005

➔ *Clinical Examples in Radiology* Spring 10:8, Winter 12:8

(Do not report 79101 in conjunction with 36400, 36410, 79403, 96360, 96374 or 96375, 96409)

(For radiolabeled monoclonal antibody by intravenous infusion, use 79403)

(For infusion or instillation of non-antibody radioelement solution that includes 3 months follow-up care, use 77750)

79200   Radiopharmaceutical therapy, by intracavitary administration

➔ *CPT Assistant* Sep 05:1, Feb 12:9; *CPT Changes: An Insider's View* 2005

79300   Radiopharmaceutical therapy, by interstitial radioactive colloid administration

➔ *CPT Assistant* Sep 05:1, Feb 12:9; *CPT Changes: An Insider's View* 2005

79403   Radiopharmaceutical therapy, radiolabeled monoclonal antibody by intravenous infusion

➔ *CPT Assistant* Sep 05:1, Feb 12:9; *CPT Changes: An Insider's View* 2004

(For pre-treatment imaging, see 78802, 78804)

(Do not report 79403 in conjunction with 79101)

79440   Radiopharmaceutical therapy, by intra-articular administration

➔ *CPT Assistant* Sep 05:1, Feb 12:9; *CPT Changes: An Insider's View* 2005

79445   Radiopharmaceutical therapy, by intra-arterial particulate administration

➔ *CPT Assistant* Sep 05:1, Dec 06:10, Feb 12:9; *CPT Changes: An Insider's View* 2005

(Do not report 79445 in conjunction with 96373, 96420)

(Use appropriate procedural and radiological supervision and interpretation codes for the angiographic and interventional procedures provided prerequisite to intra-arterial radiopharmaceutical therapy)

79999   Radiopharmaceutical therapy, unlisted procedure

➔ *CPT Assistant* Mar 05:11, Sep 05:1, Jan 07:30, Feb 12:9; *CPT Changes: An Insider's View* 2005

➔ *Clinical Examples in Radiology* Winter 12:8

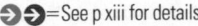

Pathology and Laboratory Guidelines

Pathology and Laboratory

The following is a listing of headings and subheadings that appear within the Pathology and Laboratory section of the CPT codebook. The subheadings or subsections denoted with asterisks (*) below have special instructions unique to that section. Where these are indicated, special "notes" or guidelines will be presented preceding those procedural terminology listings, referring to that subsection specifically.

Table of Drugs and the Appropriate Qualitative Screening, Confirmatory, and Quantitative Codes

Drug Qualitative	Multiple Drug Class Method	Single Drug Class Method	Confirmation	Quantitative
Alcohols	80100[a]	80101[b]	80102[c]	82055 or 82075[d]
Amphetamines	80100[a]	80101[b]	80102[c]	82145
Barbiturates	80100[a]	80101[b]	80102[c]	80184 or 82205[e]
Benzodiazepines	80100[a]	80101[b]	80102[c]	80154
Cocaine and metabolites	80100[a]	80101[b]	80102[c]	82520
Methadone	80100[a]	80101[b]	80102[c]	83840
Methaqualone	80100[a]	80101[b]	80102[c]	80299 or 82491[f]
Opiates	80100[a]	80101[b]	80102[c]	83925
Phencyclidine	80100[a]	80101[b]	80102[c]	83992
Phenothiazines	80100[a]	80101[b]	80102[c]	84022
Propoxyphene	80100[a]	80101[b]	80102[c]	80299 or 82491[f]
Tetrahydrocan-nabinoids	80100[a]	80101[b]	80102[c]	80299 or 82491[f]
Tricyclic antidepressants	80100[a]	80101[b]	80102[c]	80152, 80160, 80166, 80174, 80182[g], 80299 or 82491

[a] Use code **80100** for each combination of mobile phase with stationary phase.

[b] Use code **80101** for each single drug class tested and reported.

[c] Use code **80102** for each combination of mobile phase with stationary phase used for drug confirmation.

[d] Code **82055** for "Alcohol (ethanol); any specimen except breath," and code **82075** for "Alcohol (ethanol); breath."

[e] Code **80184** for "Phenobarbital," **80188** for "Primidone," and **82205** for "Barbiturates, not elsewhere specified."

[f] If there is no appropriate quantitative code for the drug listed, use code **82491** for chromatographic determination or **80299** for other methods.

[g] Code **80152** "Amitriptyline," **80160** for "Desipramine," **80166** for "Doxepin," **80174** for "Imipramine," or **80182** for "Nortriptyline."

Pathology and Laboratory Guidelines

►Guidelines to direct general reporting of services are presented in the **Introduction.** Some of the commonalities are repeated here for the convenience of those referring to this section on **Pathology and Laboratory.** Other definitions and items unique to Pathology and Laboratory are also listed.◄

Services in Pathology and Laboratory

Services in Pathology and Laboratory are provided by a physician or by technologists under responsible supervision of a physician.

Separate or Multiple Procedures

It is appropriate to designate multiple procedures that are rendered on the same date by separate entries.

Unlisted Service or Procedure

A service or procedure may be provided that is not listed in this edition of the CPT codebook. When reporting such a service, the appropriate "Unlisted Procedure" code may be used to indicate the service, identifying it by "Special Report" as discussed below. The "Unlisted Procedures" and accompanying codes for **Pathology and Laboratory** are as follows:

81099	Unlisted urinalysis procedure
● 81479	Unlisted molecular pathology procedure
● 81599	Unlisted multianalyte assay with algorithmic analysis
84999	Unlisted chemistry procedure
85999	Unlisted hematology and coagulation procedure
86486	unlisted antigen, each
86849	Unlisted immunology procedure
86999	Unlisted transfusion medicine procedure
87999	Unlisted microbiology procedure
88099	Unlisted necropsy (autopsy) procedure
88199	Unlisted cytopathology procedure
88299	Unlisted cytogenetic study

88399	Unlisted surgical pathology procedure
88749	Unlisted in vivo (eg, transcutaneous) laboratory service
89240	Unlisted miscellaneous pathology test
89398	Unlisted reproductive medicine laboratory procedure

Special Report

A service that is rarely provided, unusual, variable, or new may require a special report. Pertinent information should include an adequate definition or description of the nature, extent, and need for the procedure; and the time, effort, and equipment necessary to provide the service.

Pathology and Laboratory

Organ or Disease-Oriented Panels

These panels were developed for coding purposes only and should not be interpreted as clinical parameters. The tests listed with each panel identify the defined components of that panel.

These panel components are not intended to limit the performance of other tests. If one performs tests in addition to those specifically indicated for a particular panel, those tests should be reported separately in addition to the panel code.

Do not report two or more panel codes that include any of the same constituent tests performed from the same patient collection. If a group of tests overlaps two or more panels, report the panel that incorporates the greater number of tests to fulfill the code definition and report the remaining tests using individual test codes (eg, do not report 80047 in conjunction with 80053)

80047 Basic metabolic panel (Calcium, ionized)

This panel must include the following:

Calcium, ionized (82330)

Carbon dioxide (bicarbonate) (82374)

Chloride (82435)

Creatinine (82565)

Glucose (82947)

Potassium (84132)

Sodium (84295)

Urea Nitrogen (BUN) (84520)

➔ *CPT Assistant* Apr 08:5; *CPT Changes: An Insider's View* 2008

80048 Basic metabolic panel (Calcium, total)

This panel must include the following:

Calcium, total (82310)

Carbon dioxide (bicarbonate) (82374)

Chloride (82435)

Creatinine (82565)

Glucose (82947)

Potassium (84132)

Sodium (84295)

Urea nitrogen (BUN) (84520)

➔ *CPT Assistant* Jan 98:6, Sep 99:11, Nov 99:44, Jan 00:7, Aug 05:9; *CPT Changes: An Insider's View* 2000, 2008, 2009

80050 General health panel

This panel must include the following:

Comprehensive metabolic panel (80053)

Blood count, complete (CBC), automated and automated differential WBC count (85025 or 85027 and 85004)

OR

Blood count, complete (CBC), automated (85027) and appropriate manual differential WBC count (85007 or 85009)

Thyroid stimulating hormone (TSH) (84443)

➔ *CPT Assistant* Winter 92:14, Summer 93:14, Jun 97:10, Nov 97:28, Jan 98:6, Sep 99:11; *CPT Changes: An Insider's View* 2001, 2004

80051 Electrolyte panel

This panel must include the following:

Carbon dioxide (bicarbonate) (82374)

Chloride (82435)

Potassium (84132)

Sodium (84295)

➔ *CPT Assistant* Nov 97:28, Jan 98:7, Sep 99:11

80053 Comprehensive metabolic panel

This panel must include the following:

Albumin (82040)

Bilirubin, total (82247)

Calcium, total (82310)

Carbon dioxide (bicarbonate) (82374)

Chloride (82435)

Creatinine (82565)

Glucose (82947)

Phosphatase, alkaline (84075)

Potassium (84132)

Protein, total (84155)

Sodium (84295)

Transferase, alanine amino (ALT) (SGPT) (84460)

Transferase, aspartate amino (AST) (SGOT) (84450)

Urea nitrogen (BUN) (84520)

➔ *CPT Assistant* Jan 98:6, Nov 98:23, Sep 99:11, Nov 99:44, May 00:11, Jan 05:46, Apr 08:5, Apr 10:11; *CPT Changes: An Insider's View* 2000, 2009

80055   Obstetric panel

This panel must include the following:

Blood count, complete (CBC), automated and automated differential WBC count (85025 or 85027 and 85004)

OR

Blood count, complete (CBC), automated (85027) and appropriate manual differential WBC count (85007 or 85009)

Hepatitis B surface antigen (HBsAg) (87340)

Antibody, rubella (86762)

Syphilis test, non-treponemal antibody; qualitative (eg, VDRL, RPR, ART) (86592)

Antibody screen, RBC, each serum technique (86850)

Blood typing, ABO (86900) AND

Blood typing, Rh (D) (86901)

➔ *CPT Assistant* Winter 92:14, Summer 93:14, Jun 97:10, Apr 99:6, Sep 99:11; *CPT Changes: An Insider's View* 2004

(When syphilis screening is performed using a treponemal antibody approach [86780], do not use 80055. Use the individual codes for the tests performed in the obstetric panel)

80061   Lipid panel

This panel must include the following:

Cholesterol, serum, total (82465)

Lipoprotein, direct measurement, high density cholesterol (HDL cholesterol) (83718)

Triglycerides (84478)

➔ *CPT Assistant* Winter 92:14, Summer 93:14, Jun 97:10, Sep 99:11, Mar 00:11, Feb 05:9

80069   Renal function panel

This panel must include the following:

Albumin (82040)

Calcium, total (82310)

Carbon dioxide (bicarbonate) (82374)

Chloride (82435)

Creatinine (82565)

Glucose (82947)

Phosphorus inorganic (phosphate) (84100)

Potassium (84132)

Sodium (84295)

Urea nitrogen (BUN) (84520)

➔ *CPT Assistant* Sep 99:11, Nov 99:44; *CPT Changes: An Insider's View* 2000, 2009

80074   Acute hepatitis panel

This panel must include the following:

Hepatitis A antibody (HAAb), IgM antibody (86709)

Hepatitis B core antibody (HBcAb), IgM antibody (86705)

Hepatitis B surface antigen (HBsAg) (87340)

Hepatitis C antibody (86803)

➔ *CPT Assistant* Sep 99:11, Nov 99:45; *CPT Changes: An Insider's View* 2000

80076   Hepatic function panel

This panel must include the following:

Albumin (82040)

Bilirubin, total (82247)

Bilirubin, direct (82248)

Phosphatase, alkaline (84075)

Protein, total (84155)

Transferase, alanine amino (ALT) (SGPT) (84460)

Transferase, aspartate amino (AST) (SGOT) (84450)

➔ *CPT Assistant* Winter 92:14, Summer 93:14, Jun 97:10, Jan 98:6, Apr 99:6, Sep 99:11, Nov 99:45, Jan 00:7, Aug 05:9; *CPT Changes: An Insider's View* 2000

Drug Testing

The following list contains examples of drugs or classes of drugs that are commonly assayed by qualitative screen, followed by confirmation with a second method:

- Alcohols
- Amphetamines
- Barbiturates
- Benzodiazepines
- Cocaine and metabolites
- Methadones
- Methaqualones
- Opiates
- Phencyclidines
- Phenothiazines
- Propoxyphenes
- Tetrahydrocannabinoids
- Tricyclic antidepressants

Confirmed drugs may also be quantitated.

Use 80100 for each multiple drug class chromatographic procedure. Use 80102 for each procedure necessary for confirmation. For chromatography, each combination of stationary and mobile phase is to be counted as one procedure. For example, if detection of three drugs by chromatography requires one stationary phase with three mobile phases, use 80100 three times. However, if multiple drugs can be detected using a single analysis (eg, one stationary phase with one mobile phase), use 80100 only once.

For quantitation of drugs screened, use appropriate code in **Chemistry** section (82000-84999) or **Therapeutic Drug Assay** section (80150-80299).

80100 Drug screen, qualitative; multiple drug classes chromatographic method, each procedure

➔ *CPT Assistant* Fall 93:26, Mar 00:2, Aug 05:9, Oct 10:7, Dec 10:7; *CPT Changes: An Insider's View* 2001

80101 single drug class method (eg, immunoassay, enzyme assay), each drug class

➔ *CPT Assistant* Fall 93:26, Mar 00:2, Nov 06:22, Oct 10:7, Dec 10:7; *CPT Changes: An Insider's View* 2001

(For qualitative analysis by multiplexed screening kit for multiple drugs or drug classes, use 80104)

 # 80104 multiple drug classes other than chromatographic method, each procedure

➔ *CPT Assistant* Oct 10:7, Dec 10:3; *CPT Changes: An Insider's View* 2011

80102 Drug confirmation, each procedure

➔ *CPT Assistant* Fall 93:26, Mar 00:2; *CPT Changes: An Insider's View* 2001

80103 Tissue preparation for drug analysis

➔ *CPT Assistant* Aug 05:9

80104 Code is out of numerical sequence. See 80100-80103

Therapeutic Drug Assays

The material for examination may be from any source. Examination is quantitative. For nonquantitative testing, see Drug Testing (80100-80104).

80150 Amikacin

➔ *CPT Assistant* Aug 05:9, Oct 10:7, Dec 10:7, Mar 11:10

80152 Amitriptyline

➔ *CPT Assistant* Oct 10:7, Mar 11:10

80154 Benzodiazepines

➔ *CPT Assistant* Oct 10:7, Mar 11:10

80156 Carbamazepine; total

➔ *CPT Assistant* Oct 10:7, Mar 11:10; *CPT Changes: An Insider's View* 2001

80157 free

➔ *CPT Assistant* Oct 10:7, Mar 11:10; *CPT Changes: An Insider's View* 2001

80158 Cyclosporine

➔ *CPT Assistant* Oct 10:7, Mar 11:10

80160 Desipramine

➔ *CPT Assistant* Oct 10:7, Mar 11:10

80162 Digoxin

➔ *CPT Assistant* Oct 10:7, Mar 11:10

80164 Dipropylacetic acid (valproic acid)

➔ *CPT Assistant* Oct 10:7, Mar 11:10

80166 Doxepin

➔ *CPT Assistant* Oct 10:7, Mar 11:10

80168 Ethosuximide

➔ *CPT Assistant* Oct 10:7, Mar 11:10

80170 Gentamicin

➔ *CPT Assistant* Oct 10:7, Mar 11:10

80172 Gold

➔ *CPT Assistant* Oct 10:7, Mar 11:10

80173 Haloperidol

➔ *CPT Assistant* Oct 10:7, Mar 11:10; *CPT Changes: An Insider's View* 2001

80174 Imipramine

➔ *CPT Assistant* Oct 10:7, Mar 11:10

80176 Lidocaine

➔ *CPT Assistant* Oct 10:7, Mar 11:10

80178 Lithium

➔ *CPT Assistant* Oct 10:7, Mar 11:10

80182 Nortriptyline

➔ *CPT Assistant* Oct 10:7, Mar 11:10

80184 Phenobarbital

➔ *CPT Assistant* Oct 10:7, Mar 11:10

80185 Phenytoin; total

➔ *CPT Assistant* Oct 10:7, Mar 11:10

80186 free

➔ *CPT Assistant* Oct 10:7, Mar 11:10

80188 Primidone

➔ *CPT Assistant* Oct 10:7, Mar 11:10

80190 Procainamide;

➔ *CPT Assistant* Oct 10:7, Mar 11:10

80192 with metabolites (eg, n-acetyl procainamide)

➔ *CPT Assistant* Oct 10:7, Mar 11:10

80194 Quinidine

➔ *CPT Assistant* Oct 10:7, Mar 11:10

80195 Sirolimus

➔ *CPT Assistant* Mar 06:6, Oct 10:7, Mar 11:10; *CPT Changes: An Insider's View* 2006

80196 Salicylate

➔ *CPT Assistant* Oct 10:7, Mar 11:10

80197 Tacrolimus

➔ *CPT Assistant* Oct 10:7, Mar 11:10

80198 Theophylline

➔ *CPT Assistant* Oct 10:7, Mar 11:10

80200 Tobramycin

➔ *CPT Assistant* Oct 10:7, Mar 11:10

80201 Topiramate

➔ *CPT Assistant* Nov 97:28, Oct 10:7, Mar 11:10

80202   Vancomycin

→ *CPT Assistant* Oct 10:7, Mar 11:10

80299   Quantitation of drug, not elsewhere specified

→ *CPT Assistant* Mar 00:3, Oct 04:14, Aug 05:9, Oct 10:7, Dec 10:3, Mar 11:10

Evocative/Suppression Testing

►The following test panels involve the administration of evocative or suppressive agents and the baseline and subsequent measurement of their effects on chemical constituents. These codes are to be used for the reporting of the laboratory component of the overall testing protocol. For the administration of the evocative or suppressive agents, see Hydration, Therapeutic, Prophylactic, Diagnostic Injections and Infusions, and Chemotherapy and Other Highly Complex Drug or Highly Complex Biologic Agent Administration (eg, 96365, 96366, 96367, 96368, 96372, 96374, 96375, 96376). In the code descriptors where reference is made to a particular analyte (eg, Cortisol: 82533 x 2) the "x 2" refers to the number of times the test for that particular analyte is performed.◄

80400   ACTH stimulation panel; for adrenal insufficiency

This panel must include the following:

Cortisol (82533 x 2)

→ *CPT Assistant* Summer 94:1, Fall 94:10, Aug 05:9

80402   for 21 hydroxylase deficiency

This panel must include the following:

Cortisol (82533 x 2)

17 hydroxyprogesterone (83498 x 2)

→ *CPT Assistant* Summer 94:1, Fall 94:10

80406   for 3 beta-hydroxydehydrogenase deficiency

This panel must include the following:

Cortisol (82533 x 2)

17 hydroxypregnenolone (84143 x 2)

→ *CPT Assistant* Summer 94:1, Fall 94:10

80408   Aldosterone suppression evaluation panel (eg, saline infusion)

This panel must include the following:

Aldosterone (82088 x 2)

Renin (84244 x 2)

→ *CPT Assistant* Summer 94:1, Fall 94:10

80410   Calcitonin stimulation panel (eg, calcium, pentagastrin)

This panel must include the following:

Calcitonin (82308 x 3)

→ *CPT Assistant* Summer 94:1, Fall 94:11

80412   Corticotropic releasing hormone (CRH) stimulation panel

This panel must include the following:

Cortisol (82533 x 6)

Adrenocorticotropic hormone (ACTH) (82024 x 6)

→ *CPT Assistant* Summer 94:1, Fall 94:11

80414   Chorionic gonadotropin stimulation panel; testosterone response

This panel must include the following:

Testosterone (84403 x 2 on 3 pooled blood samples)

→ *CPT Assistant* Summer 94:1, Fall 94:11; *CPT Changes: An Insider's View* 2009

80415   estradiol response

This panel must include the following:

Estradiol (82670 x 2 on 3 pooled blood samples)

→ *CPT Assistant* Summer 94:1, Fall 94:11; *CPT Changes: An Insider's View* 2009

80416   Renal vein renin stimulation panel (eg, captopril)

This panel must include the following:

Renin (84244 x 6)

→ *CPT Assistant* Summer 94:1

80417   Peripheral vein renin stimulation panel (eg, captopril)

This panel must include the following:

Renin (84244 x 2)

80418   Combined rapid anterior pituitary evaluation panel

This panel must include the following:

Adrenocorticotropic hormone (ACTH) (82024 x 4)

Luteinizing hormone (LH) (83002 x 4)

Follicle stimulating hormone (FSH) (83001 x 4)

Prolactin (84146 x 4)

Human growth hormone (HGH) (83003 x 4)

Cortisol (82533 x 4)

Thyroid stimulating hormone (TSH) (84443 x 4)

→ *CPT Assistant* Summer 94:1, Fall 94:13

80420   Dexamethasone suppression panel, 48 hour

This panel must include the following:

Free cortisol, urine (82530 x 2)

Cortisol (82533 x 2)

Volume measurement for timed collection (81050 x 2)

→ *CPT Assistant* Fall 94:13

(For single dose dexamethasone, use 82533)

80422   Glucagon tolerance panel; for insulinoma

This panel must include the following:

Glucose (82947 x 3)

Insulin (83525 x 3)

→ *CPT Assistant* Summer 94:1, Fall 94:13

▲=Revised code   ●=New code   ►◄=Contains new or revised text   ⊘=Modifier 51 exempt

80424   for pheochromocytoma

This panel must include the following:

Catecholamines, fractionated (82384 x 2)
➔ *CPT Assistant* Summer 94:1, Fall 94:14

80426   Gonadotropin releasing hormone stimulation panel

This panel must include the following:

Follicle stimulating hormone (FSH) (83001 x 4)

Luteinizing hormone (LH) (83002 x 4)
➔ *CPT Assistant* Summer 94:1, Fall 94:14

80428   Growth hormone stimulation panel (eg, arginine infusion, l-dopa administration)

This panel must include the following:

Human growth hormone (HGH) (83003 x 4)
➔ *CPT Assistant* Summer 94:1, Fall 94:14

80430   Growth hormone suppression panel (glucose administration)

This panel must include the following:

Glucose (82947 x 3)

Human growth hormone (HGH) (83003 x 4)
➔ *CPT Assistant* Summer 94:1, Fall 94:14

80432   Insulin-induced C-peptide suppression panel

This panel must include the following:

Insulin (83525)

C-peptide (84681 x 5)

Glucose (82947 x 5)
➔ *CPT Assistant* Summer 94:1, Fall 94:15

80434   Insulin tolerance panel; for ACTH insufficiency

This panel must include the following:

Cortisol (82533 x 5)

Glucose (82947 x 5)
➔ *CPT Assistant* Summer 94:1, Fall 94:15

80435   for growth hormone deficiency

This panel must include the following:

Glucose (82947 x 5)

Human growth hormone (HGH) (83003 x 5)
➔ *CPT Assistant* Summer 94:1, Fall 94:15

80436   Metyrapone panel

This panel must include the following:

Cortisol (82533 x 2)

11 deoxycortisol (82634 x 2)
➔ *CPT Assistant* Summer 94:1, Fall 94:16

80438   Thyrotropin releasing hormone (TRH) stimulation panel; 1 hour

This panel must include the following:

Thyroid stimulating hormone (TSH) (84443 x 3)
➔ *CPT Assistant* Summer 94:1, Fall 94:16

80439   2 hour

This panel must include the following:

Thyroid stimulating hormone (TSH) (84443 x 4)
➔ *CPT Assistant* Summer 94:1, Fall 94:16

80440   for hyperprolactinemia

This panel must include the following:

Prolactin (84146 x 3)
➔ *CPT Assistant* Summer 94:1, Fall 94:16, Aug 05:9

Consultations (Clinical Pathology)

▶A clinical pathology consultation is a service, including a written report, rendered by the pathologist in response to a request from a physician or qualified health care professional in relation to a test result(s) requiring additional medical interpretive judgment.◀

Reporting of a test result(s) without medical interpretive judgment is not considered a clinical pathology consultation.

80500   Clinical pathology consultation; limited, without review of patient's history and medical records
➔ *CPT Assistant* Apr 97:9, Nov 02:9, Aug 05:9

80502   comprehensive, for a complex diagnostic problem, with review of patient's history and medical records
➔ *CPT Assistant* Apr 97:9, Nov 02:9, Aug 05:9

(These codes may also be used for pharmacokinetic consultations)

(For consultations involving the examination and evaluation of the patient, see 99241-99255)

Urinalysis

For specific analyses, see appropriate section.

81000   Urinalysis, by dip stick or tablet reagent for bilirubin, glucose, hemoglobin, ketones, leukocytes, nitrite, pH, protein, specific gravity, urobilinogen, any number of these constituents; non-automated, with microscopy
➔ *CPT Assistant* Winter 91:10, Fall 93:25, Aug 05:9

81001   automated, with microscopy

81002   non-automated, without microscopy
➔ *CPT Assistant* Mar 98:3, Apr 07:1

81003   automated, without microscopy
➔ *CPT Assistant* Apr 07:1

81005   Urinalysis; qualitative or semiquantitative, except immunoassays
➔ *CPT Assistant* Winter 91:10, Fall 93:25

(For non-immunoassay reagent strip urinalysis, see 81000, 81002)

(For immunoassay, qualitative or semiquantitative, use 83518)

(For microalbumin, see 82043, 82044)

81007   bacteriuria screen, except by culture or dipstick
⮕ *CPT Changes: An Insider's View* 2001

(For culture, see 87086-87088)

(For dipstick, use 81000 or 81002)

81015   microscopic only

(For sperm evaluation for retrograde ejaculation, use 89331)

81020   2 or 3 glass test
⮕ *CPT Assistant* Winter 91:10

81025   Urine pregnancy test, by visual color comparison methods
⮕ *CPT Assistant* Mar 98:3

81050   Volume measurement for timed collection, each

81099   Unlisted urinalysis procedure
⮕ *CPT Assistant* Aug 05:9

Molecular Pathology

Molecular pathology procedures are medical laboratory procedures involving the analyses of nucleic acid to detect variants in genes that may be indicative of germline (eg, constitutional disorders) or somatic (eg, neoplasia) conditions, or to test for histocompatibility antigens (eg, HLA). Code selection is typically based on the specific gene(s) that is being analyzed. Genes are described using Human Genome Organization (HUGO) approved gene names and are italicized in the code descriptors. Gene names were taken from tables of the HUGO Gene Nomenclature Commmittee (HGNC) at the time the CPT codes were developed. For the most part, Human Genome Variation Society (HGVS) recommendations were followed for the names of specific molecular variants. The familiar name is used for some variants because defined criteria were not in place when the variant was first described or because HGVS recommendations were changed over time (eg, intronic variants, processed proteins). When the gene name is represented by an abbreviation, the abbreviation is listed first, followed by the full gene name italicized in parentheses (eg, "F5 *[coagulation Factor V]*"), except for the HLA series of codes. Proteins or diseases commonly associated with the genes are listed as examples in the code descriptors. The examples do not represent all conditions in which testing of the gene may be indicated.

Codes that describe tests to assess for the presence of gene variants (see definitions) use common gene variant names. Typically, all of the listed variants would be tested. However, these lists are not exclusive. If other variants are also tested in the analysis, they would be included in the procedure and not reported separately. Full gene sequencing should not be reported using codes that assess for the presence of gene variants unless specifically stated in the code descriptor.

The molecular pathology codes include all analytical services performed in the test (eg, cell lysis, nucleic acid stabilization, extraction, digestion, amplification, and detection). Any procedures required prior to cell lysis (eg, microdissection, codes 88380 and 88381) should be reported separately.

The results of the procedure may require interpretation by a physician or other qualified health care professional. When only the interpretation and report are performed, modifier 26 may be appended to the specific molecular pathology code.

All analyses are qualitative unless otherwise noted.

For microbial identification, see 87149-87153 and 87470-87801, and 87900-87904. For in situ hybridization analyses, see 88271-88275 and 88365-88368.

▶Molecular pathology procedures that are not specified in 81200-81383 should be reported using either the appropriate Tier 2 code (81400-81408) or the unlisted molecular pathology procedure code, 81479.◀

Definitions

For purposes of CPT reporting, the following definitions apply:

Abnormal allele: an alternative form of a gene that contains a disease-related variation from the normal sequence.

Breakpoint: the region at which a chromosome breaks during a translocation (defined elsewhere). These regions are often consistent for a given translocation.

Codon: a discrete unit of three nucleotides of a DNA or mRNA sequence that encodes a specific amino acid within, or signals the termination of, a polypeptide.

Common variants: variants (as defined elsewhere) that are associated with compromised gene function and are interrogated in a single round of laboratory testing (in a single, typically multiplex, assay format or using more than one assay to encompass all variants to be tested). These variants typically fit the definition of a "mutation," and are usually the predominant ones causing disease. Testing for additional uncommon variants may provide additional limited value in assessment of a patient. Often there are professional society recommendations or guidelines for which variants are most appropriate to test (eg, American College of Medical Genetics/American College of Obstetrics and Gynecology guidelines for variants used in population screening for cystic fibrosis).

Constitutional: synonymous with germline, often used in reference to the genetic code that is present at birth.

Cytogenomic: chromosome analysis using molecular techniques.

Duplication/Deletion (Dup/Del): terms that are usually used together with the "/" to refer to molecular testing, which assesses the dosage of a particular genomic region. The region tested is typically of modest to substantial size - from several dozen to several million or more nucleotides. Normal gene dosage is two copies per cell, except for the sex chromosomes (X and Y). Thus, zero or one copy represents a deletion, and three (or more) copies represent a duplication.

Dynamic mutation: polynucleotide (eg, trinucleotide) repeats that are in or associated with genes that can undergo disease-producing increases or decreases in the numbers of repeats within tissues and across generations.

Exon: typically, one of multiple nucleic acid sequences used to encode information for a gene product (polypeptide or protein). Exons are separated from each other by non-protein-coding sequences known as introns. Exons at the respective ends of a gene also contain nucleic acid sequence that does not code for the gene's protein product.

Gene: a nucleic acid sequence that typically contains information for coding a protein as well as for the regulated expression of that protein. Human genes usually contain multiple protein coding regions (exons) separated by non-protein coding regions (introns). See also *exon*, *intron*, and *polypeptide*.

Intron: a nucleic acid sequence found between exons in human genes. An intron contains essential sequences for its proper removal (by a process known as *splicing*) to join exons together and thus facilitate production of a functional protein from a gene. An intron is sometimes referred to as an intervening sequence (IVS).

▶**Inversion:** A defect in a chromosome in which a segment breaks and reinserts in the same place but in the opposite orientation.

Loss of heterozygosity (LOH, allelic imbalance): An event that can occur in dividing cells that are heterozygous for one or more alleles, in which a daughter cell becomes hemizygous or homozygous, for the allele(s) through mitotic recombination, deletion, or other chromosomal event.◀

Microarray: surface(s) on which multiple specific nucleic acid sequences are attached in a known arrangement. Sometimes referred to as a 'gene chip'. Examples of uses of microarrays include evaluation of a patient specimen for gains or losses of DNA sequences (copy number variants, CNVs), identification of the presence of specific nucleotide sequence variants (also known as single nucleotide polymorphisms, SNPs), mRNA expression levels, or DNA sequence analysis.

Mutations: typically are variants associated with altered gene function that lead to functional deficits or disease (pathogenic).

Mutation scanning: a technique (eg, single strand conformation polymorphism, temperature gradient gel electrophoresis, etc.) typically employed on multiple PCR amplicons to indicate the presence of DNA sequence variants by differences in physical properties compared to normal. Variants are then further characterized by DNA sequence analysis only in amplicons which demonstrate differences.

Polymorphisms: typically are variants that do not compromise gene function or produce disease (benign).

Polypeptide: a sequence of amino acids covalently linked in a specified order. Polypeptides alone or in combination with other polypeptide subunits are the building blocks of proteins.

Short Tandem Repeat (STR): a region of DNA where a pattern of two or more nucleotides are repeated. The number of repeating segments can be used as genetic markers for human identity testing.

Single-nucleotide polymorphism (SNP): a DNA sequence variation existing at a significant frequency in the population, in which a single nucleotide (A, T, C, or G) differs between individuals and/or within an individual's paired chromosomes,

Somatic: synonymous with acquired, referring to genetic code alterations that develop after birth (eg, occurring in neoplastic cells)

Translocation: an abnormality resulting from the breakage of a chromosome and the relocation of a portion of that chromosome's DNA sequence to the same or another chromosome. Most common translocations involve a reciprocal exchange of DNA sequences between two differently numbered (ie, non-homologous) chromosomes, with or without a clinically significant loss of DNA.

▶**Uniparental disomy (UPD):** Abnormal inheritance of both members of a chromosome pair from one parent, with absence of the other parent's chromosome for the pair.◀

Variant: a nucleotide sequence difference from the "normal" (predominant) sequence for a given region. Variants are typically of two types: substitutions of one nucleotide for another, and deletions or insertions of nucleotides. Occasionally, variants reflect several nucleotide sequence changes in reasonably close proximity on the same chromosomal strand of DNA (a haplotype). These nucleotide sequence variants often result in amino acid changes in the protein made by the gene. The term *variant* does not itself carry a functional implication for those protein changes.

Variants in introns are typically described in one of two ways. The altered nucleotide(s) within a defined intervening sequence (eg, IVS3-2A>G) of a gene is listed with a "+" or "-" sign, which indicates the position relative to the first or last nucleotide of the intron. Or, the variant position is indicated relative to the last nucleotide of the preceding exon or first nucleotide of the following exon (eg, c.171+1G>A c.172-1G>T are single nucleotide changes at the first and last nucleotide of a given intron for a specific gene).

The majority of the variants described here are listed by the amino acid change using the single letter amino acid code for the original amino acid followed by the numerical position in the protein product and the amino acid substitution, eg, for *ASPA* E285A, Glutamic acid (E) at position 285 is replaced with an alanine (A). A few of the variants are described by the DNA change using the numerical position followed by the original nucleotide, a greater than sign (>) and the new nucleotide, eg, *MTHFR.* 677C>T.

A known familial variant is a specific mutation that has previously been identified within a patient's family.

Tier 1 Molecular Pathology Procedures

The following codes represent gene-specific and genomic procedures:

81200   *ASPA (aspartoacylase)* (eg, Canavan disease) gene analysis, common variants (eg, E285A, Y231X)
> *CPT Assistant* May 12:4; *CPT Changes: An Insider's View* 2012

● **81201**   APC (adenomatous polyposis coli) (eg, familial adenomatosis polyposis [FAP], attenuated FAP) gene analysis; full gene sequence
> *CPT Assistant* May 12:4; *CPT Changes: An Insider's View* 2013

● **81202**   known familial variants
> *CPT Assistant* May 12:4; *CPT Changes: An Insider's View* 2013

● **81203**   duplication/deletion variants
> *CPT Assistant* May 12:4; *CPT Changes: An Insider's View* 2013

81205   *BCKDHB (branched-chain keto acid dehydrogenase E1, beta polypeptide)* (eg, Maple syrup urine disease) gene analysis, common variants (eg, R183P, G278S, E422X)
> *CPT Assistant* May 12:4; *CPT Changes: An Insider's View* 2012

81206   *BCR/ABL1 (t(9;22))* (eg, chronic myelogenous leukemia) translocation analysis; major breakpoint, qualitative or quantitative
> *CPT Assistant* May 12:4; *CPT Changes: An Insider's View* 2012

81207   minor breakpoint, qualitative or quantitative
> *CPT Assistant* May 12:4; *CPT Changes: An Insider's View* 2012

81208   other breakpoint, qualitative or quantitative
> *CPT Assistant* May 12:4; *CPT Changes: An Insider's View* 2012

81209   *BLM (Bloom syndrome, RecQ helicase-like)* (eg, Bloom syndrome) gene analysis, 2281del6ins7 variant
> *CPT Assistant* May 12:4; *CPT Changes: An Insider's View* 2012

81210   *BRAF (v-raf murine sarcoma viral oncogene homolog B1)* (eg, colon cancer), gene analysis, V600E variant
> *CPT Assistant* May 12:4; *CPT Changes: An Insider's View* 2012

81211   *BRCA1, BRCA2 (breast cancer 1 and 2)* (eg, hereditary breast and ovarian cancer) gene analysis; full sequence analysis and common duplication/deletion variants in BRCA1 (ie, exon 13 del 3.835kb, exon 13 dup 6kb, exon 14-20 del 26kb, exon 22 del 510bp, exon 8-9 del 7.1kb)
> *CPT Assistant* May 12:4; *CPT Changes: An Insider's View* 2012

81212   185delAG, 5385insC, 6174delT variants
> *CPT Assistant* May 12:4; *CPT Changes: An Insider's View* 2012

81213   uncommon duplication/deletion variants
> *CPT Assistant* May 12:4; *CPT Changes: An Insider's View* 2012

81214   *BRCA1 (breast cancer 1)* (eg, hereditary breast and ovarian cancer) gene analysis; full sequence analysis and common duplication/deletion variants (ie, exon 13 del 3.835kb, exon 13 dup 6kb, exon 14-20 del 26kb, exon 22 del 510bp, exon 8-9 del 7.1kb)
> *CPT Assistant* May 12:4; *CPT Changes: An Insider's View* 2012

(When performing *BRCA1* full sequence analysis with *BRCA2* full sequence analysis, use 81211)

81215   known familial variant
> *CPT Assistant* May 12:4; *CPT Changes: An Insider's View* 2012

81216   *BRCA2 (breast cancer 2)* (eg, hereditary breast and ovarian cancer) gene analysis; full sequence analysis
> *CPT Assistant* May 12:4; *CPT Changes: An Insider's View* 2012

(When performing *BRCA2* full sequence analysis with *BRCA1* full sequence analysis, use 81211)

81217   known familial variant
> *CPT Assistant* May 12:4; *CPT Changes: An Insider's View* 2012

81220   *CFTR (cystic fibrosis transmembrane conductance regulator)* (eg, cystic fibrosis) gene analysis; common variants (eg, ACMG/ACOG guidelines)
> *CPT Assistant* May 12:4; *CPT Changes: An Insider's View* 2012

(When Intron 8 poly-T analysis is performed in conjunction with 81220 in a R117H positive patient, do not report 81224)

81221   known familial variants
> *CPT Assistant* May 12:4; *CPT Changes: An Insider's View* 2012

81222   duplication/deletion variants
> *CPT Assistant* May 12:4; *CPT Changes: An Insider's View* 2012

81223   full gene sequence
> *CPT Assistant* May 12:4; *CPT Changes: An Insider's View* 2012

81224   intron 8 poly-T analysis (eg, male infertility)
> *CPT Assistant* May 12:4; *CPT Changes: An Insider's View* 2012

81225   *CYP2C19 (cytochrome P450, family 2, subfamily C, polypeptide 19)* (eg, drug metabolism), gene analysis, common variants (eg, *2, *3, *4, *8, *17)
> *CPT Assistant* May 12:4; *CPT Changes: An Insider's View* 2012

81226   *CYP2D6 (cytochrome P450, family 2, subfamily D, polypeptide 6)* (eg, drug metabolism), gene analysis, common variants (eg, *2, *3, *4, *5, *6, *9, *10, *17, *19, *29, *35, *41, *1XN, *2XN, *4XN)

➔ *CPT Assistant* May 12:4; *CPT Changes: An Insider's View* 2012

81227   *CYP2C9 (cytochrome P450, family 2, subfamily C, polypeptide 9)* (eg, drug metabolism), gene analysis, common variants (eg, *2, *3, *5, *6)

➔ *CPT Assistant* May 12:4; *CPT Changes: An Insider's View* 2012

81228   Cytogenomic constitutional (genome-wide) microarray analysis; interrogation of genomic regions for copy number variants (eg, Bacterial Artificial Chromosome [BAC] or oligo-based comparative genomic hybridization [CGH] microarray analysis)

➔ *CPT Assistant* May 12:4; *CPT Changes: An Insider's View* 2012

81229   interrogation of genomic regions for copy number and single nucleotide polymorphism (SNP) variants for chromosomal abnormalities

➔ *CPT Assistant* May 12:4; *CPT Changes: An Insider's View* 2012

(Do not report 81228 in conjunction with 81229)

● **81235**   *EGFR (epidermal growth factor receptor)* (eg, non-small cell lung cancer) gene analysis, common variants (eg, exon 19 LREA deletion, L858R, T790M, G719A, G719S, L861Q)

➔ *CPT Changes: An Insider's View* 2013

81240   *F2 (prothrombin, coagulation factor II)* (eg, hereditary hypercoagulability) gene analysis, 20210G>A variant

➔ *CPT Assistant* May 12:4; *CPT Changes: An Insider's View* 2012

81241   *F5 (coagulation Factor V)* (eg, hereditary hypercoagulability) gene analysis, Leiden variant

➔ *CPT Assistant* May 12:4; *CPT Changes: An Insider's View* 2012

81242   *FANCC (Fanconi anemia, complementation group C)* (eg, Fanconi anemia, type C) gene analysis, common variant (eg, IVS4+4A>T)

➔ *CPT Assistant* May 12:4; *CPT Changes: An Insider's View* 2012

81243   *FMR1 (Fragile X mental retardation 1)* (eg, fragile X mental retardation) gene analysis; evaluation to detect abnormal (eg, expanded) alleles

➔ *CPT Assistant* May 12:4; *CPT Changes: An Insider's View* 2012

(For evaluation to detect and characterize abnormal alleles, see 81243, 81244)

(For evaluation to detect and characterize abnormal alleles using a single assay [eg, PCR], use 81243)

81244   characterization of alleles (eg, expanded size and methylation status)

➔ *CPT Assistant* May 12:4; *CPT Changes: An Insider's View* 2012

81245   *FLT3 (fms-related tyrosine kinase 3)* (eg, acute myeloid leukemia), gene analysis, internal tandem duplication (ITD) variants (ie, exons 14, 15)

➔ *CPT Assistant* May 12:4; *CPT Changes: An Insider's View* 2012

81250   *G6PC (glucose-6-phosphatase, catalytic subunit)* (eg, Glycogen storage disease, Type 1a, von Gierke disease) gene analysis, common variants (eg, R83C, Q347X)

➔ *CPT Assistant* May 12:4; *CPT Changes: An Insider's View* 2012

81251   *GBA (glucosidase, beta, acid)* (eg, Gaucher disease) gene analysis, common variants (eg, N370S, 84GG, L444P, IVS2+1G>A)

➔ *CPT Assistant* May 12:4; *CPT Changes: An Insider's View* 2012

● **81252**   *GJB2 (gap junction protein, beta 2, 26kDa; connexin 26)* (eg, nonsyndromic hearing loss) gene analysis; full gene sequence

➔ *CPT Changes: An Insider's View* 2013

● **81253**   known familial variants

➔ *CPT Changes: An Insider's View* 2013

● **81254**   *GJB6 (gap junction protein, beta 6, 30kDa, connexin 30)* (eg, nonsyndromic hearing loss) gene analysis, common variants (eg, 309kb [del(GJB6-D13S1830)] and 232kb [del(GJB6-D13S1854)])

➔ *CPT Changes: An Insider's View* 2013

81255   *HEXA (hexosaminidase A [alpha polypeptide])* (eg, Tay-Sachs disease) gene analysis, common variants (eg, 1278insTATC, 1421+1G>C, G269S)

➔ *CPT Assistant* May 12:4; *CPT Changes: An Insider's View* 2012

81256   *HFE (hemochromatosis)* (eg, hereditary hemochromatosis) gene analysis, common variants (eg, C282Y, H63D)

➔ *CPT Assistant* May 12:4; *CPT Changes: An Insider's View* 2012

81257   *HBA1/HBA2 (alpha globin 1 and alpha globin 2)* (eg, alpha thalassemia, Hb Bart hydrops fetalis syndrome, HbH disease), gene analysis, for common deletions or variant (eg, Southeast Asian, Thai, Filipino, Mediterranean, alpha3.7, alpha4.2, alpha20.5, and Constant Spring)

➔ *CPT Assistant* May 12:4; *CPT Changes: An Insider's View* 2012

81260   *IKBKAP (inhibitor of kappa light polypeptide gene enhancer in B-cells, kinase complex-associated protein)* (eg, familial dysautonomia) gene analysis, common variants (eg, 2507+6T>C, R696P)

➔ *CPT Assistant* May 12:4; *CPT Changes: An Insider's View* 2012

81261   *IGH@ (Immunoglobulin heavy chain locus)* (eg, leukemias and lymphomas, B-cell), gene rearrangement analysis to detect abnormal clonal population(s); amplified methodology (eg, polymerase chain reaction)

➔ *CPT Assistant* May 12:4; *CPT Changes: An Insider's View* 2012

81262   direct probe methodology (eg, Southern blot)

➔ *CPT Assistant* May 12:4; *CPT Changes: An Insider's View* 2012

81263   *IGH@ (Immunoglobulin heavy chain locus)* (eg, leukemia and lymphoma, B-cell), variable region somatic mutation analysis

➔ *CPT Assistant* May 12:4; *CPT Changes: An Insider's View* 2012

81264   *IGK@ (Immunoglobulin kappa light chain locus)* (eg, leukemia and lymphoma, B-cell), gene rearrangement analysis, evaluation to detect abnormal clonal population(s)

➔ *CPT Assistant* May 12:4; *CPT Changes: An Insider's View* 2012

▶(For immunoglobulin lambda gene *[IGL@]* rearrangement or immunoglobulin kappa deleting element, *[IGKDEL]* analysis, use 81479)◀

81265   Comparative analysis using Short Tandem Repeat (STR) markers; patient and comparative specimen (eg, pre-transplant recipient and donor germline testing, post-transplant non-hematopoietic recipient germline [eg, buccal swab or other germline tissue sample] and donor testing, twin zygosity testing, or maternal cell contamination of fetal cells)
➡ *CPT Assistant* May 12:4; *CPT Changes: An Insider's View* 2012

+ 81266   each additional specimen (eg, additional cord blood donor, additional fetal samples from different cultures, or additional zygosity in multiple birth pregnancies) (List separately in addition to code for primary procedure)
➡ *CPT Assistant* May 12:4; *CPT Changes: An Insider's View* 2012

(Use 81266 in conjunction with 81265)

81267   Chimerism (engraftment) analysis, post transplantation specimen (eg, hematopoietic stem cell), includes comparison to previously performed baseline analyses; without cell selection
➡ *CPT Assistant* May 12:4; *CPT Changes: An Insider's View* 2012

81268   with cell selection (eg, CD3, CD33), each cell type
➡ *CPT Assistant* May 12:4; *CPT Changes: An Insider's View* 2012

(If comparative STR analysis of recipient [using buccal swab or other germline tissue sample] and donor are performed after hematopoietic stem cell transplantation, report 81265, 81266 in conjunction with 81267, 81268 for chimerism testing)

81270   JAK2 (Janus kinase 2) (eg, myeloproliferative disorder) gene analysis, p.Val617Phe (V617F) variant
➡ *CPT Assistant* May 12:4; *CPT Changes: An Insider's View* 2012

81275   KRAS (v-Ki-ras2 Kirsten rat sarcoma viral oncogene) (eg, carcinoma) gene analysis, variants in codons 12 and 13
➡ *CPT Assistant* May 12:4; *CPT Changes: An Insider's View* 2012

81280   Long QT syndrome gene analyses (eg, KCNQ1, KCNH2, SCN5A, KCNE1, KCNE2, KCNJ2, CACNA1C, CAV3, SCN4B, AKAP, SNTA1, and ANK2); full sequence analysis
➡ *CPT Assistant* May 12:4; *CPT Changes: An Insider's View* 2012

81281   known familial sequence variant
➡ *CPT Assistant* May 12:4; *CPT Changes: An Insider's View* 2012

81282   duplication/deletion variants
➡ *CPT Assistant* May 12:4; *CPT Changes: An Insider's View* 2012

81290   MCOLN1 (mucolipin 1) (eg, Mucolipidosis, type IV) gene analysis, common variants (eg, IVS3-2A>G, del6.4kb)
➡ *CPT Assistant* May 12:4; *CPT Changes: An Insider's View* 2012

81291   MTHFR (5,10-methylenetetrahydrofolate reductase) (eg, hereditary hypercoagulability) gene analysis, common variants (eg, 677T, 1298C)
➡ *CPT Assistant* May 12:4; *CPT Changes: An Insider's View* 2012

81292   MLH1 (mutL homolog 1, colon cancer, nonpolyposis type 2) (eg, hereditary non-polyposis colorectal cancer, Lynch syndrome) gene analysis; full sequence analysis
➡ *CPT Assistant* May 12:4; *CPT Changes: An Insider's View* 2012

81293   known familial variants
➡ *CPT Assistant* May 12:4; *CPT Changes: An Insider's View* 2012

81294   duplication/deletion variants
➡ *CPT Assistant* May 12:4; *CPT Changes: An Insider's View* 2012

81295   MSH2 (mutS homolog 2, colon cancer, nonpolyposis type 1) (eg, hereditary non-polyposis colorectal cancer, Lynch syndrome) gene analysis; full sequence analysis
➡ *CPT Assistant* May 12:4; *CPT Changes: An Insider's View* 2012

81296   known familial variants
➡ *CPT Assistant* May 12:4; *CPT Changes: An Insider's View* 2012

81297   duplication/deletion variants
➡ *CPT Assistant* May 12:4; *CPT Changes: An Insider's View* 2012

81298   MSH6 (mutS homolog 6 [E. coli]) (eg, hereditary non-polyposis colorectal cancer, Lynch syndrome) gene analysis; full sequence analysis
➡ *CPT Assistant* May 12:4; *CPT Changes: An Insider's View* 2012

81299   known familial variants
➡ *CPT Assistant* May 12:4; *CPT Changes: An Insider's View* 2012

81300   duplication/deletion variants
➡ *CPT Assistant* May 12:4; *CPT Changes: An Insider's View* 2012

81301   Microsatellite instability analysis (eg, hereditary non-polyposis colorectal cancer, Lynch syndrome) of markers for mismatch repair deficiency (eg, BAT25, BAT26), includes comparison of neoplastic and normal tissue, if performed
➡ *CPT Assistant* May 12:4; *CPT Changes: An Insider's View* 2012

81302   MECP2 (methyl CpG binding protein 2) (eg, Rett syndrome) gene analysis; full sequence analysis
➡ *CPT Assistant* May 12:4; *CPT Changes: An Insider's View* 2012

81303   known familial variant
➡ *CPT Assistant* May 12:4; *CPT Changes: An Insider's View* 2012

81304   duplication/deletion variants
➡ *CPT Assistant* May 12:4; *CPT Changes: An Insider's View* 2012

81310   NPM1 (nucleophosmin) (eg, acute myeloid leukemia) gene analysis, exon 12 variants
➡ *CPT Assistant* May 12:4; *CPT Changes: An Insider's View* 2012

81315   PML/RARalpha, (t(15;17)), (promyelocytic leukemia/ retinoic acid receptor alpha) (eg, promyelocytic leukemia) translocation analysis; common breakpoints (eg, intron 3 and intron 6), qualitative or quantitative
➡ *CPT Assistant* May 12:4; *CPT Changes: An Insider's View* 2012

81316   single breakpoint (eg, intron 3, intron 6 or exon 6), qualitative or quantitative
➡ *CPT Assistant* May 12:4; *CPT Changes: An Insider's View* 2012

(For intron 3 and intron 6 [including exon 6 if performed] analysis, use 81315)

(If both intron 6 and exon 6 are analyzed, without intron 3, use one unit of 81316)

81317   PMS2 (postmeiotic segregation increased 2 [S. cerevisiae]) (eg, hereditary non-polyposis colorectal cancer, Lynch syndrome) gene analysis; full sequence analysis
➡ *CPT Assistant* May 12:4; *CPT Changes: An Insider's View* 2012

81318   known familial variants
➡ *CPT Assistant* May 12:4; *CPT Changes: An Insider's View* 2012

Pathology and Laboratory

81319 duplication/deletion variants
➜ *CPT Assistant* May 12:4; *CPT Changes: An Insider's View* 2012

● **81321** *PTEN (phosphatase and tensin homolog)* (eg, Cowden syndrome, *PTEN* hamartoma tumor syndrome) gene analysis; full sequence analysis
➜ *CPT Changes: An Insider's View* 2013

● **81322** known familial variant
➜ *CPT Changes: An Insider's View* 2013

● **81323** duplication/deletion variant
➜ *CPT Changes: An Insider's View* 2013

● **81324** *PMP22 (peripheral myelin protein 22)* (eg, Charcot-Marie-Tooth, hereditary neuropathy with liability to pressure palsies) gene analysis; duplication/deletion analysis
➜ *CPT Changes: An Insider's View* 2013

● **81325** full sequence analysis
➜ *CPT Changes: An Insider's View* 2013

● **81326** known familial variant
➜ *CPT Changes: An Insider's View* 2013

81330 *SMPD1(sphingomyelin phosphodiesterase 1, acid lysosomal)* (eg, Niemann-Pick disease, Type A) gene analysis, common variants (eg, R496L, L302P, fsP330)
➜ *CPT Assistant* May 12:4; *CPT Changes: An Insider's View* 2012

81331 *SNRPN/UBE3A (small nuclear ribonucleoprotein polypeptide N and ubiquitin protein ligase E3A)* (eg, Prader-Willi syndrome and/or Angelman syndrome), methylation analysis
➜ *CPT Assistant* May 12:4; *CPT Changes: An Insider's View* 2012

81332 *SERPINA1 (serpin peptidase inhibitor, clade A, alpha-1 antiproteinase, antitrypsin, member 1)* (eg, alpha-1-antitrypsin deficiency), gene analysis, common variants (eg, *S and *Z)
➜ *CPT Assistant* May 12:4; *CPT Changes: An Insider's View* 2012

81340 *TRB@ (T cell antigen receptor, beta)* (eg, leukemia and lymphoma), gene rearrangement analysis to detect abnormal clonal population(s); using amplification methodology (eg, polymerase chain reaction)
➜ *CPT Assistant* May 12:4; *CPT Changes: An Insider's View* 2012

81341 using direct probe methodology (eg, Southern blot)
➜ *CPT Assistant* May 12:4; *CPT Changes: An Insider's View* 2012

81342 *TRG@ (T cell antigen receptor, gamma)* (eg, leukemia and lymphoma), gene rearrangement analysis, evaluation to detect abnormal clonal population(s)
➜ *CPT Assistant* May 12:4; *CPT Changes: An Insider's View* 2012

▶(For T cell antigen alpha [*TRA@*] gene rearrangement analysis, use 81479)◀

(For T cell antigen delta [*TRD@*] gene rearrangement analysis, use 81402)

81350 *UGT1A1 (UDP glucuronosyltransferase 1 family, polypeptide A1)* (eg, irinotecan metabolism), gene analysis, common variants (eg, *28, *36, *37)
➜ *CPT Assistant* May 12:4; *CPT Changes: An Insider's View* 2012

81355 *VKORC1 (vitamin K epoxide reductase complex, subunit 1)* (eg, warfarin metabolism), gene analysis, common variants (eg, -1639/3673)
➜ *CPT Assistant* May 12:4; *CPT Changes: An Insider's View* 2012

Human Leukocyte Antigen (HLA) typing is performed to assess compatibility of recipients and potential donors as a part of solid organ and hematopoietic stem cell pretransplant testing. HLA testing is also performed to identify HLA alleles and allele groups (antigen equivalents) associated with specific diseases and individualized responses to drug therapy (eg, HLA-B*27 and ankylosing spondylitis and HLA-B*57:01 and abacavir hypersensitivity), as well as other clinical uses. One or more HLA genes may be tested in specific clinical situations (eg, HLA-DQB1 for narcolepsy and HLA-A, -B, -C, -DRB1, and -DQB1 for kidney transplantation). Each HLA gene typically has multiple variant alleles or allele groups that can be identified by typing. For HLA result reporting, a low resolution HLA type is denoted by a two digit HLA name (eg, A*02) and intermediate resolution typing by a string of alleles or an NMDP (National Marrow Donor Program) code (eg, B*14:01/07N/08/12/14, B*39CKGN). Both low and intermediate resolution are considered low resolution for code assignment. High resolution typing resolves the common well defined (CWD) alleles and is usually denoted by at least 4 digits (eg, A*02:02, *03:01:01:01, A*26:01:01G, and C*03:04P), however, high resolution typing may include some ambiguities for rare alleles, which may be reported as a string of alleles or an NMDP code.

If additional testing is required to resolve ambiguous allele combinations for high resolution typing, this is included in the base HLA typing codes below. The gene names have been italicized similar to the other molecular pathology codes.

(For HLA antigen typing by non-molecular pathology techniques, see 86812-86822)

81370 HLA Class I and II typing, low resolution (eg, antigen equivalents); *HLA-A, -B, -C, -DRB1/3/4/5*, and *-DQB1*
➜ *CPT Assistant* May 12:4; *CPT Changes: An Insider's View* 2012

81371 *HLA-A, -B, and -DRB1/3/4/5* (eg, verification typing)
➜ *CPT Assistant* May 12:4; *CPT Changes: An Insider's View* 2012

81372 HLA Class I typing, low resolution (eg, antigen equivalents); complete *(ie, HLA-A, -B, and -C)*
➜ *CPT Assistant* May 12:4; *CPT Changes: An Insider's View* 2012

(When performing both Class I and II low resolution *HLA typing for HLA-A,-B,-C, -DRB1/3/4/5, and -DQB1*, use 81370)

81373 one locus *(eg, HLA-A, -B, or -C)*, each
➜ *CPT Assistant* May 12:4, Jun 12:16; *CPT Changes: An Insider's View* 2012

(When performing a complete Class I *[HLA-A,-B, and -C]* low resolution HLA typing, use 81372)

(When the presence or absence of a single antigen equivalent is reported using low resolution testing, use 81374)

81374   one antigen equivalent (eg, *B*27*), each

→ *CPT Assistant* May 12:4, Jun 12:16; *CPT Changes: An Insider's View* 2012

(When testing for presence or absence of more than 2 antigen equivalents at a locus, use 81373 for each locus tested)

81375   HLA Class II typing, low resolution (eg, antigen equivalents); *HLA-DRB1/3/4/5* and *-DQB1*

→ *CPT Assistant* May 12:4; *CPT Changes: An Insider's View* 2012

(When performing both Class I and II low resolution HLA typing *for HLA-A,-B,-C, -DRB1/3/4/5,* and *-DQB1*, use 81370)

81376   one locus (eg, *HLA-DRB1/3/4/5, -DQB1, -DQA1, -DPB1,* or *-DPA1*), each

→ *CPT Assistant* May 12:4, Jun 12:16; *CPT Changes: An Insider's View* 2012

(When low resolution typing is performed for *HLA-DRB1/3/4/5* and *-DQB1*, use 81375)

(For low resolution typing, *HLA-DRB1/3/4/5* should be treated as a single locus)

81377   one antigen equivalent, each

→ *CPT Assistant* May 12:4, Jun 12:16; *CPT Changes: An Insider's View* 2012

(When testing for presence or absence of more than 2 antigen equivalents at a locus, use 81376 for each locus)

81378   HLA Class I and II typing, high resolution (ie, alleles or allele groups), *HLA-A, -B, -C,* and *-DRB1*

→ *CPT Assistant* May 12:4, Jun 12:16; *CPT Changes: An Insider's View* 2012

81379   HLA Class I typing, high resolution (ie, alleles or allele groups); complete (ie, *HLA-A, -B,* and *-C*)

→ *CPT Assistant* May 12:4; *CPT Changes: An Insider's View* 2012

81380   one locus (eg, *HLA-A, -B,* or *-C*), each

→ *CPT Assistant* May 12:4, Jun 12:16; *CPT Changes: An Insider's View* 2012

(When a complete Class I high resolution typing for *HLA-A,-B,* and *-C* is performed, use 81379)

(When the presence or absence of a single allele or allele group is reported using high resolution testing, use 81381)

81381   one allele or allele group (eg, *B*57:01P*), each

→ *CPT Assistant* May 12:4, Jun 12:16; *CPT Changes: An Insider's View* 2012

(When testing for the presence or absence of more than 2 alleles or allele groups at a locus, use 81380 for each locus)

81382   HLA Class II typing, high resolution (ie, alleles or allele groups); one locus (eg, *HLA-DRB1, -DRB3, -DRB4, -DRB5, -DQB1, -DQA1, -DPB1,* or *-DPA1*), each

→ *CPT Assistant* May 12:4, Jun 12:16; *CPT Changes: An Insider's View* 2012

(When only the presence or absence of a single allele or allele group is reported using high resolution testing, use 81383)

81383   one allele or allele group (eg, *HLA-DQB1*06:02P*), each

→ *CPT Assistant* May 12:4, Jun 12:16; *CPT Changes: An Insider's View* 2012

(When testing for the presence or absence of more than 2 alleles or allele groups at a locus, use 81382 for each locus)

Tier 2 Molecular Pathology Procedures

The following molecular pathology procedure (Tier 2) codes are used to report procedures not listed in the Tier 1 molecular pathology codes (81200-81383). They represent medically useful procedures that are generally performed in lower volumes than Tier 1 procedures (eg, the incidence of the disease being tested is rare). They are arranged by level of technical resources and interpretive work by the physician or other qualified health care professional. The individual analyses listed under each code (ie, level of procedure) utilize the definitions and coding principles as described in the introduction preceding the Tier 1 molecular pathology codes. The parenthetical examples of methodologies presented near the beginning of each code provide general guidelines used to group procedures for a given level and are not all-inclusive.

►Use the appropriate molecular pathology procedure level code that includes the specific analyte listed after the code descriptor. If the analyte tested is not listed under one of the Tier 2 codes or is not represented by a Tier 1 code, use the unlisted molecular pathology procedure code, 81479.◄

▲ **81400**   Molecular pathology procedure, Level 1 *(eg, identification of single germline variant [eg, SNP] by techniques such as restriction enzyme digestion or melt curve analysis)*

►*ABCC8 (ATP-binding cassette, sub-family C [CFTR/MRP], member 8) (eg, familial hyperinsulinism), F1388del variant*◄

ACADM (acyl-CoA dehydrogenase, C-4 to C-12 straight chain, MCAD) (eg, medium chain acyl dehydrogenase deficiency), K304E variant

ACE (angiotensin converting enzyme) (eg, hereditary blood pressure regulation), insertion/deletion variant

AGTR1 (angiotensin II receptor, type 1) (eg, essential hypertension), 1166A>C variant

CCR5 (chemokine C-C motif receptor 5) (eg, HIV resistance), 32-bp deletion mutation/794 825del32 deletion

►*CLRN1 (clarin 1) (eg, Usher syndrome, type 3), N48K variant*◄

DPYD (dihydropyrimidine dehydrogenase) (eg, 5-fluorouracil/5-FU and capecitabine drug metabolism), IVS14+1G>A variant

F2 (coagulation factor 2) (eg, hereditary hypercoagulability), 1199G>A variant

F5 (coagulation factor V) (eg, hereditary hypercoagulability), HR2 variant

F7 (coagulation factor VII [serum prothrombin conversion accelerator]) (eg, hereditary hypercoagulability), R353Q variant

F13B (coagulation factor XIII, B polypeptide) (eg, hereditary hypercoagulability), V34L variant

FGB (fibrinogen beta chain) (eg, hereditary ischemic heart disease), -455G>A variant

▶ *FGFR3 (fibroblast growth factor receptor 3) (eg, Muenke syndrome), P250R variant*◀

Human Platelet Antigen 1 genotyping (HPA-1), ITGB3 (integrin, beta 3 [platelet glycoprotein IIIa], antigen CD61 [GPIIIa]) (eg, neonatal alloimmune thrombocytopenia [NAIT], post-transfusion purpura), HPA-1a/b (L33P)

Human Platelet Antigen 2 genotyping (HPA-2), GP1BA (glycoprotein Ib [platelet], alpha polypeptide [GPIba]) (eg, neonatal alloimmune thrombocytopenia [NAIT], post-transfusion purpura), HPA-2a/b (T145M)

Human Platelet Antigen 3 genotyping (HPA-3), ITGA2B (integrin, alpha 2b [platelet glycoprotein IIb of IIb/IIIa complex], antigen CD41 [GPIIb]) (eg, neonatal alloimmune thrombocytopenia [NAIT], post-transfusion purpura), HPA-3a/b (I843S)

Human Platelet Antigen 4 genotyping (HPA-4), ITGB3 (integrin, beta 3 [platelet glycoprotein IIIa], antigen CD61 [GPIIIa]) (eg, neonatal alloimmune thrombocytopenia [NAIT], post-transfusion purpura), HPA-4a/b (R143Q)

Human Platelet Antigen 5 genotyping (HPA-5), ITGA2 (integrin, alpha 2 [CD49B, alpha 2 subunit of VLA-2 receptor] [GPIa]) (eg, neonatal alloimmune thrombocytopenia [NAIT], post-transfusion purpura), HPA-5a/b (K505E)

Human Platelet Antigen 6 genotyping (HPA-6w), ITGB3 (integrin, beta 3 [platelet glycoprotein IIIa, antigen CD61] [GPIIIa]) (eg, neonatal alloimmune thrombocytopenia [NAIT], post-transfusion purpura), HPA-6a/b (R489Q)

Human Platelet Antigen 9 genotyping (HPA-9w), ITGA2B (integrin, alpha 2b [platelet glycoprotein IIb of IIb/IIIa complex, antigen CD41] [GPIIb]) (eg, neonatal alloimmune thrombocytopenia [NAIT], post-transfusion purpura), HPA-9a/b (V837M)

Human Platelet Antigen 15 genotyping (HPA-15), CD109 (CD109 molecule) (eg, neonatal alloimmune thrombocytopenia [NAIT], post-transfusion purpura), HPA-15a/b (S682Y)

▶ *IVD (isovaleryl-CoA dehydrogenase) (eg, isovaleric acidemia), A282V variant*

SERPINE1 (serpine peptidase inhibitor clade E, member 1, plasminogen activator inhibitor -1, PAI-1) (eg, thrombophilia), 4G variant

SHOC2 (soc-2 suppressor of clear homolog) (eg, Noonan-like syndrome with loose anagen hair), S2G variant

SMN1 (survival of motor neuron 1, telomeric) (eg, spinal muscular atrophy), exon 7 deletion

SRY (sex determining region Y) (eg, 46,XX testicular disorder of sex development, gonadal dysgenesis), gene analysis

TOR1A (torsin family 1, member A [torsin A]) (eg, early-onset primary dystonia [DYT1]), 907_909delGAG (904_906delGAG) variant◀

➔ *CPT Assistant May 12:4; CPT Changes: An Insider's View 2012, 2013*

▲ **81401**   Molecular pathology procedure, Level 2 (eg, 2-10 SNPs, 1 methylated variant, or 1 somatic variant [typically using nonsequencing target variant analysis], or detection of a dynamic mutation disorder/triplet repeat)

ABL (c-abl oncogene 1, receptor tyrosine kinase) (eg, acquired imatinib resistance), T315I variant

ACADM (acyl-CoA dehydrogenase, C-4 to C-12 straight chain, MCAD) (eg, medium chain acyl dehydrogenase deficiency), commons variants (eg, K304E, Y42H)

ADRB2 (adrenergic beta-2 receptor surface) (eg, drug metabolism), common variants (eg, G16R, Q27E) APOB (apolipoprotein B) (eg, familial hypercholesterolemia type B), common variants (eg, R3500Q, R3500W)

APOE (apolipoprotein E) (eg, hyperlipoproteinemia type III, cardiovascular disease, Alzheimer disease), common variants (eg, *2, *3, *4)

AR (androgen receptor) (eg, spinal and bulbar muscular atrophy, Kennedy disease, X chromosome inactivation), characterization of alleles (eg, expanded size or methylation status)

ATN1 (atrophin 1) (eg, dentatorubral-pallidoluysian atrophy), evaluation to detect abnormal (eg, expanded) alleles

CBFB/MYH11 (inv(16)) (eg, acute myeloid leukemia), qualitative, and quantitative, if performed

CBS (cystathionine-beta-synthase) (eg, homocystinuria, cystathionine beta-synthase deficiency), common variants (eg, I278T, G307S)

CCND1/IGH (BCL1/IgH, t(11;14)) (eg, mantle cell lymphoma) translocation analysis, major breakpoint, qualitative, and quantitative, if performed

CFH/ARMS2 (complement factor H/age-related maculopathy susceptibility 2) (eg, macular degeneration), common variants (eg, Y402H [CFH], A69S [ARMS2])

CYP3A4 (cytochrome P450, family 3, subfamily A, polypeptide 4) (eg, drug metabolism), common variants (eg, *2, *3, *4, *5, *6)

CYP3A5 (cytochrome P450, family 3, subfamily A, polypeptide 5) (eg, drug metabolism), common variants (eg, *2, *3, *4, *5, *6)

DMPK (dystrophia myotonica-protein kinase) (eg, myotonic dystrophy, type 1), evaluation to detect abnormal (eg, expanded) alleles

E2A/PBX1 (t(1;19)) (eg, acute lymphocytic leukemia), translocation analysis, qualitative, and quantitative, if performed

Pathology and Laboratory

EML4/ALK (inv(2)) (eg, non-small cell lung cancer), translocation or inversion analysis

ETV6/RUNX1 (t(12;21)) (eg, acute lymphocytic leukemia), translocation analysis, qualitative, and quantitative, if performed

EWSR1/ERG (t(21;22)) (eg, Ewing sarcoma/peripheral neuroectodermal tumor), translocation analysis, qualitative, and quantitative, if performed

EWSR1/FLI1 (t(11;22)) (eg, Ewing sarcoma/peripheral neuroectodermal tumor), translocation analysis, qualitative, and quantitative, if performed

F11 (coagulation factor XI) (eg, coagulation disorder), common variants (eg, E117X [Type II], F283L [Type III], IVS14del14, and IVS14+1G>A [Type I])

FGFR3 (fibroblast growth factor receptor 3) (eg, achondroplasia, hypochondroplasia), common variants (eg, 1138G>A, 1138G>C, 1620C>A, 1620C>G)

FIP1L1/PDGFRA (del[4q12]) (eg, imatinib-sensitive chronic eosinophilic leukemia), qualitative, and quantitative, if performed

FOXO1/PAX3 (t(1;13)) (eg, Ewing sarcoma/peripheral neuroectodermal tumor), translocation analysis, qualitative, and quantitative, if performed

FOXO1/PAX7 (t(2;13)) (eg, Ewing sarcoma/peripheral neuroectodermal tumor), translocation analysis, qualitative, and quantitative, if performed

FXN (frataxin) (eg, Friedreich ataxia), evaluation to detect abnormal (expanded) alleles

GALT (galactose-1-phosphate uridylyltransferase) (eg, galactosemia), common variants (eg, Q188R, S135L, K285N, T138M, L195P, Y209C, IVS2-2A>G, P171S, del5kb, N314D, L218L/N314D)

H19 (imprinted maternally expressed transcript [non-protein coding]) (eg, Beckwith-Wiedemann syndrome), methylation analysis

HBB (hemoglobin, beta) (eg, sickle cell anemia, hemoglobin C, hemoglobin E), common variants (eg, HbS, HbC, HbE)

HTT (huntingtin) (eg, Huntington disease), evaluation to detect abnormal (eg, expanded) alleles

KCNQ1OT1 (KCNQ1 overlapping transcript 1 [non-protein coding]) (eg, Beckwith-Wiedemann syndrome), methylation analysis

MEG3/DLK1 (maternally expressed 3 [non-protein coding]/delta-like 1 homolog [Drosophila]) (eg, intrauterine growth retardation), methylation analysis

MLL/AFF1 (t(4;11)) (eg, acute lymphoblastic leukemia), translocation analysis, qualitative, and quantitative, if performed

MLL/MLLT3 (t(9;11)) (eg, acute myeloid leukemia), translocation analysis, qualitative, and quantitative, if performed

MT-RNR1 (mitochondrially encoded 12S RNA) (eg, nonsyndromic hearing loss), common variants (eg, m.1555A>G, m.1494C>T)

MUTYH (mutY homolog [E. coli]) (eg, MYH-associated polyposis), common variants (eg, Y165C, G382D)

MT-ATP6 (mitochondrially encoded ATP synthase 6) (eg, neuropathy with ataxia and retinitis pigmentosa [NARP], Leigh syndrome), common variants (eg, m.8993T>G, m.8993T>C)

MT-ND4, MT-ND6 (mitochondrially encoded NADH dehydrogenase 4, mitochondrially encoded NADH dehydrogenase 6) (eg, Leber hereditary optic neuropathy [LHON]), common variants (eg, m.11778G>A, m.3460G>A, m.14484T>C)

MT-TK (mitochondrially encoded tRNA lysine) (eg, myoclonic epilepsy with ragged-red fibers [MERRF]), common variants (eg, m.8344A>G, m.8356T>C)

MT-TL1 (mitochondrially encoded tRNA leucine 1 [UUA/G]) (eg, diabetes and hearing loss), common variants (eg, m.3243A>G, m.14709 T>C) MT-TL1,

MT-ND5 (mitochondrially encoded tRNA leucine 1 [UUA/G], mitochondrially encoded NADH dehydrogenase 5) (eg, mitochondrial encephalopathy with lactic acidosis and stroke-like episodes [MELAS]), common variants (eg, m.3243A>G, m.3271T>C, m.3252A>G, m.13513G>A)

MT-TS1, MT-RNR1 (mitochondrially encoded tRNA serine 1 [UCN], mitochondrially encoded 12S RNA) (eg, nonsyndromic sensorineural deafness [including aminoglycoside-induced nonsyndromic deafness]), common variants (eg, m.7445A>G, m.1555A>G)

NPM1/ALK (t(2;5)) (eg, anaplastic large cell lymphoma), translocation analysis

PAX8/PPARG (t(2;3) (q13;p25)) (eg, follicular thyroid carcinoma), translocation analysis

PRSS1 (protease, serine, 1 [trypsin 1]) (eg, hereditary pancreatitis), common variants (eg, N29I, A16V, R122H)

PYGM (phosphorylase, glycogen, muscle) (eg, glycogen storage disease type V, McArdle disease), common variants (eg, R50X, G205S)

RUNX1/RUNX1T1 (t(8;21)) (eg, acute myeloid leukemia) translocation analysis, qualitative, and quantitative, if performed

SEPT9 (Septin 9) (eg, colon cancer), methylation analysis

SMN1/SMN2 (survival of motor neuron 1, telomeric/ survival of motor neuron 2, centromeric) (eg, spinal muscular atrophy), dosage analysis (eg, carrier testing)

TPMT (thiopurine S-methyltransferase) (eg, drug metabolism), common variants (eg, *2, *3)

TYMS (thymidylate synthetase) (eg, 5-fluorouracil/5-FU drug metabolism), tandem repeat variant

VWF (von Willebrand factor) (eg, von Willebrand disease type 2N), common variants (eg, T791M, R816W, R854Q)

➔ *CPT Assistant* May 12:4; *CPT Changes: An Insider's View* 2012, 2013

Pathology and Laboratory

▲ **81402** Molecular pathology procedure, Level 3 (eg, >10 SNPs, 2-10 methylated variants, or 2-10 somatic variants [typically using non-sequencing target variant analysis], immunoglobulin and T-cell receptor gene rearrangements, duplication/deletion variants of 1 exon, loss of heterozygosity [LOH], uniparental disomy [UPD])

► Chromosome 18q- (eg, D18S55, D18S58, D18S61, D18S64, and D18S69) (eg, colon cancer), allelic imbalance assessment (ie, loss of heterozygosity) ◄

CYP21A2 (cytochrome P450, family 21, subfamily A, polypeptide 2) (eg, congenital adrenal hyperplasia, 21-hydroxylase deficiency), common variants (eg, IVS2-13G, P30L, I172N, exon 6 mutation cluster [I235N, V236E, M238K], V281L, L307FfsX6, Q318X, R356W, P453S, G110VfsX21, 30-kb deletion variant)

ESR1/PGR (receptor 1/progesterone receptor) ratio (eg, breast cancer)

KIT (v-kit Hardy-Zuckerman 4 feline sarcoma viral oncogene homolog) (eg, mastocytosis), common variants (eg, D816V, D816Y, D816F)

MEFV (Mediterranean fever) (eg, familial Mediterranean fever), common variants (eg, E148Q, P369S, F479L, M680I, I692del, M694V, M694I, K695R, V726A, A744S, R761H)

MPL (myeloproliferative leukemia virus oncogene, thrombopoietin receptor, TPOR) (eg, myeloproliferative disorder), common variants (eg, W515A, W515K, W515L, W515R)

TCD@ (T cell antigen receptor, delta) (eg, leukemia and lymphoma), gene rearrangement analysis, evaluation to detect abnormal clonal population

► Uniparental disomy (UPD) (eg, Russell-Silver syndrome, Prader-Willi/Angelman syndrome), short tandem repeat (STR) analysis ◄

➔ *CPT Assistant* May 12:4; *CPT Changes: An Insider's View* 2012, 2013

▲ **81403** Molecular pathology procedure, Level 4 (eg, analysis of single exon by DNA sequence analysis, analysis of >10 amplicons using multiplex PCR in 2 or more independent reactions, mutation scanning or duplication/deletion variants of 2-5 exons)

ABL1 (c-abl oncogene 1, receptor tyrosine kinase) (eg, acquired imatinib tyrosine kinase inhibitor resistance), variants in the kinase domain

► *ANG (angiogenin, ribonuclease, RNase A family, 5)* (eg, amyotrophic lateral sclerosis), full gene sequence

CEBPA (CCAAT/enhancer binding protein [C/EBP], alpha) (eg, acute myeloid leukemia), full gene sequence

CEL (carboxyl ester lipase [bile salt-stimulated lipase]) (eg, maturity-onset diabetes of the young [MODY]), targeted sequence analysis of exon 11 (eg, c.1785delC, c.1686delT) ◄

DAZ/SRY (deleted in azoospermia and sex determining region Y) (eg, male infertility), common deletions (eg, AZFa, AZFb, AZFc, AZFd)

► *F8 (coagulation factor VIII)* (eg, hemophilia A), inversion analysis, intron 1 and intron 22A

FGFR3 (fibroblast growth factor receptor 3) (eg, isolated craniosynostosis), targeted sequence analysis (eg, exon 7)

(For targeted sequence analysis of multiple FGFR3 exons, use 81404) ◄

GJB1 (gap junction protein, beta 1) (eg, Charcot-Marie-Tooth X-linked), full gene sequence

► *HBB (hemoglobin, beta, beta-globin)* (eg, beta thalassemia), duplication/deletion analysis

HRAS (v-Ha-ras Harvey rat sarcoma viral oncogene homolog) (eg, Costello syndrome), exon 2 sequence

IDH1 (isocitrate dehydrogenase 1 [NADP+], soluble) (eg, glioma), common exon 4 variants (eg, R132H, R132C)

IDH2 (isocitrate dehydrogenase 2 [NADP+], mitochondrial) (eg, glioma), common exon 4 variants (eg, R140W, R172M) ◄

JAK2 (Janus kinase 2) (eg, myeloproliferative disorder), exon 12 sequence and exon 13 sequence, if performed

► Known familial variant not otherwise specified, for gene listed in Tier 1 or Tier 2, DNA sequence analysis, each variant exon

(For a known familial variant that is considered a common variant, use specific common variant Tier 1 or Tier 2 code)

KRAS (v-Ki-ras2 Kirsten rat sarcoma viral oncogene) (eg, carcinoma), gene analysis, variant(s) in exon 3 (eg, codon 61) ◄

MPL (myeloproliferative leukemia virus oncogene, thrombopoietin receptor, TPOR) (eg, myeloproliferative disorder), exon 10 sequence

► *MT-RNR1 (mitochondrially encoded 12S RNA)* (eg, nonsyndromic hearing loss), full gene sequence

MT-TS1 (mitochondrially encoded tRNA serine 1) (eg, nonsyndromic hearing loss), full gene sequence

SMN1 (survival of motor neuron 1, telomeric) (eg, spinal muscular atrophy), known familial sequence variant(s) ◄

VHL (von Hippel-Lindau tumor suppressor) (eg, von Hippel-Lindau familial cancer syndrome), deletion/duplication analysis

VWF (von Willebrand factor) (eg, von Willebrand disease types 2A, 2B, 2M), targeted sequence analysis (eg, exon 28)

➔ *CPT Assistant* May 12:4; *CPT Changes: An Insider's View* 2012, 2013

▲ **81404** Molecular pathology procedure, Level 5 (eg, analysis of 2-5 exons by DNA sequence analysis, mutation scanning or duplication/deletion variants of 6-10 exons, or characterization of a dynamic mutation disorder/triplet repeat by Southern blot analysis)

► *ACADS (acyl-CoA dehydrogenase, C-2 to C-3 short chain)* (eg, short chain acyl-CoA dehydrogenase deficiency), targeted sequence analysis (eg, exons 5 and 6)

⊙ =Moderate sedation ✚ =Add-on code ✗ =FDA approval pending # =Resequenced code ○ =Recycled/reinstated code ➔➔ =See p xiii for details

AQP2 (aquaporin 2 [collecting duct]) (eg, nephrogenic diabetes insipidus), full gene sequence

ARX (aristaless related homeobox) (eg, X-linked lissencephaly with ambiguous genitalia, X-linked mental retardation), full gene sequence◄

BTD (biotinidase) (eg, biotinidase deficiency), full gene sequence

►*CAV3 (caveolin 3)* (eg, CAV3-related distal myopathy, limb-girdle muscular dystrophy type 1C), full gene sequence

CDKN2A (cyclin-dependent kinase inhibitor 2A) (eg, CDKN2A-related cutaneous malignant melanoma, familial atypical mole-malignant melanoma syndrome), full gene sequence

CLRN1 (clarin 1) (eg, Usher syndrome, type 3), full gene sequence

CPT2 (carnitine palmitoyltransferase 2) (eg, carnitine palmitoyltransferase II deficiency), full gene sequence◄

CYP1B1 (cytochrome P450, family 1, subfamily B, polypeptide 1) (eg, primary congenital glaucoma), full gene sequence

DMPK (dystrophia myotonica-protein kinase) (eg, myotonic dystrophy type 1), characterization of abnormal (eg, expanded) alleles

EGR2 (early growth response 2) (eg, Charcot-Marie-Tooth), full gene sequence

►*FGFR2 (fibroblast growth factor receptor 2)* (eg, craniosynostosis, Apert syndrome, Crouzon syndrome), targeted sequence analysis (eg, exons 8, 10)

FGFR3 (fibroblast growth factor receptor 3) (eg, achondroplasia, hypochondroplasia), targeted sequence analysis (eg, exons 8, 11, 12, 13)◄

FKRP (Fukutin related protein) (eg, congenital muscular dystrophy type 1C [MDC1C], limb-girdle muscular dystrophy [LGMD] type 2I), full gene sequence

FOXG1 (forkhead box G1) (eg, Rett syndrome), full gene sequence

FSHMD1A (facioscapulohumeral muscular dystrophy 1A) (eg, facioscapulohumeral muscular dystrophy), evaluation to detect abnormal (eg, deleted) alleles

FSHMD1A (facioscapulohumeral muscular dystrophy 1A) (eg, facioscapulohumeral muscular dystrophy), characterization of haplotype(s) (ie, chromosome 4A and 4B haplotypes)

►*FXN (frataxin)* (eg, Friedreich ataxia), full gene sequence◄

HBA1/HBA2 (alpha globin 1 and alpha globin 2) (eg, alpha thalassemia), duplication/deletion analysis

(For common deletion variants of alpha globin 1 and alpha globin 2 genes, use 81257)

HBB (hemoglobin, beta, Beta-Globin) (eg, thalassemia), full gene sequence

►*HNF1B (HNF1 homeobox B)* (eg, maturity-onset diabetes of the young [MODY]), duplication/deletion analysis

HRAS (v-Ha-ras Harvey rat sarcoma viral oncogene homolog) (eg, Costello syndrome), full gene sequence◄

KCNJ10 (potassium inwardly-rectifying channel, subfamily J, member 10) (eg, SeSAME syndrome, EAST syndrome, sensorineural hearing loss), full gene sequence

KIT (C-kit) (v-kit Hardy-Zuckerman 4 feline sarcoma viral oncogene homolog) (eg, GIST, acute myeloid leukemia, melanoma), targeted gene analysis (eg, exons 8, 11, 13, 17, 18)

LITAF (lipopolysaccharide-induced TNF factor) (eg, Charcot-Marie-Tooth), full gene sequence

MEFV (Mediterranean fever) (eg, familial Mediterranean fever), full gene sequence

►*MEN1 (multiple endocrine neoplasia I)* (eg, multiple endocrine neoplasia type 1, Wermer syndrome), duplication/deletion analysis◄

NRAS (neuroblastoma RAS viral oncogene homolog) (eg, colorectal carcinoma), exon 1 and exon 2 sequences

PDGFRA (platelet-derived growth factor receptor alpha polypeptide) (eg, gastrointestinal stromal tumor), targeted sequence analysis (eg, exons 12, 18)

►*PDX1 (pancreatic and duodenal homeobox 1)* (eg, maturity-onset diabetes of the young [MODY]), full gene sequence

PRNP (prion protein) (eg, genetic prion disease), full gene sequence

PRSS1 (protease, serine, 1 [trypsin 1]) (eg, hereditary pancreatitis), full gene sequence

RAF1 (v-raf-1 murine leukemia viral oncogene homolog 1) (eg, LEOPARD syndrome), targeted sequence analysis (eg, exons 7, 12, 14, 17)◄

RET (ret proto-oncogene) (eg, multiple endocrine neoplasia, type 2B and familial medullary thyroid carcinoma), common variants (eg, M918T, 2647_2648delinsTT, A883F)

SDHD (succinate dehydrogenase complex, subunit D, integral membrane protein) (eg, hereditary paraganglioma), full gene sequence

►*SLC25A4 (solute carrier family 25 [mitochondrial carrier; adenine nucleotide translocator], member 4)* (eg, progressive external ophthalmoplegia), full gene sequence

TP53 (tumor protein 53) (eg, tumor samples), targeted sequence analysis of 2-5 exons

TTR (transthyretin) (eg, familial transthyretin amyloidosis), full gene sequence

TYR (tyrosinase [oculocutaneous albinism IA]) (eg, oculocutaneous albinism IA), full gene sequence

USH1G (Usher syndrome 1G [autosomal recessive]) (eg, Usher syndrome, type 1), full gene sequence◄

VHL (von Hippel-Lindau tumor suppressor) (eg, von Hippel-Lindau familial cancer syndrome), full gene sequence

VWF (von Willebrand factor) (eg, von Willebrand disease type 1C), targeted sequence analysis (eg, exons 26, 27, 37)

> ➔ *CPT Assistant* May 12:4; *CPT Changes: An Insider's View* 2012, 2013

▲ **81405** *Molecular pathology procedure, Level 6* (eg, analysis of 6-10 exons by DNA sequence analysis, mutation scanning or duplication/deletion variants of 11-25 exons)

► *ABCD1 (ATP-binding cassette, sub-family D [ALD], member 1)* (eg, adrenoleukodystrophy), full gene sequence

ACADS (acyl-CoA dehydrogenase, C-2 to C-3 short chain) (eg, short chain acyl-CoA dehydrogenase deficiency), full gene sequence

ACTC1 (actin, alpha, cardiac muscle 1) (eg, familial hypertrophic cardiomyopathy), full gene sequence

APTX (aprataxin) (eg, ataxia with oculomotor apraxia 1), full gene sequence

AR (androgen receptor) (eg, androgen insensitivity syndrome), full gene sequence

CHRNA4 (cholinergic receptor, nicotinic, alpha 4) (eg, nocturnal frontal lobe epilepsy), full gene sequence

CHRNB2 (cholinergic receptor, nicotinic, beta 2 [neuronal]) (eg, nocturnal frontal lobe epilepsy), full gene sequence◄

CYP21A2 (cytochrome P450, family 21, subfamily A, polypeptide2) (eg, steroid 21-hydroxylase isoform, congenital adrenal hyperplasia), full gene sequence

► *DFNB59 (deafness, autosomal recessive 59)* (eg, autosomal recessive nonsyndromic hearing impairment), full gene sequence

DHCR7 (7-dehydrocholesterol reductase) (eg, Smith-Lemli-Opitz syndrome), full gene sequence

EYA1 (eyes absent homolog 1 [Drosophila]) (eg, branchio-oto-renal [BOR] spectrum disorders), duplication/deletion analysis

F9 (coagulation factor IX) (eg, hemophilia B), full gene sequence

FH (fumarate hydratase) (eg, fumarate hydratase deficiency, hereditary leiomyomatosis with renal cell cancer), full gene sequence◄

FKTN (fukutin) (eg, limb-girdle muscular dystrophy [LGMD] type 2M or 2L), full gene sequence

► *GFAP (glial fibrillary acidic protein)* (eg, Alexander disease), full gene sequence

GLA (galactosidase, alpha) (eg, Fabry disease), full gene sequence

HBA1/HBA2 (alpha globin 1 and alpha globin 2) (eg, thalassemia), full gene sequence

HNF1A (HNF1 homeobox A) (eg, maturity-onset diabetes of the young [MODY]), full gene sequence

HNF1B (HNF1 homeobox B) (eg, maturity-onset diabetes of the young [MODY]), full gene sequence

KRAS (v-Ki-ras2 Kirsten rat sarcoma viral oncogene homolog) (eg, Noonan syndrome), full gene sequence

LAMP2 (lysosomal-associated membrane protein 2) (eg, Danon disease), full gene sequence

MEN1 (multiple endocrine neoplasia I) (eg, multiple endocrine neoplasia type 1, Wermer syndrome), full gene sequence

MPZ (myelin protein zero) (eg, Charcot-Marie-Tooth), full gene sequence

MYL2 (myosin, light chain 2, regulatory, cardiac, slow) (eg, familial hypertrophic cardiomyopathy), full gene sequence

MYL3 (myosin, light chain 3, alkali, ventricular, skeletal, slow) (eg, familial hypertrophic cardiomyopathy), full gene sequence

MYOT (myotilin) (eg, limb-girdle muscular dystrophy), full gene sequence

NEFL (neurofilament, light polypeptide) (eg, Charcot-Marie-Tooth), full gene sequence

NF2 (neurofibromin 2 [merlin]) (eg, neurofibromatosis, type 2), duplication/deletion analysis

NSD1 (nuclear receptor binding SET domain protein 1) (eg, Sotos syndrome), duplication/deletion analysis

OTC (ornithine carbamoyltransferase) (eg, ornithine transcarbamylase deficiency), full gene sequence◄

PDHB (pyruvate dehydrogenase [lipoamide] beta) (eg, lactic acidosis), full gene sequence

PSEN1 (presenilin 1) (eg, Alzheimer disease), full gene sequence

► *RET (ret proto-oncogene)* (eg, multiple endocrine neoplasia, type 2A and familial medullary thyroid carcinoma), targeted sequence analysis (eg, exons 10, 11, 13-16)◄

SDHB (succinate dehydrogenase complex, subunit B, iron sulfur) (eg, hereditary paraganglioma), full gene sequence

► *SDHC (succinate dehydrogenase complex, subunit C, integral membrane protein, 15kDa)* (eg, hereditary paraganglioma-pheochromocytoma syndrome), full gene sequence

SGCA (sarcoglycan, alpha [50kDa dystrophin-associated glycoprotein]) (eg, limb-girdle muscular dystrophy), full gene sequence

SGCB (sarcoglycan, beta [43kDa dystrophin-associated glycoprotein]) (eg, limb-girdle muscular dystrophy), full gene sequence

SGCD (sarcoglycan, delta [35kDa dystrophin-associated glycoprotein]) (eg, limb-girdle muscular dystrophy), full gene sequence

SGCG (sarcoglycan, gamma [35kDa dystrophin-associated glycoprotein]) (eg, limb-girdle muscular dystrophy), full gene sequence

SHOC2 (soc-2 suppressor of clear homolog) (eg, Noonan-like syndrome with loose anagen hair), full gene sequence

SMN1 (survival of motor neuron 1, telomeric) (eg, spinal muscular atrophy), full gene sequence

SPRED1 (sprouty-related, EVH1 domain containing 1) (eg, Legius syndrome), full gene sequence ◄

TGFBR1 (transforming growth factor, beta receptor 1) (eg, Marfan syndrome), full gene sequence

TGFBR2 (transforming growth factor, beta receptor 2) (eg, Marfan syndrome), full gene sequence

THRB (thyroid hormone receptor, beta) (eg, thyroid hormone resistance, thyroid hormone beta receptor deficiency), full gene sequence or targeted sequence analysis of >5 exons

► *TNNI3 (troponin I, type 3 [cardiac])* (eg, familial hypertrophic cardiomyopathy), full gene sequence

TP53 (tumor protein 53) (eg, Li-Fraumeni syndrome, tumor samples), full gene sequence or targeted sequence analysis of >5 exons

TPM1 (tropomyosin 1 [alpha]) (eg, familial hypertrophic cardiomyopathy), full gene sequence

TSC1 (tuberous sclerosis 1) (eg, tuberous sclerosis), duplication/deletion analysis ◄

VWF (von Willebrand factor) (eg, von Willebrand disease type 2N), targeted sequence analysis (eg, exons 18-20, 23-25)

➔ *CPT Assistant* May 12:4; *CPT Changes: An Insider's View* 2012, 2013

▲ **81406**   Molecular pathology procedure, Level 7 (eg, analysis of 11-25 exons by DNA sequence analysis, mutation scanning or duplication/deletion variants of 26-50 exons, cytogenomic array analysis for neoplasia)

► *ACADVL (acyl-CoA dehydrogenase, very long chain)* (eg, very long chain acyl-coenzyme A dehydrogenase deficiency), full gene sequence

ACTN4 (actinin, alpha 4) (eg, focal segmental glomerulosclerosis), full gene sequence

ANO5 (anoctamin 5) (eg, limb-girdle muscular dystrophy), full gene sequence

APP (amyloid beta [A4] precursor protein) (eg, Alzheimer disease), full gene sequence

ATP7B (ATPase, Cu++ transporting, beta polypeptide) (eg, Wilson disease), full gene sequence

BRAF (v-raf murine sarcoma viral oncogene homolog B1) (eg, Noonan syndrome), full gene sequence ◄

CAPN3 (Calpain 3) (eg, limb-girdle muscular dystrophy [LGMD] type 2A, calpainopathy), full gene sequence

► *CBS (cystathionine-beta-synthase)* (eg, homocystinuria, cystathionine beta-synthase deficiency), full gene sequence

CDH1 (cadherin 1, type 1, E-cadherin [epithelial]) (eg, hereditary diffuse gastric cancer), full gene sequence

CDKL5 (cyclin-dependent kinase-like 5) (eg, early infantile epileptic encephalopathy), full gene sequence ◄

Cytogenomic microarray analysis, neoplasia (eg, interrogation of copy number, and loss-of-heterozygosity via single nucleotide polymorphism [SNP]-based comparative genomic hybridization [CGH] microarray analysis)

► *DLAT (dihydrolipoamide S-acetyltransferase)* (eg, pyruvate dehydrogenase E2 deficiency), full gene sequence

DLD (dihydrolipoamide dehydrogenase) (eg, maple syrup urine disease, type III), full gene sequence

EYA1 (eyes absent homolog 1 [Drosophila]) (eg, branchio-oto-renal [BOR] spectrum disorders), full gene sequence

F8 (coagulation factor VIII) (eg, hemophilia A), duplication/deletion analysis

GAA (glucosidase, alpha; acid) (eg, glycogen storage disease type II [Pompe disease]), full gene sequence ◄

GALT (galactose-1-phosphate uridylyltransferase) (eg, galactosemia), full gene sequence

► *GCDH (glutaryl-CoA dehydrogenase)* (eg, glutaricacidemia type 1), full gene sequence

GCK (glucokinase [hexokinase 4]) (eg, maturity-onset diabetes of the young [MODY]), full gene sequence

HADHA (hydroxyacyl-CoA dehydrogenase/3-ketoacyl-CoA thiolase/enoyl-CoA hydratase [trifunctional protein] alpha subunit) (eg, long chain acyl-coenzyme A dehydrogenase deficiency), full gene sequence ◄

HEXA (hexosaminidase A, alpha polypeptide) (eg, Tay-Sachs disease), full gene sequence

► *HNF4A (hepatocyte nuclear factor 4, alpha)* (eg, maturity-onset diabetes of the young [MODY]), full gene sequence

IVD (isovaleryl-CoA dehydrogenase) (eg, isovaleric acidemia), full gene sequence

JAG1 (jagged 1) (eg, Alagille syndrome), duplication/deletion analysis

LDB3 (LIM domain binding 3) (eg, familial dilated cardiomyopathy, myofibrillar myopathy), full gene sequence ◄

LMNA (lamin A/C) (eg, Emery-Dreifuss muscular dystrophy [EDMD1, 2 and 3] limb-girdle muscular dystrophy [LGMD] type 1B, dilated cardiomyopathy [CMD1A], familial partial lipodystrophy [FPLD2]), full gene sequence

Pathology and Laboratory

▶*MAP2K1 (mitogen-activated protein kinase 1)*(eg, cardiofaciocutaneous syndrome), full gene sequence

MAP2K2 (mitogen-activated protein kinase 2)(eg, cardiofaciocutaneous syndrome), full gene sequence

MCCC2 (methylcrotonoyl-CoA carboxylase 2 [beta])(eg, 3-methylcrotonyl carboxylase deficiency), full gene sequence

MUTYH (mutY homolog [E. coli])(eg, MYH-associated polyposis), full gene sequence

NF2 (neurofibromin 2 [merlin])(eg, neurofibromatosis, type 2), full gene sequence

NOTCH3 (notch 3)(eg, cerebral autosomal dominant arteriopathy with subcortical infarcts and leukoencephalopathy [CADASIL]), targeted sequence analysis (eg, exons 1-23)

NSD1 (nuclear receptor binding SET domain protein 1) (eg, Sotos syndrome), full gene sequence

OPA1 (optic atrophy 1)(eg, optic atrophy), duplication/deletion analysis

PAH (phenylalanine hydroxylase)(eg, phenylketonuria), full gene sequence

PALB2 (partner and localizer of BRCA2)(eg, breast and pancreatic cancer), full gene sequence

PAX2 (paired box 2)(eg, renal coloboma syndrome), full gene sequence

PC (pyruvate carboxylase)(eg, pyruvate carboxylase deficiency), full gene sequence

PCCB (propionyl CoA carboxylase, beta polypeptide)(eg, propionic acidemia), full gene sequence

PDHA1 (pyruvate dehydrogenase [lipoamide] alpha 1)(eg, lactic acidosis), full gene sequence

PDHX (pyruvate dehydrogenase complex, component X) (eg, lactic acidosis), full gene sequence◀

POLG (polymerase [DNA directed], gamma)(eg, Alpers-Huttenlocher syndrome, autosomal dominant progressive external ophthalmoplegia), full gene sequence

POMGNT1 (protein O-linked mannose beta1,2-N acetylglucosaminyltransferase)(eg, muscle-eye-brain disease, Walker-Warburg syndrome), full gene sequence

POMT1 (protein-O-mannosyltransferase 1)(eg, limb-girdle muscular dystrophy [LGMD] type 2K, Walker-Warburg syndrome), full gene sequence

POMT2 (protein-O-mannosyltransferase 2)(eg, limb-girdle muscular dystrophy [LGMD] type 2N, Walker-Warburg syndrome), full gene sequence

▶*PRKAG2 (protein kinase, AMP-activated, gamma 2 non-catalytic subunit)*(eg, familial hypertrophic cardiomyopathy with Wolff-Parkinson-White syndrome, lethal congenital glycogen storage disease of heart), full gene sequence

PSEN2 (presenilin 2 [Alzheimer disease 4])(eg, Alzheimer disease), full gene sequence

PTPN11 (protein tyrosine phosphatase, non-receptor type 11)(eg, Noonan syndrome, LEOPARD syndrome), full gene sequence

PYGM (phosphorylase, glycogen, muscle)(eg, glycogen storage disease type V, McArdle disease), full gene sequence

RAF1 (v-raf-1 murine leukemia viral oncogene homolog 1) (eg, LEOPARD syndrome), full gene sequence

RET (ret proto-oncogene)(eg, Hirschsprung disease), full gene sequence◀

RYR1 (ryanodine receptor 1, skeletal)(eg, malignant hyperthermia), targeted sequence analysis of exons with functionally-confirmed mutations

▶*SLC9A6 (solute carrier family 9 [sodium/hydrogen exchanger], member 6)*(eg, Christianson syndrome), full gene sequence

SLC26A4 (solute carrier family 26, member 4)(eg, Pendred syndrome), full gene sequence

SOS1 (son of sevenless homolog 1)(eg, Noonan syndrome, gingival fibromatosis), full gene sequence

TAZ (tafazzin)(eg, methylglutaconic aciduria type 2, Barth syndrome), full gene sequence

TNNT2 (troponin T, type 2 [cardiac])(eg, familial hypertrophic cardiomyopathy), full gene sequence

TSC1 (tuberous sclerosis 1)(eg, tuberous sclerosis), full gene sequence

TSC2 (tuberous sclerosis 2)(eg, tuberous sclerosis), duplication/deletion analysis

UBE3A (ubiquitin protein ligase E3A)(eg, Angelman syndrome), full gene sequence◀

VWF (von Willebrand factor)(von Willebrand disease type 2A), extended targeted sequence analysis (eg, exons 11-16, 24-26, 51, 52)

➔ *CPT Assistant* May 12:4; *CPT Changes: An Insider's View* 2012, 2013

▲ **81407** Molecular pathology procedure, Level 8 (eg, analysis of 26-50 exons by DNA sequence analysis, mutation scanning or duplication/deletion variants of >50 exons, sequence analysis of multiple genes on one platform)

▶*ABCC8 (ATP-binding cassette, sub-family C [CFTR/ MRP], member 8)*(eg, familial hyperinsulinism), full gene sequence

CHD7 (chromodomain helicase DNA binding protein 7) (eg, CHARGE syndrome), full gene sequence

F8 (coagulation factor VIII)(eg, hemophilia A), full gene sequence

JAG1 (jagged 1)(eg, Alagille syndrome), full gene sequence

MYBPC3 (myosin binding protein C, cardiac)(eg, familial hypertrophic cardiomyopathy), full gene sequence

MYH6 (myosin, heavy chain 6, cardiac muscle, alpha) (eg, familial dilated cardiomyopathy), full gene sequence

MYH7 (myosin, heavy chain 7, cardiac muscle, beta) (eg, familial hypertrophic cardiomyopathy, Liang distal myopathy), full gene sequence

MYO7A (myosin VIIA) (eg, Usher syndrome, type 1), full gene sequence

NOTCH1 (notch 1) (eg, aortic valve disease), full gene sequence

OPA1 (optic atrophy 1) (eg, optic atrophy), full gene sequence

PCDH15 (protocadherin-related 15) (eg, Usher syndrome, type 1), full gene sequence

SCN1A (sodium channel, voltage-gated, type 1, alpha subunit) (eg, generalized epilepsy with febrile seizures), full gene sequence

SCN5A (sodium channel, voltage-gated, type V, alpha subunit) (eg, familial dilated cardiomyopathy), full gene sequence

TSC2 (tuberous sclerosis 2) (eg, tuberous sclerosis), full gene sequence◄

USH1C (Usher syndrome 1C [autosomal recessive, severe]) (eg, Usher syndrome, type 1), full gene sequence

➔ *CPT Assistant* May 12:4; *CPT Changes: An Insider's View* 2012, 2013

▲ **81408**   Molecular pathology procedure, Level 9 (eg, analysis of >50 exons in a single gene by DNA sequence analysis)

►*ATM (ataxia telangiectasia mutated)* (eg, ataxia telangiectasia), full gene sequence

CDH23 (cadherin-related 23) (eg, Usher syndrome, type 1), full gene sequence

COL1A1 (collagen, type I, alpha 1) (eg, osteogenesis imperfecta, type I), full gene sequence

COL1A2 (collagen, type I, alpha 2) (eg, osteogenesis imperfecta, type I), full gene sequence

DYSF (dysferlin, limb girdle muscular dystrophy 2B [autosomal recessive]) (eg, limb-girdle muscular dystrophy), full gene sequence◄

FBN1 (fibrillin 1) (eg, Marfan syndrome), full gene sequence

NF1 (neurofibromin 1) (eg, neurofibromatosis, type 1), full gene sequence

RYR1 (ryanodine receptor 1, skeletal) (eg, malignant hyperthermia), full gene sequence

►*USH2A (Usher syndrome 2A [autosomal recessive, mild])* (eg, Usher syndrome, type 2), full gene sequence◄

VWF (von Willebrand factor) (eg, von Willebrand disease types 1 and 3), full gene sequence

➔ *CPT Assistant* May 12:4; *CPT Changes: An Insider's View* 2012, 2013

● **81479**   Unlisted molecular pathology procedure
➔ *CPT Changes: An Insider's View* 2013

►Multianalyte Assays with Algorithmic Analyses◄

►Multianalyte Assays with Algorithmic Analyses (MAAAs) are procedures that utilize multiple results derived from assays of various types, including molecular pathology assays, fluorescent in situ hybridization assays and nonnucleic acid–based assays (eg, proteins, polypeptides, lipids, carbohydrates). Algorithmic analysis using the results of these assays as well as other patient information (if used) is then performed, and reported typically as a numeric score(s) or as a probability. MAAAs are typically unique to a single clinical laboratory or manufacturer. The results of individual component procedure(s) that are inputs to the MAAAs may be provided on the associated laboratory report, however these assays are not reported separately using additional codes.

The format for the code descriptors of MAAAs usually include (in order):

• Disease type (eg, oncology, autoimmune, tissue rejection),

• Material(s) analyzed (eg, DNA, RNA, protein, antibody),

• Number of markers (eg, number of genes, number of proteins),

• Methodology(ies) (eg, microarray, real-time [RT]-PCR, in situ hybridization [ISH], enzyme linked immunosorbent assays [ELISA]),

• Number of functional domains (if indicated),

• Specimen type (eg, blood, fresh tissue, formalin-fixed paraffin embedded),

• Algorithm result type (eg, prognostic, diagnostic),

• Report (eg, probability index, risk score)

MAAAs, including those that do not have a Category I code, may be found in Appendix O. MAAAs that do not have a Category I code are identified in Appendix O by a four-digit number followed by the letter "M." The Category I MAAA codes that are included in this subsection are also included in Appendix O. All MAAA codes are listed in Appendix O along with the procedure's proprietary name.

When a specific MAAA procedure is not listed below or in Appendix O, the procedure must be reported using the Category I MAAA unlisted code (81599).

These codes encompass all analytical services required (eg, cell lysis, nucleic acid stabilization, extraction, digestion, amplification, hybridization, and detection) in addition to the algorithmic analysis itself. Procedures that are

Pathology and Laboratory

required prior to cell lysis (eg, microdissection, codes 88380 and 88381) should be reported separately.◄

● **81500** Oncology (ovarian), biochemical assays of two proteins (CA-125 and HE4), utilizing serum, with menopausal status, algorithm reported as a risk score

➔ *CPT Changes: An Insider's View* 2013

►(Do not report 81500 in conjunction with 86304, 86305)◄

● **81503** Oncology (ovarian), biochemical assays of five proteins (CA-125, apoliproprotein A1, beta-2 microglobulin, transferrin, and pre-albumin), utilizing serum, algorithm reported as a risk score

➔ *CPT Changes: An Insider's View* 2013

►(Do not report 81503 in conjunction with 82172, 82232, 83695, 83700, 84134, 84466, 86304)◄

● **81506** Endocrinology (type 2 diabetes), biochemical assays of seven analytes (glucose, HbA1c, insulin, hs-CRP, adoponectin, ferritin, interleukin 2-receptor alpha), utilizing serum or plasma, algorithm reporting a risk score

➔ *CPT Changes: An Insider's View* 2013

►(Do not report 81506 in conjunction with constituent components [ie, 82728, 82947, 83036, 83525, 86141], 84999 [for adopectin], and 83520 [for interleukin 2-receptor alpha])◄

● **81508** Fetal congenital abnormalities, biochemical assays of two proteins (PAPP-A, hCG [any form]), utilizing maternal serum, algorithm reported as a risk score

➔ *CPT Changes: An Insider's View* 2013

►(Do not report 81508 in conjunction with 84163, 84702)◄

● **81509** Fetal congenital abnormalities, biochemical assays of three proteins (PAPP-A, hCG [any form], DIA), utilizing maternal serum, algorithm reported as a risk score

➔ *CPT Changes: An Insider's View* 2013

►(Do not report 81509 in conjunction with 84163, 84702, 86336)◄

● **81510** Fetal congenital abnormalities, biochemical assays of three analytes (AFP, uE3, hCG [any form]), utilizing maternal serum, algorithm reported as a risk score

➔ *CPT Changes: An Insider's View* 2013

►(Do not report 81510 in conjunction with 82105, 82677, 84702)◄

● **81511** Fetal congenital abnormalities, biochemical assays of four analytes (AFP, uE3, hCG [any form], DIA) utilizing maternal serum, algorithm reported as a risk score (may include additional results from previous biochemical testing)

➔ *CPT Changes: An Insider's View* 2013

►(Do not report 81511 in conjunction with 82105, 82677, 84702, 86336)◄

● **81512** Fetal congenital abnormalities, biochemical assays of five analytes (AFP, uE3, total hCG, hyperglycosylated hCG, DIA) utilizing maternal serum, algorithm reported as a risk score

➔ *CPT Changes: An Insider's View* 2013

►(Do not report 81512 in conjunction with 82105, 82677, 84702, 86336◄

● **81599** Unlisted multianalyte assay with algorithmic analysis

➔ *CPT Changes: An Insider's View* 2013

►(Do not use 81599 for multianalyte assays with algorithmic analyses listed in Appendix O)◄

Chemistry

The material for examination may be from any source unless otherwise specified in the code descriptor. When an analyte is measured in multiple specimens from different sources, or in specimens that are obtained at different times, the analyte is reported separately for each source and for each specimen. The examination is quantitative unless specified. To report an organ or disease oriented panel, see codes 80048-80076.

When a code describes a method where measurement of multiple analytes may require one or several procedures, each procedure is coded separately (eg, 82491-82492, 82541-82544). For example, if two analytes are measured using column chromatography using a single stationary or mobile phase, use 82492. If the same two analytes are measured using different stationary or mobile phase conditions, 82491 would be used twice. If a total of four analytes are measured where two analytes are measured with a single stationary and mobile phase, and the other two analytes are measured using a different stationary and mobile phase, use 82492 twice. If a total of three analytes are measured where two analytes are measured using a single stationary or mobile phase condition, and the third analyte is measured separately using a different stationary or mobile phase procedure, use 82492 once for the two analytes measured under the same condition, and use 82491 once for the third analyte measured separately.

►Clinical information or mathematically calculated values, which are not specifically requested by the ordering physician and are derived from the results of other ordered or performed laboratory tests, are considered part of the ordered test procedure(s) and therefore are not separately reportable service(s).

When the requested analyte result is derived using a calculation that requires values from nonrequested laboratory analyses, only the requested analyte code should be reported.

When the calculated analyte determination requires values derived from other requested and nonrequested laboratory analyses, the requested analyte codes (including those calculated) should be reported.

An exception to the above is when an analyte (eg, urinary creatinine) is performed to compensate for variations in urine concentration (eg, microalbumin, thromboxane metabolites) in random urine samples; the appropriate CPT code is reported for both the ordered analyte and the additional required analyte. When the calculated result(s) represent an algorithmically derived numeric score or probability, see the appropriate multianalyte assay with algorithmic analyses (MAAA) code or the MAAA unlisted code (81599).◄

82000   Acetaldehyde, blood
➔ *CPT Assistant* Aug 05:9, Oct 10:7, Dec 10:7

82003   Acetaminophen

▲ **82009**   Ketone body(s) (eg, acetone, acetoacetic acid, beta-hydroxybutyrate); qualitative
➔ *CPT Assistant* Oct 11:11; *CPT Changes: An Insider's View* 2013

▲ **82010**   quantitative
➔ *CPT Assistant* Oct 11:11; *CPT Changes: An Insider's View* 2013

82013   Acetylcholinesterase

(For gastric acid analysis, use 82930)

(Acid phosphatase, see 84060-84066)

82016   Acylcarnitines; qualitative, each specimen
➔ *CPT Assistant* Nov 98:23

82017   quantitative, each specimen
➔ *CPT Assistant* Nov 98:23; *CPT Changes: An Insider's View* 2000

(For carnitine, use 82379)

82024   Adrenocorticotropic hormone (ACTH)

82030   Adenosine, 5-monophosphate, cyclic (cyclic AMP)

82040   Albumin; serum, plasma or whole blood
➔ *CPT Assistant* Dec 99:2; *CPT Changes: An Insider's View* 2009

82042   urine or other source, quantitative, each specimen
➔ *CPT Changes: An Insider's View* 2001

82043   urine, microalbumin, quantitative
➔ *CPT Assistant* Summer 94:2

82044   urine, microalbumin, semiquantitative (eg, reagent strip assay)
➔ *CPT Assistant* Summer 94:2, Mar 98:3, Sep 02:10

(For prealbumin, use 84134)

82045   ischemia modified
➔ *CPT Changes: An Insider's View* 2005

82055   Alcohol (ethanol); any specimen except breath

(For other volatiles, alcohol, use 84600)

82075   breath

82085   Aldolase

82088   Aldosterone
➔ *CPT Assistant* Oct 10:7

(Alkaline phosphatase, see 84075, 84080)

82101   Alkaloids, urine, quantitative
➔ *CPT Assistant* Aug 05:9, Oct 10:7

(Alphaketoglutarate, see 82009, 82010)

(Alpha tocopherol [Vitamin E], use 84446)

82103   Alpha-1-antitrypsin; total

82104   phenotype

82105   Alpha-fetoprotein (AFP); serum

82106   amniotic fluid

82107   AFP-L3 fraction isoform and total AFP (including ratio)
➔ *CPT Changes: An Insider's View* 2007

82108   Aluminum

82120   Amines, vaginal fluid, qualitative
➔ *CPT Assistant* Nov 99:45; *CPT Changes: An Insider's View* 2000

(For combined pH and amines test for vaginitis, use 82120 and 83986)

82127   Amino acids; single, qualitative, each specimen
➔ *CPT Assistant* Nov 98:24

82128   multiple, qualitative, each specimen
➔ *CPT Assistant* Nov 98:24

82131   single, quantitative, each specimen
➔ *CPT Assistant* May 98:11, Nov 98:24

82135   Aminolevulinic acid, delta (ALA)

82136   Amino acids, 2 to 5 amino acids, quantitative, each specimen
➔ *CPT Assistant* Nov 98:24

82139   Amino acids, 6 or more amino acids, quantitative, each specimen
➔ *CPT Assistant* Nov 98:24

82140   Ammonia

82143   Amniotic fluid scan (spectrophotometric)

(For L/S ratio, use 83661)

(Amobarbital, see 80100-80103 for qualitative analysis, 82205 for quantitative analysis)

82145   Amphetamine or methamphetamine

(For qualitative analysis, see 80100-80103)

82150   Amylase

82154   Androstanediol glucuronide
➔ *CPT Assistant* Summer 94:5

82157   Androstenedione

82160   Androsterone

82163   Angiotensin II

82164   Angiotensin I - converting enzyme (ACE)

(Antidiuretic hormone (ADH), use 84588)

(Antimony, use 83015)

(Antitrypsin, alpha-1-, see 82103, 82104)

82172   Apolipoprotein, each

82175   Arsenic

(For heavy metal screening, use 83015)

82180   Ascorbic acid (Vitamin C), blood

(Aspirin, see acetylsalicylic acid, 80196)

Pathology and Laboratory

(Atherogenic index, blood, ultracentrifugation, quantitative, use 83701)

82190 Atomic absorption spectroscopy, each analyte
➔ *CPT Assistant* Oct 10:7

82205 Barbiturates, not elsewhere specified
➔ *CPT Assistant* Jul 03:7, Aug 05:9, Oct 10:7

(For qualitative analysis, see 80100-80103)

(For B-Natriuretic peptide, use 83880)

82232 Beta-2 microglobulin

(Bicarbonate, use 82374)

82239 Bile acids; total

82240   cholylglycine

(For bile pigments, urine, see 81000-81005)

82247 Bilirubin; total
➔ *CPT Assistant* Nov 98:24, Apr 99:6, Dec 99:1, Jan 00:7, Dec 08:5, Apr 10:11

82248   direct
➔ *CPT Assistant* Nov 98:24, Apr 99:6, Dec 99:1, Apr 10:11

82252   feces, qualitative

82261 Biotinidase, each specimen
➔ *CPT Assistant* Nov 98:24

82270 Blood, occult, by peroxidase activity (eg, guaiac), qualitative; feces, consecutive collected specimens with single determination, for colorectal neoplasm screening (ie, patient was provided 3 cards or single triple card for consecutive collection)
➔ *CPT Assistant* Sep 03:15, Feb 06:7, Apr 08:5; *CPT Changes: An Insider's View* 2002, 2006

82271   other sources
➔ *CPT Assistant* Feb 06:7; *CPT Changes: An Insider's View* 2006

82272 Blood, occult, by peroxidase activity (eg, guaiac), qualitative, feces, 1-3 simultaneous determinations, performed for other than colorectal neoplasm screening
➔ *CPT Assistant* Feb 06:7, Apr 08:5, Jun 09:10; *CPT Changes: An Insider's View* 2006, 2008

(Blood urea nitrogen [BUN], see 84520, 84525)

82274 Blood, occult, by fecal hemoglobin determination by immunoassay, qualitative, feces, 1-3 simultaneous determinations
➔ *CPT Changes: An Insider's View* 2002

82286 Bradykinin
➔ *CPT Assistant* Oct 10:7

82300 Cadmium
➔ *CPT Assistant* Aug 05:9, Oct 10:7

82306 Vitamin D; 25 hydroxy, includes fraction(s), if performed
➔ *CPT Changes: An Insider's View* 2010

\# **82652**   1, 25 dihydroxy, includes fraction(s), if performed
➔ *CPT Changes: An Insider's View* 2010

(82307 has been deleted. For 25 hydroxy vitamin D, use 82306)

82308 Calcitonin

82310 Calcium; total
➔ *CPT Assistant* Dec 99:2

82330   ionized

82331   after calcium infusion test

82340   urine quantitative, timed specimen

82355 Calculus; qualitative analysis
➔ *CPT Changes: An Insider's View* 2002

82360   quantitative analysis, chemical

82365   infrared spectroscopy

82370   X-ray diffraction
➔ *CPT Changes: An Insider's View* 2001

(Carbamates, see individual listings)

82373 Carbohydrate deficient transferrin
➔ *CPT Changes: An Insider's View* 2001

82374 Carbon dioxide (bicarbonate)
➔ *CPT Assistant* Dec 99:2

(See also 82803)

82375 Carboxyhemoglobin; quantitative
➔ *CPT Changes: An Insider's View* 2009

82376   qualitative
➔ *CPT Changes: An Insider's View* 2009

(For transcutaneous measurement of carboxyhemoglobin, use 88740)

82378 Carcinoembryonic antigen (CEA)
➔ *CPT Assistant* Fall 93:25, Aug 96:11

82379 Carnitine (total and free), quantitative, each specimen
➔ *CPT Assistant* Nov 98:24

(For acylcarnitine, see 82016, 82017)

82380 Carotene

82382 Catecholamines; total urine

82383   blood

82384   fractionated

(For urine metabolites, see 83835, 84585)

82387 Cathepsin-D

82390 Ceruloplasmin

82397 Chemiluminescent assay
➔ *CPT Assistant* Fall 93:25, Oct 10:7

82415 Chloramphenicol
➔ *CPT Assistant* Aug 05:9, Oct 10:7

82435 Chloride; blood
➔ *CPT Assistant* Dec 99:2

82436   urine

82438   other source
➔ *CPT Assistant* Jul 03:7

(For sweat collection by iontophoresis, use 89230)

82441   Chlorinated hydrocarbons, screen

(Chlorpromazine, use 84022)

(Cholecalciferol [Vitamin D], use 82306)

82465   Cholesterol, serum or whole blood, total
➔ *CPT Assistant* Dec 99:2, Mar 00:11, Feb 05:9; *CPT Changes: An Insider's View* 2001

(For high density lipoprotein [HDL], use 83718)

82480   Cholinesterase; serum

82482   RBC

82485   Chondroitin B sulfate, quantitative

(Chorionic gonadotropin, see gonadotropin, 84702, 84703)

82486   Chromatography, qualitative; column (eg, gas liquid or HPLC), analyte not elsewhere specified
➔ *CPT Assistant* Nov 98:24-25

82487   paper, 1-dimensional, analyte not elsewhere specified

82488   paper, 2-dimensional, analyte not elsewhere specified

82489   thin layer, analyte not elsewhere specified

82491   Chromatography, quantitative, column (eg, gas liquid or HPLC); single analyte not elsewhere specified, single stationary and mobile phase
➔ *CPT Assistant* Fall 93:25, Nov 98:24-25, Mar 00:3, Mar 11:10

82492   multiple analytes, single stationary and mobile phase
➔ *CPT Assistant* Nov 98:24-25, Mar 00:3, Mar 11:10

82495   Chromium
➔ *CPT Assistant* Oct 10:7

82507   Citrate
➔ *CPT Assistant* Aug 05:9, Oct 10:7

82520   Cocaine or metabolite

(Cocaine, qualitative analysis, see 80100-80103)

(Codeine, qualitative analysis, see 80100-80103)

(Codeine, quantitative analysis, see 82101)

(Complement, see 86160-86162)

82523   Collagen cross links, any method

82525   Copper

(Coproporphyrin, see 84119, 84120)

(Corticosteroids, use 83491)

82528   Corticosterone

82530   Cortisol; free
➔ *CPT Assistant* Summer 94:3

82533   total
➔ *CPT Assistant* Summer 94:3

(C-peptide, use 84681)

82540   Creatine

82541   Column chromatography/mass spectrometry (eg, GC/MS, or HPLC/MS), analyte not elsewhere specified; qualitative, single stationary and mobile phase
➔ *CPT Assistant* Nov 98:24-25

82542   quantitative, single stationary and mobile phase
➔ *CPT Assistant* Nov 98:24-25

82543   stable isotope dilution, single analyte, quantitative, single stationary and mobile phase
➔ *CPT Assistant* Nov 98:24-25

82544   stable isotope dilution, multiple analytes, quantitative, single stationary and mobile phase
➔ *CPT Assistant* Nov 98:24-25, Dec 99:7

82550   Creatine kinase (CK), (CPK); total
➔ *CPT Assistant* Feb 98:1, Dec 99:2

82552   isoenzymes
➔ *CPT Assistant* Feb 98:1

82553   MB fraction only
➔ *CPT Assistant* Feb 98:1

82554   isoforms
➔ *CPT Assistant* Feb 98:1

82565   Creatinine; blood
➔ *CPT Assistant* Dec 99:2

82570   other source

82575   clearance

82585   Cryofibrinogen

82595   Cryoglobulin, qualitative or semi-quantitative (eg, cryocrit)
➔ *CPT Assistant* Oct 10:7; *CPT Changes: An Insider's View* 2001

(For quantitative, cryoglobulin, see 82784, 82785)

(Crystals, pyrophosphate vs urate, use 89060)

82600   Cyanide
➔ *CPT Assistant* Aug 05:9, Oct 10:7

82607   Cyanocobalamin (Vitamin B-12);

82608   unsaturated binding capacity

(Cyclic AMP, use 82030)

(Cyclic GMP, use 83008)

(Cyclosporine, use 80158)

82610   Cystatin C
➔ *CPT Assistant* Apr 08:5, Aug 08:13; *CPT Changes: An Insider's View* 2008

82615   Cystine and homocystine, urine, qualitative

82626   Dehydroepiandrosterone (DHEA)
➔ *CPT Assistant* Summer 94:4

82627   Dehydroepiandrosterone-sulfate (DHEA-S)
➔ *CPT Assistant* Summer 94:4

(Delta-aminolevulinic acid (ALA), use 82135)

82633   Desoxycorticosterone, 11-

▲=Revised code   ●=New code   ▶ ◀=Contains new or revised text   ⊘=Modifier 51 exempt

82634 Deoxycortisol, 11-

(Dexamethasone suppression test, use 80420)

(Diastase, urine, use 82150)

82638 Dibucaine number

(Dichloroethane, use 84600)

(Dichloromethane, use 84600)

(Diethylether, use 84600)

82646 Dihydrocodeinone

(For qualitative analysis, see 80100-80103)

82649 Dihydromorphinone

(For qualitative analysis, see 80100-80103)

82651 Dihydrotestosterone (DHT)

82652 Code is out of numerical sequence. See 82000-84999

82654 Dimethadione

(For qualitative analysis, see 80100-80103)

(Diphenylhydantoin, use 80185)

(Dipropylacetic acid, use 80164)

(Dopamine, see 82382-82384)

(Duodenal contents, see individual enzymes; for intubation and collection, see 43756, 43757)

82656 Elastase, pancreatic (EL-1), fecal, qualitative or semi-quantitative
➔ *CPT Assistant* Sep 05:9; *CPT Changes: An Insider's View* 2005

82657 Enzyme activity in blood cells, cultured cells, or tissue, not elsewhere specified; nonradioactive substrate, each specimen
➔ *CPT Assistant* Nov 98:25

82658 radioactive substrate, each specimen
➔ *CPT Assistant* Nov 98:25

82664 Electrophoretic technique, not elsewhere specified

(Endocrine receptor assays, see 84233-84235)

82666 Epiandrosterone

(Epinephrine, see 82382-82384)

82668 Erythropoietin

82670 Estradiol

82671 Estrogens; fractionated

82672 total

(Estrogen receptor assay, use 84233)

82677 Estriol

82679 Estrone

(Ethanol, see 82055 and 82075)

82690 Ethchlorvynol

(Ethyl alcohol, see 82055 and 82075)

82693 Ethylene glycol

82696 Etiocholanolone
➔ *CPT Assistant* Oct 10:7

(For fractionation of ketosteroids, use 83593)

82705 Fat or lipids, feces; qualitative
➔ *CPT Assistant* Aug 05:9, Oct 10:7

82710 quantitative

82715 Fat differential, feces, quantitative

82725 Fatty acids, nonesterified

82726 Very long chain fatty acids
➔ *CPT Assistant* Nov 98:25

(For long-chain [C20-22] omega-3 fatty acids in red blood cell [RBC] membranes, use Category III code 0111T)

82728 Ferritin

(Fetal hemoglobin, see hemoglobin 83030, 83033, and 85460)

(Fetoprotein, alpha-1, see 82105, 82106)

82731 Fetal fibronectin, cervicovaginal secretions, semi-quantitative
➔ *CPT Assistant* Nov 98:25

82735 Fluoride

82742 Flurazepam

(For qualitative analysis, see 80100-80103)

(Foam stability test, use 83662)

82746 Folic acid; serum

82747 RBC

(Follicle stimulating hormone [FSH], use 83001)

82757 Fructose, semen

(Fructosamine, use 82985)

(Fructose, TLC screen, use 84375)

82759 Galactokinase, RBC

82760 Galactose

82775 Galactose-1-phosphate uridyl transferase; quantitative

82776 screen

● **82777** Galectin-3
➔ *CPT Changes: An Insider's View* 2013

82784 Gammaglobulin (immunoglobulin); IgA, IgD, IgG, IgM, each
➔ *CPT Assistant* Spring 94:31, Aug 00:11; *CPT Changes: An Insider's View* 2010

82785 IgE
➔ *CPT Assistant* Spring 94:31; *CPT Changes: An Insider's View* 2010

(For allergen specific IgE, see 86003, 86005)

82787 immunoglobulin subclasses (eg, IgG1, 2, 3, or 4), each
➔ *CPT Assistant* Oct 10:7; *CPT Changes: An Insider's View* 2001, 2010

(Gamma-glutamyltransferase [GGT], use 82977)

82800   Gases, blood, pH only
> *CPT Assistant* Aug 05:9, Oct 10:7

82803   Gases, blood, any combination of pH, pCO$_2$, pO$_2$, CO$_2$, HCO$_3$ (including calculated O$_2$ saturation);

(Use 82803 for 2 or more of the above listed analytes)

82805   with O$_2$ saturation, by direct measurement, except pulse oximetry

82810   Gases, blood, O$_2$ saturation only, by direct measurement, except pulse oximetry

(For pulse oximetry, use 94760)

82820   Hemoglobin-oxygen affinity (pO$_2$ for 50% hemoglobin saturation with oxygen)
> *CPT Assistant* Oct 10:7

(82926, 82928 have been deleted)

(For gastric acid analysis, use 82930)

82930   Gastric acid analysis, includes pH if performed, each specimen
> *CPT Assistant* Oct 10:7, Dec 10:7, Sep 11:3; *CPT Changes: An Insider's View* 2011

82938   Gastrin after secretin stimulation

82941   Gastrin
> *CPT Assistant* Aug 05:9

(Gentamicin, use 80170)

(GGT, use 82977)

(GLC, gas liquid chromatography, use 82486)

82943   Glucagon

82945   Glucose, body fluid, other than blood
> *CPT Changes: An Insider's View* 2001

82946   Glucagon tolerance test

82947   Glucose; quantitative, blood (except reagent strip)
> *CPT Assistant* Summer 93:14, Summer 94:5, Sep 99:10, Dec 99:2, Jun 02:3, Feb 05:9; *CPT Changes: An Insider's View* 2001

82948   blood, reagent strip
> *CPT Assistant* Summer 94:5, Jan 99:10, Nov 10:10, Oct 11:8

82950   post glucose dose (includes glucose)
> *CPT Assistant* Sep 99:10, Jun 02:3, Feb 05:9

82951   tolerance test (GTT), 3 specimens (includes glucose)
> *CPT Assistant* Feb 01:10, Feb 05:9, Oct 10:7

+ 82952   tolerance test, each additional beyond 3 specimens (List separately in addition to code for primary procedure)
> *CPT Assistant* Feb 01:10, Oct 10:7, Dec 10:7; *CPT Changes: An Insider's View* 2011

(Use 82952 in conjunction with 82951)

82953   tolbutamide tolerance test

(For insulin tolerance test, see 80434, 80435)

(For leucine tolerance test, use 80428)

(For semiquantitative urine glucose, see 81000, 81002, 81005, 81099)

82955   Glucose-6-phosphate dehydrogenase (G6PD); quantitative

82960   screen

(For glucose tolerance test with medication, use 96374 in addition)

82962   Glucose, blood by glucose monitoring device(s) cleared by the FDA specifically for home use
> *CPT Assistant* Summer 94:4, Jan 99:10, Nov 10:10, Oct 11:8

82963   Glucosidase, beta

82965   Glutamate dehydrogenase

82975   Glutamine (glutamic acid amide)

82977   Glutamyltransferase, gamma (GGT)
> *CPT Assistant* Dec 99:1

82978   Glutathione

82979   Glutathione reductase, RBC

82980   Glutethimide

(Glycohemoglobin, use 83036)

82985   Glycated protein
> *CPT Assistant* Summer 94:2, Oct 10:7

(Gonadotropin, chorionic, see 84702, 84703)

83001   Gonadotropin; follicle stimulating hormone (FSH)
> *CPT Assistant* Aug 05:9, Oct 10:7

83002   luteinizing hormone (LH)

(For luteinizing releasing factor [LRH], use 83727)

83003   Growth hormone, human (HGH) (somatotropin)

(For antibody to human growth hormone, use 86277)

83008   Guanosine monophosphate (GMP), cyclic

83009   Helicobacter pylori, blood test analysis for urease activity, non-radioactive isotope (eg, C-13)
> *CPT Changes: An Insider's View* 2005

(For H. pylori, breath test analysis for urease activity, see 83013, 83014)

83010   Haptoglobin; quantitative

83012   phenotypes

83013   Helicobacter pylori; breath test analysis for urease activity, non-radioactive isotope (eg, C-13)
> *CPT Assistant* Nov 98:25, Feb 99:8, Nov 99:45; *CPT Changes: An Insider's View* 2001, 2002, 2005

83014   drug administration
> *CPT Assistant* Nov 98:25, Feb 99:8, Nov 99:45; *CPT Changes: An Insider's View* 2005

(For H. pylori, stool, use 87338. For H. pylori, liquid scintillation counter, see 78267, 78268. For H. pylori, enzyme immunoassay, use 87339)

(For H. pylori, blood test analysis for urease activity, use 83009)

Pathology and Laboratory

83015 Heavy metal (eg, arsenic, barium, beryllium, bismuth, antimony, mercury); screen

83018   quantitative, each

83020 Hemoglobin fractionation and quantitation; electrophoresis (eg, A2, S, C, and/or F)
➔ *CPT Assistant* Nov 98:25

83021   chromatography (eg, A2, S, C, and/or F)
➔ *CPT Assistant* Nov 98:25, Dec 99:7

(For glycosylated [A1c] hemoglobin analysis, by chromatography, in the absence of an identified hemoglobin variant, use 83036)

83026 Hemoglobin; by copper sulfate method, non-automated

83030   F (fetal), chemical

83033   F (fetal), qualitative
➔ *CPT Changes: An Insider's View* 2001

83036   glycosylated (A1C)
➔ *CPT Assistant* Summer 94:2, Feb 06:7, Oct 06:15; *CPT Changes: An Insider's View* 2006

(For glycosylated [A1c] hemoglobin analysis, by chromatography, in the setting of an identified hemoglobin variant, use 83021)

(For fecal hemoglobin detection by immunoassay, use 82274)

83037   glycosylated (A1C) by device cleared by FDA for home use
➔ *CPT Assistant* Feb 06:7, Oct 06:15; *CPT Changes: An Insider's View* 2006

83045   methemoglobin, qualitative

83050   methemoglobin, quantitative

(For transcutaneous quantitative methemoglobin determination, use 88741)

83051   plasma

83055   sulfhemoglobin, qualitative

83060   sulfhemoglobin, quantitative

83065   thermolabile

83068   unstable, screen

83069   urine

83070 Hemosiderin; qualitative

83071   quantitative

(Heroin, see 80100-80103)

(HIAA, use 83497)

(High performance liquid chromatography [HPLC], use 82486)

83080 b-Hexosaminidase, each assay
➔ *CPT Assistant* Nov 98:25

83088 Histamine

(Hollander test, see 43754, 43755)

83090 Homocysteine
➔ *CPT Assistant* Jan 01:13, Oct 10:7; *CPT Changes: An Insider's View* 2001

83150 Homovanillic acid (HVA)
➔ *CPT Assistant* Aug 05:9, Oct 10:7

(Hormones, see individual alphabetic listings in **Chemistry** section)

(Hydrogen breath test, use 91065)

83491 Hydroxycorticosteroids, 17- (17-OHCS)
➔ *CPT Assistant* Aug 05:9, Oct 10:7

(For cortisol, see 82530, 82533. For deoxycortisol, use 82634)

83497 Hydroxyindolacetic acid, 5-(HIAA)

(For urine qualitative test, use 81005)

(5-Hydroxytryptamine, use 84260)

83498 Hydroxyprogesterone, 17-d

83499 Hydroxyprogesterone, 20-
➔ *CPT Assistant* Oct 10:7

83500 Hydroxyproline; free
➔ *CPT Assistant* Aug 05:9, Oct 10:7

83505   total

83516 Immunoassay for analyte other than infectious agent antibody or infectious agent antigen; qualitative or semiquantitative, multiple step method
➔ *CPT Assistant* Nov 98:25; *CPT Changes: An Insider's View* 2010

83518   qualitative or semiquantitative, single step method (eg, reagent strip)
➔ *CPT Assistant* Fall 93:26; *CPT Changes: An Insider's View* 2010

83519   quantitative, by radioimmunoassay (eg, RIA)
➔ *CPT Assistant* Fall 93:26, Summer 94:2; *CPT Changes: An Insider's View* 2010

83520   quantitative, not otherwise specified
➔ *CPT Assistant* Fall 93:26; *CPT Changes: An Insider's View* 2010

(For immunoassays for antibodies to infectious agent antigens, see analyte and method specific codes in the **Immunology** section)

(For immunoassay of tumor antigen not elsewhere specified, use 86316)

(Immunoglobulins, see 82784, 82785)

83525 Insulin; total

(For proinsulin, use 84206)

83527   free
➔ *CPT Assistant* Summer 94:5

83528 Intrinsic factor

(For intrinsic factor antibodies, use 86340)

83540 Iron
➔ *CPT Assistant* Fall 93:25

83550 Iron binding capacity

83570 Isocitric dehydrogenase (IDH)

(Isonicotinic acid hydrazide, INH, see code for specific method)

(Isopropyl alcohol, use 84600)

83582 Ketogenic steroids, fractionation

(Ketone bodies, for serum, see 82009, 82010; for urine, see 81000-81003)

83586 Ketosteroids, 17- (17-KS); total

83593   fractionation
> *CPT Assistant* Oct 10:7

83605 Lactate (lactic acid)
> *CPT Assistant* Aug 05:9, Oct 10:7

83615 Lactate dehydrogenase (LD), (LDH);
> *CPT Assistant* Fall 93:25, Feb 98:1, Dec 99:2

83625   isoenzymes, separation and quantitation
> *CPT Assistant* Fall 93:25, Feb 98:1

83630 Lactoferrin, fecal; qualitative
> *CPT Assistant* Feb 06:7; *CPT Changes: An Insider's View* 2005, 2006

83631   quantitative
> *CPT Assistant* Feb 06:7, Jan 07:29; *CPT Changes: An Insider's View* 2006

83632 Lactogen, human placental (HPL) human chorionic somatomammotropin

83633 Lactose, urine; qualitative

83634   quantitative

(For tolerance, see 82951, 82952)

(For breath hydrogen test for lactase deficiency, use 91065)

83655 Lead

83661 Fetal lung maturity assessment; lecithin sphingomyelin (L/S) ratio
> *CPT Changes: An Insider's View* 2001

83662   foam stability test

83663   fluorescence polarization
> *CPT Changes: An Insider's View* 2001

83664   lamellar body density
> *CPT Changes: An Insider's View* 2001

(For phosphatidylglycerol, use 84081)

83670 Leucine aminopeptidase (LAP)

83690 Lipase

83695 Lipoprotein (a)
> *CPT Assistant* Feb 06:7; *CPT Changes: An Insider's View* 2006

83698 Lipoprotein-associated phospholipase A_2 (Lp-PLA$_2$)
> *CPT Assistant* Oct 10:7; *CPT Changes: An Insider's View* 2007

83700 Lipoprotein, blood; electrophoretic separation and quantitation
> *CPT Assistant* Feb 06:7, Oct 10:7; *CPT Changes: An Insider's View* 2006

83701   high resolution fractionation and quantitation of lipoproteins including lipoprotein subclasses when performed (eg, electrophoresis, ultracentrifugation)
> *CPT Assistant* Feb 06:7; *CPT Changes: An Insider's View* 2006

83704   quantitation of lipoprotein particle numbers and lipoprotein particle subclasses (eg, by nuclear magnetic resonance spectroscopy)
> *CPT Assistant* Feb 06:7; *CPT Changes: An Insider's View* 2006

83718 Lipoprotein, direct measurement; high density cholesterol (HDL cholesterol)
> *CPT Assistant* Oct 99:11, Mar 00:11, Feb 05:9

83719   VLDL cholesterol
> *CPT Assistant* Oct 99:11

83721   LDL cholesterol
> *CPT Assistant* Nov 98:25, Oct 99:11

(For fractionation by high resolution electrophoresis or ultracentrifugation, use 83701)

(For lipoprotein particle numbers and subclasses analysis by nuclear magnetic resonance spectroscopy, use 83704)

83727 Luteinizing releasing factor (LRH)

(Luteinizing hormone [LH], use 83002)

(For qualitative analysis, see 80100-80103)

(Macroglobulins, alpha-2, use 86329)

83735 Magnesium

83775 Malate dehydrogenase

(Maltose tolerance, see 82951, 82952)

(Mammotropin, use 84146)

83785 Manganese

(Marijuana, see 80100-80103)

83788 Mass spectrometry and tandem mass spectrometry (MS, MS/MS), analyte not elsewhere specified; qualitative, each specimen
> *CPT Assistant* Nov 98:26

83789   quantitative, each specimen
> *CPT Assistant* Nov 98:26, Oct 10:7

83805 Meprobamate
> *CPT Assistant* Aug 05:9, Oct 10:7

(For qualitative analysis, see 80100-80103)

83825 Mercury, quantitative

(Mercury screen, use 83015)

83835 Metanephrines

(For catecholamines, see 82382-82384)

83840	Methadone

(For methadone qualitative analysis, see 80100-80103)

(Methamphetamine, see 80100-80103, 82145)

(Methanol, use 84600)

83857	Methemalbumin

(Methemoglobin, see hemoglobin 83045, 83050)

83858	Methsuximide

(Methyl alcohol, use 84600)

(Microalbumin, see 82043 for quantitative, see 82044 for semiquantitative)

83861 Microfluidic analysis utilizing an integrated collection and analysis device, tear osmolarity

➔ *CPT Assistant* Oct 10:7, Dec 10:7; *CPT Changes: An Insider's View* 2011

(Microglobulin, beta-2, use 82232)

(For microfluidic tear osmolarity of both eyes, report 83861 twice)

83864 Mucopolysaccharides, acid; quantitative

83866 screen

83872 Mucin, synovial fluid (Ropes test)

83873 Myelin basic protein, cerebrospinal fluid

➔ *CPT Changes: An Insider's View* 2002

(For oligoclonal bands, use 83916)

83874 Myoglobin

➔ *CPT Assistant* Feb 98:1

(Nalorphine, use 83925)

83876 Myeloperoxidase (MPO)

➔ *CPT Changes: An Insider's View* 2009

83880 Natriuretic peptide

➔ *CPT Assistant* Jul 03:7; *CPT Changes: An Insider's View* 2003

83883 Nephelometry, each analyte not elsewhere specified

83885 Nickel

83887 Nicotine

▶(83890-83914 have been deleted. To report, see 81200-81479)◀

83915 Nucleotidase 5'-

83916 Oligoclonal immune (oligoclonal bands)

➔ *CPT Changes: An Insider's View* 2002

83918 Organic acids; total, quantitative, each specimen

➔ *CPT Assistant* Mar 96:11, Nov 98:26; *CPT Changes: An Insider's View* 2001

83919 qualitative, each specimen

➔ *CPT Assistant* Nov 98:26

83921 Organic acid, single, quantitative

➔ *CPT Changes: An Insider's View* 2001

83925 Opiate(s), drug and metabolites, each procedure

➔ *CPT Changes: An Insider's View* 2009

83930 Osmolality; blood

83935 urine

(For tear osmolarity using microfluidic analysis, use 83861)

83937 Osteocalcin (bone g1a protein)

➔ *CPT Assistant* Summer 94:5

83945 Oxalate

83950 Oncoprotein; HER-2/neu

➔ *CPT Changes: An Insider's View* 2002, 2009

(For tissue, see 88342, 88365)

83951 des-gamma-carboxy-prothrombin (DCP)

➔ *CPT Changes: An Insider's View* 2009

83970 Parathormone (parathyroid hormone)

(Pesticide, quantitative, see code for specific method. For screen for chlorinated hydrocarbons, use 82441)

83986 pH; body fluid, not otherwise specified

➔ *CPT Changes: An Insider's View* 2010

83987 exhaled breath condensate

➔ *CPT Changes: An Insider's View* 2010

(For blood pH, see 82800, 82803)

83992 Phencyclidine (PCP)

(For qualitative analysis, see 80100-80103)

(Phenobarbital, use 80184)

83993 Calprotectin, fecal

➔ *CPT Assistant* Apr 08:5, Oct 10:7; *CPT Changes: An Insider's View* 2008

84022 Phenothiazine

➔ *CPT Assistant* Aug 05:9, Oct 10:7

(For qualitative analysis, see 80100, 80101)

84030 Phenylalanine (PKU), blood

(Phenylalanine-tyrosine ratio, see 84030, 84510)

84035 Phenylketones, qualitative

84060 Phosphatase, acid; total

84061 forensic examination

84066 prostatic

84075 Phosphatase, alkaline;

➔ *CPT Assistant* Dec 99:2

84078 heat stable (total not included)

84080 isoenzymes

84081 Phosphatidylglycerol

(Phosphates inorganic, use 84100)

(Phosphates, organic, see code for specific method. For cholinesterase, see 82480, 82482)

84085 Phosphogluconate, 6-, dehydrogenase, RBC

84087 Phosphohexose isomerase

➔ *CPT Assistant* Oct 10:7

84100 Phosphorus inorganic (phosphate);
➜ *CPT Assistant* Dec 99:2, Aug 05:9, Oct 10:7

84105 urine

(Pituitary gonadotropins, see 83001-83002)

(PKU, see 84030, 84035)

84106 Porphobilinogen, urine; qualitative

84110 quantitative

84112 Placental alpha microglobulin-1 (PAMG-1), cervicovaginal secretion, qualitative
➜ *CPT Assistant* Oct 10:8, Dec 10:8; *CPT Changes: An Insider's View* 2011

84119 Porphyrins, urine; qualitative

84120 quantitation and fractionation

84126 Porphyrins, feces; quantitative

84127 qualitative

(Porphyrin precursors, see 82135, 84106, 84110)

(For protoporphyrin, RBC, see 84202, 84203)

84132 Potassium; serum, plasma or whole blood
➜ *CPT Assistant* Dec 99:2, Jun 02:3; *CPT Changes: An Insider's View* 2009

84133 urine

84134 Prealbumin

(For microalbumin, see 82043, 82044)

84135 Pregnanediol

84138 Pregnanetriol

84140 Pregnenolone
➜ *CPT Assistant* Summer 94:6

84143 17-hydroxypregnenolone
➜ *CPT Assistant* Summer 94:6

84144 Progesterone

(Progesterone receptor assay, use 84234)

(For proinsulin, use 84206)

84145 Procalcitonin (PCT)
➜ *CPT Changes: An Insider's View* 2010

84146 Prolactin

84150 Prostaglandin, each

84152 Prostate specific antigen (PSA); complexed (direct measurement)
➜ *CPT Changes: An Insider's View* 2001

84153 total
➜ *CPT Assistant* Fall 93:26, May 96:10, Aug 96:10, Jan 97:10, Nov 98:26, Aug 99:5, Dec 99:10

84154 free
➜ *CPT Assistant* Nov 98:26, Aug 99:5, Dec 99:10

84155 Protein, total, except by refractometry; serum, plasma or whole blood
➜ *CPT Assistant* Dec 99:2, Jan 00:7; *CPT Changes: An Insider's View* 2004, 2009

84156 urine
➜ *CPT Changes: An Insider's View* 2004

84157 other source (eg, synovial fluid, cerebrospinal fluid)
➜ *CPT Changes: An Insider's View* 2004

84160 Protein, total, by refractometry, any source
➜ *CPT Changes: An Insider's View* 2004

(For urine total protein by dipstick method, use 81000-81003)

84163 Pregnancy-associated plasma protein-A (PAPP-A)
➜ *CPT Changes: An Insider's View* 2005

84165 Protein; electrophoretic fractionation and quantitation, serum
➜ *CPT Changes: An Insider's View* 2004, 2005

84166 electrophoretic fractionation and quantitation, other fluids with concentration (eg, urine, CSF)
➜ *CPT Changes: An Insider's View* 2005

84181 Western Blot, with interpretation and report, blood or other body fluid

84182 Western Blot, with interpretation and report, blood or other body fluid, immunological probe for band identification, each
➜ *CPT Assistant* Oct 10:7

(For Western Blot tissue analysis, use 88371)

84202 Protoporphyrin, RBC; quantitative
➜ *CPT Assistant* Aug 05:9, Oct 10:7

84203 screen

84206 Proinsulin

(Pseudocholinesterase, use 82480)

84207 Pyridoxal phosphate (Vitamin B-6)

84210 Pyruvate

84220 Pyruvate kinase

84228 Quinine

84233 Receptor assay; estrogen

84234 progesterone

84235 endocrine, other than estrogen or progesterone (specify hormone)

84238 non-endocrine (specify receptor)
➜ *CPT Assistant* Nov 05:14; *CPT Changes: An Insider's View* 2006

84244 Renin

84252 Riboflavin (Vitamin B-2)

(Salicylates, use 80196)

(Secretin test, see 99070, 43756, 43757 and appropriate analyses)

84255 Selenium

84260 Serotonin

(For urine metabolites (HIAA), use 83497)

84270 Sex hormone binding globulin (SHBG)
➔ *CPT Assistant* Summer 94:4

84275 Sialic acid

(Sickle hemoglobin, use 85660)

84285 Silica

84295 Sodium; serum, plasma or whole blood
➔ *CPT Assistant* Dec 99:2, Oct 10:7; *CPT Changes: An Insider's View* 2009

84300   urine
➔ *CPT Assistant* Aug 05:9, Oct 10:7

84302   other source
➔ *CPT Assistant* Jul 03:7; *CPT Changes: An Insider's View* 2003

(Somatomammotropin, use 83632)

(Somatotropin, use 83003)

84305 Somatomedin
➔ *CPT Assistant* Summer 94:4

84307 Somatostatin
➔ *CPT Assistant* Summer 94:4

84311 Spectrophotometry, analyte not elsewhere specified

84315 Specific gravity (except urine)

(For specific gravity, urine, see 81000-81003)

(Stone analysis, see 82355-82370)

84375 Sugars, chromatographic, TLC or paper chromatography

84376 Sugars (mono-, di-, and oligosaccharides); single qualitative, each specimen
➔ *CPT Assistant* Nov 98:26-27, Dec 99:7

84377   multiple qualitative, each specimen
➔ *CPT Assistant* Nov 98:26-27, Jul 03:7

84378   single quantitative, each specimen
➔ *CPT Assistant* Nov 98:26-27

84379   multiple quantitative, each specimen
➔ *CPT Assistant* Nov 98:26-27, Dec 99:7, Jul 03:7

84392 Sulfate, urine
➔ *CPT Assistant* Oct 10:7

(Sulfhemoglobin, see hemoglobin, 83055, 83060)

(T-3, see 84479-84481)

(T-4, see 84436-84439)

84402 Testosterone; free
➔ *CPT Assistant* Aug 05:9, Oct 10:7

84403   total

84425 Thiamine (Vitamin B-1)

84430 Thiocyanate

84431 Thromboxane metabolite(s), including thromboxane if performed, urine
➔ *CPT Changes: An Insider's View* 2010

(For concurrent urine creatinine determination, use 84431 in conjunction with 82570)

84432 Thyroglobulin
➔ *CPT Assistant* Summer 94:2

(Thyroglobulin, antibody, use 86800)

(Thyrotropin releasing hormone [TRH] test, see 80438, 80439)

84436 Thyroxine; total
➔ *CPT Assistant* Fall 93:25, Summer 94:3

84437   requiring elution (eg, neonatal)

84439   free

84442 Thyroxine binding globulin (TBG)

84443 Thyroid stimulating hormone (TSH)
➔ *CPT Assistant* Summer 94:3

84445 Thyroid stimulating immune globulins (TSI)
➔ *CPT Assistant* Summer 94:3; *CPT Changes: An Insider's View* 2002

(Tobramycin, use 80200)

84446 Tocopherol alpha (Vitamin E)

(Tolbutamide tolerance, use 82953)

84449 Transcortin (cortisol binding globulin)
➔ *CPT Assistant* Summer 94:6

84450 Transferase; aspartate amino (AST) (SGOT)
➔ *CPT Assistant* Dec 99:2

84460   alanine amino (ALT) (SGPT)
➔ *CPT Assistant* Dec 99:2

84466 Transferrin
➔ *CPT Assistant* Summer 94:4

(Iron binding capacity, use 83550)

84478 Triglycerides
➔ *CPT Assistant* Dec 99:2, Mar 00:11, Feb 05:9

84479 Thyroid hormone (T3 or T4) uptake or thyroid hormone binding ratio (THBR)
➔ *CPT Assistant* Fall 93:25, Summer 94:3

84480 Triiodothyronine T3; total (TT-3)

84481   free

84482   reverse
➔ *CPT Assistant* Summer 94:2

84484 Troponin, quantitative
➔ *CPT Assistant* Nov 97:29, Jan 98:6, Feb 98:1

(For troponin, qualitative assay, use 84512)

84485 Trypsin; duodenal fluid

84488   feces, qualitative

84490   feces, quantitative, 24-hour collection
➔ *CPT Assistant* Oct 10:7

84510 Tyrosine
➔ *CPT Assistant* Oct 10:7

(Urate crystal identification, use 89060)

84512   Troponin, qualitative
> *CPT Assistant* Nov 97:29, Jan 98:6, Feb 98:1

(For troponin, quantitative assay, use 84484)

84520   Urea nitrogen; quantitative
> *CPT Assistant* Dec 99:2

84525   semiquantitative (eg, reagent strip test)
> *CPT Assistant* Mar 98:3

84540   Urea nitrogen, urine

84545   Urea nitrogen, clearance

84550   Uric acid; blood
> *CPT Assistant* Dec 99:2

84560   other source

84577   Urobilinogen, feces, quantitative

84578   Urobilinogen, urine; qualitative

84580   quantitative, timed specimen

84583   semiquantitative

(Uroporphyrins, use 84120)

(Valproic acid [dipropylacetic acid], use 80164)

84585   Vanillylmandelic acid (VMA), urine

84586   Vasoactive intestinal peptide (VIP)
> *CPT Assistant* Summer 94:6

84588   Vasopressin (antidiuretic hormone, ADH)

84590   Vitamin A
> *CPT Assistant* Aug 05:9

(Vitamin B-1, use 84425)

(Vitamin B-2, use 84252)

(Vitamin B-6, use 84207)

(Vitamin B-12, use 82607)

(Vitamin B-12, absorption (Schilling), see 78270, 78271)

(Vitamin C, use 82180)

(Vitamin D, see 82306, 82652)

(Vitamin E, use 84446)

84591   Vitamin, not otherwise specified
> *CPT Changes: An Insider's View* 2001

84597   Vitamin K
> *CPT Assistant* Oct 10:7

(VMA, use 84585)

84600   Volatiles (eg, acetic anhydride, carbon tetrachloride, dichloroethane, dichloromethane, diethylether, isopropyl alcohol, methanol)
> *CPT Assistant* Aug 05:9, Oct 10:7

(For acetaldehyde, use 82000)

(Volume, blood, RISA or Cr-51, see 78110, 78111)

84620   Xylose absorption test, blood and/or urine

(For administration, use 99070)

84630   Zinc

84681   C-peptide
> *CPT Assistant* Oct 10:7

84702   Gonadotropin, chorionic (hCG); quantitative
> *CPT Assistant* Oct 10:7

84703   qualitative

(For urine pregnancy test by visual color comparison, use 81025)

84704   free beta chain
> *CPT Assistant* Apr 08:5, Aug 08:13, Oct 10:7; *CPT Changes: An Insider's View* 2008

84830   Ovulation tests, by visual color comparison methods for human luteinizing hormone
> *CPT Assistant* Oct 10:7

84999   Unlisted chemistry procedure
> *CPT Assistant* Oct 00:24, Aug 05:9, Oct 10:7, Dec 10:7

Hematology and Coagulation

(For blood banking procedures, see **Transfusion Medicine**)

(Agglutinins, see **Immunology**)

(Antiplasmin, use 85410)

(Antithrombin III, see 85300, 85301)

85002   Bleeding time
> *CPT Assistant* Aug 05:9

85004   Blood count; automated differential WBC count
> *CPT Assistant* Jan 04:26; *CPT Changes: An Insider's View* 2003

85007   blood smear, microscopic examination with manual differential WBC count
> *CPT Assistant* Jul 03:7, Jan 04:26; *CPT Changes: An Insider's View* 2003

85008   blood smear, microscopic examination without manual differential WBC count
> *CPT Assistant* Jul 03:8, Jan 04:26; *CPT Changes: An Insider's View* 2003

(For other fluids [eg, CSF], see 89050, 89051)

85009   manual differential WBC count, buffy coat
> *CPT Assistant* Jul 03:7, Jan 04:26; *CPT Changes: An Insider's View* 2003

(Eosinophils, nasal smear, use 89190)

85013   spun microhematocrit

85014   hematocrit (Hct)
> *CPT Assistant* Jul 03:7; *CPT Changes: An Insider's View* 2003

85018   hemoglobin (Hgb)
> *CPT Assistant* Jul 03:8; *CPT Changes: An Insider's View* 2003

(For other hemoglobin determination, see 83020-83069)

(For immunoassay, hemoglobin, fecal, use 82274)

(For transcutaneous hemoglobin measurement, use 88738)

85025   complete (CBC), automated (Hgb, Hct, RBC, WBC and platelet count) and automated differential WBC count
➔ *CPT Assistant* Jul 00:11, Jul 03:7, Jan 04:26, Jul 11:16; *CPT Changes: An Insider's View* 2003

85027   complete (CBC), automated (Hgb, Hct, RBC, WBC and platelet count)
➔ *CPT Assistant* Jul 03:8, Jan 04:26; *CPT Changes: An Insider's View* 2003

85032   manual cell count (erythrocyte, leukocyte, or platelet) each
➔ *CPT Assistant* Jul 03:8, Nov 03:15; *CPT Changes: An Insider's View* 2003

85041   red blood cell (RBC), automated
➔ *CPT Assistant* Jul 03:8; *CPT Changes: An Insider's View* 2003

(Do not report code 85041 in conjunction with 85025 or 85027)

85044   reticulocyte, manual
➔ *CPT Assistant* Jul 03:8; *CPT Changes: An Insider's View* 2003

85045   reticulocyte, automated
➔ *CPT Assistant* Jul 03:8; *CPT Changes: An Insider's View* 2003

85046   reticulocytes, automated, including 1 or more cellular parameters (eg, reticulocyte hemoglobin content [CHr], immature reticulocyte fraction [IRF], reticulocyte volume [MRV], RNA content), direct measurement
➔ *CPT Assistant* Nov 98:27; *CPT Changes: An Insider's View* 2005

85048   leukocyte (WBC), automated
➔ *CPT Assistant* Jul 03:8; *CPT Changes: An Insider's View* 2003

85049   platelet, automated
➔ *CPT Changes: An Insider's View* 2003

85055   Reticulated platelet assay
➔ *CPT Changes: An Insider's View* 2004

85060   Blood smear, peripheral, interpretation by physician with written report

85097   Bone marrow, smear interpretation
➔ *CPT Assistant* Winter 92:17, Jul 98:4, Mar 03:22; *CPT Changes: An Insider's View* 2002

(For special stains, see 88312, 88313)

(For bone biopsy, see 20220, 20225, 20240, 20245, 20250, 20251)

85130   Chromogenic substrate assay
➔ *CPT Assistant* Aug 05:9

(Circulating anti-coagulant screen [mixing studies], see 85611, 85732)

85170   Clot retraction

85175   Clot lysis time, whole blood dilution

(Clotting factor I [fibrinogen], see 85384, 85385)

85210   Clotting; factor II, prothrombin, specific
➔ *CPT Assistant* Aug 05:9

(See also 85610-85613)

85220   factor V (AcG or proaccelerin), labile factor

85230   factor VII (proconvertin, stable factor)

85240   factor VIII (AHG), 1-stage

85244   factor VIII related antigen

85245   factor VIII, VW factor, ristocetin cofactor

85246   factor VIII, VW factor antigen

85247   factor VIII, von Willebrand factor, multimetric analysis

85250   factor IX (PTC or Christmas)

85260   factor X (Stuart-Prower)

85270   factor XI (PTA)

85280   factor XII (Hageman)

85290   factor XIII (fibrin stabilizing)

85291   factor XIII (fibrin stabilizing), screen solubility

85292   prekallikrein assay (Fletcher factor assay)

85293   high molecular weight kininogen assay (Fitzgerald factor assay)

85300   Clotting inhibitors or anticoagulants; antithrombin III, activity
➔ *CPT Assistant* Aug 05:9

85301   antithrombin III, antigen assay

85302   protein C, antigen

85303   protein C, activity

85305   protein S, total

85306   protein S, free

85307   Activated Protein C (APC) resistance assay
➔ *CPT Changes: An Insider's View* 2001

85335   Factor inhibitor test

85337   Thrombomodulin

(For mixing studies for inhibitors, use 85732)

85345   Coagulation time; Lee and White

85347   activated

85348   other methods

(Differential count, see 85007 et seq)

(Duke bleeding time, use 85002)

(Eosinophils, nasal smear, use 89190)

85360   Euglobulin lysis

(Fetal hemoglobin, see 83030, 83033, 85460)

85362   Fibrin(ogen) degradation (split) products (FDP) (FSP); agglutination slide, semiquantitative

(Immunoelectrophoresis, use 86320)

85366   paracoagulation

85370   quantitative

85378   Fibrin degradation products, D-dimer; qualitative or semiquantitative
→ *CPT Assistant* Jul 03:8; *CPT Changes: An Insider's View* 2003

85379   quantitative

(For ultrasensitive and standard sensitivity quantitative D-dimer, use 85379)

85380   ultrasensitive (eg, for evaluation for venous thromboembolism), qualitative or semiquantitative
→ *CPT Assistant* Jul 03:8; *CPT Changes: An Insider's View* 2003

85384   Fibrinogen; activity

85385   antigen

85390   Fibrinolysins or coagulopathy screen, interpretation and report

85396   Coagulation/fibrinolysis assay, whole blood (eg, viscoelastic clot assessment), including use of any pharmacologic additive(s), as indicated, including interpretation and written report, per day
→ *CPT Changes: An Insider's View* 2004

85397   Coagulation and fibrinolysis, functional activity, not otherwise specified (eg, ADAMTS-13), each analyte
→ *CPT Changes: An Insider's View* 2009

85400   Fibrinolytic factors and inhibitors; plasmin
→ *CPT Assistant* Aug 05:9

85410   alpha-2 antiplasmin

85415   plasminogen activator

85420   plasminogen, except antigenic assay

85421   plasminogen, antigenic assay

(Fragility, red blood cell, see 85547, 85555-85557)

85441   Heinz bodies; direct

85445   induced, acetyl phenylhydrazine

(Hematocrit [PCV], see 85014, 85025, 85027)

(Hemoglobin, see 83020-83068, 85018, 85025, 85027)

85460   Hemoglobin or RBCs, fetal, for fetomaternal hemorrhage; differential lysis (Kleihauer-Betke)
→ *CPT Assistant* Fall 93:25

(See also 83030, 83033)

(Hemolysins, see 86940, 86941)

85461   rosette

85475   Hemolysin, acid

(See also 86940, 86941)

85520   Heparin assay
→ *CPT Assistant* Aug 05:9

85525   Heparin neutralization

85530   Heparin-protamine tolerance test

85536   Iron stain, peripheral blood
→ *CPT Changes: An Insider's View* 2001

(For iron stains on bone marrow or other tissues with physician evaluation, use 88313)

85540   Leukocyte alkaline phosphatase with count

85547   Mechanical fragility, RBC

85549   Muramidase

(Nitroblue tetrazolium dye test, use 86384)

85555   Osmotic fragility, RBC; unincubated

85557   incubated

(Packed cell volume, use 85013)

(Partial thromboplastin time, see 85730, 85732)

(Parasites, blood [eg, malaria smears], use 87207)

(Plasmin, use 85400)

(Plasminogen, use 85420)

(Plasminogen activator, use 85415)

85576   Platelet, aggregation (in vitro), each agent
→ *CPT Assistant* Jul 96:10; *CPT Changes: An Insider's View* 2003

(For thromboxane metabolite[s], including thromboxane, if performed, measurement[s] in urine, use 84431)

85597   Phospholipid neutralization; platelet
→ *CPT Assistant* Oct 10:8, Dec 10:8, Apr 11:9; *CPT Changes: An Insider's View* 2011

85598   hexagonal phospholipid
→ *CPT Assistant* Oct 10:8, Dec 10:8, Apr 11:9; *CPT Changes: An Insider's View* 2011

85610   Prothrombin time;
→ *CPT Assistant* Aug 05:9

85611   substitution, plasma fractions, each

85612   Russell viper venom time (includes venom); undiluted

85613   diluted

(Red blood cell count, see 85025, 85027, 85041)

85635   Reptilase test

(Reticulocyte count, see 85044, 85045)

85651   Sedimentation rate, erythrocyte; non-automated

85652   automated

85660   Sickling of RBC, reduction

(Hemoglobin electrophoresis, use 83020)

(Smears [eg, for parasites, malaria], use 87207)

85670   Thrombin time; plasma

85675   titer

85705   Thromboplastin inhibition, tissue
→ *CPT Assistant* Aug 05:9

Pathology and Laboratory

(For individual clotting factors, see 85245-85247)

85730   Thromboplastin time, partial (PTT); plasma or whole blood

85732   substitution, plasma fractions, each
➔ *CPT Assistant* Apr 11:9

85810   Viscosity

(von Willebrand factor assay, see 85245-85247)

(WBC count, see 85025, 85027, 85048, 89050)

85999   Unlisted hematology and coagulation procedure
➔ *CPT Assistant* Aug 05:9, Oct 09:12

Immunology

(Acetylcholine receptor antibody, see 83519, 86255, 86256)

(Actinomyces, antibodies to, use 86602)

(Adrenal cortex antibodies, see 86255, 86256)

86000   Agglutinins, febrile (eg, Brucella, Francisella, Murine typhus, Q fever, Rocky Mountain spotted fever, scrub typhus), each antigen
➔ *CPT Assistant* Aug 05:9

(For antibodies to infectious agents, see 86602-86804)

86001   Allergen specific IgG quantitative or semiquantitative, each allergen
➔ *CPT Changes: An Insider's View* 2001

(Agglutinins and autohemolysins, see 86940, 86941)

86003   Allergen specific IgE; quantitative or semiquantitative, each allergen
➔ *CPT Assistant* Spring 94:31

(For total quantitative IgE, use 82785)

86005   qualitative, multiallergen screen (dipstick, paddle, or disk)
➔ *CPT Assistant* Spring 94:31

(For total qualitative IgE, use 83518)

(Alpha-1 antitrypsin, see 82103, 82104)

(Alpha-1 feto-protein, see 82105, 82106)

(Anti-AChR [acetylcholine receptor] antibody titer, see 86255, 86256)

(Anticardiolipin antibody, use 86147)

(Anti-DNA, use 86225)

(Anti-deoxyribonuclease titer, use 86215)

86021   Antibody identification; leukocyte antibodies

86022   platelet antibodies

86023   platelet associated immunoglobulin assay

86038   Antinuclear antibodies (ANA);

86039   titer

(Antistreptococcal antibody, ie, anti-DNAse, use 86215)

(Antistreptokinase titer, use 86590)

86060   Antistreptolysin 0; titer

(For antibodies to infectious agents, see 86602-86804)

86063   screen

(For antibodies to infectious agents, see 86602-86804)

(Blastomyces, antibodies to, use 86612)

86077   Blood bank physician services; difficult cross match and/or evaluation of irregular antibody(s), interpretation and written report

86078   investigation of transfusion reaction including suspicion of transmissible disease, interpretation and written report

86079   authorization for deviation from standard blood banking procedures (eg, use of outdated blood, transfusion of Rh incompatible units), with written report

(Brucella, antibodies to, use 86622)

(Candida, antibodies to, use 86628. For skin testing, use 86485)

86140   C-reactive protein;
➔ *CPT Assistant* Aug 05:9; *CPT Changes: An Insider's View* 2002

(Candidiasis, use 86628)

86141   high sensitivity (hsCRP)
➔ *CPT Changes: An Insider's View* 2002

86146   Beta 2 Glycoprotein I antibody, each
➔ *CPT Changes: An Insider's View* 2001

86147   Cardiolipin (phospholipid) antibody, each Ig class
➔ *CPT Changes: An Insider's View* 2001

#● 86152   Cell enumeration using immunologic selection and identification in fluid specimen (eg, circulating tumor cells in blood);
➔ *CPT Changes: An Insider's View* 2013

▶(For physician interpretation and report, use 86153. For cell enumeration with interpretation and report, use 86152 and 86153)◀

#● 86153   physician interpretation and report, when required
➔ *CPT Changes: An Insider's View* 2013

▶(For cell enumeration, use 86152. For cell enumeration with interpretation and report, use 86152 and 86153)

▶(For flow cytometric immunophenotyping, see 88184-88189)◀

▶(For flow cytometric quantitation, see 86355, 86356, 86357, 86359, 86360, 86361, 86367)◀

86148   Anti-phosphatidylserine (phospholipid) antibody
➔ *CPT Assistant* Nov 97:30, Jul 03:8, Nov 03:5

▶(To report antiprothrombin [phospholipid cofactor] antibody, use 86849)◀

86152   Code is out of numerical sequence. See 86000-86804

86153   Code is out of numerical sequence. See 86000-86804

86155   Chemotaxis assay, specify method

(Clostridium difficile toxin, use 87230)

(Coccidioides, antibodies to, see 86635. For skin testing, use 86490)

86156   Cold agglutinin; screen

86157   titer

86160   Complement; antigen, each component

86161   functional activity, each component

86162   total hemolytic (CH50)

86171   Complement fixation tests, each antigen

(Coombs test, see 86880-86886)

86185   Counterimmunoelectrophoresis, each antigen

(Cryptococcus, antibodies to, use 86641)

86200   Cyclic citrullinated peptide (CCP), antibody
➔ *CPT Assistant* Mar 06:6; *CPT Changes: An Insider's View* 2006

86215   Deoxyribonuclease, antibody
➔ *CPT Assistant* Aug 05:9

86225   Deoxyribonucleic acid (DNA) antibody; native or double stranded

(Echinococcus, antibodies to, see code for specific method)

(For HIV antibody tests, see 86701-86703)

86226   single stranded

(Anti D.S., DNA, IFA, eg, using C.Lucilae, see 86255 and 86266)

86235   Extractable nuclear antigen, antibody to, any method (eg, nRNP, SS-A, SS-B, Sm, RNP, Sc170, J01), each antibody

86243   Fc receptor

(Filaria, antibodies to, see code for specific method)

86255   Fluorescent noninfectious agent antibody; screen, each antibody
➔ *CPT Assistant* Nov 98:27

86256   titer, each antibody

(Fluorescent technique for antigen identification in tissue, use 88346; for indirect fluorescence, use 88347)

(FTA, use 86780)

(Gel [agar] diffusion tests, use 86331)

86277   Growth hormone, human (HGH), antibody

86280   Hemagglutination inhibition test (HAI)

(For rubella, use 86762)

(For antibodies to infectious agents, see 86602-86804)

86294   Immunoassay for tumor antigen, qualitative or semiquantitative (eg, bladder tumor antigen)
➔ *CPT Changes: An Insider's View* 2001

(For qualitative NMP22 protein, use 86386)

86300   Immunoassay for tumor antigen, quantitative; CA 15-3 (27.29)
➔ *CPT Assistant* Aug 05:9; *CPT Changes: An Insider's View* 2001

86301   CA 19-9
➔ *CPT Changes: An Insider's View* 2001

86304   CA 125
➔ *CPT Changes: An Insider's View* 2001

(For measurement of serum HER-2/neu oncoprotein, see 83950)

(For hepatitis delta agent, antibody, use 86692)

86305   Human epididymis protein 4 (HE4)
➔ *CPT Changes: An Insider's View* 2010

86308   Heterophile antibodies; screening

(For antibodies to infectious agents, see 86602-86804)

86309   titer

(For antibodies to infectious agents, see 86602-86804)

86310   titers after absorption with beef cells and guinea pig kidney

(Histoplasma, antibodies to, use 86698. For skin testing, use 86510)

(For antibodies to infectious agents, see 86602-86804)

(Human growth hormone antibody, use 86277)

86316   Immunoassay for tumor antigen, other antigen, quantitative (eg, CA 50, 72-4, 549), each
➔ *CPT Assistant* May 96:11, Aug 96:11, Apr 98:15, Aug 99:5, Dec 99:10; *CPT Changes: An Insider's View* 2001

86317   Immunoassay for infectious agent antibody, quantitative, not otherwise specified
➔ *CPT Assistant* Nov 97:30-31

(For immunoassay techniques for antigens, see 83516, 83518, 83519, 83520, 87301-87450, 87810-87899)

(For particle agglutination procedures, use 86403)

86318   Immunoassay for infectious agent antibody, qualitative or semiquantitative, single step method (eg, reagent strip)
➔ *CPT Assistant* Mar 07:10

86320   Immunoelectrophoresis; serum

86325   other fluids (eg, urine, cerebrospinal fluid) with concentration
➔ *CPT Changes: An Insider's View* 2002

86327   crossed (2-dimensional assay)

86329   Immunodiffusion; not elsewhere specified
➔ *CPT Assistant* Aug 00:11

86331   gel diffusion, qualitative (Ouchterlony), each antigen or antibody

86332   Immune complex assay

86334   Immunofixation electrophoresis; serum
➔ *CPT Changes: An Insider's View* 2005

Pathology and Laboratory

86335   other fluids with concentration (eg, urine, CSF)
→ *CPT Changes: An Insider's View* 2005

86336   Inhibin A
→ *CPT Changes: An Insider's View* 2002

86337   Insulin antibodies

86340   Intrinsic factor antibodies

(Leptospira, antibodies to, use 86720)

(Leukoagglutinins, use 86021)

86341   Islet cell antibody
→ *CPT Assistant* Summer 94:6

86343   Leukocyte histamine release test (LHR)

86344   Leukocyte phagocytosis

86352   Cellular function assay involving stimulation (eg, mitogen or antigen) and detection of biomarker (eg, ATP)
→ *CPT Changes: An Insider's View* 2010

86353   Lymphocyte transformation, mitogen (phytomitogen) or antigen induced blastogenesis

(Malaria antibodies, use 86750)

(For cellular function assay involving stimulation and detection of biomarker, use 86352)

86355   B cells, total count
→ *CPT Assistant* Mar 06:6, Apr 08:5; *CPT Changes: An Insider's View* 2006

86356   Mononuclear cell antigen, quantitative (eg, flow cytometry), not otherwise specified, each antigen
→ *CPT Assistant* Apr 08:5; *CPT Changes: An Insider's View* 2008

(Do not report 88187-88189 for interpretation of 86355, 86356, 86357, 86359, 86360, 86361, 86367)

86357   Natural killer (NK) cells, total count
→ *CPT Assistant* Mar 06:6, Apr 08:5; *CPT Changes: An Insider's View* 2006

86359   T cells; total count
→ *CPT Assistant* Nov 97:30, Apr 08:5

86360   absolute CD4 and CD8 count, including ratio
→ *CPT Assistant* Nov 97:30, Jan 07:29, Apr 08:5

86361   absolute CD4 count
→ *CPT Assistant* Nov 97:30, Apr 08:5

86367   Stem cells (ie, CD34), total count
→ *CPT Assistant* Mar 06:6, Apr 08:5; *CPT Changes: An Insider's View* 2006

(For flow cytometric immunophenotyping for the assessment of potential hematolymphoid neoplasia, see 88184-88189)

86376   Microsomal antibodies (eg, thyroid or liver-kidney), each

86378   Migration inhibitory factor test (MIF)

(Mitochondrial antibody, liver, see 86255, 86256)

(Mononucleosis, see 86308-86310)

86382   Neutralization test, viral

86384   Nitroblue tetrazolium dye test (NTD)

86386   Nuclear Matrix Protein 22 (NMP22), qualitative
→ *CPT Changes: An Insider's View* 2012

(Ouchterlony diffusion, use 86331)

(Platelet antibodies, see 86022, 86023)

86403   Particle agglutination; screen, each antibody
→ *CPT Assistant* Aug 05:9

86406   titer, each antibody

(Pregnancy test, see 84702, 84703)

(Rapid plasma reagin test (RPR), see 86592, 86593)

86430   Rheumatoid factor; qualitative

86431   quantitative

(Serologic test for syphilis, see 86592, 86593)

86480   Tuberculosis test, cell mediated immunity antigen response measurement; gamma interferon
→ *CPT Assistant* Mar 06:6, Oct 10:7, Dec 10:8; *CPT Changes: An Insider's View* 2006, 2011

86481   enumeration of gamma interferon-producing T-cells in cell suspension
→ *CPT Assistant* Oct 10:8, Dec 10:8; *CPT Changes: An Insider's View* 2011

86485   Skin test; candida

(For antibody, candida, use 86628)

86486   unlisted antigen, each
→ *CPT Changes: An Insider's View* 2008

86490   coccidioidomycosis

86510   histoplasmosis
→ *CPT Assistant* Aug 05:9

(For histoplasma, antibody, use 86698)

86580   tuberculosis, intradermal

(For tuberculosis test, cell mediated immunity measurement of gamma interferon antigen response, use 86480)

►(For skin tests for allergy, see 95012-95199)◄

(Smooth muscle antibody, see 86255, 86256)

(Sporothrix, antibodies to, see code for specific method)

(For skin testing, unlisted antigen, use 86486. For flow cytometry, quantitative, not otherwise specified, use 86356)

86590   Streptokinase, antibody

(For antibodies to infectious agents, see 86602-86804)

(Streptolysin O antibody, see antistreptolysin O, 86060, 86063)

86592   Syphilis test, non-treponemal antibody; qualitative (eg, VDRL, RPR, ART)
→ *CPT Changes: An Insider's View* 2010

(For antibodies to infectious agents, see 86602-86804)

Pathology and Laboratory

86593   quantitative
> *CPT Changes: An Insider's View* 2010

(For antibodies to infectious agents, see 86602-86804)

(Tetanus antibody, use 86774)

(Thyroglobulin antibody, use 86800)

(Thyroglobulin, use 84432)

(Thyroid microsomal antibody, use 86376)

(For toxoplasma antibody, see 86777-86778)

The following codes (86602-86804) are qualitative or semiquantitative immunoassays performed by multiple-step methods for the detection of antibodies to infectious agents. For immunoassays by single-step method (eg, reagent strips), use code 86318. Procedures for the identification of antibodies should be coded as precisely as possible. For example, an antibody to a virus could be coded with increasing specificity for virus, family, genus, species, or type. In some cases, further precision may be added to codes by specifying the class of immunoglobulin being detected. When multiple tests are done to detect antibodies to organisms classified more precisely than the specificity allowed by available codes, it is appropriate to code each as a separate service. For example, a test for antibody to an enterovirus is coded as 86658. Coxsackie viruses are enteroviruses, but there are no codes for the individual species of enterovirus. If assays are performed for antibodies to coxsackie A and B species, each assay should be separately coded. Similarly, if multiple assays are performed for antibodies of different immunoglobulin classes, each assay should be coded separately. When a coding option exists for reporting IgM specific antibodies (eg, 86632), the corresponding nonspecific code (eg, 86631) may be reported for performance of either an antibody analysis not specific for a particular immunoglobulin class or for an IgG analysis.

(For the detection of antibodies other than those to infectious agents, see specific antibody [eg, 86021-86023, 86376, 86800, 86850-86870] or specific method [eg, 83516, 86255, 86256]).

(For infectious agent/antigen detection, see 87260-87899)
> *CPT Assistant* Fall 93:26

86602   Antibody; actinomyces
> *CPT Assistant* Aug 05:9

86603   adenovirus

86606   Aspergillus

86609   bacterium, not elsewhere specified

86611   Bartonella
> *CPT Changes: An Insider's View* 2001

86612   Blastomyces

86615   Bordetella

86617   Borrelia burgdorferi (Lyme disease) confirmatory test (eg, Western Blot or immunoblot)

86618   Borrelia burgdorferi (Lyme disease)

86619   Borrelia (relapsing fever)

86622   Brucella

86625   Campylobacter

86628   Candida

(For skin test, candida, use 86485)

86631   Chlamydia

86632   Chlamydia, IgM
> *CPT Assistant* Nov 97:31

(For chlamydia antigen, see 87270, 87320. For fluorescent antibody technique, see 86255, 86256)

86635   Coccidioides

86638   Coxiella burnetii (Q fever)

86641   Cryptococcus

86644   cytomegalovirus (CMV)

86645   cytomegalovirus (CMV), IgM
> *CPT Assistant* Jul 03:7

86648   Diphtheria

86651   encephalitis, California (La Crosse)

86652   encephalitis, Eastern equine

86653   encephalitis, St. Louis

86654   encephalitis, Western equine

86658   enterovirus (eg, coxsackie, echo, polio)

(Trichinella, antibodies to, use 86784)

(Trypanosoma, antibodies to, see code for specific method)

(Tuberculosis, use 86580 for skin testing)

(Viral antibodies, see code for specific method)

86663   Epstein-Barr (EB) virus, early antigen (EA)

86664   Epstein-Barr (EB) virus, nuclear antigen (EBNA)

86665   Epstein-Barr (EB) virus, viral capsid (VCA)

86666   Ehrlichia
> *CPT Changes: An Insider's View* 2001

86668   Francisella tularensis

86671   fungus, not elsewhere specified

86674   Giardia lamblia

86677   Helicobacter pylori
> *CPT Assistant* Jan 98:6

86682   helminth, not elsewhere specified

86684   Haemophilus influenza

86687   HTLV-I

86688   HTLV-II

86689 HTLV or HIV antibody, confirmatory test (eg, Western Blot)
➔ *CPT Assistant* Mar 08:3

86692 hepatitis, delta agent
➔ *CPT Assistant* Nov 97:31

(For hepatitis delta agent, antigen, use 87380)

86694 herpes simplex, non-specific type test

86695 herpes simplex, type 1

86696 herpes simplex, type 2
➔ *CPT Changes: An Insider's View* 2001

86698 histoplasma

86701 HIV-1
➔ *CPT Assistant* Aug 05:9, Mar 08:3, Apr 08:5

86702 HIV-2
➔ *CPT Assistant* Mar 08:3, Apr 08:5

86703 HIV-1 and HIV-2, single result
➔ *CPT Assistant* Nov 97:31, Mar 08:3, Apr 08:5; *CPT Changes: An Insider's View* 2012

(For HIV-1 antigen(s) with HIV-1 and HIV-2 antibodies, single result, use 87389)

(When HIV immunoassay [HIV testing 86701-86703 or 87389] is performed using a kit or transportable instrument that wholly or in part consists of a single use, disposable analytical chamber, the service may be identified by adding modifier 92 to the usual code)

(For HIV-1 antigen, use 87390)

(For HIV-2 antigen, use 87391)

(For confirmatory test for HIV antibody (eg, Western Blot), use 86689)

86704 Hepatitis B core antibody (HBcAb); total
➔ *CPT Assistant* Nov 97:31-32; *CPT Changes: An Insider's View* 2001

86705 IgM antibody
➔ *CPT Assistant* Nov 97:31-32

86706 Hepatitis B surface antibody (HBsAb)
➔ *CPT Assistant* Nov 97:31-32

86707 Hepatitis Be antibody (HBeAb)
➔ *CPT Assistant* Nov 97:31-32

86708 Hepatitis A antibody (HAAb); total
➔ *CPT Assistant* Nov 97:31-32, Jun 00:11; *CPT Changes: An Insider's View* 2001

86709 IgM antibody
➔ *CPT Assistant* Nov 97:31-32, Jun 00:11

86710 Antibody; influenza virus

● **86711** JC (John Cunningham) virus
➔ *CPT Changes: An Insider's View* 2013

86713 Legionella

86717 Leishmania

86720 Leptospira

86723 Listeria monocytogenes

86727 lymphocytic choriomeningitis

86729 lymphogranuloma venereum

86732 mucormycosis

86735 mumps

86738 mycoplasma

86741 Neisseria meningitidis

86744 Nocardia

86747 parvovirus

86750 Plasmodium (malaria)

86753 protozoa, not elsewhere specified

86756 respiratory syncytial virus

86757 Rickettsia
➔ *CPT Changes: An Insider's View* 2001

86759 rotavirus

86762 rubella

86765 rubeola

86768 Salmonella

86771 Shigella

86774 tetanus

86777 Toxoplasma

86778 Toxoplasma, IgM

86780 Treponema pallidum
➔ *CPT Changes: An Insider's View* 2010

(86781 has been deleted)

(For syphilis testing by non-treponemal antibody analysis, see 86592-86593)

86784 Trichinella

86787 varicella-zoster

86788 West Nile virus, IgM
➔ *CPT Changes: An Insider's View* 2007

86789 West Nile virus
➔ *CPT Changes: An Insider's View* 2007

86790 virus, not elsewhere specified

86793 Yersinia

86800 Thyroglobulin antibody
➔ *CPT Assistant* Aug 05:9

(For thyroglobulin, use 84432)

86803 Hepatitis C antibody;
➔ *CPT Assistant* Nov 97:31-32

86804 confirmatory test (eg, immunoblot)
➔ *CPT Assistant* Nov 97:31-32

Tissue Typing

86805 Lymphocytotoxicity assay, visual crossmatch; with titration

86806 without titration

86807 Serum screening for cytotoxic percent reactive antibody (PRA); standard method
➔ *CPT Assistant* Jun 01:11

86808 quick method
➔ *CPT Assistant* Jun 01:11

86812 HLA typing; A, B, or C (eg, A10, B7, B27), single antigen
➔ *CPT Assistant* Mar 03:23, Jun 06:17

86813 A, B, or C, multiple antigens
➔ *CPT Assistant* Mar 03:23, Jun 06:17

86816 DR/DQ, single antigen
➔ *CPT Assistant* Mar 03:23

86817 DR/DQ, multiple antigens
➔ *CPT Assistant* Mar 03:23

86821 lymphocyte culture, mixed (MLC)
➔ *CPT Assistant* Mar 03:23

86822 lymphocyte culture, primed (PLC)
➔ *CPT Assistant* Mar 03:23

(For HLA typing by molecular pathology techniques, see 81370-81383)

86825 Human leukocyte antigen (HLA) crossmatch, non-cytotoxic (eg, using flow cytometry); first serum sample or dilution
➔ *CPT Changes: An Insider's View* 2010

+ 86826 each additional serum sample or sample dilution (List separately in addition to primary procedure)
➔ *CPT Changes: An Insider's View* 2010

(Use 86826 in conjunction with 86825)

(Do not report 86825, 86826 in conjunction with 86355, 86359, 88184-88189 for antibody surface markers integral to crossmatch testing)

(For autologous HLA crossmatch, see 86825, 86826)

(For lymphocytotoxicity visual crossmatch, see 86805, 86806)

● 86828 Antibody to human leukocyte antigens (HLA), solid phase assays (eg, microspheres or beads, ELISA, flow cytometry); qualitative assessment of the presence or absence of antibody(ies) to HLA Class I and Class II HLA antigens
➔ *CPT Changes: An Insider's View* 2013

● 86829 qualitative assessment of the presence or absence of antibody(ies) to HLA Class I or Class II HLA antigens
➔ *CPT Changes: An Insider's View* 2013

►(If solid phase testing is performed to assess presence or absence of antibody to both HLA classes, use 86828)◄

● 86830 antibody identification by qualitative panel using complete HLA phenotypes, HLA Class I
➔ *CPT Changes: An Insider's View* 2013

● 86831 antibody identification by qualitative panel using complete HLA phenotypes, HLA Class II
➔ *CPT Changes: An Insider's View* 2013

● 86832 high definition qualitative panel for identification of antibody specificities (eg, individual antigen per bead methodology), HLA Class I
➔ *CPT Changes: An Insider's View* 2013

● 86833 high definition qualitative panel for identification of antibody specificities (eg, individual antigen per bead methodology), HLA Class II
➔ *CPT Changes: An Insider's View* 2013

►(If solid phase testing is performed to test for HLA Class I or II antibody after treatment [eg, to remove IgM antibodies or other interfering substances], report 86828-86833 once for each panel with the untreated serum and once for each panel with the treated serum)◄

● 86834 semi-quantitative panel (eg, titer), HLA Class I
➔ *CPT Changes: An Insider's View* 2013

● 86835 semi-quantitative panel (eg, titer), HLA Class II
➔ *CPT Changes: An Insider's View* 2013

86849 Unlisted immunology procedure
➔ *CPT Assistant* Mar 98:10

Transfusion Medicine

(For apheresis, use 36511, 36512)

(For therapeutic phlebotomy, use 99195)

86850 Antibody screen, RBC, each serum technique
➔ *CPT Assistant* Fall 93:25, Aug 05:9, Apr 08:5

86860 Antibody elution (RBC), each elution

86870 Antibody identification, RBC antibodies, each panel for each serum technique
➔ *CPT Assistant* Fall 93:25, Mar 01:10

86880 Antihuman globulin test (Coombs test); direct, each antiserum

86885 indirect, qualitative, each reagent red cell
➔ *CPT Assistant* Apr 08:5; *CPT Changes: An Insider's View* 2008

86886 indirect, each antibody titer
➔ *CPT Assistant* Apr 08:5; *CPT Changes: An Insider's View* 2008

(For indirect antihuman globulin [Coombs] test for RBC antibody screening, use 86850)

(For indirect antihuman globulin [Coombs] test for RBC antibody identification using reagent red cell panels, use 86870)

Pathology and Laboratory

86890   Autologous blood or component, collection processing and storage; predeposited
→ *CPT Assistant* Apr 96:2

86891   intra- or postoperative salvage

(For physician services to autologous donors, see 99201-99204)

86900   Blood typing; ABO
→ *CPT Assistant* Aug 05:9

86901   Rh (D)
→ *CPT Assistant* Fall 93:25

86902   antigen testing of donor blood using reagent serum, each antigen test
→ *CPT Assistant* Oct 10:8, Dec 10:8; *CPT Changes: An Insider's View* 2011

(If multiple blood units are tested for the same antigen, 86902 should be reported once for each antigen for each unit tested)

(86903 has been deleted. To report, use 86902)

86904   antigen screening for compatible unit using patient serum, per unit screened

86905   RBC antigens, other than ABO or Rh (D), each

86906   Rh phenotyping, complete

86910   Blood typing, for paternity testing, per individual; ABO, Rh and MN

86911   each additional antigen system

86920   Compatibility test each unit; immediate spin technique
→ *CPT Assistant* Mar 06:6

86921   incubation technique
→ *CPT Assistant* Mar 06:6

86922   antiglobulin technique
→ *CPT Assistant* Mar 06:6

86923   electronic
→ *CPT Assistant* Mar 06:6; *CPT Changes: An Insider's View* 2006

(Do not use 86923 in conjunction with 86920-86922 for same unit crossmatch)

86927   Fresh frozen plasma, thawing, each unit

86930   Frozen blood, each unit; freezing (includes preparation)
→ *CPT Assistant* Apr 96:2, Jul 03:8; *CPT Changes: An Insider's View* 2003

86931   thawing
→ *CPT Assistant* Jul 03:8; *CPT Changes: An Insider's View* 2003

86932   freezing (includes preparation) and thawing
→ *CPT Assistant* Jul 03:8; *CPT Changes: An Insider's View* 2003

86940   Hemolysins and agglutinins; auto, screen, each

86941   incubated

86945   Irradiation of blood product, each unit
→ *CPT Assistant* Dec 07:14

86950   Leukocyte transfusion
►(For allogeneic lymphocyte infusion, use 38242)◄

(For leukapheresis, use 36511)

86960   Volume reduction of blood or blood product (eg, red blood cells or platelets), each unit
→ *CPT Assistant* Mar 06:6; *CPT Changes: An Insider's View* 2006

86965   Pooling of platelets or other blood products
→ *CPT Assistant* Oct 10:8, Dec 10:8

(For injection(s) of platelet rich plasma, use 0232T)

86970   Pretreatment of RBCs for use in RBC antibody detection, identification, and/or compatibility testing; incubation with chemical agents or drugs, each

86971   incubation with enzymes, each

86972   by density gradient separation

86975   Pretreatment of serum for use in RBC antibody identification; incubation with drugs, each

86976   by dilution

86977   incubation with inhibitors, each

86978   by differential red cell absorption using patient RBCs or RBCs of known phenotype, each absorption

86985   Splitting of blood or blood products, each unit
→ *CPT Assistant* Apr 96:2, May 12:11

86999   Unlisted transfusion medicine procedure
→ *CPT Assistant* Aug 05:9, Nov 05:14, Mar 09:10, Apr 09:9, May 12:11

Microbiology

Includes bacteriology, mycology, parasitology, and virology.

►Presumptive identification of microorganisms is defined as identification by colony morphology, growth on selective media, Gram stains, or up to three tests (eg, catalase, oxidase, indole, urease). Definitive identification of microorganisms is defined as an identification to the genus or species level that requires additional tests (eg, biochemical panels, slide cultures). If additional studies involve molecular probes, nucleic acid sequencing, chromatography, or immunologic techniques, these should be separately coded using 87140-87158, in addition to definitive identification codes. The molecular diagnostic codes (eg, 81200-81408) are not to be used in combination with or instead of the procedures represented by 87140-87158. For multiple specimens/sites use modifier 59. For repeat laboratory tests performed on the same day, use modifier 91.◄

87001   Animal inoculation, small animal; with observation
→ *CPT Assistant* Aug 05:9

87003   with observation and dissection

87015   Concentration (any type), for infectious agents
→ *CPT Changes: An Insider's View* 2001

(Do not report 87015 in conjunction with 87177)

87040   Culture, bacterial; blood, aerobic, with isolation and presumptive identification of isolates (includes anaerobic culture, if appropriate)

➔ *CPT Assistant* Aug 97:18, Jun 02:2, Oct 10:17, Dec 10:17; *CPT Changes: An Insider's View* 2001, 2004

87045   stool, aerobic, with isolation and preliminary examination (eg, KIA, LIA), Salmonella and Shigella species

➔ *CPT Changes: An Insider's View* 2001, 2002, 2004

87046   stool, aerobic, additional pathogens, isolation and presumptive identification of isolates, each plate

➔ *CPT Changes: An Insider's View* 2001, 2002, 2004, 2005

87070   any other source except urine, blood or stool, aerobic, with isolation and presumptive identification of isolates

➔ *CPT Assistant* Aug 97:18, Nov 01:10, Oct 03:10, Nov 11:11; *CPT Changes: An Insider's View* 2001, 2004

(For urine, use 87088)

87071   quantitative, aerobic with isolation and presumptive identification of isolates, any source except urine, blood or stool

➔ *CPT Assistant* Jun 02:3, Sep 03:3; *CPT Changes: An Insider's View* 2001

(For urine, use 87088)

87073   quantitative, anaerobic with isolation and presumptive identification of isolates, any source except urine, blood or stool

➔ *CPT Assistant* Jun 02:3; *CPT Changes: An Insider's View* 2001

(For definitive identification of isolates, use 87076 or 87077. For typing of isolates see 87140-87158)

87075   any source, except blood, anaerobic with isolation and presumptive identification of isolates

➔ *CPT Changes: An Insider's View* 2001, 2004

87076   anaerobic isolate, additional methods required for definitive identification, each isolate

➔ *CPT Changes: An Insider's View* 2001

87077   aerobic isolate, additional methods required for definitive identification, each isolate

➔ *CPT Assistant* Nov 01:10, Nov 11:10; *CPT Changes: An Insider's View* 2001

87081   Culture, presumptive, pathogenic organisms, screening only;

➔ *CPT Assistant* Nov 01:10; *CPT Changes: An Insider's View* 2001

87084   with colony estimation from density chart

87086   Culture, bacterial; quantitative colony count, urine

➔ *CPT Assistant* Nov 11:10; *CPT Changes: An Insider's View* 2001

87088   with isolation and presumptive identification of each isolate, urine

➔ *CPT Assistant* Nov 11:10; *CPT Changes: An Insider's View* 2001, 2007

87101   Culture, fungi (mold or yeast) isolation, with presumptive identification of isolates; skin, hair, or nail

➔ *CPT Assistant* Sep 99:10, Aug 05:9; *CPT Changes: An Insider's View* 2001

87102   other source (except blood)

87103   blood

87106   Culture, fungi, definitive identification, each organism; yeast

➔ *CPT Changes: An Insider's View* 2001

87107   mold

➔ *CPT Changes: An Insider's View* 2001

87109   Culture, mycoplasma, any source

87110   Culture, chlamydia, any source

➔ *CPT Changes: An Insider's View* 2001

(For immunofluorescence staining of shell vials, use 87140)

87116   Culture, tubercle or other acid-fast bacilli (eg, TB, AFB, mycobacteria) any source, with isolation and presumptive identification of isolates

➔ *CPT Changes: An Insider's View* 2001

(For concentration, use 87015)

87118   Culture, mycobacterial, definitive identification, each isolate

➔ *CPT Changes: An Insider's View* 2001

87140   Culture, typing; immunofluorescent method, each antiserum

➔ *CPT Assistant* Nov 01:10, Sep 03:3; *CPT Changes: An Insider's View* 2001

87143   gas liquid chromatography (GLC) or high pressure liquid chromatography (HPLC) method

➔ *CPT Changes: An Insider's View* 2001

87147   immunologic method, other than immunofluoresence (eg, agglutination grouping), per antiserum

➔ *CPT Assistant* Apr 02:18, Oct 03:10; *CPT Changes: An Insider's View* 2001

87149   identification by nucleic acid (DNA or RNA) probe, direct probe technique, per culture or isolate, each organism probed

➔ *CPT Assistant* Nov 01:10, May 12:5; *CPT Changes: An Insider's View* 2001, 2010

►(Do not report 87149 in conjunction with 81200-81408)◄

87150   identification by nucleic acid (DNA or RNA) probe, amplified probe technique, per culture or isolate, each organism probed

➔ *CPT Assistant* May 12:5; *CPT Changes: An Insider's View* 2010

►(Do not report 87150 in conjunction with 81200-81408)◄

87152   identification by pulse field gel typing

➔ *CPT Assistant* May 12:5; *CPT Changes: An Insider's View* 2001

►(Do not report 87152 in conjunction with 81200-81408)◄

87153   identification by nucleic acid sequencing method, each isolate (eg, sequencing of the 16S rRNA gene)
➔ *CPT Changes: An Insider's View* 2010

87158   other methods
➔ *CPT Assistant* Nov 01:10, Sep 03:3

87164   Dark field examination, any source (eg, penile, vaginal, oral, skin); includes specimen collection

87166   without collection

87168   Macroscopic examination; arthropod
➔ *CPT Changes: An Insider's View* 2001

87169   parasite
➔ *CPT Changes: An Insider's View* 2001

87172   Pinworm exam (eg, cellophane tape prep)
➔ *CPT Changes: An Insider's View* 2001

87176   Homogenization, tissue, for culture
➔ *CPT Changes: An Insider's View* 2001

87177   Ova and parasites, direct smears, concentration and identification
➔ *CPT Assistant* Jul 03:8, Nov 03:15, Mar 06:6

(Do not report 87177 in conjunction with 87015)

(For direct smears from a primary source, use 87207)

(For coccidia or microsporidia exam, use 87207)

(For complex special stain (trichrome, iron hematoxylin), use 87209)

(For nucleic acid probes in cytologic material, use 88365)

87181   Susceptibility studies, antimicrobial agent; agar dilution method, per agent (eg, antibiotic gradient strip)
➔ *CPT Assistant* Nov 01:10; *CPT Changes: An Insider's View* 2001

87184   disk method, per plate (12 or fewer agents)
➔ *CPT Assistant* Nov 01:10; *CPT Changes: An Insider's View* 2001

87185   enzyme detection (eg, beta lactamase), per enzyme
➔ *CPT Assistant* Nov 01:10; *CPT Changes: An Insider's View* 2001

87186   microdilution or agar dilution (minimum inhibitory concentration [MIC] or breakpoint), each multi-antimicrobial, per plate
➔ *CPT Assistant* Nov 01:10; *CPT Changes: An Insider's View* 2001

+ 87187   microdilution or agar dilution, minimum lethal concentration (MLC), each plate (List separately in addition to code for primary procedure)
➔ *CPT Assistant* Nov 01:10; *CPT Changes: An Insider's View* 2001

(Use 87187 in conjunction with 87186 or 87188)

87188   macrobroth dilution method, each agent
➔ *CPT Assistant* Nov 01:10; *CPT Changes: An Insider's View* 2001

87190   mycobacteria, proportion method, each agent
➔ *CPT Changes: An Insider's View* 2001

(For other mycobacterial susceptibility studies, see 87181, 87184, 87186, or 87188)

87197   Serum bactericidal titer (Schlicter test)

87205   Smear, primary source with interpretation; Gram or Giemsa stain for bacteria, fungi, or cell types
➔ *CPT Assistant* Aug 05:9, Oct 09:12; *CPT Changes: An Insider's View* 2001

87206   fluorescent and/or acid fast stain for bacteria, fungi, parasites, viruses or cell types
➔ *CPT Changes: An Insider's View* 2001

87207   special stain for inclusion bodies or parasites (eg, malaria, coccidia, microsporidia, trypanosomes, herpes viruses)
➔ *CPT Assistant* Jul 03:8, Mar 06:6; *CPT Changes: An Insider's View* 2001, 2003

(For direct smears with concentration and identification, use 87177)

(For thick smear preparation, use 87015)

(For fat, meat, fibers, nasal eosinophils, and starch, see miscellaneous section)

87209   complex special stain (eg, trichrome, iron hemotoxylin) for ova and parasites
➔ *CPT Assistant* Mar 06:6; *CPT Changes: An Insider's View* 2006

87210   wet mount for infectious agents (eg, saline, India ink, KOH preps)
➔ *CPT Changes: An Insider's View* 2001

(For KOH examination of skin, hair or nails, see 87220)

87220   Tissue examination by KOH slide of samples from skin, hair, or nails for fungi or ectoparasite ova or mites (eg, scabies)
➔ *CPT Changes: An Insider's View* 2001

87230   Toxin or antitoxin assay, tissue culture (eg, Clostridium difficile toxin)

87250   Virus isolation; inoculation of embryonated eggs, or small animal, includes observation and dissection
➔ *CPT Changes: An Insider's View* 2001

87252   tissue culture inoculation, observation, and presumptive identification by cytopathic effect
➔ *CPT Changes: An Insider's View* 2001

87253   tissue culture, additional studies or definitive identification (eg, hemabsorption, neutralization, immunofluoresence stain), each isolate
➔ *CPT Changes: An Insider's View* 2001

(Electron microscopy, use 88348)

(Inclusion bodies in tissue sections, see 88304-88309; in smears, see 87207-87210; in fluids, use 88106)

87254   centrifuge enhanced (shell vial) technique, includes identification with immunofluorescence stain, each virus
➔ *CPT Assistant* Jul 03:8; *CPT Changes: An Insider's View* 2001, 2003

(Report 87254 in addition to 87252 as appropriate)

87255   including identification by non-immunologic method, other than by cytopathic effect (eg, virus specific enzymatic activity)
→ *CPT Assistant* Jul 03:9; *CPT Changes: An Insider's View* 2003

►These codes are intended for primary source only. For similar studies on culture material, refer to codes 87140-87158. Infectious agents by antigen detection, immunofluorescence microscopy, or nucleic acid probe techniques should be reported as precisely as possible. The molecular pathology procedures codes (81200-81408) are not to be used in combination with or instead of the procedures represented by 87470-87801. The most specific code possible should be reported. If there is no specific agent code, the general methodology code (eg, 87299, 87449, 87450, 87797, 87798, 87799, 87899) should be used. For identification of antibodies to many of the listed infectious agents, see 86602-86804. When separate results are reported for different species or strain of organisms, each result should be coded separately. Use modifier 59 when separate results are reported for different species or strains that are described by the same code.◄

87260   Infectious agent antigen detection by immunofluorescent technique; adenovirus
→ *CPT Assistant* Nov 97:32; *CPT Changes: An Insider's View* 2001

87265   Bordetella pertussis/parapertussis
→ *CPT Assistant* Nov 97:32

87267   Enterovirus, direct fluorescent antibody (DFA)
→ *CPT Assistant* Jul 03:8

87269   giardia
→ *CPT Changes: An Insider's View* 2004

87270   Chlamydia trachomatis
→ *CPT Assistant* Nov 97:32

87271   Cytomegalovirus, direct fluorescent antibody (DFA)
→ *CPT Assistant* Jul 03:7

87272   cryptosporidium
→ *CPT Assistant* Nov 97:32; *CPT Changes: An Insider's View* 2004

87273   Herpes simplex virus type 2
→ *CPT Changes: An Insider's View* 2001

87274   Herpes simplex virus type 1
→ *CPT Assistant* Nov 97:32; *CPT Changes: An Insider's View* 2001

87275   influenza B virus
→ *CPT Changes: An Insider's View* 2001

87276   influenza A virus
→ *CPT Assistant* Nov 97:32, May 09:6

87277   Legionella micdadei
→ *CPT Changes: An Insider's View* 2001

87278   Legionella pneumophila
→ *CPT Assistant* Nov 97:32

87279   Parainfluenza virus, each type
→ *CPT Changes: An Insider's View* 2001

87280   respiratory syncytial virus
→ *CPT Assistant* Nov 97:32

87281   Pneumocystis carinii
→ *CPT Changes: An Insider's View* 2001

87283   Rubeola
→ *CPT Changes: An Insider's View* 2001

87285   Treponema pallidum
→ *CPT Assistant* Nov 97:32

87290   Varicella zoster virus
→ *CPT Assistant* Nov 97:32

87299   not otherwise specified, each organism
→ *CPT Assistant* Nov 97:32, Nov 01:10; *CPT Changes: An Insider's View* 2001

87300   Infectious agent antigen detection by immunofluorescent technique, polyvalent for multiple organisms, each polyvalent antiserum
→ *CPT Assistant* Aug 05:9; *CPT Changes: An Insider's View* 2001

(For physician evaluation of infectious disease agents by immunofluorescence, use 88346)

87301   Infectious agent antigen detection by enzyme immunoassay technique, qualitative or semiquantitative, multiple-step method; adenovirus enteric types 40/41
→ *CPT Assistant* Nov 97:32, Nov 99:46

87305   Aspergillus
→ *CPT Changes: An Insider's View* 2007

87320   Chlamydia trachomatis
→ *CPT Assistant* Nov 97:32

87324   Clostridium difficile toxin(s)
→ *CPT Assistant* Nov 97:32; *CPT Changes: An Insider's View* 2001

87327   Cryptococcus neoformans
→ *CPT Changes: An Insider's View* 2001

(For Cryptococcus latex agglutination, use 86403)

87328   cryptosporidium
→ *CPT Assistant* Nov 97:32; *CPT Changes: An Insider's View* 2004

87329   giardia
→ *CPT Changes: An Insider's View* 2004

87332   cytomegalovirus
→ *CPT Assistant* Nov 97:32

87335   Escherichia coli O157
→ *CPT Assistant* Nov 97:32

(For giardia antigen, use 87329)

87336   Entamoeba histolytica dispar group
→ *CPT Changes: An Insider's View* 2001

87337   Entamoeba histolytica group
→ *CPT Changes: An Insider's View* 2001

87338 Helicobacter pylori, stool
> *CPT Assistant* Nov 99:46; *CPT Changes: An Insider's View* 2000

87339 Helicobacter pylori
> *CPT Changes: An Insider's View* 2001

(For H. pylori, stool, use 87338. For H. pylori, breath and blood by mass spectrometry, see 83013, 83014. For H. pylori, liquid scintillation counter, see 78267, 78268)

87340 hepatitis B surface antigen (HBsAg)
> *CPT Assistant* Nov 97:32, Jan 00:11

87341 hepatitis B surface antigen (HBsAg) neutralization
> *CPT Changes: An Insider's View* 2001

87350 hepatitis Be antigen (HBeAg)
> *CPT Assistant* Nov 97:32

87380 hepatitis, delta agent
> *CPT Assistant* Nov 97:32

87385 Histoplasma capsulatum
> *CPT Assistant* Nov 97:32

87389 HIV-1 antigen(s), with HIV-1 and HIV-2 antibodies, single result
> *CPT Changes: An Insider's View* 2012

87390 HIV-1
> *CPT Assistant* Nov 97:32

87391 HIV-2
> *CPT Assistant* Nov 97:32

87400 Influenza, A or B, each
> *CPT Assistant* Jun 01:11, Dec 01:6, Aug 05:9, May 09:6; *CPT Changes: An Insider's View* 2001

87420 respiratory syncytial virus
> *CPT Assistant* Nov 97:32

87425 rotavirus
> *CPT Assistant* Nov 97:32

87427 Shiga-like toxin
> *CPT Changes: An Insider's View* 2001

87430 Streptococcus, group A
> *CPT Assistant* Nov 97:32

87449 Infectious agent antigen detection by enzyme immunoassay technique qualitative or semiquantitative; multiple step method, not otherwise specified, each organism
> *CPT Assistant* Nov 97:32, Jan 00:11, Nov 01:10; *CPT Changes: An Insider's View* 2001

87450 single step method, not otherwise specified, each organism
> *CPT Assistant* Nov 97:33; *CPT Changes: An Insider's View* 2001

87451 multiple step method, polyvalent for multiple organisms, each polyvalent antiserum
> *CPT Changes: An Insider's View* 2001

87470 Infectious agent detection by nucleic acid (DNA or RNA); Bartonella henselae and Bartonella quintana, direct probe technique
> *CPT Assistant* Nov 97:33-34

87471 Bartonella henselae and Bartonella quintana, amplified probe technique

87472 Bartonella henselae and Bartonella quintana, quantification

87475 Borrelia burgdorferi, direct probe technique

87476 Borrelia burgdorferi, amplified probe technique

87477 Borrelia burgdorferi, quantification

87480 Candida species, direct probe technique

87481 Candida species, amplified probe technique

87482 Candida species, quantification

87485 Chlamydia pneumoniae, direct probe technique

87486 Chlamydia pneumoniae, amplified probe technique

87487 Chlamydia pneumoniae, quantification

87490 Chlamydia trachomatis, direct probe technique

87491 Chlamydia trachomatis, amplified probe technique

87492 Chlamydia trachomatis, quantification

87493 Clostridium difficile, toxin gene(s), amplified probe technique
> *CPT Assistant* Sep 10:8; *CPT Changes: An Insider's View* 2010

87495 cytomegalovirus, direct probe technique

87496 cytomegalovirus, amplified probe technique

87497 cytomegalovirus, quantification

▲ **87498** enterovirus, reverse transcription and amplified probe technique
> *CPT Changes: An Insider's View* 2007, 2013

87500 vancomycin resistance (eg, enterococcus species van A, van B), amplified probe technique
> *CPT Assistant* Apr 08:5; *CPT Changes: An Insider's View* 2008

87501 influenza virus, reverse transcription and amplified probe technique, each type or subtype
> *CPT Assistant* Oct 10:8, Dec 10:8; *CPT Changes: An Insider's View* 2011

87502 influenza virus, for multiple types or sub-types, multiplex reverse transcription and amplified probe technique, first 2 types or sub-types
> *CPT Assistant* Oct 10:8, Dec 10:8; *CPT Changes: An Insider's View* 2011, 2012

+ **87503** influenza virus, for multiple types or sub-types, multiplex reverse transcription and amplified probe technique, each additional influenza virus type or sub-type beyond 2 (List separately in addition to code for primary procedure)
> *CPT Assistant* Oct 10:8, Dec 10:8; *CPT Changes: An Insider's View* 2011

(Use 87503 in conjunction with 87502)

87510 Gardnerella vaginalis, direct probe technique
> *CPT Assistant* Aug 05:9

87511 Gardnerella vaginalis, amplified probe technique

⊙ =Moderate sedation   ✚ =Add-on code   ⚲ =FDA approval pending   # =Resequenced code   ○ =Recycled/reinstated code   ➜➜ =See p xiii for details

87512	Gardnerella vaginalis, quantification	87562	Mycobacteria avium-intracellulare, quantification
87515	hepatitis B virus, direct probe technique	87580	Mycoplasma pneumoniae, direct probe technique
87516	hepatitis B virus, amplified probe technique	87581	Mycoplasma pneumoniae, amplified probe technique
87517	hepatitis B virus, quantification	87582	Mycoplasma pneumoniae, quantification
87520	hepatitis C, direct probe technique	87590	Neisseria gonorrhoeae, direct probe technique

▲ 87521 hepatitis C, reverse transcription and amplified probe technique
> → *CPT Changes: An Insider's View* 2013

87591 Neisseria gonorrhoeae, amplified probe technique

87592 Neisseria gonorrhoeae, quantification

▲ 87522 hepatitis C, reverse transcription and quantification
> → *CPT Changes: An Insider's View* 2013

87620 papillomavirus, human, direct probe technique
> → *CPT Assistant* Feb 02:10, Aug 05:9

87525 hepatitis G, direct probe technique

87621 papillomavirus, human, amplified probe technique

87526 hepatitis G, amplified probe technique

87622 papillomavirus, human, quantification

87527 hepatitis G, quantification

● 87631 respiratory virus (eg, adenovirus, influenza virus, coronavirus, metapneumovirus, parainfluenza virus, respiratory syncytial virus, rhinovirus), multiplex reverse transcription and amplified probe technique, multiple types or subtypes, 3-5 targets
> → *CPT Changes: An Insider's View* 2013

87528 Herpes simplex virus, direct probe technique

87529 Herpes simplex virus, amplified probe technique

87530 Herpes simplex virus, quantification

87531 Herpes virus-6, direct probe technique

● 87632 respiratory virus (eg, adenovirus, influenza virus, coronavirus, metapneumovirus, parainfluenza virus, respiratory syncytial virus, rhinovirus), multiplex reverse transcription and amplified probe technique, multiple types or subtypes, 6-11 targets
> → *CPT Changes: An Insider's View* 2013

87532 Herpes virus-6, amplified probe technique

87533 Herpes virus-6, quantification

87534 HIV-1, direct probe technique

▲ 87535 HIV-1, reverse transcription and amplified probe technique
> → *CPT Assistant* Mar 08:3; *CPT Changes: An Insider's View* 2013

● 87633 respiratory virus (eg, adenovirus, influenza virus, coronavirus, metapneumovirus, parainfluenza virus, respiratory syncytial virus, rhinovirus), multiplex reverse transcription and amplified probe technique, multiple types or subtypes, 12-25 targets
> → *CPT Changes: An Insider's View* 2013

▲ 87536 HIV-1, reverse transcription and quantification
> → *CPT Changes: An Insider's View* 2013

87537 HIV-2, direct probe technique

►(Use 87631-87633 for nucleic acid assays which detect multiple respiratory viruses in a multiplex reaction [ie, single procedure with multiple results])◄

▲ 87538 HIV-2, reverse transcription and amplified probe technique
> → *CPT Changes: An Insider's View* 2013

►(For assays that are used to type or subtype influenza viruses only, see 87501-87503)◄

▲ 87539 HIV-2, reverse transcription and quantification
> → *CPT Changes: An Insider's View* 2013

►(For assays that include influenza viruses with additional respiratory viruses, see 87631-87633)◄

87540 Legionella pneumophila, direct probe technique

►(For detection of multiple infectious agents not otherwise specified which report a single result, see 87800, 87801)◄

87541 Legionella pneumophila, amplified probe technique

87542 Legionella pneumophila, quantification

87640 Staphylococcus aureus, amplified probe technique
> → *CPT Assistant* Aug 07:7; *CPT Changes: An Insider's View* 2007

87550 Mycobacteria species, direct probe technique

87551 Mycobacteria species, amplified probe technique

87552 Mycobacteria species, quantification

87641 Staphylococcus aureus, methicillin resistant, amplified probe technique
> → *CPT Assistant* Aug 07:7; *CPT Changes: An Insider's View* 2007

87555 Mycobacteria tuberculosis, direct probe technique

87556 Mycobacteria tuberculosis, amplified probe technique

87557 Mycobacteria tuberculosis, quantification

87560 Mycobacteria avium-intracellulare, direct probe technique

(For assays that detect methicillin resistance and identify Staphylococcus aureus using a single nucleic acid sequence, use 87641)

87650 Streptococcus, group A, direct probe technique

87561 Mycobacteria avium-intracellulare, amplified probe technique

87651 Streptococcus, group A, amplified probe technique

Pathology and Laboratory

87652   Streptococcus, group A, quantification

87653   Streptococcus, group B, amplified probe technique

→ *CPT Assistant* Aug 07:7; *CPT Changes: An Insider's View* 2007

87660   Trichomonas vaginalis, direct probe technique

→ *CPT Changes: An Insider's View* 2004

87797   Infectious agent detection by nucleic acid (DNA or RNA), not otherwise specified; direct probe technique, each organism

→ *CPT Assistant* Nov 97:34, Nov 01:10, Aug 05:9; *CPT Changes: An Insider's View* 2001

87798   amplified probe technique, each organism

→ *CPT Assistant* Nov 97:34, Nov 01.10, Aug 07:7; *CPT Changes: An Insider's View* 2001

87799   quantification, each organism

→ *CPT Assistant* Nov 97:34; *CPT Changes: An Insider's View* 2001

87800   Infectious agent detection by nucleic acid (DNA or RNA), multiple organisms; direct probe(s) technique

→ *CPT Assistant* Aug 05:9; *CPT Changes: An Insider's View* 2001

87801   amplified probe(s) technique

→ *CPT Assistant* May 12:5; *CPT Changes: An Insider's View* 2001

(For each specific organism nucleic acid detection from a primary source, see 87470-87660. For detection of specific infectious agents not otherwise specified, see 87797, 87798, or 87799 1 time for each agent)

►(For detection of multiple infectious agents not otherwise specified which report a single result, see 87800, 87801)◄

►(Do not use 87801 for nucleic acid assays that detect multiple respiratory viruses in a multiplex reaction [ie, single procedure with multiple results], see 87631-87633)◄

87802   Infectious agent antigen detection by immunoassay with direct optical observation; Streptococcus, group B

→ *CPT Assistant* Jun 03:12; *CPT Changes: An Insider's View* 2002

87803   Clostridium difficile toxin A

→ *CPT Assistant* Jun 03:12; *CPT Changes: An Insider's View* 2002

87804   Influenza

→ *CPT Assistant* Jun 03:11-12, May 09:6; *CPT Changes: An Insider's View* 2002

87807   respiratory syncytial virus

→ *CPT Changes: An Insider's View* 2005

87808   Trichomonas vaginalis

→ *CPT Changes: An Insider's View* 2007

87809   adenovirus

→ *CPT Assistant* Apr 08:5; *CPT Changes: An Insider's View* 2008

87810   Chlamydia trachomatis

→ *CPT Assistant* Nov 97:34, Jan 98:6; *CPT Changes: An Insider's View* 2009

87850   Neisseria gonorrhoeae

→ *CPT Assistant* Nov 97:34, Jan 98:6

87880   Streptococcus, group A

→ *CPT Assistant* Nov 97:34, Jan 98:6, Dec 98:8

87899   not otherwise specified

→ *CPT Assistant* Jan 98:6, Jun 01:11

87900   Infectious agent drug susceptibility phenotype prediction using regularly updated genotypic bioinformatics

→ *CPT Assistant* Mar 06:6, May 12:5; *CPT Changes: An Insider's View* 2006

#● **87910**   Infectious agent genotype analysis by nucleic acid (DNA or RNA); cytomegalovirus

→ *CPT Changes: An Insider's View* 2013

▲ **87901**   HIV-1, reverse transcriptase and protease regions

→ *CPT Assistant* Aug 05:9, Mar 06:6, Oct 10:9, Dec 10:9, May 12:5; *CPT Changes: An Insider's View* 2001, 2002, 2011, 2013

87906   HIV-1, other region (eg, integrase, fusion)

→ *CPT Assistant* Oct 10:8, Dec 10:8; *CPT Changes: An Insider's View* 2011

(For infectious agent drug susceptibility phenotype prediction for HIV-1, use 87900)

#● **87912**   Hepatitis B virus

→ *CPT Changes: An Insider's View* 2013

87902   Hepatitis C virus

→ *CPT Assistant* May 12:5; *CPT Changes: An Insider's View* 2002

87903   Infectious agent phenotype analysis by nucleic acid (DNA or RNA) with drug resistance tissue culture analysis, HIV 1; first through 10 drugs tested

→ *CPT Assistant* Apr 04:15, Mar 06:6, May 12:3; *CPT Changes: An Insider's View* 2001, 2002

+ **87904**   each additional drug tested (List separately in addition to code for primary procedure)

→ *CPT Assistant* Apr 04:15, Mar 06:6, May 12:3; *CPT Changes: An Insider's View* 2001, 2002, 2006

(Use 87904 in conjunction with 87903)

87905   Infectious agent enzymatic activity other than virus (eg, sialidase activity in vaginal fluid)

→ *CPT Changes: An Insider's View* 2009

(For virus isolation including identification by non-immunologic method, other than by cytopathic effect, use 87255)

87906   ►Code is out of numerical sequence. See 87001-87999◄

87910   ►Code is out of numerical sequence. See 87001-87999◄

87912   ►Code is out of numerical sequence. See 87001-87999◄

87999   Unlisted microbiology procedure

→ *CPT Assistant* Aug 05:9

Anatomic Pathology

Postmortem Examination

Procedures 88000 through 88099 represent physician services only. Use modifier 90 for outside laboratory services.

→ *CPT Assistant* Fall 93:26

88000   Necropsy (autopsy), gross examination only; without CNS
→ *CPT Assistant* Aug 05:9

88005   with brain

88007   with brain and spinal cord

88012   infant with brain

88014   stillborn or newborn with brain

88016   macerated stillborn

88020   Necropsy (autopsy), gross and microscopic; without CNS

88025   with brain

88027   with brain and spinal cord

88028   infant with brain

88029   stillborn or newborn with brain

88036   Necropsy (autopsy), limited, gross and/or microscopic; regional

88037   single organ

88040   Necropsy (autopsy); forensic examination

88045   coroner's call

88099   Unlisted necropsy (autopsy) procedure

Cytopathology

88104   Cytopathology, fluids, washings or brushings, except cervical or vaginal; smears with interpretation
→ *CPT Assistant* Spring 91:6, Fall 94:3, Aug 05:9

88106   simple filter method with interpretation
→ *CPT Assistant* Fall 94:3; *CPT Changes: An Insider's View* 2007

(Do not report 88106 in conjunction with 88104)

(88107 has been deleted. To report smears and simple filter preparation, see 88104, 88106)

(For nongynecological selective cellular enhancement including filter transfer techniques, use 88112)

88108   Cytopathology, concentration technique, smears and interpretation (eg, Saccomanno technique)
→ *CPT Assistant* Fall 94:3, Nov 97:34, Jan 98:6

(For cervical or vaginal smears, see 88150-88155)

(For gastric intubation with lavage, see 43754, 43755)

(For x-ray localization, use 74340)

88112   Cytopathology, selective cellular enhancement technique with interpretation (eg, liquid based slide preparation method), except cervical or vaginal
→ *CPT Changes: An Insider's View* 2004

(Do not report 88112 with 88108)

88120   Cytopathology, in situ hybridization (eg, FISH), urinary tract specimen with morphometric analysis, 3-5 molecular probes, each specimen; manual
→ *CPT Assistant* Oct 10:9, Dec 10:9; *CPT Changes: An Insider's View* 2011

88121   using computer-assisted technology
→ *CPT Assistant* Oct 10:9, Dec 10:9; *CPT Changes: An Insider's View* 2011

(For morphometric in situ hybridization on cytologic specimens other than urinary tract, see 88367, 88368)

(For more than 5 probes, use 88399)

88125   Cytopathology, forensic (eg, sperm)

88130   Sex chromatin identification; Barr bodies

88140   peripheral blood smear, polymorphonuclear drumsticks
→ *CPT Assistant* Nov 98:27-28, Mar 06:6

(For Guard stain, use 88313)

Codes 88141-88155, 88164-88167, 88174-88175 are used to report cervical or vaginal screening by various methods and to report physician interpretation services. Use codes 88150-88154 to report conventional Pap smears that are examined using non-Bethesda reporting. Use codes 88164-88167 to report conventional Pap smears that are examined using the Bethesda System of reporting. Use codes 88142-88143 to report liquid-based specimens processed as thin-layer preparations that are examined using any system of reporting (Bethesda or non-Bethesda). Use codes 88174-88175 to report automated screening of liquid-based specimens that are examined using any system of reporting (Bethesda or non-Bethesda). Within each of these three code families choose the one code that describes the screening method(s) used. Codes 88141 and 88155 should be reported in addition to the screening code chosen when the additional services are provided. Manual rescreening requires a complete visual reassessment of the entire slide initially screened by either an automated or manual process. Manual review represents an assessment of selected cells or regions of a slide identified by initial automated review.

88141   Cytopathology, cervical or vaginal (any reporting system), requiring interpretation by physician
→ *CPT Assistant* Nov 97:35, Jan 98:6, Jan 99:11, May 99:6, Nov 99:46, Mar 04:6, Mar 05:16, May 11:10, Dec 11:17

(Use 88141 in conjunction with 88142-88154, 88164-88167, 88174-88175)

Pathology and Laboratory

88142   Cytopathology, cervical or vaginal (any reporting system), collected in preservative fluid, automated thin layer preparation; manual screening under physician supervision
→ *CPT Assistant* Nov 97:34-35, Jan 98:6, Nov 98:28, May 99:6, Jul 03:7, Mar 04:4

88143   with manual screening and rescreening under physician supervision
→ *CPT Assistant* Nov 97:34-35, Nov 98:28, May 99:6, Jul 03:7, Mar 04:4, Mar 05:16

(For automated screening of automated thin layer preparation, see 88174, 88175)

88147   Cytopathology smears, cervical or vaginal; screening by automated system under physician supervision
→ *CPT Assistant* Nov 97:35, Nov 98:28, Jan 99:11, May 99:6, Nov 99:46, Mar 04:6

88148   screening by automated system with manual rescreening under physician supervision
→ *CPT Assistant* Jan 99:1, May 99:6, Nov 99:46, Mar 04:6; *CPT Changes: An Insider's View* 2000

88150   Cytopathology, slides, cervical or vaginal; manual screening under physician supervision
→ *CPT Assistant* Winter 91:19, Nov 97:34-35, Nov 98:28, May 99:6, Mar 04:5

88152   with manual screening and computer-assisted rescreening under physician supervision
→ *CPT Assistant* Nov 97:35, Jan 98:6, May 99:6, Mar 04:5

88153   with manual screening and rescreening under physician supervision
→ *CPT Assistant* Nov 97:34-35, Nov 98:28, May 99:6, Mar 04:5, Mar 05:16

88154   with manual screening and computer-assisted rescreening using cell selection and review under physician supervision
→ *CPT Assistant* Nov 97:34-35, Nov 98:28, May 99:6, Mar 04:5

+ 88155   Cytopathology, slides, cervical or vaginal, definitive hormonal evaluation (eg, maturation index, karyopyknotic index, estrogenic index) (List separately in addition to code[s] for other technical and interpretation services)
→ *CPT Assistant* Nov 97:35, Nov 98:28, May 99:6, Nov 99:46, Mar 04:5, May 11:10

(Use 88155 in conjunction with 88142-88154, 88164-88167, 88174-88175)

88160   Cytopathology, smears, any other source; screening and interpretation
→ *CPT Assistant* Jan 98:6

88161   preparation, screening and interpretation
→ *CPT Assistant* Aug 97:18, Jan 98:6

88162   extended study involving over 5 slides and/or multiple stains

(For aerosol collection of sputum, use 89220)

(For special stains, see 88312-88314)

88164   Cytopathology, slides, cervical or vaginal (the Bethesda System); manual screening under physician supervision
→ *CPT Assistant* Nov 98:28, May 99:6, Mar 04:5

88165   with manual screening and rescreening under physician supervision
→ *CPT Assistant* Nov 98:28, May 99:6, Mar 04:5, Mar 05:16

88166   with manual screening and computer-assisted rescreening under physician supervision
→ *CPT Assistant* Nov 98:28, May 99:6, Mar 04:5

88167   with manual screening and computer-assisted rescreening using cell selection and review under physician supervision
→ *CPT Assistant* Nov 98:28, May 99:6, Jul 03:7, Mar 04:5

(To report collection of specimen via fine needle aspiration, see 10021, 10022)

88172   Cytopathology, evaluation of fine needle aspirate; immediate cytohistologic study to determine adequacy for diagnosis, first evaluation episode, each site
→ *CPT Assistant* Fall 93:26, Fall 94:2, Dec 98:8, Aug 07:15, Oct 10:9, Dec 10:9; *CPT Changes: An Insider's View* 2001, 2011

(The evaluation episode represents a complete set of cytologic material submitted for evaluation and is independent of the number of needle passes or slides prepared. A separate evaluation episode occurs if the proceduralist provider obtains additional material from the same site, based on the prior immediate adequacy assessment, or a separate lesion is aspirated)

88173   interpretation and report
→ *CPT Assistant* Fall 93:26, Fall 94:2, Dec 98:8, Oct 10:9, Dec 10:9

(Report one unit of 88173 for the interpretation and report from each anatomic site, regardless of the number of passes or evaluation episodes performed during the aspiration procedure)

(For fine needle aspirate, see 10021, 10022)

(Do not report 88172, 88173 in conjunction with 88333 and 88334 for the same specimen)

#+ 88177   immediate cytohistologic study to determine adequacy for diagnosis, each separate additional evaluation episode, same site (List separately in addition to code for primary procedure)
→ *CPT Assistant* Oct 10:9, Dec 10:9; *CPT Changes: An Insider's View* 2011

(When repeat immediate evaluation episode(s) is required on subsequent cytologic material from the same site, eg, following determination the prior sampling that was not adequate for diagnosis, use 1 unit of 88177 for each additional evaluation episode)

(Use 88177 in conjunction with 88172)

88174   Cytopathology, cervical or vaginal (any reporting system), collected in preservative fluid, automated thin layer preparation; screening by automated system, under physician supervision
→ *CPT Assistant* Jul 03:9, Mar 04:4; *CPT Changes: An Insider's View* 2003

88175   with screening by automated system and manual rescreening or review, under physician supervision

> *CPT Assistant* Jul 03:9, Mar 04:4, Mar 06:6, May 11:10; *CPT Changes: An Insider's View* 2003, 2006

(For manual screening, see 88142, 88143)

88177   Code is out of numerical sequence. See 88104-88199

88182   Flow cytometry, cell cycle or DNA analysis

(For DNA ploidy analysis by morphometric technique, use 88358)

88184   Flow cytometry, cell surface, cytoplasmic, or nuclear marker, technical component only; first marker

> *CPT Assistant* Dec 07:14; *CPT Changes: An Insider's View* 2005

+ 88185   each additional marker (List separately in addition to code for first marker)

> *CPT Assistant* Dec 07:14; *CPT Changes: An Insider's View* 2005

(Report 88185 in conjunction with 88184)

88187   Flow cytometry, interpretation; 2 to 8 markers

> *CPT Assistant* Apr 05:14; *CPT Changes: An Insider's View* 2005

88188   9 to 15 markers

> *CPT Assistant* Apr 05:14; *CPT Changes: An Insider's View* 2005

88189   16 or more markers

> *CPT Assistant* Apr 05:14; *CPT Changes: An Insider's View* 2005

(Do not report 88187-88189 for interpretation of 86355, 86356, 86357, 86359, 86360, 86361, 86367)

▶(For assessment of circulating antibodies by flow cytometric techniques, see analyte and method-specific codes in the Chemistry section [83516-83520] or Immunology section [86000-86849])◀

(For cell enumeration using immunologic selection and identification in fluid specimen [eg, circulating tumor cells in blood], see 0279T, 0280T)

88199   Unlisted cytopathology procedure

(For electron microscopy, see 88348, 88349)

Cytogenetic Studies

▶Molecular pathology procedures should be reported using either the appropriate Tier 1 (81200-81383), Tier 2 (81400-81408), or the unlisted molecular pathology procedure code, 81479.◀

(For acetylcholinesterase, use 82013)

(For alpha-fetoprotein, serum or amniotic fluid, see 82105, 82106)

(For laser microdissection of cells from tissue sample, see 88380)

88230   Tissue culture for non-neoplastic disorders; lymphocyte

> *CPT Assistant* Nov 98:29, Oct 99:2, Aug 05:9, May 08:5

88233   skin or other solid tissue biopsy

> *CPT Assistant* Nov 98:29, Oct 99:2, May 08:5

88235   amniotic fluid or chorionic villus cells

> *CPT Assistant* Nov 98:29, Oct 99:2, May 08:5

88237   Tissue culture for neoplastic disorders; bone marrow, blood cells

> *CPT Assistant* Nov 98:29, Oct 99:2, May 08:5

88239   solid tumor

> *CPT Assistant* Nov 98:29, Oct 99:2, May 08:5

88240   Cryopreservation, freezing and storage of cells, each cell line

> *CPT Assistant* Nov 98:29, Oct 99:2, Jul 03:9, May 08:5

(For therapeutic cryopreservation and storage, use 38207)

88241   Thawing and expansion of frozen cells, each aliquot

> *CPT Assistant* Nov 98:29, Oct 99:2, Jul 03:9, May 08:5

(For therapeutic thawing of previous harvest, use 38208)

88245   Chromosome analysis for breakage syndromes; baseline Sister Chromatid Exchange (SCE), 20-25 cells

> *CPT Assistant* Nov 98:29, Oct 99:2, Jul 05:1, May 08:5

88248   baseline breakage, score 50-100 cells, count 20 cells, 2 karyotypes (eg, for ataxia telangiectasia, Fanconi anemia, fragile X)

> *CPT Assistant* Nov 98:29, Oct 99:2, Jul 05:1, May 08:5

88249   score 100 cells, clastogen stress (eg, diepoxybutane, mitomycin C, ionizing radiation, UV radiation)

> *CPT Assistant* Nov 98:29, Oct 99:2, Jul 05:1, May 08:5

88261   Chromosome analysis; count 5 cells, 1 karyotype, with banding

> *CPT Assistant* Nov 98:29, Oct 99:2, Jul 05:1, May 08:5

88262   count 15-20 cells, 2 karyotypes, with banding

> *CPT Assistant* Nov 98:29, Oct 99:2, May 08:5, May 11:10

88263   count 45 cells for mosaicism, 2 karyotypes, with banding

> *CPT Assistant* Nov 98:29, Oct 99:2, Jul 05:1, May 08:5

88264   analyze 20-25 cells

> *CPT Assistant* Nov 98:29, Oct 99:2, Jul 05:1, May 08:5

88267   Chromosome analysis, amniotic fluid or chorionic villus, count 15 cells, 1 karyotype, with banding

> *CPT Assistant* Jul 05:1

88269   Chromosome analysis, in situ for amniotic fluid cells, count cells from 6-12 colonies, 1 karyotype, with banding

> *CPT Assistant* Jul 05:1

88271   Molecular cytogenetics; DNA probe, each (eg, FISH)

> *CPT Assistant* Nov 98:29, Mar 99:10, Oct 99:3, Jun 02:11, Jul 05:1, May 08:5, May 12:5

88272   chromosomal in situ hybridization, analyze 3-5 cells (eg, for derivatives and markers)

> *CPT Assistant* Nov 98:29, Mar 99:10, Oct 99:3, Jun 02:11, Jul 05:1, May 08:5, May 12:5

Pathology and Laboratory

88273   chromosomal in situ hybridization, analyze 10-30 cells (eg, for microdeletions)
> *CPT Assistant* Nov 98:29, Mar 99:10, Oct 99:3, Jun 02:11, Jul 05:1, May 08:5, May 12:5

88274   interphase in situ hybridization, analyze 25-99 cells
> *CPT Assistant* Nov 98:29, Mar 99:10, Oct 99:3, Jun 02:11, Jul 05:1, May 08:5, May 12:5

88275   interphase in situ hybridization, analyze 100-300 cells
> *CPT Assistant* Nov 98:29, Mar 99:10, Oct 99:3, Jun 02:11, Jul 05:1, May 08:5, May 12:5

88280   Chromosome analysis; additional karyotypes, each study
> *CPT Assistant* Jul 05:1, May 08:5

88283   additional specialized banding technique (eg, NOR, C-banding)
> *CPT Assistant* Jul 05:1, May 08:5

88285   additional cells counted, each study
> *CPT Assistant* Jul 05:1, Dec 07:14, May 08:5, May 11:10

88289   additional high resolution study
> *CPT Assistant* Oct 99:3, Jul 05:1

88291   Cytogenetics and molecular cytogenetics, interpretation and report
> *CPT Assistant* Nov 98:29, Oct 99:3, Jul 05:1, May 08:5

88299   Unlisted cytogenetic study
> *CPT Assistant* Oct 99:3

Surgical Pathology

Services 88300 through 88309 include accession, examination, and reporting. They do not include the services designated in codes 88311 through 88365 and 88399, which are coded in addition when provided.

The unit of service for codes 88300 through 88309 is the specimen.

A specimen is defined as tissue or tissues that is (are) submitted for individual and separate attention, requiring individual examination and pathologic diagnosis. Two or more such specimens from the same patient (eg, separately identified endoscopic biopsies, skin lesions) are each appropriately assigned an individual code reflective of its proper level of service.

Service code 88300 is used for any specimen that in the opinion of the examining pathologist can be accurately diagnosed without microscopic examination. Service code 88302 is used when gross and microscopic examination is performed on a specimen to confirm identification and the absence of disease. Service codes 88304 through 88309 describe all other specimens requiring gross and microscopic examination, and represent additional ascending levels of physician work. Levels 88302 through 88309 are specifically defined by the assigned specimens.

Any unlisted specimen should be assigned to the code which most closely reflects the physician work involved when compared to other specimens assigned to that code.

(Do not report 88302-88309 on the same specimen as part of Mohs surgery)

88300   **Level I** - Surgical pathology, gross examination only
> *CPT Assistant* Winter 91:18, Sep 00:10, Aug 05:9

88302   **Level II** - Surgical pathology, gross and microscopic examination

Appendix, incidental

Fallopian tube, sterilization

Fingers/toes, amputation, traumatic

Foreskin, newborn

Hernia sac, any location

Hydrocele sac

Nerve

Skin, plastic repair

Sympathetic ganglion

Testis, castration

Vaginal mucosa, incidental

Vas deferens, sterilization
> *CPT Assistant* Winter 91:18, Sep 00:10, Nov 06:1, Jan 07:29, Dec 11:17

88304   **Level III** - Surgical pathology, gross and microscopic examination

Abortion, induced

Abscess

Aneurysm - arterial/ventricular

Anus, tag

Appendix, other than incidental

Artery, atheromatous plaque

Bartholin's gland cyst

Bone fragment(s), other than pathologic fracture

Bursa/synovial cyst

Carpal tunnel tissue

Cartilage, shavings

Cholesteatoma

Colon, colostomy stoma

Conjunctiva - biopsy/pterygium

Cornea

Diverticulum - esophagus/small intestine

Dupuytren's contracture tissue

Femoral head, other than fracture

Fissure/fistula

Foreskin, other than newborn

Gallbladder

Ganglion cyst

Hematoma

Hemorrhoids

Hydatid of Morgagni

Intervertebral disc

Joint, loose body

Meniscus

Mucocele, salivary

Neuroma - Morton's/traumatic

Pilonidal cyst/sinus

Polyps, inflammatory - nasal/sinusoidal

Skin - cyst/tag/debridement

Soft tissue, debridement

Soft tissue, lipoma

Spermatocele

Tendon/tendon sheath

Testicular appendage

Thrombus or embolus

Tonsil and/or adenoids

Varicocele

Vas deferens, other than sterilization

Vein, varicosity

➔ *CPT Assistant* Spring 91:2, Winter 91:18, Aug 97:18, Sep 00:10, Jan 07:29, Dec 11:17; *CPT Changes: An Insider's View* 2002

88305 **Level IV** - Surgical pathology, gross and microscopic examination

Abortion - spontaneous/missed

Artery, biopsy

Bone marrow, biopsy

Bone exostosis

Brain/meninges, other than for tumor resection

Breast, biopsy, not requiring microscopic evaluation of surgical margins

Breast, reduction mammoplasty

Bronchus, biopsy

Cell block, any source

Cervix, biopsy

Colon, biopsy

Duodenum, biopsy

Endocervix, curettings/biopsy

Endometrium, curettings/biopsy

Esophagus, biopsy

Extremity, amputation, traumatic

Fallopian tube, biopsy

Fallopian tube, ectopic pregnancy

Femoral head, fracture

Fingers/toes, amputation, non-traumatic

Gingiva/oral mucosa, biopsy

Heart valve

Joint, resection

Kidney, biopsy

Larynx, biopsy

Leiomyoma(s), uterine myomectomy - without uterus

Lip, biopsy/wedge resection

Lung, transbronchial biopsy

Lymph node, biopsy

Muscle, biopsy

Nasal mucosa, biopsy

Nasopharynx/oropharynx, biopsy

Nerve, biopsy

Odontogenic/dental cyst

Omentum, biopsy

Ovary with or without tube, non-neoplastic

Ovary, biopsy/wedge resection

Parathyroid gland

Peritoneum, biopsy

Pituitary tumor

Placenta, other than third trimester

Pleura/pericardium - biopsy/tissue

Polyp, cervical/endometrial

Polyp, colorectal

Polyp, stomach/small intestine

Prostate, needle biopsy

Prostate, TUR

Salivary gland, biopsy

Sinus, paranasal biopsy

Skin, other than cyst/tag/debridement/plastic repair

Small intestine, biopsy

Soft tissue, other than tumor/mass/lipoma/debridement

Spleen

Stomach, biopsy

Synovium

Testis, other than tumor/biopsy/castration

Thyroglossal duct/brachial cleft cyst

Tongue, biopsy

Tonsil, biopsy

Trachea, biopsy

Ureter, biopsy

Urethra, biopsy

Urinary bladder, biopsy

Uterus, with or without tubes and ovaries, for prolapse

Vagina, biopsy

Vulva/labia, biopsy

➡ *CPT Assistant* Winter 90:2, Spring 91:6, Winter 91:18, Winter 92:17, Aug 97:18, Jul 98:4, Nov 98:29-30, Jul 00:4, Sep 00:10, Dec 00:15, Jul 05:13, Nov 06:1, Jan 07:29, Dec 11:17; *CPT Changes: An Insider's View* 2002

88307 **Level V** - Surgical pathology, gross and microscopic examination

Adrenal, resection

Bone - biopsy/curettings

Bone fragment(s), pathologic fracture

Brain, biopsy

Brain/meninges, tumor resection

Breast, excision of lesion, requiring microscopic evaluation of surgical margins

Breast, mastectomy - partial/simple

Cervix, conization

Colon, segmental resection, other than for tumor

Extremity, amputation, non-traumatic

Eye, enucleation

Kidney, partial/total nephrectomy

Larynx, partial/total resection

Liver, biopsy - needle/wedge

Liver, partial resection

Lung, wedge biopsy

Lymph nodes, regional resection

Mediastinum, mass

Myocardium, biopsy

Odontogenic tumor

Ovary with or without tube, neoplastic

Pancreas, biopsy

Placenta, third trimester

Prostate, except radical resection

Salivary gland

Sentinel lymph node

Small intestine, resection, other than for tumor

Soft tissue mass (except lipoma) - biopsy/simple excision

Stomach - subtotal/total resection, other than for tumor

Testis, biopsy

Thymus, tumor

Thyroid, total/lobe

Ureter, resection

Urinary bladder, TUR

Uterus, with or without tubes and ovaries, other than neoplastic/prolapse

➡ *CPT Assistant* Winter 91.18, Winter 92:18, Jul 98:4, Nov 98:29-30, Jul 99:10, Jul 00:4, Sep 00:10, Dec 00:15, Dec 03:11, Nov 06:1, Jan 07:29, Dec 11:17; *CPT Changes: An Insider's View* 2001

88309 **Level VI** - Surgical pathology, gross and microscopic examination

Bone resection

Breast, mastectomy - with regional lymph nodes

Colon, segmental resection for tumor

Colon, total resection

Esophagus, partial/total resection

Extremity, disarticulation

Fetus, with dissection

Larynx, partial/total resection - with regional lymph nodes

Lung - total/lobe/segment resection

Pancreas, total/subtotal resection

Prostate, radical resection

Small intestine, resection for tumor

Soft tissue tumor, extensive resection

Stomach - subtotal/total resection for tumor

Testis, tumor

Tongue/tonsil - resection for tumor

Urinary bladder, partial/total resection

Uterus, with or without tubes and ovaries, neoplastic

Vulva, total/subtotal resection

➡ *CPT Assistant* Spring 91:2, Winter 91:18, Fall 93:2, 26, Jul 00:4, Sep 00:10, Dec 03:11, Nov 06:1, Jan 07:29, Dec 11:18

(For fine needle aspiration, see 10021, 10022)

(For evaluation of fine needle aspirate, see 88172-88173)

(Do not report 88302-88309 on the same specimen as part of Mohs surgery)

+ **88311** Decalcification procedure (List separately in addition to code for surgical pathology examination)

➡ *CPT Assistant* Winter 92:18, Jul 98:4, Jun 02:11, Nov 02:7, Nov 06:1, Dec 11:18

88312   Special stain including interpretation and report; Group I
for microorganisms (eg, acid fast, methenamine silver)
➔ *CPT Assistant* Winter 91:19, Jun 02:11, Nov 02:7, Nov 06:1,
Dec 11:18; *CPT Changes: An Insider's View* 2004, 2010, 2012

(Report one unit of 88312 for each special stain, on each
surgical pathology block, cytologic specimen, or
hematologic smear)

88313   Group II, all other (eg, iron, trichrome), except stain
for microorganisms, stains for enzyme constituents,
or immunocytochemistry and immunohistochemistry
➔ *CPT Assistant* Jun 02:11, Nov 02:7, Mar 03:22, Nov 03:15,
Jun 06:17, Nov 06:1, Dec 11:18; *CPT Changes: An Insider's
View* 2010, 2012

(Report one unit of 88313 for each special stain, on each
surgical pathology block, cytologic specimen, or
hematologic smear)

(For immunocytochemistry and immunohistochemistry,
use 88342)

+ 88314   histochemical stain on frozen tissue block (List
separately in addition to code for primary procedure)
➔ *CPT Assistant* Nov 02:7, Nov 06:1, Dec 11:18; *CPT Changes:
An Insider's View* 2010, 2012

(Use 88314 in conjunction with 17311-17315, 88302-
88309, 88331, 88332)

(Do not report 88314 with 17311-17315 for routine frozen
section stain [eg, hematoxylin and eosin, toluidine blue],
performed during Mohs surgery. When a nonroutine
histochemical stain on frozen tissue during Mohs surgery
is utilized, report 88314 with modifier 59)

(Report one unit of 88314 for each special stain on each
frozen surgical pathology block)

(For a special stain performed on frozen tissue section
material to identify enzyme constituents, use 88319)

(88318 has been deleted)

(For determinative histochemistry to identify chemical
components, use 88313)

88319   Group III, for enzyme constituents
➔ *CPT Assistant* Dec 11:18; *CPT Changes: An Insider's View*
2012

(For each stain on each surgical pathology block,
cytologic specimen, or hematologic smear, use one unit
of 88319)

(For detection of enzyme constituents by
immunohistochemical or immunocytochemical technique,
use 88342)

88321   Consultation and report on referred slides prepared
elsewhere
➔ *CPT Assistant* Winter 91:19, Apr 97:9, Oct 00:7, Dec 02:10,
Jan 10:11, Dec 11:18

88323   Consultation and report on referred material requiring
preparation of slides
➔ *CPT Assistant* Winter 91:19, Apr 97:9, Oct 00:7, Dec 02:10,
Dec 11:18

88325   Consultation, comprehensive, with review of records and
specimens, with report on referred material
➔ *CPT Assistant* Winter 91:19, Apr 97:9, Dec 02:10, Dec 11:18

88329   Pathology consultation during surgery;
➔ *CPT Assistant* Winter 91:19, Apr 97:12, Aug 97:18, Jan 07:29,
Dec 11:18

88331   first tissue block, with frozen section(s), single
specimen
➔ *CPT Assistant* Spring 91:2, Winter 91:19, Apr 97:12,
Aug 97:18, Jul 00:4, Nov 02:7, Mar 06:6, Nov 06:1,
Jan 07:29, Oct 10:9, Dec 10:9, Dec 11:18; *CPT Changes: An
Insider's View* 2001

+ 88332   each additional tissue block with frozen section(s)
(List separately in addition to code for primary
procedure)
➔ *CPT Assistant* Winter 91:19, Apr 97:12, Aug 97:18, Jul 00:4,
Mar 06:6, Jan 07:29, Oct 10:9, Dec 10:9, Dec 11:18; *CPT
Changes: An Insider's View* 2011

(Use 88332 in conjunction with 88331)

88333   cytologic examination (eg, touch prep, squash prep),
initial site
➔ *CPT Assistant* Mar 06:6, Jan 07:29, Jun 08:15, Dec 10:9,
Dec 11:18; *CPT Changes: An Insider's View* 2006

+ 88334   cytologic examination (eg, touch prep, squash prep),
each additional site (List separately in addition to
code for primary procedure)
➔ *CPT Assistant* Mar 06:6, Jan 07:29, Oct 10:9, Dec 11:18; *CPT
Changes: An Insider's View* 2006, 2011

(Use 88334 in conjunction with 88331, 88333)

(For intraoperative consultation on a specimen requiring
both frozen section and cytologic evaluation, use 88331
and 88334)

(For percutaneous needle biopsy requiring intraprocedural
cytologic examination, use 88333)

(Do not report 88333 and 88334 for non-intraoperative
cytologic examination, see 88160-88162)

(Do not report 88333 and 88334 for intraprocedural
cytologic evaluation of fine needle aspirate, see 88172)

88342   Immunohistochemistry (including tissue
immunoperoxidase), each antibody
➔ *CPT Assistant* Winter 91:17, Jul 00:10, Nov 02:6-7, Nov 06:1,
Dec 11:18; *CPT Changes: An Insider's View* 2004

(Do not report 88342 in conjunction with 88360 or 88361
for the same antibody)

(For quantitative or semiquantitative
immunohistochemistry, see 88360, 88361)

88346   Immunofluorescent study, each antibody; direct method
➔ *CPT Assistant* Dec 11:18

88347   indirect method
➔ *CPT Assistant* Dec 11:18

88348   Electron microscopy; diagnostic
➔ *CPT Assistant* Dec 11:18

88349   scanning
➔ *CPT Assistant* Dec 11:18

Pathology and Laboratory

88355   Morphometric analysis; skeletal muscle
➔ *CPT Assistant* Dec 11:18

88356   nerve
➔ *CPT Assistant* Dec 11:18

88358   tumor (eg, DNA ploidy)
➔ *CPT Assistant* Jul 98:4, Jul 99:11, Jun 02:11, Jun 06:17, Dec 11:18; *CPT Changes: An Insider's View* 2004

(Do not report 88358 with 88313 unless each procedure is for a different special stain)

88360   Morphometric analysis, tumor immunohistochemistry (eg, Her-2/neu, estrogen receptor/progesterone receptor), quantitative or semiquantitative, each antibody; manual
➔ *CPT Assistant* Dec 11:18; *CPT Changes: An Insider's View* 2005

88361   using computer-assisted technology
➔ *CPT Assistant* Dec 11:18; *CPT Changes: An Insider's View* 2004, 2005

(Do not report 88360, 88361 with 88342 unless each procedure is for a different antibody)

(For morphometric analysis using in situ hybridization techniques, see 88367, 88368)

(When semi-thin plastic-embedded sections are performed in conjunction with morphometric analysis, only the morphometric analysis should be reported; if performed as an independent procedure, see codes 88300-88309 for surgical pathology.)

88362   Nerve teasing preparations
➔ *CPT Assistant* Dec 11:18

88363   Examination and selection of retrieved archival (ie, previously diagnosed) tissue(s) for molecular analysis (eg, KRAS mutational analysis)
➔ *CPT Assistant* Oct 10:10, Dec 10:10, Dec 11:18; *CPT Changes: An Insider's View* 2011

88365   In situ hybridization (eg, FISH), each probe
➔ *CPT Assistant* Jun 02:11, Mar 05:16, Dec 11:18, May 12:3; *CPT Changes: An Insider's View* 2005

(Do not report 88365 in conjunction with 88367, 88368 for the same probe)

88367   Morphometric analysis, in situ hybridization (quantitative or semi-quantitative) each probe; using computer-assisted technology
➔ *CPT Assistant* Mar 05:16, Oct 10:9, Dec 11:18; *CPT Changes: An Insider's View* 2005

88368   manual
➔ *CPT Assistant* Mar 05:16, Oct 10:9, Dec 11:18, May 12:5; *CPT Changes: An Insider's View* 2005

(For morphometric in situ hybridization evaluation of urinary tract cytologic specimens, see 88120, 88121)

88371   Protein analysis of tissue by Western Blot, with interpretation and report;
➔ *CPT Assistant* Dec 11:18

88372   immunological probe for band identification, each
➔ *CPT Assistant* Dec 11:8

● 88375   Optical endomicroscopic image(s), interpretation and report, real-time or referred, each endoscopic session
➔ *CPT Changes: An Insider's View* 2013

▶(Do not report 88375 in conjunction with 43206 or 43252)◀

88380   Microdissection (ie, sample preparation of microscopically identified target); laser capture
➔ *CPT Assistant* Apr 02:17, Apr 08:5, Dec 11:18, May 12:8, 10; *CPT Changes: An Insider's View* 2002, 2008

88381   manual
➔ *CPT Assistant* Apr 08:5, Dec 11:18, May 12:8, 10, *CPT Changes: An Insider's View* 2008

(Do not report 88380 in conjunction with 88381)

▶(88384-88386 have been deleted. To report, see 81200-81479)◀

88387   Macroscopic examination, dissection, and preparation of tissue for non-microscopic analytical studies (eg, nucleic acid-based molecular studies); each tissue preparation (eg, a single lymph node)
➔ *CPT Assistant* Dec 11:18; *CPT Changes: An Insider's View* 2010

(Do not report 88387 for tissue preparation for microbiologic cultures or flow cytometric studies)

(Do not report 88387 in conjunction with 88388, 88329-88334)

+ 88388   in conjunction with a touch imprint, intraoperative consultation, or frozen section, each tissue preparation (eg, a single lymph node) (List separately in addition to code for primary procedure)
➔ *CPT Assistant* Dec 11:18; *CPT Changes: An Insider's View* 2010

(Use 88388 in conjunction with 88329-88334)

(Do not report 88387 or 88388 for tissue preparation for microbiologic cultures or flow cytometric studies)

88399   Unlisted surgical pathology procedure

(88400 has been deleted. To report, use 88720)

In Vivo (eg, Transcutaneous) Laboratory Procedures

(For all in vivo measurements not specifically listed, use 88749)

(For wavelength fluorescent spectroscopy of advanced glycation end products (skin), use 0233T)

(For transcutaneous oxyhemoglobin measurement in a lower extremity wound by near infrared spectroscopy, use 0286T)

88720   Bilirubin, total, transcutaneous
➔ *CPT Assistant* Dec 10:10; *CPT Changes: An Insider's View* 2009

(For transdermal oxygen saturation, see 94760-94762)

⊙=Moderate sedation   ✚=Add-on code   ✗=FDA approval pending   #=Resequenced code   ○=Recycled/reinstated code   ➔➔=See p xiii for details

88738   Hemoglobin (Hgb), quantitative, transcutaneous
→ *CPT Changes: An Insider's View* 2010

(For in vitro hemoglobin measurement, use 85018)

88740   Hemoglobin, quantitative, transcutaneous, per day; carboxyhemoglobin
→ *CPT Changes: An Insider's View* 2009

(For in vitro carboxyhemoglobin measurement, use 82375)

88741   methemoglobin
→ *CPT Changes: An Insider's View* 2009

(For in vitro quantitative methemoglobin determination, use 83050)

88749   Unlisted in vivo (eg, transcutaneous) laboratory service
→ *CPT Assistant* Oct 10:10, Dec 10:10; *CPT Changes: An Insider's View* 2011

Other Procedures

89049   Caffeine halothane contracture test (CHCT) for malignant hyperthermia susceptibility, including interpretation and report
→ *CPT Assistant* Mar 06:6, May 06:19, Sep 11:4; *CPT Changes: An Insider's View* 2006

89050   Cell count, miscellaneous body fluids (eg, cerebrospinal fluid, joint fluid), except blood;
→ *CPT Assistant* Aug 05:9, Sep 11:4; *CPT Changes: An Insider's View* 2002

89051   with differential count
→ *CPT Assistant* Sep 11:4

89055   Leukocyte assessment, fecal, qualitative or semiquantitative
→ *CPT Assistant* Jul 03:9, Sep 11:4; *CPT Changes: An Insider's View* 2003, 2004

89060   Crystal identification by light microscopy with or without polarizing lens analysis, tissue or any body fluid (except urine)
→ *CPT Assistant* Sep 11:4; *CPT Changes: An Insider's View* 2007

(Do not report 89060 for crystal identification on paraffin-embedded tissue)

(89100, 89105 have been deleted. To report, see 43756, 43757)

89125   Fat stain, feces, urine, or respiratory secretions
→ *CPT Assistant* Sep 11:4; *CPT Changes: An Insider's View* 2001

(89130-89141 have been deleted. To report, see 43754, 43755)

89160   Meat fibers, feces
→ *CPT Assistant* Sep 11:4

89190   Nasal smear for eosinophils
→ *CPT Assistant* Sep 11:4

(Occult blood, feces, use 82270)

(Paternity tests, use 86910)

89220   Sputum, obtaining specimen, aerosol induced technique (separate procedure)
→ *CPT Assistant* Aug 05:9, Sep 11:4; *CPT Changes: An Insider's View* 2004

(89225 has been deleted)

89230   Sweat collection by iontophoresis
→ *CPT Assistant* Sep 11:4; *CPT Changes: An Insider's View* 2004

(89235 has been deleted)

89240   Unlisted miscellaneous pathology test
→ *CPT Assistant* Nov 05:14, Jan 07:30, Sep 11:4; *CPT Changes: An Insider's View* 2004

Reproductive Medicine Procedures

89250   Culture of oocyte(s)/embryo(s), less than 4 days;
→ *CPT Assistant* Nov 97:35-36, Jan 98:6, Oct 98:1, Apr 04:2, May 04:16, Jun 04:9, Sep 11:4; *CPT Changes: An Insider's View* 2004

89251   with co-culture of oocyte(s)/embryos
→ *CPT Assistant* Nov 97:35-36, Jan 98:6, Oct 98:1, Apr 04:2; *CPT Changes: An Insider's View* 2004

(For extended culture of oocyte[s]/embryo[s], see 89272)

89253   Assisted embryo hatching, microtechniques (any method)
→ *CPT Assistant* Nov 97:35-36, Jan 98:6, Oct 98:1, Apr 04:2, May 04:16, Jun 04:9

89254   Oocyte identification from follicular fluid
→ *CPT Assistant* Nov 97:35-36, Jan 98:6, Oct 98:1, Apr 04:2, May 04:16, Jun 04:9

89255   Preparation of embryo for transfer (any method)
→ *CPT Assistant* Nov 97:35-36, Jan 98:6, Oct 98:1, Apr 04:2, May 04:16, Jun 04:9

89257   Sperm identification from aspiration (other than seminal fluid)
→ *CPT Assistant* Nov 97:35-36, Jan 98:6, Oct 98:1, Nov 98:30, Apr 04:2

(For semen analysis, see 89300-89320)

(For sperm identification from testis tissue, use 89264)

89258   Cryopreservation; embryo(s)
→ *CPT Assistant* Nov 97:36, Jan 98:6, Oct 98:1, Apr 04:2, 4; *CPT Changes: An Insider's View* 2004

89259   sperm
→ *CPT Assistant* Nov 97:36, Jan 98:6, Oct 98:1, Apr 04:2, 4

(For cryopreservation of reproductive tissue, testicular, use 89335)

89260   Sperm isolation; simple prep (eg, sperm wash and swim-up) for insemination or diagnosis with semen analysis
→ *CPT Assistant* Nov 97:36, Jan 98:6, Oct 98:1, Apr 04:3-4

89261   complex prep (eg, Percoll gradient, albumin gradient) for insemination or diagnosis with semen analysis
→ *CPT Assistant* Nov 97:36, Jan 98:6, Oct 98:1, Apr 04:3-4

▲=Revised code   ●=New code   ▶◀=Contains new or revised text   ⊘=Modifier 51 exempt   American Medical Association   **471**

(For semen analysis without sperm wash or swim-up, use 89320)

89264 Sperm identification from testis tissue, fresh or cryopreserved

➜ *CPT Assistant* Nov 98:30, Apr 04:3-4

(For biopsy of testis, see 54500, 54505)

(For sperm identification from aspiration, use 89257)

(For semen analysis, see 89300-89320)

89268 Insemination of oocytes

➜ *CPT Assistant* Apr 04:3-4; *CPT Changes: An Insider's View* 2004

89272 Extended culture of oocyte(s)/embryo(s), 4-7 days

➜ *CPT Assistant* Apr 04:3-4; *CPT Changes: An Insider's View* 2004

89280 Assisted oocyte fertilization, microtechnique; less than or equal to 10 oocytes

➜ *CPT Assistant* Apr 04:3-4; *CPT Changes: An Insider's View* 2004

89281   greater than 10 oocytes

➜ *CPT Assistant* Apr 04:3-4; *CPT Changes: An Insider's View* 2004

89290 Biopsy, oocyte polar body or embryo blastomere, microtechnique (for pre-implantation genetic diagnosis); less than or equal to 5 embryos

➜ *CPT Assistant* Apr 04:5; *CPT Changes: An Insider's View* 2004

89291   greater than 5 embryos

➜ *CPT Assistant* Apr 04:3, 5; *CPT Changes: An Insider's View* 2004

89300 Semen analysis; presence and/or motility of sperm including Huhner test (post coital)

➜ *CPT Assistant* Nov 97:36, Jul 98:10, Oct 98:4, Apr 04:3, Aug 05:9

89310   motility and count (not including Huhner test)

➜ *CPT Assistant* Jul 03:9, Apr 04:3; *CPT Changes: An Insider's View* 2003

89320   volume, count, motility, and differential

➜ *CPT Assistant* Apr 04:3, Apr 08:5; *CPT Changes: An Insider's View* 2008

▶(Skin tests, see 86485-86580 and 95012-95199)◀

89321   sperm presence and motility of sperm, if performed

➜ *CPT Changes: An Insider's View* 2001, 2008

(To report Hyaluronan binding assay [HBA], use 89398)

89322   volume, count, motility, and differential using strict morphologic criteria (eg, Kruger)

➜ *CPT Assistant* Apr 08:5; *CPT Changes: An Insider's View* 2008

89325 Sperm antibodies

(For medicolegal identification of sperm, use 88125)

89329 Sperm evaluation; hamster penetration test

89330   cervical mucus penetration test, with or without spinnbarkeit test

➜ *CPT Assistant* Nov 05:14

89331 Sperm evaluation, for retrograde ejaculation, urine (sperm concentration, motility, and morphology, as indicated)

➜ *CPT Assistant* Apr 08:5; *CPT Changes: An Insider's View* 2008

(For semen analysis on concurrent semen specimen, see 89300-89322 in conjunction with 89331)

(For detection of sperm in urine, use 81015)

89335 Cryopreservation, reproductive tissue, testicular

➜ *CPT Assistant* Apr 04:5; *CPT Changes: An Insider's View* 2004

(For cryopreservation of embryo[s], use 89258. For cryopreservation of sperm, use 89259)

(For cryopreservation, ovarian reproductive tissue, oocytes, use 89240)

89342 Storage (per year); embryo(s)

➜ *CPT Assistant* Apr 04:5; *CPT Changes: An Insider's View* 2004

89343   sperm/semen

➜ *CPT Assistant* Apr 04:5; *CPT Changes: An Insider's View* 2004

89344   reproductive tissue, testicular/ovarian

➜ *CPT Assistant* Apr 04:5; *CPT Changes: An Insider's View* 2004

89346   oocyte(s)

➜ *CPT Assistant* Apr 04:5; *CPT Changes: An Insider's View* 2004, 2005

89352 Thawing of cryopreserved; embryo(s)

➜ *CPT Assistant* Apr 04:5; *CPT Changes: An Insider's View* 2004

89353   sperm/semen, each aliquot

➜ *CPT Assistant* Apr 04:5; *CPT Changes: An Insider's View* 2004

89354   reproductive tissue, testicular/ovarian

➜ *CPT Assistant* Apr 04:5; *CPT Changes: An Insider's View* 2004

89356   oocytes, each aliquot

➜ *CPT Assistant* Apr 04:5, Aug 05:9; *CPT Changes: An Insider's View* 2004

89398 Unlisted reproductive medicine laboratory procedure

➜ *CPT Changes: An Insider's View* 2010

Medicine Guidelines

Medicine

The following is a listing of headings and subheadings that appear within the Medicine section of the CPT codebook. The subheadings or subsections denoted with asterisks (*) below have special instructions unique to that section. Where these are indicated, special "notes" or guidelines will be presented preceding those procedural terminology listings, referring to that subsection specifically.

Medicine Guidelines

In addition to the definitions and commonly used terms presented in the **Introduction**, several other items unique to this section on **Medicine** are defined or identified here.

Add-on Codes

Some of the listed procedures are commonly carried out in addition to the primary procedure performed. All add-on codes found in the CPT codebook are exempt from the multiple procedure concept. They are exempt from the use of modifier 51, as these procedures are not reported as stand-alone codes. These additional or supplemental procedures are designated as "add-on" codes. Add-on codes in the CPT codebook can be readily identified by specific descriptor nomenclature which includes phrases such as "each additional" or "(List separately in addition to primary procedure)."

Separate Procedures

Some of the procedures or services listed in the CPT codebook that are commonly carried out as an integral component of a total service or procedure have been identified by the inclusion of the term "separate procedure." The codes designated as "separate procedure" should not be reported in addition to the code for the total procedure or service of which it is considered an integral component.

However, when a procedure or service that is designated as a "separate procedure" is carried out independently or considered to be unrelated or distinct from other procedures/services provided at that time, it may be reported by itself, or in addition to other procedures/services by appending modifier 59 to the specific "separate procedure" code to indicate that the procedure is not considered to be a component of another procedure, but is a distinct, independent procedure. This may represent a different session or patient encounter, different procedure or surgery, different site or organ system, separate incision/excision, separate lesion, or separate injury (or area of injury in extensive injuries).

Unlisted Service or Procedure

A service or procedure may be provided that is not listed in this edition of the CPT codebook. When reporting such a service, the appropriate "Unlisted Procedure" code may be used to indicate the service, identifying it by "Special Report" as discussed on this page. The "Unlisted Procedures" and accompanying codes for **Medicine** are as follows:

90399	Unlisted immune globulin
90749	Unlisted vaccine/toxoid
90899	Unlisted psychiatric service or procedure
90999	Unlisted dialysis procedure, inpatient or outpatient
91299	Unlisted diagnostic gastroenterology procedure
92499	Unlisted ophthalmological service or procedure
92700	Unlisted otorhinolaryngological service or procedure
93799	Unlisted cardiovascular service or procedure
93998	Unlisted noninvasive vascular diagnostic study
94799	Unlisted pulmonary service or procedure
95199	Unlisted allergy/clinical immunologic service or procedure
95999	Unlisted neurological or neuromuscular diagnostic procedure
96379	Unlisted therapeutic, prophylactic, or diagnostic intravenous or intra-arterial injection or infusion
96549	Unlisted chemotherapy procedure
96999	Unlisted special dermatological service or procedure
97039	Unlisted modality (specify type and time if constant attendance)
97139	Unlisted therapeutic procedure (specify)
97799	Unlisted physical medicine/rehabilitation service or procedure
99199	Unlisted special service, procedure or report
99600	Unlisted home visit service or procedure

Special Report

A service that is rarely provided, unusual, variable, or new may require a special report. Pertinent information should include an adequate definition or description of the nature, extent, and need for the procedure; and the time, effort, and equipment necessary to provide the service.

▶Supplied Materials◀

▶Supplies and materials (eg, trays, drug supplies, and materials) over and above those usually included with the procedure(s) rendered are reported separately using code 99070 or a specific supply code.◀

Medicine

Immune Globulins, Serum or Recombinant Products

Codes 90281-90399 identify the serum globulins, extracted from human blood; or recombinant immune globulin products created in a laboratory through genetic modification of human and/or animal proteins. Both are reported in addition to the administration codes 96365-96368, 96372, 96374, 96375 as appropriate. Modifier 51 should not be reported with this section of products codes when performed with another procedure. The serum or recombinant globulin products listed here include broad-spectrum anti-infective immune globulins, antitoxins, various isoantibodies, and monoclonal antibodies.

90281 Immune globulin (Ig), human, for intramuscular use
➔ *CPT Assistant* Nov 98:30, Jan 99:3, Sep 99:10; *CPT Changes: An Insider's View* 2008

90283 Immune globulin (IgIV), human, for intravenous use
➔ *CPT Assistant* Nov 98:30, Jan 99:3; *CPT Changes: An Insider's View* 2008

90284 Immune globulin (SCIg), human, for use in subcutaneous infusions, 100 mg, each
➔ *CPT Changes: An Insider's View* 2008

90287 Botulinum antitoxin, equine, any route
➔ *CPT Assistant* Nov 98:30, Jan 99:3; *CPT Changes: An Insider's View* 2008

90288 Botulism immune globulin, human, for intravenous use
➔ *CPT Assistant* Nov 98:30, Jan 99:3; *CPT Changes: An Insider's View* 2008

90291 Cytomegalovirus immune globulin (CMV-IgIV), human, for intravenous use
➔ *CPT Assistant* Nov 98:30, Jan 99:3; *CPT Changes: An Insider's View* 2008

90296 Diphtheria antitoxin, equine, any route
➔ *CPT Assistant* Nov 98:30, Jan 99:3; *CPT Changes: An Insider's View* 2008

90371 Hepatitis B immune globulin (HBIg), human, for intramuscular use
➔ *CPT Assistant* Nov 98:30, Jan 99:3; *CPT Changes: An Insider's View* 2008

90375 Rabies immune globulin (RIg), human, for intramuscular and/or subcutaneous use
➔ *CPT Assistant* Nov 98:30, Jan 99:3; *CPT Changes: An Insider's View* 2008

90376 Rabies immune globulin, heat-treated (RIg-HT), human, for intramuscular and/or subcutaneous use
➔ *CPT Assistant* Nov 98:30, Jan 99:3; *CPT Changes: An Insider's View* 2008

90378 Respiratory syncytial virus, monoclonal antibody, recombinant, for intramuscular use, 50 mg, each
➔ *CPT Assistant* Jan 99:3, Nov 99:47, Jun 00:10; *CPT Changes: An Insider's View* 2000, 2001, 2008, 2010

(90379 has been deleted)

90384 Rho(D) immune globulin (RhIg), human, full-dose, for intramuscular use
➔ *CPT Assistant* Nov 98:30, Jan 99:3; *CPT Changes: An Insider's View* 2008

90385 Rho(D) immune globulin (RhIg), human, mini-dose, for intramuscular use
➔ *CPT Assistant* Nov 98:30, Jan 99:3; *CPT Changes: An Insider's View* 2008

90386 Rho(D) immune globulin (RhIgIV), human, for intravenous use
➔ *CPT Assistant* Nov 98:30, Jan 99:3; *CPT Changes: An Insider's View* 2008

90389 Tetanus immune globulin (TIg), human, for intramuscular use
➔ *CPT Assistant* Nov 98:30, Jan 99:3; *CPT Changes: An Insider's View* 2008

90393 Vaccinia immune globulin, human, for intramuscular use
➔ *CPT Assistant* Nov 98:30, Jan 99:3; *CPT Changes: An Insider's View* 2008

90396 Varicella-zoster immune globulin, human, for intramuscular use
➔ *CPT Assistant* Nov 98:30, Jan 99:3; *CPT Changes: An Insider's View* 2008

90399 Unlisted immune globulin
➔ *CPT Assistant* Nov 98:30, Jan 99:3, Feb 99:11, Sep 99:10; *CPT Changes: An Insider's View* 2008

Immunization Administration for Vaccines/Toxoids

Report vaccine immunization administration codes 90460, 90461, 90471-90474 in addition to the vaccine and toxoid code(s) 90476-90749.

▶Report codes 90460 and 90461 only when the physician or qualified health care professional provides face-to-face counseling of the patient/family during the administration of a vaccine. For immunization administration of any vaccine that is not accompanied by face-to-face physician or qualified health care professional counseling to the patient/family or for administration of vaccines to patients over 18 years of age, report codes 90471-90474. (See also Instructions for Use of the CPT Codebook for definition of reporting qualifications).

If a significant separately identifiable Evaluation and Management service (eg, new or established patient office or other outpatient services [99201-99215], office or other outpatient consultations [99241-99245], emergency department services [99281-99285], preventive medicine services [99381-99429]) is performed, the appropriate E/M service code should be reported in addition to the vaccine and toxoid administration codes.◄

A component refers to all antigens in a vaccine that prevent disease(s) caused by one organism (90460 and 90461). Multi-valent antigens or multiple serotypes of antigens against a single organism are considered a single component of vaccines. Combination vaccines are those vaccines that contain multiple vaccine components. Conjugates or adjuvants contained in vaccines are not considered to be component parts of the vaccine as defined above.

(For allergy testing, see 95004 et seq)

(For skin testing of bacterial, viral, fungal extracts, see 86485-86580)

(For therapeutic or diagnostic injections, see 96372-96379)

90460 Immunization administration through 18 years of age via any route of administration, with counseling by physician or other qualified health care professional; first or only component of each vaccine or toxoid administered
➜ *CPT Assistant* Mar 11:3, Jun 11:14, Jan 12:43, Jul 12:7; *CPT Changes: An Insider's View* 2011, 2012

+ 90461 each additional vaccine or toxoid component administered (List separately in addition to code for primary procedure)
➜ *CPT Assistant* Mar 11:3, Jun 11:14, Jan 12:43, Jul 12:7; *CPT Changes: An Insider's View* 2011, 2012

(Use 90460 for each vaccine administered. For vaccines with multiple components [combination vaccines], report 90460 in conjunction with 90461 for each additional component in a given vaccine)

(90465-90468 have been deleted. To report, see 90460, 90461, 90471-90474)

(90470 has been deleted)

90471 Immunization administration (includes percutaneous, intradermal, subcutaneous, or intramuscular injections); 1 vaccine (single or combination vaccine/toxoid)
➜ *CPT Assistant* Nov 98:31, Jan 99:2, Apr 99:10, Oct 99:9, Nov 99:47-48, Nov 00:10, Feb 01:5, Jul 01:2, Nov 02:11, Mar 04:11, Apr 04:14, Apr 05:1-3, 5, Nov 05:1, Jan 09:8, Jul 09:7, Aug 09:9, Sep 09:7, Oct 09:3, Mar 11:3, Jun 11:14, Jul 12:7; *CPT Changes: An Insider's View* 2002, 2005

(Do not report 90471 in conjunction with 90473)

+ 90472 each additional vaccine (single or combination vaccine/toxoid) (List separately in addition to code for primary procedure)
➜ *CPT Assistant* Nov 98:31, Jan 99:2, Apr 99:10, Oct 99:9, Nov 99:47-48, Nov 00:10, Feb 01:5, Jul 01:2, Nov 02:11, Mar 04:11, Apr 04:14, Apr 05:1-3, Nov 05:1, Jan 09:3, 8, Jul 09:7, Aug 09:9, Sep 09:7, Oct 09:3, Mar 11:3, Jun 11:14, Jul 12:7; *CPT Changes: An Insider's View* 2000

►(Use 90472 in conjunction with 90460, 90471, 90473)◄

(For administration of immune globulins, see 90281-90399, 96360, 96361, 96365-96368, 96374)

(For intravesical administration of BCG vaccine, see 51720, 90586)

90473 Immunization administration by intranasal or oral route; 1 vaccine (single or combination vaccine/toxoid)
➜ *CPT Assistant* Feb 01:5, Nov 02:11, Apr 04:14, Apr 05:1-3, Jan 09:3, 8, Jul 09:7, Aug 09:9, Oct 09:3, Mar 11:3, Jun 11:14, Jul 12:7; *CPT Changes: An Insider's View* 2002

(Do not report 90473 in conjunction with 90471)

+ 90474 each additional vaccine (single or combination vaccine/toxoid) (List separately in addition to code for primary procedure)
➜ *CPT Assistant* Feb 01:5, Nov 02:11, Apr 04:14, Apr 05:1-3, Jan 09:3, 8, Jul 09:7, Aug 09:9, Oct 09:3, Mar 11:3, Jun 11:14, Jul 12:7; *CPT Changes: An Insider's View* 2002

►(Use 90474 in conjunction with 90460, 90471, 90473)◄

Vaccines, Toxoids

To assist users to report the most recent new or revised vaccine product codes, the American Medical Association (AMA) currently uses the CPT Website, which features updates of CPT Editorial Panel actions regarding these products. Once approved by the CPT Editorial Panel, these codes will be made available for release on a semi-annual (twice a year: July 1 and January 1) basis. As part of the electronic distribution, there is a six-month implementation period from the initial release date (ie, codes released on January 1 are eligible for use on July 1 and codes released on July 1 are eligible for use January 1).

The CPT Editorial Panel, in recognition of the public health interest in vaccine products, has chosen to publish new vaccine product codes prior to approval by the U. S. Food and Drug Administration (FDA). These codes are indicated with the ∕ symbol and will be tracked by the AMA to monitor FDA approval status. Once the FDA status changes to approval, the ∕ symbol will be removed. CPT users should refer to the AMA Internet site (www.ama-assn.org/ama/pub/category/10902.html) for the most up-to-date information on codes with the ∕ symbol.

Codes 90476-90748 identify the vaccine product **only.** To report the administration of a vaccine/toxoid, the vaccine/toxoid product codes 90476-90749 must be used in addition to an immunization administration code(s) 90460-90474. Modifier 51 should not be reported for the vaccines, toxoids when performed with these administration procedures.

If a significantly separately identifiable Evaluation and Management (E/M) service (eg, office or other outpatient services, preventive medicine services) is performed, the appropriate E/M service code should be reported in addition to the vaccine and toxoid administration codes.

To meet the reporting requirements of immunization registries, vaccine distribution programs, and reporting systems (eg, Vaccine Adverse Event Reporting System) the exact vaccine product administered needs to be reported. Multiple codes for a particular vaccine are provided in the CPT codebook when the schedule (number of doses or timing) differs for two or more products of the same vaccine type (eg, hepatitis A, Hib) or the vaccine product is available in more than one chemical formulation, dosage, or route of administration.

The "when administered to" age descriptions included in CPT vaccine codes are not intended to identify a product's licensed age indication. The term "preservative free" includes use for vaccines that contain no preservative and vaccines that contain trace amounts of preservative agents that are not present in a sufficient concentration for the purpose of preserving the final vaccine formulation. The absence of a designation regarding a preservative does not necessarily indicate the presence or absence of preservative in the vaccine. Refer to the product's prescribing information (PI) for the licensed age indication before administering vaccine to a patient.

Separate codes are available for combination vaccines (eg, DTP-Hib, DtaP-Hib, HepB-Hib). It is inappropriate to code each component of a combination vaccine separately. If a specific vaccine code is not available, the unlisted procedure code should be reported, until a new code becomes available.

(For immune globulins, see codes 90281-90399, 96365-96368, 96372-96375 for administration of immune globulins)

➜ *CPT Assistant* Nov 99:48

90476   Adenovirus vaccine, type 4, live, for oral use

➜ *CPT Assistant* Nov 98:31-33, Jan 99:2, Sep 99:10, Oct 99:9, Nov 99:48, Mar 11:4; *CPT Changes: An Insider's View* 2008

90477   Adenovirus vaccine, type 7, live, for oral use

➜ *CPT Assistant* Nov 98:31-33, Jan 99:2, Oct 99:9, Mar 11:4; *CPT Changes: An Insider's View* 2008

90581   Anthrax vaccine, for subcutaneous or intramuscular use

➜ *CPT Assistant* Nov 98:31-33, Jan 99:2, Oct 99:9, Mar 11:4; *CPT Changes: An Insider's View* 2008, 2012

90585   Bacillus Calmette-Guerin vaccine (BCG) for tuberculosis, live, for percutaneous use

➜ *CPT Assistant* Nov 98:31-33, Jan 99:2, Oct 99:9, Mar 11:4; *CPT Changes: An Insider's View* 2008

90586   Bacillus Calmette-Guerin vaccine (BCG) for bladder cancer, live, for intravesical use

➜ *CPT Assistant* Nov 98:31-33, Jan 99:2, Oct 99:9, Nov 02:11, Mar 11:4; *CPT Changes: An Insider's View* 2008

90632   Hepatitis A vaccine, adult dosage, for intramuscular use

➜ *CPT Assistant* Nov 98:31-33, Jan 99:2, Oct 99:9, Mar 11:4; *CPT Changes: An Insider's View* 2008

90633   Hepatitis A vaccine, pediatric/adolescent dosage-2 dose schedule, for intramuscular use

➜ *CPT Assistant* Nov 98:31-33, Jan 99:2, Oct 99:9, Mar 11:4; *CPT Changes: An Insider's View* 2008

90634   Hepatitis A vaccine, pediatric/adolescent dosage-3 dose schedule, for intramuscular use

➜ *CPT Assistant* Nov 98:31-33, Jan 99:2, Oct 99:9, Mar 11:4; *CPT Changes: An Insider's View* 2008

90636   Hepatitis A and hepatitis B vaccine (HepA-HepB), adult dosage, for intramuscular use

➜ *CPT Assistant* Nov 98:31-33, Jan 99:2, Oct 99:9, Mar 11:4; *CPT Changes: An Insider's View* 2008

90644   Meningococcal conjugate vaccine, serogroups C & Y and Hemophilus influenza B vaccine (Hib-MenCY), 4 dose schedule, when administered to children 2-15 months of age, for intramuscular use

➜ *CPT Assistant* Mar 11:4; *CPT Changes: An Insider's View* 2011, 2012

90645   Hemophilus influenza b vaccine (Hib), HbOC conjugate (4 dose schedule), for intramuscular use

➜ *CPT Assistant* Nov 98:31-33, Jan 99:2, Oct 99:9, Mar 11:4; *CPT Changes: An Insider's View* 2008

90646   Hemophilus influenza b vaccine (Hib), PRP-D conjugate, for booster use only, intramuscular use

➜ *CPT Assistant* Nov 98:31-33, Jan 99:2, Oct 99:9, Mar 11:4; *CPT Changes: An Insider's View* 2008

90647   Hemophilus influenza b vaccine (Hib), PRP-OMP conjugate (3 dose schedule), for intramuscular use

➜ *CPT Assistant* Nov 98:31-33, Jan 99:2, Oct 99:9, Mar 11:4; *CPT Changes: An Insider's View* 2008

90648   Hemophilus influenza b vaccine (Hib), PRP-T conjugate (4 dose schedule), for intramuscular use

➜ *CPT Assistant* Nov 98:31-33, Jan 99:2, Oct 99:9, Sep 09:7, Mar 11:4; *CPT Changes: An Insider's View* 2008

90649   Human Papilloma virus (HPV) vaccine, types 6, 11, 16, 18 (quadrivalent), 3 dose schedule, for intramuscular use

➜ *CPT Assistant* Dec 05:9, Jun 06:8, Sep 06:14, Jul 07:13, Mar 11:4; *CPT Changes: An Insider's View* 2006, 2008

90650   Human Papilloma virus (HPV) vaccine, types 16, 18, bivalent, 3 dose schedule, for intramuscular use

➜ *CPT Assistant* Mar 11:4; *CPT Changes: An Insider's View* 2009, 2011

⚡● **90653**   Influenza vaccine, inactivated, subunit, adjuvanted, for intramuscular use

➜ *CPT Changes: An Insider's View* 2013

90654   Influenza virus vaccine, split virus, preservative-free, for intradermal use

➜ *CPT Changes: An Insider's View* 2012

▲ **90655**   Influenza virus vaccine, trivalent, split virus, preservative free, when administered to children 6-35 months of age, for intramuscular use

➜ *CPT Assistant* Oct 99:9, Feb 04:2, Apr 07:12, Apr 08:8, Oct 09:3, Mar 11:4; *CPT Changes: An Insider's View* 2004, 2007, 2008, 2013

▲ **90656**   Influenza virus vaccine, trivalent, split virus, preservative free, when administered to individuals 3 years and older, for intramuscular use

➜ *CPT Assistant* Apr 08:8, Oct 09:3, Mar 11:4; *CPT Changes: An Insider's View* 2005, 2007, 2008, 2013

▲ **90657**   Influenza virus vaccine, trivalent, split virus, when administered to children 6-35 months of age, for intramuscular use

➜ *CPT Assistant* Nov 98:31-33, Jan 99:2, Oct 99:9, Feb 02:10, Feb 04:2, Apr 05:5, Apr 08:8, Oct 09:3, Mar 11:4; *CPT Changes: An Insider's View* 2004, 2007, 2008, 2013

▲ **90658**   Influenza virus vaccine, trivalent, split virus, when administered to individuals 3 years of age and older, for intramuscular use

➜ *CPT Assistant* Nov 98:31-33, Jan 99:2, Oct 99:9, Feb 04:2, Apr 07:12, Apr 08:8, Oct 09:3, Mar 11:4; *CPT Changes: An Insider's View* 2004, 2007, 2008, 2013

▲ **90660**   Influenza virus vaccine, trivalent, live, for intranasal use

➜ *CPT Assistant* Nov 98:31-33, Jan 99:2, Oct 99:9, Mar 04:11, Apr 04:14, Oct 09:3, Mar 11:4; *CPT Changes: An Insider's View* 2008, 2013

#● **90672**   Influenza virus vaccine, quadrivalent, live, for intranasal use

➜ *CPT Changes: An Insider's View* 2013

∕ **90661**   Influenza virus vaccine, derived from cell cultures, subunit, preservative and antibiotic free, for intramuscular use

➜ *CPT Assistant* Apr 08:8, Oct 09:3, Mar 11:4; *CPT Changes: An Insider's View* 2008

90662   Influenza virus vaccine, split virus, preservative free, enhanced immunogenicity via increased antigen content, for intramuscular use

➜ *CPT Assistant* Apr 08:8, Oct 09:3, 6, Mar 11:4; *CPT Changes: An Insider's View* 2008, 2011

(90663 has been deleted)

90664   Influenza virus vaccine, pandemic formulation, live, for intranasal use

➜ *CPT Assistant* Mar 11:4; *CPT Changes: An Insider's View* 2011

►(90665 has been deleted)◄

∕ **90666**   Influenza virus vaccine, pandemic formulation, split virus, preservative free, for intramuscular use

➜ *CPT Assistant* Mar 11:4; *CPT Changes: An Insider's View* 2011

∕ **90667**   Influenza virus vaccine, pandemic formulation, split virus, adjuvanted, for intramuscular use

➜ *CPT Assistant* Mar 11:4; *CPT Changes: An Insider's View* 2011

∕ **90668**   Influenza virus vaccine, pandemic formulation, split virus, for intramuscular use

➜ *CPT Assistant* Mar 11:4; *CPT Changes: An Insider's View* 2011

90669   Pneumococcal conjugate vaccine, 7 valent, for intramuscular use

➜ *CPT Assistant* Nov 98:31-33, Jan 99:2, Oct 99:9, Jun 00:10, Mar 11:4; *CPT Changes: An Insider's View* 2001, 2007, 2008, 2010

90670   Pneumococcal conjugate vaccine, 13 valent, for intramuscular use

➜ *CPT Assistant* Mar 11:4; *CPT Changes: An Insider's View* 2010, 2011

90672   Code is out of numerical sequence. See 90476-90749

90675   Rabies vaccine, for intramuscular use

➜ *CPT Assistant* Nov 98:31-33, Jan 99:2, Oct 99:9, Mar 11:4; *CPT Changes: An Insider's View* 2008

90676   Rabies vaccine, for intradermal use

➜ *CPT Assistant* Nov 98:31-33, Jan 99:2, Oct 99:9, Mar 11:4, Jul 12:7; *CPT Changes: An Insider's View* 2008

90680   Rotavirus vaccine, pentavalent, 3 dose schedule, live, for oral use

➜ *CPT Assistant* Nov 98:31-33, Jan 99:2, Oct 99:9, Jun 05:6, Dec 05:9, Jun 06:8, Mar 11:4; *CPT Changes: An Insider's View* 2006, 2008

90681   Rotavirus vaccine, human, attenuated, 2 dose schedule, live, for oral use

➜ *CPT Assistant* Mar 11:4, Jul 12:7; *CPT Changes: An Insider's View* 2009

90690   Typhoid vaccine, live, oral

➜ *CPT Assistant* Nov 98:31-33, Jan 99:2, Oct 99:9, Mar 11:4; *CPT Changes: An Insider's View* 2008

90691   Typhoid vaccine, Vi capsular polysaccharide (ViCPs), for intramuscular use

➜ *CPT Assistant* Nov 98:31-33, Jan 99:2, Oct 99:9, Mar 11:4; *CPT Changes: An Insider's View* 2008

90692   Typhoid vaccine, heat- and phenol-inactivated (H-P), for subcutaneous or intradermal use

➜ *CPT Assistant* Nov 98:31-33, Jan 99:2, Oct 99:9, Jan 08:4, Mar 11:4; *CPT Changes: An Insider's View* 2008

90693   Typhoid vaccine, acetone-killed, dried (AKD), for subcutaneous use (U.S. military)

➜ *CPT Assistant* Nov 98:31-33, Jan 99:2, Oct 99:9, Mar 11:4; *CPT Changes: An Insider's View* 2004, 2008

90696   Diphtheria, tetanus toxoids, acellular pertussis vaccine and poliovirus vaccine, inactivated (DTaP-IPV), when administered to children 4 through 6 years of age, for intramuscular use

➜ *CPT Assistant* Mar 11:4; *CPT Changes: An Insider's View* 2009

90698   Diphtheria, tetanus toxoids, acellular pertussis vaccine, haemophilus influenza Type B, and poliovirus vaccine, inactivated (DTaP - Hib - IPV), for intramuscular use

➜ *CPT Assistant* Oct 99:9, Dec 05:9, Jun 06:8, Mar 11:4; *CPT Changes: An Insider's View* 2008, 2009

90700   Diphtheria, tetanus toxoids, and acellular pertussis vaccine (DTaP), when administered to individuals younger than 7 years, for intramuscular use

➜ *CPT Assistant* Jan 96:5, Apr 97:10, Nov 98:31-33, Jan 99:2, Oct 99:9, Nov 03:13, Mar 11:4, Jul 12:7; *CPT Changes: An Insider's View* 2005, 2007, 2008

►(90701 has been deleted)◄

90702   Diphtheria and tetanus toxoids (DT) adsorbed when administered to individuals younger than 7 years, for intramuscular use

➜ *CPT Assistant* Jan 96:6, Aug 96:10, Apr 97:10, Nov 98:31-33, Jan 99:2, Sep 99:10, Oct 99:9, Jun 00:10, Feb 07:11, Mar 11:4; *CPT Changes: An Insider's View* 2001, 2007, 2008

90703   Tetanus toxoid adsorbed, for intramuscular use

➜ *CPT Assistant* Jan 96:6, Apr 97:10, Nov 98:31-33, Jan 99:2, Sep 99:10, Oct 99:9, Mar 11:4; *CPT Changes: An Insider's View* 2004, 2008

Medicine

Medicine

90704 Mumps virus vaccine, live, for subcutaneous use

→ *CPT Assistant* Apr 97:10, Nov 98:31-33, Jan 99:2, Oct 99:9, Mar 11:4; *CPT Changes: An Insider's View* 2004, 2008

90705 Measles virus vaccine, live, for subcutaneous use

→ *CPT Assistant* Apr 97:10, Nov 98:31-33, Jan 99:2, Oct 99:9, Mar 11:4; *CPT Changes: An Insider's View* 2004, 2008

90706 Rubella virus vaccine, live, for subcutaneous use

→ *CPT Assistant* Apr 97:10, Nov 98:31-33, Jan 99:2, Oct 99:9, Mar 11:4; *CPT Changes: An Insider's View* 2004, 2008

90707 Measles, mumps and rubella virus vaccine (MMR), live, for subcutaneous use

→ *CPT Assistant* Jan 96:6, May 96:10, Apr 97:10, Nov 98:31-33, Jan 99:2, Oct 99:9, Apr 05:1, 5, Mar 11:4, Jul 12:7; *CPT Changes: An Insider's View* 2004, 2008

90708 Measles and rubella virus vaccine, live, for subcutaneous use

→ *CPT Assistant* Apr 97:10, Nov 98:31-33, Jan 99:2, Oct 99:9, Mar 11:4; *CPT Changes: An Insider's View* 2004, 2008

90710 Measles, mumps, rubella, and varicella vaccine (MMRV), live, for subcutaneous use

→ *CPT Assistant* May 96:10, Apr 97:10, Nov 98:31-33, Jan 99:2, Oct 99:9, Dec 05:9, Jun 06:8, Mar 11:4; *CPT Changes: An Insider's View* 2008

90712 Poliovirus vaccine, (any type[s]) (OPV), live, for oral use

→ *CPT Assistant* Jan 96:6, Apr 97:10, Nov 98:31-33, Jan 99:2, Oct 99:9, Nov 09:10, Mar 11:4; *CPT Changes: An Insider's View* 2008

90713 Poliovirus vaccine, inactivated (IPV), for subcutaneous or intramuscular use

→ *CPT Assistant* Apr 97:10, Nov 98:31-33, Jan 99:2, Oct 99:9, Jun 05:6, Mar 11:4; *CPT Changes: An Insider's View* 2006, 2008

90714 Tetanus and diphtheria toxoids (Td) adsorbed, preservative free, when administered to individuals 7 years or older, for intramuscular use

→ *CPT Assistant* Jun 05:6, Mar 11:4; *CPT Changes: An Insider's View* 2006, 2007, 2008

90715 Tetanus, diphtheria toxoids and acellular pertussis vaccine (Tdap), when administered to individuals 7 years or older, for intramuscular use

→ *CPT Assistant* Oct 99:9, Jun 05:6, Dec 05:9, Jun 06:8, Mar 11:4; *CPT Changes: An Insider's View* 2006, 2007, 2008

90716 Varicella virus vaccine, live, for subcutaneous use

→ *CPT Assistant* Jan 96:6, May 96:10, Apr 97:10, Nov 98:31-33, Jan 99:2, Oct 99:9, Mar 11:4; *CPT Changes: An Insider's View* 2008

90717 Yellow fever vaccine, live, for subcutaneous use

→ *CPT Assistant* Apr 97:10, Nov 98:31-33, Jan 99:2, Oct 99:9, Mar 11:4; *CPT Changes: An Insider's View* 2008

►(90718 has been deleted)◄

90719 Diphtheria toxoid, for intramuscular use

→ *CPT Assistant* Apr 97:10, Nov 98:31-33, Jan 99:2, Sep 99:10, Oct 99:9, Mar 11:4; *CPT Changes: An Insider's View* 2008

90720 Diphtheria, tetanus toxoids, and whole cell pertussis vaccine and Hemophilus influenza B vaccine (DTP-Hib), for intramuscular use

→ *CPT Assistant* Jan 96:5, Apr 97:10, Nov 98:31-33, Jan 99:2, Oct 99:9, Mar 11:4; *CPT Changes: An Insider's View* 2008

90721 Diphtheria, tetanus toxoids, and acellular pertussis vaccine and Hemophilus influenza B vaccine (DtaP-Hib), for intramuscular use

→ *CPT Assistant* Jan 96:5, Apr 97:10, Nov 98:31-33, Jan 99:2, Oct 99:9, Mar 11:4; *CPT Changes: An Insider's View* 2000, 2008

90723 Diphtheria, tetanus toxoids, acellular pertussis vaccine, Hepatitis B, and poliovirus vaccine, inactivated (DtaP-HepB-IPV), for intramuscular use

→ *CPT Assistant* Apr 97:10, Oct 99:9, Mar 11:4; *CPT Changes: An Insider's View* 2001, 2008

90725 Cholera vaccine for injectable use

→ *CPT Assistant* Apr 97:10, Nov 98:31-33, Jan 99:2, Oct 99:9, Mar 11:4; *CPT Changes: An Insider's View* 2008

90727 Plague vaccine, for intramuscular use

→ *CPT Assistant* Apr 97:10, Nov 98:31-33, Jan 99:2, Oct 99:9, Mar 11:4; *CPT Changes: An Insider's View* 2004, 2008

90732 Pneumococcal polysaccharide vaccine, 23-valent, adult or immunosuppressed patient dosage, when administered to individuals 2 years or older, for subcutaneous or intramuscular use

→ *CPT Assistant* Apr 97:10, Nov 98:31-33, Jan 99:2, Oct 99:9, Mar 11:4; *CPT Changes: An Insider's View* 2002, 2007, 2008

90733 Meningococcal polysaccharide vaccine (any group(s)), for subcutaneous use

→ *CPT Assistant* Apr 97:10, Nov 98:31-33, Jan 99:2, Oct 99:9, Dec 99:7, Mar 11:4; *CPT Changes: An Insider's View* 2001, 2004, 2008

90734 Meningococcal conjugate vaccine, serogroups A, C, Y and W-135 (tetravalent), for intramuscular use

→ *CPT Assistant* Oct 99:9, Mar 11:4; *CPT Changes: An Insider's View* 2008

90735 Japanese encephalitis virus vaccine, for subcutaneous use

→ *CPT Assistant* Apr 97:10, Nov 98:31-33, Jan 99:2, Oct 99:9, Mar 11:4; *CPT Changes: An Insider's View* 2008

90736 Zoster (shingles) vaccine, live, for subcutaneous injection

→ *CPT Assistant* Dec 05:9, Jun 06:8, Jul 07:13, Mar 11:4; *CPT Changes: An Insider's View* 2006, 2008

90738 Japanese encephalitis virus vaccine, inactivated, for intramuscular use

→ *CPT Assistant* Mar 11:4; *CPT Changes: An Insider's View* 2009, 2010

✗● **90739** Hepatitis B vaccine, adult dosage (2 dose schedule), for intramuscular use

→ *CPT Changes: An Insider's View* 2013

90740 Hepatitis B vaccine, dialysis or immunosuppressed patient dosage (3 dose schedule), for intramuscular use

→ *CPT Assistant* Apr 97:10, Oct 99:9, Apr 01:10, Mar 11:4; *CPT Changes: An Insider's View* 2001, 2008

90743 Hepatitis B vaccine, adolescent (2 dose schedule), for intramuscular use

→ *CPT Assistant* Apr 97:10, Oct 99:9, Mar 11:4; *CPT Changes: An Insider's View* 2001, 2008

90744 Hepatitis B vaccine, pediatric/adolescent dosage (3 dose schedule), for intramuscular use

→ *CPT Assistant* Jan 96:5, Apr 97:10, Jun 97:10, Nov 98:31-33, Jan 99:2, Oct 99:9, Nov 99:48-49, Jun 00:10, Mar 11:4; *CPT Changes: An Insider's View* 2000, 2001, 2008

▲ **90746**   Hepatitis B vaccine, adult dosage (3 dose schedule), for
             intramuscular use
             ➲ *CPT Assistant* Jan 96:5, Apr 97:10, Nov 98:31-33, Jan 99:2,
               Oct 99:9, Mar 11:4; *CPT Changes: An Insider's View* 2008, 2013

90747   Hepatitis B vaccine, dialysis or immunosuppressed
           patient dosage (4 dose schedule), for intramuscular use
           ➲ *CPT Assistant* Jan 96:5, Apr 97:10, Jun 97:10, Nov 98:31-33,
             Jan 99:2, Oct 99:9, Jun 00:10, Apr 01:10, Mar 11:4; *CPT
             Changes: An Insider's View* 2001, 2008

90748   Hepatitis B and Hemophilus influenza b vaccine (HepB-
           Hib), for intramuscular use
           ➲ *CPT Assistant* Apr 97:10, Nov 97:37, Nov 98:31-33, Jan 99:2,
             Sep 99:10, Oct 99:9, Mar 11:4, Jul 12:7; *CPT Changes: An
             Insider's View* 2008

90749   Unlisted vaccine/toxoid
           ➲ *CPT Assistant* Jan 96:6, Apr 97:10, Jun 97:10, Nov 98:31-33,
             Jan 99:2, Oct 99:9, Nov 02:11, Mar 11:4; *CPT Changes: An
             Insider's View* 2008

Psychiatry

►Psychiatry services include diagnostic services, psychotherapy, and other services to an individual, family, or group. Patient condition, characteristics, or situational factors may require services described as being with interactive complexity. Services may be provided to a patient in crisis. Services are provided in all settings of care and psychiatry services codes are reported without regard to setting. Services may be provided by a physician or other qualified health care professional. Some psychiatry services may be reported with **Evaluation and Management Services** (99201-99255, 99281-99285, 99304-99337, 99341-99350) or other services when performed. **Evaluation and Management Services** (99201-99285, 99304-99337, 99341-99350) may be reported for treatment of psychiatric conditions, rather than using **Psychiatry Services** codes, when appropriate.

Hospital care in treating a psychiatric inpatient or partial hospitalization may be initial or subsequent in nature (see 99221-99233).

Some patients receive hospital evaluation and management services only and others receive hospital evaluation and management services and other procedures. If other procedures such as electroconvulsive therapy or psychotherapy are rendered in addition to hospital evaluation and management services, these may be listed separately (eg, hospital care services [99221-99223, 99231-99233] plus electroconvulsive therapy [90870]), or when psychotherapy is done, with appropriate code(s) defining psychotherapy services.

Consultation for psychiatric evaluation of a patient includes examination of a patient and exchange of information with the primary physician and other informants such as nurses or family members, and preparation of a report. These services may be reported using consultation codes (see **Consultations**).◄

►Interactive Complexity◄

►Code 90785 is an add-on code for interactive complexity to be reported in conjunction with codes for diagnostic psychiatric evaluation (90791, 90792), psychotherapy (90832, 90834, 90837), psychotherapy when performed with an evaluation and management service (90833, 90836, 90838, 99201-99255, 99304-99337, 99341-99350), and group psychotherapy (90853).

Interactive complexity refers to specific communication factors that complicate the delivery of a psychiatric procedure. Common factors include more difficult communication with discordant or emotional family members and engagement of young and verbally undeveloped or impaired patients. Typical patients are those who have third parties, such as parents, guardians, other family members, interpreters, language translators, agencies, court officers, or schools involved in their psychiatric care.

These factors are typically present with patients who:

■ Have other individuals legally responsible for their care, such as minors or adults with guardians, or

■ Request others to be involved in their care during the visit, such as adults accompanied by one or more participating family members or interpreter or language translator, or

■ Require the involvement of other third parties, such as child welfare agencies, parole or probation officers, or schools.

Psychiatric procedures may be reported "with interactive complexity" when at least one of the following is present:

1. The need to manage maladaptive communication (related to, eg, high anxiety, high reactivity, repeated questions, or disagreement) among participants that complicates delivery of care.

2. Caregiver emotions or behavior that interferes with the caregiver's understanding and ability to assist in the implementation of the treatment plan.

3. Evidence or disclosure of a sentinel event and mandated report to third party (eg, abuse or neglect with report to state agency) with initiation of discussion of the sentinel event and/or report with patient and other visit participants.

4. Use of play equipment, other physical devices, interpreter, or translator to communicate with the patient to overcome barriers to therapeutic or diagnostic interaction between the physician or other qualified health care professional and a patient who:

■ Is not fluent in the same language as the physician or other qualified health care professional, or

■ Has not developed, or has lost, either the expressive language communication skills to explain his/her symptoms and response to treatment, or the receptive communication skills to understand the physician or other qualified health care professional if he/she were to use typical language for communication.

When provided in conjunction with the psychotherapy services (90832-90838), the amount of time spent by a physician or other qualified health care professional providing interactive complexity services should be reflected in the timed service code for psychotherapy (90832, 90834, 90837) or the psychotherapy add-on code performed with an evaluation and management service (90833, 90836, 90838) and must relate to the psychotherapy service only. Interactive complexity is not a factor for evaluation and management services selection (99201-99255, 99281-99285, 99304-99337, 99341-99350), except as it directly affects key components as defined in the Evaluation and Management Services Guidelines (ie, history, examination, and medical decision making).◄

+● 90785   Interactive complexity (List separately in addition to the code for primary procedure)

➔ *CPT Changes: An Insider's View* 2013

►(Use 90785 in conjunction with codes for diagnostic psychiatric evaluation [90791, 90792], psychotherapy [90832, 90834, 90837], psychotherapy when performed with an evaluation and management service [90833, 90836, 90838, 99201-99255, 99304-99337, 99341-99350], and group psychotherapy [90853])◄

►(Do not report 90785 in conjunction with 90839, 90840, or in conjunction with E/M services when no psychotherapy service is also reported)◄

►Psychiatric Diagnostic Procedures◄

►Psychiatric diagnostic evaluation is an integrated biopsychosocial assessment, including history, mental status, and recommendations. The evaluation may include communication with family or other sources and review and ordering of diagnostic studies.

Psychiatric diagnostic evaluation with medical services is an integrated biopsychosocial and medical assessment, including history, mental status, other physical examination elements as indicated, and recommendations. The evaluation may include communication with family or other sources, prescription of medications, and review and ordering of laboratory or other diagnostic studies.

In certain circumstances one or more other informants (family members, guardians, or significant others) may be seen in lieu of the patient. Codes 90791, 90792 may be reported more than once for the patient when separate diagnostic evaluations are conducted with the patient and other informants. Report services as being provided to the patient and not the informant or other party in such circumstances. Codes 90791, 90792 may be reported once per day and not on the same day as an evaluation and management service performed by the same individual for the same patient.

The psychiatric diagnostic evaluation may include interactive complexity services when factors exist that complicate the delivery of the psychiatric procedure. These services should be reported with add-on code 90785 used in conjunction with the diagnostic psychiatric evaluation codes 90791, 90792.

Codes 90791, 90792 are used for the diagnostic assessment(s) or reassessment(s), if required, and do not include psychotherapeutic services. Psychotherapy services, including for crisis, may not be reported on the same day.◄

● 90791   Psychiatric diagnostic evaluation

➔ *CPT Changes: An Insider's View* 2013

● 90792   Psychiatric diagnostic evaluation with medical services

➔ *CPT Changes: An Insider's View* 2013

►(Do not report 90791 or 90792 in conjunction with 99201-99337, 99341-99350, 99366-99368, 99401-99444)◄

►(Use 90785 in conjunction with 90791, 90792 when the diagnostic evaluation includes interactive complexity services)◄

►(90801 and 90802 have been deleted. To report diagnostic evaluations, see 90791, 90792)◄

►(90804, 90805, 90806, 90807, 90808, 90809 have been deleted. To report, see psychotherapy codes 90832, 90834, 90837 or psychotherapy add-on codes when performed with an evaluation and management service [90833, 90836, 90838, 99201-99255, 99304-99337, 99341-99350])◄

►(90810, 90811, 90812, 90813, 90814, 90815 have been deleted. To report interactive psychotherapy, report 90785 in conjunction with psychotherapy codes 90832, 90834, 90837 or psychotherapy add-on codes when performed with an evaluation and management service [90833, 90836, 90838, 99201-99255, 99304-99337, 99341-99350])◄

►(90816, 90817, 90818, 90819, 90821, 90822 have been deleted. To report, see psychotherapy codes 90832, 90834, 90837 or psychotherapy add-on codes when performed with an evaluation and management service [90833, 90836, 90838, 99201-99255, 99304-99337, 99341-99350])◄

►(90823, 90824, 90826, 90827, 90828, 90829 have been deleted. To report interactive psychotherapy, report 90785 in conjunction with psychotherapy codes 90832, 90834, 90837 or psychotherapy add-on codes when performed with an evaluation and management service [90833, 90836, 90838, 99201-99255, 99304-99337, 99341-99350])◄

►Psychotherapy◄

►Psychotherapy is the treatment of mental illness and behavioral disturbances in which the physician or other qualified health care professional, through definitive therapeutic communication, attempts to alleviate the emotional disturbances, reverse or change maladaptive patterns of behavior, and encourage personality growth and development.

The psychotherapy service codes 90832-90838 include ongoing assessment and adjustment of psychotherapeutic interventions, and may include involvement of family member(s) or others in the treatment process.

Psychotherapy times are for face-to-face services with patient and/or family member. The patient must be present for all or some of the service. For family psychotherapy without the patient present, use 90846. In reporting, choose the code closest to the actual time (ie, 16-37 minutes for 90832 and 90833, 38-52 minutes for 90834 and 90836, and 53 or more minutes for 90837 and 90838). Do not report psychotherapy of less than 16 minutes duration. (See instructions for the usage of time in the Introduction of the CPT code set).

Psychotherapy provided to a patient in a crisis state is reported with codes 90839 and 90840 and cannot be reported in addition to the psychotherapy codes 90832-90838. For psychotherapy for crisis, see "Other Psychotherapy."

Code 90785 is an add-on code to report interactive complexity services when provided in conjunction with the psychotherapy codes 90832-90838. The amount of time spent by a physician or other qualified health care professional providing interactive complexity services should be reflected in the timed service code for psychotherapy (90832, 90834, 90837) or the psychotherapy add-on code performed with an evaluation and management service (90833, 90836, 90838).

Some psychiatric patients receive a medical evaluation and management (E/M) service on the same day as a psychotherapy service by the same physician or other qualified health care professional. To report both E/M and psychotherapy, the two services must be significant and separately identifiable. These services are reported by using codes specific for psychotherapy when performed with evaluation and management services (90833, 90836, and 90838) as add-on codes to the evaluation and management service.

Medical symptoms and disorders inform treatment choices of psychotherapeutic interventions, and data from therapeutic communication are used to evaluate the presence, type, and severity of medical symptoms and disorders. For the purposes of reporting, the medical and psychotherapeutic components of the service may be separately identified as follows:

1. The type and level of E/M service is selected first based upon the key components of history, examination, and medical decision-making.

2. Time associated with activities used to meet criteria for the E/M service is not included in the time used for reporting the psychotherapy service (ie, time spent on history, examination and medical decision making **when used for the E/M service** is not psychotherapy time). Time may not be used as the basis of E/M code selection and Prolonged Services may not be reported when psychotherapy with E/M (90833, 90836, 90838) are reported.

3. A separate diagnosis is not required for the reporting of E/M and psychotherapy on the same date of service.◄

● **90832**   Psychotherapy, 30 minutes with patient and/or family member
➔ *CPT Changes: An Insider's View* 2013

+● **90833**   Psychotherapy, 30 minutes with patient and/or family member when performed with an evaluation and management service (List separately in addition to the code for primary procedure)
➔ *CPT Changes: An Insider's View* 2013

►(Use 90833 in conjunction with 99201-99255, 99304-99337, 99341-99350)◄

● **90834**   Psychotherapy, 45 minutes with patient and/or family member
➔ *CPT Changes: An Insider's View* 2013

+● **90836**   Psychotherapy, 45 minutes with patient and/or family member when performed with an evaluation and management service (List separately in addition to the code for primary procedure)
➔ *CPT Changes: An Insider's View* 2013

►(Use 90836 in conjunction with 99201-99255, 99304-99337, 99341-99350)◄

● **90837**   Psychotherapy, 60 minutes with patient and/or family member
➔ *CPT Changes: An Insider's View* 2013

+● **90838**   Psychotherapy, 60 minutes with patient and/or family member when performed with an evaluation and management service (List separately in addition to the code for primary procedure)
➔ *CPT Changes: An Insider's View* 2013

►(Use 90838 in conjunction with 99201-99255, 99304-99337, 99341-99350)◄

►(Use the appropriate prolonged services code [99354-99357] for psychotherapy services 68 minutes or longer)◄

►(Use 90785 in conjunction with 90832, 90833, 90834, 90836, 90837, 90838 when psychotherapy includes interactive complexity services)◄

Medicine

Other Psychotherapy

►Psychotherapy for Crisis◄

►Psychotherapy for crisis is an urgent assessment and history of a crisis state, a mental status exam, and a disposition. The treatment includes psychotherapy, mobilization of resources to defuse the crisis and restore safety, and implementation of psychotherapeutic interventions to minimize the potential for psychological trauma. The presenting problem is typically life threatening or complex and requires immediate attention to a patient in high distress.

Codes 90839, 90840 are used to report the total duration of time face-to-face with the patient and/or family spent by the physician or other qualified health care professional providing psychotherapy for crisis, even if the time spent on that date is not continuous. For any given period of time spent providing psychotherapy for crisis state, the physician or other qualified health care professional must devote his or her full attention to the patient and, therefore, cannot provide services to any other patient during the same time period. The patient must be present for all or some of the service. Do not report with 90791 or 90792.

Code 90839 is used to report the first 30-74 minutes of psychotherapy for crisis on a given date. It should be used only once per date even if the time spent by the physician or other health care professional is not continuous on that date. Psychotherapy for crisis of less than 30 minutes total duration on a given date should be reported with 90832 or 90833 (when provided with evaluation and management services). Code 90840 is used to report additional block(s) of time, of up to 30 minutes each beyond the first 74 minutes.◄

● **90839** Psychotherapy for crisis; first 60 minutes
> *CPT Changes: An Insider's View* 2013

+● **90840** each additional 30 minutes (List separately in addition to code for primary service)
> *CPT Changes: An Insider's View* 2013

►(Use 90840 in conjunction with 90839)◄

►(Do not report 90839, 90840 in conjunction with 90791, 90792, psychotherapy codes 90832-90838 or other psychiatric services, or 90785-90899)◄

90845 Psychoanalysis
> *CPT Assistant* Summer 92:15, Nov 97:40-41, Mar 01:8, Mar 02:4, May 05:1, Feb 06:15, Mar 10:6

90846 Family psychotherapy (without the patient present)
> *CPT Assistant* Summer 92:15, Nov 97:40-41, Mar 01:8, Mar 02:4, May 05:1, Sep 09:11, Mar 10:6

90847 Family psychotherapy (conjoint psychotherapy) (with patient present)
> *CPT Assistant* Summer 92:15, Nov 97:40-41, Mar 01:5, Mar 02:4, May 05:1, Mar 10:6

90849 Multiple-family group psychotherapy
> *CPT Assistant* Summer 92:15, Nov 97:40-41, Mar 01:5, Mar 02:4, May 05:1, Mar 10:6

90853 Group psychotherapy (other than of a multiple-family group)
> *CPT Assistant* Summer 92:15, Nov 97:40-41, Mar 01:8, Mar 02:4, May 05:1, Mar 10:6

►(Use 90853 in conjunction with 90785 for the specified patient when group psychotherapy includes interactive complexity)◄

►(90857 has been deleted. To report, use 90785 in conjunction with 90853)◄

►Other Psychiatric Services or Procedures◄

(For analysis/programming of neurostimulators used for vagus nerve stimulation therapy, see 95970, 95974, 95975)

►(90862 has been deleted. To report, see 90863 or evaluation and management services codes 99201-99255, 99281-99285, 99304-99337, 99341-99350)◄

+● **90863** Pharmacologic management, including prescription and review of medication, when performed with psychotherapy services (List separately in addition to the code for primary procedure)
> *CPT Changes: An Insider's View* 2013

►(Use 90863 in conjunction with 90832, 90834, 90837)◄

►(For pharmacologic management with psychotherapy services performed by a physician or other qualified health care professional who may report evaluation and management codes, use the appropriate evaluation and management codes 99201-99255, 99281-99285, 99304-99337, 99341-99350 and the appropriate psychotherapy with evaluation and management service 90833, 90836, 90838)◄

►(Do not count time spent on providing pharmacologic management services in the time used for selection of the psychotherapy service)◄

90865 Narcosynthesis for psychiatric diagnostic and therapeutic purposes (eg, sodium amobarbital (Amytal) interview)
> *CPT Assistant* Nov 97:41, Mar 01:5, Mar 02:4, May 05:1

90867 Therapeutic repetitive transcranial magnetic stimulation (TMS) treatment; initial, including cortical mapping, motor threshold determination, delivery and management
> *CPT Changes: An Insider's View* 2011, 2012

(Report only once per course of treatment)

►(Do not report 90867 in conjunction with 90868, 90869, 95860-95870, 95928, 95929, 95939)◄

90868 subsequent delivery and management, per session
> *CPT Changes: An Insider's View* 2011, 2012

90869 subsequent motor threshold re-determination with delivery and management
> *CPT Changes: An Insider's View* 2012

►(Do not report 90869 in conjunction with 90867, 90868, 95860-95870, 95928, 95929, 95939)◄

►(If a significant, separately identifiable evaluation and management, medication management, or psychotherapy service is performed, the appropriate E/M or psychotherapy code, may be reported in addition to 90867-90869. Evaluation and management activities directly related to cortical mapping, motor threshold determination, delivery and management of TMS are not separately reported)◄

►(For transcranial magnetic stimulation motor function mapping for therapeutic planning other than for repetitive transcranial magnetic stimulation, use 0310T)◄

►(Do not count time spent on providing pharmacologic management services in the time used for selection of the psychotherapy service)◄

90870 Electroconvulsive therapy (includes necessary monitoring)

➜ *CPT Assistant* Summer 92:16, Mar 01:5, Mar 02:4, May 05:1, Mar 10:6; *CPT Changes: An Insider's View* 2006

▲ **90875** Individual psychophysiological therapy incorporating biofeedback training by any modality (face-to-face with the patient), with psychotherapy (eg, insight oriented, behavior modifying or supportive psychotherapy); 30 minutes

➜ *CPT Assistant* Nov 96:15, Sep 97:11, Nov 97:41, Apr 98:14, Jun 99:5, Mar 01:5, Mar 02:4, Mar 05:16, May 05:1; *CPT Changes: An Insider's View* 2013

▲ **90876** 45 minutes

➜ *CPT Assistant* Nov 96:15, Sep 97:11, Nov 97:41, Jun 99:5, Mar 01:5, Mar 05:16, May 05:1; *CPT Changes: An Insider's View* 2013

90880 Hypnotherapy

➜ *CPT Assistant* Summer 92:16, Nov 97:41, Mar 01:5, Mar 02:4, May 05:1

90882 Environmental intervention for medical management purposes on a psychiatric patient's behalf with agencies, employers, or institutions

➜ *CPT Assistant* Summer 92:16, Mar 01:5, Mar 02:4, May 05:1

90885 Psychiatric evaluation of hospital records, other psychiatric reports, psychometric and/or projective tests, and other accumulated data for medical diagnostic purposes

➜ *CPT Assistant* Nov 97:41, Mar 01:5, Mar 02:4, Oct 04:10, May 05:1

90887 Interpretation or explanation of results of psychiatric, other medical examinations and procedures, or other accumulated data to family or other responsible persons, or advising them how to assist patient

➜ *CPT Assistant* Summer 92:17, Mar 01:5, Mar 02:4, Oct 02:11, May 05:1

▲ **90889** Preparation of report of patient's psychiatric status, history, treatment, or progress (other than for legal or consultative purposes) for other individuals, agencies, or insurance carriers

➜ *CPT Assistant* Summer 92:17, Mar 01:5, Mar 02:4, May 05:1; *CPT Changes: An Insider's View* 2013

90899 Unlisted psychiatric service or procedure

➜ *CPT Assistant* Mar 01:5, Mar 02:4, May 05:1, Jan 10:11

Biofeedback

(For psychophysiological therapy incorporating biofeedback training, see 90875, 90876)

90901 Biofeedback training by any modality

➜ *CPT Assistant* Sep 97:11, Apr 98:14, Jun 98:10, Jun 99:5, May 02:18, Sep 04:13, Mar 05:16

90911 Biofeedback training, perineal muscles, anorectal or urethral sphincter, including EMG and/or manometry

➜ *CPT Assistant* Sep 97:11, Nov 97:41, Jun 98:10, Jun 99:5

(For testing of rectal sensation, tone and compliance, use 91120)

(For incontinence treatment by pulsed magnetic neuromodulation, use 53899)

Dialysis

(90918, 90922 have been deleted. To report ESRD-related services for patients younger than 2 years of age, see 90951-90953, 90963, 90967)

(90919, 90923 have been deleted. To report ESRD-related services for patients between 2 and 11 years of age, see 90954-90956, 90964, 90968)

(90920, 90924 have been deleted. To report ESRD-related services for patients between 12 and 19 years of age, see 90957-90959, 90965, 90969)

(90921, 90925 have been deleted. To report ESRD-related services for patients 20 years of age and older, see 90960-90962, 90966, 90970)

Hemodialysis

►Codes 90935, 90937 are reported to describe the hemodialysis procedure with all evaluation and management services related to the patient's renal disease on the day of the hemodialysis procedure. These codes are used for inpatient ESRD and non-ESRD procedures or for outpatient non-ESRD dialysis services. Code 90935 is reported if only one evaluation of the patient is required related to that hemodialysis procedure. Code 90937 is reported when patient re-evaluation(s) is required during a hemodialysis procedure. Use modifier 25 with evaluation and management codes, including new or established patient office or other outpatient services (99201-99215), office or other outpatient consultations (99241-99245), observation care (99217-99220, 99224-99226), observation or inpatient care including admission and discharge (99234-99236), initial hospital care (99221-99226, 99231-99239), new or established patient emergency department services (99281-99285), critical care services (99291, 99292), inpatient neonatal intensive care services and pediatric and neonatal critical care services (99466-99480), nursing facility services (99304-99318), domiciliary, rest home services, or custodial care (99324-99337), and home services (99341-99350), for separately identifiable services unrelated to the dialysis procedure or renal failure which cannot be rendered during the dialysis session.◄

(For home visit hemodialysis services performed by a non-physician health care professional, use 99512)

(For cannula declotting, see 36831, 36833, 36860, 36861)

(For declotting of implanted vascular access device or catheter by thrombolytic agent, use 36593)

(For collection of blood specimen from a partially or completely implantable venous access device, use 36591)

►(For prolonged attendance by a physician or other qualified health care professional, see 99354-99360)◄

▲ **90935** Hemodialysis procedure with single evaluation by a physician or other qualified health care professional

➔ *CPT Assistant* Fall 93:2, May 02:17, Jan 03:22; *CPT Changes: An Insider's View* 2013

90937 Hemodialysis procedure requiring repeated evaluation(s) with or without substantial revision of dialysis prescription

➔ *CPT Assistant* Fall 93:2, May 02:17, Jan 03:22

90940 Hemodialysis access flow study to determine blood flow in grafts and arteriovenous fistulae by an indicator method

➔ *CPT Assistant* Jan 03:22, May 06:18; *CPT Changes: An Insider's View* 2001, 2006

➔ *Clinical Examples in Radiology* Summer 06:7, 12

(For duplex scan of hemodialysis access, use 93990)

Miscellaneous Dialysis Procedures

►Codes 90945, 90947 describe dialysis procedures other than hemodialysis (eg, peritoneal dialysis, hemofiltration or continuous renal replacement therapies), and all evaluation and management services related to the patient's renal disease on the day of the procedure. Code 90945 is reported if only one evaluation of the patient is required related to that procedure. Code 90947 is reported when patient re-evaluation(s) is required during a procedure. Use modifier 25 with evaluation and management codes, including office or other outpatient services (99201-99215), office or other outpatient consultations (99241-99245), observation care (99217-99220, 99224-99226), observation or inpatient care including admission and discharge (99234-99239), hospital care (99221-99226, 99231-99239), new or established patient emergency department services (99281-99285), critical care services (99291, 99292), inpatient neonatal intensive care services and pediatric and neonatal critical care services (99466-99480), nursing facility services (99304-99318), domiciliary, rest home, or custodial care services (99324-99337), and home services (99341-99350) for separately identifiable services

unrelated to the procedure or the renal failure which cannot be rendered during the dialysis session.◄

(For percutaneous insertion of intraperitoneal tunneled catheter, use 49418. For open insertion of tunneled intraperitoneal catheter, use 49421)

►(For prolonged attendance by a physician or other qualified health care professional, see 99354-99360)◄

▲ **90945** Dialysis procedure other than hemodialysis (eg, peritoneal dialysis, hemofiltration, or other continuous renal replacement therapies), with single evaluation by a physician or other qualified health care professional

➔ *CPT Assistant* Fall 93:2, Nov 97:41, Jul 98:10, Oct 01:11, Jan 03:22; *CPT Changes: An Insider's View* 2001, 2013

(For home infusion of peritoneal dialysis, use 99601, 99602)

▲ **90947** Dialysis procedure other than hemodialysis (eg, peritoneal dialysis, hemofiltration, or other continuous renal replacement therapies) requiring repeated evaluation by a physician or other qualified health care professional, with or without substantial revision of dialysis prescription

➔ *CPT Assistant* Fall 93:2, Nov 97:41, Jul 98:10, Oct 01:11, Jan 03:22; *CPT Changes: An Insider's View* 2001, 2013

End-Stage Renal Disease Services

►Codes 90951-90962 are reported **once** per month to distinguish age-specific services related to the patient's end-stage renal disease (ESRD) performed in an outpatient setting with three levels of service based on the number of face-to-face visits. ESRD-related services by a physician or other qualified health care professional include establishment of a dialyzing cycle, outpatient evaluation and management of the dialysis visits, telephone calls, and patient management during the dialysis provided during a full month. In circumstances in which the patient has had a complete assessment visit during the month and services are provided over a period of less than a month, 90951-90962 may be used according to the number of visits performed.◄

Codes 90963-90966 are reported once per month for a full month of service to distinguish age-specific services for end-stage renal disease (ESRD) services for home dialysis patients.

For ESRD and non-ESRD dialysis services performed in an inpatient setting, and for non-ESRD dialysis services performed in an outpatient setting, see 90935-90937 and 90945-90947.

Evaluation and management services unrelated to ESRD services that cannot be performed during the dialysis session may be reported separately.

Codes 90967-90970 are reported to distinguish age-specific services for end-stage renal disease (ESRD) services for less than a full month of service, per day, for services provided under the following circumstances:

home dialysis patients less than a full month, transient patients, partial month where there was one or more face-to-face visits without the complete assessment, the patient was hospitalized before a complete assessment was furnished, dialysis was stopped due to recovery or death, or the patient received a kidney transplant. For reporting purposes, each month is considered 30 days.

Examples:

ESRD-related services:

►ESRD-related services are initiated on July 1 for a 57-year-old male. On July 11, he is admitted to the hospital as an inpatient and is discharged on July 27. He has had a complete assessment and the physician or other qualified health care professional has performed two face-to-face visits prior to admission. Another face-to-face visit occurs after discharge during the month.◄

In this example, 90961 is reported for the three face-to-face outpatient visits. Report inpatient E/M services as appropriate. Dialysis procedures rendered during the hospitalization (July 11-27) should be reported as appropriate (90935-90937, 90945-90947).

If the patient did not have a complete assessment during the month or was a transient or dialysis was stopped due to recovery or death, 90970 would be used to report each day outside the inpatient hospitalization as described in the home dialysis example below.

ESRD-related services for the home dialysis patient:

Home ESRD-related services are initiated on July 1 for a 57-year-old male. On July 11, he is admitted to the hospital as an inpatient and is discharged on July 27.

In this example, 90970 should be reported for each day outside of the inpatient hospitalization (30 days/month less 17 days/hospitalization = 13 days). Report inpatient E/M services as appropriate. Dialysis procedures rendered during the hospitalization (July 11-27) should be reported as appropriate (90935-90937, 90945-90947).

►(Do not report 90951-90970 during the same month in conjuction with 99487-99489)◄

►(Do not report 90951-90970 during the service time of 99495-99496)◄

▲ **90951** End-stage renal disease (ESRD) related services monthly, for patients younger than 2 years of age to include monitoring for the adequacy of nutrition, assessment of growth and development, and counseling of parents; with 4 or more face-to-face visits by a physician or other qualified health care professional per month
➜ *CPT Changes: An Insider's View* 2009, 2013

▲ **90952** with 2-3 face-to-face visits by a physician or other qualified health care professional per month
➜ *CPT Changes: An Insider's View* 2009, 2013

▲ **90953** with 1 face-to-face visit by a physician or other qualified health care professional per month
➜ *CPT Changes: An Insider's View* 2009, 2013

▲ **90954** End-stage renal disease (ESRD) related services monthly, for patients 2-11 years of age to include monitoring for the adequacy of nutrition, assessment of growth and development, and counseling of parents; with 4 or more face-to-face visits by a physician or other qualified health care professional per month
➜ *CPT Changes: An Insider's View* 2009, 2013

▲ **90955** with 2-3 face-to-face visits by a physician or other qualified health care professional per month
➜ *CPT Changes: An Insider's View* 2009, 2013

▲ **90956** with 1 face-to-face visit by a physician or other qualified health care professional per month
➜ *CPT Changes: An Insider's View* 2009, 2013

▲ **90957** End-stage renal disease (ESRD) related services monthly, for patients 12-19 years of age to include monitoring for the adequacy of nutrition, assessment of growth and development, and counseling of parents; with 4 or more face-to-face visits by a physician or other qualified health care professional per month
➜ *CPT Changes: An Insider's View* 2009, 2013

▲ **90958** with 2-3 face-to-face visits by a physician or other qualified health care professional per month
➜ *CPT Changes: An Insider's View* 2009, 2013

▲ **90959** with 1 face-to-face visit by a physician or other qualified health care professional per month
➜ *CPT Changes: An Insider's View* 2009, 2013

▲ **90960** End-stage renal disease (ESRD) related services monthly, for patients 20 years of age and older; with 4 or more face-to-face visits by a physician or other qualified health care professional per month
➜ *CPT Changes: An Insider's View* 2009, 2013

▲ **90961** with 2-3 face-to-face visits by a physician or other qualified health care professional per month
➜ *CPT Changes: An Insider's View* 2009, 2013

▲ **90962** with 1 face-to-face visit by a physician or other qualified health care professional per month
➜ *CPT Changes: An Insider's View* 2009, 2013

90963 End-stage renal disease (ESRD) related services for home dialysis per full month, for patients younger than 2 years of age to include monitoring for the adequacy of nutrition, assessment of growth and development, and counseling of parents
➜ *CPT Changes: An Insider's View* 2009

90964 End-stage renal disease (ESRD) related services for home dialysis per full month, for patients 2-11 years of age to include monitoring for the adequacy of nutrition, assessment of growth and development, and counseling of parents
➜ *CPT Changes: An Insider's View* 2009

90965 End-stage renal disease (ESRD) related services for home dialysis per full month, for patients 12-19 years of age to include monitoring for the adequacy of nutrition, assessment of growth and development, and counseling of parents
➜ *CPT Changes: An Insider's View* 2009

Medicine

90966 End-stage renal disease (ESRD) related services for home dialysis per full month, for patients 20 years of age and older
> *CPT Changes: An Insider's View* 2009

90967 End-stage renal disease (ESRD) related services for dialysis less than a full month of service, per day; for patients younger than 2 years of age
> *CPT Changes: An Insider's View* 2009

90968   for patients 2-11 years of age
> *CPT Changes: An Insider's View* 2009

90969   for patients 12-19 years of age
> *CPT Changes: An Insider's View* 2009

90970   for patients 20 years of age and older
> *CPT Changes: An Insider's View* 2009

Other Dialysis Procedures

90989 Dialysis training, patient, including helper where applicable, any mode, completed course
> *CPT Assistant* Fall 93:5, Jun 01:10

90993 Dialysis training, patient, including helper where applicable, any mode, course not completed, per training session
> *CPT Assistant* Winter 90:11, Fall 93:5, Jun 01:10

90997 Hemoperfusion (eg, with activated charcoal or resin)

90999 Unlisted dialysis procedure, inpatient or outpatient

Gastroenterology

(For duodenal intubation and aspiration, see 43756, 43757)

(For gastrointestinal radiologic procedures, see 74210-74363)

▶(For esophagoscopy procedures, see 43200-43228; upper GI endoscopy 43235-43259; endoscopy, small intestine and stomal 44360-44393; proctosigmoidoscopy 45300-45321; sigmoidoscopy 45330-45339; colonoscopy 45355-45385; anoscopy 46600-46615)◀

(91000 has been deleted)

91010 Esophageal motility (manometric study of the esophagus and/or gastroesophageal junction) study with interpretation and report;
> *CPT Assistant* Nov 97:42; *CPT Changes: An Insider's View* 2011, 2012

(91011, 91012 have been deleted. To report esophageal motility studies with stimulant or perfusion, use 91013 in conjunction with 91010)

+ 91013   with stimulation or perfusion (eg, stimulant, acid or alkali perfusion) (List separately in addition to code for primary procedure)
> *CPT Changes: An Insider's View* 2011, 2012

(Use 91013 in conjunction with 91010)

(Do not report 91013 more than once per session)

(To report esophageal motility studies with high resolution esophageal pressure topography, use 0240T and with stimulant or perfusion, use 0241T)

91020 Gastric motility (manometric) studies
> *CPT Assistant* Nov 97:42

91022 Duodenal motility (manometric) study
> *CPT Changes: An Insider's View* 2006

(If gastrointestinal endoscopy is performed, use 43235)

(If fluoroscopy is performed, use 76000)

(If gastric motility study is performed, use 91020)

▶(Do not report 91020, 91022 in conjunction with 91112)◀

91030 Esophagus, acid perfusion (Bernstein) test for esophagitis

91034 Esophagus, gastroesophageal reflux test; with nasal catheter pH electrode(s) placement, recording, analysis and interpretation
> *CPT Assistant* May 05:3; *CPT Changes: An Insider's View* 2005

Esophageal Acid Reflux Test
91034

A catheter with a pH electrode is placed into the esophagus, either through the nares or swallowed, to measure intraesophageal pH (an indicator of gastric reflux).

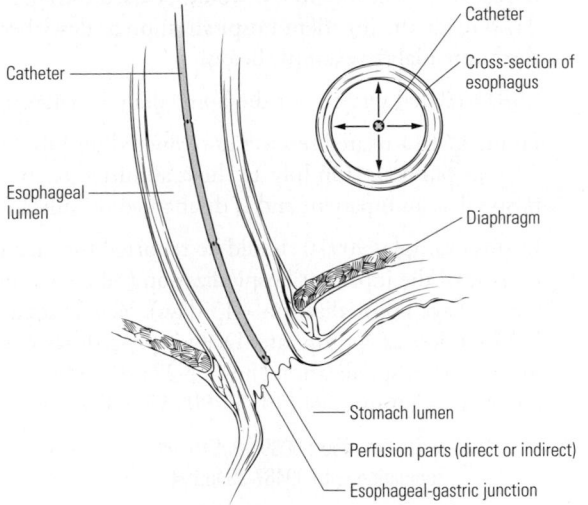

91035   with mucosal attached telemetry pH electrode placement, recording, analysis and interpretation
> *CPT Assistant* May 05:3; *CPT Changes: An Insider's View* 2005

91037 Esophageal function test, gastroesophageal reflux test with nasal catheter intraluminal impedance electrode(s) placement, recording, analysis and interpretation;
> *CPT Assistant* May 05:3; *CPT Changes: An Insider's View* 2005

91038   prolonged (greater than 1 hour, up to 24 hours)
> *CPT Assistant* May 05:3; *CPT Changes: An Insider's View* 2005

91040 Esophageal balloon distension provocation study
> *CPT Assistant* May 05:3; *CPT Changes: An Insider's View* 2005

(For balloon dilatation with endoscopy, see 43220, 43249, 43456, or 43458)

(91052, 91055 have been deleted. To report, see 43754, 43755)

91065   Breath hydrogen test (eg, for detection of lactase deficiency, fructose intolerance, bacterial overgrowth, or oro-cecal gastrointestinal transit)

➔ *CPT Assistant* May 05:3; *CPT Changes: An Insider's View* 2005

(For H. pylori breath test analysis, use 83013 for non-radioactive (C-13) isotope or 78268 for radioactive (C-14) isotope)

(91100 has been deleted)

(To report placement of an esophageal tamponade tube for management of variceal bleeding, use 43460. To report placement of a long intestinal Miller-Abbott tube, use 44500)

(91105 has been deleted. To report, use 43753)

(For cholangiography, see 47500, 74320)

(For abdominal paracentesis, see 49082, 49083, 49084; with instillation of medication, see 96440, 96446)

(For peritoneoscopy, use 49320; with biopsy, use 49321)

(For peritoneoscopy and guided transhepatic cholangiography, use 47560; with biopsy, use 47561)

(For splenoportography, see 38200, 75810)

▲ **91110**   Gastrointestinal tract imaging, intraluminal (eg, capsule endoscopy), esophagus through ileum, with interpretation and report

➔ *CPT Assistant* Oct 04:15, Aug 05:14, May 09:8; *CPT Changes: An Insider's View* 2004, 2013

(Visualization of the colon is not reported separately)

(Append modifier 52 if the ileum is not visualized)

▲ **91111**   Gastrointestinal tract imaging, intraluminal (eg, capsule endoscopy), esophagus with interpretation and report

➔ *CPT Changes: An Insider's View* 2007, 2013

(Do not report 91111 in conjunction with 91110)

►(For measurement of gastrointestinal tract transit times or pressure using wireless capsule, use 91112)◄

● **91112**   Gastrointestinal transit and pressure measurement, stomach through colon, wireless capsule, with interpretation and report

➔ *CPT Changes: An Insider's View* 2013

►(Do not report 91112 in conjunction with 83986, 91020, 91022, 91117)◄

91117   Colon motility (manometric) study, minimum 6 hours continuous recording (including provocation tests, eg, meal, intracolonic balloon distension, pharmacologic agents, if performed), with interpretation and report

➔ *CPT Changes: An Insider's View* 2011

►(For wireless capsule pressure measurements, use 91112)◄

(Do not report 91117 in conjunction with 91120, 91122)

91120   Rectal sensation, tone, and compliance test (ie, response to graded balloon distention)

➔ *CPT Assistant* May 05:3; *CPT Changes: An Insider's View* 2005

(For biofeedback training, use 90911)

(For anorectal manometry, use 91122)

91122   Anorectal manometry

(Do not report 91120, 91122 in conjunction with 91117)

(91123 has been deleted)

Gastric Physiology

91132   Electrogastrography, diagnostic, transcutaneous;

➔ *CPT Changes: An Insider's View* 2001

91133   with provocative testing

➔ *CPT Changes: An Insider's View* 2001

Other Procedures

91299   Unlisted diagnostic gastroenterology procedure

➔ *CPT Assistant* Aug 05:14

Ophthalmology

(For surgical procedures, see **Surgery,** Eye and Ocular Adnexa, 65091 et seq)

Definitions

Intermediate ophthalmological services describes an evaluation of a new or existing condition complicated with a new diagnostic or management problem not necessarily relating to the primary diagnosis, including history, general medical observation, external ocular and adnexal examination and other diagnostic procedures as indicated; may include the use of mydriasis for ophthalmoscopy.

For example:

a. Review of history, external examination, ophthalmoscopy, biomicroscopy for an acute complicated condition (eg, iritis) not requiring comprehensive ophthalmological services.

b. Review of interval history, external examination, ophthalmoscopy, biomicroscopy and tonometry in established patient with known cataract not requiring comprehensive ophthalmological services.

Comprehensive ophthalmological services describes a general evaluation of the complete visual system. The comprehensive services constitute a single service entity but need not be performed at one session. The service includes history, general medical observation, external and ophthalmoscopic examinations, gross visual fields and basic sensorimotor examination. It often includes, as indicated: biomicroscopy, examination with cycloplegia or mydriasis and tonometry. It always includes initiation of diagnostic and treatment programs.

Medicine

Intermediate and comprehensive ophthalmological services constitute integrated services in which medical decision making cannot be separated from the examining techniques used. Itemization of service components, such as slit lamp examination, keratometry, routine ophthalmoscopy, retinoscopy, tonometry, or motor evaluation is not applicable.

For example:

The comprehensive services required for diagnosis and treatment of a patient with symptoms indicating possible disease of the visual system, such as glaucoma, cataract or retinal disease, or to rule out disease of the visual system, new or established patient.

Initiation of diagnostic and treatment program includes the prescription of medication, and arranging for special ophthalmological diagnostic or treatment services, consultations, laboratory procedures and radiological services.

Special ophthalmological services describes services in which a special evaluation of part of the visual system is made, which goes beyond the services included under general ophthalmological services, or in which special treatment is given. Special ophthalmological services may be reported in addition to the general ophthalmological services or evaluation and management services.

For example:

Fluorescein angioscopy, quantitative visual field examination, refraction or extended color vision examination (such as Nagel's anomaloscope) should be separately reported.

Prescription of lenses, when required, is included in 92015. It includes specification of lens type (monofocal, bifocal, other), lens power, axis, prism, absorptive factor, impact resistance, and other factors.

▶Interpretation and report by the physician or other qualified health care professional is an integral part of special ophthalmological services where indicated. Technical procedures (which may or may not be performed personally) are often part of the service, but should not be mistaken to constitute the service itself.◀

General Ophthalmological Services

New Patient

▶(For distinguishing between new and established patients, see **Evaluation and Management** guidelines)◀

92002 Ophthalmological services: medical examination and evaluation with initiation of diagnostic and treatment program; intermediate, new patient
➜ *CPT Assistant* Feb 97:6, Aug 98:3, Jun 05:11, Dec 05:10, Jan 07:30, Jan 08:1, Sep 08:7, Feb 11:10

92004 comprehensive, new patient, 1 or more visits
➜ *CPT Assistant* Feb 97:6, Aug 98:3, Jun 05:11, Dec 05:10, Jan 07:30, Jan 08:1, Sep 08:7, Nov 10:8, Jan 11:9, Feb 11:10

Established Patient

▶(For distinguishing between new and established patients, see **Evaluation and Management** guidelines)◀

92012 Ophthalmological services: medical examination and evaluation, with initiation or continuation of diagnostic and treatment program; intermediate, established patient
➜ *CPT Assistant* Feb 97:6, Aug 98:3, Jun 05:11, Dec 05:10, Jan 07:30, Jan 08:1, Sep 08:7, Feb 11:10

92014 comprehensive, established patient, 1 or more visits
➜ *CPT Assistant* Feb 97:6, Aug 98:3, Dec 99:10, Jun 05:11, Dec 05:10, Jan 07:30, Jan 08:1, Sep 08:7, Nov 10:8, Jan 11:9, Feb 11:10

(For surgical procedures, see **Surgery,** Eye and Ocular Adnexa, 65091 et seq)

Special Ophthalmological Services

92015 Determination of refractive state
➜ *CPT Assistant* Mar 96:11, Feb 97:6, Aug 98:3, Aug 06:11

▶(For instrument based ocular screening, use 99174)◀

92018 Ophthalmological examination and evaluation, under general anesthesia, with or without manipulation of globe for passive range of motion or other manipulation to facilitate diagnostic examination; complete
➜ *CPT Assistant* Feb 97:6, Aug 98:3

92019 limited
➜ *CPT Assistant* Feb 97:6, Aug 98:3

92020 Gonioscopy (separate procedure)
➜ *CPT Assistant* Feb 97:6, Aug 98:3

(For gonioscopy under general anesthesia, use 92018)

92025 Computerized corneal topography, unilateral or bilateral, with interpretation and report
➜ *CPT Assistant* Oct 10:10; *CPT Changes: An Insider's View* 2007

(Do not report 92025 in conjunction with 65710-65771)

(92025 is not used for manual keratoscopy, which is part of a single system Evaluation and Management or ophthalmological service)

92060 Sensorimotor examination with multiple measurements of ocular deviation (eg, restrictive or paretic muscle with diplopia) with interpretation and report (separate procedure)
➜ *CPT Assistant* Feb 97:6, Aug 98:3

92065 Orthoptic and/or pleoptic training, with continuing medical direction and evaluation
➜ *CPT Assistant* Feb 97:6, Jun 98:10, Aug 98:3

(92070 has been deleted. To report, see 92071, 92072)

92071 Fitting of contact lens for treatment of ocular surface disease
➜ *CPT Changes: An Insider's View* 2012

(Do not report 92071 in conjunction with 92072)

(Report supply of lens separately with 99070 or appropriate supply code)

92072   Fitting of contact lens for management of keratoconus, initial fitting

➔ *CPT Changes: An Insider's View* 2012

(For subsequent fittings, report using evaluation and management services or general ophthalmological services)

(Do not report 92072 in conjunction with 92071)

(Report supply of lens separately with 99070 or appropriate supply code)

92081   Visual field examination, unilateral or bilateral, with interpretation and report; limited examination (eg, tangent screen, Autoplot, arc perimeter, or single stimulus level automated test, such as Octopus 3 or 7 equivalent)

➔ *CPT Assistant* Feb 97:6, Aug 98:3, Sep 10:10

92082   intermediate examination (eg, at least 2 isopters on Goldmann perimeter, or semiquantitative, automated suprathreshold screening program, Humphrey suprathreshold automatic diagnostic test, Octopus program 33)

➔ *CPT Assistant* Feb 97:6, Aug 98:3

92083   extended examination (eg, Goldmann visual fields with at least 3 isopters plotted and static determination within the central 30°, or quantitative, automated threshold perimetry, Octopus program G-1, 32 or 42, Humphrey visual field analyzer full threshold programs 30-2, 24-2, or 30/60-2)

➔ *CPT Assistant* Feb 97:6, Aug 98:3

(Gross visual field testing (eg, confrontation testing) is a part of general ophthalmological services and is not reported separately)

92100   Serial tonometry (separate procedure) with multiple measurements of intraocular pressure over an extended time period with interpretation and report, same day (eg, diurnal curve or medical treatment of acute elevation of intraocular pressure)

➔ *CPT Assistant* Feb 97:6, Jun 98:10, Aug 98:3

(92120, 92130 have been deleted)

(Ocular blood flow measurements are reported with 0198T. Single-episode tonometry is a component of general ophthalmological service or E/M service)

92132   Scanning computerized ophthalmic diagnostic imaging, anterior segment, with interpretation and report, unilateral or bilateral

➔ *CPT Assistant* Feb 11:6; *CPT Changes: An Insider's View* 2011

▶(For specular microscopy and endothelial cell analysis, use 92286)◀

92133   Scanning computerized ophthalmic diagnostic imaging, posterior segment, with interpretation and report, unilateral or bilateral; optic nerve

➔ *CPT Assistant* Feb 11:6; *CPT Changes: An Insider's View* 2011

92134   retina

➔ *CPT Assistant* Feb 11:6; *CPT Changes: An Insider's View* 2011

(Do not report 92133 and 92134 at the same patient encounter)

(92135 has been deleted)

(For scanning computerized ophthalmic diagnostic imaging of the optic nerve and retina, see 92133, 92134)

92136   Ophthalmic biometry by partial coherence interferometry with intraocular lens power calculation

➔ *CPT Assistant* Aug 98:3, Apr 02:18, Sep 09:5; *CPT Changes: An Insider's View* 2002

92140   Provocative tests for glaucoma, with interpretation and report, without tonography

➔ *CPT Assistant* Feb 97:6, Aug 98:3

Ophthalmoscopy

Routine ophthalmoscopy is part of general and special ophthalmologic services whenever indicated. It is a non-itemized service and is not reported separately.

92225   Ophthalmoscopy, extended, with retinal drawing (eg, for retinal detachment, melanoma), with interpretation and report; initial

➔ *CPT Assistant* Feb 97:6, Aug 98:2, Dec 99:10, Feb 11:6

92226   subsequent

➔ *CPT Assistant* Feb 97:6, Aug 98:2, Feb 11:6

92227   Remote imaging for detection of retinal disease (eg, retinopathy in a patient with diabetes) with analysis and report under physician supervision, unilateral or bilateral

➔ *CPT Assistant* Feb 11:7, May 11:9; *CPT Changes: An Insider's View* 2011

(Do not report 92227 in conjunction with 92002-92014, 92133, 92134, 92250, 92228 or with the evaluation and management of the single organ system, the eye, 99201-99350)

92228   Remote imaging for monitoring and management of active retinal disease (eg, diabetic retinopathy) with physician review, interpretation and report, unilateral or bilateral

➔ *CPT Assistant* Feb 11:7, May 11:9; *CPT Changes: An Insider's View* 2011

(Do not report 92228 in conjunction with 92002-92014, 92133, 92134, 92250, 92227 or with the evaluation and management of the single organ system, the eye, 99201-99350)

92230   Fluorescein angioscopy with interpretation and report

➔ *CPT Assistant* Feb 97:6, Feb 11:6

Medicine

Extended Ophthalmoscopy
92225, 92226

Illustration of retinal structures to document for comparison with future examinations

Ophthalmoscopic appearance of retina

92235 Fluorescein angiography (includes multiframe imaging) with interpretation and report

→ *CPT Assistant* Feb 97:6, Feb 11:6

92240 Indocyanine-green angiography (includes multiframe imaging) with interpretation and report

→ *CPT Assistant* Feb 11:6

92250 Fundus photography with interpretation and report

→ *CPT Assistant* Feb 97:6, Apr 99:10, Feb 11:6

92260 Ophthalmodynamometry

→ *CPT Assistant* Feb 97:6, Feb 11:6

(For ophthalmoscopy under general anesthesia, use 92018)

Fluorescein Angiography
92235

Fluorescein dye is injected in a peripheral vein to enhance imaging. Serial multiframe angiography is performed to evaluate choroidal and retinal circulation. In this illustration, arteries display an even fluorescence, while veins appear striped from the laminar dye flow.

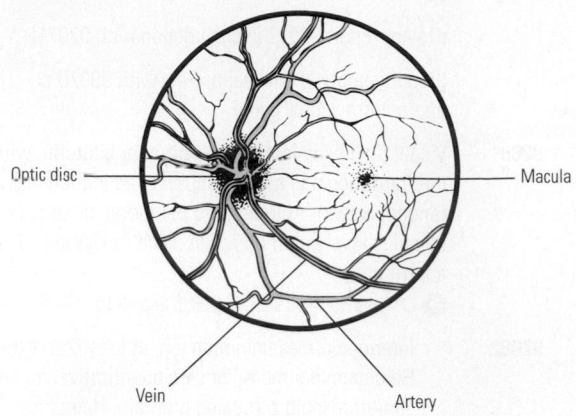

Other Specialized Services

For prescription, fitting, and/or medical supervision of ocular prosthetic (artificial eye) adaptation by a physician, see evaluation and management services including office or other outpatient services (99201-99215), office or other outpatient consultations (99241-99245), or general ophthalmological service codes 92002-92014.

92265 Needle oculoelectromyography, 1 or more extraocular muscles, 1 or both eyes, with interpretation and report

→ *CPT Assistant* Feb 97:6

92270 Electro-oculography with interpretation and report

→ *CPT Assistant* Feb 97:6, Aug 08:12, May 09:9

92275 Electroretinography with interpretation and report

→ *CPT Assistant* Feb 97:6

(For electronystagmography for vestibular function studies, see 92541 et seq)

(For ophthalmic echography (diagnostic ultrasound), see 76511-76529)

92283 Color vision examination, extended, eg, anomaloscope or equivalent

→ *CPT Assistant* Feb 97:6

(Color vision testing with pseudoisochromatic plates [such as HRR or Ishihara] is not reported separately. It is included in the appropriate general or ophthalmological service, or 99172)

92284 Dark adaptation examination with interpretation and report

→ *CPT Assistant* Feb 97:6

92285 External ocular photography with interpretation and report for documentation of medical progress (eg, close-up photography, slit lamp photography, goniophotography, stereo-photography)

→ *CPT Assistant* Feb 97:6, Sep 97:10

▲ **92286**   Anterior segment imaging with interpretation and report; with specular microscopy and endothelial cell analysis
➔ *CPT Assistant* Feb 97:6; *CPT Changes: An Insider's View* 2013

▲ **92287**   with fluorescein angiography
➔ *CPT Assistant* Feb 97:6; *CPT Changes: An Insider's View* 2013

Contact Lens Services

The prescription of contact lens includes specification of optical and physical characteristics (such as power, size, curvature, flexibility, gas-permeability). It is **not** a part of the general ophthalmological services.

The fitting of contact lens includes instruction and training of the wearer and incidental revision of the lens during the training period.

Follow-up of successfully fitted extended wear lenses is reported as part of a general ophthalmological service (92012 et seq).

The supply of contact lenses may be reported as part of the service of fitting. It may also be reported separately by using the appropriate supply codes.

(For therapeutic or surgical use of contact lens, see 68340, 92071, 92072)

92310   Prescription of optical and physical characteristics of and fitting of contact lens, with medical supervision of adaptation; corneal lens, both eyes, except for aphakia
➔ *CPT Assistant* Feb 97:6

(For prescription and fitting of 1 eye, add modifier 52)

92311   corneal lens for aphakia, 1 eye
➔ *CPT Assistant* Feb 97:6

92312   corneal lens for aphakia, both eyes
➔ *CPT Assistant* Feb 97:6

92313   corneoscleral lens
➔ *CPT Assistant* Feb 97:7, Mar 03:1

92314   Prescription of optical and physical characteristics of contact lens, with medical supervision of adaptation and direction of fitting by independent technician; corneal lens, both eyes except for aphakia
➔ *CPT Assistant* Feb 97:7

(For prescription and fitting of 1 eye, add modifier 52)

92315   corneal lens for aphakia, 1 eye
➔ *CPT Assistant* Feb 97:7

92316   corneal lens for aphakia, both eyes
➔ *CPT Assistant* Feb 97:7

92317   corneoscleral lens
➔ *CPT Assistant* Feb 97:7

92325   Modification of contact lens (separate procedure), with medical supervision of adaptation
➔ *CPT Assistant* Feb 97:7

92326   Replacement of contact lens
➔ *CPT Assistant* Feb 97:7

Spectacle Services (Including Prosthesis for Aphakia)

Prescription of lenses, when required, is included in 92015 Determination of refractive state. It includes specification of lens type (monofocal, bifocal, other), lens power, axis, prism, absorptive factor, impact resistance, and other factors.

▶When provided, fitting of spectacles is a separate service and is reported as indicated by 92340-92371.

Fitting includes measurement of anatomical facial characteristics, the writing of laboratory specifications, and the final adjustment of the spectacles to the visual axes and anatomical topography. Presence of the physician or other qualified health care professional is not required.◀

Supply of materials is a separate service component; it is not part of the service of fitting spectacles.

92340   Fitting of spectacles, except for aphakia; monofocal
➔ *CPT Assistant* Feb 97:7, Aug 98:4

92341   bifocal
➔ *CPT Assistant* Feb 97:7, Aug 98:4

92342   multifocal, other than bifocal
➔ *CPT Assistant* Feb 97:7, Aug 98:4

92352   Fitting of spectacle prosthesis for aphakia; monofocal
➔ *CPT Assistant* Feb 97:7, Aug 98:4

92353   multifocal
➔ *CPT Assistant* Feb 97:7, Aug 98:4

92354   Fitting of spectacle mounted low vision aid; single element system
➔ *CPT Assistant* Feb 97:7, Aug 98:4

92355   telescopic or other compound lens system
➔ *CPT Assistant* Feb 97:7, Aug 98:4

92358   Prosthesis service for aphakia, temporary (disposable or loan, including materials)
➔ *CPT Assistant* Feb 97:7, Aug 98:4

92370   Repair and refitting spectacles; except for aphakia
➔ *CPT Assistant* Feb 97:7

92371   spectacle prosthesis for aphakia
➔ *CPT Assistant* Feb 97:7, Aug 98:4

Other Procedures

92499   Unlisted ophthalmological service or procedure
➔ *CPT Assistant* Feb 97:7

Special Otorhinolaryngologic Services

Diagnostic or treatment procedures that are reported as evaluation and management services (eg, otoscopy, anterior rhinoscopy, tuning fork test, removal of non-impacted cerumen) are not reported separately.

▶Special otorhinolaryngologic services are those diagnostic and treatment services not included in an evaluation and management service, including office or other outpatient services (99201-99215), or office or other outpatient consultations (99241-99245).◀

Code 92506 is used to report evaluation of speech production, receptive language, and expressive language abilities. Tests may examine speech sound production, articulatory movements of oral musculature, the patient's ability to understand the meaning and intent of written and verbal expressions, and the appropriate formulation and utterance of expressive thought. In contrast, 92626 and 92627 are reported for an evaluation of auditory rehabilitation status determining the patient's ability to use residual hearing in order to identify the acoustic characteristics of sounds associated with speech communication.

(For laryngoscopy with stroboscopy, use 31579)

92502   Otolaryngologic examination under general anesthesia

92504   Binocular microscopy (separate diagnostic procedure)
➔ CPT Assistant Jul 05:14, Oct 11:10

92506   Evaluation of speech, language, voice, communication, and/or auditory processing
➔ CPT Assistant Sep 04:13, Dec 04:14, Mar 05:7, Jan 06:7, Mar 09:11; CPT Changes: An Insider's View 2006

92507   Treatment of speech, language, voice, communication, and/or auditory processing disorder; individual
➔ CPT Assistant Dec 04:14, Jan 06:7; CPT Changes: An Insider's View 2006

92508   group, 2 or more individuals
➔ CPT Assistant Dec 04:14

(For auditory rehabilitation, prelingual hearing loss, use 92630)

(For auditory rehabilitation, postlingual hearing loss, use 92633)

(For cochlear implant programming, see 92601-92604)

92511   Nasopharyngoscopy with endoscope (separate procedure)

92512   Nasal function studies (eg, rhinomanometry)

92516   Facial nerve function studies (eg, electroneuronography)

92520   Laryngeal function studies (ie, aerodynamic testing and acoustic testing)
➔ CPT Assistant Dec 04:17, Jan 06:7; CPT Changes: An Insider's View 2006

(For performance of a single test, use modifier 52)

(To report flexible fiberoptic laryngeal evaluation of swallowing and laryngeal sensory testing, see 92611-92617)

(To report other testing of laryngeal function (eg, electroglottography), use 92700)

92526   Treatment of swallowing dysfunction and/or oral function for feeding

Vestibular Function Tests, Without Electrical Recording

92531   Spontaneous nystagmus, including gaze

92532   Positional nystagmus test
➔ CPT Changes: An Insider's View 2002

▶(Do not report 92531, 92532 with evaluation and management services including office or other outpatient services [99201-99215], observation care [99218-99220, 99224-99226], observation or inpatient care including admission and discharge [99234-99236], hospital care [99221-99223, 99231-99233], office or other outpatient consultations [99241-99245], nursing facility services [99304-99318], and domiciliary, rest home, or custodial care services [99324-99337])◀

92533   Caloric vestibular test, each irrigation (binaural, bithermal stimulation constitutes 4 tests)
➔ CPT Assistant May 96:5

92534   Optokinetic nystagmus test
➔ CPT Changes: An Insider's View 2002

Vestibular Function Tests, With Recording (eg, ENG)

92540   Basic vestibular evaluation, includes spontaneous nystagmus test with eccentric gaze fixation nystagmus, with recording, positional nystagmus test, minimum of 4 positions, with recording, optokinetic nystagmus test, bidirectional foveal and peripheral stimulation, with recording, and oscillating tracking test, with recording
➔ CPT Changes: An Insider's View 2010

(Do not report 92540 in conjunction with 92541, 92542, 92544, or 92545)

92541   Spontaneous nystagmus test, including gaze and fixation nystagmus, with recording
➔ CPT Assistant Feb 05:13, Aug 08:12, May 11:10

(Do not report 92541 in conjunction with 92540 or the set of 92542, 92544, 92545)

92542   Positional nystagmus test, minimum of 4 positions, with recording
➔ CPT Assistant Feb 05:13, Aug 08:12, Sep 10:9

(Do not report 92542 in conjunction with 92540 or the set of 92541, 92544, and 92545)

92543   Caloric vestibular test, each irrigation (binaural, bithermal stimulation constitutes 4 tests), with recording
➔ CPT Assistant May 96:5, Oct 04:10, Feb 05:13, Sep 06:13, Aug 08:12

92544   Optokinetic nystagmus test, bidirectional, foveal or peripheral stimulation, with recording
➔ CPT Assistant Feb 05:13, Aug 08:12

(Do not report 92544 in conjunction with 92540 or the set of 92541, 92542, and 92545)

92545   Oscillating tracking test, with recording
➔ CPT Assistant Feb 05:13, Aug 08:12, May 11:10

(Do not report 92545 in conjunction with 92540 or the set of 92541, 92542, and 92544)

92546   Sinusoidal vertical axis rotational testing
➔ *CPT Assistant* Sep 04:13, Feb 05:13, Aug 08:12, May 11:10

+ 92547   Use of vertical electrodes (List separately in addition to code for primary procedure)
➔ *CPT Assistant* May 04:14, Feb 05:13, Aug 08:12

(Use 92547 in conjunction with 92540-92546)

(For unlisted vestibular tests, use 92700)

92548   Computerized dynamic posturography
➔ *CPT Assistant* May 11:10

Audiologic Function Tests

The audiometric tests listed below require the use of calibrated electronic equipment, recording of results and a report with interpretation. Hearing tests (such as whispered voice, tuning fork) that are otorhinolaryngologic Evaluation and Management services are not reported separately. All services include testing of both ears. Use modifier 52 if a test is applied to one ear instead of two ears. All codes (except 92559) apply to testing of individuals. For testing of groups, use 92559 and specify test(s) used.

(For evaluation of speech, language and/or hearing problems through observation and assessment of performance, use 92506)

92550   Tympanometry and reflex threshold measurements
➔ *CPT Changes: An Insider's View* 2010

(Do not report 92550 in conjunction with 92567, 92568)

92551   Screening test, pure tone, air only

92552   Pure tone audiometry (threshold); air only

92553   air and bone
➔ *CPT Assistant* Mar 11:8

92555   Speech audiometry threshold;

92556   with speech recognition
➔ *CPT Assistant* Mar 11:8

92557   Comprehensive audiometry threshold evaluation and speech recognition (92553 and 92556 combined)
➔ *CPT Assistant* Sep 07:11, Mar 11:8

(For hearing aid evaluation and selection, see 92590-92595)

(For automated audiometry, see 0208T-0212T)

―― *Coding Tip* ――

Instructions for Reporting Group Testing

For testing of groups, use 92559 and specify test(s) used.

CPT Coding Guidelines, Special Otorhinolaryngologic Service, Audiologic Function Tests

92558   Code is out of numerical sequence. See 92550-92597

92559   Audiometric testing of groups

92560   Bekesy audiometry; screening

92561   diagnostic

92562   Loudness balance test, alternate binaural or monaural
➔ *CPT Assistant* Mar 05:7, 9

92563   Tone decay test

92564   Short increment sensitivity index (SISI)
➔ *CPT Assistant* Oct 96:9

92565   Stenger test, pure tone

92567   Tympanometry (impedance testing)
➔ *CPT Assistant* Winter 90:11

92568   Acoustic reflex testing, threshold
➔ *CPT Assistant* Jan 06:7, Sep 07:11, Jun 09:10; *CPT Changes: An Insider's View* 2006, 2010

(92569 has been deleted. For acoustic reflex decay testing performed in conjunction with tympanometry, use 92570)

92570   Acoustic immittance testing, includes tympanometry (impedance testing), acoustic reflex threshold testing, and acoustic reflex decay testing
➔ *CPT Changes: An Insider's View* 2010

(Do not report 92570 in conjunction with 92567, 92568)

92571   Filtered speech test
➔ *CPT Assistant* Mar 05:7

92572   Staggered spondaic word test
➔ *CPT Assistant* Mar 05:7

92575   Sensorineural acuity level test

92576   Synthetic sentence identification test
➔ *CPT Assistant* Mar 05:7

92577   Stenger test, speech

92579   Visual reinforcement audiometry (VRA)

92582   Conditioning play audiometry

92583   Select picture audiometry

92584   Electrocochleography
➔ *CPT Assistant* Jul 11:17

92585   Auditory evoked potentials for evoked response audiometry and/or testing of the central nervous system; comprehensive
➔ *CPT Assistant* Winter 90:11; *CPT Changes: An Insider's View* 2001

92586   limited
➔ *CPT Changes: An Insider's View* 2001

 # 92558   Evoked otoacoustic emissions, screening (qualitative measurement of distortion product or transient evoked otoacoustic emissions), automated analysis
➔ *CPT Changes: An Insider's View* 2012

92587 Distortion product evoked otoacoustic emissions; limited evaluation (to confirm the presence or absence of hearing disorder, 3-6 frequencies) or transient evoked otoacoustic emissions, with interpretation and report

➔ *CPT Assistant* Sep 07:11; *CPT Changes: An Insider's View* 2012

92588 comprehensive diagnostic evaluation (quantitative analysis of outer hair cell function by cochlear mapping, minimum of 12 frequencies), with interpretation and report

➔ *CPT Changes: An Insider's View* 2012

(For central auditory function evaluation, see 92620, 92621)

92590 Hearing aid examination and selection; monaural

92591 binaural

92592 Hearing aid check; monaural

92593 binaural

92594 Electroacoustic evaluation for hearing aid; monaural

92595 binaural

92596 Ear protector attenuation measurements

92597 Evaluation for use and/or fitting of voice prosthetic device to supplement oral speech

(To report augmentative and alternative communication device services, see 92605, 92607, 92608)

Evaluative and Therapeutic Services

Codes 92601 and 92603 describe post-operative analysis and fitting of previously placed external devices, connection to the cochlear implant, and programming of the stimulator. Codes 92602 and 92604 describe subsequent sessions for measurements and adjustment of the external transmitter and re-programming of the internal stimulator.

(For placement of cochlear implant, use 69930)

92601 Diagnostic analysis of cochlear implant, patient younger than 7 years of age; with programming

➔ *CPT Assistant* Mar 03:1, Jan 06:7, Jul 11:17; *CPT Changes: An Insider's View* 2003

92602 subsequent reprogramming

➔ *CPT Assistant* Mar 03:1, 21, Jan 06:7; *CPT Changes: An Insider's View* 2003

(Do not report 92602 in addition to 92601)

(For aural rehabilitation services following cochlear implant, including evaluation of rehabilitation status, see 92626-92627, 92630-92633)

92603 Diagnostic analysis of cochlear implant, age 7 years or older; with programming

➔ *CPT Assistant* Mar 03:2, 4, Jan 06:7, Jul 11:17; *CPT Changes: An Insider's View* 2003

92604 subsequent reprogramming

➔ *CPT Assistant* Mar 03:2, 21, Jan 06:7, Jul 11:17; *CPT Changes: An Insider's View* 2003

(Do not report 92604 in addition to 92603)

A View of the Outer Cochlear Implant
92601-92604

An example of the elements that are addressed in the diagnostic analysis and reprogramming of the cochlear implant

— Transmitting coil

— Headset with microphone

— Cord to speech processor

92605 Evaluation for prescription of non-speech-generating augmentative and alternative communication device, face-to-face with the patient; first hour

➔ *CPT Assistant* Mar 03:2, 4; *CPT Changes: An Insider's View* 2003, 2012

#+ 92618 each additional 30 minutes (List separately in addition to code for primary procedure)

➔ *CPT Changes: An Insider's View* 2012

(Use 92618 in conjunction with 92605)

92606 Therapeutic service(s) for the use of non-speech-generating device, including programming and modification

➔ *CPT Assistant* Mar 03:2, 4; *CPT Changes: An Insider's View* 2003

92607 Evaluation for prescription for speech-generating augmentative and alternative communication device, face-to-face with the patient; first hour

➔ *CPT Assistant* Mar 03:2, 4, Dec 04:16; *CPT Changes: An Insider's View* 2003

(For evaluation for prescription of a non-speech-generating device, use 92605)

+ 92608 each additional 30 minutes (List separately in addition to code for primary procedure)

➔ *CPT Assistant* Mar 03:2, 5, Dec 04:16; *CPT Changes: An Insider's View* 2003

(Use 92608 in conjunction with 92607)

92609 Therapeutic services for the use of speech-generating device, including programming and modification

➔ *CPT Assistant* Mar 03:2, 4, Dec 04:16; *CPT Changes: An Insider's View* 2003

(For therapeutic service(s) for the use of a non-speech-generating device, use 92606)

92610 Evaluation of oral and pharyngeal swallowing function

➔ *CPT Assistant* Mar 03:2, 5, Dec 04:17; *CPT Changes: An Insider's View* 2003

(For motion fluoroscopic evaluation of swallowing function, use 92611)

(For flexible endoscopic examination, use 92612-92617)

92611 Motion fluoroscopic evaluation of swallowing function by cine or video recording
→ *CPT Assistant* Mar 03:2, 5, Dec 04:17, Jan 06:7; *CPT Changes: An Insider's View* 2003
→ *Clinical Examples in Radiology* Summer 06:4-5

(For radiological supervision and interpretation, use 74230)

(For evaluation of oral and pharyngeal swallowing function, use 92610)

(For flexible fiberoptic diagnostic laryngoscopy, use 31575. Do not report 31575 in conjunction with 92612-92617)

92612 Flexible fiberoptic endoscopic evaluation of swallowing by cine or video recording;
→ *CPT Assistant* Mar 03:6, Jan 06:7; *CPT Changes: An Insider's View* 2003

(If flexible fiberoptic or endoscopic evaluation of swallowing is performed without cine or video recording, use 92700)

▲ **92613** interpretation and report only
→ *CPT Assistant* Jan 06:7; *CPT Changes: An Insider's View* 2003, 2013

(To report an evaluation of oral and pharyngeal swallowing function, use 92610)

(To report motion fluoroscopic evaluation of swallowing function, use 92611)

92614 Flexible fiberoptic endoscopic evaluation, laryngeal sensory testing by cine or video recording;
→ *CPT Assistant* Mar 03:6, Jan 06:7; *CPT Changes: An Insider's View* 2003

(If flexible fiberoptic or endoscopic evaluation of swallowing is performed without cine or video recording, use 92700)

▲ **92615** interpretation and report only
→ *CPT Assistant* Mar 03:6, Jan 06:7; *CPT Changes: An Insider's View* 2003, 2013

92616 Flexible fiberoptic endoscopic evaluation of swallowing and laryngeal sensory testing by cine or video recording;
→ *CPT Assistant* Mar 03:6, Jan 06:7; *CPT Changes: An Insider's View* 2003

(If flexible fiberoptic or endoscopic evaluation of swallowing is performed without cine or video recording, use 92700)

▲ **92617** interpretation and report only
→ *CPT Assistant* Mar 03:6, Jan 06:7; *CPT Changes: An Insider's View* 2003, 2013

92618 Code is out of numerical sequence. See 92601-92633

92620 Evaluation of central auditory function, with report; initial 60 minutes
→ *CPT Assistant* Mar 05:7-8; *CPT Changes: An Insider's View* 2005

+ **92621** each additional 15 minutes (List separately in addition to code for primary procedure)
→ *CPT Assistant* Mar 05:7; *CPT Changes: An Insider's View* 2005, 2012

(Use 92621 in conjunction with 92620)

(Do not report 92620, 92621 in conjunction with 92506)

92625 Assessment of tinnitus (includes pitch, loudness matching, and masking)
→ *CPT Assistant* Mar 05:7-10; *CPT Changes: An Insider's View* 2005

(Do not report 92625 in conjunction with 92562)

(For unilateral assessment, use modifier 52)

92626 Evaluation of auditory rehabilitation status; first hour
→ *CPT Assistant* Jan 06:7; *CPT Changes: An Insider's View* 2006

+ **92627** each additional 15 minutes (List separately in addition to code for primary procedure)
→ *CPT Assistant* Jan 06:7; *CPT Changes: An Insider's View* 2006

(Use 92627 in conjunction with 92626)

(When reporting 92626, 92627, use the face-to-face time with the patient or family)

92630 Auditory rehabilitation; prelingual hearing loss
→ *CPT Assistant* Jan 06:7; *CPT Changes: An Insider's View* 2006

92633 postlingual hearing loss
→ *CPT Assistant* Jan 06:7; *CPT Changes: An Insider's View* 2006

Special Diagnostic Procedures

92640 Diagnostic analysis with programming of auditory brainstem implant, per hour
→ *CPT Changes: An Insider's View* 2007

(Report nonprogramming services separately [eg, cardiac monitoring])

Other Procedures

92700 Unlisted otorhinolaryngological service or procedure
→ *CPT Assistant* Sep 04:14, Oct 04:10, Jan 06:7, Sep 06:13, Sep 07:11, Mar 11:10, Jul 11:17; *CPT Changes: An Insider's View* 2003

Cardiovascular

Therapeutic Services and Procedures

92920 ► Code is out of numerical sequence. See 92998-93000 ◄

92921 ► Code is out of numerical sequence. See 92998-93000 ◄

92924 ► Code is out of numerical sequence. See 92998-93000 ◄

92925 ► Code is out of numerical sequence. See 92998-93000 ◄

92928 ► Code is out of numerical sequence. See 92998-93000 ◄

▲=Revised code   ●=New code   ►◄=Contains new or revised text   ⊘=Modifier 51 exempt

Medicine

92929 ►Code is out of numerical sequence. See 92998-93000◄

92933 ►Code is out of numerical sequence. See 92998-93000◄

92934 ►Code is out of numerical sequence. See 92998-93000◄

92937 ►Code is out of numerical sequence. See 92998-93000◄

92938 ►Code is out of numerical sequence. See 92998-93000◄

92941 ►Code is out of numerical sequence. See 92998-93000◄

92943 ►Code is out of numerical sequence. See 92998-93000◄

92944 ►Code is out of numerical sequence. See 92998-93000◄

►Other Therapeutic Services and Procedures◄

92950 Cardiopulmonary resuscitation (eg, in cardiac arrest)
➔ *CPT Assistant* Jan 96:7, Oct 04:14, Nov 07:5, Jul 12:13

(See also critical care services, 99291, 99292)

⊙ **92953** Temporary transcutaneous pacing
➔ *CPT Assistant* Nov 99:49, Feb 07:10, Jul 07:1

►(For direction of ambulance or rescue personnel outside the hospital by a physician or other qualified health care professional, use 99288)◄

⊙ **92960** Cardioversion, elective, electrical conversion of arrhythmia; external
➔ *CPT Assistant* Summer 93:13, Nov 99:49, Jun 00:5, Nov 00:9, Jul 01:11, Jan 12:13; *CPT Changes: An Insider's View* 2000

⊙ **92961** internal (separate procedure)
➔ *CPT Assistant* Summer 93:13, Nov 99:49, Jun 00:5, Jul 00:5, Nov 00:9; *CPT Changes: An Insider's View* 2000

►(Do not report 92961 in conjunction with 93282-93284, 93287, 93289, 93295, 93296, 93618-93624, 93631, 93640-93642, 93650, 93653-93657, 93662)◄

92970 Cardioassist-method of circulatory assist; internal

92971 external

(For balloon atrial-septostomy, use 92992)

(For placement of catheters for use in circulatory assist devices such as intra-aortic balloon pump, use 33970)

92973 ►Code is out of numerical sequence. See 92998-93000◄

92974 ►Code is out of numerical sequence. See 92998-93000◄

92975 ►Code is out of numerical sequence. See 92998-93000◄

92977 ►Code is out of numerical sequence. See 92998-93000◄

92978 ►Code is out of numerical sequence. See 92998-93000◄

92979 ►Code is out of numerical sequence. See 92998-93000◄

►(92980, 92981, 92982, 92984 have been deleted. To report, see 92920-92944)◄

⊙ **92986** Percutaneous balloon valvuloplasty; aortic valve

⊙ **92987** mitral valve

92990 pulmonary valve
➔ *CPT Assistant* Winter 91:3

92992 Atrial septectomy or septostomy; transvenous method, balloon (eg, Rashkind type) (includes cardiac catheterization)
➔ *CPT Assistant* Nov 97:44, Apr 98:3, 10, Nov 07:9

92993 blade method (Park septostomy) (includes cardiac catheterization)
➔ *CPT Assistant* Apr 98:10

►(92995, 92996 have been deleted. To report, see 92924, 92925, 92933-92944)◄

92997 Percutaneous transluminal pulmonary artery balloon angioplasty; single vessel
➔ *CPT Assistant* Nov 97:44

+ **92998** each additional vessel (List separately in addition to code for primary procedure)
➔ *CPT Assistant* Nov 97:44

(Use 92998 in conjunction with 92997)

►Coronary Therapeutic Services and Procedures◄

►Codes 92920-92944 describe percutaneous revascularization services performed for occlusive disease of the coronary vessels (major coronary arteries, coronary artery branches, or coronary artery bypass grafts). These percutaneous coronary intervention (PCI) codes are built on progressive hierarchies with more intensive services inclusive of lesser intensive services. These PCI codes all include the work of accessing and selectively catheterizing the vessel, traversing the lesion, radiological supervision and interpretation directly related to the intervention(s) performed, closure of the arteriotomy when performed through the access sheath, and imaging performed to document completion of the intervention in addition to the intervention(s) performed. These codes include angioplasty (eg, balloon, cutting balloon, wired balloons, cryoplasty), atherectomy (eg, directional, rotational, laser), and stenting (eg, balloon expandable, self-expanding, bare metal, drug eluting, covered). Each code in this family includes balloon angioplasty, when performed. Diagnostic coronary angiography may be reported separately under specific circumstances.

Diagnostic coronary angiography codes (93454-93461) and injection procedure codes (93563-93564) should not be used with percutaneous coronary revascularization services (92920-92944) to report:

1. Contrast injections, angiography, roadmapping, and/or fluoroscopic guidance for the coronary intervention,

2. Vessel measurement for the coronary intervention, or

3. Post-coronary angioplasty/stent/atherectomy angiography, as this work is captured in the percutaneous coronary revascularization services codes (92920-92944).

Diagnostic angiography performed at the time of a coronary interventional procedure may be separately reportable if:

1. No prior catheter-based coronary angiography study is available, and a full diagnostic study is performed, and a decision to intervene is based on the diagnostic angiography, **or**

2. A prior study is available, but as documented in the medical record:

   a. The patient's condition with respect to the clinical indication has changed since the prior study, **or**

   b. There is inadequate visualization of the anatomy and/or pathology, **or**

   c. There is a clinical change during the procedure that requires new evaluation outside the target area of intervention.

Diagnostic coronary angiography performed at a separate session from an interventional procedure is separately reportable.

Major coronary arteries: The major coronary arteries are the left main, left anterior descending, left circumflex, right, and ramus intermedius arteries. All PCI procedures performed in all segments (proximal, mid, distal) of a single major coronary artery through the native coronary circulation are reported with one code. When one segment of a major coronary artery is treated through the native circulation and treatment of another segment of the same artery requires access through a coronary artery bypass graft, the intervention through the bypass graft is reported separately.

Coronary artery branches: Up to two coronary artery branches of the left anterior descending (diagonals), left circumflex (marginals), and right (posterior descending, posterolaterals) coronary arteries are recognized. The left main and ramus intermedius coronary arteries do not have recognized branches for reporting purposes. All PCI(s) performed in any segment (proximal, mid, distal) of a coronary artery branch is reported with one code. PCI is reported for up to two branches of a major coronary artery. Additional PCI in a third branch of the same major coronary artery is not separately reportable.

Coronary artery bypass grafts: Each coronary artery bypass graft represents a coronary vessel. A sequential bypass graft with more than one distal anastomosis represents only one graft. A branching bypass graft (eg, Y graft) represents a coronary vessel for the main graft, and each branch off the main graft constitutes an additional coronary vessel. PCI performed on major coronary arteries or coronary artery branches by access through a bypass graft is reported using the bypass graft PCI codes. All bypass graft PCI codes include the use of coronary artery embolic protection devices when performed.

Only one base code from this family may be reported for revascularization of a major coronary artery and its recognized branches. Only one base code should be reported for revascularization of a coronary artery bypass graft, its subtended coronary artery, and recognized branches of the subtended coronary artery. If one segment of a major coronary artery and its recognized branches is treated through the native circulation, and treatment of another segment of the same vessel requires access through a coronary artery bypass graft, an additional base code is reported to describe the intervention performed through the bypass graft. The PCI base codes are 92920, 92924, 92928, 92933, 92937, 92941, and 92943. The PCI base code that includes the most intensive service provided for the target vessel should be reported. The hierarchy of these services is built on an intensity of service ranked from highest to lowest as 92943 = 92941 = 92933 > 92924 > 92937 = 92928 > 92920.

PCI performed during the same session in additional recognized branches of the target vessel should be reported using the applicable add-on code(s). The add-on codes are 92921, 92925, 92929, 92934, 92938, and 92944 and follow the same principle in regard to reporting the most intensive service provided. The intensity of service is ranked from highest to lowest as 92944 = 92938 > 92934 > 92925 > 92929 > 92921.

PCI performed during the same session in additional major coronary or in additional coronary artery bypass grafts should be reported using the applicable additional base code(s). PCI performed during the same session in additional coronary artery branches should be reported using the applicable additional add-on code(s).

If a single lesion extends from one target vessel (major coronary artery, coronary artery bypass graft, or coronary artery branch) into another target vessel, but can be revascularized with a single intervention bridging the two vessels, this PCI should be reported with a single code despite treating more than one vessel. For example, if a left main coronary lesion extends into the proximal left circumflex coronary artery and a single stent is placed to treat the entire lesion, this PCI should be reported as a single vessel stent (92928). In this example, a code for additional vessel treatment (92929) would not be additionally reported.

When bifurcation lesions are treated, PCI is reported for both vessels treated. For example, when a bifurcation lesion involving the left anterior descending artery and the first diagonal artery is treated by stenting both vessels, 92928 and 92929 are both reported.

Target vessel PCI for acute myocardial infarction is inclusive of all balloon angioplasty, atherectomy, stenting, manual aspiration thrombectomy, distal protection, and intracoronary rheolytic agent administration performed. Mechanical thrombectomy is reported separately.

Chronic total occlusion of a coronary vessel is present when there is no antegrade flow through the true lumen, accompanied by suggestive angiographic and clinical criteria (eg, antegrade "bridging" collaterals present, calcification at the occlusion site, no current presentation with ST elevation or Q wave acute myocardial infarction attributable to the occluded target lesion). Current presentation with ST elevation or Q wave acute myocardial infarction attributable to the occluded target lesion, subtotal occlusion, and occlusion with dye staining at the site consistent with fresh thrombus are not considered chronic total occlusion.

Codes 92973 (percutaneous transluminal coronary thrombectomy, mechanical), 92974 (coronary brachytherapy), 92978 and 92979 (intravascular ultrasound), and 93571 and 93572 (intravascular Doppler velocity and/or pressure [fractional flow reserve (FFR) or coronary flow reserve (CFR)]) are add-on codes for reporting procedures performed in addition to coronary and bypass graft diagnostic and interventional services, unless included in the base code. Non-mechanical, aspiration thrombectomy is not reported with 92973, and is included in the PCI code for acute myocardial infarction (92941), when performed.◄

►(To report transcatheter placement of radiation delivery device for coronary intravascular brachytherapy, use 92974)◄

►(For intravascular radioelement application, see 77785-77787)◄

(For nonsurgical septal reduction therapy [eg, alcohol ablation], use 93799)

#⊙● 92920 Percutaneous transluminal coronary angioplasty; single major coronary artery or branch

➔ *CPT Changes: An Insider's View* 2013

#⊙+● 92921 each additional branch of a major coronary artery (List separately in addition to code for primary procedure)

➔ *CPT Changes: An Insider's View* 2013

►(Use 92921 in conjunction with 92920, 92924, 92928, 92933, 92937, 92941, 92943)◄

#⊙● 92924 Percutaneous transluminal coronary atherectomy, with coronary angioplasty when performed; single major coronary artery or branch

➔ *CPT Changes: An Insider's View* 2013

#⊙+● 92925 each additional branch of a major coronary artery (List separately in addition to code for primary procedure)

➔ *CPT Changes: An Insider's View* 2013

►(Use 92925 in conjunction with 92924, 92928, 92933, 92937, 92941, 92943)◄

#⊙● 92928 Percutaneous transcatheter placement of intracoronary stent(s), with coronary angioplasty when performed; single major coronary artery or branch

➔ *CPT Changes: An Insider's View* 2013

#⊙+● 92929 each additional branch of a major coronary artery (List separately in addition to code for primary procedure)

➔ *CPT Changes: An Insider's View* 2013

►(Use 92929 in conjunction with 92928, 92933, 92937, 92941, 92943)◄

#⊙● 92933 Percutaneous transluminal coronary atherectomy, with intracoronary stent, with coronary angioplasty when performed; single major coronary artery or branch

➔ *CPT Changes: An Insider's View* 2013

#⊙+● 92934 each additional branch of a major coronary artery (List separately in addition to code for primary procedure)

➔ *CPT Changes: An Insider's View* 2013

►(Use 92934 in conjunction with 92933, 92937, 92941, 92943)◄

#⊙● 92937 Percutaneous transluminal revascularization of or through coronary artery bypass graft (internal mammary, free arterial, venous), any combination of intracoronary stent, atherectomy and angioplasty, including distal protection when performed; single vessel

➔ *CPT Changes: An Insider's View* 2013

#⊙+● 92938 each additional branch subtended by the bypass graft (List separately in addition to code for primary procedure)

➔ *CPT Changes: An Insider's View* 2013

►(Use 92938 in conjunction with 92937)◄

#⊙● 92941 Percutaneous transluminal revascularization of acute total/subtotal occlusion during acute myocardial infarction, coronary artery or coronary artery bypass graft, any combination of intracoronary stent, atherectomy and angioplasty, including aspiration thrombectomy when performed, single vessel

➔ *CPT Changes: An Insider's View* 2013

►(For additional vessels treated, see 92920-92938, 92943, 92944)◄

#⊙● 92943 Percutaneous transluminal revascularization of chronic total occlusion, coronary artery, coronary artery branch, or coronary artery bypass graft, any combination of intracoronary stent, atherectomy and angioplasty; single vessel

➔ *CPT Changes: An Insider's View* 2013

#⊙+● 92944 each additional coronary artery, coronary artery branch, or bypass graft (List separately in addition to code for primary procedure)

➔ *CPT Changes: An Insider's View* 2013

►(Use 92944 in conjunction with 92924, 92928, 92933, 92937, 92941, 92943)◄

►(To report transcatheter placement of radiation delivery device for coronary intravascular brachytherapy, use 92974)◄

►(For intravascular radioelement application, see 77785-77787)◄

#⊙+▲ 92973 Percutaneous transluminal coronary thrombectomy mechanical (List separately in addition to code for primary procedure)

➔ *CPT Assistant* Mar 02:2, 10, Mar 04:10; *CPT Changes: An Insider's View* 2002, 2013

►(Use 92973 in conjunction with 92920, 92924, 92928, 92933, 92937, 92941, 92943, 92975, 93454-93461, 93563, 93564)◄

⊙=Moderate sedation +=Add-on code ∕=FDA approval pending #=Resequenced code ○=Recycled/reinstated code ➔➔=See p xiii for details

▶(Do not report 92973 for aspiration thrombectomy)◀

#⊙✛ **92974**   Transcatheter placement of radiation delivery device for subsequent coronary intravascular brachytherapy (List separately in addition to code for primary procedure)

➡ *CPT Assistant* Mar 02:2; *CPT Changes: An Insider's View* 2002

▶(Use 92974 in conjunction with 92920, 92924, 92928, 92933, 92937, 92941, 92943, 93454-93461)◀

(For intravascular radioelement application, see 77785-77787)

#⊙ **92975**   Thrombolysis, coronary; by intracoronary infusion, including selective coronary angiography

92977   by intravenous infusion

▶(For thrombolysis of vessels other than coronary, see 37211-37214)◀

(For cerebral thrombolysis, use 37195)

#⊙✛ **92978**   Intravascular ultrasound (coronary vessel or graft) during diagnostic evaluation and/or therapeutic intervention including imaging supervision, interpretation and report; initial vessel (List separately in addition to code for primary procedure)

➡ *CPT Assistant* Nov 97:43-44, Nov 99:49; *CPT Changes: An Insider's View* 2000

▶(Use 92978 in conjunction with 92975, 92920, 92924, 92928, 92933, 92937, 92941, 92943, 93454-93461, 93563, 93564)◀

Intravascular Ultrasound (Coronary Vessel or Graft) 92978

A catheter with a transducer at its tip is inserted and threaded through a selected coronary artery(s) or coronary bypass graft(s).

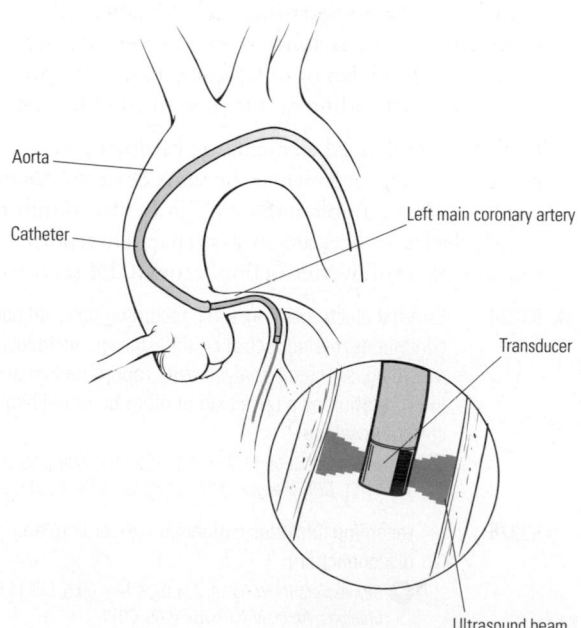

Aorta

Catheter

Left main coronary artery

Transducer

Ultrasound beam

#⊙✛ **92979**   each additional vessel (List separately in addition to code for primary procedure)

➡ *CPT Assistant* Nov 97:43-44, Nov 99:49; *CPT Changes: An Insider's View* 2000

(Use 92979 in conjunction with 92978)

(Intravascular ultrasound services include all transducer manipulations and repositioning within the specific vessel being examined, both before and after therapeutic intervention [eg, stent placement])

(For intravascular spectroscopy, use 0205T)

▶(For intravascular optical coherence tomography, see 0291T, 0292T)◀

Cardiography

Codes 93040-93042 are appropriate when an order for the test is triggered by an event, the rhythm strip is used to help diagnose the presence or absence of an arrhythmia, and a report is generated. There must be a specific order for an electrocardiogram or rhythm strip followed by a separate, signed, written, and retrievable report. It is not appropriate to use these codes for reviewing the telemetry monitor strips taken from a monitoring system. The need for an electrocardiogram or rhythm strip should be supported by documentation in the patient medical record.

(For echocardiography, see 93303-93350)

▶(For electrocardiogram, 64 leads or greater, with graphic presentation and analysis, use 93799)◀

(For acoustic cardiography services, see 0223T-0225T)

93000   Electrocardiogram, routine ECG with at least 12 leads; with interpretation and report

➡ *CPT Assistant* Aug 97:9, Feb 05:9, Mar 05:1, 11, Jul 08:3

93005   tracing only, without interpretation and report

➡ *CPT Assistant* Aug 97:9, Mar 05:1

93010   interpretation and report only

➡ *CPT Assistant* Aug 97:9, Mar 05:1, Apr 07:1

(For ECG monitoring, see 99354-99360)

--- *Coding Tip* ---

Instructions for Reporting Electrocardiographic Recording

Do not report 93268-93272 when performing 93279-93289, 93291-93296 or 93298-93299. Do not report 93040-93042 when performing 93279-93289, 93291-93296 or 93298-93299.

CPT Coding Guidelines, Cardiovascular, Cardiography Implantable and Wearable Cardiac Device Evaluations

---

(93012, 93014 have been deleted. To report telephonic transmission of post-symptom electrocardiogram rhythm strips, see 93268-93272)

Medicine

▲ **93015** Cardiovascular stress test using maximal or submaximal treadmill or bicycle exercise, continuous electrocardiographic monitoring, and/or pharmacological stress; with supervision, interpretation and report
> *CPT Assistant* Apr 96:11, Jun 96:10, Aug 02:10, Jul 08:3, Jan 10:8, May 10:6; *CPT Changes: An Insider's View* 2013
> *Clinical Examples in Radiology* Winter 10:12

▲ **93016** supervision only, without interpretation and report
> *CPT Assistant* Apr 96:11, Aug 02:10, Jul 08:3, Jan 10:8, May 10:6; *CPT Changes: An Insider's View* 2013
> *Clinical Examples in Radiology* Winter 10:12

93017 tracing only, without interpretation and report
> *CPT Assistant* Aug 02:10, Jul 08:3, Jan 10:8, May 10:6
> *Clinical Examples in Radiology* Winter 10:12

93018 interpretation and report only
> *CPT Assistant* Apr 96:11, Jun 96:10, Jul 08:3, Jan 10:8, May 10:6
> *Clinical Examples in Radiology* Winter 10:12

93024 Ergonovine provocation test

93025 Microvolt T-wave alternans for assessment of ventricular arrhythmias
> *CPT Assistant* Mar 02:3; *CPT Changes: An Insider's View* 2002

--- *Coding Tip* ---

Instructions for Reporting Electrocardiographic Recording

Codes 93040-93042 are appropriate when an order for the test is triggered by an event, the rhythm strip is used to help diagnose the presence or absence of an arrhythmia, and a report is generated. There must be a specific order for an electrocardiogram or rhythm strip followed by a separate, signed, written, and retrievable report. It is not appropriate to use these codes for reviewing the telemetry monitor strips taken from a monitoring system. The need for an electrocardiogram or rhythm strip should be supported by documentation in the patient medical record.

CPT Coding Guidelines, Cardiovascular, Cardiography

93040 Rhythm ECG, 1-3 leads; with interpretation and report
> *CPT Assistant* Apr 04:8, Oct 10:10

93041 tracing only without interpretation and report
> *CPT Assistant* Apr 04:8, Oct 10:10

93042 interpretation and report only
> *CPT Assistant* Apr 04:8, Oct 10:10, Oct 11:7

Cardiovascular Monitoring Services

Cardiovascular monitoring services are diagnostic medical procedures using in-person and remote technology to assess cardiovascular rhythm (ECG) data. Holter monitors (93224-93227) include up to 48 hours of continuous recording. Mobile cardiac telemetry monitors (93228, 93229) have the capability of transmitting a tracing at any time, always have internal ECG analysis algorithms designed to detect major arrhythmias, and

transmit to an attended surveillance center. Event monitors (93268-93272) record segments of ECGs with recording initiation triggered either by patient activation or by an internal automatic, pre-programmed detection algorithm (or both) and transmit the recorded electrocardiographic data when requested (but cannot transmit immediately based upon the patient or algorithmic activation rhythm) and require attended surveillance.

Attended surveillance: is the immediate availability of a remote technician to respond to rhythm or device alert transmissions from a patient, either from an implanted or wearable monitoring or therapy device, as they are generated and transmitted to the remote surveillance location or center.

Electrocardiographic rhythm derived elements: elements derived from recordings of the electrical activation of the heart including, but not limited to heart rhythm, rate, ST analysis, heart rate variability, T-wave alternans.

▶*Mobile cardiovascular telemetry (MCT):* continuously records the electrocardiographic rhythm from external electrodes placed on the patient's body. Segments of the ECG data are automatically (without patient intervention) transmitted to a remote surveillance location by cellular or landline telephone signal. The segments of the rhythm, selected for transmission, are triggered automatically (MCT device algorithm) by rapid and slow heart rates or by the patient during a symptomatic episode. There is continuous real time data analysis by preprogrammed algorithms in the device and attended surveillance of the transmitted rhythm segments by a surveillance center technician to evaluate any arrhythmias and to determine signal quality. The surveillance center technician reviews the data and notifies the physician or other qualified health care professional depending on the prescribed criteria.◀

ECG rhythm derived elements are distinct from physiologic data, even when the same device is capable of producing both. Implantable cardiovascular monitor (ICM) device services are always separately reported from implantable cardioverter-defibrillator (ICD) service.

▲ **93224** External electrocardiographic recording up to 48 hours by continuous rhythm recording and storage; includes recording, scanning analysis with report, review and interpretation by a physician or other qualified health care professional
> *CPT Assistant* Oct 05:14, Apr 07:3, Mar 08:4, Mar 09:5, Oct 11:5, Nov 11:11; *CPT Changes: An Insider's View* 2009, 2011, 2013

93225 recording (includes connection, recording, and disconnection)
> *CPT Assistant* Oct 05:14, Apr 07:3, Mar 09:5, Oct 11:5; *CPT Changes: An Insider's View* 2009, 2011

93226 scanning analysis with report
> *CPT Assistant* Oct 05:14, Apr 07:3, Mar 09:5, Oct 11:5; *CPT Changes: An Insider's View* 2009, 2011

▲ **93227** review and interpretation by a physician or other qualified health care professional

→ *CPT Assistant* Apr 07:3, Mar 09:5, Apr 09:7, Oct 11:5; *CPT Changes: An Insider's View* 2009, 2011, 2013

(For less than 12 hours of continuous recording, use modifier 52)

►(For greater than 48 hours of monitoring, see Category III codes 0295T-0298T)◄

▲ **93228** External mobile cardiovascular telemetry with electrocardiographic recording, concurrent computerized real time data analysis and greater than 24 hours of accessible ECG data storage (retrievable with query) with ECG triggered and patient selected events transmitted to a remote attended surveillance center for up to 30 days; review and interpretation with report by a physician or other qualified health care professional

→ *CPT Assistant* Oct 11:5; *CPT Changes: An Insider's View* 2009, 2011, 2013

(Report 93228 only once per 30 days)

(Do not report 93228 in conjunction with 93224, 93227)

▲ **93229** technical support for connection and patient instructions for use, attended surveillance, analysis and transmission of daily and emergent data reports as prescribed by a physician or other qualified health care professional

→ *CPT Assistant* Oct 11:5; *CPT Changes: An Insider's View* 2009, 2011, 2013

(Report 93229 only once per 30 days)

(Do not report 93229 in conjunction with 93224, 93226)

(For external cardiovascular monitors that do not perform automatic ECG triggered transmissions to an attended surveillance center, see 93224-93227, 93268-93272)

(93230-93237 have been deleted. To report external electrocardiographic rhythm derived monitoring for up to 48 hours, see 93224-93227)

▲ **93268** External patient and, when performed, auto activated electrocardiographic rhythm derived event recording with symptom-related memory loop with remote download capability up to 30 days, 24-hour attended monitoring; includes transmission, review and interpretation by a physician or other qualified health care professional

→ *CPT Assistant* Jun 96:2, Nov 99:49-50, Oct 05:14, Apr 07:3, Mar 08:4, Mar 09:5, Oct 11:5; *CPT Changes: An Insider's View* 2003, 2009, 2011, 2013

93270 recording (includes connection, recording, and disconnection)

→ *CPT Assistant* Jun 96:2, Oct 05:14, Apr 07:3, Mar 09:5, Aug 10:13, Oct 11:5; *CPT Changes: An Insider's View* 2009, 2011

93271 transmission and analysis

→ *CPT Assistant* Jun 96:2, Oct 05:14, Apr 07:3, Mar 09:5, Oct 11:5; *CPT Changes: An Insider's View* 2009, 2011

▲ **93272** review and interpretation by a physician or other qualified health care professional

→ *CPT Assistant* Jun 96:2, Apr 98:14, Nov 99:49-50, Oct 05:14, Apr 07:3, Mar 09:5, Apr 09:7, Oct 11:5; *CPT Changes: An Insider's View* 2009, 2011, 2013

(For implanted patient activated cardiac event recording, see 33282, 93285, 93291, 93298)

93278 Signal-averaged electrocardiography (SAECG), with or without ECG

→ *CPT Assistant* Oct 11:5

(For interpretation and report only, use 93278 with modifier 26)

(For unlisted cardiographic procedure, use 93799)

Implantable and Wearable Cardiac Device Evaluations

►Cardiac device evaluation services are diagnostic medical procedures using in-person and remote technology to assess device therapy and cardiovascular physiologic data. Codes 93279-93299 describe this technology and technical/professional and service center practice. Codes 93279-93292 are reported per procedure. Codes 93293-93296 are reported no more than **once** every 90 days. Do not report 93293-93296 if the monitoring period is less than 30 days. Codes 93297, 93298 are reported no more than **once** up to every 30 days. Do not report 93297-93299 if the monitoring period is less than 10 days.

A service center may report 93296 or 93299 during a period in which a physician or other qualified health care professional performs an in-person interrogation device evaluation. The same individual may not report an in-person and remote interrogation of the same device during the same period. Report only remote services when an in-person interrogation device evaluation is performed during a period of remote interrogation device evaluation. A period is established by the initiation of the remote monitoring or the 91st day of a pacemaker or implantable cardioverter-defibrillator (ICD) monitoring or the 31st day of an implantable loop recorder (ILR) or implantable cardiovascular monitor (ICM) monitoring and extends for the subsequent 90 or 30 days, respectively, for which remote monitoring is occurring. Programming device evaluations and in-person interrogation device evaluations may not be reported on the same date by the same individual. Programming device evaluations and remote interrogation device evaluations may both be reported during the remote interrogation device evaluation period.◄

For monitoring by wearable devices, see 93224-93272.

ECG rhythm derived elements are distinct from physiologic data, even when the same device is capable of producing both. ICM device services are always separately reported from ICD services. When ILR data is derived from an ICD or pacemaker, do not report ILR services with pacemaker or ICD services.

Do not report 93268-93272 when performing 93279-93289, 93291-93296 or 93298-93299. Do not report 93040-93042 when performing 93279-93289, 93291-93296, or 93298-93299.

▶The pacemaker and ICD interrogation device evaluations, peri-procedural device evaluations and programming, and programming device evaluations may not be reported in conjunction with pacemaker or ICD device and/or lead insertion or revision services by the same individual.◄

The following definitions and instructions apply to codes 93279-93299:

Attended surveillance: the immediate availability of a remote technician to respond to rhythm or device alert transmissions from a patient, either from an implanted or wearable monitoring or therapy device, as they are generated and transmitted to the remote surveillance location or center.

Device, single lead: a pacemaker or implantable cardioverter-defibrillator with pacing and sensing function in only one chamber of the heart.

Device, dual lead: a pacemaker or implantable cardioverter-defibrillator with pacing and sensing function in only two chambers of the heart.

Device, multiple lead: a pacemaker or implantable cardioverter-defibrillator with pacing and sensing function in three or more chambers of the heart.

Electrocardiographic rhythm derived elements: elements derived from recordings of the electrical activation of the heart including, but not limited to heart rhythm, rate, ST analysis, heart rate variability, T-wave alternans.

▶*Implantable cardiovascular monitor (ICM):* an implantable cardiovascular device used to assist the physician in the management of non-rhythm related cardiac conditions such as heart failure. The device collects longitudinal physiologic cardiovascular data elements from one or more internal sensors (such as right ventricular pressure, left atrial pressure or an index of lung water) and/or external sensors (such as blood pressure or body weight) for patient assessment and management. The data are stored and transmitted by either local telemetry or remotely to an Internet-based file server or surveillance technician. The function of the ICM may be an additional function of an implantable cardiac device (eg, implantable cardioverter-defibrillator) or a function of a stand-alone device. When ICM functionality is included in an ICD device or pacemaker, the ICM data and the ICD or pacemaker, heart rhythm data such as sensing, pacing, and tachycardia detection therapy are distinct and therefore, the monitoring processes are distinct.◄

Implantable cardioverter-defibrillator (ICD): an implantable device that provides high-energy and low-energy stimulation to one or more chambers of the heart to terminate rapid heart rhythms called tachycardia or fibrillation. ICDs also have pacemaker functions to treat slow heart rhythms called bradycardia. In addition to the tachycardia and bradycardia functions, the ICD may or may not include the functionality of an implantable cardiovascular monitor or an implantable loop recorder.

▶*Implantable loop recorder (ILR):* an implantable device that continuously records the electrocardiographic rhythm triggered automatically by rapid and slow heart rates or by the patient during a symptomatic episode. The ILR function may be the only function of the device or it may be part of a pacemaker or implantable cardioverter-defibrillator device. The data are stored and transmitted by either local telemetry or remotely to an Internet-based file server or surveillance technician. Extraction of data and compilation or report for physician or qualified health care professional interpretation is usually performed in the office setting.◄

Interrogation device evaluation: an evaluation of an implantable device such as a cardiac pacemaker, implantable cardioverter-defibrillator, implantable cardiovascular monitor, or implantable loop recorder. Using an office, hospital, or emergency room instrument or via a remote interrogation system, stored and measured information about the lead(s) when present, sensor(s) when present, battery and the implanted device function, as well as data collected about the patient's heart rhythm and heart rate is retrieved. The retrieved information is evaluated to determine the current programming of the device and to evaluate certain aspects of the device function such as battery voltage, lead impedance, tachycardia detection settings, and rhythm treatment settings.

The components that must be evaluated for the various types of implantable cardiac devices are listed below. (The required components for both remote and in-person interrogations are the same.)

Pacemaker: Programmed parameters, lead(s), battery, capture and sensing function and heart rhythm.

Implantable cardioverter-defibrillator: Programmed parameters, lead(s), battery, capture and sensing function, presence or absence of therapy for ventricular tachyarrhythmias and underlying heart rhythm.

Implantable cardiovascular monitor: Programmed parameters and analysis of at least one recorded physiologic cardiovascular data element from either internal or external sensors.

Implantable loop recorder: Programmed parameters and the heart rate and rhythm during recorded episodes from both patient initiated and device algorithm detected events, when present.

Interrogation device evaluation (remote): a procedure performed for patients with pacemakers, implantable cardioverter-defibrillators or implantable loop recorders using data obtained remotely. All device functions, including the programmed parameters, lead(s), battery, capture and sensing function, presence or absence of therapy for ventricular tachyarrhythmias (for ICDs) and underlying heart rhythm are evaluated.

The components that must be evaluated for the various types of implantable cardiac devices are listed below. (The required components for both remote and in person interrogations are the same.)

Pacemaker: Programmed parameters, lead(s), battery, capture and sensing function, and heart rhythm.

Implantable cardioverter-defibrillator: Programmed parameters, lead(s), battery, capture and sensing function, presence or absence of therapy for ventricular tachyarrhythmias, and underlying heart rhythm.

Implantable cardiovascular monitor: Programmed parameters and analysis of at least one recorded physiologic cardiovascular data element from either internal or external sensors.

Implantable loop recorder: Programmed parameters and the heart rate and rhythm during recorded episodes from both patient-initiated and device algorithm detected events, when present.

Pacemaker: an implantable device that provides low energy localized stimulation to one or more chambers of the heart to initiate contraction in that chamber.

►*Peri-procedural device evaluation and programming:* an evaluation of an implantable device system (either a pacemaker or implantable cardioverter defibrillator) to adjust the device to settings appropriate for the patient prior to a surgery, procedure, or test. The device system data are interrogated to evaluate the lead(s), sensor(s), and battery in addition to review of stored information, including patient and system measurements. The device is programmed to settings appropriate for the surgery, procedure, or test, as required. A second evaluation and programming are performed after the surgery, procedure, or test to provide settings appropriate to the post procedural situation, as required. If one performs both the pre- and post-evaluation and programming service, the appropriate code, either 93286 or 93287, would be reported two times. If one performs the pre-surgical service and a separate individual performs the post-surgical service, each reports either 93286 or 93287 only one time.◄

Physiologic cardiovascular data elements: data elements from one or more internal sensors (such as right ventricular pressure, left atrial pressure or an index of lung water) and/or external sensors (such as blood pressure or body weight) for patient assessment and management. It does not include ECG rhythm derived data elements.

Programming device evaluation (in person): a procedure performed for patients with a pacemaker, implantable cardioverter-defibrillator, or implantable loop recorder. All device functions, including the battery, programmable settings and lead(s), when present, are evaluated. To assess capture thresholds, iterative adjustments (eg, progressive changes in pacing output of

a pacing lead) of the programmable parameters are conducted. The iterative adjustments provide information that permits the operator to assess and select the most appropriate final program parameters to provide for consistent delivery of the appropriate therapy and to verify the function of the device. The final program parameters may or may not change after evaluation.

The programming device evaluation includes all of the components of the interrogation device evaluation (remote) or the interrogation device evaluation (in person), and it includes the selection of patient specific programmed parameters depending on the type of device.

The components that must be evaluated for the various types of programming device evaluations are listed below. (See also required interrogation device evaluation [remote and in person] components above.)

Pacemaker: Programmed parameters, lead(s), battery, capture and sensing function, and heart rhythm. Often, but not always, the sensor rate response, lower and upper heart rates, AV intervals, pacing voltage and pulse duration, sensing value, and diagnostics will be adjusted during a programming evaluation.

Implantable cardioverter-defibrillator: Programmed parameters, lead(s), battery, capture and sensing function, presence or absence of therapy for ventricular tachyarrhythmias and underlying heart rhythm. Often, but not always, the sensor rate response, lower and upper heart rates, AV intervals, pacing voltage and pulse duration, sensing value, and diagnostics will be adjusted during a programming evaluation. In addition, ventricular tachycardia detection and therapies are sometimes altered depending on the interrogated data, patient's rhythm, symptoms, and condition.

Implantable loop recorder: Programmed parameters and the heart rhythm during recorded episodes from both patient initiated and device algorithm detected events. Often, but not always, the tachycardia and bradycardia detection criteria will be adjusted during a programming evaluation.

Transtelephonic rhythm strip pacemaker evaluation: service of transmission of an electrocardiographic rhythm strip over the telephone by the patient using a transmitter and recorded by a receiving location using a receiver/recorder (also commonly known as transtelephonic pacemaker monitoring). The electrocardiographic rhythm strip is recorded both with and without a magnet applied over the pacemaker. The rhythm strip is evaluated for heart rate and rhythm, atrial and ventricular capture (if observed) and atrial and ventricular sensing (if observed). In addition, the battery status of the pacemaker is determined by measurement of the paced rate on the electrocardiographic rhythm strip recorded with the magnet applied.

▲ 93279   Programming device evaluation (in person) with iterative adjustment of the implantable device to test the function of the device and select optimal permanent programmed values with analysis, review and report by a physician or other qualified health care professional; single lead pacemaker system
➜ *CPT Assistant* Jun 12:4; *CPT Changes: An Insider's View* 2009, 2010, 2013

(Do not report 93279 in conjunction with 93286, 93288)

▲ 93280   dual lead pacemaker system
➜ *CPT Assistant* Jun 12:4; *CPT Changes: An Insider's View* 2009, 2010, 2013

(Do not report 93280 in conjunction with 93286, 93288)

▲ 93281   multiple lead pacemaker system
➜ *CPT Assistant* Jun 12:4; *CPT Changes: An Insider's View* 2009, 2010, 2013

(Do not report 93281 in conjunction with 93286, 93288)

▲ 93282   single lead implantable cardioverter-defibrillator system
➜ *CPT Changes: An Insider's View* 2009, 2010, 2013

(Do not report 93282 in conjunction with 93287, 93289, 93745)

▲ 93283   dual lead implantable cardioverter-defibrillator system
➜ *CPT Changes: An Insider's View* 2009, 2010, 2013

(Do not report 93283 in conjunction with 93287, 93289)

▲ 93284   multiple lead implantable cardioverter-defibrillator system
➜ *CPT Changes: An Insider's View* 2009, 2010, 2013

(Do not report 93284 in conjunction with 93287, 93289)

▲ 93285   implantable loop recorder system
➜ *CPT Changes: An Insider's View* 2009, 2010, 2013

(Do not report 93285 in conjunction with 33282, 93279-93284, 93291)

▲ 93286   Peri-procedural device evaluation (in person) and programming of device system parameters before or after a surgery, procedure, or test with analysis, review and report by a physician or other qualified health care professional; single, dual, or multiple lead pacemaker system
➜ *CPT Changes: An Insider's View* 2009, 2010, 2013

(Report 93286 once before and once after surgery, procedure, or test, when device evaluation and programming is performed before and after surgery, procedure, or test)

(Do not report 93286 in conjunction with 93279-93281, 93288)

▲ 93287   single, dual, or multiple lead implantable cardioverter-defibrillator system
➜ *CPT Changes: An Insider's View* 2009, 2010, 2013

(Report 93287 once before and once after surgery, procedure, or test, when device evaluation and programming is performed before and after surgery, procedure, or test)

(Do not report 93287 in conjunction with 93282-93284, 93289)

▲ 93288   Interrogation device evaluation (in person) with analysis, review and report by a physician or other qualified health care professional, includes connection, recording and disconnection per patient encounter; single, dual, or multiple lead pacemaker system
➜ *CPT Assistant* Jun 12:4; *CPT Changes: An Insider's View* 2009, 2013

(Do not report 93288 in conjunction with 93279-93281, 93286, 93294, 93296)

▲ 93289   single, dual, or multiple lead implantable cardioverter-defibrillator system, including analysis of heart rhythm derived data elements
➜ *CPT Changes: An Insider's View* 2009, 2013

(For monitoring physiologic cardiovascular data elements derived from an ICD, use 93290)

(Do not report 93289 in conjunction with 93282-93284, 93287, 93295, 93296)

▲ 93290   implantable cardiovascular monitor system, including analysis of 1 or more recorded physiologic cardiovascular data elements from all internal and external sensors
➜ *CPT Assistant* Feb 10:13; *CPT Changes: An Insider's View* 2009, 2013

(For heart rhythm derived data elements, use 93289)

(Do not report 93290 in conjunction with 93297, 93299)

▲ 93291   implantable loop recorder system, including heart rhythm derived data analysis
➜ *CPT Changes: An Insider's View* 2009, 2013

(Do not report 93291 in conjunction with 33282, 93288-93290, 93298, 93299)

▲ 93292   wearable defibrillator system
➜ *CPT Changes: An Insider's View* 2009, 2013

--- *Coding Tip* ---

Instructions for Reporting Pacemaker and Interrogation Device Evaluations

Codes 93293-93296 are reported no more than once every 90 days. Do not report 93293-93296 if the monitoring period is less than 30 days.

CPT Coding Guidelines, Cardiovascular, Cardiography Implantable and Wearable Cardiac Device Evaluations

(Do not report 93292 in conjunction with 93745)

⊙=Moderate sedation   ✚=Add-on code   ✎=FDA approval pending   #=Resequenced code   ○=Recycled/reinstated code   ➜➜=See p xiii for details

▲ **93293**   Transtelephonic rhythm strip pacemaker evaluation(s) single, dual, or multiple lead pacemaker system, includes recording with and without magnet application with analysis, review and report(s) by a physician or other qualified health care professional, up to 90 days

➔ *CPT Changes: An Insider's View* 2009, 2013

(Do not report 93293 in conjunction with 93294)

(For in person evaluation, see 93040, 93041, 93042)

(Report 93293 only once per 90 days)

▲ **93294**   Interrogation device evaluation(s) (remote), up to 90 days; single, dual, or multiple lead pacemaker system with interim analysis, review(s) and report(s) by a physician or other qualified health care professional

➔ *CPT Assistant* Jun 12:4; *CPT Changes: An Insider's View* 2009, 2013

(Do not report 93294 in conjunction with 93288, 93293)

(Report 93294 only once per 90 days)

▲ **93295**   single, dual, or multiple lead implantable cardioverter-defibrillator system with interim analysis, review(s) and report(s) by a physician or other qualified health care professional

➔ *CPT Changes: An Insider's View* 2009, 2013

(For remote monitoring of physiologic cardiovascular data elements derived from an ICD, use 93297)

(Do not report 93295 in conjunction with 93289)

(Report 93295 only once per 90 days)

93296   single, dual, or multiple lead pacemaker system or implantable cardioverter-defibrillator system, remote data acquisition(s), receipt of transmissions and technician review, technical support and distribution of results

➔ *CPT Changes: An Insider's View* 2009

(Do not report 93296 in conjunction with 93288, 93289, 93299)

(Report 93296 only once per 90 days)

▲ **93297**   Interrogation device evaluation(s), (remote) up to 30 days; implantable cardiovascular monitor system, including analysis of 1 or more recorded physiologic cardiovascular data elements from all internal and external sensors, analysis, review(s) and report(s) by a physician or other qualified health care professional

➔ *CPT Changes: An Insider's View* 2009, 2013

(For heart rhythm derived data elements, use 93295)

(Do not report 93297 in conjunction with 93290, 93298)

(Report 93297 only once per 30 days)

▲ **93298**   implantable loop recorder system, including analysis of recorded heart rhythm data, analysis, review(s) and report(s) by a physician or other qualified health care professional

➔ *CPT Changes: An Insider's View* 2009, 2013

(Do not report 93298 in conjunction with 33282, 93291, 93297)

(Report 93298 only once per 30 days)

93299   implantable cardiovascular monitor system or implantable loop recorder system, remote data acquisition(s), receipt of transmissions and technician review, technical support and distribution of results

➔ *CPT Changes: An Insider's View* 2009

(Do not report 93299 in conjunction with 93290, 93291, 93296)

(Report 93299 only once per 30 days)

Echocardiography

Echocardiography includes obtaining ultrasonic signals from the heart and great vessels, with real time image and/or Doppler ultrasonic signal documentation, with interpretation and report. When interpretation is performed separately, use modifier 26.

A complete transthoracic echocardiogram without spectral or color flow Doppler (93307) is a comprehensive procedure that includes 2-dimensional and, when performed, selected M-mode examination of the left and right atria, left and right ventricles, the aortic, mitral, and tricuspid valves, the pericardium, and adjacent portions of the aorta. Multiple views are required to obtain a complete functional and anatomic evaluation, and appropriate measurements are obtained and recorded. Despite significant effort, identification and measurement of some structures may not always be possible. In such instances, the reason that an element could not be visualized must be documented. Additional structures that may be visualized (eg, pulmonary veins, pulmonary artery, pulmonic valve, inferior vena cava) would be included as part of the service.

A complete transthoracic echocardiogram with spectral and color flow Doppler (93306) is a comprehensive procedure that includes spectral Doppler and color flow Doppler in addition to the 2-dimensional and selected M-mode examinations, when performed. Spectral Doppler (93320, 93321) and color flow Doppler (93325) provide information regarding intracardiac blood flow and hemodynamics.

A follow-up or limited echocardiographic study (93308) is an examination that does not evaluate or document the attempt to evaluate all the structures that comprise the complete echocardiographic exam. This is typically limited to, or performed in follow-up of a focused clinical concern.

In stress echocardiography, echocardiographic images are recorded from multiple cardiac windows before, after, and in some protocols, during stress. The stress is achieved by (1) walking on a treadmill; (2) using a bicycle (supine or upright); or (3) the administration of pharmacological agents that either simulate exercise (by increasing heart rate, blood pressure, or myocardial contractility) or alter coronary flow (vasodilation). The patient's ECG, heart rate, and blood pressure are monitored at baseline, throughout the procedure and during recovery. Reports are prepared to evaluate (1) the duration of stress, the reason for stopping, and the hemodynamic response to stress; (2) the electrocardiographic response to stress; and (3) the echocardiographic response to stress.

▶When a stress echocardiogram is performed with a complete cardiovascular stress test (continuous electrocardiographic monitoring, supervision, interpretation and report by a physician or other qualified health care professional), use 93351. When only the professional components of a complete stress test and a stress echocardiogram are provided (eg, in a facility setting) by the same physician, use 93351 with modifier 26. When all professional services of a stress test are not performed by the same physician performing the stress echocardiogram, use 93350 in conjunction with the appropriate codes (93016-93018) for the components of the cardiovascular stress test that are provided.◀

When left ventricular endocardial borders cannot be adequately identified by standard echocardiographic imaging, echocardiographic contrast may be infused intravenously both at rest and with stress to achieve that purpose. Code 93352 is used to report the administration of echocardiographic contrast agent in conjunction with the stress echocardiography codes (93350 or 93351). Supply of contrast agent and/or drugs used for pharmacological stress is reported separately in addition to the procedure code.

Report of an echocardiographic study, whether complete or limited, includes an interpretation of all obtained information, documentation of all clinically relevant findings including quantitative measurements obtained, plus a description of any recognized abnormalities. Pertinent images, videotape, and/or digital data are archived for permanent storage and are available for subsequent review. Use of echocardiography not meeting these criteria is not separately reportable.

Use of ultrasound, without thorough evaluation of organ(s) or anatomic region, image documentation and final, written report, is not separately reportable.

(For fetal echocardiography, see 76825-76828)

93303 Transthoracic echocardiography for congenital cardiac anomalies; complete

➔ *CPT Assistant* Nov 97:44, Dec 97:5, Sep 05:10-11, Mar 08:4, Oct 10:17, Dec 10:17

➔ *Clinical Examples in Radiology* Fall 06:9-10

93304 follow-up or limited study

➔ *CPT Assistant* Nov 97:44, Dec 97:5, Jan 10:8, Oct 10:17, Dec 10:17

➔ *Clinical Examples in Radiology* Fall 06:9-10

93306 Echocardiography, transthoracic, real-time with image documentation (2D), includes M-mode recording, when performed, complete, with spectral Doppler echocardiography, and with color flow Doppler echocardiography

➔ *CPT Assistant* Oct 10:17, Dec 10:17; *CPT Changes: An Insider's View* 2009

(For transthoracic echocardiography without spectral and color Doppler, use 93307)

93307 Echocardiography, transthoracic, real-time with image documentation (2D), includes M-mode recording, when performed, complete, without spectral or color Doppler echocardiography

➔ *CPT Assistant* Dec 97:5, Sep 05:11, Oct 10:17, Dec 10:17; *CPT Changes: An Insider's View* 2009

➔ *Clinical Examples in Radiology* Fall 06:9-10

(Do not report 93307 in conjunction with 93320, 93321, 93325)

93308 Echocardiography, transthoracic, real-time with image documentation (2D), includes M-mode recording, when performed, follow-up or limited study

➔ *CPT Assistant* Dec 97:5, Sep 05:11, Jan 10:8, Oct 10:17, Dec 10:17, Mar 12:10; *CPT Changes: An Insider's View* 2009

➔ *Clinical Examples in Radiology* Fall 06:9-10

⊙ **93312** Echocardiography, transesophageal, real-time with image documentation (2D) (with or without M-mode recording); including probe placement, image acquisition, interpretation and report

➔ *CPT Assistant* Dec 97:5, Jan 00:10, Jan 10:8

Transesophageal Echocardiography (TEE)
93312-93318

An endoscopic ultrasound transducer is passed through the mouth into the esophagus and 2-dimensional images are obtained from the posterior aspect of the heart.

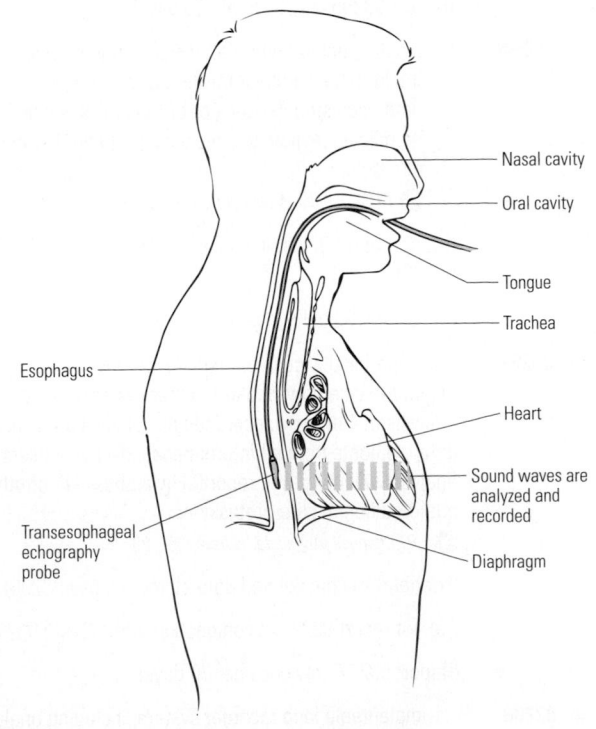

⊙ **93313** placement of transesophageal probe only

➔ *CPT Assistant* Dec 97:5, Mar 08:4, Jan 10:8

⊙ **93314** image acquisition, interpretation and report only

➔ *CPT Assistant* Dec 97:5, Jan 00:10, Jan 10:8

⊙ **93315**   Transesophageal echocardiography for congenital cardiac anomalies; including probe placement, image acquisition, interpretation and report

→ *CPT Assistant* Nov 97:44, Dec 97:5, Jan 10:8

⊙ **93316**   placement of transesophageal probe only

→ *CPT Assistant* Nov 97:44, Dec 97:5, Jan 10:8

⊙ **93317**   image acquisition, interpretation and report only

→ *CPT Assistant* Nov 97:44, Dec 97:5, Jan 10:8

⊙ **93318**   Echocardiography, transesophageal (TEE) for monitoring purposes, including probe placement, real time 2-dimensional image acquisition and interpretation leading to ongoing (continuous) assessment of (dynamically changing) cardiac pumping function and to therapeutic measures on an immediate time basis

→ *CPT Assistant* Jan 10:8, Apr 10:6; *CPT Changes: An Insider's View* 2001

+ **93320**   Doppler echocardiography, pulsed wave and/or continuous wave with spectral display (List separately in addition to codes for echocardiographic imaging); complete

→ *CPT Assistant* Nov 97:44, Dec 97:5

→ *Clinical Examples in Radiology* Fall 06:9-10

(Use 93320 in conjunction with 93303, 93304, 93312, 93314, 93315, 93317, 93350, 93351)

+ **93321**   follow-up or limited study (List separately in addition to codes for echocardiographic imaging)

→ *CPT Assistant* Nov 97:44, Dec 97:5, Jan 10:8

→ *Clinical Examples in Radiology* Fall 06:9-10

(Use 93321 in conjunction with 93303, 93304, 93308, 93312, 93314, 93315, 93317, 93350, 93351)

+ **93325**   Doppler echocardiography color flow velocity mapping (List separately in addition to codes for echocardiography)

→ *CPT Assistant* Nov 97:44, Dec 97:5

→ *Clinical Examples in Radiology* Fall 06:9-10

(Use 93325 in conjunction with 76825, 76826, 76827, 76828, 93303, 93304, 93308, 93312, 93314, 93315, 93317, 93350, 93351)

93350   Echocardiography, transthoracic, real-time with image documentation (2D), includes M-mode recording, when performed, during rest and cardiovascular stress test using treadmill, bicycle exercise and/or pharmacologically induced stress, with interpretation and report;

→ *CPT Assistant* Aug 02:11, Jan 10:8, Oct 10:17, Dec 10:17; *CPT Changes: An Insider's View* 2009

(Stress testing codes 93016-93018 should be reported, when appropriate, in conjunction with 93350 to capture the cardiovascular stress portion of the study)

(Do not report 93350 in conjunction with 93015)

▲ **93351**   including performance of continuous electrocardiographic monitoring, with supervision by a physician or other qualified health care professional

→ *CPT Assistant* Jan 10:8, Oct 10:17, Dec 10:17; *CPT Changes: An Insider's View* 2009, 2013

(Do not report 93351 in conjunction with 93015-93018, 93350. Do not report 93351-26 in conjunction with 93016, 93018, 93350-26)

+ **93352**   Use of echocardiographic contrast agent during stress echocardiography (List separately in addition to code for primary procedure)

→ *CPT Assistant* Jan 10:8, Oct 10:17, Dec 10:17; *CPT Changes: An Insider's View* 2009

(Do not report 93352 more than once per stress echocardiogram)

(Use 93352 in conjunction with 93350, 93351)

Cardiac Catheterization

Cardiac catheterization is a diagnostic medical procedure which includes introduction, positioning and repositioning, when necessary, of catheter(s), within the vascular system, recording of intracardiac and/or intravascular pressure(s), and final evaluation and report of procedure. There are two code families for cardiac catheterization: one for congenital heart disease and one for all other conditions. Anomalous coronary arteries, patent foramen ovale, mitral valve prolapse, and bicuspid aortic valve are to be reported with 93451-93464, 93566-93568.

▶Right heart catheterization includes catheter placement in one or more right-sided cardiac chamber(s) or structures (ie, the right atrium, right ventricle, pulmonary artery, pulmonary wedge), obtaining blood samples for measurement of blood gases, and cardiac output measurements (Fick or other method), when performed. Left heart catheterization involves catheter placement in a left-sided (systemic) cardiac chamber(s) (left ventricle or left atrium) and includes left ventricular injection(s) when performed. Do not report 93503 in conjunction with other diagnostic cardiac catheterization codes. When right heart catheterization is performed in conjunction with other cardiac catheterization services, report 93453, 93456, 93457, 93460, or 93461. For placement of a flow directed catheter (eg, Swan-Ganz) performed for hemodynamic monitoring purposes not in conjunction with other catheterization services, use 93503. Right heart catheterization does not include right ventricular or right atrial angiography (93566). When left heart catheterization is performed using either transapical puncture of the left ventricle or transseptal puncture of an intact septum, report 93462 in conjunction with 93452, 93453, 93458-93461, 93653, 93654. Catheter placement(s) in coronary artery(ies) involves selective engagement of the origins of the native coronary artery(ies) for the purpose of coronary angiography. Catheter placement(s) in bypass graft(s) (venous, internal mammary, free arterial graft[s]) involve selective engagement of the origins of the graft(s) for the purpose of bypass angiography. It is typically performed only in conjunction with coronary angiography of native vessels.◀

The cardiac catheterization codes (93452-93461), other than those for congenital heart disease, include contrast injection(s), imaging supervision, interpretation, and report for imaging typically performed. Codes for left heart catheterization (93452, 93453, 93458-93461), other than those for congenital heart disease, include intraprocedural injection(s) for left ventricular/left atrial angiography, imaging supervision, and interpretation, when performed. Codes for coronary catheter placement(s) (93454-93461), other than those for congenital heart disease, include intraprocedural injection(s) for coronary angiography, imaging supervision, and interpretation. Codes for catheter placement(s) in bypass graft(s) (93455, 93457, 93459, 93461), other than those for congenital heart disease, include intraprocedural injection(s) for bypass graft angiography, imaging supervision, and interpretation. Do not report 93563-93565 in conjunction with 93452-93461.

For cardiac catheterization for congenital cardiac anomalies, see 93530-93533. When contrast injection(s) are performed in conjunction with cardiac catheterization for congenital anomalies, see 93563-93568.

Cardiac catheterization (93451-93461) includes all roadmapping angiography in order to place the catheters, including any injections and imaging supervision, interpretation, and report. It does not include contrast injection(s) and imaging supervision, interpretation, and report for imaging that is separately identified by specific procedure code(s). For right ventricular or right atrial angiography performed in conjunction with cardiac catheterization for congenital or noncongenital heart disease (93451-93461, 93530-93533), use 93566. For aortography, use 93567. For pulmonary angiography, use 93568. For angiography of noncoronary arteries and veins, performed as a distinct service, use appropriate codes from the Radiology section and the Vascular Injection Procedures section.

►When cardiac catheterization is combined with pharmacologic agent administration with the specific purpose of repeating hemodynamic measurements to evaluate hemodynamic response, use 93463 in conjunction with 93451-93453 and 93456-93461. Do not report 93463 for intracoronary administration of pharmacologic agents during percutaneous coronary interventional procedures, during intracoronary assessment of coronary pressure, flow or resistance, or during intracoronary imaging procedures. Do not report 93463 in conjunction with 92920-92944, 92975, 92977.◄

When cardiac catheterization is combined with exercise (eg, walking or arm or leg ergometry protocol) with the specific purpose of repeating hemodynamic measurements to evaluate hemodynamic response, report 93464 in conjunction with 93451-93453, 93456-93461, and 93530-93533.

Contrast injection to image the access site(s) for the specific purpose of placing a closure device is inherent to the catheterization procedure and not separately

reportable. Closure device placement at the vascular access site is inherent to the catheterization procedure and not separately reportable.

Modifier 51 should not be appended to 93451, 93456, 93503.

Please see the cardiac catheterization table located following 93571.

⊙⊘ **93451**   Right heart catheterization including measurement(s) of oxygen saturation and cardiac output, when performed
➔ *CPT Assistant* Aug 11:5, Mar 12:10; *CPT Changes: An Insider's View* 2011

(Do not report 93451 in conjunction with 93453, 93456, 93457, 93460, 93461)

Right Heart Catheterization
93451

The physician introduces a cardiac catheter into the venous system. The catheter is directed into the right atrium, right ventricle, and pulmonary artery.

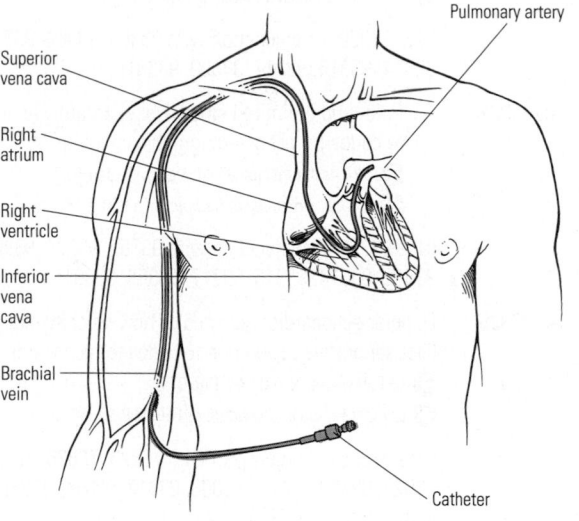

⊙ **93452**   Left heart catheterization including intraprocedural injection(s) for left ventriculography, imaging supervision and interpretation, when performed
➔ *CPT Assistant* Aug 11:3, Mar 12:10; *CPT Changes: An Insider's View* 2011

(Do not report 93452 in conjunction with 93453, 93458-93461)

⊙ **93453**   Combined right and left heart catheterization including intraprocedural injection(s) for left ventriculography, imaging supervision and interpretation, when performed
➔ *CPT Assistant* Aug 11:3, Mar 12:10; *CPT Changes: An Insider's View* 2011

(Do not report 93453 in conjunction with 93451, 93452, 93456-93461)

Right Heart Catheterization – Infant

Catheter is advanced retrograde through the arterial system to the ascending aorta; pressures are measured in the aortic root; the catheter is manipulated using fluoroscopic guidance into the ostium of a coronary artery, arterial bypass conduit, or venous coronary bypass graft.

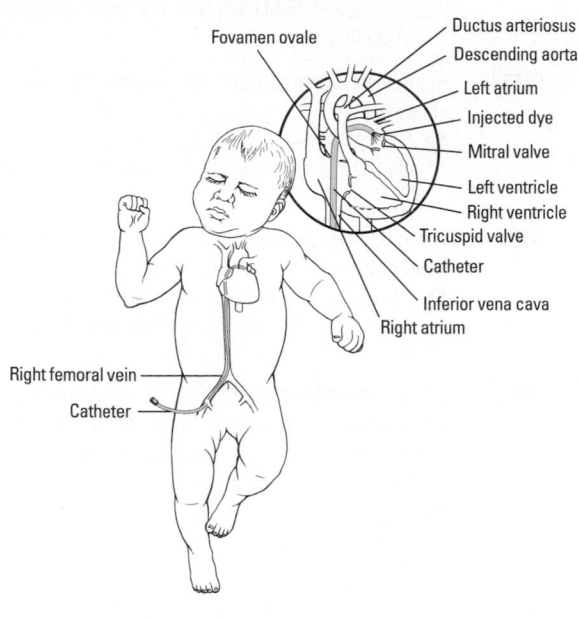

Left Heart Catheterization
93452

A catheter is inserted into the arterial system and then into the left ventricle.

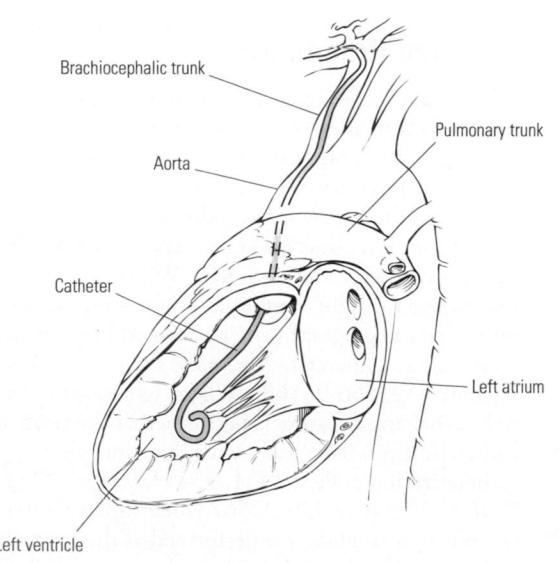

⊙ **93454**   Catheter placement in coronary artery(s) for coronary angiography, including intraprocedural injection(s) for coronary angiography, imaging supervision and interpretation;

➔ *CPT Assistant* Aug 11:3, Mar 12:10; *CPT Changes: An Insider's View* 2011

Coronary Angiography Without Concomitant Left Heart Catheterization
93454

Cardiac catheterization procedure performed wherein the catheter does not cross the aortic valve into the left ventricle (left heart catheterization).

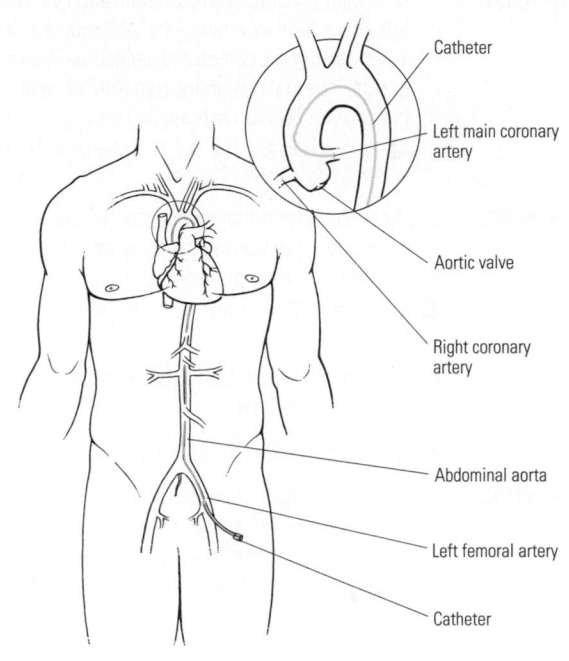

⊙ **93455**   with catheter placement(s) in bypass graft(s) (internal mammary, free arterial, venous grafts) including intraprocedural injection(s) for bypass graft angiography

➔ *CPT Assistant* Aug 11:3, Dec 11:9, Mar 12:10; *CPT Changes: An Insider's View* 2011

⊙⊘ **93456**   with right heart catheterization

➔ *CPT Assistant* Aug 11:3, Mar 12:10; *CPT Changes: An Insider's View* 2011

⊙ **93457**   with catheter placement(s) in bypass graft(s) (internal mammary, free arterial, venous grafts) including intraprocedural injection(s) for bypass graft angiography and right heart catheterization

➔ *CPT Assistant* Aug 11:3, Dec 11:9, Mar 12:10; *CPT Changes: An Insider's View* 2011

⊙ **93458**   with left heart catheterization including intraprocedural injection(s) for left ventriculography, when performed

➔ *CPT Assistant* Aug 11:3, Mar 12:10; *CPT Changes: An Insider's View* 2011

⊙ **93459**   with left heart catheterization including intraprocedural injection(s) for left ventriculography, when performed, catheter placement(s) in bypass graft(s) (internal mammary, free arterial, venous grafts) with bypass graft angiography

➔ *CPT Assistant* Aug 11:3, Dec 11:11, Mar 12:10; *CPT Changes: An Insider's View* 2011

⊙ **93460** with right and left heart catheterization including intraprocedural injection(s) for left ventriculography, when performed

→ *CPT Assistant* Aug 11:3, Mar 12:10; *CPT Changes: An Insider's View* 2011

⊙ **93461** with right and left heart catheterization including intraprocedural injection(s) for left ventriculography, when performed, catheter placement(s) in bypass graft(s) (internal mammary, free arterial, venous grafts) with bypass graft angiography

→ *CPT Assistant* Aug 11:3, Dec 11:9, Mar 12:10; *CPT Changes: An Insider's View* 2011

⊙+ **93462** Left heart catheterization by transseptal puncture through intact septum or by transapical puncture (List separately in addition to code for primary procedure)

→ *CPT Assistant* Aug 11:3, Mar 12:10; *CPT Changes: An Insider's View* 2011

▶(Use 93462 in conjunction with 93452, 93453, 93458-93461, 93653, 93654)◀

▶(Do not report 93462 in conjunction with 93656)◀

⊙+ **93463** Pharmacologic agent administration (eg, inhaled nitric oxide, intravenous infusion of nitroprusside, dobutamine, milrinone, or other agent) including assessing hemodynamic measurements before, during, after and repeat pharmacologic agent administration, when performed (List separately in addition to code for primary procedure)

→ *CPT Assistant* Aug 11:3, Mar 12:10; *CPT Changes: An Insider's View* 2011

▶(Use 93463 in conjunction with 93451-93453, 93456-93461, 93563, 93564, 93580, 93581)◀

(Report 93463 only once per catheterization procedure)

▶(Do not report 93463 for pharmacologic agent administration in conjunction with coronary interventional procedure codes 92920-92944, 92975, 92977)◀

⊙+ **93464** Physiologic exercise study (eg, bicycle or arm ergometry) including assessing hemodynamic measurements before and after (List separately in addition to code for primary procedure)

→ *CPT Assistant* Aug 11:3, Mar 12:10; *CPT Changes: An Insider's View* 2011

(Use 93464 in conjunction with 93451-93453, 93456-93461, 93530-93533)

(Report 93464 only once per catheterization procedure)

(For pharmacologic agent administration, use 93463)

(For bundle of His recording, use 93600)

⊘ **93503** Insertion and placement of flow directed catheter (eg, Swan-Ganz) for monitoring purposes

→ *CPT Assistant* Winter 91:3, Fall 95:8, Feb 97:5, Apr 98:2, Mar 08:4, Aug 11:3, Dec 11:18

(For subsequent monitoring, see 99356-99357)

⊙ **93505** Endomyocardial biopsy

→ *CPT Assistant* Apr 98:2, Apr 00:10, Aug 11:3; *CPT Changes: An Insider's View* 2008

(To report transcatheter placement of radiation delivery device for coronary intravascular brachytherapy, use 92974)

(For intravascular radioelement application, see 77785-77787)

(93501, 93508-93529 have been deleted. To report, see 93451-93461)

⊙ **93530** Right heart catheterization, for congenital cardiac anomalies

→ *CPT Assistant* Nov 97:45, Jan 98:11, Mar 98:11, Apr 98:3, 6-7, Aug 11:3, Dec 11:11, Mar 12:10; *CPT Changes: An Insider's View* 2008

93531 Combined right heart catheterization and retrograde left heart catheterization, for congenital cardiac anomalies

→ *CPT Assistant* Nov 97:45, Jan 98:11, Mar 98:11, Apr 98:8, 10-11, Aug 11:3, Dec 11:11, Mar 12:10; *CPT Changes: An Insider's View* 2008

93532 Combined right heart catheterization and transseptal left heart catheterization through intact septum with or without retrograde left heart catheterization, for congenital cardiac anomalies

→ *CPT Assistant* Nov 97:45, Jan 98:11, Mar 98:11, Apr 98:10-11, Aug 11:3, Dec 11:11, Mar 12:10; *CPT Changes: An Insider's View* 2008

93533 Combined right heart catheterization and transseptal left heart catheterization through existing septal opening, with or without retrograde left heart catheterization, for congenital cardiac anomalies

→ *CPT Assistant* Nov 97:45, Jan 98:11, Mar 98:11, Apr 98:12-13, Aug 11:3, Dec 11:11, Mar 12:10; *CPT Changes: An Insider's View* 2008

Injection Procedures

All injection codes include radiological supervision, interpretation, and report. Cardiac catheterization codes (93452-93461), other than those for congenital heart disease, include contrast injection(s) for imaging typically performed during these procedures (see Cardiac Catheterization above). Do not report 93563-93565 in conjunction with 93452-93461. When injection procedures for right ventricular, right atrial, aortic, or pulmonary angiography are performed in conjunction with cardiac catheterization, these services are reported separately (93566-93568). When right ventricular or right atrial angiography is performed at the time of heart catheterization, use 93566 with the appropriate catheterization code (93451, 93453, 93456, 93457, 93460, or 93461). Use 93567 when supravalvular ascending aortography is performed at the time of heart catheterization. Use 93568 with the appropriate right heart catheterization code when pulmonary angiography is performed. Separately reported injection procedures do not include introduction of catheters but do include repositioning of catheters when necessary and use of automatic power injectors, when performed.

When contrast injection(s) are performed in conjunction with cardiac catheterization for congenital cardiac anomalies (93530-93533), see 93563-93568. Injection procedure codes 93563-93568 include imaging supervision, interpretation, and report.

Injection procedures 93563-93568 represent separate identifiable services and may be coded in conjunction with one another when appropriate. The technical details of angiography, supervision of filming and processing, interpretation, and report are included.

(93539-93545 have been deleted. To report, see 93451-93461, 93563-93568)

(93555, 93556 have been deleted. See introductory guidelines for Cardiac Catheterization and Injection Procedures)

⊙ **93561** Indicator dilution studies such as dye or thermodilution, including arterial and/or venous catheterization; with cardiac output measurement (separate procedure)
→ *CPT Assistant* Winter 91:25, Summer 95:2, Aug 00:2, Feb 07:10, Jul 07:1, Aug 11:3; *CPT Changes: An Insider's View* 2012

⊙ **93562** subsequent measurement of cardiac output
→ *CPT Assistant* Winter 91:25, Summer 95:2, Aug 00:2, Feb 07:10, Jul 07:1, Aug 11:3; *CPT Changes: An Insider's View* 2012

(Do not report 93561, 93562 in conjunction with 93451-93462)

(For radioisotope method of cardiac output, see 78472, 78473, or 78481)

⊙+ **93563** Injection procedure during cardiac catheterization including imaging supervision, interpretation, and report; for selective coronary angiography during congenital heart catheterization (List separately in addition to code for primary procedure)
→ *CPT Assistant* Aug 11:3, Dec 11:11; *CPT Changes: An Insider's View* 2011

⊙+ **93564** for selective opacification of aortocoronary venous or arterial bypass graft(s) (eg, aortocoronary saphenous vein, free radial artery, or free mammary artery graft) to one or more coronary arteries and in situ arterial conduits (eg, internal mammary), whether native or used for bypass to one or more coronary arteries during congenital heart catheterization, when performed (List separately in addition to code for primary procedure)
→ *CPT Assistant* Aug 11:3, Dec 11:11; *CPT Changes: An Insider's View* 2011

⊙+ **93565** for selective left ventricular or left atrial angiography (List separately in addition to code for primary procedure)
→ *CPT Assistant* Aug 11:3, Dec 11:9, *CPT Changes: An Insider's View* 2011

(Do not report 93563-93565 in conjunction with 93452-93461)

(Use 93563-93565 in conjunction with 93530-93533)

⊙+ **93566** for selective right ventricular or right atrial angiography (List separately in addition to code for primary procedure)
→ *CPT Assistant* Aug 11:3, Dec 11:9; *CPT Changes: An Insider's View* 2011

▶(Use 93566 in conjunction with 93451, 93453, 93456, 93457, 93460, 93461, 93530-93533)◀

⊙+ **93567** for supravalvular aortography (List separately in addition to code for primary procedure)
→ *CPT Assistant* Aug 11:3, Dec 11:9; *CPT Changes: An Insider's View* 2011

▶(Use 93567 in conjunction with 93451-93461, 93530-93533)◀

▶(For non-supravalvular thoracic aortography or abdominal aortography performed at the time of cardiac catheterization, use the appropriate radiological supervision and interpretation codes [36221, 75600-75630])◀

⊙+ **93568** for pulmonary angiography (List separately in addition to code for primary procedure)
→ *CPT Assistant* Aug 11:3, Dec 11:9; *CPT Changes: An Insider's View* 2011

▶(Use 93568 in conjunction with 93451, 93453, 93456, 93457, 93460, 93461, 93530-93533)◀

⊙+ **93571** Intravascular Doppler velocity and/or pressure derived coronary flow reserve measurement (coronary vessel or graft) during coronary angiography including pharmacologically induced stress; initial vessel (List separately in addition to code for primary procedure)
→ *CPT Assistant* Nov 98:33, Apr 00:2, Mar 08:4, Aug 11:3

▶(Use 93571 in conjunction with 92920, 92924, 92928, 92933, 92937, 92941, 92943, 92975, 93454-93461, 93563, 93564)◀

Intravascular Distal Blood Flow Velocity
93571

A Doppler guidewire is positioned in a proximal coronary artery with the transducer beam parallel to blood flow to measure blood flow velocity.

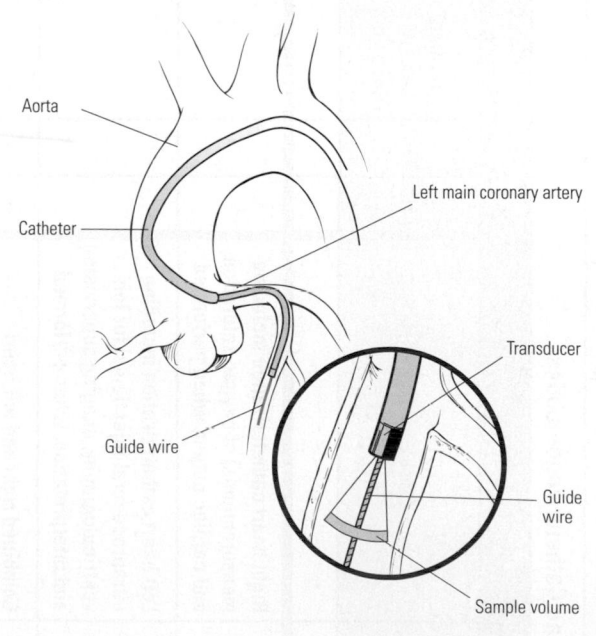

Cardiac Catheterization Codes

CPT Code	Code Descriptor	Catheter Placement Type				Add-on Procedures (Can Be Reported Separately)					
		RHC	LHC	Coronary Artery Placement	Bypass Graft(s)	With Transseptal or Transapical Puncture — 93462	With Pharmacological Study — 93463	With Exercise Study — 93464	Injection Procedure for Selective Right Ventricular or Right Atrial Angiography — 93566	Injection Procedure for Supravalvular Aortography — 93567	Injection Procedure for Pulmonary Angiography — 93568
93451	Right heart catheterization including measurement(s) of oxygen saturation and cardiac output, when performed	X					X	X	X		X
93452	Left heart catheterization including intraprocedural injection(s) for left ventriculography, imaging supervision and interpretation, when performed		X			X	X	X		X	
93453	Combined right and left heart catheterization including intraprocedural injection(s) for left ventriculography, imaging supervision and interpretation, when performed	X	X			X	X	X	X	X	X
93454	Catheter placement in coronary artery(s) for coronary angiography, including intraprocedural injection(s) for coronary angiography, imaging supervision and interpretation;			X						X	
93455	Catheter placement in coronary artery(s) for coronary angiography, including intraprocedural injection(s) for coronary angiography, imaging supervision and interpretation; with catheter placement(s) in bypass graft(s), (internal mammary, free arterial, venous grafts) including intraprocedural injection(s) for bypass graft angiography			X	X					X	

Cardiac Catheterization Codes, *continued*

CPT Code	Code Descriptor	Catheter Placement Type				Add-on Procedures (Can Be Reported Separately)					
		RHC	LHC	Coronary Artery Placement	Bypass Graft(s)	With Transseptal or Transapical Puncture 93462	With Pharmacological Study 93463	With Exercise Study 93464	Injection Procedure for Selective Right Ventricular or Right Atrial Angiography 93566	Injection Procedure for Supravalvular Aortography 93567	Injection Procedure for Pulmonary Angiography 93568
93456	Catheter placement in coronary artery(s) for coronary angiography, including intraprocedural injection(s) for coronary angiography, imaging supervision and interpretation; **with right heart catheterization**	X		X			X	X	X	X	X
93457	Catheter placement in coronary artery(s) for coronary angiography, including intraprocedural injection(s) for coronary angiography, imaging supervision and interpretation; **with catheter placement(s) in bypass graft(s) (internal mammary, free arterial, venous grafts) including intraprocedural injection(s) for bypass graft angiography and right heart catheterization**	X		X	X		X	X	X	X	X
93458	Catheter placement in coronary artery(s) for coronary angiography, including intraprocedural injection(s) for coronary angiography, imaging supervision and interpretation; **with left heart catheterization including intraprocedural injection(s) for left ventriculography, when performed**		X	X		X	X	X		X	

Medicine

Cardiac Catheterization Codes, *continued*

CPT Code	Code Descriptor	Catheter Placement Type				Add-on Procedures (Can Be Reported Separately)					
		RHC	LHC	Coronary Artery Placement	Bypass Graft(s)	With Transseptal or Transapical Puncture 93462	With Pharmacological Study 93463	With Exercise Study 93464	Injection Procedure for Selective Right Ventricular or Right Atrial Angiography 93566	Injection Procedure for Supravalvular Aortography 93567	Injection Procedure for Pulmonary Angiography 93568
93459	Catheter placement in coronary artery(s) for coronary angiography, including intraprocedural injection(s) for coronary angiography, imaging supervision and interpretation; **with left heart catheterization including intraprocedural injection(s) for left ventriculography, when performed, catheter placement(s) in bypass graft(s) (internal mammary, free arterial, venous grafts) with bypass graft angiography**		X	X	X	X	X	X		X	
93460	Catheter placement in coronary artery(s) for coronary angiography, including intraprocedural injection(s) for coronary angiography, imaging supervision and interpretation; **with right and left heart catheterization including intraprocedural injection(s) for left ventriculography, when performed**	X	X	X		X	X	X	X	X	X
93461	Catheter placement in coronary artery(s) for coronary angiography, including intraprocedural injection(s) for coronary angiography, imaging supervision and interpretation; **with right and left heart catheterization including intraprocedural injection(s) for left ventriculography, when performed, catheter placement(s) in bypass graft(s) (internal mammary, free arterial, venous grafts) with bypass graft angiography**	X	X	X	X	X	X	X	X	X	X

⊙**+ 93572**   each additional vessel (List separately in addition to code for primary procedure)

→ *CPT Assistant* Nov 98:34, Apr 00:2, Aug 11:5

►(Use 93572 in conjunction with 93571)◄

(Intravascular distal coronary blood flow velocity measurements include all Doppler transducer manipulations and repositioning within the specific vessel being examined, during coronary angiography or therapeutic intervention [eg, angioplasty])

(For unlisted cardiac catheterization procedure, use 93799)

Repair of Septal Defect

93580   Percutaneous transcatheter closure of congenital interatrial communication (ie, Fontan fenestration, atrial septal defect) with implant

→ *CPT Assistant* Mar 03:23; *CPT Changes: An Insider's View* 2003

(Percutaneous transcatheter closure of atrial septal defect includes a right heart catheterization procedure. Code 93580 includes injection of contrast for atrial and ventricular angiograms. Codes 93451-93453, 93455-93461, 93530-93533, 93564-93566 should not be reported separately in addition to code 93580)

93581   Percutaneous transcatheter closure of a congenital ventricular septal defect with implant

→ *CPT Assistant* Mar 03:23, Mar 08:4; *CPT Changes: An Insider's View* 2003

(Percutaneous transcatheter closure of ventricular septal defect includes a right heart catheterization procedure. Code 93581 includes injection of contrast for atrial and ventricular angingrams. Codes 93451-93453, 93455-93461, 93530-93533, 93564-93566 should not be reported separately in addition to code 93581)

(For echocardiographic services performed in addition to 93580, 93581, see 93303-93317, 93662 as appropriate)

Intracardiac Electrophysiological Procedures/Studies

►Intracardiac electrophysiologic studies (EPS) are invasive diagnostic medical procedures which include the insertion and repositioning of electrode catheters, recording of electrograms before and during pacing, programmed stimulation of multiple locations in the heart, analysis of recorded information, and report of the procedure. In many circumstances, patients with arrhythmias are evaluated and treated at the same encounter. In this situation, a diagnostic *electrophysiologic study* is performed, induced tachycardia(s) are *mapped*, and on the basis of the diagnostic and mapping information, the tissue is *ablated*.◄

Definitions

►*Arrhythmia Induction*: In most electrophysiologic studies, an attempt is made to induce arrhythmia(s) from single or multiple sites within the heart. Arrhythmia induction may be achieved by multiple techniques, eg, by performing pacing at different rates or programmed stimulation (introduction of critically timed electrical impulses). Because arrhythmia induction occurs via the same catheter(s) inserted for the electrophysiologic study(ies), catheter insertion and temporary pacemaker codes are not additionally reported. Codes 93600-93603, 93610, 93612, and 93618 are used to describe unusual situations where there may be recording, pacing, or an attempt at arrhythmia induction from only one site in the heart. Code 93619 describes only evaluation of the sinus node, atrioventricular node, and His-Purkinje conduction system, without arrhythmia induction. Codes 93620-93624, 93640-93642, 93653, 93654, and 93656 all include recording, pacing, and attempted arrhythmia induction from one or more site(s) in the heart.

Mapping: When a tachycardia is induced, the site of tachycardia origination or its electrical path through the heart is often defined by mapping. Mapping creates a multidimensional depiction of a tachycardia by recording multiple electrograms obtained sequentially or simultaneously from multiple catheter sites in the heart. Depending upon the technique, certain types of mapping catheters may be repositioned from point-to-point within the heart, allowing sequential recording from the various sites to construct maps. Other types of mapping catheters allow mapping without a point-to-point technique by allowing simultaneous recording from many electrodes on the same catheter and computer-assisted three-dimensional reconstruction of the tachycardia activation sequence.

Mapping is a distinct procedure performed in addition to a diagnostic electrophysiologic study or ablation procedure and may be separately reported using 93609 or 93613. Do not report standard mapping (93609) in addition to 3-dimensional mapping (93613).

Ablation: Once the part of the heart involved in the tachycardia is localized, the tachycardia may be treated by ablation (the delivery of a radiofrequency or cryo-energy to the area to selectively destroy cardiac tissue). Ablation procedures (93653-93657) are performed at the same session as electrophysiology studies and therefore represent a combined code description. When reporting ablation therapy codes (93653-93657), the single site electrophysiology studies (93600-93603, 93610, 93612, 93618) and the comprehensive electrophysiology studies (93619, 93620) may not be reported separately. Codes 93622 and 93623 may be reported separately with 93656 for treatment of atrial fibrillation. However, 93621 for left atrial pacing and recording from coronary sinus or left atrium should not be reported in conjunction with 93656 as this is a component of 93656.

The differences in the techniques involved for ablation of supraventricular arrhythmias, ventricular arrhythmias, and atrial fibrillation are reflected within the descriptions for 93653-93657. Code 93653 is a primary code for catheter ablation for treatment of supraventricular tachycardia caused by dual atrioventricular nodal pathways, accessory atrioventricular connections, or other atrial foci. Code 93654 describes catheter ablation for treatment of ventricular tachycardia or focus of ventricular ectopy. Code 93656 is a primary code for reporting treatment of atrial fibrillation by ablation to achieve complete pulmonary vein electrical isolation. Codes 93653, 93654, and 93656 are distinct primary procedure codes and may not be reported together.

Codes 93655 and 93657 are add-on codes listed in addition to the primary ablation code to report ablation of sites distinct from the primary ablation site. After ablation of the primary target site, post-ablation electrophysiologic evaluation is performed as part of those ablation services (93653, 93654, 93656) and additional mechanisms of tachycardia may be identified. For example, if the primary tachycardia ablated was atrioventricular nodal reentrant tachycardia and during post-ablation testing an atrial tachycardia, atrial flutter, or accessory pathway with orthodromic reentry tachycardia was identified, this would be considered a separate mechanism of tachycardia. Pacing maneuvers are performed to define the mechanism(s) of the new tachycardia(s). Catheter ablation of this distinct mechanism of tachycardia is then performed at the newly discovered atrial or ventricular origin. Appropriate post-ablation attempts at re-induction and observation are again performed. Code 93655 is listed in conjunction with 93653 when repeat ablation is for treatment of an additional supraventricular tachycardia mechanism and with 93654 when the repeat ablation is for treatment of an additional ventricular tachycardia mechanism. Code 93655 may be reported with 93656 when an additional non-atrial fibrillation tachycardia is separately diagnosed after pulmonary vein isolation. Code 93657 is reported in conjunction with 93656 when successful pulmonary vein isolation is achieved, attempts at re-induction of atrial fibrillation identify an additional left or right atrial focus for atrial fibrillation, and further ablation of this new focus is performed.

In certain circumstances, depending on the chamber of origin, a catheter or catheters may be maneuvered into the left ventricle to facilitate arrhythmia diagnosis. This may be accomplished via a retrograde aortic approach by means of the arterial access or through a transseptal puncture. For ablation treatment of supraventricular tachycardia (93653) and ventricular tachycardia (93654), the left heart catheterization by transseptal puncture through intact septum (93462) may be reported separately as an add-on code. However, for ablation treatment of atrial fibrillation (93656), the transseptal puncture (93462) is a standard component of the procedure and may not be reported separately. Do not report 93462 in conjunction with 93656.◄

Modifier 51 should not be appended to 93600-93603, 93610, 93612, 93615-93618, 93631.

⊘ **93600** Bundle of His recording
➔ *CPT Assistant* Summer 94:12, Aug 97:9, Apr 04:9, Jul 04:13, Aug 05:13, Dec 07:16, Mar 08:4

⊘ **93602** Intra-atrial recording
➔ *CPT Assistant* Summer 94:12, Aug 97:9, Apr 04:9, Jul 04:13, Aug 05:13

⊘ **93603** Right ventricular recording
➔ *CPT Assistant* Summer 94:12, Aug 97:9, Apr 04:9, Jul 04:13, Aug 05:13

⊙+ **93609** Intraventricular and/or intra-atrial mapping of tachycardia site(s) with catheter manipulation to record from multiple sites to identify origin of tachycardia (List separately in addition to code for primary procedure)
➔ *CPT Assistant* Summer 94:12, Aug 97:9, Apr 04:9, Aug 05:13; *CPT Changes: An Insider's View* 2002

▶(Use 93609 in conjunction with 93620, 93653)◄

▶(Do not report 93609 in conjunction with 93613, 93654)◄

⊘ **93610** Intra-atrial pacing
➔ *CPT Assistant* Summer 94:12, Aug 97:9, Apr 04:9, Jul 04:13

⊘ **93612** Intraventricular pacing
➔ *CPT Assistant* Summer 94:12, Aug 97:9, Apr 04:9, Jul 04:13

(Do not report 93612 in conjunction with 93620-93622)

⊙+ **93613** Intracardiac electrophysiologic 3-dimensional mapping (List separately in addition to code for primary procedure)
➔ *CPT Assistant* Apr 04:8, Aug 05:13; *CPT Changes: An Insider's View* 2002

▶(Use 93613 in conjunction with 93620, 93653)◄

▶(Do not report 93613 in conjunction with 93609, 93654)◄

⊙⊘ **93615** Esophageal recording of atrial electrogram with or without ventricular electrogram(s);
➔ *CPT Assistant* Summer 94:12, Aug 97:9, Apr 04:9, Aug 05:13

⊙⊘ **93616** with pacing
➔ *CPT Assistant* Summer 94:12, Aug 97:9, Apr 04:9, Aug 05:13

⊙⊘ **93618** Induction of arrhythmia by electrical pacing
➔ *CPT Assistant* Summer 94:12, Aug 97:9, Oct 97:10, Apr 99:10, Jun 00:5, Nov 00:9, Apr 04:9, Jul 04:13, Aug 05:13, Dec 07:16

(For intracardiac phonocardiogram, use 93799)

⊙ **93619** Comprehensive electrophysiologic evaluation with right atrial pacing and recording, right ventricular pacing and recording, His bundle recording, including insertion and repositioning of multiple electrode catheters, without induction or attempted induction of arrhythmia
➔ *CPT Assistant* Aug 97:9, Oct 97:10, Nov 00:9, Apr 04:9, Jul 04:13, Aug 05:13, Dec 07:16; *CPT Changes: An Insider's View* 2002, 2008

(Do not report 93619 in conjunction with 93600, 93602, 93610, 93612, 93618, or 93620-93622)

⊙ **93620** Comprehensive electrophysiologic evaluation including insertion and repositioning of multiple electrode catheters with induction or attempted induction of arrhythmia; with right atrial pacing and recording, right ventricular pacing and recording, His bundle recording
➔ *CPT Assistant* Summer 94:12, Aug 97:9, Oct 97:10, Jul 98:10, Aug 98:7, Nov 00:9, Apr 04:9, Jul 04:13, Aug 05:13, Dec 07:16, Oct 08:10; *CPT Changes: An Insider's View* 2002, 2003, 2008

(Do not report 93620 in conjunction with 93600, 93602, 93610, 93612, 93618 or 93619)

⊙+ 93621 with left atrial pacing and recording from coronary sinus or left atrium (List separately in addition to code for primary procedure)

→ *CPT Assistant* Summer 94:12, Aug 97:9, Oct 97:10, Jul 98:10, Aug 98:7, Nov 98:34, Nov 00:9, Apr 04:9, Jul 04:13, Aug 05:13, Dec 07:16, Oct 08:10; *CPT Changes: An Insider's View* 2002

(Use 93621 in conjunction with 93620)

►(Do not report 93621 in conjunction with 93656)◄

⊙+ 93622 with left ventricular pacing and recording (List separately in addition to code for primary procedure)

→ *CPT Assistant* Summer 94:14, Aug 97:9, Oct 97:10, Jul 98:10, Aug 98:7, Nov 98:34, Nov 00:9, Apr 04:9, Jul 04:13, Aug 05:13, Dec 07:16, Mar 08:4; *CPT Changes: An Insider's View* 2002

(Use 93622 in conjunction with 93620)

+ 93623 Programmed stimulation and pacing after intravenous drug infusion (List separately in addition to code for primary procedure)

→ *CPT Assistant* Summer 94:14, Aug 97:9, Nov 00:9, Aug 05:13, Dec 07:16, Oct 08:10

(Use 93623 in conjunction with 93619, 93620)

⊙ 93624 Electrophysiologic follow-up study with pacing and recording to test effectiveness of therapy, including induction or attempted induction of arrhythmia

→ *CPT Assistant* Summer 94:14, Aug 97:9, Nov 00:9, Aug 05:13, Dec 07:16; *CPT Changes: An Insider's View* 2008

⊘ 93631 Intra-operative epicardial and endocardial pacing and mapping to localize the site of tachycardia or zone of slow conduction for surgical correction

→ *CPT Assistant* Summer 94:14, Aug 97:9, Nov 00:9, Aug 05:13, Dec 07:16

►(For operative ablation of an arrhythmogenic focus or pathway by a separate individual, see 33250-33261)◄

⊙ 93640 Electrophysiologic evaluation of single or dual chamber pacing cardioverter-defibrillator leads including defibrillation threshold evaluation (induction of arrhythmia, evaluation of sensing and pacing for arrhythmia termination) at time of initial implantation or replacement;

→ *CPT Assistant* Summer 94:14, Aug 97:9, Apr 99:10, Nov 99:50, Nov 00:9, Aug 05:13, Jun 12:3; *CPT Changes: An Insider's View* 2000, 2008

⊙ 93641 with testing of single or dual chamber pacing cardioverter-defibrillator pulse generator

→ *CPT Assistant* Summer 94:14, Aug 97:9, Apr 99:10, Nov 99:50, Jun 00:5, Jul 00:5, Nov 00:9, Aug 05:13, Jun 12:3; *CPT Changes: An Insider's View* 2000, 2008

(For subsequent or periodic electronic analysis and/or reprogramming of single or dual chamber pacing cardioverter-defibrillators, see 93282, 93283, 93289, 93292, 93295, 93642)

⊙ 93642 Electrophysiologic evaluation of single or dual chamber pacing cardioverter-defibrillator (includes defibrillation threshold evaluation, induction of arrhythmia, evaluation of sensing and pacing for arrhythmia termination, and programming or reprogramming of sensing or therapeutic parameters)

→ *CPT Assistant* Summer 94:14, Aug 97:9, Nov 99:50, Jun 00:5, Nov 00:9, Aug 05:13; *CPT Changes: An Insider's View* 2000, 2008

⊙ 93650 Intracardiac catheter ablation of atrioventricular node function, atrioventricular conduction for creation of complete heart block, with or without temporary pacemaker placement

→ *CPT Assistant* Summer 94:15, Aug 97:9, Nov 00:9, Aug 05:13, Apr 12:18, May 12:15; *CPT Changes: An Insider's View* 2008

►(93651, 93652 have been deleted. To report, see 93653-93657)◄

⊙● 93653 Comprehensive electrophysiologic evaluation including insertion and repositioning of multiple electrode catheters with induction or attempted induction of an arrhythmia with right atrial pacing and recording, right ventricular pacing and recording, His recording with intracardiac catheter ablation of arrhythmogenic focus; with treatment of supraventricular tachycardia by ablation of fast or slow atrioventricular pathway, accessory atrioventricular connection, cavo-tricuspid isthmus or other single atrial focus or source of atrial re-entry

→ *CPT Changes: An Insider's View* 2013

►(Do not report 93653 in conjunction with 93600-93603, 93610, 93612, 93618-93620, 93642, 93654)◄

⊙● 93654 with treatment of ventricular tachycardia or focus of ventricular ectopy including intracardiac electrophysiologic 3D mapping, when performed, and left ventricular pacing and recording, when performed

→ *CPT Changes: An Insider's View* 2013

►(Do not report 93654 in conjunction with 93279-93284, 93286-93289, 93600-93603, 93609, 93610, 93612, 93613, 93618-93620, 93622, 93642, 93653)◄

⊙+● 93655 Intracardiac catheter ablation of a discrete mechanism of arrhythmia which is distinct from the primary ablated mechanism, including repeat diagnostic maneuvers, to treat a spontaneous or induced arrhythmia (List separately in addition to code for primary procedure)

→ *CPT Changes: An Insider's View* 2013

►(Use 93655 in conjunction with 93653, 93654, 93656)◄

⊙● 93656 Comprehensive electrophysiologic evaluation including transseptal catheterizations, insertion and repositioning of multiple electrode catheters with induction or attempted induction of an arrhythmia with atrial recording and pacing, when possible, right ventricular pacing and recording, His bundle recording with intracardiac catheter ablation of arrhythmogenic focus, with treatment of atrial fibrillation by ablation by pulmonary vein isolation

→ *CPT Changes: An Insider's View* 2013

Medicine

►(Do not report 93656 in conjunction with 93279-93284, 93286-93289, 93462, 93600, 93602, 93603, 93610, 93612, 93618, 93619, 93620, 93621, 93653, 93654)◄

⊙+● **93657**   Additional linear or focal intracardiac catheter ablation of the left or right atrium for treatment of atrial fibrillation remaining after completion of pulmonary vein isolation (List separately in addition to code for primary procedure)
➔ *CPT Changes: An Insider's View* 2013

►(Use 93657 in conjunction with 93656)◄

93660   Evaluation of cardiovascular function with tilt table evaluation, with continuous ECG monitoring and intermittent blood pressure monitoring, with or without pharmacological intervention
➔ *CPT Changes: An Insider's View* 2008

►(For testing of autonomic nervous system function, see 95921, 95924, 95943)◄

+ 93662   Intracardiac echocardiography during therapeutic/ diagnostic intervention, including imaging supervision and interpretation (List separately in addition to code for primary procedure)
➔ *CPT Assistant* Mar 03:23; *CPT Changes: An Insider's View* 2001

►(Use 93662 in conjunction with 92987, 93453, 93460-93462, 93532, 93580, 93581, 93621, 93622, 93653, 93654, 93656 as appropriate)◄

(Do not report 92961 in addition to 93662)

Peripheral Arterial Disease Rehabilitation

►Peripheral arterial disease (PAD) rehabilitative physical exercise consists of a series of sessions, lasting 45-60 minutes per session, involving use of either a motorized treadmill or a track to permit each patient to achieve symptom-limited claudication. Each session is supervised by an exercise physiologist or nurse. The supervising provider monitors the individual patient's claudication threshold and other cardiovascular limitations for adjustment of workload. During this supervised rehabilitation program, the development of new arrhythmias, symptoms that might suggest angina or the continued inability of the patient to progress to an adequate level of exercise may require review and examination of the patient by a physician or other qualified health care professional. These services would be separately reported with an appropriate level E/M service code including office or other outpatient services (99201-99215), initial hospital care (99221-99223), subsequent hospital care (99231-99233), critical care services (99291-99292).◄

93668   Peripheral arterial disease (PAD) rehabilitation, per session
➔ *CPT Changes: An Insider's View* 2001

Noninvasive Physiologic Studies and Procedures

(For arterial cannulization and recording of direct arterial pressure, use 36620)

(For radiographic injection procedures, see 36000-36299)

(For vascular cannulization for hemodialysis, see 36800-36821)

(For chemotherapy for malignant disease, see 96409-96549)

(For penile plethysmography, use 54240)

93701   Bioimpedance-derived physiologic cardiovascular analysis
➔ *CPT Assistant* Mar 02:3, Mar 08:4; *CPT Changes: An Insider's View* 2002, 2010

(For left ventricular filling pressure indirect measurement by computerized calibration of the arterial waveform response to Valsalva, use 93799)

(93720-93722 have been deleted. To report, use 94726)

93724   Electronic analysis of antitachycardia pacemaker system (includes electrocardiographic recording, programming of device, induction and termination of tachycardia via implanted pacemaker, and interpretation of recordings)
➔ *CPT Assistant* Summer 94:23

(93727 has been deleted. For programming of implantable loop recorder, use 93285. For interrogation of implantable loop recorder, see 93291, 93298)

(93731, 93732 have been deleted. For interrogation of dual lead pacemaker, see 93288, 93294. For programming of dual chamber pacemaker, use 93280)

(93733 has been deleted. For transtelephonic rhythm strip pacemaker, single and dual, or multiple lead pacemaker evaluation, use 93293)

(93734, 93735 have been deleted. For interrogation of single lead pacemaker, see 93288, 93294. For programming of single lead pacemaker, use 93279)

(93736 has been deleted. For transtelephonic rhythm strip pacemaker, single and dual, or multiple lead pacemaker evaluation, use 93293)

93740   Temperature gradient studies

(93741, 93742 have been deleted. For interrogation of single implantable cardioverter-defibrillator [ICD], see 93289, 93295. For programming of single ICD, use 93282. For interrogation of wearable cardioverter-defibrillator, use 93292)

(93743, 93744 have been deleted. For interrogation of dual implantable cardioverter-defibrillator [ICD], see 93289, 93295. For programming of dual ICD, use 93283)

▲ **93745**　Initial set-up and programming by a physician or other qualified health care professional of wearable cardioverter-defibrillator includes initial programming of system, establishing baseline electronic ECG, transmission of data to data repository, patient instruction in wearing system and patient reporting of problems or events
　　➔ *CPT Changes: An Insider's View* 2005, 2013

　　(Do not report 93745 in conjunction with 93282, 93292)

▲ **93750**　Interrogation of ventricular assist device (VAD), in person, with physician or other qualified health care professional analysis of device parameters (eg, drivelines, alarms, power surges), review of device function (eg, flow and volume status, septum status, recovery), with programming, if performed, and report
　　➔ *CPT Assistant* Apr 10:6; *CPT Changes: An Insider's View* 2010, 2013

　　(Do not report 93750 in conjunction with 33975, 33976, 33979, 33981-33983)

　　(93760, 93762 have been deleted)

93770　Determination of venous pressure

　　(For central venous cannulization see 36555-36556, 36500)

93784　Ambulatory blood pressure monitoring, utilizing a system such as magnetic tape and/or computer disk, for 24 hours or longer; including recording, scanning analysis, interpretation and report

93786　recording only

93788　scanning analysis with report

▲ **93790**　review with interpretation and report
　　➔ *CPT Changes: An Insider's View* 2013

Other Procedures

▲ **93797**　Physician or other qualified health care professional services for outpatient cardiac rehabilitation; without continuous ECG monitoring (per session)
　　➔ *CPT Changes: An Insider's View* 2013

▲ **93798**　with continuous ECG monitoring (per session)
　　➔ *CPT Changes: An Insider's View* 2013

93799　Unlisted cardiovascular service or procedure
　　➔ *CPT Assistant* Mar 98:11, Mar 02:10, Nov 05:15, Apr 09:9, Jul 10:10, Oct 11:7, Nov 11:11

Noninvasive Vascular Diagnostic Studies

Vascular studies include patient care required to perform the studies, supervision of the studies and interpretation of study results with copies for patient records of hard copy output with analysis of all data, including bidirectional vascular flow or imaging when provided.

The use of a simple hand-held or other Doppler device that does not produce hard copy output, or that produces a record that does not permit analysis of bidirectional vascular flow, is considered to be part of the physical examination of the vascular system and is not separately reported. The Ankle-Brachial Index (or ABI) is reportable with 93922 or 93923 as long as simultaneous Doppler recording and analysis of bidirectional blood flow, volume plethysmography, or transcutaneous oxygen tension measurements are also performed.

Duplex scan (eg, 93880, 93882) describes an ultrasonic scanning procedure for characterizing the pattern and direction of blood flow in arteries or veins with the production of real-time images integrating B-mode two-dimensional vascular structure, Doppler spectral analysis, and color flow Doppler imaging.

Physiologic studies Noninvasive physiologic studies are performed using equipment separate and distinct from the duplex ultrasound imager. Codes 93922, 93923, 93924, and 93965 describe the evaluation of non-imaging physiologic recordings of pressures with Doppler analysis of bi-directional blood flow, plethysmography, and/or oxygen tension measurements appropriate for the anatomic area studied.

Limited studies for lower extremity require either:

(1) ankle/brachial indices at distal posterior tibial and anterior tibial/dorsalis pedis arteries plus bidirectional Doppler waveform recording and analysis at 1-2 levels; or (2) ankle/brachial indices at distal posterior tibial and anterior tibial/dorsalis pedis arteries plus volume plethysmography at 1-2 levels; or (3) ankle/brachial indices at distal posterior tibial and anterior tibial/dorsalis pedis arteries with transcutaneous oxygen tension measurements at 1-2 levels. Potential levels include high thigh, low thigh, calf, ankle, metatarsal and toes.

Limited studies for upper extremity require either:

(1) Doppler-determined systolic pressures and bidirectional Doppler waveform recording and analysis at 1-2 levels; or (2) Doppler-determined systolic pressures and volume plethysmography at 1-2 levels; or (3) Doppler-determined systolic pressures and transcutaneous oxygen tension measurements at 1-2 levels. Potential levels include arm, forearm, wrist, and digits.

Complete studies for lower extremity require either:

(1) ankle/brachial indices at distal posterior tibial and anterior tibial/dorsalis pedis arteries plus bidirectional Doppler waveform recording and analysis at 3 or more levels; or (2) ankle/brachial indices at distal posterior tibial and anterior tibial/dorsalis pedis arteries plus volume plethysmography at 3 or more levels; or (3) ankle/brachial indices at distal posterior tibial and anterior tibial/dorsalis pedis arteries with transcutaneous oxygen tension measurements at 3 or more levels. Alternatively, a complete study may be reported with measurements at a single level if provocative functional maneuvers (eg, measurements with postural provocative tests, or measurements with reactive hyperemia) are performed.

Complete studies for upper extremity require either:

(1) Doppler-determined systolic pressures and bidirectional Doppler waveform recording and analysis at 3 or more levels; or (2) Doppler-determined systolic pressures and volume plethysmography at 3 or more levels; or (3) Doppler-determined systolic pressures and transcutaneous oxygen tension measurements at 3 or more levels. Potential levels include arm, forearm, wrist, and digits. Alternatively, a complete study may be reported with measurements at a single level if provocative functional maneuvers (eg, measurements with postural provocative tests, or measurements with cold stress) are performed.

Cerebrovascular Arterial Studies

A complete transcranial Doppler (TCD) study (93886) includes ultrasound evaluation of the right and left anterior circulation territories and the posterior circulation territory (to include vertebral arteries and basilar artery). In a limited TCD study (93888) there is ultrasound evaluation of two or fewer of these territories. For TCD, ultrasound evaluation is a reasonable and concerted attempt to identify arterial signals through an acoustic window.

(93875 has been deleted)

93880 Duplex scan of extracranial arteries; complete bilateral study

➔ *CPT Assistant* Jun 96:9, Dec 05:3

➔ *Clinical Examples in Radiology* Fall 07:6, Winter 09:2

93882 unilateral or limited study

➔ *CPT Assistant* Jun 96:9, Dec 05:3

➔ *Clinical Examples in Radiology* Fall 07:6, Winter 09:2

(To report common carotid intima-media thickness (IMT) study for evaluation of atherosclerotic burden or coronary heart disease risk factor assessment, use Category III code 0126T)

93886 Transcranial Doppler study of the intracranial arteries; complete study

➔ *CPT Assistant* Jun 96:9, Dec 05:3

93888 limited study

➔ *CPT Assistant* Jun 96:9, Dec 05:3

93890 vasoreactivity study

➔ *CPT Assistant* Dec 05:3; *CPT Changes: An Insider's View* 2005

93892 emboli detection without intravenous microbubble injection

➔ *CPT Assistant* Dec 05:3; *CPT Changes: An Insider's View* 2005

93893 emboli detection with intravenous microbubble injection

➔ *CPT Assistant* Dec 05:3; *CPT Changes: An Insider's View* 2005

(Do not report 93890-93893 in conjunction with 93888)

Extremity Arterial Studies (Including Digits)

93922 Limited bilateral noninvasive physiologic studies of upper or lower extremity arteries, (eg, for lower extremity: ankle/brachial indices at distal posterior tibial and anterior tibial/dorsalis pedis arteries plus bidirectional, Doppler waveform recording and analysis at 1-2 levels, or ankle/brachial indices at distal posterior tibial and anterior tibial/dorsalis pedis arteries plus volume plethysmography at 1-2 levels, or ankle/brachial indices at distal posterior tibial and anterior tibial/dorsalis pedis arteries with, transcutaneous oxygen tension measurement at 1-2 levels)

➔ *CPT Assistant* Jun 96:9, Dec 05:3, Aug 09:3, Jun 12:16; *CPT Changes: An Insider's View* 2011

➔ *Clinical Examples in Radiology* Spring 11:5, 6, Summer 11:11

(When only 1 arm or leg is available for study, report 93922 with modifier 52 for a unilateral study when recording 1-2 levels. Report 93922 when recording 3 or more levels or performing provocative functional maneuvers)

(Report 93922 only once in the upper extremity(s) and/or once in the lower extremity(s). When both the upper and lower extremities are evaluated in the same setting, 93922 may be reported twice by adding modifier 59 to the second procedure)

(For transcutaneous oxyhemoglobin measurement in a lower extremity wound by near infrared spectroscopy, use 0286T)

93923 Complete bilateral noninvasive physiologic studies of upper or lower extremity arteries, 3 or more levels (eg, for lower extremity: ankle/brachial indices at distal posterior tibial and anterior tibial/dorsalis pedis arteries plus segmental blood pressure measurements with bidirectional Doppler waveform recording and analysis, at 3 or more levels, or ankle/brachial indices at distal posterior tibial and anterior tibial/dorsalis pedis arteries plus segmental volume plethysmography at 3 or more levels, or ankle/brachial indices at distal posterior tibial and anterior tibial/dorsalis pedis arteries plus segmental transcutaneous oxygen tension measurements at 3 or more levels), or single level study with provocative functional maneuvers (eg, measurements with postural provocative tests, or measurements with reactive hyperemia)

➔ *CPT Assistant* Jun 96:9, Jun 01:10, Dec 05:3, Aug 09:3, Jun 12:16; *CPT Changes: An Insider's View* 2011

➔ *Clinical Examples in Radiology* Spring 11:5, 6, Summer 11:11

(When only 1 arm or leg is available for study, report 93922 for a unilateral study when recording 3 or more levels or when performing provocative functional maneuvers)

(Report 93923 only once in the upper extremity(s) and/or once in the lower extremity(s). When both the upper and lower extremities are evaluated in the same setting, 93923 may be reported twice by adding modifier 59 to the second procedure)

(For transcutaneous oxyhemoglobin measurement in a lower extremity wound by near infrared spectroscopy, use 0286T)

93924 Noninvasive physiologic studies of lower extremity arteries, at rest and following treadmill stress testing, (ie, bidirectional Doppler waveform or volume plethysmography recording and analysis at rest with ankle/brachial indices immediately after and at timed intervals following performance of a standardized protocol on a motorized treadmill plus recording of time of onset of claudication or other symptoms, maximal walking time, and time to recovery) complete bilateral study

➔ *CPT Assistant* Jun 96:9, Dec 05:3, Aug 09:3, Jun 12:16; *CPT Changes: An Insider's View* 2011

➔ *Clinical Examples in Radiology* Spring 11:5, 6

(Do not report 93924 in conjunction with 93922, 93923)

93925 Duplex scan of lower extremity arteries or arterial bypass grafts; complete bilateral study

➔ *CPT Assistant* Jun 96:9, Dec 05:3

93926 unilateral or limited study

➔ *CPT Assistant* Jun 96:9, Oct 01:2, Dec 05:3

➔ *Clinical Examples in Radiology* Fall 09:4, 5

93930 Duplex scan of upper extremity arteries or arterial bypass grafts; complete bilateral study

➔ *CPT Assistant* Jun 96:9, Dec 05:3

93931 unilateral or limited study

➔ *CPT Assistant* Jun 96:9, Oct 01:2, Dec 05:3

Extremity Venous Studies (Including Digits)

93965 Noninvasive physiologic studies of extremity veins, complete bilateral study (eg, Doppler waveform analysis with responses to compression and other maneuvers, phleborheography, impedance plethysmography)

➔ *CPT Assistant* Jun 96:9, Dec 05:3; *CPT Changes: An Insider's View* 2007

➔ *Clinical Examples in Radiology* Spring 12:8

93970 Duplex scan of extremity veins including responses to compression and other maneuvers; complete bilateral study

➔ *CPT Assistant* Jun 96:9, Dec 05:3, Jan 12:13, Feb 12:11

➔ *Clinical Examples in Radiology* Spring 12:8

93971 unilateral or limited study

➔ *CPT Assistant* Jun 96:9, Oct 01:2, Mar 03:21, Dec 05:3, Jul 10:6, Apr 11:13, Jan 12:13, Feb 12:11

➔ *Clinical Examples in Radiology* Winter 08:11, Fall 09:4, 5

Visceral and Penile Vascular Studies

93975 Duplex scan of arterial inflow and venous outflow of abdominal, pelvic, scrotal contents and/or retroperitoneal organs; complete study

➔ *CPT Assistant* Apr 96:11, Jun 96:9, Dec 05:3

➔ *Clinical Examples in Radiology* Spring 08:9, Winter 08:10, Summer 09:12

93976 limited study

➔ *CPT Assistant* Apr 96:11, Jun 96:9, Dec 05:3

➔ *Clinical Examples in Radiology* Spring 08:10, Summer 09:12

93978 Duplex scan of aorta, inferior vena cava, iliac vasculature, or bypass grafts; complete study

➔ *CPT Assistant* Jun 96:9, Dec 05:3

➔ *Clinical Examples in Radiology* Spring 07:5-6

93979 unilateral or limited study

➔ *CPT Assistant* Jun 96:9, Dec 05:3

93980 Duplex scan of arterial inflow and venous outflow of penile vessels; complete study

➔ *CPT Assistant* Jun 96:9, Dec 05:3

93981 follow-up or limited study

➔ *CPT Assistant* Jun 96:9, Dec 05:3

93982 Noninvasive physiologic study of implanted wireless pressure sensor in aneurysmal sac following endovascular repair, complete study including recording, analysis of pressure and waveform tracings, interpretation and report

➔ *CPT Changes: An Insider's View* 2008

(Do not report 93982 in conjunction with 34806)

Extremity Arterial-Venous Studies

93990 Duplex scan of hemodialysis access (including arterial inflow, body of access and venous outflow)

➔ *CPT Assistant* Jun 96:9, Dec 05:3

➔ *Clinical Examples in Radiology* Spring 07:5-6

(For measurement of hemodialysis access flow using indicator dilution methods, use 90940)

Other Noninvasive Vascular Diagnostic Studies

93998 Unlisted noninvasive vascular diagnostic study

➔ *CPT Changes: An Insider's View* 2012

Pulmonary

Ventilator Management

94002 Ventilation assist and management, initiation of pressure or volume preset ventilators for assisted or controlled breathing; hospital inpatient/observation, initial day

➔ *CPT Assistant* Feb 07:10, Mar 07:10, Apr 07:3, Jul 07:1, Nov 08:5; *CPT Changes: An Insider's View* 2007

94003 hospital inpatient/observation, each subsequent day

➔ *CPT Assistant* Feb 07:10, Apr 07:3, Jul 07:1, Nov 08:5; *CPT Changes: An Insider's View* 2007

94004 nursing facility, per day

➔ *CPT Assistant* Feb 07:10, Apr 07:3, Jul 07:1, Nov 08:5; *CPT Changes: An Insider's View* 2007

(Do not report 94002-94004 in conjunction with Evaluation and Management services 99201-99499)

94005   Home ventilator management care plan oversight of a patient (patient not present) in home, domiciliary or rest home (eg, assisted living) requiring review of status, review of laboratories and other studies and revision of orders and respiratory care plan (as appropriate), within a calendar month, 30 minutes or more

➔ *CPT Assistant* Mar 07:11, Apr 07:3, Nov 08:5; *CPT Changes: An Insider's View* 2007

(Do not report 94005 in conjunction with 99339, 99340, 99374-99378)

▶(Ventilator management care plan oversight is reported separately from home or domiciliary, rest home [eg, assisted living] services. A physician or other qualified health care professional may report 94005, when performed, including when a different individual reports 99339, 99340, 99374-99378 for the same 30 days)◀

Pulmonary Diagnostic Testing and Therapies

▶Codes 94010-94799 include laboratory procedure(s) and interpretation of test results. If a separate identifiable evaluation and management service is performed, the appropriate E/M service code including new or established patient office or other outpatient services (99201-99215), office or other outpatient consultations (99241-99245), emergency department services (99281-99285), nursing facility services (99304-99318), domiciliary, rest home, or custodial care services (99324-99337), and home services (99341-99350) may be reported in addition to 94010-94799.◀

Spirometry (94010) measures expiratory airflow and volumes and forms the basis of most pulmonary function testing. When spirometry is performed before and after administration of a bronchodilator, report 94060. Measurement of vital capacity (94150) is a component of spirometry and is only reported when performed alone. The flow-volume loop (94375) is used to identify patterns of inspiratory and/or expiratory obstruction in central or peripheral airways. Spirometry (94010, 94060) includes maximal breathing capacity (94200) and flow-volume loop (94375), when performed.

Measurement of lung volumes may be performed using plethysmography, helium dilution or nitrogen washout. Plethysmography (94726) is utilized to determine total lung capacity, residual volume, functional residual capacity, and airway resistance. Nitrogen washout or helium dilution (94727) may be used to measure lung volumes, distribution of ventilation and closing volume. Impulse oscillometry (94728) assesses airway resistance and may be reported in addition to gas dilution techniques. Spirometry (94010, 94060) and bronchial provocation (94070) are not included in 94726 and 94727 and may be reported separately.

Diffusing capacity (94729) is most commonly performed in conjunction with lung volumes or spirometry and is an add-on code to 94726-94728, 94010, 94060, 94070, and 94375.

Pulmonary function tests (94011-94013) are reported for measurements in infants and young children through 2 years of age.

Pulmonary function testing measurements are reported as actual values and as a percent of predicted values by age, gender, height, and race.

94010   Spirometry, including graphic record, total and timed vital capacity, expiratory flow rate measurement(s), with or without maximal voluntary ventilation

➔ *CPT Assistant* Summer 91:16, Summer 95:4, Feb 96:9, Mar 96:10, Nov 97:45, Nov 98:35, Jan 99:8, Feb 99:9, Aug 03:15, Jul 05:11, Nov 08:5, Oct 10:15, Dec 10:15

(Do not report 94010 in conjunction with 94150, 94200, 94375, 94728)

⊙ **94011**   Measurement of spirometric forced expiratory flows in an infant or child through 2 years of age

➔ *CPT Assistant* May 10:7; *CPT Changes: An Insider's View* 2010

⊙ **94012**   Measurement of spirometric forced expiratory flows, before and after bronchodilator, in an infant or child through 2 years of age

➔ *CPT Assistant* May 10:7; *CPT Changes: An Insider's View* 2010

⊙ **94013**   Measurement of lung volumes (ie, functional residual capacity [FRC], forced vital capacity [FVC], and expiratory reserve volume [ERV]) in an infant or child through 2 years of age

➔ *CPT Assistant* May 10:7; *CPT Changes: An Insider's View* 2010

▲ **94014**   Patient-initiated spirometric recording per 30-day period of time; includes reinforced education, transmission of spirometric tracing, data capture, analysis of transmitted data, periodic recalibration and review and interpretation by a physician or other qualified health care professional

➔ *CPT Assistant* Summer 95:4, Nov 98:34, Jan 99:8, Jul 05:11, Nov 08:5; *CPT Changes: An Insider's View* 2000, 2013

94015   recording (includes hook-up, reinforced education, data transmission, data capture, trend analysis, and periodic recalibration)

➔ *CPT Assistant* Summer 95:4, Nov 98:34, Jan 99:8, Jul 05:11, Nov 08:5

▲ **94016**   review and interpretation only by a physician or other qualified health care professional

➔ *CPT Assistant* Summer 95:4, Nov 98:34, Jan 99:8, Jul 05:11, Nov 08:5; *CPT Changes: An Insider's View* 2013

94060   Bronchodilation responsiveness, spirometry as in 94010, pre- and post-bronchodilator administration

➔ *CPT Assistant* Summer 95:4, Feb 96:9, Feb 97:10, Nov 98:34, Jan 99:8, Feb 99:9, Jul 05:11, Nov 08:5, Dec 10:15; *CPT Changes: An Insider's View* 2005

(Do not report 94060 in conjunction with 94150, 94200, 94375, 94728)

(Report bronchodilator supply separately with 99070 or appropriate supply code)

(For prolonged exercise test for bronchospasm with pre- and post-spirometry, use 94620)

94070 Bronchospasm provocation evaluation, multiple spirometric determinations as in 94010, with administered agents (eg, antigen[s], cold air, methacholine)

➔ *CPT Assistant* Summer 91:16, Summer 95:4, Feb 96:9, Nov 97:45, Jan 99:8, Jul 05:11, Nov 08:5; *CPT Changes: An Insider's View* 2005

(Report antigen[s] administration separately with 99070 or appropriate supply code)

94150 Vital capacity, total (separate procedure)

➔ *CPT Assistant* Summer 95:4, Feb 96:9, Jul 05:11, Nov 08:5, Dec 10:15

(Do not report 94150 in conjunction with 94010, 94060, 94728. To report thoracic gas volumes, see 94726, 94727)

94200 Maximum breathing capacity, maximal voluntary ventilation

➔ *CPT Assistant* Summer 95:4, Feb 96:9, Aug 03:15, Jul 05:11, Nov 08:5, Dec 10:15

(Do not report 94200 in conjunction with 94010, 94060)

(94240 has been deleted. To report thoracic gas volumes, see 94726, 94727)

94250 Expired gas collection, quantitative, single procedure (separate procedure)

➔ *CPT Assistant* Summer 95:4, Feb 96:9, Jul 05:11, Nov 08:5

(94260 has been deleted. To report thoracic gas volumes, see 94726, 94727)

(94350 has been deleted. To report, use 94727)

(94360 has been deleted. To report, see 94726, 94728)

(94370 has been deleted. To report, see 94726, 94727)

94375 Respiratory flow volume loop

➔ *CPT Assistant* Summer 95:4, Feb 96:9, Oct 03:2, Jul 05:11, Jul 06:4, Jul 07:1, Nov 08:5

(Do not report 94375 in conjunction with 94010, 94060, 94728)

94400 Breathing response to CO_2 (CO_2 response curve)

➔ *CPT Assistant* Summer 95:4, Feb 96:9, Jul 05:11, Nov 08:5, Dec 10:15

94450 Breathing response to hypoxia (hypoxia response curve)

➔ *CPT Assistant* Summer 95:4, Feb 96:9, Jul 05:11, Nov 08:5

(For high altitude simulation test [HAST], see 94452, 94453)

▲ **94452** High altitude simulation test (HAST), with interpretation and report by a physician or other qualified health care professional;

➔ *CPT Assistant* Jul 05:11, Nov 08:5; *CPT Changes: An Insider's View* 2005, 2013

(For obtaining arterial blood gases, use 36600)

(Do not report 94452 in conjunction with 94453, 94760, 94761)

▲ **94453** with supplemental oxygen titration

➔ *CPT Assistant* Jul 05:11, Nov 08:5; *CPT Changes: An Insider's View* 2005, 2013

(For obtaining arterial blood gases, use 36600)

(Do not report 94453 in conjunction with 94452, 94760, 94761)

⊘▲ **94610** Intrapulmonary surfactant administration by a physician or other qualified health care professional through endotracheal tube

➔ *CPT Assistant* Apr 07:3, Jul 08:7, Nov 08:5, Dec 10:15; *CPT Changes: An Insider's View* 2007, 2013

(Do not report 94610 in conjunction with 99468-99472)

(For endotracheal intubation, use 31500)

(Report 94610 once per dosing episode)

94620 Pulmonary stress testing; simple (eg, 6-minute walk test, prolonged exercise test for bronchospasm with pre- and post-spirometry and oximetry)

➔ *CPT Assistant* Summer 95:4, Feb 96:9, Nov 98:35, Jan 99:8, Mar 04:10, Jul 05:11, 13, Apr 07:3, Jun 07:11, Nov 08:5; *CPT Changes: An Insider's View* 2007

94621 complex (including measurements of CO_2 production, O_2 uptake, and electrocardiographic recordings)

➔ *CPT Assistant* Summer 95:4, Nov 98:35, Jan 99:8, Aug 02:10, Jul 05:11, Nov 08:5

94640 Pressurized or nonpressurized inhalation treatment for acute airway obstruction or for sputum induction for diagnostic purposes (eg, with an aerosol generator, nebulizer, metered dose inhaler or intermittent positive pressure breathing [IPPB] device)

➔ *CPT Assistant* Summer 95:4, Feb 96:9, May 98:10, Apr 00:11, Jul 05:11, Apr 07:3, Nov 08:5, Sep 10:3; *CPT Changes: An Insider's View* 2003

(For more than 1 inhalation treatment performed on the same date, append modifier 76)

(For continuous inhalation treatment of 1 hour or more, see 94644, 94645)

94642 Aerosol inhalation of pentamidine for pneumocystis carinii pneumonia treatment or prophylaxis

➔ *CPT Assistant* Summer 95:4, Feb 96:9, Jul 05:11, Nov 08:5

94644 Continuous inhalation treatment with aerosol medication for acute airway obstruction; first hour

➔ *CPT Assistant* Apr 07:3, Nov 08:5; *CPT Changes: An Insider's View* 2007

(For services of less than 1 hour, use 94640)

+ **94645** each additional hour (List separately in addition to code for primary procedure)

➔ *CPT Assistant* Apr 07:3, Nov 08:5; *CPT Changes: An Insider's View* 2007

(Use 94645 in conjunction with 94644)

94660 Continuous positive airway pressure ventilation (CPAP), initiation and management

➔ *CPT Assistant* Fall 92:30, Spring 95:4, Summer 95:4, Feb 96:9, Jan 99:10, Aug 00:2, Oct 03:2, Jul 05:11, Jul 06:4, Feb 07:10, Jul 07:1, Nov 08:5

94662 Continuous negative pressure ventilation (CNP), initiation and management

➔ *CPT Assistant* Fall 92:30, Spring 94:4, Summer 95:4, Feb 96:9, Aug 00:2, Jul 05:11, Feb 07:10, Jul 07:1, Nov 08:5

Medicine

Medicine

94664 Demonstration and/or evaluation of patient utilization of an aerosol generator, nebulizer, metered dose inhaler or IPPB device

→ *CPT Assistant* Summer 95:4, Feb 96:9, May 98:10, Apr 00:11, Jul 05:11, Nov 08:5, Sep 10:3; *CPT Changes: An Insider's View* 2003

(94664 can be reported 1 time only per day of service)

94667 Manipulation chest wall, such as cupping, percussing, and vibration to facilitate lung function; initial demonstration and/or evaluation

→ *CPT Assistant* Summer 95:4, Feb 96:9, Jul 05:11, Nov 08:5, Sep 10:3

94668 subsequent

→ *CPT Assistant* Summer 95:4, Feb 96:9, Jul 05:11, Sep 10:3

94680 Oxygen uptake, expired gas analysis; rest and exercise, direct, simple

→ *CPT Assistant* Summer 95:4, Feb 96:9, Jul 05:11

94681 including CO_2 output, percentage oxygen extracted

→ *CPT Assistant* Summer 95:4, Feb 96:9, Jul 05:11

94690 rest, indirect (separate procedure)

→ *CPT Assistant* Summer 95:4, Feb 96:9, Jul 05:11

(For single arterial puncture, use 36600)

(94720, 94725 have been deleted. To report, see 94729)

94726 Plethysmography for determination of lung volumes and, when performed, airway resistance

→ *CPT Assistant* Jan 12:3; *CPT Changes: An Insider's View* 2012

(Do not report 94726 in conjunction with 94727, 94728)

94727 Gas dilution or washout for determination of lung volumes and, when performed, distribution of ventilation and closing volumes

→ *CPT Assistant* Jan 12:3; *CPT Changes: An Insider's View* 2012

(Do not report 94727 in conjunction with 94726)

94728 Airway resistance by impulse oscillometry

→ *CPT Assistant* Jan 12:3; *CPT Changes: An Insider's View* 2012

(Do not report 94728 in conjunction with 94010, 94060, 94070, 94375, 94726)

+ 94729 Diffusing capacity (eg, carbon monoxide, membrane) (List separately in addition to code for primary procedure)

→ *CPT Assistant* Jan 12:3; *CPT Changes: An Insider's View* 2012

(Report 94729 in conjunction with 94010, 94060, 94070, 94375, 94726-94728)

94750 Pulmonary compliance study (eg, plethysmography, volume and pressure measurements)

→ *CPT Assistant* Summer 95:4, Feb 96:9, Jul 05:11; *CPT Changes: An Insider's View* 2002

94760 Noninvasive ear or pulse oximetry for oxygen saturation; single determination

→ *CPT Assistant* Summer 95:4, Feb 96:9, Feb 97:10, Jul 98:2, Oct 03:2, Jul 05:11, Feb 06:9, Jul 06:4, Feb 07:10, Apr 07:1, Jul 07:1, Dec 10:15

(For blood gases, see 82803-82810)

94761 multiple determinations (eg, during exercise)

→ *CPT Assistant* Summer 95:4, Feb 96:9, Jul 98:2, Jun 99:10, Jul 05:11, Feb 06:9, Jul 06:4, Feb 07:10, Apr 07:1, Jun 07:11, Jul 07:1, Dec 08:5

94762 by continuous overnight monitoring (separate procedure)

→ *CPT Assistant* Summer 95:4, Feb 96:9, Jul 98:2, Oct 03:2, Jul 05:11, Feb 06:9, Jul 06:4, Feb 07:10, Apr 07:1, Jul 07:1, Dec 08:5

(For other in vivo laboratory procedures, see 88720-88741)

94770 Carbon dioxide, expired gas determination by infrared analyzer

→ *CPT Assistant* Summer 95:4, Feb 96:9, Jul 05:11

►(For bronchoscopy, see 31622-31646)◄

(For placement of flow directed catheter, use 93503)

(For venipuncture, use 36410)

(For central venous catheter placement, see 36555-36556)

(For arterial puncture, use 36600)

(For arterial catheterization, use 36620)

►(For thoracentesis, see 32554, 32555)◄

(For phlebotomy, therapeutic, use 99195)

(For lung biopsy, needle, use 32405)

(For intubation, orotracheal or nasotracheal, use 31500)

94772 Circadian respiratory pattern recording (pediatric pneumogram), 12-24 hour continuous recording, infant

→ *CPT Assistant* Summer 95:4, Feb 96:9, Jul 05:11

(Separate procedure codes for electromyograms, EEG, ECG, and recordings of respiration are excluded when 94772 is reported)

▲ **94774** Pediatric home apnea monitoring event recording including respiratory rate, pattern and heart rate per 30-day period of time; includes monitor attachment, download of data, review, interpretation, and preparation of a report by a physician or other qualified health care professional

→ *CPT Assistant* Apr 07:3, Mar 08:4; *CPT Changes: An Insider's View* 2007, 2013

(Do not report 94774 in conjunction with 94775-94777 during the same reporting period)

94775 monitor attachment only (includes hook-up, initiation of recording and disconnection)

→ *CPT Assistant* Apr 07:3, Mar 08:4; *CPT Changes: An Insider's View* 2007

94776 monitoring, download of information, receipt of transmission(s) and analyses by computer only

→ *CPT Assistant* Apr 07:3, Mar 08:4; *CPT Changes: An Insider's View* 2007

▲ **94777**   review, interpretation and preparation of report only by a physician or other qualified health care professional

→ *CPT Assistant* Apr 07:3, Mar 08:4; *CPT Changes: An Insider's View* 2007, 2013

(When oxygen saturation monitoring is used in addition to heart rate and respiratory monitoring, it is not reported separately)

(Do not report 94774-94777 in conjunction with 93224-93272)

(Do not report apnea recording device separately)

(For sleep study, see 95805-95811)

94780   Car seat/bed testing for airway integrity, neonate, with continual nursing observation and continuous recording of pulse oximetry, heart rate and respiratory rate, with interpretation and report; 60 minutes

→ *CPT Changes: An Insider's View* 2012

(Do not report 94780 for less than 60 minutes)

(Do not report 94780 in conjunction with 93040-93042, 94760, 94761, 99468-99472, 99477-99480)

+ **94781**   each additional full 30 minutes (List separately in addition to code for primary procedure)

→ *CPT Changes: An Insider's View* 2012

(Use 94781 in conjunction with 94780)

94799   Unlisted pulmonary service or procedure

→ *CPT Assistant* Summer 95:4, Feb 96:9, Mar 96:10, Jul 05:11, Dec 10:15

Allergy and Clinical Immunology

Definitions

Immunotherapy (desensitization, hyposensitization): is the parenteral administration of allergenic extracts as antigens at periodic intervals, usually on an increasing dosage scale to a dosage which is maintained as maintenance therapy. Indications for immunotherapy are determined by appropriate diagnostic procedures coordinated with clinical judgment and knowledge of the natural history of allergic diseases.

▶ ***Other therapy:*** for medical conferences on the use of mechanical and electronic devices (precipitators, air conditioners, air filters, humidifiers, dehumidifiers), climatotherapy, physical therapy, occupational and recreational therapy, see **Evaluation and Management** services.

Do not report Evaluation and Management (E/M) services for test interpretation and report. If a significant separately identifiable E/M service is performed, the appropriate E/M service code, which may include new or established patient office or other outpatient services (99201-99215), hospital observation services (99217-

99220, 99224-99226), hospital care (99221-99223, 99231-99233), consultations (99241-99255), emergency department services (99281-99285), nursing facility services (99304-99318), domiciliary, rest home, or custodial care services (99324-99337), home services (99341-99350), or preventive medicine services (99381-99429) should be reported using modifier 25.◀

Allergy Testing

(For allergy laboratory tests, see 86000-86999)

▶(For administration of medications [eg, epinephrine, steroidal agents, antihistamines] for therapy for severe or intractable allergic reaction, use 96372)◀

▲ **95004**   Percutaneous tests (scratch, puncture, prick) with allergenic extracts, immediate type reaction, including test interpretation and report, specify number of tests

→ *CPT Assistant* Summer 91:15, May 10:3; *CPT Changes: An Insider's View* 2007, 2008, 2013

95012   Nitric oxide expired gas determination

→ *CPT Assistant* Mar 07:11, Apr 07:6; *CPT Changes: An Insider's View* 2007

▶(95010 and 95015 have been deleted. To report, see 95017 and 95018)◀

● **95017**   Allergy testing, any combination of percutaneous (scratch, puncture, prick) and intracutaneous (intradermal), sequential and incremental, with venoms, immediate type reaction, including test interpretation and report, specify number of tests

→ *CPT Changes: An Insider's View* 2013

● **95018**   Allergy testing, any combination of percutaneous (scratch, puncture, prick) and intracutaneous (intradermal), sequential and incremental, with drugs or biologicals, immediate type reaction, including test interpretation and report, specify number of tests

→ *CPT Changes: An Insider's View* 2013

▲ **95024**   Intracutaneous (intradermal) tests with allergenic extracts, immediate type reaction, including test interpretation and report, specify number of tests

→ *CPT Assistant* Summer 91:15, May 10:3; *CPT Changes: An Insider's View* 2003, 2008, 2013

▲ **95027**   Intracutaneous (intradermal) tests, sequential and incremental, with allergenic extracts for airborne allergens, immediate type reaction, including test interpretation and report, specify number of tests

→ *CPT Assistant* Summer 91:15, Jun 97:10, Dec 07:9, May 10:3; *CPT Changes: An Insider's View* 2003, 2008, 2013

95028   Intracutaneous (intradermal) tests with allergenic extracts, delayed type reaction, including reading, specify number of tests

→ *CPT Assistant* Summer 91:14, May 10:3; *CPT Changes: An Insider's View* 2003

95044   Patch or application test(s) (specify number of tests)

→ *CPT Assistant* Summer 91:15, Spring 94:31

95052   Photo patch test(s) (specify number of tests)

→ *CPT Assistant* Spring 94:31

95056 Photo tests
→ *CPT Assistant* Summer 91:16

95060 Ophthalmic mucous membrane tests
→ *CPT Assistant* Summer 91:16

95065 Direct nasal mucous membrane test
→ *CPT Assistant* Summer 91:15

95070 Inhalation bronchial challenge testing (not including necessary pulmonary function tests); with histamine, methacholine, or similar compounds
→ *CPT Assistant* Summer 91:16

95071 with antigens or gases, specify
→ *CPT Assistant* Summer 91:16

(For pulmonary function tests, see 94060, 94070)

►(95075 has been deleted. For ingestion challenge testing, see 95076, 95079)◄

►Ingestion Challenge Testing◄

►Codes 95076 and 95079 are used to report ingestion challenge testing. Report 95076 for initial 120 minutes of testing time (ie, not physician face-to-face time). Report 95079 for each additional 60 minutes of testing time (ie, not physician face-to-face time). For total testing time less than 61 minutes (eg, positive challenge resulting in cessation of testing), report an evaluation and management service, if appropriate. Patient assessment/monitoring activities for allergic reaction (eg, blood pressure testing, peak flow meter testing) are not separately reported. Intervention therapy (eg, injection of steroid or epinephrine) may be reported separately as appropriate.

For purposes of reporting testing times, if an evaluation and management service is required, then testing time ends.◄

● **95076** Ingestion challenge test (sequential and incremental ingestion of test items, eg, food, drug or other substance); initial 120 minutes of testing
→ *CPT Changes: An Insider's View* 2013

+● **95079** each additional 60 minutes of testing (List separately in addition to code for primary procedure)
→ *CPT Changes: An Insider's View* 2013

►(Use 95079 in conjunction with 95076)◄

Allergen Immunotherapy

Codes 95115-95199 include the professional services necessary for allergen immunotherapy. Office visit codes may be used in addition to allergen immunotherapy if other identifiable services are provided at that time.

95115 Professional services for allergen immunotherapy not including provision of allergenic extracts; single injection
→ *CPT Assistant* Fall 91:19, Spring 94:30, Summer 95:4, May 96:1, Nov 98:35, Apr 00:4, Feb 05:10-12, Nov 05:1, Nov 06:23, Dec 07:9

95117 2 or more injections
→ *CPT Assistant* Fall 91:19, Spring 94:30, Summer 95:4, May 96:1, Aug 96:10, Nov 98:35, Apr 00:4, Feb 05:10-12, Nov 05:1, Nov 06:23, Dec 07:9

▲ **95120** Professional services for allergen immunotherapy in the office or institution of the prescribing physician or other qualified health care professional, including provision of allergenic extract; single injection
→ *CPT Assistant* Fall 91:19, Spring 94:30, Summer 95:4, May 96:2, Nov 98:35, Feb 05:10-12; *CPT Changes: An Insider's View* 2013

▲ **95125** 2 or more injections
→ *CPT Assistant* Fall 91:19, Spring 94:30, Summer 95:4, May 96:2, Aug 96:10, Nov 98:35, Feb 05:10, 12; *CPT Changes: An Insider's View* 2013

▲ **95130** single stinging insect venom
→ *CPT Assistant* Fall 91:19, Summer 95:4, May 96:2, Jun 96:10, Nov 98:35, Sep 99:10, Feb 05:10, 12; *CPT Changes: An Insider's View* 2013

▲ **95131** 2 stinging insect venoms
→ *CPT Assistant* Fall 91:19, Summer 95:4, May 96:2, Jun 96:10, Nov 98:35, Sep 99:10, Feb 05:10, 12; *CPT Changes: An Insider's View* 2013

▲ **95132** 3 stinging insect venoms
→ *CPT Assistant* Fall 91:19, Summer 95:4, May 96:2, Nov 98:35, Sep 99:11, Feb 05:10, 12; *CPT Changes: An Insider's View* 2013

▲ **95133** 4 stinging insect venoms
→ *CPT Assistant* Fall 91:19, Summer 95:4, May 96:2, Nov 98:35, Sep 99:11, Feb 05:10, 12; *CPT Changes: An Insider's View* 2013

▲ **95134** 5 stinging insect venoms
→ *CPT Assistant* Fall 91:19, Summer 95:4, May 96:2, Nov 98:35, Sep 99:11, Feb 05:10, 12; *CPT Changes: An Insider's View* 2013

95144 Professional services for the supervision of preparation and provision of antigens for allergen immunotherapy, single dose vial(s) (specify number of vials)
→ *CPT Assistant* Fall 91:19, Spring 94:30, Summer 95:4, May 96:11, Nov 98:35, Feb 05:10-11; *CPT Changes: An Insider's View* 2002

(A single dose vial contains a single dose of antigen administered in 1 injection)

95145 Professional services for the supervision of preparation and provision of antigens for allergen immunotherapy (specify number of doses); single stinging insect venom
→ *CPT Assistant* Fall 91:19, Summer 95:4, May 96:11, Nov 98:35, Feb 05:10-12; *CPT Changes: An Insider's View* 2002

95146 2 single stinging insect venoms
→ *CPT Assistant* Fall 91:19, Summer 95:4, May 96:11, Nov 98:35, Feb 05:10-12

95147 3 single stinging insect venoms
→ *CPT Assistant* Fall 91:19, Summer 95:4, May 96:11, Nov 98:35, Feb 05:10-12

95148 4 single stinging insect venoms
→ *CPT Assistant* Fall 91:19, Summer 95:4, May 96:11, Nov 98:35, Feb 05:10-12

95149 5 single stinging insect venoms
→ *CPT Assistant* Fall 91:19, Summer 95:4, May 96:11, Nov 98:35, Feb 05:10-12

95165   Professional services for the supervision of preparation and provision of antigens for allergen immunotherapy; single or multiple antigens (specify number of doses)

➔ *CPT Assistant* Fall 91:19, Spring 94:30, Summer 95:4, May 96:11, Nov 98:35, Apr 00:4, Apr 01:11, Feb 05:10-12, Jun 05:9; *CPT Changes: An Insider's View* 2002

95170   whole body extract of biting insect or other arthropod (specify number of doses)

➔ *CPT Assistant* Fall 91:19, Spring 94:30, Summer 95:4, May 96:12, Apr 01:11, Feb 05:10-12, Jun 05:9

(For allergy immunotherapy reporting, a dose is the amount of antigen[s] administered in a single injection from a multiple dose vial)

95180   Rapid desensitization procedure, each hour (eg, insulin, penicillin, equine serum)

➔ *CPT Assistant* Summer 95:4; *CPT Changes: An Insider's View* 2002

95199   Unlisted allergy/clinical immunologic service or procedure

➔ *CPT Assistant* Summer 95:4, Nov 98:35

(For skin testing of bacterial, viral, fungal extracts, see 86485-86580, 95028)

(For special reports on allergy patients, use 99080)

(For testing procedures such as radioallergosorbent testing [RAST], rat mast cell technique [RMCT], mast cell degranulation test [MCDT], lymphocytic transformation test [LTT], leukocyte histamine release [LHR], migration inhibitory factor test [MIF], transfer factor test [TFT], nitroblue tetrazolium dye test [NTD], see Immunology section in **Pathology** or use 95199)

Endocrinology

95250   Ambulatory continuous glucose monitoring of interstitial tissue fluid via a subcutaneous sensor for a minimum of 72 hours; sensor placement, hook-up, calibration of monitor, patient training, removal of sensor, and printout of recording

➔ *CPT Changes: An Insider's View* 2002, 2006, 2009

(Do not report 95250 more than once per month)

(Do not report 95250 in conjunction with 99091)

95251   interpretation and report

➔ *CPT Changes: An Insider's View* 2006, 2009

(Do not report 95251 more than once per month)

(Do not report 95251 in conjunction with 99091)

Neurology and Neuromuscular Procedures

Neurologic services are typically consultative, and any of the levels of consultation (99241-99255) may be appropriate.

In addition, services and skills outlined under **Evaluation and Management** levels of service appropriate to neurologic illnesses should be reported similarly.

▶The EEG, autonomic function, evoked potential, reflex tests, EMG, NCV, and MEG services (95812-95829 and 95860-95967) include recording, interpretation, and report by a physician or other qualified health care professional. For interpretation only, use modifier 26. For EMG guidance, see 95873, 95874.

Codes 95812-95822, 95950-95953 and 95956 use recording time as a basis for code use. Recording time is when the recording is underway and data is being collected. Recording time excludes set up and take down time. Codes 95961-95962 use physician or other qualified health care professional attendance time as a basis for code use.◀

(Do not report codes 95860-95875 in addition to 96000-96004)

Sleep Medicine Testing

Sleep medicine services include procedures that evaluate adult and pediatric patients for a variety of sleep disorders. Sleep medicine testing services are diagnostic procedures using in-laboratory and portable technology to assess physiologic data and therapy.

▶All sleep services (95800-95811) include recording, interpretation, and report. (Report with modifier 52 if less than 6 hours of recording for 95800, 95801 and 95806, 95807, 95810, 95811; if less than 7 hours of recording for 95782, 95783, or if less than four nap opportunities are recorded for 95805).◀

Definitions

For purposes of CPT reporting of sleep medicine testing services, the following definitions apply:

Actigraphy: the use of a portable, non-invasive, device that continuously records gross motor movement over an extended period of time. The periods of activity and rest are indirect parameters for estimates of the periods of wakefulness and sleep of an individual.

Attended: a technologist or qualified health care professional is physically present (ie, sufficient proximity such that the qualified health care professional can physically respond to emergencies, to other appropriate patient needs or to technical problems at the bedside) throughout the recording session.

Electrooculogram (EOG): a recording of electrical activity indicative of eye movement.

Maintenance of wakefulness test (MWT): a standardized objective test used to determine a person's ability to stay awake. MWT requires sleep staging of the trials that are performed at defined intervals and is attended by a qualified health care professional.

Multiple sleep latency test (MSLT): a standardized objective test of the tendency to fall asleep. MSLT requires sleep staging of the nap opportunities that are performed at defined intervals and is attended by a technologist or qualified health care professional.

Peripheral arterial tonometry (PAT): a plethysmography technique that continuously measures pulsatile volume changes in a digit. This reflects the relative change of blood volume as an indirect measure of sympathetic nervous system activity which is used in respiratory analysis.

Physiological measurements of sleep as used in 95805: the parameters measured are a frontal, central and occipital lead of EEG (3 leads), submental EMG lead and a left and right EOG. These parameters are used together for staging sleep.

Polysomnography: a sleep test involving the continuous, simultaneous, recording of physiological parameters for a period of at least 6 hours that is performed in a sleep laboratory and attended by a technologist or qualified health care professional. The parameters measured are a frontal, central and occipital lead of EEG (3 leads), submental EMG lead and a left and right EOG, (from which sleep is staged), plus four or more additional parameters. The additional parameters typically required in polysomnography are listed below:

a. Electrocardiogram (ECG)

b. Nasal and/or oral airflow

c. Respiratory effort

d. Oxyhemoglobin saturation, SpO2

e. Bilateral anterior tibialis EMG

Positive airway pressure (PAP): a device used to treat sleep-related breathing disorders with the use of non-invasive delivery of positive pressure to the airway. Examples include but are not limited to: CPAP (continuous positive airway pressure), bilevel PAP, AutoPAP (autotitrating or adjusting PAP), ASV (adaptive-servo ventilation).

Remote: the site of service is distant from the monitoring center. Neither a technologist nor a qualified health care professional is physically present at the testing site.

Respiratory airflow (ventilation): the movement of air during inhaled and exhaled breaths. This is typically assessed using thermistor and nasal pressure sensors.

Respiratory analysis: generation of derived parameters that describe components of respiration obtained by using direct or indirect parameters, eg, by airflow or peripheral arterial tone.

Respiratory effort: contraction of the diaphragmatic and/or intercostal muscles to cause (or attempt to cause) respiratory airflow. This is typically measured using transducers that estimate motion of the thorax and abdomen such as respiratory inductive plethysmography, transducers that estimate pressures generated by breathing muscles such as esophageal monometry, or by contraction of breathing muscles, such as diaphragmatic/intercostal EMG.

Respiratory (thoracoabdominal) movement: movement of the chest and abdomen during respiratory effort.

Sleep latency: the length of time it takes to transition from wakefulness to sleep. In the sleep laboratory it is the time from "lights out" to the first epoch scored as any stage of sleep.

Sleep staging: the delineation of the distinct sleep levels through the simultaneous evaluation of physiologic measures including a frontal, central and occipital lead of EEG (3 leads), submental EMG lead and a left and right EOG.

Sleep testing (or sleep study): the continuous, simultaneous monitoring of physiological parameters during sleep (eg, polysomnography, EEG).

Total sleep time: a derived parameter obtained by sleep staging or may be estimated indirectly using actigraphy or other methods.

Unattended: a technologist or qualified health care professional is not physically present with the patient during the recording session.

(Report with modifier 52 if less than 6 hours of recording or in other cases of reduced services as appropriate)

(For unattended sleep study, use 95806)

95782 ▶Code is out of numerical sequence. See 95803-95783◀

95783 ▶Code is out of numerical sequence. See 95803-95783◀

95800 ▶Code is out of numerical sequence. See 95803-95811◀

95801 ▶Code is out of numerical sequence. See 95800-95811◀

95803 Actigraphy testing, recording, analysis, interpretation, and report (minimum of 72 hours to 14 consecutive days of recording)

➔ *CPT Assistant* Nov 11:3; *CPT Changes: An Insider's View* 2009

(Do not report 95803 more than once in any 14 day period)

(Do not report 95803 in conjunction with 95806-95811)

95805 Multiple sleep latency or maintenance of wakefulness testing, recording, analysis and interpretation of physiological measurements of sleep during multiple trials to assess sleepiness

➔ *CPT Assistant* Nov 97:45-46, Nov 98:35, Dec 01:3, Sep 02:2-3, Mar 08:4, Nov 11:3

95806 Sleep study, unattended, simultaneous recording of, heart rate, oxygen saturation, respiratory airflow, and respiratory effort (eg, thoracoabdominal movement)

➔ *CPT Assistant* Nov 97:45-46, Aug 98:10, Nov 98:35, Jan 11:7, Nov 11:3; *CPT Changes: An Insider's View* 2010

(Do not report 95806 in conjunction with 93041-93227, 93228, 93229, 93268-93272, 95800, 95801)

(For unattended sleep study that measures heart rate, oxygen saturation, respiratory analysis, and sleep time, use 95800)

(For unattended sleep study that measures a minimum heart rate, oxygen saturation, and respiratory analysis, use 95801)

 # 95800 Sleep study, unattended, simultaneous recording; heart rate, oxygen saturation, respiratory analysis (eg, by airflow or peripheral arterial tone), and sleep time
> *CPT Assistant* Jan 11:6, Nov 11:3; *CPT Changes: An Insider's View* 2011

(Do not report 95800 in conjunction with 93041-93227, 93228, 93229, 93268-93272, 95801, 95803, 95806)

(For unattended sleep study that measures a minimum of heart rate, oxygen saturation, and respiratory analysis, use 95801)

 # 95801 minimum of heart rate, oxygen saturation, and respiratory analysis (eg, by airflow or peripheral arterial tone)
> *CPT Assistant* Jan 11:7, Nov 11:3; *CPT Changes: An Insider's View* 2011

(Do not report 95801 in conjunction with 93041-93227, 93228, 93229, 93268-93272, 95800, 95806)

(For unattended sleep study that measures heart rate, oxygen saturation, respiratory analysis and sleep time, use 95800)

95807 Sleep study, simultaneous recording of ventilation, respiratory effort, ECG or heart rate, and oxygen saturation, attended by a technologist
> *CPT Assistant* Nov 97:46, Nov 98:35, Mar 08:4, Nov 11:3

▲ 95808 Polysomnography; any age, sleep staging with 1-3 additional parameters of sleep, attended by a technologist
> *CPT Assistant* Sep 96:11, Nov 97:46, Feb 98:6, Nov 98:35, Sep 02:2-3, Mar 08:4, Nov 11:3; *CPT Changes: An Insider's View* 2013

▲ 95810 age 6 years or older, sleep staging with 4 or more additional parameters of sleep, attended by a technologist
> *CPT Assistant* Feb 98:6, Nov 98:35, Sep 02:2-3, Nov 11:3; *CPT Changes: An Insider's View* 2013

▲ 95811 age 6 years or older, sleep staging with 4 or more additional parameters of sleep, with initiation of continuous positive airway pressure therapy or bilevel ventilation, attended by a technologist
> *CPT Assistant* Nov 97:46, Feb 98:6, Nov 98:35, Sep 02:2-3, Mar 08:4, Nov 11:3; *CPT Changes: An Insider's View* 2013

#● 95782 younger than 6 years, sleep staging with 4 or more additional parameters of sleep, attended by a technologist
> *CPT Changes: An Insider's View* 2013

#● 95783 younger than 6 years, sleep staging with 4 or more additional parameters of sleep, with initiation of continuous positive airway pressure therapy or bi-level ventilation, attended by a technologist
> *CPT Changes: An Insider's View* 2013

Routine Electroencephalography (EEG)

EEG codes 95812-95822 include hyperventilation and/or photic stimulation when appropriate. Routine EEG codes 95816-95822 include 20 to 40 minutes of recording. Extended EEG codes 95812-95813 include reporting times longer than 40 minutes.

95812 Electroencephalogram (EEG) extended monitoring; 41-60 minutes
> *CPT Assistant* Winter 94:18, Nov 98:35, May 11:3, 10; *CPT Changes: An Insider's View* 2003

95813 greater than 1 hour
> *CPT Assistant* Winter 94:18, Nov 98:35, May 11:3, 10

95816 Electroencephalogram (EEG); including recording awake and drowsy
> *CPT Assistant* Sep 96:11, Nov 98:35, Nov 99:51, Jul 00:1, 11:3; *CPT Changes: An Insider's View* 2000, 2003

95819 including recording awake and asleep
> *CPT Assistant* Nov 98:35, Nov 99:51, Jul 00:1, 11:3; *CPT Changes: An Insider's View* 2000, 2003

95822 recording in coma or sleep only
> *CPT Assistant* Nov 98:35, 11:3; *CPT Changes: An Insider's View* 2003

95824 cerebral death evaluation only
> *CPT Assistant* Nov 98:35

95827 all night recording
> *CPT Assistant* Nov 98:35; *CPT Changes: An Insider's View* 2003

(For 24-hour EEG monitoring, see 95950-95953 or 95956)

(For EEG during nonintracranial surgery, use 95955)

(For Wada test, use 95958)

(For digital analysis of EEG, use 95957)

95829 Electrocorticogram at surgery (separate procedure)
> *CPT Assistant* Nov 98:35

▲ 95830 Insertion by physician or other qualified health care professional of sphenoidal electrodes for electroencephalographic (EEG) recording
> *CPT Changes: An Insider's View* 2013

Muscle and Range of Motion Testing

95831 Muscle testing, manual (separate procedure) with report; extremity (excluding hand) or trunk
> *CPT Assistant* Nov 99:51, Dec 99:10, Mar 00:11, Jul 00:2, Nov 01:5, Apr 03:28, Dec 03:7, Feb 04:5, May 08:9; *CPT Changes: An Insider's View* 2000

95832 hand, with or without comparison with normal side
> *CPT Assistant* Nov 99:51, Dec 99:10, Mar 00:11, Jul 00:2, Nov 01:5, Apr 03:28, Dec 03:7, Feb 04:5, May 08:9

Medicine

Medicine

95833   total evaluation of body, excluding hands
> *CPT Assistant* Nov 99:51, Dec 99:10, Jul 00:2, Nov 01:5, Jul 02:2, Apr 03:28, Dec 03:7, Feb 04:5, May 08:9

95834   total evaluation of body, including hands
> *CPT Assistant* Nov 99:51, Dec 99:10, Jul 00:2, Nov 01:5, Apr 03:28, Dec 03:7, Feb 04:5, May 08:9

95851   Range of motion measurements and report (separate procedure); each extremity (excluding hand) or each trunk section (spine)
> *CPT Assistant* Sep 99:10, Nov 01:5, Apr 03:28, Dec 03:7, Feb 04:5, Dec 07:16, May 08:9

95852   hand, with or without comparison with normal side
> *CPT Assistant* Nov 01:5, Apr 03:28, Dec 03:7, May 08:9

95857   Cholinesterase inhibitor challenge test for myasthenia gravis
> *CPT Assistant* Feb 11:3; *CPT Changes: An Insider's View* 2011

Electromyography

Needle electromyographic (EMG) procedures include the interpretation of electrical waveforms measured by equipment that produces both visible and audible components of electrical signals recorded from the muscle(s) studied by the needle electrode.

Use 95870 or 95885 when four or fewer muscles are tested in an extremity. Use 95860-95864 or 95886 when five or more muscles are tested in an extremity.

►Use EMG codes (95860-95864 and 95867-95870) when no nerve conduction studies (95907-95913) are performed on that day. Use 95885, 95886, and 95887 for EMG services when nerve conduction studies (95907-95913) are performed in conjunction with EMG on the same day.◄

Report either 95885 or 95886 once per extremity. Codes 95885 and 95886 can be reported together up to a combined total of four units of service per patient when all four extremities are tested.

95860   Needle electromyography; 1 extremity with or without related paraspinal areas
> *CPT Assistant* Nov 97:46, Jul 00:2, Apr 02:2, May 03:20, Jun 03:3, Feb 04:4, Jul 04:6, Oct 04:15, Jun 06:8, Sep 06:5, Aug 08:12, Jan 09:8, Oct 10:15, Dec 10:15, Feb 12:8; *CPT Changes: An Insider's View* 2003

95861   2 extremities with or without related paraspinal areas
> *CPT Assistant* Nov 97:46, Jul 00:2, Apr 02:2, May 03:20, Jun 03:3, Feb 04:4, Jul 04:6, Oct 04:15, Jun 05:9, Jun 06:8, Sep 06:5, Aug 08:12, Jan 09:8, Oct 10:15, Dec 10:15, Feb 12:8; *CPT Changes: An Insider's View* 2003

(For dynamic electromyography performed during motion analysis studies, see 96002-96003)

95863   3 extremities with or without related paraspinal areas
> *CPT Assistant* Nov 97:46, Jul 00:2, Apr 02:2, May 03:20, Jun 03:3, Feb 04:4, Jul 04:6, Oct 04:15, Jun 06:8, Sep 06:5, Oct 10:15, Dec 10:15, Feb 12:8; *CPT Changes: An Insider's View* 2003

95864   4 extremities with or without related paraspinal areas
> *CPT Assistant* Nov 97:46, Jul 00:2, Jan 02:11, Apr 02:2, May 03:20, Jun 03:3, Feb 04:4, Jul 04:6, Oct 04:15, Jun 06:8, Sep 06:5, Aug 08:12, Jan 09:8, Oct 10:15, Dec 10:15, Feb 12:8; *CPT Changes: An Insider's View* 2003

95865   larynx
> *CPT Assistant* Sep 06:5, Dec 07:16, Jan 09:8; *CPT Changes: An Insider's View* 2006

(Do not report modifier 50 in conjunction with 95865)

(For unilateral procedure, report modifier 52 in conjunction with 95865)

95866   hemidiaphragm
> *CPT Changes: An Insider's View* 2006

95867   cranial nerve supplied muscle(s), unilateral
> *CPT Assistant* Apr 02:2, May 03:20, Jun 03:3, Jun 06:8, Sep 06:5, Dec 07:16, Aug 08:12, Jan 09:8, Feb 12:8; *CPT Changes: An Insider's View* 2003

95868   cranial nerve supplied muscles, bilateral
> *CPT Assistant* Apr 02:2, May 03:20, Jun 03:3, Jun 06:8, Sep 06:5, Dec 07:16, Jan 09:8, Feb 12:8; *CPT Changes: An Insider's View* 2003

95869   thoracic paraspinal muscles (excluding T1 or T12)
> *CPT Assistant* Nov 97:46, Apr 02:2, May 03:20, Jun 03:3, Feb 04:4, Jun 06:8, Sep 06:5, Jan 09:8, May 10:9, Feb 12:8; *CPT Changes: An Insider's View* 2003

95870   limited study of muscles in 1 extremity or non-limb (axial) muscles (unilateral or bilateral), other than thoracic paraspinal, cranial nerve supplied muscles, or sphincters
> *CPT Assistant* Nov 97:46, Nov 99:51, Jul 00:2, Apr 02:2, May 03:20, Jun 03:3, Feb 04:4, Jul 04:6, Jun 05:9, Jun 06:8, Sep 06:5, Jan 09:8, Feb 12:8; *CPT Changes: An Insider's View* 2000

(To report a complete study of the extremities, see 95860-95864)

(For anal or urethral sphincter, detrusor, urethra, perineum musculature, see 51785-51792)

(For eye muscles, use 92265)

95872   Needle electromyography using single fiber electrode, with quantitative measurement of jitter, blocking and/or fiber density, any/all sites of each muscle studied
> *CPT Assistant* Apr 02:2, May 03:20, Jun 03:3, Sep 06:5, Jan 09:8

#+ **95885**   Needle electromyography, each extremity, with related paraspinal areas, when performed, done with nerve conduction, amplitude and latency/velocity study; limited (List separately in addition to code for primary procedure)
> *CPT Assistant* Feb 12:8; *CPT Changes: An Insider's View* 2012

#+ **95886**   complete, five or more muscles studied, innervated by three or more nerves or four or more spinal levels (List separately in addition to code for primary procedure)
> *CPT Assistant* Feb 12:8; *CPT Changes: An Insider's View* 2012

►(Use 95885, 95886 in conjunction with 95907-95913)◄

(Do not report 95885, 95886 in conjunction with 95860-95864, 95870, 95905)

#+ 95887   Needle electromyography, non-extremity (cranial nerve supplied or axial) muscle(s) done with nerve conduction, amplitude and latency/velocity study (List separately in addition to code for primary procedure)

> ➔ *CPT Assistant* Feb 12:8, Jul 12:12; *CPT Changes: An Insider's View* 2012

▶(Use 95887 in conjunction with 95907-95913)◀

(Do not report 95887 in conjunction with 95867-95870, 95905)

Guidance for Chemodenervation and Ischemic Muscle Testing

+ 95873   Electrical stimulation for guidance in conjunction with chemodenervation (List separately in addition to code for primary procedure)

> ➔ *CPT Changes: An Insider's View* 2006

+ 95874   Needle electromyography for guidance in conjunction with chemodenervation (List separately in addition to code for primary procedure)

> ➔ *CPT Changes: An Insider's View* 2006

(Use 95873, 95874 in conjunction with 64612-64614)

(Do not report 95874 in conjunction with 95873)

(Do not report 95873, 95874 in conjunction with 95860-95870)

95875   Ischemic limb exercise test with serial specimen(s) acquisition for muscle(s) metabolite(s)

> ➔ *CPT Assistant* Jun 03:3; *CPT Changes: An Insider's View* 2002, 2003

(For listing of nerves considered for separate study, see **Appendix J**)

95885   Code is out of numerical sequence. See 95860-95887

95886   Code is out of numerical sequence. See 95860-95887

95887   Code is out of numerical sequence. See 95860-95887

Nerve Conduction Tests

▶The following applies to nerve conduction tests (95907-95913): Codes 95907-95913 describe nerve conduction tests when performed with individually placed stimulating, recording, and ground electrodes. The stimulating, recording, and ground electrode placement and the test design must be individualized to the patient's unique anatomy. Nerves tested must be limited to the specific nerves and conduction studies needed for the particular clinical question being investigated. The stimulating electrode must be placed directly over the nerve to be tested, and stimulation parameters properly adjusted to avoid stimulating other nerves or nerve branches. In most motor nerve conduction studies, and in some sensory and mixed nerve conduction studies, both proximal and distal stimulation will be used. Motor nerve conduction study recordings must be made from electrodes placed directly over the motor point of the specific muscle to be tested. Sensory nerve conduction study recordings must be made from electrodes placed directly over the specific nerve to be tested. Waveforms must be reviewed on site in real time, and the technique (stimulus site, recording site, ground site, filter settings) must be adjusted, as appropriate, as the test proceeds in order to minimize artifact, and to minimize the chances of unintended stimulation of adjacent nerves and the unintended recording from adjacent muscles or nerves. Reports must be prepared on site by the examiner, and consist of the work product of the interpretation of numerous test results, using well-established techniques to assess the amplitude, latency, and configuration of waveforms elicited by stimulation at each site of each nerve tested. This includes the calculation of nerve conduction velocities, sometimes including specialized F-wave indices, along with comparison to normal values, summarization of clinical and electrodiagnostic data, and physician or other qualified health care professional interpretation. Codes 95907-95913 describe one or more nerve conduction studies. For the purposes of coding, a single conduction study is defined as a sensory conduction test, a motor conduction test with or without an F wave test, or an H-reflex test. Each type of study (sensory, motor with or without F wave, H-reflex) for each nerve includes all orthodromic and antidromic impulses associated with that nerve and constitutes a distinct study when determining the number of studies in each grouping (eg, 1-2 or 3-4 nerve conduction studies). Each type of nerve conduction study is counted only once when multiple sites on the same nerve are stimulated or recorded. The numbers of these separate tests should be added to determine which code to use. For a list of nerves, see Appendix J. Use 95885-95887 in conjunction with 95907-95913 when performing electromyography with nerve conduction studies.◀

Code 95905 describes nerve conduction tests when performed with preconfigured electrodes customized to a specific anatomic site.

▶(95900, 95903, 95904 have been deleted. For nerve conduction studies, see 95907-95913)◀

⊘ 95905   Motor and/or sensory nerve conduction, using preconfigured electrode array(s), amplitude and latency/velocity study, each limb, includes F-wave study when performed, with interpretation and report;

> ➔ *CPT Changes: An Insider's View* 2010

(Report 95905 only once per limb studied)

▶(Do not report 95905 in conjunction with 95885, 95886, 95907-95913)◀

● 95907   Nerve conduction studies; 1-2 studies

> ➔ *CPT Changes: An Insider's View* 2013

● 95908   3-4 studies

> ➔ *CPT Changes: An Insider's View* 2013

● 95909   5-6 studies

> ➔ *CPT Changes: An Insider's View* 2013

● **95910** 7-8 studies
  ➔ *CPT Changes: An Insider's View* 2013

● **95911** 9-10 studies
  ➔ *CPT Changes: An Insider's View* 2013

● **95912** 11-12 studies
  ➔ *CPT Changes: An Insider's View* 2013

● **95913** 13 or more studies
  ➔ *CPT Changes: An Insider's View* 2013

Intraoperative Neurophysiology

▶Codes 95940, 95941 describe ongoing neurophysiologic monitoring, testing, and data interpretation distinct from performance of specific type(s) of baseline neurophysiologic study(s) performed during surgical procedures. When the service is performed by the surgeon or anesthesiologist, the professional services are included in the surgeon's or anesthesiologist's primary service code(s) for the procedure and are not reported separately. Do not report these codes for automated monitoring devices that do not require continuous attendance by a professional qualified to interpret the testing and monitoring.

Recording and testing are performed either personally or by a technologist who is physically present with the patient during the service. Supervision is performed either in the operating room or by real time connection outside the operating room. The monitoring professional must be solely dedicated to performing the intraoperative neurophysiologic monitoring and must be available to intervene at all times during the service as necessary, for the reported time period(s). For any given period of time spent providing these services, the service takes full attention and, therefore, other clinical activities beyond providing and interpreting of monitoring cannot be provided during the same period of time.

Throughout the monitoring, there must be provisions for continuous and immediate communication directly with the operating room team in the surgical suite. One or more simultaneous cases may be reported (95941). When monitoring more than one procedure, there must be the immediate ability to transfer patient monitoring to another monitoring professional during the surgical procedure should that individual's exclusive attention be required for another procedure. Report 95941 for all remote or non-one-on-one monitoring time connected to each case regardless of overlap with other cases.

Codes 95940, 95941 include only the ongoing neurophysiologic monitoring time distinct from performance of specific type(s) of baseline neurophysiologic study(s), or other services such as intraoperative functional cortical or subcortical mapping. Codes 95940 and 95941 are reported based upon the time spent monitoring only, and not the number of baseline tests performed or parameters monitored. The time spent performing or interpreting the baseline

neurophysiologic study(ies) should not be counted as intraoperative monitoring, but represents separately reportable procedures. When reporting 95940 and 95941, the same neurophysiologic study(ies) performed at baseline should be reported not more than once per operative session. Baseline study reporting is based upon the total unique studies performed. For example, if during the course of baseline testing and one-on-one monitoring, two separate nerves have motor testing performed in conjunction with limited single extremity EMG, then 95885 and 95907 would be reported in addition to 95940. For procedures that last beyond midnight, report services using the day on which the monitoring began and using the total time monitored.

Code 95940 is reported per 15 minutes of service. Code 95940 requires reporting only the portion of time the monitoring professional was physically present in the operating room providing one-on-one patient monitoring, and no other cases may be monitored at the same time. Report continuous intraoperative neurophysiologic monitoring in the operating room (95940) in addition to the services related to monitoring from outside the operating room (95941).

Code 95941 should be used once per hour even if multiple methods of neurophysiologic monitoring are used during the time. Code 95941 requires the monitoring of neurophysiological data that is collected from the operating room continuously on-line in real time via a secure data link. When reporting 95941, real-time ability must be available through sufficient data bandwidth transfer rates to view and interrogate the neurophysiologic data contemporaneously.

Report 95941 for all cases in which there was no physical presence by the monitoring professional in the operating room during the monitoring time or when monitoring more than one case in an operating room. It is also used to report the time of monitoring physically performed outside of the operating room in those cases where monitoring occurred both within and outside the operating room. Do not report 95941 if the monitoring lasts 30 minutes or less.

Intraoperative neurophysiology monitoring codes 95940 and 95941 are each used to report the total duration of respective time spent providing each service, even if that time is not in a single continuous block.◀

▶(95920 has been deleted. To report, see 95940, 95941)◀

#✚● **95940** Continuous intraoperative neurophysiology monitoring in the operating room, one on one monitoring requiring personal attendance, each 15 minutes (List separately in addition to code for primary procedure)
  ➔ *CPT Changes: An Insider's View* 2013

▶(Use 95940 in conjunction with the study performed, 92585, 95822, 95860-95870, 95907-95913, 95925, 95926, 95927, 95928, 95929, 95930-95937, 95938, 95939)◀

#+● **95941** Continuous intraoperative neurophysiology monitoring, from outside the operating room (remote or nearby) or for monitoring of more than one case while in the operating room, per hour (List separately in addition to code for primary procedure)

➜ *CPT Changes: An Insider's View* 2013

▶(Use 95941 in conjunction with the study performed, 92585, 95822, 95860-95870, 95907-95913, 95925, 95926, 95927, 95928, 95929, 95930-95937, 95938, 95939)◀

(For time spent waiting on standby before monitoring, use 99360)

(For electrocorticography, use 95829)

(For intraoperative EEG during nonintracranial surgery, use 95955)

(For intraoperative functional cortical or subcortical mapping, see 95961-95962)

(For intraoperative neurostimulator programming and analysis, see 95970-95975)

Autonomic Function Tests

▶The purpose of autonomic nervous system function testing is to determine the presence of autonomic dysfunction, the site of autonomic dysfunction, and the various autonomic subsystems that may be disordered.

Code 95921 should be reported only when electrocardiographic monitoring of heart rate derived from the time elapsing between two consecutive R waves in the electrocardiogram, or the R-R interval, is displayed on a monitor and stored for subsequent analysis of waveforms. Testing is typically performed in the prone position. A tilt table may be used, but is not required equipment for testing of the parasympathetic function. At least two of the following components need to be included in testing:

1. Heart rate response to deep breathing derived from a visual quantitative analysis of recordings with subject breathing at a rate of 5-6 breaths per minute.

2. Valsalva ratio determined by dividing the maximum heart rate by the lowest heart rate. The initial heart rate responses to sustained oral pressure (blowing into a tube with an open glottis) consist of tachycardia followed by a bradycardia at 15-45 seconds after the Valsalva pressure has been released. A minimum of two Valsalva maneuvers are to be performed. The initial cardioacceleration is an exercise reflex while the subsequent tachycardia and bradycardia are baroreflex-mediated.

3. A 30:15 ratio (R-R interval at beat 30)/(R-R interval at beat 15) used as an index of cardiovascular function.

Code 95922 should be reported only when all of the following components are included in testing:

1. Continuous recording of beat-to-beat BP and heart rate. The heart rate needs to be derived from an electrocardiogram (ECG) unit such that an accurate quantitative graphical measurement of the R-R interval is obtained.

2. A period of supine rest of at least 20 minutes prior to testing.

3. The performance and recording of beat-to-beat blood pressure and heart rate during a minimum of two (2) Valsalva maneuvers.

4. The performance of passive head-up tilt with continuous recording of beat-to-beat blood pressure and heart rate for a minimum of five minutes, followed by passive tilt-back to the supine position. This must be performed using a tilt table.

Code 95924 should be reported only when both the parasympathetic function and the adrenergic function are tested together with the use of a tilt table.◀

▶(To report autonomic function testing that does not include beat-to-beat recording or for testing without use of a tilt table, use 95943)◀

95921 Testing of autonomic nervous system function; cardiovagal innervation (parasympathetic function), including 2 or more of the following: heart rate response to deep breathing with recorded R-R interval, Valsalva ratio, and 30:15 ratio

➜ *CPT Assistant* Nov 98:35-36, Apr 02:2, Oct 03:11, Feb 06:15

95922 vasomotor adrenergic innervation (sympathetic adrenergic function), including beat-to-beat blood pressure and R-R interval changes during Valsalva maneuver and at least 5 minutes of passive tilt

➜ *CPT Assistant* Nov 98:35-36, Apr 02:2, Jun 03:11, Feb 06:15, Nov 06:23, Dec 08:4

▶(Do not report 95922 in conjunction with 95921)◀

95923 sudomotor, including 1 or more of the following: quantitative sudomotor axon reflex test (QSART), silastic sweat imprint, thermoregulatory sweat test, and changes in sympathetic skin potential

➜ *CPT Assistant* Nov 98:35-36, Apr 02:2, Feb 06:15

● **95924** combined parasympathetic and sympathetic adrenergic function testing with at least 5 minutes of passive tilt

➜ *CPT Changes: An Insider's View* 2013

▶(Do not report 95924 in conjunction with 95921 or 95922)◀

#● **95943** Simultaneous, independent, quantitative measures of both parasympathetic function and sympathetic function, based on time-frequency analysis of heart rate variability concurrent with time-frequency analysis of continuous respiratory activity, with mean heart rate and blood pressure measures, during rest, paced (deep) breathing, Valsalva maneuvers, and head-up postural change

➜ *CPT Changes: An Insider's View* 2013

▶(Do not report 95943 in conjunction with 93040, 95921, 95922, 95924)◀

Evoked Potentials and Reflex Tests

95925 Short-latency somatosensory evoked potential study, stimulation of any/all peripheral nerves or skin sites, recording from the central nervous system; in upper limbs
> ➔ *CPT Assistant* Nov 98:35-36, Apr 02:2, Apr 12:17

(Do not report 95925 in conjunction with 95926)

95926   in lower limbs
> ➔ *CPT Assistant* May 01:11, Apr 02:2, Apr 12:17

(Do not report 95926 in conjunction with 95925)

 # 95938   in upper and lower limbs
> ➔ *CPT Assistant* Apr 12:17, 18; *CPT Changes: An Insider's View* 2012

(Do not report 95938 in conjunction with 95925, 95926)

95927   in the trunk or head
> ➔ *CPT Assistant* Apr 02:2

(To report a unilateral study, use modifier 52)

(For auditory evoked potentials, use 92585)

95928 Central motor evoked potential study (transcranial motor stimulation); upper limbs
> ➔ *CPT Changes: An Insider's View* 2005

(Do not report 95928 in conjunction with 95929)

95929   lower limbs
> ➔ *CPT Changes: An Insider's View* 2005

(Do not report 95929 in conjunction with 95928)

 # 95939   in upper and lower limbs
> ➔ *CPT Assistant* Apr 12:17, 18; *CPT Changes: An Insider's View* 2012

(Do not report 95939 in conjunction with 95928, 95929)

95930 Visual evoked potential (VEP) testing central nervous system, checkerboard or flash

95933 Orbicularis oculi (blink) reflex, by electrodiagnostic testing
> ➔ *CPT Assistant* Nov 98:35-36

▶(95934, 95936 have been deleted. To report H-reflex testing, see 95907-95913)◀

95937 Neuromuscular junction testing (repetitive stimulation, paired stimuli), each nerve, any 1 method
> ➔ *CPT Assistant* Nov 98:35-36, Apr 02:2, Jun 06:8

95938 ▶Code is out of numerical sequence. See 95925-95939◀

95939 ▶Code is out of numerical sequence. See 95925-95939◀

95940 ▶Code is out of numerical sequence. See 95921-95943◀

95941 ▶Code is out of numerical sequence. See 95921-95943◀

95943 ▶Code is out of numerical sequence. See 95921-95943◀

Special EEG Tests

Codes 95950-95953 and 95956 are used per 24 hours of recording. For recording more than 12 hours, do not use modifier 52. For recording 12 hours or less, use modifier 52. Codes 95951 and 95956 are used for recordings in which interpretations can be made throughout the recording time, with interventions to alter or end the recording or to alter the patient care during the recordings as needed.

▶Codes 95961 and 95962 use physician or other qualified health care professional time as a basis for unit of service. Report 95961 for the first hour of attendance. Use modifier 52 with 95961 for 30 minutes or less. Report 95962 for each additional hour of attendance.◀

95950 Monitoring for identification and lateralization of cerebral seizure focus, electroencephalographic (eg, 8 channel EEG) recording and interpretation, each 24 hours
> ➔ *CPT Assistant* Nov 98:35, Feb 11:3

95951 Monitoring for localization of cerebral seizure focus by cable or radio, 16 or more channel telemetry, combined electroencephalographic (EEG) and video recording and interpretation (eg, for presurgical localization), each 24 hours
> ➔ *CPT Assistant* Nov 98:35, Mar 03:21, Dec 04:18, Dec 09:3, Nov 10:6, Feb 11:3

Electroencephalographic (EEG) Monitoring and Video Recording
95951

Video-EEG monitoring

95953 Monitoring for localization of cerebral seizure focus by computerized portable 16 or more channel EEG, electroencephalographic (EEG) recording and interpretation, each 24 hours, unattended
➔ *CPT Assistant* Nov 98:35, Dec 09:3, Feb 11:3; *CPT Changes: An Insider's View* 2011

▲ **95954** Pharmacological or physical activation requiring physician or other qualified health care professional attendance during EEG recording of activation phase (eg, thiopental activation test)
➔ *CPT Assistant* Winter 94:18, Nov 98:35; *CPT Changes: An Insider's View* 2013

95955 Electroencephalogram (EEG) during nonintracranial surgery (eg, carotid surgery)
➔ *CPT Assistant* Nov 98:35

95956 Monitoring for localization of cerebral seizure focus by cable or radio, 16 or more channel telemetry, electroencephalographic (EEG) recording and interpretation, each 24 hours, attended by a technologist or nurse
➔ *CPT Assistant* Nov 98:35, Dec 09:3, Feb 11:3; *CPT Changes: An Insider's View* 2011

95957 Digital analysis of electroencephalogram (EEG) (eg, for epileptic spike analysis)
➔ *CPT Assistant* Winter 94:18, Nov 98:35, Nov 10:6

95958 Wada activation test for hemispheric function, including electroencephalographic (EEG) monitoring
➔ *CPT Assistant* Nov 98:35

▲ **95961** Functional cortical and subcortical mapping by stimulation and/or recording of electrodes on brain surface, or of depth electrodes, to provoke seizures or identify vital brain structures; initial hour of attendance by a physician or other qualified health care professional
➔ *CPT Assistant* Winter 94:18, Nov 98:35, Nov 99:52-53, Apr 10:10, Aug 10:13, Feb 11:3; *CPT Changes: An Insider's View* 2000, 2013

+▲ **95962** each additional hour of attendance by a physician or other qualified health care professional (List separately in addition to code for primary procedure)
➔ *CPT Assistant* Winter 94:18, Nov 98:35, Nov 99:52-53, Apr 10:10, Aug 10:13, Feb 11:3; *CPT Changes: An Insider's View* 2013

(Use 95962 in conjunction with 95961)

95965 Magnetoencephalography (MEG), recording and analysis; for spontaneous brain magnetic activity (eg, epileptic cerebral cortex localization)
➔ *CPT Changes: An Insider's View* 2002

95966 for evoked magnetic fields, single modality (eg, sensory, motor, language, or visual cortex localization)
➔ *CPT Changes: An Insider's View* 2002

+ **95967** for evoked magnetic fields, each additional modality (eg, sensory, motor, language, or visual cortex localization) (List separately in addition to code for primary procedure)
➔ *CPT Changes: An Insider's View* 2002

(Use 95967 in conjunction with 95966)

(For electroencephalography performed in addition to magnetoencephalography, see 95812-95827)

(For somatosensory evoked potentials, auditory evoked potentials, and visual evoked potentials performed in addition to magnetic evoked field responses, see 92585, 95925, 95926, and/or 95930)

(For computerized tomography performed in addition to magnetoencephalography, see 70450-70470, 70496)

(For magnetic resonance imaging performed in addition to magnetoencephalography, see 70551-70553)

Neurostimulators, Analysis-Programming

Simple intraoperative or subsequent programming of the neurostimulator pulse generator/transmitter (95971) includes changes to three or fewer of the following parameters: rate, pulse amplitude, pulse duration, pulse frequency, eight or more electrode contacts, cycling, stimulation train duration, train spacing, number of programs, number of channels, alternating electrode polarities, dose time (stimulation parameters changing in time periods of minutes including dose lockout times), more than one clinical feature (eg, rigidity, dyskinesia, tremor). Complex intraoperative or subsequent programming (95972-95979) includes changes to more than three of the above.

Code 95970 describes subsequent electronic analysis of a previously-implanted simple or complex brain, spinal cord, or peripheral neurostimulator pulse generator system, without reprogramming. Code 95971 describes intraoperative or subsequent electronic analysis of an implanted simple spinal cord, or peripheral (ie, peripheral nerve, autonomic nerve, neuromuscular) neurostimulator pulse generator system, with programming. Codes 95972 and 95973 describe intraoperative (at initial insertion/revision) or subsequent electronic analysis of an implanted complex spinal cord or peripheral (except cranial nerve) neurostimulator pulse generator system, with programming. Codes 95974 and 95975 describe intraoperative (at initial insertion/revision) or subsequent electronic analysis of an implanted complex cranial nerve neurostimulator pulse generator system, with programming. Codes 95978 and 95979 describe initial or subsequent electronic analysis of an implanted brain neurostimulator pulse generator system, with programming.

Code 95980 describes intraoperative electronic analysis of an implanted gastric neurostimulator pulse generator system, with programming; code 95981 describes subsequent analysis of the device; code 95982 describes subsequent analysis and reprogramming. For electronic analysis and reprogramming of gastric neurostimulator, lesser curvature, see 95980-95982.

For 95972, 95974, and 95978, use modifier 52 if less than 31 minutes in duration.

Medicine

(For electronic analysis and reprogramming of a peripheral subcutaneous field stimulation pulse generator, use 0285T)

(For insertion of neurostimulator pulse generator, see 61885, 63685, 64590)

(For revision or removal of neurostimulator pulse generator or receiver, see 61888, 63688, 64595)

(For implantation of neurostimulator electrodes, see 43647, 43881, 61850-61875, 63650-63655, 64553-64580. For revision or removal of neurostimulator electrodes, see 43648, 43882, 61880, 63661-63664, 64585)

95970 Electronic analysis of implanted neurostimulator pulse generator system (eg, rate, pulse amplitude, pulse duration, configuration of wave form, battery status, electrode selectability, output modulation, cycling, impedance and patient compliance measurements); simple or complex brain, spinal cord, or peripheral (ie, cranial nerve, peripheral nerve, sacral nerve, neuromuscular) neurostimulator pulse generator/transmitter, without reprogramming

> *CPT Assistant* Nov 98:36-37, Sep 99:1, Nov 99:53-54, Aug 05:7, Sep 05:10; *CPT Changes: An Insider's View* 2000, 2012

95971 simple spinal cord, or peripheral (ie, peripheral nerve, sacral nerve, neuromuscular) neurostimulator pulse generator/transmitter, with intraoperative or subsequent programming

> *CPT Assistant* Nov 98:36-37, Sep 99:1, Nov 99:53-54, Aug 05:7, Oct 10:14, Dec 10:14, Apr 11:11; *CPT Changes: An Insider's View* 2000, 2005, 2012

95972 complex spinal cord, or peripheral (ie, peripheral nerve, sacral nerve, neuromuscular) (except cranial nerve) neurostimulator pulse generator/transmitter, with intraoperative or subsequent programming, first hour

> *CPT Assistant* Nov 98:36-37, Sep 99:1, Nov 99:53-54, Aug 05:7, Apr 11:10; *CPT Changes: An Insider's View* 2000, 2005, 2012

+ 95973 complex spinal cord, or peripheral (ie, peripheral nerve, sacral nerve, neuromuscular) (except cranial nerve) neurostimulator pulse generator/transmitter, with intraoperative or subsequent programming, each additional 30 minutes after first hour (List separately in addition to code for primary procedure)

> *CPT Assistant* Nov 98:36-37, Sep 99:1, Nov 99:53-54, Aug 05:7, Apr 11:11; *CPT Changes: An Insider's View* 2000, 2005, 2012

(Use 95973 in conjunction with 95972)

95974 complex cranial nerve neurostimulator pulse generator/transmitter, with intraoperative or subsequent programming, with or without nerve interface testing, first hour

> *CPT Assistant* Nov 98:36-37, Sep 99:1, Nov 99:53-54, Sep 05:10, Apr 11:11; *CPT Changes: An Insider's View* 2012

+ 95975 complex cranial nerve neurostimulator pulse generator/transmitter, with intraoperative or subsequent programming, each additional 30 minutes after first hour (List separately in addition to code for primary procedure)

> *CPT Assistant* Nov 98:36-37, Sep 99:1, Nov 99:53-54, Sep 05:10, Apr 11:11; *CPT Changes: An Insider's View* 2012

(Use 95975 in conjunction with 95974)

95978 Electronic analysis of implanted neurostimulator pulse generator system (eg, rate, pulse amplitude and duration, battery status, electrode selectability and polarity, impedance and patient compliance measurements), complex deep brain neurostimulator pulse generator/transmitter, with initial or subsequent programming; first hour

> *CPT Assistant* Aug 05:7; *CPT Changes: An Insider's View* 2005

+ 95979 each additional 30 minutes after first hour (List separately in addition to code for primary procedure)

> *CPT Assistant* Aug 05:7; *CPT Changes: An Insider's View* 2005

(Use 95979 in conjunction with 95978)

95980 Electronic analysis of implanted neurostimulator pulse generator system (eg, rate, pulse amplitude and duration, configuration of wave form, battery status, electrode selectability, output modulation, cycling, impedance and patient measurements) gastric neurostimulator pulse generator/transmitter; intraoperative, with programming

> *CPT Assistant* Jan 08:8, Nov 10:8; *CPT Changes: An Insider's View* 2008

95981 subsequent, without reprogramming

> *CPT Assistant* Jan 08:8; *CPT Changes: An Insider's View* 2008

95982 subsequent, with reprogramming

> *CPT Assistant* Jan 08:8; *CPT Changes: An Insider's View* 2008

►(For intraoperative or subsequent analysis, with programming, when performed, of vagus nerve trunk stimulator used for blocking therapy [morbid obesity], see 0312T, 0317T)◄

Other Procedures

95990 Refilling and maintenance of implantable pump or reservoir for drug delivery, spinal (intrathecal, epidural) or brain (intraventricular), includes electronic analysis of pump, when performed;

> *CPT Assistant* Nov 02:4, Nov 05:1, Jul 06:1, Jul 12:6; *CPT Changes: An Insider's View* 2003, 2012

▲ 95991 requiring skill of a physician or other qualified health care professional

> *CPT Assistant* Nov 05:1, Jul 06:1, Jul 12:6; *CPT Changes: An Insider's View* 2004, 2012, 2013

(Do not report 95990, 95991 in conjunction with 62367-62370. For analysis and/or reprogramming of implantable infusion pump, see 62367-62370)

(For refill and maintenance of implanted infusion pump or reservoir for systemic drug therapy [eg, chemotherapy], use 96522)

— *Coding Tip* —

Instructions for Use of the CPT Codebook

When advanced practice nurses and physician assistants are working with physicians, they are considered as working in the exact same specialty and exact same subspecialties as the physician. A "physician or other qualified health care professional" is an individual who is qualified by education, training, licensure/regulation (when applicable), and facility privileging (when applicable) who performs a professional service within his or her scope of practice and independently reports that professional service. These professionals are distinct from "clinical staff." A clinical staff member is a person who works under the supervision of a physician or other qualified health care professional, and who is allowed by law, regulation and facility policy to perform or assist in the performance of a specific professional service, but does not individually report that professional service. Other policies may also affect who may report specific services.

CPT Coding Guidelines, Introduction, Instructions for Use of the CPT Codebook

---

⊘ **95992**   Canalith repositioning procedure(s) (eg, Epley maneuver, Semont maneuver), per day

→ *CPT Changes: An Insider's View* 2009

(Do not report 95992 in conjunction with 92531, 92532)

95999   Unlisted neurological or neuromuscular diagnostic procedure

→ *CPT Assistant* Feb 99:11, Jan 02:11, Mar 07:4, Apr 07:7, Dec 08:10

Motion Analysis

Codes 96000-96004 describe services performed as part of a major therapeutic or diagnostic decision making process. Motion analysis is performed in a dedicated motion analysis laboratory (ie, a facility capable of performing videotaping from the front, back and both sides, computerized 3D kinematics, 3D kinetics, and dynamic electromyography). Code 96000 may include 3D kinetics and stride characteristics. Codes 96002-96003 describe dynamic electromyography.

Code 96004 should only be reported once regardless of the number of study(ies) reviewed/interpreted.

▶(For performance of needle electromyography procedures, see 95860-95870, 95872, 95885-95887)◀

(For gait training, use 97116)

96000   Comprehensive computer-based motion analysis by video-taping and 3D kinematics;

→ *CPT Assistant* Aug 02:5, Jun 03:2; *CPT Changes: An Insider's View* 2002

96001   with dynamic plantar pressure measurements during walking

→ *CPT Assistant* Aug 02:5, Jun 03:2; *CPT Changes: An Insider's View* 2002

96002   Dynamic surface electromyography, during walking or other functional activities, 1-12 muscles

→ *CPT Assistant* Aug 02:5, Jun 03:3; *CPT Changes: An Insider's View* 2002

96003   Dynamic fine wire electromyography, during walking or other functional activities, 1 muscle

→ *CPT Assistant* Aug 02:5, Jun 03:3; *CPT Changes: An Insider's View* 2002

▶(Do not report 96002, 96003 in conjunction with 95860-95866, 95869-95872, 95885-95887)◀

▲ **96004**   Review and interpretation by physician or other qualified health care professional of comprehensive computer-based motion analysis, dynamic plantar pressure measurements, dynamic surface electromyography during walking or other functional activities, and dynamic fine wire electromyography, with written report

→ *CPT Assistant* Aug 02:5, Jun 03:3; *CPT Changes: An Insider's View* 2002, 2013

Functional Brain Mapping

Code 96020 includes selection and administration of testing of language, memory, cognition, movement, sensation, and other neurological functions when conducted in association with functional neuroimaging, monitoring of performance of this testing, and determination of validity of neurofunctional testing relative to separately interpreted functional magnetic resonance images.

▲ **96020**   Neurofunctional testing selection and administration during noninvasive imaging functional brain mapping, with test administered entirely by a physician or other qualified health care professional (ie, psychologist), with review of test results and report

→ *CPT Assistant* Feb 07:6; *CPT Changes: An Insider's View* 2007, 2013

(For functional magnetic resonance imaging [fMRI], brain, use 70555)

(Do not report 96020 in conjunction with 96101-96103, 96116-96120)

(Do not report 96020 in conjunction with 70554)

(Evaluation and Management services codes should not be reported on the same day as 96020)

Medical Genetics and Genetic Counseling Services

These services are provided by trained genetic counselors and may include obtaining a structured family genetic history, pedigree construction, analysis for genetic risk assessment, and counseling of the patient and family.

These activities may be provided during one or more sessions and may include review of medical data and family information, face-to-face interviews, and counseling services.

Code 96040 is reported for each 30-minute increment of face-to-face time. Do not report 96040 for 15 minutes or less of face-to-face time. Report 96040 once for 16 to 30 minutes of face-to-face time.

96040 Medical genetics and genetic counseling services, each 30 minutes face-to-face with patient/family

➲ *CPT Assistant* Aug 07:9; *CPT Changes: An Insider's View* 2007

▶(For genetic counseling and education provided to an individual by a physician or other qualified health care professional who may report evaluation and management services, see the appropriate Evaluation and Management codes)◀

▶(For genetic counseling and education to a group by a physician or other qualified health care professional, use 99078)◀

(For education regarding genetic risks by a nonphysician to a group, see 98961, 98962)

▶(For genetic counseling and/or risk factor reduction intervention provided to patient(s) without symptoms or established disease, by a physician or other qualified health care professional who may report evaluation and management services, see 99401-99412)◀

Central Nervous System Assessments/Tests (eg, Neuro-Cognitive, Mental Status, Speech Testing)

The following codes are used to report the services provided during testing of the cognitive function of the central nervous system. The testing of cognitive processes, visual motor responses, and abstractive abilities is accomplished by the combination of several types of testing procedures. It is expected that the administration of these tests will generate material that will be formulated into a report. A minimum of 31 minutes must be provided to report any per hour code. Services 96101, 96116, 96118, and 96125 report time as face-to-face time with the patient and the time spent interpreting and preparing the report.

(For development of cognitive skills, see 97532, 97533)

(For mini-mental status examination performed by a physician, see **Evaluation and Management** services codes)

96101 Psychological testing (includes psychodiagnostic assessment of emotionality, intellectual abilities, personality and psychopathology, eg, MMPI, Rorschach, WAIS), per hour of the psychologist's or physician's time, both face-to-face time administering tests to the patient and time interpreting these test results and preparing the report

➲ *CPT Assistant* Sep 10:9, Oct 11:4; *CPT Changes: An Insider's View* 2006, 2008

(96101 is also used in those circumstances when additional time is necessary to integrate other sources of clinical data, including previously completed and reported technician- and computer-administered tests)

(Do not report 96101 for the interpretation and report of 96102, 96103)

96102 Psychological testing (includes psychodiagnostic assessment of emotionality, intellectual abilities, personality and psychopathology, eg, MMPI and WAIS), with qualified health care professional interpretation and report, administered by technician, per hour of technician time, face-to-face

➲ *CPT Changes: An Insider's View* 2006

96103 Psychological testing (includes psychodiagnostic assessment of emotionality, intellectual abilities, personality and psychopathology, eg, MMPI), administered by a computer, with qualified health care professional interpretation and report

➲ *CPT Assistant* Oct 11:10; *CPT Changes: An Insider's View* 2006

96105 Assessment of aphasia (includes assessment of expressive and receptive speech and language function, language comprehension, speech production ability, reading, spelling, writing, eg, by Boston Diagnostic Aphasia Examination) with interpretation and report, per hour

➲ *CPT Assistant* Jul 96:8, May 05:1, Nov 09:10

96110 Developmental screening, with interpretation and report, per standardized instrument form

➲ *CPT Assistant* Jul 96:9, May 05:1, Nov 09:10; *CPT Changes: An Insider's View* 2012

96111 Developmental testing, (includes assessment of motor, language, social, adaptive, and/or cognitive functioning by standardized developmental instruments) with interpretation and report

➲ *CPT Assistant* Jul 96:9, May 05:1, Nov 09:10; *CPT Changes: An Insider's View* 2005, 2012

96116 Neurobehavioral status exam (clinical assessment of thinking, reasoning and judgment, eg, acquired knowledge, attention, language, memory, planning and problem solving, and visual spatial abilities), per hour of the psychologist's or physician's time, both face-to-face time with the patient and time interpreting test results and preparing the report

➲ *CPT Assistant* Oct 11:4; *CPT Changes: An Insider's View* 2006

96118   Neuropsychological testing (eg, Halstead-Reitan
Neuropsychological Battery, Wechsler Memory Scales
and Wisconsin Card Sorting Test), per hour of the
psychologist's or physician's time, both face-to-face time
administering tests to the patient and time interpreting
these test results and preparing the report

➔ *CPT Assistant* Sep 10:9, Oct 11:4; *CPT Changes: An Insider's
View* 2006, 2008

(96118 is also used in those circumstances when
additional time is necessary to integrate other sources of
clinical data, including previously completed and reported
technician- and computer-administered tests)

(Do not report 96118 for the interpretation and report of
96119 or 96120)

96119   Neuropsychological testing (eg, Halstead-Reitan
Neuropsychological Battery, Wechsler Memory Scales
and Wisconsin Card Sorting Test), with qualified health
care professional interpretation and report, administered
by technician, per hour of technician time, face-to-face

➔ *CPT Changes: An Insider's View* 2006

96120   Neuropsychological testing (eg, Wisconsin Card Sorting
Test), administered by a computer, with qualified health
care professional interpretation and report

➔ *CPT Changes: An Insider's View* 2006

96125   Standardized cognitive performance testing (eg, Ross
Information Processing Assessment) per hour of a
qualified health care professional's time, both face-to-
face time administering tests to the patient and time
interpreting these test results and preparing the report

➔ *CPT Assistant* Oct 11:4; *CPT Changes: An Insider's View* 2008

(For psychological and neuropsychological testing by a
physician or psychologist, see 96101-96103, 96118-
96120)

Health and Behavior
Assessment/Intervention

Health and behavior assessment procedures are used to
identify the psychological, behavioral, emotional,
cognitive, and social factors important to the prevention,
treatment, or management of physical health problems.

The focus of the assessment is not on mental health but
on the biopsychosocial factors important to physical
health problems and treatments. The focus of the
intervention is to improve the patient's health and well-
being utilizing cognitive, behavioral, social, and/or
psychophysiological procedures designed to ameliorate
specific disease-related problems.

Codes 96150-96155 describe services offered to patients
who present with primary physical illnesses, diagnoses, or
symptoms and may benefit from assessments and
interventions that focus on the biopsychosocial factors
related to the patient's health status. These services do not
represent preventive medicine counseling and risk factor
reduction interventions.

For patients that require psychiatric services (90801-
90899) as well as health and behavior assessment/
intervention (96150-96155), report the predominant
service performed. Do not report 96150-96155 in
conjunction with 90801-90899 on the same date.

Evaluation and Management services codes (including
Counseling Risk Factor Reduction and Behavior Change
Intervention [99401-99412]), should not be reported on
the same day.

▶(For health and behavior assessment and/or
intervention performed by a physician or other qualified
health care professional who may report evaluation and
management services, see evaluation and management
or preventive medicine services codes)◀

96150   Health and behavior assessment (eg, health-focused
clinical interview, behavioral observations,
psychophysiological monitoring, health-oriented
questionnaires), each 15 minutes face-to-face with the
patient; initial assessment

➔ *CPT Assistant* Mar 02:4, Feb 04:11, Mar 04:10, May 05:1,
Jun 05:10, Aug 09:9; *CPT Changes: An Insider's View* 2002

96151   re-assessment

➔ *CPT Assistant* Mar 02:4, Feb 04:11, Mar 04:10, May 05:1,
Jun 05:10, Aug 09:9; *CPT Changes: An Insider's View* 2002

96152   Health and behavior intervention, each 15 minutes, face-
to-face; individual

➔ *CPT Assistant* Mar 02:4, Feb 04:11, Mar 04:10, May 05:1,
Jun 05:10, Aug 09:9; *CPT Changes: An Insider's View* 2002

96153   group (2 or more patients)

➔ *CPT Assistant* Mar 02:4, Feb 04:11, Mar 04:10, May 05:1,
Jun 05:10, Aug 09:9; *CPT Changes: An Insider's View* 2002

96154   family (with the patient present)

➔ *CPT Assistant* Mar 02:4, Feb 04:11, Mar 04:10, May 05:1,
Jun 05:10, Aug 09:9; *CPT Changes: An Insider's View* 2002

96155   family (without the patient present)

➔ *CPT Assistant* Mar 02:4, 12, Feb 04:11, Mar 04:10,
May 05:1, Jun 05:10, Aug 09:9; *CPT Changes: An Insider's
View* 2002

Hydration, Therapeutic,
Prophylactic, Diagnostic
Injections and Infusions, and
Chemotherapy and Other
Highly Complex Drug or Highly
Complex Biologic Agent
Administration

▶Physician or other qualified health care professional
work related to hydration, injection, and infusion services
predominantly involves affirmation of treatment plan and
direct supervision of staff.◀

▲=Revised code   ●=New code   ▶ ◀=Contains new or revised text   ⊘=Modifier 51 exempt

Codes 96360-96379, 96401, 96402, 96409-96425, 96521-96523 are not intended to be reported by the physician in the facility setting. If a significant, separately identifiable office or other outpatient Evaluation and Management service is performed, the appropriate E/M service (99201-99215, 99241-99245, 99354-99355) should be reported using modifier 25 in addition to 96360-96549. For same day E/M service, a different diagnosis is not required.

If performed to facilitate the infusion or injection, the following services are included and are not reported separately:

a. Use of local anesthesia

b. IV start

c. Access to indwelling IV, subcutaneous catheter or port

d. Flush at conclusion of infusion

e. Standard tubing, syringes, and supplies

(For declotting a catheter or port, use 36593)

When multiple drugs are administered, report the service(s) and the specific materials or drugs for each.

When administering multiple infusions, injections or combinations, only one "initial" service code should be reported for a given date, unless protocol requires that two separate IV sites must be used. Do not report a second initial service on the same date due to an intravenous line requiring a re-start, an IV rate not being able to be reached without two lines, or for accessing a port of a multi-lumen catheter. If an injection or infusion is of a subsequent or concurrent nature, even if it is the first such service within that group of services, then a subsequent or concurrent code from the appropriate section should be reported (eg, the first IV push given subsequent to an initial one-hour infusion is reported using a subsequent IV push code).

▶*Initial infusion:* For physician or other qualified health care professional reporting, an initial infusion is the *key or primary reason for the encounter* reported irrespective of the temporal order in which the infusion(s) or injection(s) are administered. For facility reporting, an initial infusion is based using the hierarchy. For both physician or other qualified health care professional and facility reporting, only one *initial* service code (eg, 96365) should be reported unless the protocol or patient condition requires that two separate IV sites must be utilized. The difference in time and effort in providing this second IV site access is also reported using the *initial* service code with modifier 59 appended (eg, 96365, 96365-59).◀

Sequential infusion: A sequential infusion is an infusion or IV push of a new substance or drug following a primary or initial service. All sequential services require that there be a new substance or drug, except that facilities may report a sequential intravenous push of the same drug using 96376.

Concurrent infusion: A concurrent infusion is an infusion of a new substance or drug infused at the same time as another substance or drug. A concurrent infusion service is not time based and is only reported once per day regardless of whether an additional new drug or substance is administered concurrently. Hydration may not be reported concurrently with any other service. A separate subsequent concurrent administration of another new drug or substance (the third substance or drug) is not reported.

▶In order to determine which service should be reported as the initial service when there is more than one type of service, hierarchies have been created. These vary by whether the physician or other qualified health care professional or a facility is reporting. The order of selection for reporting is based upon the physician's or other qualified health care professional's knowledge of the clinical condition(s) and treatment(s). The hierarchy that facilities are to use is based upon a structural algorithm. When these codes are reported by the physician or other qualified health care professional, the "initial" code that best describes the key or primary reason for the encounter should always be reported irrespective of the order in which the infusions or injections occur.◀

When these codes are reported *by the facility*, the following instructions apply. The initial code should be selected using a hierarchy whereby chemotherapy services are primary to therapeutic, prophylactic, and diagnostic services which are primary to hydration services. Infusions are primary to pushes, which are primary to injections. This hierarchy is to be followed by facilities and supersedes parenthetical instructions for add-on codes that suggest an add-on of a higher hierarchical position may be reported in conjunction with a base code of a lower position. (For example, the hierarchy would not permit reporting 96376 with 96360, as 96376 is a higher order code. IV push is primary to hydration.)

When reporting multiple infusions of the same drug/substance on the same date of service, the initial code should be selected. The second and subsequent infusion(s) should be reported based on the individual time(s) of each additional infusion(s) of the same drug/substance using the appropriate add-on code.

Example: In the outpatient observation setting, a patient receives one-hour intravenous infusions of the same antibiotic every 8 hours on the same date of service through the same IV access. The hierarchy for facility reporting permits the reporting of code 96365 for the first one-hour dose administered. Add-on 96366 would be reported twice (once for the second and third one-hour infusions of the same drug).

▶When reporting codes for which infusion time is a factor, use the actual time over which the infusion is administered. Intravenous or intra-arterial push is defined as: (a) an injection in which the health care professional who administers the drug/substance is continuously present to administer the injection and observe the patient, or (b) an infusion of 15 minutes or less. If intravenous hydration (96360, 96361) is given from 11 PM to 2 AM, 96360 would be reported once and 96361 twice. For continuous services that last beyond midnight, use the date in which the service began and report the total units of time provided continuously. However, if instead of a continuous infusion, a medication was given by intravenous push at 10 PM and 2 AM, as the service was not continuous, the two administrations would be reported as an initial service (96374) and sequential (96376) as: (1) no other infusion services were performed; and (2) the push of the same drug was performed more than 30 minutes beyond the initial administration. A "keep open" infusion of any type is not separately reported.◄

Hydration

►Codes 96360-96361 are intended to report a hydration IV infusion to consist of a pre-packaged fluid and electrolytes (eg, normal saline, D5-1/2 normal saline+30mEq KCl/liter), but are not used to report infusion of drugs or other substances. Hydration IV infusions typically require direct supervision for purposes of consent, safety oversight, or intraservice supervision of staff. Typically such infusions require little special handling to prepare or dispose of, and staff that administer these do not typically require advanced practice training. After initial set-up, infusion typically entails little patient risk and thus little monitoring. These codes are not intended to be reported by the physician or other qualified health care professional in the facility setting.◄

Some chemotherapeutic agents and other therapeutic agents require pre- and/or post-hydration to be given in order to avoid specific toxicities. A minimum time duration of 31 minutes of hydration infusion is required to report the service. However, the hydration codes 96360 or 96361 are not used when the purpose of the intravenous fluid is to "keep open" an IV line prior or subsequent to a therapeutic infusion, or as a free-flowing IV during chemotherapy or other therapeutic infusion.

96360   Intravenous infusion, hydration; initial, 31 minutes to 1 hour

➔ *CPT Assistant* May 10:8, May 11:7, Oct 11:3, Dec 11:3; *CPT Changes: An Insider's View* 2009

(Do not report 96360 if performed as a concurrent infusion service)

(Do not report intravenous infusion for hydration of 30 minutes or less)

+ 96361   each additional hour (List separately in addition to code for primary procedure)

➔ *CPT Assistant* May 10:8, May 11:7, Oct 11:3, Dec 11:3; *CPT Changes: An Insider's View* 2009

(Use 96361 in conjunction with 96360)

(Report 96361 for hydration infusion intervals of greater than 30 minutes beyond 1 hour increments)

(Report 96361 to identify hydration if provided as a secondary or subsequent service after a different initial service [96360, 96365, 96374, 96409, 96413] is administered through the same IV access)

Therapeutic, Prophylactic, and Diagnostic Injections and Infusions (Excludes Chemotherapy and Other Highly Complex Drug or Highly Complex Biologic Agent Administration)

►A therapeutic, prophylactic, or diagnostic IV infusion or injection (other than hydration) is for the administration of substances/drugs. When fluids are used to administer the drug(s), the administration of the fluid is considered incidental hydration and is not separately reportable. These services typically require direct supervision for any or all purposes of patient assessment, provision of consent, safety oversight, and intra-service supervision of staff. Typically, such infusions require special consideration to prepare, dose or dispose of, require practice training and competency for staff who administer the infusions, and require periodic patient assessment with vital sign monitoring during the infusion. These codes are not intended to be reported by the physician or other qualified health care professional in the facility setting.

See codes 96401-96549 for the administration of chemotherapy or other highly complex drug or highly complex biologic agent services. These highly complex services require advanced practice training and competency for staff who provide these services; special considerations for preparation, dosage or disposal; and commonly, these services entail significant patient risk and frequent monitoring. Examples are frequent changes in the infusion rate, prolonged presence of nurse administering the solution for patient monitoring and infusion adjustments, and frequent conferring with the physician or other qualified health care professional about these issues.◄

(Do not report 96365-96379 with codes for which IV push or infusion is an inherent part of the procedure [eg, administration of contrast material for a diagnostic imaging study])

───── *Coding Tip* ─────

Instructions for Reporting Medication Administration With Chemotherapy and Other Highly Complex Drug or Highly Complex Biologic Agent Administration

The administration of medications (eg, antibiotics, steroidal agents, antiemetics, narcotics, analgesics) administered independently or sequentially as supportive management of chemotherapy administration, should be separately reported using 96360, 96361, 96365, 96379 as appropriate.

CPT Coding Guidelines, Chemotherapy and Other Highly Complex Drug or Highly Complex Biologic Agent Administration

96365 Intravenous infusion, for therapy, prophylaxis, or diagnosis (specify substance or drug); initial, up to 1 hour

➔ *CPT Assistant* May 10:8, May 11:7, Oct 11:4, Dec 11:3; *CPT Changes: An Insider's View* 2009

➔ *Clinical Examples in Radiology* Spring 10:10

+ 96366 each additional hour (List separately in addition to code for primary procedure)

➔ *CPT Assistant* May 11:7, Dec 11:3; *CPT Changes: An Insider's View* 2009

(Report 96366 in conjunction with 96365, 96367)

(Report 96366 for additional hour[s] of sequential infusion)

(Report 96366 for infusion intervals of greater than 30 minutes beyond 1 hour increments)

(Report 96366 in conjunction with 96365 to identify each second and subsequent infusions of the same drug/substance)

+ 96367 additional sequential infusion of a new drug/substance, up to 1 hour (List separately in addition to code for primary procedure)

➔ *CPT Assistant* May 11:7, Dec 11:3; *CPT Changes: An Insider's View* 2009, 2012

(Report 96367 in conjunction with 96365, 96374, 96409, 96413 to identify the infusion of a new drug/substance provided as a secondary or subsequent service after a different initial service is administered through the same IV access. Report 96367 only once per sequential infusion of same infusate mix)

+ 96368 concurrent infusion (List separately in addition to code for primary procedure)

➔ *CPT Assistant* May 10:8, May 11:7, Dec 11:3; *CPT Changes: An Insider's View* 2009

(Report 96368 only once per date of service)

(Report 96368 in conjunction with 96365, 96366, 96413, 96415, 96416)

96369 Subcutaneous infusion for therapy or prophylaxis (specify substance or drug); initial, up to 1 hour, including pump set-up and establishment of subcutaneous infusion site(s)

➔ *CPT Assistant* May 11:7; *CPT Changes: An Insider's View* 2009

(For infusions of 15 minutes or less, use 96372)

+ 96370 each additional hour (List separately in addition to code for primary procedure)

➔ *CPT Assistant* May 11:7; *CPT Changes: An Insider's View* 2009

(Use 96370 in conjunction with 96369)

(Use 96370 for infusion intervals of greater than 30 minutes beyond 1 hour increments)

+ 96371 additional pump set-up with establishment of new subcutaneous infusion site(s) (List separately in addition to code for primary procedure)

➔ *CPT Assistant* May 11:7; *CPT Changes: An Insider's View* 2009

(Use 96371 in conjunction with 96369)

(Use 96369, 96371 only once per encounter)

96372 Therapeutic, prophylactic, or diagnostic injection (specify substance or drug); subcutaneous or intramuscular

➔ *CPT Assistant* May 10:9, May 11:7; *CPT Changes: An Insider's View* 2009

(For administration of vaccines/toxoids, see 96365, 96366, 90471, 90472)

(Report 96372 for non-antineoplastic hormonal therapy injections)

(Report 96401 for anti-neoplastic nonhormonal injection therapy)

(Report 96402 for anti-neoplastic hormonal injection therapy)

▶(Do not report 96372 for injections given without direct physician or other qualified health care professional supervision. To report, use 99211. Hospitals may report 96372 when the physician or other qualified health care professional is not present)◀

(96372 does not include injections for allergen immunotherapy. For allergen immunotherapy injections, see 95115-95117)

96373 intra-arterial

➔ *CPT Assistant* May 11:7; *CPT Changes: An Insider's View* 2009

96374 intravenous push, single or initial substance/drug

➔ *CPT Assistant* May 10:8, May 11:7, Oct 11:3, Dec 11:4; *CPT Changes: An Insider's View* 2009

➔ *Clinical Examples in Radiology* Spring 10:10

+ 96375 each additional sequential intravenous push of a new substance/drug (List separately in addition to code for primary procedure)

➔ *CPT Assistant* May 10:8, May 11:7; *CPT Changes: An Insider's View* 2009

(Use 96375 in conjunction with 96365, 96374, 96409, 96413)

(Report 96375 to identify intravenous push of a new substance/drug if provided as a secondary or subsequent service after a different initial service is administered through the same IV access)

+ 96376   each additional sequential intravenous push of the same substance/drug provided in a facility (List separately in addition to code for primary procedure)
→ *CPT Assistant* May 10:6, May 11:7, Dec 11:3; *CPT Changes: An Insider's View* 2009

(Do not report 96376 for a push performed within 30 minutes of a reported push of the same substance or drug)

(96376 may be reported by facilities only)

(Report 96376 in conjunction with 96365, 96374, 96409, 96413)

96379   Unlisted therapeutic, prophylactic, or diagnostic intravenous or intra-arterial injection or infusion
→ *CPT Assistant* May 11:7, Dec 11:19; *CPT Changes: An Insider's View* 2009

(For allergy immunology, see 95004 et seq)

Chemotherapy and Other Highly Complex Drug or Highly Complex Biologic Agent Administration

▶Chemotherapy administration codes 96401-96549 apply to parenteral administration of non-radionuclide anti-neoplastic drugs; and also to anti-neoplastic agents provided for treatment of noncancer diagnoses (eg, cyclophosphamide for auto-immune conditions) or to substances such as certain monoclonal antibody agents, and other biologic response modifiers. The highly complex infusion of chemotherapy or other drug or biologic agents requires physician or other qualified health care professional work and/or clinical staff monitoring well beyond that of therapeutic drug agents (96360-96379) because the incidence of severe adverse patient reactions are typically greater. These services can be provided by any physician or other qualified health care professional. Chemotherapy services are typically highly complex and require direct supervision for any or all purposes of patient assessment, provision of consent, safety oversight, and intraservice supervision of staff. Typically, such chemotherapy services require advanced practice training and competency for staff who provide these services; special considerations for preparation, dosage, or disposal; and commonly, these services entail significant patient risk and frequent monitoring. Examples are frequent changes in the infusion rate, prolonged presence of the nurse administering the solution for patient monitoring and infusion adjustments, and frequent conferring with the physician or other qualified health care professional about these issues. When performed to facilitate the infusion of injection, preparation of chemotherapy agent(s), highly complex agent(s), or other highly complex drugs is included and is not reported separately. To report infusions that do not require this level of complexity, see 96360-96379. Codes 96401-96402, 96409-96425, 96521-96523 are not intended to be reported by the individual physician or other qualified health care professional in the facility setting.◀

The term "chemotherapy" in 96401-96549 includes other highly complex drugs or highly complex biologic agents.

Report separate codes for each parenteral method of administration employed when chemotherapy is administered by different techniques. The administration of medications (eg, antibiotics, steroidal agents, antiemetics, narcotics, analgesics) administered independently or sequentially as supportive management of chemotherapy administration, should be separately reported using 96360, 96361, 96365, 96379 as appropriate.

Report both the specific service as well as code(s) for the specific substance(s) or drug(s) provided. The fluid used to administer the drug(s) is considered incidental hydration and is not separately reportable.

Regional (isolation) chemotherapy perfusion should be reported using the codes for arterial infusion (96420-96425). Placement of the intra-arterial catheter should be reported using the appropriate code from the **Cardiovascular Surgery** section. Placement of arterial and venous cannula(s) for extracorporeal circulation via a membrane oxygenator perfusion pump should be reported using 36823. Code 36823 includes dose calculation and administration of the chemotherapy agent by injection into the perfusate. Do not report 96409-96425 in conjunction with 36823.

(For home infusion services, see 99601-99602)

Injection and Intravenous Infusion Chemotherapy and Other Highly Complex Drug or Highly Complex Biologic Agent Administration

Intravenous or intra-arterial push is defined as: (a) an injection in which the healthcare professional who administers the substance/drug is continuously present to administer the injection and observe the patient, or (b) an infusion of 15 minutes or less.

96401   Chemotherapy administration, subcutaneous or intramuscular; non-hormonal anti-neoplastic
→ *CPT Assistant* Nov 05:1, Jan 06:47, Jan 07:30, May 07:3, Jun 07:4, Feb 09:17, Aug 11:9, Dec 11:3; *CPT Changes: An Insider's View* 2006

96402   hormonal anti-neoplastic
→ *CPT Assistant* Nov 05:1, Jan 07:30, May 07:3, Feb 09:17, Dec 11:3; *CPT Changes: An Insider's View* 2006

96405   Chemotherapy administration; intralesional, up to and including 7 lesions
→ *CPT Assistant* Sep 96:5, Aug 97:19, Feb 01:10, Jul 01:2, Nov 05:1, Jan 07:30, May 07:3, Feb 09:17; *CPT Changes: An Insider's View* 2006

Medicine

96406 intralesional, more than 7 lesions

➔ *CPT Assistant* Sep 96:5, Aug 97:19, Feb 01:10, Jul 01:2, Nov 05:1, Jan 07:30, May 07:3, Feb 09:17; *CPT Changes: An Insider's View* 2006

96409 intravenous, push technique, single or initial substance/drug

➔ *CPT Assistant* Nov 05:1, Jan 07:30, May 07:3, Feb 09:17, May 10:8, May 11:17, Dec 11:3; *CPT Changes: An Insider's View* 2006

+ 96411 intravenous, push technique, each additional substance/drug (List separately in addition to code for primary procedure)

➔ *CPT Assistant* Nov 05:1, Jan 07:30, May 07:3, Feb 09:17, Dec 11:3; *CPT Changes: An Insider's View* 2006

(Use 96411 in conjunction with 96409, 96413)

96413 Chemotherapy administration, intravenous infusion technique; up to 1 hour, single or initial substance/drug

➔ *CPT Assistant* Nov 05:1, Jan 07:30, May 07:3, Sep 07:3, Dec 07:15, Feb 09:17, May 10:8, May 11:7, Dec 11:4; *CPT Changes: An Insider's View* 2006

(Report 96361 to identify hydration if administered as a secondary or subsequent service in association with 96413 through the same IV access)

(Report 96366, 96367, 96375 to identify therapeutic, prophylactic, or diagnostic drug infusion or injection, if administered as a secondary or subsequent service in association with 96413 through the same IV access)

+ 96415 each additional hour (List separately in addition to code for primary procedure)

➔ *CPT Assistant* Nov 05:1, Jan 07:30, May 07:3, Sep 07:3, Dec 07:15, Feb 09:17, Dec 11:3; *CPT Changes: An Insider's View* 2006, 2007

(Use 96415 in conjunction with 96413)

(Report 96415 for infusion intervals of greater than 30 minutes beyond 1-hour increments)

96416 initiation of prolonged chemotherapy infusion (more than 8 hours), requiring use of a portable or implantable pump

➔ *CPT Assistant* Nov 05:1, Jan 07:30, May 07:3, Sep 07:3, Dec 07:15, Feb 09:17, Dec 11:3; *CPT Changes: An Insider's View* 2006

(For refilling and maintenance of a portable pump or an implantable infusion pump or reservoir for drug delivery, see 96521-96523)

+ 96417 each additional sequential infusion (different substance/drug), up to 1 hour (List separately in addition to code for primary procedure)

➔ *CPT Assistant* Nov 05:1, Jan 07:30, May 07:3, Jun 07:4, Feb 09:17, Aug 11:9, Dec 11:3; *CPT Changes: An Insider's View* 2006

(Use 96417 in conjunction with 96413)

(Report only once per sequential infusion. Report 96415 for additional hour(s) of sequential infusion)

Intra-Arterial Chemotherapy and Other Highly Complex Drug or Highly Complex Biologic Agent Administration

96420 Chemotherapy administration, intra-arterial; push technique

➔ *CPT Assistant* Aug 97:19, Nov 98:37, Nov 99:54, Feb 01:10, Jul 01:2, Nov 05:1, Jan 07:30, May 07:3, Jun 07:4, Feb 09:17, Aug 11:9, Dec 11:3

➔ *Clinical Examples in Radiology* Summer 08:1, 2, 4

96422 infusion technique, up to 1 hour

➔ *CPT Assistant* Dec 96:10, Aug 97:19, Nov 98:37, Feb 01:10, Jul 01:2, Nov 05:1, Jan 07:30, May 07:3, Dec 07:15, Feb 09:17, Aug 11:9, Dec 11:3

+ 96423 infusion technique, each additional hour (List separately in addition to code for primary procedure)

➔ *CPT Assistant* Dec 96:10, Nov 98:37, Feb 01:10, Jul 01:2, Nov 05:1, Jan 07:30, May 07:3, Dec 07:15, Feb 09:17, Dec 11:3; *CPT Changes: An Insider's View* 2006, 2007

(Use 96423 in conjunction with 96422)

(Report 96423 for infusion intervals of greater than 30 minutes beyond 1-hour increments)

(For regional chemotherapy perfusion via membrane oxygenator perfusion pump to an extremity, use 36823)

96425 infusion technique, initiation of prolonged infusion (more than 8 hours), requiring the use of a portable or implantable pump

➔ *CPT Assistant* Nov 99:54, Feb 01:10, Jul 01:2, Nov 05:1, Jan 07:30, May 07:3, Jun 07:4, Feb 09:17, Aug 11:9, Dec 11:3

(For refilling and maintenance of a portable pump or an implantable infusion pump or reservoir for drug delivery, see 96521-96523)

Other Injection and Infusion Services

▶Code 96523 does not require direct supervision. Codes 96521-96523 may be reported when these devices are used for therapeutic drugs other than chemotherapy.◀

(For collection of blood specimen from a completely implantable venous access device, use 36591)

96440 Chemotherapy administration into pleural cavity, requiring and including thoracentesis

➔ *CPT Assistant* Feb 01:10, Jul 01:2, Nov 05:1, Jan 07:30, May 07:3, Jun 07:4, Feb 09:17

(96445 has been deleted. To report intraperitoneal chemotherapy administration, use 96446)

96446 Chemotherapy administration into the peritoneal cavity via indwelling port or catheter

➔ *CPT Assistant* Oct 10:16, Dec 10:16; *CPT Changes: An Insider's View* 2011

96450 Chemotherapy administration, into CNS (eg, intrathecal), requiring and including spinal puncture

➔ *CPT Assistant* Feb 01:10, Jul 01:2, Nov 05:1, Jan 07:30, May 07:3, Feb 09:17; *CPT Changes: An Insider's View* 2002

➔ *Clinical Examples in Radiology* Spring 11:10

(For intravesical (bladder) chemotherapy administration, use 51720)

(For insertion of subarachnoid catheter and reservoir for infusion of drug, see 62350, 62351, 62360-62362; for insertion of intraventricular catheter and reservoir, see 61210, 61215)

96521 Refilling and maintenance of portable pump
➔ *CPT Assistant* Nov 05:1, Jan 07:30, May 07:3, Feb 09:17, Dec 11:3; *CPT Changes: An Insider's View* 2006

96522 Refilling and maintenance of implantable pump or reservoir for drug delivery, systemic (eg, intravenous, intra-arterial)
➔ *CPT Assistant* Jul 06:1, Jan 07:30, May 07:3, Feb 09:17, Dec 11:3; *CPT Changes: An Insider's View* 2006

(For refilling and maintenance of an implantable infusion pump for spinal or brain drug infusion, use 95990-95991)

96523 Irrigation of implanted venous access device for drug delivery systems
➔ *CPT Assistant* Jan 07:30, May 07:3, Feb 09:17, Jul 11:16, Dec 11:3; *CPT Changes: An Insider's View* 2006

(Do not report 96523 in conjunction with other services. To report collection of blood specimen, use 36591)

96542 Chemotherapy injection, subarachnoid or intraventricular via subcutaneous reservoir, single or multiple agents
➔ *CPT Assistant* Aug 97:19, Jul 01:2, Nov 05:1, Jan 07:30, May 07:3, Feb 09:17

(For radioactive isotope therapy, use 79005)

96549 Unlisted chemotherapy procedure
➔ *CPT Assistant* Aug 97:19, Jul 01:2, Nov 05:1, Jan 07:30, May 07:3, Jun 07:4, Oct 10:16, Dec 10:16

Photodynamic Therapy

(To report ocular photodynamic therapy, use 67221)

96567 Photodynamic therapy by external application of light to destroy premalignant and/or malignant lesions of the skin and adjacent mucosa (eg, lip) by activation of photosensitive drug(s), each phototherapy exposure session
➔ *CPT Assistant* Aug 03:15, Aug 09:7, Mar 10:10; *CPT Changes: An Insider's View* 2002

+ 96570 Photodynamic therapy by endoscopic application of light to ablate abnormal tissue via activation of photosensitive drug(s); first 30 minutes (List separately in addition to code for endoscopy or bronchoscopy procedures of lung and gastrointestinal tract)
➔ *CPT Assistant* Nov 99:54, Sep 00:5, Oct 11:11; *CPT Changes: An Insider's View* 2000, 2010

(Report 96570 with modifier 52 for service of less than 23 minutes with report)

+ 96571 each additional 15 minutes (List separately in addition to code for endoscopy or bronchoscopy procedures of lung and gastrointestinal tract)
➔ *CPT Assistant* Nov 99:54, Sep 00:5, Oct 11:11; *CPT Changes: An Insider's View* 2000, 2010

(For 23-37 minutes of service, use 96570. For 38-52 minutes of service, use 96570 in conjunction with 96571)

(96570, 96571 are to be used in addition to bronchoscopy, endoscopy codes)

(Use 96570, 96571 in conjunction with 31641, 43228 as appropriate)

Special Dermatological Procedures

▶See the **Evaluation and Management coding guidelines** for further instructions on reporting that is appropriate for management of dermatologic illnesses.◀

(For intralesional injections, see 11900, 11901)

(For Tzanck smear, see 88160-88161)

96900 Actinotherapy (ultraviolet light)
➔ *CPT Assistant* Jul 12:9

(For rhinophototherapy, intranasal application of ultraviolet and visible light, use 30999)

96902 Microscopic examination of hairs plucked or clipped by the examiner (excluding hair collected by the patient) to determine telogen and anagen counts, or structural hair shaft abnormality
➔ *CPT Assistant* Nov 97:46-47

96904 Whole body integumentary photography, for monitoring of high risk patients with dysplastic nevus syndrome or a history of dysplastic nevi, or patients with a personal or familial history of melanoma
➔ *CPT Changes: An Insider's View* 2007

96910 Photochemotherapy; tar and ultraviolet B (Goeckerman treatment) or petrolatum and ultraviolet B
➔ *CPT Assistant* Jul 12:9

96912 psoralens and ultraviolet A (PUVA)
➔ *CPT Assistant* Jul 12:9

96913 Photochemotherapy (Goeckerman and/or PUVA) for severe photoresponsive dermatoses requiring at least 4-8 hours of care under direct supervision of the physician (includes application of medication and dressings)

96920 Laser treatment for inflammatory skin disease (psoriasis); total area less than 250 sq cm
➔ *CPT Assistant* Oct 10:9, Jul 12:9; *CPT Changes: An Insider's View* 2003

96921 250 sq cm to 500 sq cm
➔ *CPT Assistant* Oct 10:9, Jul 12:9; *CPT Changes: An Insider's View* 2003

96922 over 500 sq cm
➔ *CPT Assistant* Oct 10:9, Jul 12:9; *CPT Changes: An Insider's View* 2003

(For laser destruction of premalignant lesions, see 17000-17004)

(For laser destruction of cutaneous vascular proliferative lesions, see 17106-17108)

(For laser destruction of benign lesions, see 17110-17111)

(For laser destruction of malignant lesions, see 17260-17286)

96999 Unlisted special dermatological service or procedure

➥ *CPT Assistant* Jul 12:9

Physical Medicine and Rehabilitation

Codes 97001-97755 should be used to report each distinct procedure performed. Do not append modifier 51 to 97001-97755.

▶The work of the physician or other qualified health care professional consists of face-to-face time with the patient (and caregiver, if applicable) delivering skilled services. For the purpose of determining the total time of a service, incremental intervals of treatment at the same visit may be accumulated.◀

(For muscle testing, range of joint motion, electromyography, see 95831 et seq)

(For biofeedback training by EMG, use 90901)

(For transcutaneous nerve stimulation (TNS), use 64550)

97001 Physical therapy evaluation

➥ *CPT Assistant* Nov 97:47, Feb 00:11, Sep 01:10, Oct 02:11, Dec 03:4, Feb 04:5, Apr 05:13, Aug 06:11, May 08:9

97002 Physical therapy re-evaluation

➥ *CPT Assistant* Nov 97:47, Feb 00:11, Sep 01:10, Oct 02:11, Dec 03:4, Feb 04:5, May 08:9

97003 Occupational therapy evaluation

➥ *CPT Assistant* Nov 97:47, Oct 02:11, Feb 04:5, Aug 06:11, May 08:9

97004 Occupational therapy re-evaluation

➥ *CPT Assistant* Nov 97:47, Oct 02:11, Feb 04:5, May 08:9

97005 Athletic training evaluation

➥ *CPT Assistant* Jun 02:9, Feb 04:5; *CPT Changes: An Insider's View* 2002

97006 Athletic training re-evaluation

➥ *CPT Assistant* Jun 02:9, Feb 04:5; *CPT Changes: An Insider's View* 2002

Modalities

Any physical agent applied to produce therapeutic changes to biologic tissue; includes but not limited to thermal, acoustic, light, mechanical, or electric energy.

Supervised

▶The application of a modality that does not require direct (one-on-one) patient contact.◀

97010 Application of a modality to 1 or more areas; hot or cold packs

➥ *CPT Assistant* Summer 95:5, Apr 96:11, Nov 97:47, Dec 98:1, Nov 01:5, Aug 02:11, Aug 06:11, Nov 09:10, Jun 10:8, Aug 10:13, Nov 10:8

97012 traction, mechanical

➥ *CPT Assistant* Summer 95:5, Apr 96:11, Nov 97:47, Dec 98:1, May 99:11, Nov 01:5, Aug 02:11, Dec 03:4, Oct 04:9, Jun 10:8, Aug 10:13, Nov 10:8

97014 electrical stimulation (unattended)

➥ *CPT Assistant* Summer 95:5, Apr 96:11, Nov 97:47, May 98:10, Nov 01:5, Jan 02:11, Apr 02:18, Aug 02:11, Dec 03:4, Nov 09:10, Jun 10:8, Aug 10:13, Nov 10:8, Aug 11:6

(For acupuncture with electrical stimulation, see 97813, 97814)

97016 vasopneumatic devices

➥ *CPT Assistant* Summer 95:6, Apr 96:11, Dec 98:1, Nov 01:5, Aug 02:11, May 05:14, Jun 10:8, Aug 10:13, Nov 10:8

97018 paraffin bath

➥ *CPT Assistant* Summer 95:6, Apr 96:11, Dec 98:1, Nov 01:5, Aug 02:11, Nov 09:10, Jun 10:8, Aug 10:13, Nov 10:8

97022 whirlpool

➥ *CPT Assistant* Summer 95:6, Apr 96:11, May 98:10, Dec 98:1, Nov 01:5, Aug 02:11, Nov 09:10, Jun 10:8, Aug 10:13, Nov 10:8

97024 diathermy (eg, microwave)

➥ *CPT Assistant* Summer 95:6, Apr 96:11, Dec 98:1, Nov 01:5, Aug 02:11, Nov 09:10, Jun 10:8, Aug 10:13, Nov 10:8; *CPT Changes: An Insider's View* 2006

97026 infrared

➥ *CPT Assistant* Summer 95:6, Apr 96:11, Dec 98:1, Nov 01:5, Aug 02:11, Nov 09:10, Feb 10:12, Jun 10:8, Aug 10:13, Nov 10:8

97028 ultraviolet

➥ *CPT Assistant* Summer 95:6, Apr 96:11, Dec 98:1, Nov 01:5, Aug 02:11, Nov 09:10, Jun 10:8, Aug 10:13, Nov 10:8

Constant Attendance

▶The application of a modality that requires direct (one-on-one) patient contact.◀

97032 Application of a modality to 1 or more areas; electrical stimulation (manual), each 15 minutes

➥ *CPT Assistant* Summer 95:6, Dec 98:1, Nov 01:5, Apr 02:18, Jul 04:14, Nov 09:10, Jun 10:8, Aug 10:13, Nov 10:8

(For transcutaneous electrical modulation pain reprocessing [TEMPR/scrambler therapy], use 0278T)

97033 iontophoresis, each 15 minutes

➥ *CPT Assistant* Summer 95:7, Dec 98:1, Nov 01:5, Nov 09:10, Jun 10:8, Aug 10:13, Nov 10:8

97034   contrast baths, each 15 minutes

> *CPT Assistant* Summer 95:7, Dec 98:1, Nov 01:5, Jun 10:8, Aug 10:13, Nov 10:8

97035   ultrasound, each 15 minutes

> *CPT Assistant* Summer 95:7, Sep 96:10, Dec 98:1, Nov 01:5, Nov 09:10, Jun 10:8, Aug 10:13, Nov 10:8

97036   Hubbard tank, each 15 minutes

> *CPT Assistant* Summer 95:7, Dec 98:1, Nov 01:5, Nov 09:10, Jun 10:8, Aug 10:13, Nov 10:8

97039   Unlisted modality (specify type and time if constant attendance)

> *CPT Assistant* Summer 95:7, May 98:10, Dec 98:1, Jan 00:10, Nov 01:5, May 05:14, Nov 09:10, Feb 10:12, Jun 10:8, Aug 10:13, Nov 10:8

Therapeutic Procedures

A manner of effecting change through the application of clinical skills and/or services that attempt to improve function.

►Physician or other qualified health care professional (ie, therapist) required to have direct (one-on-one) patient contact.◄

97110   Therapeutic procedure, 1 or more areas, each 15 minutes; therapeutic exercises to develop strength and endurance, range of motion and flexibility

> *CPT Assistant* Summer 95:7, Feb 97:10, Nov 98:37, Dec 99:11, Mar 05:11, Apr 05:14, Aug 05:11, Dec 05:8, Mar 06:15, Aug 06:11, May 08:13, Dec 09:15, May 10:9, Mar 12:9

97112   neuromuscular reeducation of movement, balance, coordination, kinesthetic sense, posture, and/or proprioception for sitting and/or standing activities

> *CPT Assistant* Summer 95:7, Feb 97:10, Apr 05:14, Aug 05:11, Mar 06:15, Aug 06:11, May 08:13, Oct 09:10, May 10:9, Mar 12:9; *CPT Changes: An Insider's View* 2002

97113   aquatic therapy with therapeutic exercises

> *CPT Assistant* Summer 95:7, Feb 97:10, Apr 05:14, Mar 06:15, Aug 06:11, Oct 09:10, May 10:9

97116   gait training (includes stair climbing)

> *CPT Assistant* Summer 95:8, Sep 96:7, Feb 97:10, Jun 03:3, Apr 05:14, Mar 06:15, Aug 06:11, Oct 09:10, May 10:9

(Use 96000-96003 to report comprehensive gait and motion analysis procedures)

97124   massage, including effleurage, petrissage and/or tapotement (stroking, compression, percussion)

> *CPT Assistant* Summer 95:8, May 96:10, Feb 97:10, Dec 99:7, Apr 05:14, May 05:14, Mar 06:15, Aug 06:11, Oct 09:10, May 10:9

(For myofascial release, use 97140)

97139   Unlisted therapeutic procedure (specify)

> *CPT Assistant* Summer 95:8, Feb 97:10, Apr 05:14, Aug 06:11

97140   Manual therapy techniques (eg, mobilization/manipulation, manual lymphatic drainage, manual traction), 1 or more regions, each 15 minutes

> *CPT Assistant* Nov 98:37, Feb 99:10, Mar 99:1, Jul 99:11, Aug 01:10, Dec 03:5, May 09:9, Oct 09:10

(Do not report 97140 in conjunction with 29581-29584)

97150   Therapeutic procedure(s), group (2 or more individuals)

> *CPT Assistant* Summer 95:8, Dec 96:10, Feb 97:10, Oct 99:10, Nov 99:54-55, Dec 99:11, Apr 05:14, Aug 06:11

(Report 97150 for each member of group)

►(Group therapy procedures involve constant attendance of the physician or other qualified health care professional [ie, therapist], but by definition do not require one-on-one patient contact by the same physician or other qualified health care professional)◄

(For manipulation under general anesthesia, see appropriate anatomic section in **Musculoskeletal System**)

(For osteopathic manipulative treatment [OMT], see 98925-98929)

▲ **97530**   Therapeutic activities, direct (one-on-one) patient contact (use of dynamic activities to improve functional performance), each 15 minutes

> *CPT Assistant* Summer 95:9, Dec 01:6, Apr 03:26, Jul 03:15, Aug 05:11, May 08:13; *CPT Changes: An Insider's View* 2013

▲ **97532**   Development of cognitive skills to improve attention, memory, problem solving (includes compensatory training), direct (one-on-one) patient contact, each 15 minutes

> *CPT Assistant* Dec 01:1; *CPT Changes: An Insider's View* 2001, 2013

▲ **97533**   Sensory integrative techniques to enhance sensory processing and promote adaptive responses to environmental demands, direct (one-on-one) patient contact, each 15 minutes

> *CPT Assistant* Dec 01:1; *CPT Changes: An Insider's View* 2001, 2013

▲ **97535**   Self-care/home management training (eg, activities of daily living (ADL) and compensatory training, meal preparation, safety procedures, and instructions in use of assistive technology devices/adaptive equipment) direct one-on-one contact, each 15 minutes

> *CPT Assistant* Sep 96:7, Apr 00:11, Dec 03:6; *CPT Changes: An Insider's View* 2002, 2013

▲ **97537**   Community/work reintegration training (eg, shopping, transportation, money management, avocational activities and/or work environment/modification analysis, work task analysis, use of assistive technology device/adaptive equipment), direct one-on-one contact, each 15 minutes

> *CPT Assistant* Sep 96:7, Dec 03:6; *CPT Changes: An Insider's View* 2004, 2013

(For wheelchair management/propulsion training, use 97542)

97542   Wheelchair management (eg, assessment, fitting, training), each 15 minutes

> *CPT Assistant* Sep 96:8; *CPT Changes: An Insider's View* 2006

97545   Work hardening/conditioning; initial 2 hours

Medicine

+ 97546   each additional hour (List separately in addition to code for primary procedure)

(Use 97546 in conjunction with 97545)

Active Wound Care Management

►Active wound care procedures are performed to remove devitalized and/or necrotic tissue and promote healing. Services require direct (one-on-one) contact with the patient.◄

(Do not report 97597-97602 in conjunction with 11042-11047 for the same wound)

(For debridement of burn wounds, see 16020-16030)

97597   Debridement (eg, high pressure waterjet with/without suction, sharp selective debridement with scissors, scalpel and forceps), open wound, (eg, fibrin, devitalized epidermis and/or dermis, exudate, debris, biofilm), including topical application(s), wound assessment, use of a whirlpool, when performed and instruction(s) for ongoing care, per session, total wound(s) surface area; first 20 sq cm or less

➔ *CPT Assistant* Jun 05:1, 10, Nov 09:10, Jun 10:8, Nov 10:9, May 11:3, Sep 11:11, Jan 12:8, Mar 12:3; *CPT Changes: An Insider's View* 2005, 2011

+ 97598   each additional 20 sq cm, or part thereof (List separately in addition to code for primary procedure)

➔ *CPT Assistant* Jun 05:1, 10, May 11:3, Sep 11:11, Jan 12:8, Mar 12:3; *CPT Changes: An Insider's View* 2005, 2011

(Use 97598 in conjunction with 97597)

97602   Removal of devitalized tissue from wound(s), non-selective debridement, without anesthesia (eg, wet-to-moist dressings, enzymatic, abrasion), including topical application(s), wound assessment, and instruction(s) for ongoing care, per session

➔ *CPT Assistant* May 02:5, Jun 05:1, 10, Sep 08:11, May 11:4, Aug 11:7, Jan 12:9, Mar 12:3; *CPT Changes: An Insider's View* 2001

97605   Negative pressure wound therapy (eg, vacuum assisted drainage collection), including topical application(s), wound assessment, and instruction(s) for ongoing care, per session; total wound(s) surface area less than or equal to 50 square centimeters

➔ *CPT Assistant* Apr 05:13, Jun 05:1, 10, May 11:4; *CPT Changes: An Insider's View* 2005

97606   total wound(s) surface area greater than 50 square centimeters

➔ *CPT Assistant* Apr 05:13, Jun 05:1, 10, May 11:4; *CPT Changes: An Insider's View* 2005

Tests and Measurements

Requires direct one-on-one patient contact.

►(For muscle testing, manual or electrical, joint range of motion, electromyography, or nerve velocity determination, see 95831-95857, 95860-95872, 95885-95887, 95907-95913)◄

97750   Physical performance test or measurement (eg, musculoskeletal, functional capacity), with written report, each 15 minutes

➔ *CPT Assistant* Summer 95:5, Feb 97:10, Aug 98:11, Mar 00:11, Nov 01:5, May 02:18, Apr 03:28, Dec 03:7, Feb 04:5, Feb 07:12, May 08:9

▲ 97755   Assistive technology assessment (eg, to restore, augment or compensate for existing function, optimize functional tasks and/or maximize environmental accessibility), direct one-on-one contact, with written report, each 15 minutes

➔ *CPT Changes: An Insider's View* 2004, 2013

(To report augmentative and alternative communication devices, see 92605, 92607)

Orthotic Management and Prosthetic Management

97760   Orthotic(s) management and training (including assessment and fitting when not otherwise reported), upper extremity(s), lower extremity(s) and/or trunk, each 15 minutes

➔ *CPT Assistant* Dec 05:8, 11, Feb 07:8; *CPT Changes: An Insider's View* 2006

(Code 97760 should not be reported with 97116 for the same extremity)

97761   Prosthetic training, upper and/or lower extremity(s), each 15 minutes

➔ *CPT Assistant* Dec 05:8, 11, Feb 07:8; *CPT Changes: An Insider's View* 2006

97762   Checkout for orthotic/prosthetic use, established patient, each 15 minutes

➔ *CPT Assistant* Dec 05:8, 11, Feb 07:8; *CPT Changes: An Insider's View* 2006

Other Procedures

(For extracorporeal shock wave musculoskeletal therapy, see Category III codes 0019T, 0101T, 0102T)

97799   Unlisted physical medicine/rehabilitation service or procedure

➔ *CPT Assistant* Summer 95:5, Oct 99:10

Medical Nutrition Therapy

97802   Medical nutrition therapy; initial assessment and intervention, individual, face-to-face with the patient, each 15 minutes

➔ *CPT Assistant* Apr 03:10, Nov 03:1, Feb 09:13; *CPT Changes: An Insider's View* 2001

97803   re-assessment and intervention, individual, face-to-face with the patient, each 15 minutes

➔ *CPT Assistant* Apr 03:10, Nov 03:1, Feb 09:13; *CPT Changes: An Insider's View* 2001

97804   group (2 or more individual(s)), each 30 minutes

➔ *CPT Assistant* Apr 03:10, Nov 03:1, Feb 09:13; *CPT Changes: An Insider's View* 2001

►(Physicians and other qualified health care professionals who may report evaluation and management services should use the appropriate Evaluation and Management codes)◄

Acupuncture

Acupuncture is reported based on 15-minute increments of personal (face-to-face) contact with the patient, not the duration of acupuncture needle(s) placement.

If no electrical stimulation is used during a 15-minute increment, use 97810, 97811. If electrical stimulation of any needle is used during a 15-minute increment, use 97813, 97814.

Only one code may be reported for each 15-minute increment. Use either 97810 or 97813 for the initial 15-minute increment. Only one initial code is reported per day.

►Evaluation and management services may be reported in addition to acupuncture procedures when performed by physicians or other health care professionals, who may report evaluation and management services, including new or established patient office or other outpatient services (99201-99215), hospital observation care (99217-99220, 99224-99226), hospital care (99221-99223, 99231-99233), office or other outpatient consultations (99241-99245), inpatient consultations (99251-99255), critical care services (99291, 99292), inpatient neonatal intensive care services and pediatric and neonatal critical care services (99466-99480), emergency department services (99281-99285), nursing facility services (99304-99318), domiciliary, rest home, or custodial care services (99324-99337), and home services (99341-99350) may be reported separately using modifier 25 if the patient's condition requires a significant, separately identifiable E/M service above and beyond the usual preservice and postservice work associated with the acupuncture services. The time of the E/M service is not included in the time of the acupuncture service.◄

97810   Acupuncture, 1 or more needles; without electrical stimulation, initial 15 minutes of personal one-on-one contact with the patient
> *CPT Assistant* Jan 05:16-17, Jun 05:5, Jun 06:20, Aug 06:4; *CPT Changes: An Insider's View* 2005

(Do not report 97810 in conjunction with 97813)

+ 97811   without electrical stimulation, each additional 15 minutes of personal one-on-one contact with the patient, with re-insertion of needle(s) (List separately in addition to code for primary procedure)
> *CPT Assistant* Jan 05:16, Jun 05:5, Aug 06:4; *CPT Changes: An Insider's View* 2005, 2006

(Use 97811 in conjunction with 97810, 97813)

Acupuncture, Needle
97810-97811

Acupuncture needle

97813   with electrical stimulation, initial 15 minutes of personal one-on-one contact with the patient
> *CPT Assistant* Jan 05:16-18, Jun 05:5, Jun 06:20, Aug 06:4; *CPT Changes: An Insider's View* 2005, 2006

(Do not report 97813 in conjunction with 97810)

+ 97814   with electrical stimulation, each additional 15 minutes of personal one-on-one contact with the patient, with re-insertion of needle(s) (List separately in addition to code for primary procedure)
> *CPT Assistant* Jan 05:16, Jun 05:5, Aug 06:4; *CPT Changes: An Insider's View* 2005, 2006

(Use 97814 in conjunction with 97810, 97813)

Osteopathic Manipulative Treatment

►Osteopathic manipulative treatment (OMT) is a form of manual treatment applied by a physician or other qualified health care professional to eliminate or alleviate somatic dysfunction and related disorders. This treatment may be accomplished by a variety of techniques.

Evaluation and management services including new or established patient office or other outpatient services (99201-99215), hospital observation care (99217-99220, 99224-99226), hospital care (99221-99223, 99231-99233), critical care services (99291, 99292), observation or inpatient care services (99234-99236), office or other outpatient consultations (99241-99245), emergency department services (99281-99285), nursing facility services (99304-99318), domiciliary, rest home, or custodial care services (99324-99337), and home services (99341-99350) may be reported separately using modifier 25 if the patient's condition requires a significant, separately identifiable E/M service above and beyond the usual preservice and postservice work associated with the procedure. The E/M service may be caused or prompted by the same symptoms or condition for which the OMT service was provided. As such, different diagnoses are not required for the reporting of the OMT and E/M service on the same date.◀

Body regions referred to are: head region; cervical region; thoracic region; lumbar region; sacral region; pelvic region; lower extremities; upper extremities; rib cage region; abdomen and viscera region.

98925 Osteopathic manipulative treatment (OMT); 1-2 body regions involved
➔ *CPT Assistant* May 96:10, Jan 97:8, 10, Jul 98:10, Aug 00.11, Dec 00:15, Oct 09:10

98926 3-4 body regions involved
➔ *CPT Assistant* May 96:10, Jan 97:8, Aug 00:11, Dec 00:15, Oct 09:10

98927 5-6 body regions involved
➔ *CPT Assistant* May 96:10, Jan 97:8, Aug 00:11, Dec 00:15, Oct 09:10

98928 7-8 body regions involved
➔ *CPT Assistant* May 96:10, Jan 97:8, Aug 00:11, Dec 00:15, Oct 09:10, Mar 12:14, May 12:14

98929 9-10 body regions involved
➔ *CPT Assistant* May 96:10, Jan 97:8, 10, Aug 00:11, Oct 09:10

Chiropractic Manipulative Treatment

Chiropractic manipulative treatment (CMT) is a form of manual treatment to influence joint and neurophysiological function. This treatment may be accomplished using a variety of techniques.

▶The chiropractic manipulative treatment codes include a pre-manipulation patient assessment. Additional evaluation and management services including office or other outpatient services (99201-99215), subsequent observation care (99224-99226), subsequent hospital care (99231-99233), office or other outpatient consultations (99241-99245), subsequent nursing facility services (99307-99310), domiciliary, rest home, or custodial care services (99324-99337), and home services (99341-99350) may be reported separately using modifier 25 if the patient's condition requires a significant, separately identifiable E/M service above and beyond the usual preservice and postservice work associated with the procedure. The E/M service may be caused or prompted by the same symptoms or condition for which the CMT service was provided. As such, different diagnoses are not required for the reporting of the CMT and E/M service on the same date.◀

For purposes of CMT, the five spinal regions referred to are: cervical region (includes atlanto-occipital joint);

thoracic region (includes costovertebral and costotransverse joints); lumbar region; sacral region; and pelvic (sacro-iliac joint) region. The five extraspinal regions referred to are: head (including temporomandibular joint, excluding atlanto-occipital) region; lower extremities; upper extremities; rib cage (excluding costotransverse and costovertebral joints) and abdomen.

98940 Chiropractic manipulative treatment (CMT); spinal, 1-2 regions
➔ *CPT Assistant* Jan 97:7, 11, Feb 99:10, Dec 00:15, Mar 06:15, Dec 07:16, 17, Oct 09:10, May 10:9

98941 spinal, 3-4 regions
➔ *CPT Assistant* Jan 97:7, 11, Mar 97:10, Feb 99:10, Dec 00:15, Mar 06:15, Dec 07:16, 17, Oct 09:10, May 10:9

98942 spinal, 5 regions
➔ *CPT Assistant* Jan 97:7, 11, Feb 99:10, Dec 00:15, Mar 06:15, Dec 07:16, 17, Oct 09:10, May 10:9

98943 extraspinal, 1 or more regions
➔ *CPT Assistant* Jan 97:7, 11, Mar 97:10, Feb 99:10, Dec 00:15, Mar 06:15, Dec 07:16, 17, Oct 09:10, May 10:9

Education and Training for Patient Self-Management

▶The following codes are used to report educational and training services prescribed by a physician or other qualified health care professional and provided by a qualified, nonphysician health care professional using a standardized curriculum to an individual or a group of patients for the treatment of established illness(s)/disease(s) or to delay comorbidity(s). Education and training for patient self-management may be reported with these codes only when using a standardized curriculum as described below. This curriculum may be modified as necessary for the clinical needs, cultural norms and health literacy of the individual patient(s).◀

The purpose of the educational and training services is to teach the patient (may include caregiver[s]) how to effectively self-manage the patient's illness(s)/disease(s) or delay disease comorbidity(s) in conjunction with the patient's professional healthcare team. Education and training related to subsequent reinforcement or due to changes in the patient's condition or treatment plan are reported in the same manner as the original education and training. The type of education and training provided for the patient's clinical condition will be identified by the appropriate diagnosis code(s) reported.

The qualifications of the nonphysician healthcare professionals and the content of the educational and training program must be consistent with guidelines or standards established or recognized by a physician society, nonphysician healthcare professional society/association, or other appropriate source.

►(For counseling and education provided by a physician to an individual, see the appropriate evaluation and management codes including office or other outpatient services [99201-99215], hospital observation care [99217-99220, 99224-99226], hospital care [99221-99223, 99231-99233], new or established patient office or other outpatient consultations [99241-99245], inpatient consultations [99251-99255], emergency department services [99281-99285], nursing facility services [99304-99318], domiciliary, rest home, or custodial care services [99324-99337], home services [99341-99350], and counseling risk factor reduction and behavior change intervention [99401-99429]. See also **Instructions for Use of the CPT Codebook** for definition of reporting qualifications).◄

(For counseling and education provided by a physician to a group, use 99078)

(For counseling and/or risk factor reduction intervention provided by a physician to patient[s] without symptoms or established disease, see 99401-99412)

(For medical nutrition therapy, see 97802-97804)

(For health and behavior assessment/intervention that is not part of a standardized curriculum, see 96150-96155)

(For education provided as genetic counseling services, use 96040. For education to a group regarding genetic risks, see 98961, 98962)

98960 Education and training for patient self-management by a qualified, nonphysician health care professional using a standardized curriculum, face-to-face with the patient (could include caregiver/family) each 30 minutes; individual patient

➔ *CPT Changes: An Insider's View* 2006

98961 2-4 patients

➔ *CPT Assistant* Aug 07.9, Aug 08:3, Feb 09:13; *CPT Changes: An Insider's View* 2006

98962 5-8 patients

➔ *CPT Assistant* Aug 07:9, Aug 08:3, Feb 09:13; *CPT Changes: An Insider's View* 2006

Non-Face-to-Face Nonphysician Services

Telephone Services

Telephone services are non-face-to-face assessment and management services provided by a qualified health care professional to a patient using the telephone. These codes are used to report episodes of care by the qualified health care professional initiated by an established patient or guardian of an established patient. If the telephone service ends with a decision to see the patient within 24 hours or the next available urgent visit appointment, the code is not reported; rather the encounter is considered part of the preservice work of the subsequent assessment and management service, procedure and visit. Likewise, if

the telephone call refers to a service performed and reported by the qualified health care professional within the previous seven days (either qualified health care professional requested or unsolicited patient follow-up) or within the postoperative period of the previously completed procedure, then the service(s) are considered part of that previous service or procedure. (Do not report 98966-98969 if reporting 98966-98969 performed in the previous seven days.)

(For telephone services provided by a physician, see 99441-99443)

98966 Telephone assessment and management service provided by a qualified nonphysician health care professional to an established patient, parent, or guardian not originating from a related assessment and management service provided within the previous 7 days nor leading to an assessment and management service or procedure within the next 24 hours or soonest available appointment; 5-10 minutes of medical discussion

➔ *CPT Changes: An Insider's View* 2008

98967 11-20 minutes of medical discussion

➔ *CPT Changes: An Insider's View* 2008

98968 21-30 minutes of medical discussion

➔ *CPT Changes: An Insider's View* 2008

►(Do not report 98966-98968 during the same month with 99487-99489)◄

►(Do not report 98966-98968 when performed during the service time of codes 99495, 99496)◄

On-line Medical Evaluation

An on-line electronic medical evaluation is a non-face-to-face assessment and management service by a qualified health care professional to a patient using Internet resources in response to a patient's on-line inquiry. Reportable services involve the qualified health care professional's personal timely response to the patient's inquiry and must involve permanent storage (electronic or hard copy) of the encounter. This service is reported only once for the same episode of care during a seven-day period, although multiple qualified health care professionals could report their exchange with the same patient. If the on-line medical evaluation refers to an assessment and management service previously performed and reported by the qualified health care professional within the previous seven days (either qualified health care professional requested or unsolicited patient follow-up) or within the postoperative period of the previously completed procedure, then the service(s) are considered covered by the previous assessment and management office service or procedure. A reportable service encompasses the sum of communication (eg, related telephone calls, prescription provision, laboratory orders) pertaining to the on-line patient encounter.

(For an on-line medical evaluation provided by a physician, use 99444)

Medicine

▲ **98969** Online assessment and management service provided by a qualified nonphysician health care professional to an established patient or guardian, not originating from a related assessment and management service provided within the previous 7 days, using the Internet or similar electronic communications network
➔ *CPT Changes: An Insider's View* 2008, 2013

(Do not report 98969 when using 99339-99340, 99374-99380 for the same communication[s])

(Do not report 98969 for anticoagulation management when reporting 99363, 99364)

▶(Do not report 98969 during the same month with 99487-99489)◀

▶(Do not report 98969 when performed during the service time of codes 99495, 99496)◀

Special Services, Procedures and Reports

▶The procedures with code numbers 99000 through 99091 provide the reporting physician or other qualified health care professional with the means of identifying the completion of special reports and services that are an adjunct to the basic services rendered. The specific number assigned indicates the special circumstances under which a basic procedure is performed.

Code 99091 should be reported no more than once in a 30-day period to include the physician or other qualified health care professional time involved with data accession, review and interpretation, modification of care plan as necessary (including communication to patient and/or caregiver), and associated documentation.◀

If the services described by 99091 are provided on the same day the patient presents for an E/M service, these services should be considered part of the E/M service and not separately reported.

Do not report 99091 if it occurs within 30 days of care plan oversight services 99374-99380. Do not report 99091 if other more specific CPT codes exist (eg, 93227, 93272 for cardiographic services; 95250 for continuous glucose monitoring). Do not report 99091 for transfer and interpretation of data from hospital or clinical laboratory computers.

Codes 99050-99060 are reported in addition to an associated basic service. Do not append modifier 51 to 99050-99060. Typically only a single adjunct code from among 99050-99060 would be reported per patient encounter. However, there may be circumstances in which reporting multiple adjunct codes per patient encounter may be appropriate.

Miscellaneous Services

▲ **99000** Handling and/or conveyance of specimen for transfer from the office to a laboratory
➔ *CPT Assistant* Winter 94:26, Feb 99:10, Oct 99:11, May 02:19, Aug 06:6, Sep 06:15, Jan 07:30; *CPT Changes: An Insider's View* 2013

▲ **99001** Handling and/or conveyance of specimen for transfer from the patient in other than an office to a laboratory (distance may be indicated)
➔ *CPT Assistant* Winter 94:26, May 02:19, Aug 06:6, Sep 06:15, Jan 07:30; *CPT Changes: An Insider's View* 2013

▲ **99002** Handling, conveyance, and/or any other service in connection with the implementation of an order involving devices (eg, designing, fitting, packaging, handling, delivery or mailing) when devices such as orthotics, protectives, prosthetics are fabricated by an outside laboratory or shop but which items have been designed, and are to be fitted and adjusted by the attending physician or other qualified health care professional
➔ *CPT Assistant* Winter 94:26, May 02:19, Aug 06:6, Sep 06:15, Jan 07:30; *CPT Changes: An Insider's View* 2013

(For routine collection of venous blood, use 36415)

99024 Postoperative follow-up visit, normally included in the surgical package, to indicate that an evaluation and management service was performed during a postoperative period for a reason(s) related to the original procedure
➔ *CPT Assistant* Winter 94:26, Sep 97:10, Aug 98:5, May 02:19, Nov 03:13, Aug 06:6, Sep 06:15, Jan 07:30; *CPT Changes: An Insider's View* 2004

(As a component of a surgical "package," see **Surgery Guidelines**)

99026 Hospital mandated on call service; in-hospital, each hour
➔ *CPT Assistant* Jun 03:10, Aug 06:6, Sep 06:15, Jan 07:30; *CPT Changes: An Insider's View* 2003

99027 out-of-hospital, each hour
➔ *CPT Assistant* Jun 03:10, Aug 06:6, Sep 06:15, Jan 07:30; *CPT Changes: An Insider's View* 2003

▶(For standby services requiring prolonged attendance, use 99360, as appropriate. Time spent performing separately reportable procedure(s) or service(s) should not be included in the time reported as mandated on-call service)◀

99050 Services provided in the office at times other than regularly scheduled office hours, or days when the office is normally closed (eg, holidays, Saturday or Sunday), in addition to basic service
➔ *CPT Assistant* Winter 94:27, May 02:19, Jun 03:10, May 06:18, Aug 06:6, Sep 06:15, Jan 07:30, Aug 10:9; *CPT Changes: An Insider's View* 2004, 2006

99051 Service(s) provided in the office during regularly scheduled evening, weekend, or holiday office hours, in addition to basic service
➔ *CPT Assistant* May 06:18, Aug 06:6, Sep 06:15, Jan 07:30, Aug 10:9; *CPT Changes: An Insider's View* 2006

99053　Service(s) provided between 10:00 PM and 8:00 AM at 24-hour facility, in addition to basic service
➔ *CPT Assistant* May 06:18, Aug 06:6, Sep 06:15, Jan 07:30; *CPT Changes: An Insider's View* 2006

99056　Service(s) typically provided in the office, provided out of the office at request of patient, in addition to basic service
➔ *CPT Assistant* Winter 94:27, May 02:19, May 06:18, Aug 06:6, Sep 06:15, Jan 07:30; *CPT Changes: An Insider's View* 2006

99058　Service(s) provided on an emergency basis in the office, which disrupts other scheduled office services, in addition to basic service
➔ *CPT Assistant* Winter 94:27, May 02:19, May 06:18, Aug 06:6, Sep 06:15, Jan 07:30, Aug 10:9; *CPT Changes: An Insider's View* 2006

99060　Service(s) provided on an emergency basis, out of the office, which disrupts other scheduled office services, in addition to basic service
➔ *CPT Assistant* May 06:18, Aug 06:6, Sep 06:15, Jan 07:30; *CPT Changes: An Insider's View* 2006

▲ **99070**　Supplies and materials (except spectacles), provided by the physician or other qualified health care professional over and above those usually included with the office visit or other services rendered (list drugs, trays, supplies, or materials provided)
➔ *CPT Assistant* Winter 94:28, May 98:10, Jun 99:10, Jun 00:11, Jul 01:2, May 02:19, Aug 02:11, Jun 05:1, Jul 06:1, Aug 06:6, Sep 06:15, Jan 07:30, 31, Feb 07:8, Sep 08:11, May 09:8, Sep 09:5, May 10:10, Jun 10:8, Sep 10:11, Apr 12:10; *CPT Changes: An Insider's View* 2013

(For supply of spectacles, use the appropriate supply codes)

▲ **99071**　Educational supplies, such as books, tapes, and pamphlets, for the patient's education at cost to physician or other qualified health care professional
➔ *CPT Assistant* Winter 94:28, May 02:19, Aug 06:6, Sep 06:15, Jan 07:30; *CPT Changes: An Insider's View* 2013

99075　Medical testimony
➔ *CPT Assistant* Winter 94:28, May 02:19, Aug 06:6, Sep 06:15, Jan 07:30

▲ **99078**　Physician or other qualified health care professional qualified by education, training, licensure/regulation (when applicable) educational services rendered to patients in a group setting (eg, prenatal, obesity, or diabetic instructions)
➔ *CPT Assistant* Winter 94:28, Jan 98:12, May 02:19, Aug 06:6, Sep 06:15, Jan 07:30, Aug 07:9; *CPT Changes: An Insider's View* 2013

99080　Special reports such as insurance forms, more than the information conveyed in the usual medical communications or standard reporting form
➔ *CPT Assistant* Winter 94:28, May 02:19, Aug 06:6, Sep 06:15, Jan 07:30

(Do not report 99080 in conjunction with 99455, 99456 for the completion of Workmen's Compensation forms)

99082　Unusual travel (eg, transportation and escort of patient)
➔ *CPT Assistant* May 02:19, Jan 03:24, Nov 03:14, Aug 06:6, Sep 06:15, Jan 07:30

99090　Analysis of clinical data stored in computers (eg, ECGs, blood pressures, hematologic data)
➔ *CPT Assistant* Winter 94:28, May 02:19, Jun 03:10, Aug 06:6, Sep 06:15, Jan 07:30, Feb 07:10, Jul 07:1, Apr 09:7; *CPT Changes: An Insider's View* 2002

►(For physician/or other qualified health care professional qualified by education, training, licensure/ regulation [when applicable] collection and interpretation of physiologic data stored/transmitted by patient/ caregiver, see 99091)◄

(Do not report 99090 if other more specific CPT codes exist, eg, 93227, 93272, 0206T for cardiographic services; 95250 for continuous glucose monitoring; 97750 for musculoskeletal function testing)

▲ **99091**　Collection and interpretation of physiologic data (eg, ECG, blood pressure, glucose monitoring) digitally stored and/or transmitted by the patient and/or caregiver to the physician or other qualified health care professional, qualified by education, training, licensure/regulation (when applicable) requiring a minimum of 30 minutes of time
➔ *CPT Assistant* May 02:19, Jun 03:10, Aug 06:6, Sep 06:15, Jan 07:30, Apr 09:7, Dec 09:6; *CPT Changes: An Insider's View* 2002, 2013

Qualifying Circumstances for Anesthesia

(For explanation of these services, see **Anesthesia Guidelines**)

+ **99100**　Anesthesia for patient of extreme age, younger than 1 year and older than 70 (List separately in addition to code for primary anesthesia procedure)
➔ *CPT Assistant* Apr 08:3

(For procedure performed on infants younger than 1 year of age at time of surgery, see 00326, 00561, 00834, 00836)

+ **99116**　Anesthesia complicated by utilization of total body hypothermia (List separately in addition to code for primary anesthesia procedure)
➔ *CPT Assistant* Apr 08:3

+ **99135**　Anesthesia complicated by utilization of controlled hypotension (List separately in addition to code for primary anesthesia procedure)
➔ *CPT Assistant* Apr 08:3

+ **99140**　Anesthesia complicated by emergency conditions (specify) (List separately in addition to code for primary anesthesia procedure)
➔ *CPT Assistant* Mar 01:10, Apr 08:3

(An emergency is defined as existing when delay in treatment of the patient would lead to a significant increase in the threat to life or body part)

Moderate (Conscious) Sedation

Moderate (conscious) sedation is a drug induced depression of consciousness during which patients respond purposefully to verbal commands, either alone or accompanied by light tactile stimulation. No interventions are required to maintain a patent airway, and spontaneous ventilation is adequate. Cardiovascular function is usually maintained.

Moderate sedation does not include minimal sedation (anxiolysis), deep sedation or monitored anesthesia care (00100-01999).

When providing moderate sedation, the following services are included and **not** reported separately:

- Assessment of the patient (not included in intraservice time);

- Establishment of IV access and fluids to maintain patency, when performed;

- Administration of agent(s);

- Maintenance of sedation;

- Monitoring of oxygen saturation, heart rate and blood pressure; and

- Recovery (not included in intraservice time).

Intraservice time starts with the administration of the sedation agent(s), requires continuous face-to-face attendance, and ends at the conclusion of personal contact by the physician providing the sedation.

Do not report 99143-99150 in conjunction with 94760-94762.

Do not report 99143-99145 in conjunction with codes listed in Appendix G. Do not report 99148-99150 in conjunction with codes listed in Appendix G when performed in the nonfacility setting.

►When a second physician or other qualified health care professional other than the health care professional performing the diagnostic or therapeutic services provides moderate sedation in the facility setting (eg, hospital, outpatient hospital/ambulatory surgery center, skilled nursing facility) for the procedures listed in Appendix G, the second physician or other qualified health care professional reports 99148-99150. However, for the circumstance in which these services are performed by the second physician or other qualified health care professional in the nonfacility setting (eg, office, freestanding imaging center), codes 99148-99150 are not reported. See also **Instructions for Use of the CPT Codebook** for definition of reporting qualifications.◄

⊘▲ **99143** Moderate sedation services (other than those services described by codes 00100-01999) provided by the same physician or other qualified health care professional performing the diagnostic or therapeutic service that the sedation supports, requiring the presence of an independent trained observer to assist in the monitoring of the patient's level of consciousness and physiological status; younger than 5 years of age, first 30 minutes intra-service time

➔ *CPT Assistant* Feb 06:9, May 06:19, 20, Feb 08:5, Nov 09:11, Dec 09:10, Oct 11:4; *CPT Changes: An Insider's View* 2006, 2013

➔ *Clinical Examples in Radiology* Winter 06:18, Winter 10:14, Summer 11:2

⊘▲ **99144** age 5 years or older, first 30 minutes intra-service time

➔ *CPT Assistant* Feb 06:9, May 06:19, 20, Feb 08:5, Nov 09:11, Dec 09:10, Jul 11:17, Oct 11:4, Jul 12:13; *CPT Changes: An Insider's View* 2006, 2013

➔ *Clinical Examples in Radiology* Summer 06:1-3, Winter 06:18, Fall 07:1, 2, Spring 08:1, 2, Summer 08:1, 2, Summer 10:1, Winter 10:14, Summer 11:1

+▲ **99145** each additional 15 minutes intra-service time (List separately in addition to code for primary service)

➔ *CPT Assistant* Feb 06:9, May 06:19, 20, Feb 08:5, Nov 09:11, Dec 09:10, Jul 11:17, Oct 11:4; *CPT Changes: An Insider's View* 2006, 2013

➔ *Clinical Examples in Radiology* Summer 06:1-3, Winter 06:18, Fall 07:1, 2, Spring 08:1, 2, Summer 08:1, 2, Summer 10:1, Winter 10:14, Summer 11:1

(Use 99145 in conjunction with 99143, 99144)

▲ **99148** Moderate sedation services (other than those services described by codes 00100-01999), provided by a physician or other qualified health care professional other than the health care professional performing the diagnostic or therapeutic service that the sedation supports; younger than 5 years of age, first 30 minutes intra-service time

➔ *CPT Assistant* Feb 06:9, May 06:19, 20, Nov 09:11, Dec 09:10, Oct 11:4; *CPT Changes: An Insider's View* 2006, 2008, 2013

➔ *Clinical Examples in Radiology* Winter 06:18, Winter 10:14, Summer 11:2

▲ **99149** age 5 years or older, first 30 minutes intra-service time

➔ *CPT Assistant* Feb 06:9, May 06:19, 20, Nov 09:11, Dec 09:10, Oct 11:4; *CPT Changes: An Insider's View* 2006, 2008, 2013

➔ *Clinical Examples in Radiology* Winter 06:18, Winter 10:14, Summer 11:2

+▲ **99150** each additional 15 minutes intra-service time (List separately in addition to code for primary service)

➔ *CPT Assistant* Feb 06:9, May 06:19, 20, Nov 09:11, Dec 09:10, Oct 11:4; *CPT Changes: An Insider's View* 2006, 2013

➔ *Clinical Examples in Radiology* Winter 06:18, Winter 10:14, Summer 11:2

(Use 99150 in conjunction with 99148, 99149)

Other Services and Procedures

99170   Anogenital examination with colposcopic magnification in childhood for suspected trauma

→ *CPT Assistant* Nov 99:55, Apr 06:1

(For conscious sedation, use 99143-99150)

99172   Visual function screening, automated or semi-automated bilateral quantitative determination of visual acuity, ocular alignment, color vision by pseudoisochromatic plates, and field of vision (may include all or some screening of the determination[s] for contrast sensitivity, vision under glare)

→ *CPT Assistant* Feb 01:7, Mar 05:1, 3; *CPT Changes: An Insider's View* 2001

(This service must employ graduated visual acuity stimuli that allow a quantitative determination of visual acuity [eg, Snellen chart]. This service may not be used in addition to a general ophthalmological service or an E/M service)

(Do not report 99172 in conjunction with 99173)

99173   Screening test of visual acuity, quantitative, bilateral

→ *CPT Assistant* Nov 99:55, May 02:2, Mar 05:1, 3; *CPT Changes: An Insider's View* 2000

(The screening test used must employ graduated visual acuity stimuli that allow a quantitative estimate of visual acuity [eg, Snellen chart]. Other identifiable services unrelated to this screening test provided at the same time may be reported separately [eg, preventive medicine services]. When acuity is measured as part of a general ophthalmological service or of an E/M service of the eye, it is a diagnostic examination and not a screening test.)

(Do not report 99173 in conjunction with 99172)

▲ **99174**   Instrument-based ocular screening (eg, photoscreening, automated-refraction), bilateral

→ *CPT Changes: An Insider's View* 2008, 2013

(Do not report 99174 in conjunction with 92002-92014, 99172, 99173)

99175   Ipecac or similar administration for individual emesis and continued observation until stomach adequately emptied of poison

(For diagnostic intubation, see 43754, 43755)

(For gastric lavage for diagnostic purposes, see 43754, 43755)

▲ **99183**   Physician or other qualified health care professional attendance and supervision of hyperbaric oxygen therapy, per session

→ *CPT Assistant* Jan 03:23; *CPT Changes: An Insider's View* 2013

(Evaluation and Management services and/or procedures [eg, wound debridement] provided in a hyperbaric oxygen treatment facility in conjunction with a hyperbaric oxygen therapy session should be reported separately)

(99185, 99186 have been deleted)

99190   Assembly and operation of pump with oxygenator or heat exchanger (with or without ECG and/or pressure monitoring); each hour

99191   45 minutes

99192   30 minutes

99195   Phlebotomy, therapeutic (separate procedure)

→ *CPT Assistant* Apr 96:3, Jun 96:10

99199   Unlisted special service, procedure or report

→ *CPT Assistant* Nov 99:55, Jun 12:16; *CPT Changes: An Insider's View* 2000

Home Health Procedures/ Services

These codes are used by non-physician health care professionals. Physicians should utilize the home visit codes 99341-99350 and utilize CPT codes other than 99500-99600 for any additional procedure/service provided to a patient living in a residence.

The following codes are used to report services provided in a patient's residence (including assisted living apartments, group homes, nontraditional private homes, custodial care facilities, or schools).

Health care professionals who are authorized to use Evaluation and Management (E/M) Home Visit codes (99341-99350) may report 99500-99600 in addition to 99341-99350 if both services are performed. E/M services may be reported separately, using modifier 25, if the patient's condition requires a significant separately identifiable E/M service, above and beyond the home health service(s)/procedure(s) codes 99500-99600.

99500   Home visit for prenatal monitoring and assessment to include fetal heart rate, non-stress test, uterine monitoring, and gestational diabetes monitoring

→ *CPT Assistant* Oct 03:7, Jan 07:30; *CPT Changes: An Insider's View* 2002

99501   Home visit for postnatal assessment and follow-up care

→ *CPT Assistant* Oct 03:7, Jan 07:30; *CPT Changes: An Insider's View* 2002

99502   Home visit for newborn care and assessment

→ *CPT Assistant* Oct 03:7, Jan 07:30; *CPT Changes: An Insider's View* 2002

99503   Home visit for respiratory therapy care (eg, bronchodilator, oxygen therapy, respiratory assessment, apnea evaluation)

→ *CPT Assistant* Oct 03:7, Jan 07:30; *CPT Changes: An Insider's View* 2002

99504   Home visit for mechanical ventilation care

→ *CPT Assistant* Oct 03:7, Jan 07:30; *CPT Changes: An Insider's View* 2002, 2003

99505   Home visit for stoma care and maintenance including colostomy and cystostomy

→ *CPT Assistant* Oct 03:7, Jan 07:30; *CPT Changes: An Insider's View* 2002

Medicine

99506   Home visit for intramuscular injections
>   *CPT Assistant* Oct 03:7, Jan 07:30; *CPT Changes: An Insider's View* 2002

99507   Home visit for care and maintenance of catheter(s) (eg, urinary, drainage, and enteral)
>   *CPT Assistant* Oct 03:7, Jan 07:30; *CPT Changes: An Insider's View* 2002

99509   Home visit for assistance with activities of daily living and personal care
>   *CPT Assistant* Oct 03:7, Jan 07:30; *CPT Changes: An Insider's View* 2002

(To report self-care/home management training, see 97535)

(To report home medical nutrition assessment and intervention services, see 97802-97804)

(To report home speech therapy services, see 92507-92508)

99510   Home visit for individual, family, or marriage counseling
>   *CPT Assistant* Oct 03:7, Jan 07:30; *CPT Changes: An Insider's View* 2002

99511   Home visit for fecal impaction management and enema administration
>   *CPT Assistant* Oct 03:7, Jan 07:30; *CPT Changes: An Insider's View* 2002

99512   Home visit for hemodialysis
>   *CPT Assistant* Oct 03:7, Jan 07:30; *CPT Changes: An Insider's View* 2002, 2004

(For home infusion of peritoneal dialysis, use 99601, 99602)

99600   Unlisted home visit service or procedure
>   *CPT Assistant* Oct 03:7, Jan 07:30; *CPT Changes: An Insider's View* 2003

Home Infusion Procedures/Services

99601   Home infusion/specialty drug administration, per visit (up to 2 hours);
>   *CPT Assistant* Nov 05:1; *CPT Changes: An Insider's View* 2004

＋ 99602   each additional hour (List separately in addition to code for primary procedure)
>   *CPT Assistant* Nov 05:1; *CPT Changes: An Insider's View* 2004

(Use 99602 in conjunction with 99601)

Medication Therapy Management Services

Medication therapy management service(s) (MTMS) describe face-to-face patient assessment and intervention as appropriate, by a pharmacist, upon request. MTMS is provided to optimize the response to medications or to manage treatment-related medication interactions or complications.

MTMS includes the following documented elements: review of the pertinent patient history, medication profile (prescription and nonprescription), and recommendations for improving health outcomes and treatment compliance. These codes are not to be used to describe the provision of product-specific information at the point of dispensing or any other routine dispensing-related activities.

99605   Medication therapy management service(s) provided by a pharmacist, individual, face-to-face with patient, with assessment and intervention if provided; initial 15 minutes, new patient
>   *CPT Changes: An Insider's View* 2008

99606   initial 15 minutes, established patient
>   *CPT Changes: An Insider's View* 2008

＋ 99607   each additional 15 minutes (List separately in addition to code for primary service)
>   *CPT Changes: An Insider's View* 2008

(Use 99607 in conjunction with 99605, 99606)

Category II Codes

The following section of *Current Procedural Terminology* (CPT) contains a set of supplemental tracking codes that can be used for performance measurement. It is anticipated that the use of Category II codes for performance measurement will decrease the need for record abstraction and chart review, and thereby minimize administrative burden on physicians, other health care professionals, hospitals, and entities seeking to measure the quality of patient care. These codes are intended to facilitate data collection about the quality of care rendered by coding certain services and test results that support nationally established performance measures and that have an evidence base as contributing to quality patient care.

The use of these codes is optional. The codes are not required for correct coding and may not be used as a substitute for Category I codes.

These codes describe clinical components that may be typically included in evaluation and management services or clinical services and, therefore, do not have a relative value associated with them. Category II codes may also describe results from clinical laboratory or radiology tests and other procedures, identified processes intended to address patient safety practices, or services reflecting compliance with state or federal law.

Category II codes described in this section make use of alphabetical characters as the 5th character in the string (ie, 4 digits followed by the letter **F**). These digits are not intended to reflect the placement of the code in the regular (Category I) part of the CPT codebook. To promote understanding of these codes and their associated measures, users are referred to the Alphabetical Clinical Topics Listing, which contains information about performance measurement exclusion modifiers, measures, and the measure's source.

Cross-references to the measures associated with each Category II code and their source are included for reference in the Alphabetical Clinical Topics Listing. In addition, acronyms for the related diseases or clinical condition(s) have been added at the end of each code descriptor to identify the topic or clinical category in which that code is included. A complete listing of the diseases/clinical conditions, and their acronyms are provided in alphabetical order in the Alphabetical Clinical Topics Listing. The Alphabetical Clinical Topics Listing can be accessed on the Web site at www.ama-assn. org, under the Category II link. Users should review the complete measure(s) associated with each code prior to implementation.

Category II codes are reviewed by the Performance Measures Advisory Group (PMAG), an advisory body to the CPT Editorial Panel and the CPT/HCPAC Advisory Committee. The PMAG is comprised of performance measurement experts representing the Agency for Healthcare Research and Quality (AHRQ), the American Medical Association (AMA), the Centers for Medicare and Medicaid Services (CMS), The Joint Commission (TJC), and the Physician Consortium for Performance Improvement® (PCPI). The PMAG may seek additional expertise and/or input from other national health care organizations, as necessary, for the development of tracking codes. These may include national medical specialty societies, other national health care professional associations, accrediting bodies, and federal regulatory agencies.

The most current listing of Category II codes, including guidelines, Code Change Proposal forms, and release and implementation dates for Category II codes may be accessed at http://www.ama-assn.org/go/cpt.

> (For blood pressure measured, use 2000F)
>
> (For tobacco use cessation intervention, pharmacologic therapy, use 4001F)

The superscripted numbers included at the end of each code descriptor direct users to the footnotes. The following information identifies the name and web address of the measure developers that are associated with these footnotes:

Footnotes

[1]Physician Consortium for Performance Improvement®(PCPI), www.physicianconsortium.org.

[2]National Committee on Quality Assurance (NCQA), Health Employer Data Information Set (HEDIS®), www.ncqa.org.

[3]Joint Commission on Accreditation of Healthcare Organizations (JCAHO), ORYX Initiative Performance Measures, www.jointcommission.org/performance_measurement.aspx.

[4]National Diabetes Quality Improvement Alliance (NDQIA),www.nationaldiabetesalliance.org

[5]Joint measure from The Physician Consortium for Performance Improvement, www.physician consortium.org and National Committee on Quality Assurance (NCQA), www.ncqa.org.

[6]The Society of Thoracic Surgeons at www.sts.org and National Quality Forum, www.qualityforum.org.

[7]Ingenix, www.ingenix.com.

[8]American Academy of Neurology, www.aan.com/go/practice/quality/measurements or quality@aan.com.

[9]College of American Pathologists (CAP), www.cap.org/apps/docs/advocacy/pathology performance measurement.pdf.

[10]American Gastroenterological Association (AGA), www.gastro.org/quality

Modifiers

The following performance measurement modifiers may be used for Category II codes to indicate that a service specified in the associated measure(s) was considered but, due to either medical, patient, or system circumstance(s) documented in the medical record, the service was not provided. These modifiers serve as denominator exclusions from the performance measure. The user should note that not all listed measures provide for exclusions (see Alphabetical Clinical Topics Listing for more discussion regarding exclusion criteria).

Category II modifiers should only be reported with Category II codes—they should not be reported with Category I or Category III codes. In addition, the modifiers in the Category II section should only be used where specified in the guidelines, reporting instructions, parenthetic notes, or code descriptor language listed in the Category II section (code listing and the Alphabetical Clinical Topics Listing).

1P   Performance Measure Exclusion Modifier due to Medical Reasons

Reasons include:

■ Not indicated (absence of organ/limb, already received/performed, other)

■ Contraindicated (patient allergic history, potential adverse drug interaction, other)

■ Other medical reasons

2P   Performance Measure Exclusion Modifier due to Patient Reasons

Reasons include:

■ Patient declined

■ Economic, social, or religious reasons

■ Other patient reasons

3P   Performance Measure Exclusion Modifier due to System Reasons

Reasons include:

■ Resources to perform the services not available

■ Insurance coverage/payor-related limitations

■ Other reasons attributable to health care delivery system

Modifier 8P is intended to be used as a "reporting modifier" to allow the reporting of circumstances when an action described in a measure's numerator is not performed and the reason is not otherwise specified.

8P   Performance measure reporting modifier–action not performed, reason not otherwise specified

Composite Codes

Composite codes combine several measures grouped within a single code descriptor to facilitate reporting for a clinical condition when all components are met. If only some of the components are met or if services are provided in addition to those included in the composite code, they may be reported individually using the corresponding CPT Category II codes for those services.

0001F   Heart failure assessed (includes assessment of all the following components) (CAD)[1]:

Blood pressure measured (2000F)[1]

Level of activity assessed (1003F)[1]

Clinical symptoms of volume overload (excess) assessed (1004F)[1]

Weight, recorded (2001F)[1]

Clinical signs of volume overload (excess) assessed (2002F)[1]

➔ *CPT Assistant* Oct 05:1; *CPT Changes: An Insider's View* 2006, 2007

(To report blood pressure measured, use 2000F)

0005F   Osteoarthritis assessed (OA)[1]

Includes assessment of all the following components:

Osteoarthritis symptoms and functional status assessed (1006F)[1]

Use of anti-inflammatory or over-the-counter (OTC) analgesic medications assessed (1007F)[1]

Initial examination of the involved joint(s) (includes visual inspection, palpation, range of motion) (2004F)[1]

➔ *CPT Assistant* Oct 05:1, 6; *CPT Changes: An Insider's View* 2006, 2007, 2009

(To report tobacco use cessation intervention, use 4001F)

0012F   Community-acquired bacterial pneumonia assessment (includes all of the following components) (CAP)[1]:

Co-morbid conditions assessed (1026F)[1]

Vital signs recorded (2010F)[1]

Mental status assessed (2014F)[1]

Hydration status assessed (2018F)[1]

➔ *CPT Changes: An Insider's View* 2007

0014F   Comprehensive preoperative assessment performed for cataract surgery with intraocular lens (IOL) placement (includes assessment of all of the following components) (EC)[5]:

Dilated fundus evaluation performed within 12 months prior to cataract surgery (2020F)[5]

Pre-surgical (cataract) axial length, corneal power measurement and method of intraocular lens power calculation documented (must be performed within 12 months prior to surgery) (3073F)[5]

Preoperative assessment of functional or medical indication(s) for surgery prior to the cataract surgery with intraocular lens placement (must be performed within 12 months prior to cataract surgery) (3325F)[5]

➔ *CPT Changes: An Insider's View* 2009

0015F   Melanoma follow up completed (includes assessment of all of the following components) (ML)[5]:

History obtained regarding new or changing moles (1050F)[5]

Complete physical skin exam performed (2029F)[5]

Patient counseled to perform a monthly self skin examination (5005F)[5]

➔ *CPT Changes: An Insider's View* 2009

Patient Management

Patient management codes describe utilization measures or measures of patient care provided for specific clinical purposes (eg, prenatal care, pre- and post-surgical care).

0500F   Initial prenatal care visit (report at first prenatal encounter with health care professional providing obstetrical care. Report also date of visit and, in a separate field, the date of the last menstrual period [LMP]) (Prenatal)[2]

➔ *CPT Assistant* Oct 05:1, 6, Aug 07:1; *CPT Changes: An Insider's View* 2005

0501F   Prenatal flow sheet documented in medical record by first prenatal visit (documentation includes at minimum blood pressure, weight, urine protein, uterine size, fetal heart tones, and estimated date of delivery). Report also: date of visit and, in a separate field, the date of the last menstrual period [LMP] (Note: If reporting 0501F Prenatal flow sheet, it is not necessary to report 0500F Initial prenatal care visit) (Prenatal)[1]

➔ *CPT Assistant* Oct 05:6; *CPT Changes: An Insider's View* 2005

0502F   Subsequent prenatal care visit (Prenatal)[2]

[Excludes: patients who are seen for a condition unrelated to pregnancy or prenatal care (eg, an upper respiratory infection; patients seen for consultation only, not for continuing care)]

➔ *CPT Assistant* Oct 05:6; *CPT Changes: An Insider's View* 2005, 2007

0503F   Postpartum care visit (Prenatal)[2]

➔ *CPT Assistant* Oct 05:6; *CPT Changes: An Insider's View* 2005

0505F   Hemodialysis plan of care documented (ESRD, P-ESRD)[1]

➔ *CPT Changes: An Insider's View* 2008

0507F   Peritoneal dialysis plan of care documented (ESRD)[1]

➔ *CPT Changes: An Insider's View* 2008

0509F   Urinary incontinence plan of care documented (GER)[5]

➔ *CPT Changes: An Insider's View* 2008

0513F   Elevated blood pressure plan of care documented (CKD)[1]

➔ *CPT Changes: An Insider's View* 2009

0514F   Plan of care for elevated hemoglobin level documented for patient receiving Erythropoiesis-Stimulating Agent therapy (ESA) (CKD)[1]

➔ *CPT Changes: An Insider's View* 2009

0516F   Anemia plan of care documented (ESRD)[1]

➔ *CPT Changes: An Insider's View* 2009

0517F   Glaucoma plan of care documented (EC)[5]

➔ *CPT Changes: An Insider's View* 2009

0518F   Falls plan of care documented (GER)[5]

➔ *CPT Changes: An Insider's View* 2009

0519F   Planned chemotherapy regimen, including at a minimum: drug(s) prescribed, dose, and duration, documented prior to initiation of a new treatment regimen (ONC)[1]

➔ *CPT Changes: An Insider's View* 2009, 2010

0520F   Radiation dose limits to normal tissues established prior to the initiation of a course of 3D conformal radiation for a minimum of 2 tissue/organ (ONC)[1]

➔ *CPT Changes: An Insider's View* 2009, 2010

0521F   Plan of care to address pain documented (COA)[2] (ONC)[1]

➔ *CPT Changes: An Insider's View* 2009, 2010

0525F   Initial visit for episode (BkP)[2]

➔ *CPT Changes: An Insider's View* 2009

0526F   Subsequent visit for episode (BkP)[2]

➔ *CPT Changes: An Insider's View* 2009

0528F   Recommended follow-up interval for repeat colonoscopy of at least 10 years documented in colonoscopy report (End/Polyp)[5]

➔ *CPT Changes: An Insider's View* 2010

0529F   Interval of 3 or more years since patient's last colonoscopy, documented (End/Polyp)[5]

➔ *CPT Changes: An Insider's View* 2010

0535F   Dyspnea management plan of care, documented (Pall Cr)[5]

➔ *CPT Changes: An Insider's View* 2010

0540F   Glucorticoid Management Plan Documented (RA)[5]

➔ *CPT Changes: An Insider's View* 2010

0545F   Plan for follow-up care for major depressive disorder, documented (MDD ADOL)[1]

➔ *CPT Changes: An Insider's View* 2011

0550F   Cytopathology report on routine nongynecologic specimen finalized within two working days of accession date (PATH)[9]

➔ *CPT Changes: An Insider's View* 2012

0551F   Cytopathology report on nongynecologic specimen with documentation that the specimen was non-routine (PATH)[9]

➔ *CPT Changes: An Insider's View* 2012

0555F   Symptom management plan of care documented (HF)[1]

➔ *CPT Changes: An Insider's View* 2012

0556F   Plan of care to achieve lipid control documented (CAD)[1]

➔ *CPT Changes: An Insider's View* 2012

Category II

0557F   Plan of care to manage anginal symptoms documented (CAD)[1]

> *CPT Changes: An Insider's View* 2012

0575F   HIV RNA control plan of care, documented (HIV)[5]

> *CPT Changes: An Insider's View* 2010

Patient History

Patient history codes describe measures for select aspects of patient history or review of systems.

1000F   Tobacco use assessed (CAD, CAP, COPD, PV)[1] (DM)[4]

> *CPT Assistant* Oct 05.1, 6, *CPT Changes: An Insider's View* 2005, 2007

1002F   Anginal symptoms and level of activity assessed (NMA–No Measure Associated)

> *CPT Assistant* Oct 05:6; *CPT Changes: An Insider's View* 2005

1003F   Level of activity assessed (NMA–No Measure Associated)

> *CPT Assistant* Oct 05:6; *CPT Changes: An Insider's View* 2006

1004F   Clinical symptoms of volume overload (excess) assessed (NMA–No Measure Associated)

> *CPT Assistant* Oct 05:6; *CPT Changes: An Insider's View* 2006

▲ **1005F**   Asthma symptoms evaluated (includes documentation of numeric frequency of symptoms or patient completion of an asthma assessment tool/survey/questionnaire) (NMA–No Measure Associated)

> *CPT Assistant* Oct 05:6; *CPT Changes: An Insider's View* 2006, 2013

1006F   Osteoarthritis symptoms and functional status assessed (may include the use of a standardized scale or the completion of an assessment questionnaire, such as the SF-36, AAOS Hip & Knee Questionnaire) (OA)[1]

[Instructions: Report when osteoarthritis is addressed during the patient encounter]

> *CPT Assistant* Oct 05:6; *CPT Changes: An Insider's View* 2006

1007F   Use of anti-inflammatory or analgesic over-the-counter (OTC) medications for symptom relief assessed (OA)[1]

> *CPT Assistant* Oct 05:6; *CPT Changes: An Insider's View* 2006

1008F   Gastrointestinal and renal risk factors assessed for patients on prescribed or OTC non-steroidal anti-inflammatory drug (NSAID) (OA)[1]

> *CPT Assistant* Oct 05:6; *CPT Changes: An Insider's View* 2006

1010F   Severity of angina assessed by level of activity (CAD)[1]

> *CPT Changes: An Insider's View* 2012

1011F   Angina present (CAD)[1]

> *CPT Changes: An Insider's View* 2012

1012F   Angina absent (CAD)[1]

> *CPT Changes: An Insider's View* 2012

1015F   Chronic obstructive pulmonary disease (COPD) symptoms assessed (Includes assessment of at least 1 of the following: dyspnea, cough/sputum, wheezing), or respiratory symptom assessment tool completed (COPD)[1]

> *CPT Changes: An Insider's View* 2007

1018F   Dyspnea assessed, not present (COPD)[1]

> *CPT Changes: An Insider's View* 2007

1019F   Dyspnea assessed, present (COPD)[1]

> *CPT Changes: An Insider's View* 2007

1022F   Pneumococcus immunization status assessed (CAP, COPD)[1]

> *CPT Changes: An Insider's View* 2007

1026F   Co-morbid conditions assessed (eg, includes assessment for presence or absence of: malignancy, liver disease, congestive heart failure, cerebrovascular disease, renal disease, chronic obstructive pulmonary disease, asthma, diabetes, other co-morbid conditions) (CAP)[1]

> *CPT Changes: An Insider's View* 2007

1030F   Influenza immunization status assessed (CAP)[1]

> *CPT Changes: An Insider's View* 2007

1031F   Smoking status and exposure to second hand smoke in the home assessed (Asthma)[1]

> *CPT Changes: An Insider's View* 2012

1032F   Current tobacco smoker **or** currently exposed to secondhand smoke (Asthma)[1]

> *CPT Changes: An Insider's View* 2012

1033F   Current tobacco non-smoker **and** not currently exposed to secondhand smoke (Asthma)[1]

> *CPT Changes: An Insider's View* 2012

1034F   Current tobacco smoker (CAD, CAP, COPD, PV)[1] (DM)[4]

> *CPT Changes: An Insider's View* 2007

1035F   Current smokeless tobacco user (eg, chew, snuff) (PV)[1]

> *CPT Changes: An Insider's View* 2007

1036F   Current tobacco non-user (CAD, CAP, COPD, PV)[1] (DM)[4] (IBD)[10]

> *CPT Changes: An Insider's View* 2007

1038F   Persistent asthma (mild, moderate or severe) (Asthma)[1]

> *CPT Assistant* Jul 10:3; *CPT Changes: An Insider's View* 2007

1039F   Intermittent asthma (Asthma)[1]

> *CPT Assistant* Jul 10:3; *CPT Changes: An Insider's View* 2007

1040F   DSM-IV™ criteria for major depressive disorder documented at the initial evaluation (MDD, MDD ADOL)[1]

> *CPT Changes: An Insider's View* 2008, 2009

1050F   History obtained regarding new or changing moles (ML)[5]

> *CPT Changes: An Insider's View* 2008

● **1052F**   Type, anatomic location, and activity all assessed (IBD)[10]

> *CPT Changes: An Insider's View* 2013

1055F   Visual functional status assessed (EC)[5]

> *CPT Changes: An Insider's View* 2008

1060F   Documentation of permanent **or** persistent **or** paroxysmal atrial fibrillation (STR)[5]

> *CPT Changes: An Insider's View* 2008

1061F   Documentation of absence of permanent **and** persistent **and** paroxysmal atrial fibrillation (STR)[5]

> *CPT Changes: An Insider's View* 2008

1065F   Ischemic stroke symptom onset of less than 3 hours prior to arrival (STR)[5]
➜ *CPT Changes: An Insider's View* 2008

1066F   Ischemic stroke symptom onset greater than or equal to 3 hours prior to arrival (STR)[5]
➜ *CPT Changes: An Insider's View* 2008

1070F   Alarm symptoms (involuntary weight loss, dysphagia, or gastrointestinal bleeding) assessed; none present (GERD)[5]
➜ *CPT Changes: An Insider's View* 2008

1071F   1 or more present (GERD)[5]
➜ *CPT Changes: An Insider's View* 2008

(1080F has been deleted. To report Surrogate decision maker or advance care plan documented in the medical record, report code 1123F or 1124F.)

1090F   Presence or absence of urinary incontinence assessed (GER)[5]
➜ *CPT Changes: An Insider's View* 2008

1091F   Urinary incontinence characterized (eg, frequency, volume, timing, type of symptoms, how bothersome) (GER)[5]
➜ *CPT Changes: An Insider's View* 2008

1100F   Patient screened for future fall risk; documentation of 2 or more falls in the past year or any fall with injury in the past year (GER)[5]
➜ *CPT Changes: An Insider's View* 2008

1101F   documentation of no falls in the past year or only 1 fall without injury in the past year (GER)[5]
➜ *CPT Changes: An Insider's View* 2008

1110F   Patient discharged from an inpatient facility (eg, hospital, skilled nursing facility, or rehabilitation facility) within the last 60 days (GER)[5]
➜ *CPT Changes: An Insider's View* 2008

1111F   Discharge medications reconciled with the current medication list in outpatient medical record (COA)[2] (GER)[5]
➜ *CPT Changes: An Insider's View* 2008

1116F   Auricular or periauricular pain assessed (AOE)[1]
➜ *CPT Changes: An Insider's View* 2009

1118F   GERD symptoms assessed after 12 months of therapy (GERD)[5]
➜ *CPT Changes: An Insider's View* 2009

1119F   Initial evaluation for condition (HEP C)[1] (EPI)[8]
➜ *CPT Changes: An Insider's View* 2009

1121F   Subsequent evaluation for condition (HEP C)[1] (EPI)[8]
➜ *CPT Changes: An Insider's View* 2009

1123F   Advance Care Planning discussed and documented advance care plan or surrogate decision maker documented in the medical record (DEM)[1] (GER, Pall Cr)[5]
➜ *CPT Changes: An Insider's View* 2009

1124F   Advance Care Planning discussed and documented in the medical record, patient did not wish or was not able to name a surrogate decision maker or provide an advance care plan (DEM)[1] (GER, Pall Cr)[5]
➜ *CPT Changes: An Insider's View* 2009, 2010

1125F   Pain severity quantified; pain present (COA)[2] (ONC)[1]
➜ *CPT Changes: An Insider's View* 2009

1126F   no pain present (COA)[2] (ONC)[1]
➜ *CPT Changes: An Insider's View* 2009, 2010

1127F   New episode for condition (NMA–No Measure Associated)
➜ *CPT Changes: An Insider's View* 2009, 2012

1128F   Subsequent episode for condition (NMA–No Measure Associated)
➜ *CPT Changes: An Insider's View* 2009, 2012

1130F   Back pain and function assessed, including all of the following: Pain assessment **and** functional status **and** patient history, including notation of presence or absence of "red flags" (warning signs) **and** assessment of prior treatment and response, **and** employment status (BkP)[2]
➜ *CPT Changes: An Insider's View* 2009

1134F   Episode of back pain lasting 6 weeks or less (BkP)[2]
➜ *CPT Changes: An Insider's View* 2009

1135F   Episode of back pain lasting longer than 6 weeks (BkP)[2]
➜ *CPT Changes: An Insider's View* 2009

1136F   Episode of back pain lasting 12 weeks or less (BkP)[2]
➜ *CPT Changes: An Insider's View* 2009

1137F   Episode of back pain lasting longer than 12 weeks (BkP)[2]
➜ *CPT Changes: An Insider's View* 2009

1150F   Documentation that a patient has a substantial risk of death within 1 year (Pall Cr)[5]
➜ *CPT Changes: An Insider's View* 2010

1151F   Documentation that a patient does not have a substantial risk of death within one year (Pall Cr)[5]
➜ *CPT Changes: An Insider's View* 2010

1152F   Documentation of advanced disease diagnosis, goals of care prioritize comfort (Pall Cr)[5]
➜ *CPT Changes: An Insider's View* 2010

1153F   Documentation of advanced disease diagnosis, goals of care do not prioritize comfort (Pall Cr)[5]
➜ *CPT Changes: An Insider's View* 2010

1157F   Advance care plan or similar legal document present in the medical record (COA)[2]
➜ *CPT Changes: An Insider's View* 2010

1158F   Advance care planning discussion documented in the medical record (COA)[2]
➜ *CPT Changes: An Insider's View* 2010

1159F   Medication list documented in medical record (COA)[2]
➜ *CPT Changes: An Insider's View* 2010

1160F   Review of all medications by a prescribing practitioner or clinical pharmacist (such as, prescriptions, OTCs, herbal therapies and supplements) documented in the medical record (COA)[2]
➜ *CPT Changes: An Insider's View* 2010

1170F   Functional status assessed (COA)[2] (RA)[5]
➜ *CPT Changes: An Insider's View* 2010

1175F   Functional status for dementia assessed and results reviewed (DEM)[1]
➜ *CPT Changes: An Insider's View* 2012

▲ =Revised code   ● =New code   ▶◀ =Contains new or revised text   ⊘ =Modifier 51 exempt

Category II

Category II

1180F All specified thromboembolic risk factors assessed (AFIB)[1]
➔ *CPT Changes: An Insider's View* 2010

1181F Neuropsychiatric symptoms assessed and results reviewed (DEM)[1]
➔ *CPT Changes: An Insider's View* 2012

1182F Neuropsychiatric symptoms, one or more present (DEM)[1]
➔ *CPT Changes: An Insider's View* 2012

1183F Neuropsychiatric symptoms, absent (DEM)[1]
➔ *CPT Changes: An Insider's View* 2012

1200F Seizure type(s) and current seizure frequency(ies) documented (EPI)[8]
➔ *CPT Changes: An Insider's View* 2011

1205F Etiology of epilepsy or epilepsy syndrome(s) reviewed and documented (EPI)[8]
➔ *CPT Changes: An Insider's View* 2011

1220F Patient screened for depression (SUD)[5]
➔ *CPT Changes: An Insider's View* 2010

1400F Parkinson's disease diagnosis reviewed (Prkns)[8]
➔ *CPT Changes: An Insider's View* 2011

1450F Symptoms improved or remained consistent with treatment goals since last assessment (HF)[1]
➔ *CPT Changes: An Insider's View* 2012

1451F Symptoms demonstrated clinically important deterioration since last assessment (HF)[1]
➔ *CPT Changes: An Insider's View* 2012

1460F Qualifying cardiac event/diagnosis in previous 12 months (CAD)[1]
➔ *CPT Changes: An Insider's View* 2012

1461F No qualifying cardiac event/diagnosis in previous 12 months (CAD)[1]
➔ *CPT Changes: An Insider's View* 2012

1490F Dementia severity classified, mild (DEM)[1]
➔ *CPT Changes: An Insider's View* 2012

1491F Dementia severity classified, moderate (DEM)[1]
➔ *CPT Changes: An Insider's View* 2012

1493F Dementia severity classified, severe (DEM)[1]
➔ *CPT Changes: An Insider's View* 2012

1494F Cognition assessed and reviewed (DEM)[1]
➔ *CPT Changes: An Insider's View* 2012

Physical Examination

Physical examination codes describe aspects of physical examination or clinical assessment.

2000F Blood pressure measured (CKD)[1] (DM)[2,4]
➔ *CPT Assistant* Oct 05:1, 6, Aug 07:1; *CPT Changes: An Insider's View* 2005, 2009

2001F Weight recorded (PAG)[1]
➔ *CPT Assistant* Oct 05:6; *CPT Changes: An Insider's View* 2006

2002F Clinical signs of volume overload (excess) assessed (NMA – No Measure Associated)
➔ *CPT Assistant* Oct 05:6; *CPT Changes: An Insider's View* 2006

2004F Initial examination of the involved joint(s) (includes visual inspection, palpation, range of motion) (OA)[1]

[Instructions: Report only for initial osteoarthritis visit or for visits for new joint involvement]
➔ *CPT Assistant* Oct 05:6; *CPT Changes: An Insider's View* 2006

2010F Vital signs (temperature, pulse, respiratory rate, and blood pressure) documented and reviewed (CAP)[1] (EM)[5]
➔ *CPT Changes: An Insider's View* 2007, 2008

2014F Mental status assessed (CAP)[1] (EM)[5]
➔ *CPT Changes: An Insider's View* 2007, 2008

2015F Asthma impairment assessed (Asthma)[1]
➔ *CPT Changes: An Insider's View* 2012

2016F Asthma risk assessed (Asthma)[1]
➔ *CPT Changes: An Insider's View* 2012

2018F Hydration status assessed (normal/mildly dehydrated/ severely dehydrated) (CAP)[1]
➔ *CPT Changes: An Insider's View* 2007

2019F Dilated macular exam performed, including documentation of the presence or absence of macular thickening or hemorrhage **and** the level of macular degeneration severity (EC)[5]
➔ *CPT Changes: An Insider's View* 2008

2020F Dilated fundus evaluation performed within 12 months prior to cataract surgery (EC)[5]
➔ *CPT Changes: An Insider's View* 2008, 2009

2021F Dilated macular or fundus exam performed, including documentation of the presence or absence of macular edema **and** level of severity of retinopathy (EC)[5]
➔ *CPT Changes: An Insider's View* 2008

2022F Dilated retinal eye exam with interpretation by an ophthalmologist or optometrist documented and reviewed (DM)[2,4]
➔ *CPT Changes: An Insider's View* 2007, 2009

2024F 7 standard field stereoscopic photos with interpretation by an ophthalmologist or optometrist documented and reviewed (DM)[2,4]
➔ *CPT Changes: An Insider's View* 2007, 2009

2026F Eye imaging validated to match diagnosis from 7 standard field stereoscopic photos results documented and reviewed (DM)[2,4]
➔ *CPT Changes: An Insider's View* 2007, 2009

2027F Optic nerve head evaluation performed (EC)[5]
➔ *CPT Changes: An Insider's View* 2008

2028F Foot examination performed (includes examination through visual inspection, sensory exam with monofilament, and pulse exam – report when any of the 3 components are completed) (DM)[4]
➔ *CPT Changes: An Insider's View* 2007

2029F Complete physical skin exam performed (ML)[5]
➔ *CPT Changes: An Insider's View* 2008

2030F   Hydration status documented, normally hydrated (PAG)[1]
> *CPT Changes: An Insider's View* 2008

2031F   Hydration status documented, dehydrated (PAG)[1]
> *CPT Changes: An Insider's View* 2008

2035F   Tympanic membrane mobility assessed with pneumatic otoscopy or tympanometry (OME)[1]
> *CPT Changes: An Insider's View* 2009

2040F   Physical examination on the date of the initial visit for low back pain performed, in accordance with specifications (BkP)[2]
> *CPT Changes: An Insider's View* 2009

2044F   Documentation of mental health assessment prior to intervention (back surgery or epidural steroid injection) or for back pain episode lasting longer than 6 weeks (BkP)[2]
> *CPT Changes: An Insider's View* 2009

2050F   Wound characteristics including size **and** nature of wound base tissue **and** amount of drainage prior to debridement documented (CWC)[5]
> *CPT Changes: An Insider's View* 2010

▲ **2060F**   Patient interviewed directly on or before date of diagnosis of major depressive disorder (MDD ADOL)[1]
> *CPT Changes: An Insider's View* 2011, 2013

Diagnostic/Screening Processes or Results

Diagnostic/screening processes or results codes describe results of tests ordered (clinical laboratory tests, radiological or other procedural examinations, and conclusions of medical decision-making).

> (To report blood pressure use the corresponding systolic codes [3074F, 3075F, 3077F] and diastolic codes [3078F, 3079F, 3080F])

3006F   Chest X-ray results documented and reviewed (CAP)[1]
> *CPT Assistant* Aug 07:1; *CPT Changes: An Insider's View* 2007

3008F   Body Mass Index (BMI), documented (PV)[1]
> *CPT Changes: An Insider's View* 2011

3011F   Lipid panel results documented and reviewed (must include total cholesterol, HDL-C, triglycerides and calculated LDL-C) (CAD)[1]
> *CPT Changes: An Insider's View* 2007

3014F   Screening mammography results documented and reviewed (PV)[1,2]
> *CPT Changes: An Insider's View* 2007, 2009

3015F   Cervical cancer screening results documented and reviewed (PV)[1]
> *CPT Changes: An Insider's View* 2011

3016F   Patient screened for unhealthy alcohol use using a systematic screening method (PV)[1]
> *CPT Changes: An Insider's View* 2010

3017F   Colorectal cancer screening results documented and reviewed (PV)[1,2]
> *CPT Changes: An Insider's View* 2009

3018F   Pre-procedure risk assessment **and** depth of insertion **and** quality of the bowel prep **and** complete description of polyp(s) found, including location of each polyp, size, number and gross morphology **and** recommendations for follow-up in final colonoscopy report documented (End/Polyp)[5]
> *CPT Changes: An Insider's View* 2010

3019F   Left ventricular ejection fraction (LVEF) assessment planned post discharge (HF)[1]
> *CPT Changes: An Insider's View* 2012

3020F   Left ventricular function (LVF) assessment (eg, echocardiography, nuclear test, or ventriculography) documented in the medical record (Includes quantitative or qualitative assessment results) (NMA – No Measure Associated)
> *CPT Changes: An Insider's View* 2007

3021F   Left ventricular ejection fraction (LVEF) less than 40% or documentation of moderately or severely depressed left ventricular systolic function (CAD, HF)[1]
> *CPT Changes: An Insider's View* 2007

3022F   Left ventricular ejection fraction (LVEF) greater than or equal to 40% or documentation as normal or mildly depressed left ventricular systolic function (CAD, HF)[1]
> *CPT Changes: An Insider's View* 2007

3023F   Spirometry results documented and reviewed (COPD)[1]
> *CPT Changes: An Insider's View* 2007

3025F   Spirometry test results demonstrate FEV_1/FVC less than 70% with COPD symptoms (eg, dyspnea, cough/sputum, wheezing) (CAP, COPD)[1]
> *CPT Changes: An Insider's View* 2007

3027F   Spirometry test results demonstrate FEV_1/FVC greater than or equal to 70% or patient does not have COPD symptoms (COPD)[1]
> *CPT Changes: An Insider's View* 2007

3028F   Oxygen saturation results documented and reviewed (includes assessment through pulse oximetry or arterial blood gas measurement) (CAP, COPD)[1] (EM)[5]
> *CPT Changes: An Insider's View* 2007

3035F   Oxygen saturation less than or equal to 88% or a PaO_2 less than or equal to 55 mm Hg (COPD)[1]
> *CPT Changes: An Insider's View* 2007

3037F   Oxygen saturation greater than 88% or PaO_2 greater than 55 mm Hg (COPD)[1]
> *CPT Changes: An Insider's View* 2007

3038F   Pulmonary function test performed within 12 months prior to surgery (Lung/Esop Cx)[6]
> *CPT Changes: An Insider's View* 2011

3040F   Functional expiratory volume (FEV_1) less than 40% of predicted value (COPD)[1]
> *CPT Changes: An Insider's View* 2007

Category II

3042F   Functional expiratory volume (FEV$_1$) greater than or equal to 40% of predicted value (COPD)[1]

→ *CPT Changes: An Insider's View* 2007

3044F   Most recent hemoglobin A1c (HbA1c) level less than 7.0% (DM)[2,4]

→ *CPT Changes: An Insider's View* 2008

3045F   Most recent hemoglobin A1c (HbA1c) level 7.0–9.0% (DM)[2,4]

→ *CPT Changes: An Insider's View* 2008, 2011

3046F   Most recent hemoglobin A1c level greater than 9.0% (DM)[4]

→ *CPT Changes: An Insider's View* 2007

(To report most recent hemoglobin A1c level less than or equal to 9.0%, see codes 3044F-3045F)

3048F   Most recent LDL-C less than 100 mg/dL (CAD)[1] (DM)[4]

→ *CPT Changes: An Insider's View* 2007

3049F   Most recent LDL-C 100-129 mg/dL (CAD)[1] (DM)[4]

→ *CPT Changes: An Insider's View* 2007

3050F   Most recent LDL-C greater than or equal to 130 mg/dL (CAD)[1] (DM)[4]

→ *CPT Changes: An Insider's View* 2007

3055F   Left ventricular ejection fraction (LVEF) less than or equal to 35% (HF)[1]

→ *CPT Changes: An Insider's View* 2012

3056F   Left ventricular ejection fraction (LVEF) greater than 35% or no LVEF result available (HF)[1]

→ *CPT Changes: An Insider's View* 2012

3060F   Positive microalbuminuria test result documented and reviewed (DM)[2,4]

→ *CPT Changes: An Insider's View* 2007

3061F   Negative microalbuminuria test result documented and reviewed (DM)[2,4]

→ *CPT Changes: An Insider's View* 2007

3062F   Positive macroalbuminuria test result documented and reviewed (DM)[2,4]

→ *CPT Changes: An Insider's View* 2007

3066F   Documentation of treatment for nephropathy (eg, patient receiving dialysis, patient being treated for ESRD, CRF, ARF, or renal insufficiency, any visit to a nephrologist) (DM)[2,4]

→ *CPT Changes: An Insider's View* 2007

3072F   Low risk for retinopathy (no evidence of retinopathy in the prior year) (DM)[2,4]

→ *CPT Changes: An Insider's View* 2007

3073F   Pre-surgical (cataract) axial length, corneal power measurement and method of intraocular lens power calculation documented within 12 months prior to surgery (EC)[5]

→ *CPT Changes: An Insider's View* 2008, 2009

3074F   Most recent systolic blood pressure less than 130 mm Hg (DM)[2,4] (HTN, CKD, CAD)[1]

→ *CPT Changes: An Insider's View* 2008

3075F   Most recent systolic blood pressure 130 - 139 mm Hg (DM)[2,4] (HTN, CKD, CAD)[1]

→ *CPT Changes: An Insider's View* 2008

(To report most recent systolic blood pressure less than 140 mm Hg, see codes 3074F-3075F)

3077F   Most recent systolic blood pressure greater than or equal to 140 mm Hg (HTN, CKD, CAD)[1] (DM)[2,4]

→ *CPT Changes: An Insider's View* 2007

3078F   Most recent diastolic blood pressure less than 80 mm Hg (HTN, CKD, CAD)[1] (DM)[2,4]

→ *CPT Changes: An Insider's View* 2007

3079F   Most recent diastolic blood pressure 80-89 mm Hg (HTN, CKD, CAD)[1] (DM)[2,4]

→ *CPT Changes: An Insider's View* 2007

3080F   Most recent diastolic blood pressure greater than or equal to 90 mm Hg (HTN, CKD, CAD)[1] (DM)[2,4]

→ *CPT Changes: An Insider's View* 2007, 2012

3082F   Kt/V less than 1.2 (Clearance of urea [Kt]/volume [V]) (ESRD, P-ESRD)[1]

→ *CPT Changes: An Insider's View* 2008

3083F   Kt/V equal to or greater than 1.2 and less than 1.7 (Clearance of urea [Kt]/volume [V]) (ESRD, P-ESRD)[1]

→ *CPT Changes: An Insider's View* 2008

3084F   Kt/V greater than or equal to 1.7 (Clearance of urea [Kt]/volume [V]) (ESRD, P-ESRD)[1]

→ *CPT Changes: An Insider's View* 2008

3085F   Suicide risk assessed (MDD, MDD ADOL)[1]

→ *CPT Changes: An Insider's View* 2008

3088F   Major depressive disorder, mild (MDD)[1]

→ *CPT Changes: An Insider's View* 2008

3089F   Major depressive disorder, moderate (MDD)[1]

→ *CPT Changes: An Insider's View* 2008

3090F   Major depressive disorder, severe without psychotic features (MDD)[1]

→ *CPT Changes: An Insider's View* 2008

3091F   Major depressive disorder, severe with psychotic features (MDD)[1]

→ *CPT Changes: An Insider's View* 2008

3092F   Major depressive disorder, in remission (MDD)[1]

→ *CPT Changes: An Insider's View* 2008

3093F   Documentation of new diagnosis of initial or recurrent episode of major depressive disorder (MDD)[1]

→ *CPT Changes: An Insider's View* 2008

3095F   Central dual-energy X-ray absorptiometry (DXA) results documented (OP)[5] (IBD)[10]

→ *CPT Changes: An Insider's View* 2008

3096F   Central dual-energy X-ray absorptiometry (DXA) ordered (OP)[5] (IBD)[10]

→ *CPT Changes: An Insider's View* 2008

Category II

3100F   Carotid imaging study report (includes direct or indirect reference to measurements of distal internal carotid diameter as the denominator for stenosis measurement) (STR, RAD)[5]

➔ *CPT Changes: An Insider's View* 2008

3110F   Documentation in final CT or MRI report of presence or absence of hemorrhage and mass lesion and acute infarction (STR)[5]

➔ *CPT Changes: An Insider's View* 2008, 2011

➔ *Clinical Examples in Radiology* Winter 08:6

3111F   CT or MRI of the brain performed in the hospital within 24 hours of arrival **or** performed in an outpatient imaging center, to confirm initial diagnosis of stroke, TIA or intracranial hemorrhage (STR)[5]

➔ *CPT Changes: An Insider's View* 2008, 2011, 2012

3112F   CT or MRI of the brain performed greater than 24 hours after arrival to the hospital **or** performed in an outpatient imaging center for purpose other than confirmation of initial diagnosis of stroke, TIA, or intracranial hemorrhage (STR)[5]

➔ *CPT Changes: An Insider's View* 2008, 2011, 2012

➔ *Clinical Examples in Radiology* Winter 08:6

3115F   Quantitative results of an evaluation of current level of activity and clinical symptoms (HF)[1]

➔ *CPT Changes: An Insider's View* 2012

3117F   Heart failure disease specific structured assessment tool completed (HF)[1]

➔ *CPT Changes: An Insider's View* 2012

3118F   New York Heart Association (NYHA) Class documented (HF)[1]

➔ *CPT Changes: An Insider's View* 2012

3119F   No evaluation of level of activity or clinical symptoms (HF)[1]

➔ *CPT Changes: An Insider's View* 2012

3120F   12-Lead ECG Performed (EM)[5]

➔ *CPT Changes: An Insider's View* 2008

3125F   Esophageal biopsy report with statement about dysplasia (present, absent, or indefinite) (PATH)[9]

➔ *CPT Changes: An Insider's View* 2012

3130F   Upper gastrointestinal endoscopy performed (GERD)[5]

➔ *CPT Changes: An Insider's View* 2008

3132F   Documentation of referral for upper gastrointestinal endoscopy (GERD)[5]

➔ *CPT Changes: An Insider's View* 2008

3140F   Upper gastrointestinal endoscopy report indicates suspicion of Barrett's esophagus (GERD)[5]

➔ *CPT Changes: An Insider's View* 2008

3141F   Upper gastrointestinal endoscopy report indicates no suspicion of Barrett's esophagus (GERD)[5]

➔ *CPT Changes: An Insider's View* 2008

3142F   Barium swallow test ordered (GERD)[1]

➔ *CPT Changes: An Insider's View* 2008

(To report documentation of barium swallow study, use code 3142F)

3150F   Forceps esophageal biopsy performed (GERD)[5]

➔ *CPT Changes: An Insider's View* 2008

3155F   Cytogenetic testing performed on bone marrow at time of diagnosis or prior to initiating treatment (HEM)[1]

➔ *CPT Changes: An Insider's View* 2008

3160F   Documentation of iron stores prior to initiating erythropoietin therapy (HEM)[1]

➔ *CPT Changes: An Insider's View* 2008

3170F   Flow cytometry studies performed at time of diagnosis or prior to initiating treatment (HEM)[1]

➔ *CPT Changes: An Insider's View* 2008

3200F   Barium swallow test not ordered (GERD)[5]

➔ *CPT Changes: An Insider's View* 2008

3210F   Group A Strep Test Performed (PHAR)[2]

➔ *CPT Changes: An Insider's View* 2008

3215F   Patient has documented immunity to Hepatitis A (HEP-C)[1]

➔ *CPT Changes: An Insider's View* 2009

3216F   Patient has documented immunity to Hepatitis B (HEP-C)[1] (IBD)[10]

➔ *CPT Changes: An Insider's View* 2009

(3217F has been deleted)

3218F   RNA testing for Hepatitis C documented as performed within 6 months prior to initiation of antiviral treatment for Hepatitis C (HEP-C)[1]

➔ *CPT Changes: An Insider's View* 2009

(3219F has been deleted)

3220F   Hepatitis C quantitative RNA testing documented as performed at 12 weeks from initiation of antiviral treatment (HEP-C)[1]

➔ *CPT Changes: An Insider's View* 2009

3230F   Documentation that hearing test was performed within 6 months prior to tympanostomy tube insertion (OME)[1]

➔ *CPT Changes: An Insider's View* 2009

3250F   Specimen site other than anatomic location of primary tumor (PATH)[1]

➔ *CPT Changes: An Insider's View* 2010

3260F   pT category (primary tumor), pN category (regional lymph nodes), and histologic grade documented in pathology report (PATH)[1]

➔ *CPT Changes: An Insider's View* 2009

3265F   Ribonucleic acid (RNA) testing for Hepatitis C viremia ordered or results documented (HEP C)[1]

➔ *CPT Changes: An Insider's View* 2009

3266F   Hepatitis C genotype testing documented as performed prior to initiation of antiviral treatment for Hepatitis C (HEP C)[1]

➔ *CPT Changes: An Insider's View* 2009

3267F   Pathology report includes pT category, pN category, Gleason score, and statement about margin status (PATH)[9]

➔ *CPT Changes: An Insider's View* 2012

▲=Revised code   ●=New code   ►◄=Contains new or revised text   ⊘=Modifier 51 exempt

Category II

3268F Prostate-specific antigen (PSA), **and** primary tumor (T) stage, **and** Gleason score documented prior to initiation of treatment (PRCA)[1]
→ *CPT Changes: An Insider's View* 2009

3269F Bone scan performed prior to initiation of treatment or at any time since diagnosis of prostate cancer (PRCA)[1]
→ *CPT Changes: An Insider's View* 2009

3270F Bone scan not performed prior to initiation of treatment nor at any time since diagnosis of prostate cancer (PRCA)[1]
→ *CPT Changes: An Insider's View* 2009

3271F Low risk of recurrence, prostate cancer (PRCA)[1]
→ *CPI Changes: An Insider's View* 2009

3272F Intermediate risk of recurrence, prostate cancer (PRCA)[1]
→ *CPT Changes: An Insider's View* 2009

3273F High risk of recurrence, prostate cancer (PRCA)[1]
→ *CPT Changes: An Insider's View* 2009

3274F Prostate cancer risk of recurrence not determined or neither low, intermediate nor high (PRCA)[1]
→ *CPT Changes: An Insider's View* 2009

3278F Serum levels of calcium, phosphorus, intact Parathyroid Hormone (PTH) and lipid profile ordered (CKD)[1]
→ *CPT Changes: An Insider's View* 2009

3279F Hemoglobin level greater than or equal to 13 g/dL (CKD, ESRD)[1]
→ *CPT Changes: An Insider's View* 2009

3280F Hemoglobin level 11 g/dL to 12.9 g/dL (CKD, ESRD)[1]
→ *CPT Changes: An Insider's View* 2009

3281F Hemoglobin level less than 11 g/dL (CKD, ESRD)[1]
→ *CPT Changes: An Insider's View* 2009

3284F Intraocular pressure (IOP) reduced by a value of greater than or equal to 15% from the pre-intervention level (EC)[5]
→ *CPT Changes: An Insider's View* 2009

3285F Intraocular pressure (IOP) reduced by a value less than 15% from the pre-intervention level (EC)[5]
→ *CPT Changes: An Insider's View* 2009

3288F Falls risk assessment documented (GER)[5]
→ *CPT Changes: An Insider's View* 2009

3290F Patient is D (Rh) negative and unsensitized (Pre-Cr)[1]
→ *CPT Changes: An Insider's View* 2009

3291F Patient is D (Rh) positive or sensitized (Pre-Cr)[1]
→ *CPT Changes: An Insider's View* 2009

3292F HIV testing ordered or documented and reviewed during the first or second prenatal visit (Pre-Cr)[1]
→ *CPT Changes: An Insider's View* 2009

3293F ABO and Rh blood typing documented as performed (Pre-Cr)[7]
→ *CPT Changes: An Insider's View* 2011

3294F Group B Streptococcus (GBS) screening documented as performed during week 35-37 gestation (Pre-Cr)[7]
→ *CPT Changes: An Insider's View* 2011

3300F American Joint Committee on Cancer (AJCC) stage documented and reviewed (ONC)[1]
→ *CPT Changes: An Insider's View* 2009

3301F Cancer stage documented in medical record as metastatic and reviewed (ONC)[1]
→ *CPT Changes: An Insider's View* 2009

(Codes 3302F-3312F have been deleted)

(To report measures for cancer staging, see 3321F-3390F)

3315F Estrogen receptor (ER) or progesterone receptor (PR) positive breast cancer (ONC)[1]
→ *CPT Changes: An Insider's View* 2009

3316F Estrogen receptor (ER) and progesterone receptor (PR) negative breast cancer (ONC)[1]
→ *CPT Changes: An Insider's View* 2009

3317F Pathology report confirming malignancy documented in the medical record and reviewed prior to the initiation of chemotherapy (ONC)[1]
→ *CPT Changes: An Insider's View* 2009

3318F Pathology report confirming malignancy documented in the medical record and reviewed prior to the initiation of radiation therapy (ONC)[1]
→ *CPT Changes: An Insider's View* 2009

3319F 1 of the following diagnostic imaging studies ordered: chest x-ray, CT, Ultrasound, MRI, PET, or nuclear medicine scans (ML)[5]
→ *CPT Changes: An Insider's View* 2009, 2010

3320F None of the following diagnostic imaging studies ordered: chest X-ray, CT, Ultrasound, MRI, PET, or nuclear medicine scans (ML)[5]
→ *CPT Changes: An Insider's View* 2009

3321F AJCC Cancer Stage 0 or IA Melanoma, documented (ML)[5]
→ *CPT Changes: An Insider's View* 2010

3322F Melanoma greater than AJCC Stage 0 or IA (ML)[5]
→ *CPT Changes: An Insider's View* 2010

3323F Clinical tumor, node and metastases (TNM) staging documented and reviewed prior to surgery (Lung/Esop Cx)[6]
→ *CPT Changes: An Insider's View* 2011

3324F MRI or CT scan ordered, reviewed or requested (EPI)[8]
→ *CPT Changes: An Insider's View* 2011

3325F Preoperative assessment of functional or medical indication(s) for surgery prior to the cataract surgery with intraocular lens placement (must be performed within 12 months prior to cataract surgery) (EC)[5]
→ *CPT Changes: An Insider's View* 2009

3328F Performance status documented and reviewed within 2 weeks prior to surgery (Lung/Esop Cx)[6]
→ *CPT Changes: An Insider's View* 2011

3330F Imaging study ordered (BkP)[2]
→ *CPT Changes: An Insider's View* 2009

3331F Imaging study not ordered (BkP)[2]
→ *CPT Changes: An Insider's View* 2009

3340F   Mammogram assessment category of "incomplete: need additional imaging evaluation" documented (RAD)[5]
➔ *CPT Changes: An Insider's View* 2009

3341F   Mammogram assessment category of "negative," documented (RAD)[5]
➔ *CPT Changes: An Insider's View* 2009

3342F   Mammogram assessment category of "benign," documented (RAD)[5]
➔ *CPT Changes: An Insider's View* 2009

3343F   Mammogram assessment category of "probably benign," documented (RAD)[5]
➔ *CPT Changes: An Insider's View* 2009

3344F   Mammogram assessment category of "suspicious," documented (RAD)[5]
➔ *CPT Changes: An Insider's View* 2009

3345F   Mammogram assessment category of "highly suggestive of malignancy," documented (RAD)[5]
➔ *CPT Changes: An Insider's View* 2009

3350F   Mammogram assessment category of "known biopsy proven malignancy," documented (RAD)[5]
➔ *CPT Changes: An Insider's View* 2009

3351F   Negative screen for depressive symptoms as categorized by using a standardized depression screening/ assessment tool (MDD)[2]
➔ *CPT Changes: An Insider's View* 2009

3352F   No significant depressive symptoms as categorized by using a standardized depression assessment tool (MDD)[2]
➔ *CPT Changes: An Insider's View* 2009

3353F   Mild to moderate depressive symptoms as categorized by using a standardized depression screening/assessment tool (MDD)[2]
➔ *CPT Changes: An Insider's View* 2009

3354F   Clinically significant depressive symptoms as categorized by using a standardized depression screening/ assessment tool (MDD)[2]
➔ *CPT Changes: An Insider's View* 2009

3370F   AJCC Breast Cancer Stage 0 documented (ONC)[1]
➔ *CPT Changes: An Insider's View* 2010

3372F   AJCC Breast Cancer Stage I: T1mic, T1a or T1b (tumor size ≤ 1 cm) documented (ONC)[1]
➔ *CPT Changes: An Insider's View* 2010

3374F   AJCC Breast Cancer Stage I: T1c (tumor size > 1 cm to 2 cm) documented (ONC)[1]
➔ *CPT Changes: An Insider's View* 2010

3376F   AJCC Breast Cancer Stage II documented (ONC)[1]
➔ *CPT Changes: An Insider's View* 2010

3378F   AJCC Breast Cancer Stage III documented (ONC)[1]
➔ *CPT Changes: An Insider's View* 2010

3380F   AJCC Breast Cancer Stage IV documented (ONC)[1]
➔ *CPT Changes: An Insider's View* 2010

3382F   AJCC colon cancer, Stage 0 documented (ONC)[1]
➔ *CPT Changes: An Insider's View* 2010

3384F   AJCC colon cancer, Stage I documented (ONC)[1]
➔ *CPT Changes: An Insider's View* 2010

3386F   AJCC colon cancer, Stage II documented (ONC)[1]
➔ *CPT Changes: An Insider's View* 2010

3388F   AJCC colon cancer, Stage III documented (ONC)[1]
➔ *CPT Changes: An Insider's View* 2010

3390F   AJCC colon cancer, Stage IV documented (ONC)[1]
➔ *CPT Changes: An Insider's View* 2010

3394F   Quantitative HER2 immunohistochemistry (IHC) evaluation of breast cancer consistent with the scoring system defined in the ASCO/CAP guidelines (PATH)[9]
➔ *CPT Changes: An Insider's View* 2012

3395F   Quantitative non-HER2 immunohistochemistry (IHC) evaluation of breast cancer (eg, testing for estrogen or progesterone receptors [ER/PR]) performed (PATH)[9]
➔ *CPT Changes: An Insider's View* 2012

3450F   Dyspnea screened, no dyspnea or mild dyspnea (Pall Cr)[5]
➔ *CPT Changes: An Insider's View* 2010

3451F   Dyspnea screened, moderate or severe dyspnea (Pall Cr)[5]
➔ *CPT Changes: An Insider's View* 2010

3452F   Dyspnea not screened (Pall Cr)[5]
➔ *CPT Changes: An Insider's View* 2010

3455F   TB screening performed and results interpreted within six months prior to initiation of first-time biologic disease modifying anti-rheumatic drug therapy for RA (RA)[5]
➔ *CPT Changes: An Insider's View* 2010

3470F   Rheumatoid arthritis (RA) disease activity, low (RA)[5]
➔ *CPT Changes: An Insider's View* 2010

3471F   Rheumatoid arthritis (RA) disease activity, moderate (RA)[5]
➔ *CPT Changes: An Insider's View* 2010

3472F   Rheumatoid arthritis (RA) disease activity, high (RA)[5]
➔ *CPT Changes: An Insider's View* 2010

3475F   Disease prognosis for rheumatoid arthritis assessed, poor prognosis documented (RA)[5]
➔ *CPT Changes: An Insider's View* 2010

3476F   Disease prognosis for rheumatoid arthritis assessed, good prognosis documented (RA)[5]
➔ *CPT Changes: An Insider's View* 2010

3490F   History of AIDS-defining condition (HIV)[5]
➔ *CPT Changes: An Insider's View* 2010

3491F   HIV indeterminate (infants of undetermined HIV status born of HIV-infected mothers) (HIV)[5]
➔ *CPT Changes: An Insider's View* 2010

3492F   History of nadir CD4+ cell count < 350 cells/mm^3 (HIV)[5]
➔ *CPT Changes: An Insider's View* 2010

3493F   No history of nadir CD4+ cell count < 350 cells/mm^3 **and** no history of AIDS-defining condition (HIV)[5]
➔ *CPT Changes: An Insider's View* 2010

3494F   CD4+ cell count < 200 cells/mm^3 (HIV)[5]
➔ *CPT Changes: An Insider's View* 2010

Category II

Category II

3495F   CD4+ cell count 200 – 499 cells/mm^3 (HIV)[5]
→ *CPT Changes: An Insider's View* 2010

3496F   CD4+ cell count ≥ 500 cells/mm^3 (HIV)[5]
→ *CPT Changes: An Insider's View* 2010

3497F   CD4+ cell percentage < 15% (HIV)[5]
→ *CPT Changes: An Insider's View* 2010

3498F   CD4+ cell percentage ≥ 15% (HIV)[5]
→ *CPT Changes: An Insider's View* 2010

3500F   CD4+ cell count or CD4+ cell percentage documented as performed (HIV)[5]
→ *CPT Changes: An Insider's View* 2010

3502F   HIV RNA viral load below limits of quantification (HIV)[5]
→ *CPT Changes: An Insider's View* 2010

3503F   HIV RNA viral load not below limits of quantification (HIV)[5]
→ *CPT Changes: An Insider's View* 2010

3510F   Documentation that tuberculosis (TB) screening test performed and results interpreted (HIV)[5] (IBD)[10]
→ *CPT Changes: An Insider's View* 2010

3511F   Chlamydia and gonorrhea screenings documented as performed (HIV)[5]
→ *CPT Changes: An Insider's View* 2010

3512F   Syphilis screening documented as performed (HIV)[5]
→ *CPT Changes: An Insider's View* 2010

3513F   Hepatitis B screening documented as performed (HIV)[5]
→ *CPT Changes: An Insider's View* 2010

3514F   Hepatitis C screening documented as performed (HIV)[5]
→ *CPT Changes: An Insider's View* 2010

3515F   Patient has documented immunity to Hepatitis C (HIV)[5]
→ *CPT Changes: An Insider's View* 2010

● **3517F**   Hepatitis B Virus (HBV) status assessed and results interpreted within one year prior to receiving a first course of anti-TNF (tumor necrosis factor) therapy (IBD)[10]
→ *CPT Changes: An Insider's View* 2013

● **3520F**   Clostridium difficile testing performed (IBD)[10]
→ *CPT Changes: An Insider's View* 2013

3550F   Low risk for thromboembolism (AFIB)[1]
→ *CPT Changes: An Insider's View* 2010

3551F   Intermediate risk for thromboembolism (AFIB)[1]
→ *CPT Changes: An Insider's View* 2010

3552F   High risk for thromboembolism (AFIB)[1]
→ *CPT Changes: An Insider's View* 2010

3555F   Patient had International Normalized Ratio (INR) measurement performed (AFIB)[1]
→ *CPT Changes: An Insider's View* 2010

3570F   Final report for bone scintigraphy study includes correlation with existing relevant imaging studies (eg, x-ray, MRI, CT) corresponding to the same anatomical region in question (NUC_MED)[1]
→ *CPT Changes: An Insider's View* 2010

3572F   Patient considered to be potentially at risk for fracture in a weight-bearing site (NUC_MED)[1]
→ *CPT Changes: An Insider's View* 2010

3573F   Patient not considered to be potentially at risk for fracture in a weight-bearing site (NUC_MED)[1]
→ *CPT Changes: An Insider's View* 2010

3650F   Electroencephalogram (EEG) ordered, reviewed or requested (EPI)[8]
→ *CPT Changes: An Insider's View* 2011

3700F   Psychiatric disorders or disturbances assessed (Prkns)[8]
→ *CPT Changes: An Insider's View* 2011

3720F   Cognitive impairment or dysfunction assessed (Prkns)[8]
→ *CPT Changes: An Insider's View* 2011

3725F   Screening for depression performed (DEM)[1]
→ *CPT Changes: An Insider's View* 2012

● **3750F**   Patient not receiving dose of corticosteroids greater than or equal to 10mg/day for 60 or greater consecutive days (IBD)[10]
→ *CPT Changes: An Insider's View* 2013

Therapeutic, Preventive, or . Other Interventions

Therapeutic, preventive, or other interventions codes describe pharmacologic, procedural, or behavioral therapies, including preventive services such as patient education and counseling.

4000F   Tobacco use cessation intervention, counseling (COPD, CAP, CAD, Asthma)[1](DM)[4](PV)[2]
→ *CPT Assistant* Oct 05:1; *CPT Changes: An Insider's View* 2005

4001F   Tobacco use cessation intervention, pharmacologic therapy (COPD, CAD, CAP, PV, Asthma)[1] (DM)[4] (PV)[2]
→ *CPT Assistant* Oct 05:6; *CPT Changes: An Insider's View* 2005

(4002F has been deleted. To report statin therapy, use 4013F)

4003F   Patient education, written/oral, appropriate for patients with heart failure, performed (NMA – No measure Associated)[1]
→ *CPT Assistant* Oct 05:6; *CPT Changes: An Insider's View* 2006

4004F   Patient screened for tobacco use **and** received tobacco cessation intervention (counseling, pharmacotherapy, or both), if identified as a tobacco user (PV, CAD)[1]
→ *CPT Changes: An Insider's View* 2011, 2012

4005F   Pharmacologic therapy (other than minerals/vitamins) for osteoporosis prescribed (OP)[5] (IBD)[10]
→ *CPT Changes: An Insider's View* 2008

(4006F has been deleted. To report beta blocker therapy, use 4008F.)

(4007F has been deleted. To report age related eye disease study (AREDS) formulation prescribed or recommended, use code 4177F)

4008F   Beta-blocker therapy prescribed or currently being taken (CAD,HF)[1]

➔ *CPT Changes: An Insider's View 2012*

(4009F has been deleted. To report Angiotensin converting enzyme [ACE] inhibitor or angiotensin receptor blocker [ARB] therapy, use 4010F)

4010F   Angiotensin Converting Enzyme (ACE) Inhibitor or Angiotensin Receptor Blocker (ARB) therapy prescribed or currently being taken (CAD, CKD, HF)[1] (DM)[2]

➔ *CPT Changes: An Insider's View 2012*

4011F   Oral antiplatelet therapy prescribed (CAD)[1]

➔ *CPT Assistant Oct 05:6; CPT Changes: An Insider's View 2005, 2010*

4012F   Warfarin therapy prescribed (NMA–No Measure Associated)[1]

➔ *CPT Assistant Oct 05:6; CPT Changes: An Insider's View 2006*

4013F   Statin therapy prescribed or currently being taken (CAD)[1]

➔ *CPT Changes: An Insider's View 2012*

4014F   Written discharge instructions provided to heart failure patients discharged home (Instructions include all of the following components: activity level, diet, discharge medications, follow-up appointment, weight monitoring, what to do if symptoms worsen) (NMA–No Measure Associated)

➔ *CPT Changes: An Insider's View 2006, 2007, 2009*

4015F   Persistent asthma, preferred long term control medication or an acceptable alternative treatment, prescribed (NMA–No Measure Associated)

➔ *CPT Changes: An Insider's View 2006, 2007, 2009*

(Note: There is no medical exclusion criteria)

(Do not report modifier 1P with 4015F)

(To report patient reasons for not prescribing, use modifier 2P)

4016F   Anti-inflammatory/analgesic agent prescribed (OA)[1]

(Use for prescribed or continued medication[s], including over-the-counter medication[s])

➔ *CPT Assistant Oct 05:6; CPT Changes: An Insider's View 2006*

4017F   Gastrointestinal prophylaxis for NSAID use prescribed (OA)[1]

➔ *CPT Assistant Oct 05:6; CPT Changes: An Insider's View 2006*

4018F   Therapeutic exercise for the involved joint(s) instructed or physical or occupational therapy prescribed (OA)[1]

➔ *CPT Assistant Oct 05:6; CPT Changes: An Insider's View 2006*

4019F   Documentation of receipt of counseling on exercise **and** either both calcium and vitamin D use or counseling regarding both calcium and vitamin D use (OP)[5]

➔ *CPT Changes: An Insider's View 2008*

4025F   Inhaled bronchodilator prescribed (COPD)[1]

➔ *CPT Changes: An Insider's View 2007*

4030F   Long-term oxygen therapy prescribed (more than 15 hours per day) (COPD)[1]

➔ *CPT Changes: An Insider's View 2007*

4033F   Pulmonary rehabilitation exercise training recommended (COPD)[1]

➔ *CPT Changes: An Insider's View 2007*

(Report 4033F with 1019F)

4035F   Influenza immunization recommended (COPD)[1] (IBD)[10]

➔ *CPT Changes: An Insider's View 2007*

4037F   Influenza immunization ordered or administered (COPD, PV, CKD, ESRD)[1] (IBD)[10]

➔ *CPT Changes: An Insider's View 2007*

4040F   Pneumococcal vaccine administered or previously received (COPD)[1] (PV)[1,2] (IBD)[10]

➔ *CPT Changes: An Insider's View 2007, 2009*

4041F   Documentation of order for cefazolin OR cefuroxime for antimicrobial prophylaxis (PERI 2)[5]

➔ *CPT Changes: An Insider's View 2008*

4042F   Documentation that prophylactic antibiotics were neither given within 4 hours prior to surgical incision nor given intraoperatively (PERI 2)[5]

➔ *CPT Changes: An Insider's View 2008*

4043F   Documentation that an order was given to discontinue prophylactic antibiotics within 48 hours of surgical end time, cardiac procedures (PERI 2)[5]

➔ *CPT Changes: An Insider's View 2008*

4044F   Documentation that an order was given for venous thromboembolism (VTE) prophylaxis to be given within 24 hours prior to incision time or 24 hours after surgery end time (PERI 2)[5]

➔ *CPT Changes: An Insider's View 2008*

4045F   Appropriate empiric antibiotic prescribed (CAP)[1] (EM)[5]

➔ *CPT Changes: An Insider's View 2007, 2008*

4046F   Documentation that prophylactic antibiotics were given within 4 hours prior to surgical incision or given intraoperatively (PERI 2)[5]

➔ *CPT Changes: An Insider's View 2008*

4047F   Documentation of order for prophylactic parenteral antibiotics to be given within 1 hour (if fluoroquinolone or vancomycin, 2 hours) prior to surgical incision (or start of procedure when no incision is required) (PERI 2)[5]

➔ *CPT Changes: An Insider's View 2008, 2011*

4048F   Documentation that administration of prophylactic parenteral antibiotic was initiated within 1 hour (if fluoroquinolone or vancomycin, 2 hours) prior to surgical incision (or start of procedure when no incision is required) as ordered (PERI 2)[5]

➔ *CPT Changes: An Insider's View 2008, 2011*

4049F   Documentation that order was given to discontinue prophylactic antibiotics within 24 hours of surgical end time, non-cardiac procedure (PERI 2)[5]

➔ *CPT Changes: An Insider's View 2008*

4050F   Hypertension plan of care documented as appropriate (NMA–No Measure Associated)[1]

➔ *CPT Changes: An Insider's View 2007*

4051F   Referred for an arteriovenous (AV) fistula (ESRD, CKD)[1]

➔ *CPT Changes: An Insider's View 2008*

▲=Revised code   ●=New code   ▶◀=Contains new or revised text   ⊘=Modifier 51 exempt

4052F Hemodialysis via functioning arteriovenous (AV) fistula (ESRD)[1]

➔ *CPT Changes: An Insider's View* 2008

4053F Hemodialysis via functioning arteriovenous (AV) graft (ESRD)[1]

➔ *CPT Changes: An Insider's View* 2008

4054F Hemodialysis via catheter (ESRD)[1]

➔ *CPT Changes: An Insider's View* 2008

4055F Patient receiving peritoneal dialysis (ESRD)[1]

➔ *CPT Changes: An Insider's View* 2008

4056F Appropriate oral rehydration solution recommended (PAG)[1]

➔ *CPT Changes: An Insider's View* 2008

4058F Pediatric gastroenteritis education provided to caregiver (PAG)[1]

➔ *CPT Changes: An Insider's View* 2008

4060F Psychotherapy services provided (MDD, MDD ADOL)[1]

➔ *CPT Changes: An Insider's View* 2008, 2011

4062F Patient referral for psychotherapy documented (MDD, MDD ADOL)[1]

➔ *CPT Changes: An Insider's View* 2008

4063F Antidepressant pharmacotherapy considered and not prescribed (MDD ADOL)[1]

➔ *CPT Changes: An Insider's View* 2011

4064F Antidepressant pharmacotherapy prescribed (MDD, MDD ADOL)[1]

➔ *CPT Changes: An Insider's View* 2008

4065F Antipsychotic pharmacotherapy prescribed (MDD)[1]

➔ *CPT Changes: An Insider's View* 2008

4066F Electroconvulsive therapy (ECT) provided (MDD)[1]

➔ *CPT Changes: An Insider's View* 2008

4067F Patient referral for electroconvulsive therapy (ECT) documented (MDD)[1]

➔ *CPT Changes: An Insider's View* 2008

● **4069F** Venous thromboembolism (VTE) prophylaxis received (IBD)[10]

➔ *CPT Changes: An Insider's View* 2013

4070F Deep vein thrombosis (DVT) prophylaxis received by end of hospital day 2 (STR)[5]

➔ *CPT Changes: An Insider's View* 2008

4073F Oral antiplatelet therapy prescribed at discharge (STR)[5]

➔ *CPT Changes: An Insider's View* 2008

4075F Anticoagulant therapy prescribed at discharge (STR)[5]

➔ *CPT Changes: An Insider's View* 2008

4077F Documentation that tissue plasminogen activator (t-PA) administration was considered (STR)[5]

➔ *CPT Changes: An Insider's View* 2008

4079F Documentation that rehabilitation services were considered (STR)[5]

➔ *CPT Changes: An Insider's View* 2008

4084F Aspirin received within 24 hours before emergency department arrival or during emergency department stay (EM)[5]

➔ *CPT Changes: An Insider's View* 2008

4086F Aspirin or clopidogrel prescribed or currently being taken (CAD)[1]

➔ *CPT Changes: An Insider's View* 2012

4090F Patient receiving erythropoietin therapy (HEM)[1]

➔ *CPT Changes: An Insider's View* 2008

4095F Patient not receiving erythropoietin therapy (HEM)[1]

➔ *CPT Changes: An Insider's View* 2008

4100F Bisphosphonate therapy, intravenous, ordered or received (HEM)[1]

➔ *CPT Changes: An Insider's View* 2008

4110F Internal mammary artery graft performed for primary, isolated coronary artery bypass graft procedure (CABG)[6]

➔ *CPT Changes: An Insider's View* 2008

4115F Beta blocker administered within 24 hours prior to surgical incision (CABG)[6]

➔ *CPT Changes: An Insider's View* 2008

4120F Antibiotic prescribed or dispensed (URI, PHAR)[2] (A-BRONCH)[2]

➔ *CPT Changes: An Insider's View* 2008

4124F Antibiotic neither prescribed nor dispensed (URI, PHAR)[2] (A-BRONCH)[2]

➔ *CPT Changes: An Insider's View* 2008

4130F Topical preparations (including OTC) prescribed for acute otitis externa (AOE)[1]

➔ *CPT Changes: An Insider's View* 2009

4131F Systemic antimicrobial therapy prescribed (AOE)[1]

➔ *CPT Changes: An Insider's View* 2009

4132F Systemic antimicrobial therapy not prescribed (AOE)[1]

➔ *CPT Changes: An Insider's View* 2009

4133F Antihistamines or decongestants prescribed or recommended (OME)[1]

➔ *CPT Changes: An Insider's View* 2009

4134F Antihistamines or decongestants neither prescribed nor recommended (OME)[1]

➔ *CPT Changes: An Insider's View* 2009

4135F Systemic corticosteroids prescribed (OME)[1]

➔ *CPT Changes: An Insider's View* 2009

4136F Systemic corticosteroids not prescribed (OME)[1]

➔ *CPT Changes: An Insider's View* 2009

4140F Inhaled corticosteroids prescribed (Asthma)[1]

➔ *CPT Changes: An Insider's View* 2012

● **4142F** Corticosteroid sparing therapy prescribed (IBD)[10]

➔ *CPT Changes: An Insider's View* 2013

4144F Alternative long-term control medication prescribed (Asthma)[1]

➔ *CPT Changes: An Insider's View* 2012

4145F   Two or more anti-hypertensive agents prescribed or currently being taken (CAD, HTN)
> *CPT Changes: An Insider's View* 2012

4148F   Hepatitis A vaccine injection administered or previously received (HEP-C)[1]
> *CPT Changes: An Insider's View* 2010

4149F   Hepatitis B vaccine injection administered or previously received (HEP-C, HIV)[1] (IBD)[10]
> *CPT Changes: An Insider's View* 2010, 2012

4150F   Patient receiving antiviral treatment for Hepatitis C (HEP-C)[1]
> *CPT Changes: An Insider's View* 2009

4151F   Patient not receiving antiviral treatment for Hepatitis C (HEP-C)[1]
> *CPT Changes: An Insider's View* 2009

(Code 4152F has been deleted.)

4153F   Combination peginterferon and ribavirin therapy prescribed (HEP-C)[1]
> *CPT Changes: An Insider's View* 2009

(Code 4154F has been deleted.)

4155F   Hepatitis A vaccine series previously received (HEP-C)[1]
> *CPT Changes: An Insider's View* 2009

(Code 4156F has been deleted.)

4157F   Hepatitis B vaccine series previously received (HEP-C)[1]
> *CPT Changes: An Insider's View* 2009

4158F   Patient counseled about risks of alcohol use (HEP-C)[1]
> *CPT Changes: An Insider's View* 2009, 2010

4159F   Counseling regarding contraception received prior to initiation of antiviral treatment (HEP-C)[1]
> *CPT Changes: An Insider's View* 2009

4163F   Patient counseling at a minimum on all of the following treatment options for clinically localized prostate cancer: active surveillance, **and** interstitial prostate brachytherapy, **and** external beam radiotherapy, **and** radical prostatectomy, provided prior to initiation of treatment (PRCA)[1]
> *CPT Changes: An Insider's View* 2009

4164F   Adjuvant (ie, in combination with external beam radiotherapy to the prostate for prostate cancer) hormonal therapy (gonadotropin-releasing hormone [GnRH] agonist or antagonist) prescribed/administered (PRCA)[1]
> *CPT Changes: An Insider's View* 2009

4165F   3-dimensional conformal radiotherapy (3D-CRT) or intensity modulated radiation therapy (IMRT) received (PRCA)[1]
> *CPT Changes: An Insider's View* 2009

4167F   Head of bed elevation (30-45 degrees) on first ventilator day ordered (CRIT)[1]
> *CPT Changes: An Insider's View* 2009

4168F   Patient receiving care in the intensive care unit (ICU) and receiving mechanical ventilation, 24 hours or less (CRIT)[1]
> *CPT Changes: An Insider's View* 2009

4169F   Patient either not receiving care in the intensive care unit (ICU) OR not receiving mechanical ventilation OR receiving mechanical ventilation greater than 24 hours (CRIT)[1]
> *CPT Changes: An Insider's View* 2009

4171F   Patient receiving erythropoiesis-stimulating agents (ESA) therapy (CKD)[1]
> *CPT Changes: An Insider's View* 2009

4172F   Patient not receiving erythropoiesis-stimulating agents (ESA) therapy (CKD)[1]
> *CPT Changes: An Insider's View* 2009

4174F   Counseling about the potential impact of glaucoma on visual functioning and quality of life, and importance of treatment adherence provided to patient and/or caregiver(s) (EC)[5]
> *CPT Changes: An Insider's View* 2009

4175F   Best-corrected visual acuity of 20/40 or better (distance or near) achieved within the 90 days following cataract surgery (EC)[5]
> *CPT Changes: An Insider's View* 2009

4176F   Counseling about value of protection from UV light and lack of proven efficacy of nutritional supplements in prevention or progression of cataract development provided to patient and/or caregiver(s) (NMA–No Measure Associated)
> *CPT Changes: An Insider's View* 2009

4177F   Counseling about the benefits and/or risks of the Age-Related Eye Disease Study (AREDS) formulation for preventing progression of age-related macular degeneration (AMD) provided to patient and/or caregiver(s) (EC)[5]
> *CPT Changes: An Insider's View* 2009

4178F   Anti-D immune globulin received between 26 and 30 weeks gestation (Pre-Cr)[1]
> *CPT Changes: An Insider's View* 2009

4179F   Tamoxifen or aromatase inhibitor (AI) prescribed (ONC)[1]
> *CPT Changes: An Insider's View* 2009

4180F   Adjuvant chemotherapy referred, prescribed, or previously received for Stage III colon cancer (ONC)[1]
> *CPT Changes: An Insider's View* 2009, 2010

4181F   Conformal radiation therapy received (NMA–No Measure Associated)
> *CPT Changes: An Insider's View* 2009

4182F   Conformal radiation therapy not received (NMA–No Measure Associated)
> *CPT Changes: An Insider's View* 2009

4185F   Continuous (12-months) therapy with proton pump inhibitor (PPI) or histamine H2 receptor antagonist (H2RA) received (GERD)[5]
> *CPT Changes: An Insider's View* 2009

4186F   No continuous (12-months) therapy with either proton pump inhibitor (PPI) or histamine H2 receptor antagonist (H2RA) received (GERD)[5]
> *CPT Changes: An Insider's View* 2009

▲=Revised code   ●=New code   ►◄=Contains new or revised text   ⦵=Modifier 51 exempt

Category II

Category II

4187F Disease modifying anti-rheumatic drug therapy prescribed or dispensed (RA)[2]

➔ *CPT Changes: An Insider's View* 2009

4188F Appropriate angiotensin converting enzyme (ACE)/ angiotensin receptor blockers (ARB) therapeutic monitoring test ordered or performed (AM)[2]

➔ *CPT Changes: An Insider's View* 2009

4189F Appropriate digoxin therapeutic monitoring test ordered or performed (AM)[2]

➔ *CPT Changes: An Insider's View* 2009

4190F Appropriate diuretic therapeutic monitoring test ordered or performed (AM)[2]

➔ *CPT Changes: An Insider's View* 2009

4191F Appropriate anticonvulsant therapeutic monitoring test ordered or performed (AM)[2]

➔ *CPT Changes: An Insider's View* 2009

4192F Patient not receiving glucocorticoid therapy (RA)[5]

➔ *CPT Changes: An Insider's View* 2010

4193F Patient receiving <10 mg daily prednisone (or equivalent), or RA activity is worsening, or glucocorticoid use is for less than 6 months (RA)[5]

➔ *CPT Changes: An Insider's View* 2010

4194F Patient receiving ≥10 mg daily prednisone (or equivalent) for longer than 6 months, and improvement or no change in disease activity (RA)[5]

➔ *CPT Changes: An Insider's View* 2010

4195F Patient receiving first-time biologic disease modifying anti-rheumatic drug therapy for rheumatoid arthritis (RA)[5]

➔ *CPT Changes: An Insider's View* 2010

4196F Patient not receiving first-time biologic disease modifying anti-rheumatic drug therapy for rheumatoid arthritis (RA)[5]

➔ *CPT Changes: An Insider's View* 2010

4200F External beam radiotherapy as primary therapy to prostate with or without nodal irradiation (PRCA)[1]

➔ *CPT Changes: An Insider's View* 2009, 2010

4201F External beam radiotherapy with or without nodal irradiation as adjuvant or salvage therapy for prostate cancer patient (PRCA)[1]

➔ *CPT Changes: An Insider's View* 2009, 2010

4210F Angiotensin converting enzyme (ACE) or angiotensin receptor blockers (ARB) medication therapy for 6 months or more (MM)[2]

➔ *CPT Changes: An Insider's View* 2009

4220F Digoxin medication therapy for 6 months or more (MM)[2]

➔ *CPT Changes: An Insider's View* 2009

4221F Diuretic medication therapy for 6 months or more (MM)[2]

➔ *CPT Changes: An Insider's View* 2009

4230F Anticonvulsant medication therapy for 6 months or more (MM)[2]

➔ *CPT Changes: An Insider's View* 2009

▲ **4240F** Instruction in therapeutic exercise with follow-up provided to patients during episode of back pain lasting longer than 12 weeks (BkP)[2]

➔ *CPT Changes: An Insider's View* 2009, 2013

4242F Counseling for supervised exercise program provided to patients during episode of back pain lasting longer than 12 weeks (BkP)[2]

➔ *CPT Changes: An Insider's View* 2009

4245F Patient counseled during the initial visit to maintain or resume normal activities (BkP)[2]

➔ *CPT Changes: An Insider's View* 2009

4248F Patient counseled during the initial visit for an episode of back pain against bed rest lasting 4 days or longer (BkP)[2]

➔ *CPT Changes: An Insider's View* 2009

4250F Active warming used intraoperatively for the purpose of maintaining normothermia, **or** at least 1 body temperature equal to or greater than 36 degrees Centigrade (or 96.8 degrees Fahrenheit) recorded within the 30 minutes immediately before or the 15 minutes immediately after anesthesia end time (CRIT)[1]

➔ *CPT Changes: An Insider's View* 2009, 2010

4255F Duration of general or neuraxial anesthesia 60 minutes or longer, as documented in the anesthesia record (CRIT)[5]

➔ *CPT Changes: An Insider's View* 2011

4256F Duration of general or neuraxial anesthesia less than 60 minutes, as documented in the anesthesia record (CRIT)[5]

➔ *CPT Changes: An Insider's View* 2011

4260F Wound surface culture technique used (CWC)[5]

➔ *CPT Changes: An Insider's View* 2010

4261F Technique other than surface culture of the wound exudate used (eg, Levine/deep swab technique, semi-quantitative or quantitative swab technique) **or** wound surface culture technique not used (CWC)[5]

➔ *CPT Changes: An Insider's View* 2010

4265F Use of wet to dry dressings prescribed or recommended (CWC)[5]

➔ *CPT Changes: An Insider's View* 2010

4266F Use of wet to dry dressings neither prescribed nor recommended (CWC)[5]

➔ *CPT Changes: An Insider's View* 2010

4267F Compression therapy prescribed (CWC)[5]

➔ *CPT Changes: An Insider's View* 2010

4268F Patient education regarding the need for long term compression therapy including interval replacement of compression stockings received (CWC)[5]

➔ *CPT Changes: An Insider's View* 2010

4269F Appropriate method of offloading (pressure relief) prescribed (CWC)[5]

➔ *CPT Changes: An Insider's View* 2010

4270F Patient receiving potent antiretroviral therapy for 6 months or longer (HIV)[5]

➔ *CPT Changes: An Insider's View* 2010

4271F   Patient receiving potent antiretroviral therapy for less than 6 months or not receiving potent antiretroviral therapy (HIV)[5]
> *CPT Changes: An Insider's View* 2010

4274F   Influenza immunization administered or previously received (HIV)[5] (P-ESRD)[1]
> *CPT Changes: An Insider's View* 2010

(4275F has been deleted. To report Hepatitis B vaccine injection administered or previously received, use 4149F)

4276F   Potent antiretroviral therapy prescribed (HIV)[5]
> *CPT Changes: An Insider's View* 2010

4279F   Pneumocystis jiroveci pneumonia prophylaxis prescribed (HIV)[5]
> *CPT Changes: An Insider's View* 2010

4280F   Pneumocystis jiroveci pneumonia prophylaxis prescribed within 3 months of low CD4+ cell count or percentage (HIV)[5]
> *CPT Changes: An Insider's View* 2010

4290F   Patient screened for injection drug use (HIV)[5]
> *CPT Changes: An Insider's View* 2010

4293F   Patient screened for high-risk sexual behavior (HIV)[5]
> *CPT Changes: An Insider's View* 2010

4300F   Patient receiving warfarin therapy for nonvalvular atrial fibrillation or atrial flutter (AFIB)[1]
> *CPT Changes: An Insider's View* 2010

4301F   Patient not receiving warfarin therapy for nonvalvular atrial fibrillation or atrial flutter (AFIB)[1]
> *CPT Changes: An Insider's View* 2010

4305F   Patient education regarding appropriate foot care **and** daily inspection of the feet received (CWC)[5]
> *CPT Changes: An Insider's View* 2010

4306F   Patient counseled regarding psychosocial **and** pharmacologic treatment options for opioid addiction (SUD)[1]
> *CPT Changes: An Insider's View* 2010

4320F   Patient counseled regarding psychosocial **and** pharmacologic treatment options for alcohol dependence (SUD)[5]
> *CPT Changes: An Insider's View* 2010

4322F   Caregiver provided with education and referred to additional resources for support (DEM)[1]
> *CPT Changes: An Insider's View* 2012

4324F   Patient (or caregiver) queried about Parkinson's disease medication related motor complications (Prkns)[8]
> *CPT Changes: An Insider's View* 2011

4325F   Medical and surgical treatment options reviewed with patient (or caregiver) (Prkns)[8]
> *CPT Changes: An Insider's View* 2011

4326F   Patient (or caregiver) queried about symptoms of autonomic dysfunction (Prkns)[8]
> *CPT Changes: An Insider's View* 2011

4328F   Patient (or caregiver) queried about sleep disturbances (Prkns)[8]
> *CPT Changes: An Insider's View* 2011

4330F   Counseling about epilepsy specific safety issues provided to patient (or caregiver(s)) (EPI)[8]
> *CPT Changes: An Insider's View* 2011

4340F   Counseling for women of childbearing potential with epilepsy (EPI)[8]
> *CPT Changes: An Insider's View* 2011

4350F   Counseling provided on symptom management, end of life decisions, and palliation (DEM)[1]
> *CPT Changes: An Insider's View* 2012

4400F   Rehabilitative therapy options discussed with patient (or caregiver) (Prkns)[8]
> *CPT Changes: An Insider's View* 2011

4450F   Self-care education provided to patient (HF)[1]
> *CPT Changes: An Insider's View* 2012

4470F   Implantable cardioverter-defibrillator (ICD) counseling provided (HF)[1]
> *CPT Changes: An Insider's View* 2012

4480F   Patient receiving ACE inhibitor/ARB therapy and beta-blocker therapy for 3 months or longer (HF)[1]
> *CPT Changes: An Insider's View* 2012

4481F   Patient receiving ACE inhibitor/ARB therapy and beta-blocker therapy for less than 3 months or patient not receiving ACE inhibitor/ARB therapy and beta-blocker therapy (HF)[1]
> *CPT Changes: An Insider's View* 2012

4500F   Referred to an outpatient cardiac rehabilitation program (CAD)[1]
> *CPT Changes: An Insider's View* 2012

4510F   Previous cardiac rehabilitation for qualifying cardiac event completed (CAD)[1]
> *CPT Changes: An Insider's View* 2012

4525F   Neuropsychiatric intervention ordered (DEM)[1]
> *CPT Changes: An Insider's View* 2012

4526F   Neuropsychiatric intervention received (DEM)[1]
> *CPT Changes: An Insider's View* 2012

Follow-up or Other Outcomes

Follow-up or other outcomes codes describe review and communication of test results to patients, patient satisfaction or experience with care, patient functional status, and patient morbidity and mortality.

5005F   Patient counseled on self-examination for new or changing moles (ML)[5]
> *CPT Changes: An Insider's View* 2008

▲ **5010F**   Findings of dilated macular or fundus exam communicated to the physician or other qualified health care professional managing the diabetes care (EC)[5]
> *CPT Changes: An Insider's View* 2008, 2013

Category II

5015F Documentation of communication that a fracture occurred and that the patient was or should be tested or treated for osteoporosis (OP)[5]

➔ CPT Changes: An Insider's View 2008

▲ **5020F** Treatment summary report communicated to physician(s) or other qualified health care professional(s) managing continuing care and to the patient within 1 month of completing treatment (ONC)[1]

➔ CPT Changes: An Insider's View 2009, 2010, 2013

5050F Treatment plan communicated to provider(s) managing continuing care within 1 month of diagnosis (ML)[5]

➔ CPT Changes: An Insider's View 2009

5060F Findings from diagnostic mammogram communicated to practice managing patient's on-going care within 3 business days of exam interpretation (RAD)[5]

➔ CPT Changes: An Insider's View 2009

5062F Findings from diagnostic mammogram communicated to the patient within 5 days of exam interpretation (RAD)[5]

➔ CPT Changes: An Insider's View 2009

▲ **5100F** Potential risk for fracture communicated to the referring physician or other qualified health care professional within 24 hours of completion of the imaging study (NUC_MED)[1]

➔ CPT Changes: An Insider's View 2010, 2013

5200F Consideration of referral for a neurological evaluation of appropriateness for surgical therapy for intractable epilepsy within the past 3 years (EPI)[8]

➔ CPT Changes: An Insider's View 2011

5250F Asthma discharge plan provided to patient (Asthma)[1]

➔ CPT Changes: An Insider's View 2012

Patient Safety

Patient safety codes that describe patient safety practices.

6005F Rationale (eg, severity of illness and safety) for level of care (eg, home, hospital) documented (CAP)[1]

➔ CPT Assistant Aug 07:1; CPT Changes: An Insider's View 2007

6010F Dysphagia screening conducted prior to order for or receipt of any foods, fluids, or medication by mouth (STR)[5]

➔ CPT Changes: An Insider's View 2008

6015F Patient receiving or eligible to receive foods, fluids, or medication by mouth (STR)[5]

➔ CPT Changes: An Insider's View 2008

6020F NPO (nothing by mouth) ordered (STR)[5]

➔ CPT Changes: An Insider's View 2008

6030F All elements of maximal sterile barrier technique followed including: cap **and** mask **and** sterile gown **and** sterile gloves **and** a large sterile sheet **and** hand hygiene **and** 2% chlorhexidine for cutaneous antisepsis (or acceptable alternative antiseptics, per current guideline) (CRIT)[1]

➔ CPT Changes: An Insider's View 2009, 2010

6040F Use of appropriate radiation dose reduction devices OR manual techniques for appropriate moderation of exposure, documented (RAD)[5]

➔ CPT Changes: An Insider's View 2009

6045F Radiation exposure or exposure time in final report for procedure using fluoroscopy, documented (RAD)[5]

➔ CPT Changes: An Insider's View 2009

➔ Clinical Examples in Radiology Summer 10:1, Winter 11:2, Spring 11:2,9,10, Summer 11:2, Fall 11:2,3

6070F Patient queried and counseled about anti-epileptic drug (AED) side effects (EPI)[8]

➔ CPT Changes: An Insider's View 2011

6080F Patient (or caregiver) queried about falls (Prkns)[8]

➔ CPT Changes: An Insider's View 2011

6090F Patient (or caregiver) counseled about safety issues appropriate to patient's stage of disease (Prkns)[8]

➔ CPT Changes: An Insider's View 2011

6100F Timeout to verify correct patient, correct site, and correct procedure, documented (PATH)[9]

➔ CPT Changes: An Insider's View 2012

6101F Safety counseling for dementia provided (DEM)[1]

➔ CPT Changes: An Insider's View 2012

6102F Safety counseling for dementia ordered (DEM)[1]

➔ CPT Changes: An Insider's View 2012

6110F Counseling provided regarding risks of driving and the alternatives to driving (DEM)[1]

➔ CPT Changes: An Insider's View 2012

● **6150F** Patient not receiving a first course of anti-TNF (tumor necrosis factor) therapy (IBD)[10]

➔ CPT Changes: An Insider's View 2013

Structural Measures

Structural measures codes are used to identify measures that address the setting or system of the delivered care. These codes also address aspects of the capabilities of the organization or health care professional providing the care.

7010F Patient information entered into a recall system that includes: target date for the next exam specified **and** a process to follow up with patients regarding missed or unscheduled appointments (ML)[5]

➔ CPT Changes: An Insider's View 2009, 2011

7020F Mammogram assessment category (eg, Mammography Quality Standards Act [MQSA], Breast Imaging Reporting and Data System [BI-RADS®], or FDA approved equivalent categories) entered into an internal database to allow for analysis of abnormal interpretation (recall) rate (RAD)[5]

➔ CPT Changes: An Insider's View 2009

7025F Patient information entered into a reminder system with a target due date for the next mammogram (RAD)[5]

➔ CPT Changes: An Insider's View 2009

Category III Codes

The following section contains a set of temporary codes for emerging technology, services, and procedures. Category III codes allow data collection for these services/ procedures. Use of unlisted codes does not offer the opportunity for the collection of specific data. If a Category III code is available, this code must be reported instead of a Category I unlisted code. This is an activity that is critically important in the evaluation of health care delivery and the formation of public and private policy. The use of the codes in this section allow physicians and other qualified health care professionals, insurers, health services researchers, and health policy experts to identify emerging technology, services, and procedures for clinical efficacy, utilization and outcomes.

The inclusion of a service or procedure in this section neither implies nor endorses clinical efficacy, safety, or the applicability to clinical practice. The codes in this section may not conform to the usual requirements for CPT Category I codes established by the Editorial Panel. For Category I codes, the Panel requires that the service/ procedure be performed by many health care professionals in clinical practice in multiple locations and that FDA approval, as appropriate, has already been received. The nature of emerging technology, services, and procedures is such that these requirements may not be met. For these reasons, temporary codes for emerging technology, services, and procedures have been placed in a separate section of the CPT codebook and the codes are differentiated from Category I CPT codes by the use of alphanumeric characters.

▶ Services/procedures described in this section make use of alphanumeric characters. These codes have an alpha character as the 5th character in the string, preceded by four digits. The digits are not intended to reflect the placement of the code in the Category I section of CPT nomenclature. Codes in this section may or may not eventually receive a Category I CPT code. In either case, in general, a given Category III code will be archived five years from the date of initial publication or extension unless a modification of the archival date is specifically noted at the time of a revision or change to a code (eg, addition of parenthetical instructions, reinstatement). Services/procedures described by Category III codes which have been archived after five years, without conversion, must be reported using the Category I unlisted code unless another specific cross reference is established at the time of archiving. New or revised codes in this section are released semi annually via the AMA/ CPT Internet site, to expedite dissemination for reporting. The full set of temporary codes for emerging technology, services, and procedures are published annually in the CPT codebook. Go to www.ama-assn. org/go/cpt for the most current listing.◄

(0016T, 0017T have been deleted)

(For destruction of localized lesion of choroid by transpupillary thermotherapy, use 67299)

(For destruction of macular drusen, photocoagulation, use 67299)

0019T   Extracorporeal shock wave involving musculoskeletal system, not otherwise specified, low energy
Sunset January 2017

→ *CPT Assistant* Jun 05:6, Mar 06:1; *CPT Changes: An Insider's View* 2002, 2006

(For application of high energy extracorporeal shock wave involving musculoskeletal system not otherwise specified, use 0101T)

(For application of high energy extracorporeal shock wave involving lateral humeral epicondyle, use 0102T)

(0024T has been deleted)

(For non-surgical septal reduction therapy, use 93799)

(0026T has been deleted)

(For lipoprotein, direct measurement, intermediate density lipoproteins [IDL] [remnant lipoprotein], use 84999)

(0027T has been deleted)

(For endoscopic lysis of epidural adhesions with direct visualization using mechnical means or solution injection [eg, normal saline], use 64999)

(0028T has been deleted)

(For dual energy x-ray absorptiometry [DXA] body composition study, use 76499)

(0029T has been deleted)

(For pulsed magnetic neuromodulation incontinence treatment, use 53899)

▶(0030T has been deleted)◄

▶(To report antiprothrombin [phospholipid cofactor] antibody, use 86849)◄

(0031T, 0032T have been deleted)

(For speculoscopy, including sampling, use 58999)

(0041T has been deleted)

(For urinalysis infectious agent detection, semi-quantitative analysis of volatile compounds, use 81099)

Category III

0042T Cerebral perfusion analysis using computed tomography with contrast administration, including post-processing of parametric maps with determination of cerebral blood flow, cerebral blood volume, and mean transit time
Sunset January 2014

➜ *CPT Changes: An Insider's View* 2003

(0043T has been deleted)

(For carbon monoxide, expired gas analysis [eg, ETCO$_c$/ hemolysis breath test], use 84999)

(0046T, 0047T have been deleted)

(For mammary duct[s] catheter lavage, use 19499)

►(0048T has been deleted. To report, use 33991)◄

(0049T has been deleted)

►(0050T has been deleted. To report, see 33990-33993)◄

0051T Implantation of a total replacement heart system (artificial heart) with recipient cardiectomy
Sunset January 2014

➜ *CPT Assistant* Jun 04:7; *CPT Changes: An Insider's View* 2004

(For implantation of heart assist or ventricular assist device, see 33975, 33976)

0052T Replacement or repair of thoracic unit of a total replacement heart system (artificial heart)
Sunset January 2014

➜ *CPT Assistant* Jun 04:7; *CPT Changes: An Insider's View* 2004

(For replacement or repair of other implantable components in a total replacement heart system (artificial heart), use 0053T)

0053T Replacement or repair of implantable component or components of total replacement heart system (artificial heart), excluding thoracic unit
Sunset January 2014

➜ *CPT Assistant* Jun 04:7; *CPT Changes: An Insider's View* 2004

(For replacement or repair of a thoracic unit of a total replacement heart system (artificial heart), use 0052T)

+ 0054T Computer-assisted musculoskeletal surgical navigational orthopedic procedure, with image-guidance based on fluoroscopic images (List separately in addition to code for primary procedure)
Sunset January 2014

➜ *CPT Assistant* May 04:14, Jun 04:8; *CPT Changes: An Insider's View* 2004

+ 0055T Computer-assisted musculoskeletal surgical navigational orthopedic procedure, with image-guidance based on CT/ MRI images (List separately in addition to code for primary procedure)
Sunset January 2014

➜ *CPT Assistant* May 04:14, Jun 04:8; *CPT Changes: An Insider's View* 2004, 2005

(When CT and MRI are both performed, report 0055T only once)

(0056T has been deleted. To report, use 20985)

0058T Cryopreservation; reproductive tissue, ovarian
Sunset January 2016

➜ *CPT Changes: An Insider's View* 2004, 2011

0059T   oocyte(s)
Sunset January 2016

➜ *CPT Changes: An Insider's View* 2004, 2011

(For cryopreservation of embryo(s), sperm and testicular reproductive tissue, see 89258, 89259, 89335)

(0060T has been deleted)

(For electrical impedance breast scan, use 76499)

(0061T has been deleted)

(For destruction/reduction of malignant breast tumor, microwave phased array thermotherapy, use 19499)

(0062T, 0063T have been deleted)

(For percutaneous intradiscal annuloplasty, any method other than electrothermal, use 22899)

(For intradiscal electrothermal annuloplasty, see 22526, 22527)

(0064T has been deleted. To report, use 94799)

(0066T has been deleted)

(To report CT colon, screening, use 74263)

(0067T has been deleted)

(To report CT colon, diagnostic, see 74261-74262)

(0068T-0070T have been deleted)

(For acoustic heart sound recording and computer analysis, use 93799)

0071T Focused ultrasound ablation of uterine leiomyomata, including MR guidance; total leiomyomata volume less than 200 cc of tissue
Sunset January 2015

➜ *CPT Assistant* Mar 05:1, 5, Dec 05:3; *CPT Changes: An Insider's View* 2005

0072T   total leiomyomata volume greater or equal to 200 cc of tissue
Sunset January 2015

➜ *CPT Assistant* Mar 05:1, 5, Dec 05:3; *CPT Changes: An Insider's View* 2005

(Do not report 0071T, 0072T in conjunction with 51702 or 77022)

0073T Compensator-based beam modulation treatment delivery of inverse planned treatment using 3 or more high resolution (milled or cast) compensator convergent beam modulated fields, per treatment session
Sunset January 2015

➜ *CPT Assistant* Mar 05:1, 6, May 05:7, Nov 09:3; *CPT Changes: An Insider's View* 2005

(For treatment planning, use 77301)

(Do not report 0073T in conjunction with 77401-77416, 77418)

0075T Transcatheter placement of extracranial vertebral or intrathoracic carotid artery stent(s), including radiologic supervision and interpretation, percutaneous; initial vessel
Sunset January 2015

➔ *CPT Assistant* May 05:7; *CPT Changes: An Insider's View* 2005

+ 0076T each additional vessel (List separately in addition to code for primary procedure)
Sunset January 2015

➔ *CPT Assistant* May 05:7; *CPT Changes: An Insider's View* 2005

(Use 0076T in conjunction with 0075T)

(When the ipsilateral extracranial vertebral or intrathoracic carotid arteriogram (including imaging and selective catheterization) confirms the need for stenting, then 0075T and 0076T include all ipsilateral extracranial vertebral or intrathoracic selective carotid catheterization, all diagnostic imaging for ipsilateral extracranial vertebral or intrathoracic carotid artery stenting, and all related radiologic supervision and interpretation. If stenting is not indicated, then the appropriate codes for selective catheterization and imaging should be reported in lieu of code 0075T or 0076T.)

(0077T has been deleted. To report, see 61107, 61210)

(0078T-0081T should be reported in accordance with the Endovascular Abdominal Aneurysm Repair guidelines established for 34800-34826)

0078T Endovascular repair using prosthesis of abdominal aortic aneurysm, pseudoaneurysm or dissection, abdominal aorta involving visceral branches (superior mesenteric, celiac and/or renal artery[s])
Sunset January 2015

➔ *CPT Assistant* May 05:7, Jun 05:6, Jun 11:13, Apr 12:9; *CPT Changes: An Insider's View* 2005, 2006

➔ *Clinical Examples In Radiology* Winter 06:20

(Do not report 0078T in conjunction with 34800-34805, 35081, 35102, 35452, 35472)

(Report 0078T in conjunction with 37205-37208, 37220-37223, only when these procedures are performed outside the target zone of the endoprosthesis)

+ 0079T Placement of visceral extension prosthesis for endovascular repair of abdominal aortic aneurysm involving visceral vessels, each visceral branch (List separately in addition to code for primary procedure)
Sunset January 2015

➔ *CPT Assistant* May 05:7, Apr 12:9; *CPT Changes: An Insider's View* 2005

(Use 0079T in conjunction with 0078T)

0080T Endovascular repair using prosthesis of abdominal aortic aneurysm, pseudoaneurysm or dissection, abdominal aorta involving visceral vessels (superior mesenteric, celiac and/or renal artery[s]), radiological supervision and interpretation
Sunset January 2017

➔ *CPT Assistant* May 05:7, Apr 12:9; *CPT Changes: An Insider's View* 2005, 2012

(Do not report 0080T in conjunction with 34800-34805, 35081, 35102, 35452, 35472)

(Report 0080T in conjunction with 37205-37208, 37220-37223, only when these procedures are performed outside the target zone of the endoprosthesis)

+ 0081T Placement of visceral extension prosthesis for endovascular repair of abdominal aortic aneurysm involving visceral vessels, each visceral branch, radiological supervision and interpretation (List separately in addition to code for primary procedure)
Sunset January 2015

➔ *CPT Assistant* May 05:7, Apr 12:9; *CPT Changes: An Insider's View* 2005

(Use 0081T in conjunction with 0080T)

(0084T has been deleted. To report, use 53855)

0085T Breath test for heart transplant rejection
Sunset January 2016

➔ *CPT Assistant* May 05:7; *CPT Changes: An Insider's View* 2005

(0086T has been deleted. To report use, 93799)

(0087T has been deleted. To report, use 89398)

(0088T has been deleted. To report, use 41530)

(0089T has been deleted. For actigraphy testing, use 95803)

(0090T has been deleted. To report total disc cervical arthroplasty, use 22856)

(To report total disc lumbar arthroplasty, use 22857)

+ 0092T Total disc arthroplasty (artificial disc), anterior approach, including discectomy with end plate preparation (includes osteophytectomy for nerve root or spinal cord decompression and microdissection), each additional interspace, cervical (List separately in addition to code for primary procedure)
Sunset January 2014

➔ *CPT Assistant* Jun 05:6, Feb 06:1; *CPT Changes: An Insider's View* 2006, 2009

(Use 0092T in conjunction with 22856)

(Do not report 0092T in conjunction with 22851 when performed at the same level)

(0093T has been deleted. To report removal of total disc cervical arthroplasty, use 22864)

(To report removal of total disc lumbar arthroplasty, use 22865)

+ 0095T Removal of total disc arthroplasty (artificial disc), anterior approach, each additional interspace, cervical (List separately in addition to code for primary procedure)
Sunset January 2014

➔ *CPT Assistant* Jun 05:6, Feb 06:1; *CPT Changes: An Insider's View* 2006, 2009

(Use 0095T in conjunction with 22864)

(0096T has been deleted. To report revision of total disc cervical arthroplasty, use 22861)

(To report revision of total disc lumbar arthroplasty, use 22862)

Category III

Category III

+ **0098T** Revision including replacement of total disc arthroplasty (artificial disc), anterior approach, each additional interspace, cervical (List separately in addition to code for primary procedure)
Sunset January 2014
➜ CPT Assistant Jun 05:6, Feb 06:1; CPT Changes: An Insider's View 2006, 2009

(Use 0098T in conjunction with 22861)

(Do not report 0098T in conjunction with 0095T)

(Do not report 0098T in conjunction with 22851 when performed at the same level)

(For decompression, see 63001-63048)

0099T Implantation of intrastromal corneal ring segments
Sunset January 2016
➜ CPT Assistant Jun 05:6, Feb 06:1; CPT Changes: An Insider's View 2006

0100T Placement of a subconjunctival retinal prosthesis receiver and pulse generator, and implantation of intra-ocular retinal electrode array, with vitrectomy
Sunset January 2016
➜ CPT Assistant Jun 05:6, Feb 06:1, Jun 11:13; CPT Changes: An Insider's View 2006

0101T Extracorporeal shock wave involving musculoskeletal system, not otherwise specified, high energy
Sunset January 2016
➜ CPT Assistant Jun 05:6, Mar 06:1, Jun 11:13; CPT Changes: An Insider's View 2006

(For application of low energy musculoskeletal system extracorporeal shock wave, use 0019T)

►(For extracorporeal shock wave therapy involving integumentary system not otherwise specified, see 0299T, 0300T)◄

►(Do not report 0101T in conjunction with 0299T, 0300T when treating same area)◄

0102T Extracorporeal shock wave, high energy, performed by a physician, requiring anesthesia other than local, involving lateral humeral epicondyle
Sunset January 2016
➜ CPT Assistant Jun 05:6, Mar 06:1, Jun 11:13; CPT Changes: An Insider's View 2006

(For application of low energy musculoskeletal system extracorporeal shock wave, use 0019T)

0103T Holotranscobalamin, quantitative
Sunset January 2016
➜ CPT Assistant Jun 05:6, Mar 06:1, Jun 11:13; CPT Changes: An Insider's View 2006

(0104T, 0105T have been deleted)

(For inert gas rebreathing for cardiac output measurement during rest, use 93799)

(For inert gas rebreathing for cardiac output measurement during exercise, use 93799)

0106T Quantitative sensory testing (QST), testing and interpretation per extremity; using touch pressure stimuli to assess large diameter sensation
Sunset January 2016
➜ CPT Assistant Jun 05:6, Mar 06:1, May 11:10, Jun 11:13; CPT Changes: An Insider's View 2006

0107T using vibration stimuli to assess large diameter fiber sensation
Sunset January 2016
➜ CPT Assistant Jun 05:6, Mar 06:1, May 11:10, Jun 11:13; CPT Changes: An Insider's View 2006

0108T using cooling stimuli to assess small nerve fiber sensation and hyperalgesia
Sunset January 2016
➜ CPT Assistant Jun 05:6, Mar 06:1, May 11:10, Jun 11:13; CPT Changes: An Insider's View 2006

0109T using heat-pain stimuli to assess small nerve fiber sensation and hyperalgesia
Sunset January 2016
➜ CPT Assistant Jun 05:6, Mar 06:1, May 11:10, Jun 11:13; CPT Changes: An Insider's View 2006

0110T using other stimuli to assess sensation
Sunset January 2016
➜ CPT Assistant Jun 05:6, Mar 06:1, May 11:10, Jun 11:13; CPT Changes: An Insider's View 2006

0111T Long-chain (C20-22) omega-3 fatty acids in red blood cell (RBC) membranes
Sunset January 2016
➜ CPT Assistant Jun 05:6, Mar 06:1, Jun 11:13; CPT Changes: An Insider's View 2006

(For very long chain fatty acids, use 82726)

0123T Fistulization of sclera for glaucoma, through ciliary body
Sunset January 2016
➜ CPT Assistant Jun 11:13; CPT Changes: An Insider's View 2006

0124T Conjunctival incision with posterior extrascleral placement of pharmacological agent (does not include supply of medication)
Sunset January 2014
➜ CPT Assistant Jan 08:6; CPT Changes: An Insider's View 2006, 2009

(For suprachoroidal delivery of pharmacologic agent, use 0186T)

0126T Common carotid intima-media thickness (IMT) study for evaluation of atherosclerotic burden or coronary heart disease risk factor assessment
Sunset January 2016
➜ CPT Assistant Jun 11:13; CPT Changes: An Insider's View 2006

(0130T has been deleted)

(For validated, statistically reliable, randomized, controlled, single-patient clinical investigation of FDA approved chronic care drugs, provided by a pharmacist, interpretation and report to the prescribing health care professional, use 99199)

(0137T has been deleted. For transperineal stereotactic template guided saturation prostate biopsies, use 55706)

(0140T has been deleted. To report, use 83987)

(0141T-0143T have been deleted)

(To report pancreatic islet cell transplantation, use 48999)

(0144T-0151T have been deleted. To report, see 75571-75574)

(0155T, 0156T have been deleted)

(For laparoscopic implantation, replacement, revision, or removal of gastric stimulation electrodes, lesser curvature, use 43659)

(0157T, 0158T have been deleted)

(For open implantation, replacement, revision, or removal of gastric stimulation electrodes, lesser curvature, use 43999)

+ 0159T   Computer-aided detection, including computer algorithm analysis of MRI image data for lesion detection/characterization, pharmacokinetic analysis, with further physician review for interpretation, breast MRI (List separately in addition to code for primary procedure)
Sunset January 2017

➔ *CPT Assistant* Mar 07:7, Jul 07:6; *CPT Changes: An Insider's View* 2007

➔ *Clinical Examples in Radiology* Winter 07:9, Spring 07:8

(Use 0159T in conjunction with 77058, 77059)

(Do not report 0159T in conjunction with 76376, 76377)

(0160T, 0161T have been deleted. To report, see 90867, 90869)

(0162T has been deleted. To report, see 95980-95982)

+ 0163T   Total disc arthroplasty (artificial disc), anterior approach, including discectomy to prepare interspace (other than for decompression), each additional interspace, lumbar (List separately in addition to code for primary procedure)
Sunset January 2014

➔ *CPT Assistant* Jun 07:1; *CPT Changes: An Insider's View* 2007, 2009

(Use 0163T in conjunction with 22857)

+ 0164T   Removal of total disc arthroplasty, (artificial disc), anterior approach, each additional interspace, lumbar (List separately in addition to code for primary procedure)
Sunset January 2014

➔ *CPT Assistant* Jun 07:1; *CPT Changes: An Insider's View* 2007, 2009

(Use 0164T in conjunction with 22865)

+ 0165T   Revision including replacement of total disc arthroplasty (artificial disc), anterior approach, each additional interspace, lumbar (List separately in addition to code for primary procedure)
Sunset January 2014

➔ *CPT Assistant* Jun 07:1; *CPT Changes: An Insider's View* 2007, 2009

(Use 0165T in conjunction with 22862)

(Do not report 0163T-0165T in conjunction with 22851, 49010, when performed at the same level)

(For decompression, see 63001-63048)

(0166T, 0167T have been deleted)

(For transmyocardial transcatheter closure of ventricular septal defect, with implant, including cardiopulmonary bypass if performed, use 33999)

(0168T has been deleted)

(For rhinophototherapy, intranasal application of ultraviolet and visible light, use 30999)

0169T   Stereotactic placement of infusion catheter(s) in the brain for delivery of therapeutic agent(s), including computerized stereotactic planning and burr hole(s)
Sunset January 2017

➔ *CPT Assistant* Jul 07:6, May 08:15, Jul 08:4; *CPT Changes: An Insider's View* 2007

(Do not report code 0169T in conjunction with 20660, 61107, 61781, 61782, 61783)

(0170T has been deleted. To report, use 46707)

0171T   Insertion of posterior spinous process distraction device (including necessary removal of bone or ligament for insertion and imaging guidance), lumbar; single level
Sunset December 2017

➔ *CPT Changes: An Insider's View* 2008

+ 0172T   each additional level (List separately in addition to code for primary procedure)
Sunset December 2017

➔ *CPT Changes: An Insider's View* 2008

(Use 0172T in conjunction with 0171T)

▶ (0173T has been deleted) ◀

+ 0174T   Computer-aided detection (CAD) (computer algorithm analysis of digital image data for lesion detection) with further physician review for interpretation and report, with or without digitization of film radiographic images, chest radiograph(s), performed concurrent with primary interpretation (List separately in addition to code for primary procedure)
Sunset December 2017

➔ *CPT Changes: An Insider's View* 2008

(Use 0174T in conjunction with 71010, 71020, 71021, 71022, 71030)

0175T   Computer-aided detection (CAD) (computer algorithm analysis of digital image data for lesion detection) with further physician review for interpretation and report, with or without digitization of film radiographic images, chest radiograph(s), performed remote from primary interpretation
Sunset December 2017

➔ *CPT Changes: An Insider's View* 2008

(Do not report 0175T in conjunction with 71010, 71020, 71021, 71022, 71030)

(0176T, 0177T have been deleted. To report, see 66174, 66175)

0178T   Electrocardiogram, 64 leads or greater, with graphic presentation and analysis; with interpretation and report
Sunset January 2018

➔ *CPT Changes: An Insider's View* 2008

Category III

0179T   tracing and graphics only, without interpretation and report
              Sunset January 2018
              ➔ *CPT Changes: An Insider's View* 2008

0180T   interpretation and report only
              Sunset January 2018
              ➔ *CPT Changes: An Insider's View* 2008

              (For electrocardiogram routine, with at least 12 leads separately performed, see 93000-93010)

0181T   Corneal hysteresis determination, by air impulse stimulation, bilateral, with interpretation and report
              Sunset January 2018
              ➔ *CPT Changes: An Insider's View* 2008

0182T   High dose rate electronic brachytherapy, per fraction
              Sunset December 2017
              ➔ *CPT Changes: An Insider's View* 2008

              (Do not report 0182T in conjunction with 77761-77763, 77776-77778, 77785-77787, 77789)

0183T   Low frequency, non-contact, non-thermal ultrasound, including topical application(s), when performed, wound assessment, and instruction(s) for ongoing care, per day
              Sunset January 2017
              ➔ *CPT Changes: An Insider's View* 2008

0184T   Excision of rectal tumor, transanal endoscopic microsurgical approach (ie, TEMS), including muscularis propria (ie, full thickness)
              Sunset January 2014
              ➔ *CPT Assistant* Jun 10:3; *CPT Changes: An Insider's View* 2009, 2011

              (For non-endoscopic excision of rectal tumor, see 45160, 45171, 45172)

              (Do not report 0184T in conjunction with 45300-45327, 69990)

0185T   Multivariate analysis of patient-specific findings with quantifiable computer probability assessment, including report
              Sunset January 2014
              ➔ *CPT Changes: An Insider's View* 2009

              (Do not report 0185T in conjunction with 99090)

0186T   Suprachoroidal delivery of pharmacologic agent (does not include supply of medication)
              Sunset January 2014
              ➔ *CPT Changes: An Insider's View* 2009

              (0187T has been deleted. To report, use 92132)

Remote Real-Time Interactive Video-conferenced Critical Care Services

►Remote real-time interactive video-conferenced critical care is the direct delivery by a physician(s) or other qualified health care professional(s) of medical care for a critically ill or critically injured patient from an off-site location. Remote real-time interactive video-conferenced critical care is intended to supplement on-site critical care

services at times when a critically ill or injured patient requires additional critical care resources than are available on-site. (For definitions of critical illness or injury and critical care services, see **Critical Care Services** section).

In order to report remote real-time interactive video-conferenced critical care, the physician(s) or other qualified health care professional(s) in the remote location must have real-time access to the patient's medical record including progress notes, nursing notes, current medications, vital signs, clinical laboratory test results, other diagnostic test results, and radiographic images. The remote physician or other qualified health care professional must have real-time capability to enter electronic orders; document the remote care services provided in the hospital medical record; video conference with the on-site health care team in the patient room; assess patients in their individual rooms, using high fidelity audio and video capabilities, including clear observation of the patient, monitors, ventilators, and infusion pumps; and speak to patients and family members.

The review and/or interpretation of all diagnostic information is included in reporting remote real-time interactive video-conferenced critical care when performed during the critical period by the individual(s) providing remote real-time interactive video-conferenced critical care and should not be reported separately.

The remote real-time interactive video-conferenced critical care codes 0188T and 0189T are used to report the total duration of time spent by the individual providing remote real-time interactive video-conferenced critical care services to a critically ill or critically injured patient, even if the time spent by the individual on that date is not continuous. For any given period of time spent providing remote real-time interactive video-conferenced critical care services, the physician or other qualified health care professional must devote his or her full attention to the patient and, therefore, cannot provide services to any other patient during the same period of time.◄

Time spent with the individual patient should be recorded in the patient's record. The time that can be reported as remote real-time interactive video-conferenced critical care is the time spent engaged in work directly related to the individual patient's care. For example, time spent reviewing test results or imaging studies, discussing the critically ill patient's care with other medical staff or documenting remote real-time interactive video-conferenced critical care services in the medical record would be reported as remote real-time interactive video-conferenced critical care, even though it does not occur at the bedside. Also, when the patient is unable or lacks capacity to participate in discussions, time spent from the remote site with family members or surrogate decision makers obtaining a medical history, reviewing the patient's condition or prognosis, or discussing treatment or limitation(s) of treatment may be reported as remote real-time interactive video-conferenced critical care, provided that the conversation bears directly on the management of the patient.

▶Time spent in activities that occur away from the bedside when the individual does not have the real-time capabilities described above may not be reported as remote real-time interactive video-conferenced critical care because the individual is not immediately available to the patient. Time spent in activities that do not directly contribute to the treatment of the patient may not be reported as remote real-time interactive video-conferenced critical care, even if they are performed in the remote site (eg, participation in administrative meetings or telephone calls to discuss other patients). Only one physician or other qualified health care professional may report either critical care services (99291, 99292) or remote real-time interactive video-conferenced critical care for the same period of time. Do not report remote real-time interactive video-conferenced critical care if another individual reports pediatric or neonatal critical care or intensive care services (99468-99476).

Code 0188T is used to report the first 30 to 74 minutes of remote real-time interactive video-conferenced, critical care on a given date. It should be used only once per date even if the time spent by the physician or other qualified health care professional is not continuous on that date. Remote real-time interactive video-conferenced, critical care of less than 30 minutes total duration on a given date should not be reported.◄

Code 0189T is used to report additional block(s) of time, of up to 30 minutes each, beyond the first 74 minutes (see table below).

The following examples illustrate the correct reporting of remote critical care services:

Total Duration of Critical Care	Codes
less than 30 minutes (less than 1/2 hour)	do not report
30-74 minutes (1/2 hr. - 1 hr. 14 min.)	0188T X 1
75-104 minutes (1 hr. 15 min. - 1 hr. 44 min.)	0188T X 1 AND 0189T X 1
105-134 minutes (1 hr. 45 min. - 2 hr. 14 min.)	0188T X 1 AND 0189T X 2

0188T   Remote real-time interactive video-conferenced critical care, evaluation and management of the critically ill or critically injured patient; first 30-74 minutes
Sunset January 2014
➜ *CPT Assistant* Aug 11:10; *CPT Changes: An Insider's View* 2009

+ 0189T   each additional 30 minutes (List separately in addition to code for primary service)
Sunset January 2014
➜ *CPT Assistant* Aug 11:10; *CPT Changes: An Insider's View* 2009

(Use 0189T in conjunction with 0188T)

+ 0190T   Placement of intraocular radiation source applicator (List separately in addition to primary procedure)
Sunset January 2014
➜ *CPT Changes: An Insider's View* 2009

(Use 0190T in conjunction with 67036)

(For application of the source by radiation oncologist, see Clinical Brachytherapy section)

0191T   Insertion of anterior segment aqueous drainage device, without extraocular reservoir; internal approach, into the trabecular meshwork
Sunset January 2014
➜ *CPT Changes: An Insider's View* 2009, 2011

 # 0253T   internal approach, into the suprachoroidal space
Sunset January 2016
➜ *CPT Changes: An Insider's View* 2011

0192T   external approach
Sunset January 2014
➜ *CPT Changes: An Insider's View* 2009

(0193T has been deleted. To report, use 53860)

(0194T has been deleted. To report procalcitonin, use 84145)

▲ 0195T   Arthrodesis, pre-sacral interbody technique, disc space preparation, discectomy, without instrumentation, with image guidance, includes bone graft when performed; L5-S1 interspace
Sunset January 2014
➜ *CPT Changes: An Insider's View* 2009, 2013

+▲ 0196T   L4-L5 interspace (List separately in addition to code for primary procedure)
Sunset January 2014
➜ *CPT Changes: An Insider's View* 2009, 2013

(Use 0196T in conjunction with 0195T)

▶(Do not report 0195T, 0196T in conjunction with 20930-20938, 22558, 22840, 22845, 22848, 22851, 72275, 76000, 76380, 76496, 76497, 77002, 77003, 77011, 77012)◄

0197T   Intra-fraction localization and tracking of target or patient motion during delivery of radiation therapy (eg, 3D positional tracking, gating, 3D surface tracking), each fraction of treatment
Sunset January 2015
➜ *CPT Changes: An Insider's View* 2010

0198T   Measurement of ocular blood flow by repetitive intraocular pressure sampling, with interpretation and report
Sunset January 2015
➜ *CPT Assistant* Mar 11:10; *CPT Changes: An Insider's View* 2010

0199T   Physiologic recording of tremor using accelerometer(s) and/or gyroscope(s) (including frequency and amplitude), including interpretation and report
Sunset January 2015
➜ *CPT Changes: An Insider's View* 2010

Category III

Category III

⊙ **0200T**   Percutaneous sacral augmentation (sacroplasty), unilateral injection(s), including the use of a balloon or mechanical device, when used, 1 or more needles
Sunset January 2015
➜ *CPT Changes: An Insider's View* 2010

⊙ **0201T**   Percutaneous sacral augmentation (sacroplasty), bilateral injections, including the use of a balloon or mechanical device, when used, 2 or more needles
Sunset January 2015
➜ *CPT Changes: An Insider's View* 2010

(For radiological supervision and interpretation, see 72291, 72292)

(If bone biopsy is performed, see 20220, 20225)

0202T   Posterior vertebral joint(s) arthroplasty (eg, facet joint[s] replacement), including facetectomy, laminectomy, foraminotomy, and vertebral column fixation, injection of bone cement, when performed, including fluoroscopy, single level, lumbar spine
Sunset January 2015
➜ *CPT Changes: An Insider's View* 2010

(Do not report 0202T in conjunction with 22521, 22524, 22840, 22851, 22857, 63005, 63012, 63017, 63030, 63042, 63047, 63056 at the same level)

(0203T has been deleted. To report, use 95800)

(0204T has been deleted. To report, use 95801)

✚ **0205T**   Intravascular catheter-based coronary vessel or graft spectroscopy (eg, infrared) during diagnostic evaluation and/or therapeutic intervention including imaging supervision, interpretation, and report, each vessel (List separately in addition to code for primary procedure)
Sunset January 2015
➜ *CPT Changes: An Insider's View* 2010

▶(Use 0205T in conjunction with 92920, 92924, 92928, 92933, 92937, 92941, 92943, 92975, 93454-93461, 93563, 93564)◀

▲ **0206T**   Computerized database analysis of multiple cycles of digitized cardiac electrical data from two or more ECG leads, including transmission to a remote center, application of multiple nonlinear mathematical transformations, with coronary artery obstruction severity assessment
Sunset January 2015
➜ *CPT Changes: An Insider's View* 2010, 2013

(When a 12-lead ECG is performed, 93000-93010 may be reported, as appropriate)

0207T   Evacuation of meibomian glands, automated, using heat and intermittent pressure, unilateral
Sunset January 2015
➜ *CPT Changes: An Insider's View* 2010

0208T   Pure tone audiometry (threshold), automated; air only
Sunset January 2016
➜ *CPT Changes: An Insider's View* 2011

0209T   air and bone
Sunset January 2016
➜ *CPT Assistant* Mar 11:8; *CPT Changes: An Insider's View* 2011

0210T   Speech audiometry threshold, automated;
Sunset January 2016
➜ *CPT Changes: An Insider's View* 2011

0211T   with speech recognition
Sunset January 2016
➜ *CPT Assistant* Mar 11:8; *CPT Changes: An Insider's View* 2011

0212T   Comprehensive audiometry threshold evaluation and speech recognition (0209T, 0211T combined), automated
Sunset January 2016
➜ *CPT Assistant* Mar 11:8; *CPT Changes: An Insider's View* 2011

(For audiometric testing using audiometers performed manually by a qualified health care professional, see 92551-92557)

0213T   Injection(s), diagnostic or therapeutic agent, paravertebral facet (zygapophyseal) joint (or nerves innervating that joint) with ultrasound guidance, cervical or thoracic; single level
Sunset January 2016
➜ *CPT Assistant* Feb 11:5, Jul 11:14; *CPT Changes: An Insider's View* 2011
➜ *Clinical Examples in Radiology* Winter 10:15

(To report bilateral procedure, use 0213T with modifier 50)

✚ **0214T**   second level (List separately in addition to code for primary procedure)
Sunset January 2016
➜ *CPT Assistant* Jul 11:14; *CPT Changes: An Insider's View* 2011
➜ *Clinical Examples in Radiology* Winter 10:15

(To report bilateral procedure, use 0214T with modifier 50)

✚ **0215T**   third and any additional level(s) (List separately in addition to code for primary procedure)
Sunset January 2016
➜ *CPT Assistant* Jul 11:14; *CPT Changes: An Insider's View* 2011
➜ *Clinical Examples in Radiology* Winter 10:14

(Do not report 0215T more than once per day)

(Use 0214T, 0215T in conjunction with 0213T)

(To report bilateral procedure, use 0215T with modifier 50)

0216T   Injection(s), diagnostic or therapeutic agent, paravertebral facet (zygapophyseal) joint (or nerves innervating that joint) with ultrasound guidance, lumbar or sacral; single level
Sunset January 2016
➜ *CPT Assistant* Jul 11:14; *CPT Changes: An Insider's View* 2011
➜ *Clinical Examples in Radiology* Winter 10:14

(To report bilateral procedure, use 0216T with modifier 50)

+ 0217T   second level (List separately in addition to code for primary procedure)

Sunset January 2016

→ *CPT Assistant* Jul 11:14; *CPT Changes: An Insider's View* 2011

→ *Clinical Examples in Radiology* Winter 10:14

(To report bilateral procedure, use 0217T with modifier 50)

+ 0218T   third and any additional level(s) (List separately in addition to code for primary procedure)

Sunset January 2016

→ *CPT Assistant* Feb 11:5, Jul 11:14; *CPT Changes: An Insider's View* 2011

→ *Clinical Examples in Radiology* Winter 10:14

(Do not report 0218T more than once per day)

(Use 0217T, 0218T in conjunction with 0216T)

(If injection(s) are performed using fluoroscopy or CT, see 64490-64495)

(To report bilateral procedure, use 0218T with modifier 50)

0219T   Placement of a posterior intrafacet implant(s), unilateral or bilateral, including imaging and placement of bone graft(s) or synthetic device(s), single level; cervical

Sunset January 2016

→ *CPT Assistant* Nov 10:8, Jul 11:18; *CPT Changes: An Insider's View* 2011

0220T   thoracic

Sunset January 2016

→ *CPT Assistant* Nov 10:8, Jul 11:18; *CPT Changes: An Insider's View* 2011

0221T   lumbar

Sunset January 2016

→ *CPT Assistant* Nov 10:8, Jul 11:18; *CPT Changes: An Insider's View* 2011

(Do not report 0219T-0221T in conjunction with any radiological service)

(Do not report 0219T-0221T in conjunction with 20930, 20931, 22600-22614, 22840, 22851 at the same level)

+ 0222T   each additional vertebral segment (List separately in addition to code for primary procedure)

Sunset January 2016

→ *CPT Assistant* Nov 10:6, Jul 11:18; *CPT Changes: An Insider's View* 2011

(Use 0222T in conjunction with 0219T-0221T)

(For posterior or posterolateral arthrodesis technique, see 22600-22614)

Acoustic cardiography codes 0223T-0225T describe the evaluation and optimization of physiologic data including systolic and diastolic heart sounds and their temporal relationships to the electrocardiogram (ECG).

Codes 0224T and 0225T also include interrogation and limited reprogramming of a cardiac pacing device to ensure hemodynamic optimization (heart rate parameter and/or automated timing modes, including explicit

changes of AV/VV intervals) and facilitate device parameter optimization. Do not report 0224T or 0225T in conjunction with 93288 or 93289.

Acoustic cardiography services include a rhythm strip ECG. Do not report 93040-93042 in conjunction with 0223T-0225T.

For complete programming services as a separate procedure, see 93280, 93281, 93283, and 93284.

0223T   Acoustic cardiography, including automated analysis of combined acoustic and electrical intervals; single, with interpretation and report

Sunset January 2016

→ *CPT Changes: An Insider's View* 2011

0224T   multiple, including serial trended analysis and limited reprogramming of device parameter, AV or VV delays only, with interpretation and report

Sunset January 2016

→ *CPT Changes: An Insider's View* 2011

0225T   multiple, including serial trended analysis and limited reprogramming of device parameter, AV and VV delays, with interpretation and report

Sunset January 2016

→ *CPT Changes: An Insider's View* 2011

0226T   Anoscopy, high resolution (HRA) (with magnification and chemical agent enhancement); diagnostic, including collection of specimen(s) by brushing or washing when performed

Sunset January 2016

→ *CPT Changes: An Insider's View* 2011

0227T   with biopsy(ies)

Sunset January 2016

→ *CPT Changes: An Insider's View* 2011

0228T   Injection(s), anesthetic agent and/or steroid, transforaminal epidural, with ultrasound guidance, cervical or thoracic; single level

Sunset January 2016

→ *CPT Assistant* Feb 11:4, Jul 11:16; *CPT Changes: An Insider's View* 2011

+ 0229T   each additional level (List separately in addition to code for primary procedure)

Sunset January 2016

→ *CPT Assistant* Feb 11:4, Jul 11:16; *CPT Changes: An Insider's View* 2011

(Use 0229T in conjunction with 0228T)

0230T   Injection(s), anesthetic agent and/or steroid, transforaminal epidural, with ultrasound guidance, lumbar or sacral; single level

Sunset January 2016

→ *CPT Assistant* Feb 11:4, Jul 11:16, Nov 11:11; *CPT Changes: An Insider's View* 2011

+ 0231T   each additional level (List separately in addition to code for primary procedure)

Sunset January 2016

→ *CPT Assistant* Feb 11:4, Jul 11:16; *CPT Changes: An Insider's View* 2011

▲=Revised code   ●=New code   ▶◀=Contains new or revised text   ⊘=Modifier 51 exempt

(Use 0231T in conjunction with 0230T)

(For transforaminal epidural injections performed under fluoroscopy or CT, see 64479–64484)

(Do not report 0228T-0231T in conjunction with 76942, 76998, 76999)

0232T Injection(s), platelet rich plasma, any site, including image guidance, harvesting and preparation when performed
Sunset January 2016
➔ *CPT Assistant* Oct 10:8, Dec 10:8, May 12:11; *CPT Changes: An Insider's View* 2011

(Do not report 0232T in conjunction with 20550, 20551, 20600-20610, 20926, 76942, 77002, 77012, 77021, 86965)

▶(Do not report 38220-38230 for bone marrow aspiration for platelet rich stem cell injection. For bone marrow aspiration for platelet rich stem cell injection, use 0232T)◀

0233T Skin advanced glycation endproducts (AGE) measurement by multi-wavelength fluorescent spectroscopy
Sunset January 2016
➔ *CPT Assistant* Oct 10:10, Dec 10:10; *CPT Changes: An Insider's View* 2011

Atherectomy (Open or Percutaneous) for Supra-Inguinal Arteries

Codes 0234T-0238T describe atherectomy performed by any method (eg, directional, rotational, laser) in arteries above the inguinal ligaments. These codes are structured differently than the codes describing atherectomy performed below the inguinal ligaments (37225, 37227, 37229, 37231, 37233, 37235).

These supra-inguinal atherectomy codes all include the surgical work of performing the atherectomy plus the radiological supervision and interpretation of the atherectomy. Unlike the atherectomy codes for infra-inguinal arteries, this set of Category III codes does not include accessing and selectively catheterizing the vessel, traversing the lesion, embolic protection if used, other intervention used to treat the same or other vessels, or closure of the arteriotomy by any method. These codes describe endovascular procedures performed percutaneously and/or through an open surgical exposure.

0234T Transluminal peripheral atherectomy, open or percutaneous, including radiological supervision and interpretation; renal artery
Sunset January 2016
➔ *CPT Assistant* Jul 11:3; *CPT Changes: An Insider's View* 2011
➔ *Clinical Examples in Radiology* Spring 11:3

0235T visceral artery (except renal), each vessel
Sunset January 2016
➔ *CPT Assistant* Jul 11:3; *CPT Changes: An Insider's View* 2011
➔ *Clinical Examples in Radiology* Spring 11:3

0236T abdominal aorta
Sunset January 2016
➔ *CPT Assistant* Jul 11:3; *CPT Changes: An Insider's View* 2011
➔ *Clinical Examples in Radiology* Spring 11:3

0237T brachiocephalic trunk and branches, each vessel
Sunset January 2016
➔ *CPT Assistant* Jul 11:3; *CPT Changes: An Insider's View* 2011
➔ *Clinical Examples in Radiology* Spring 11:3

0238T iliac artery, each vessel
Sunset January 2016
➔ *CPT Assistant* Jul 11:3; *CPT Changes: An Insider's View* 2011
➔ *Clinical Examples in Radiology* Spring 11:3

0239T Bioimpedance spectroscopy (BIS), measuring 100 frequencies or greater, direct measurement of extracellular fluid differences between the limbs
Sunset January 2016
➔ *CPT Changes: An Insider's View* 2011

0240T Esophageal motility (manometric study of the esophagus and/or gastroesophageal junction) study with interpretation and report; with high resolution esophageal pressure topography
Sunset January 2016
➔ *CPT Changes: An Insider's View* 2011, 2012

(Do not report 0240T in conjunction with 91010 or 91013)

+ 0241T with stimulation or perfusion during high resolution esophageal pressure topography study (eg, stimulant, acid or alkali perfusion) (List separately in addition to code for primary procedure)
Sunset January 2016
➔ *CPT Changes: An Insider's View* 2011, 2012

(Use 0241T in conjunction with 0240T)

(Do not report 0241T in conjunction with 91010 or 91013)

(Do not report 0241T more than once per session)

(To report esophageal motility studies without high resolution esophageal pressure topography, use 91010 and with stimulant or perfusion, use 91013)

▶(0242T has been deleted. To report, use 91112)◀

0243T Intermittent measurement of wheeze rate for bronchodilator or bronchial-challenge diagnostic evaluation(s), with interpretation and report
Sunset January 2016
➔ *CPT Changes: An Insider's View* 2011

(Use 0243T once per 24 hour period)

(Do not report 0243T in conjunction with 0244T for the same 24 hour period)

0244T Continuous measurement of wheeze rate during treatment assessment or during sleep for documentation of nocturnal wheeze and cough for diagnostic evaluation 3 to 24 hours, with interpretation and report
Sunset January 2016
➔ *CPT Changes: An Insider's View* 2011

Category III

0245T   Open treatment of rib fracture requiring internal fixation, unilateral; 1-2 ribs
Sunset January 2016
➔ *CPT Changes: An Insider's View* 2011

0246T   3-4 ribs
Sunset January 2016
➔ *CPT Changes: An Insider's View* 2011

0247T   5-6 ribs
Sunset January 2016
➔ *CPT Changes: An Insider's View* 2011

0248T   7 or more ribs
Sunset January 2016
➔ *CPT Changes: An Insider's View* 2011

0249T   Ligation, hemorrhoidal vascular bundle(s), including ultrasound guidance
Sunset January 2016
➔ *CPT Changes: An Insider's View* 2011

(Do not report 0249T in conjunction with 46020, 46221, 46250-46262, 46600, 46945, 46946, 76872, 76942, 76998)

▶(0250T-0252T have been deleted. For airway sizing and insertion and removal of bronchial valve[s], see 31647-31649)◀

0253T   Code is out of numerical sequence. See 0188T-0254T

0254T   Endovascular repair of iliac artery bifurcation (eg, aneurysm, pseudoaneurysm, arteriovenous malformation, trauma) using bifurcated endoprosthesis from the common iliac artery into both the external and internal iliac artery, unilateral;
Sunset January 2016
➔ *CPT Changes: An Insider's View* 2011

0255T   radiological supervision and interpretation
Sunset January 2016
➔ *CPT Changes: An Insider's View* 2011

▶(0256T has been deleted. To report, see 33361-33364)◀

▶(0257T has been deleted. To report, see 33365, 0318T)◀

▶(0258T has been deleted. To report, see 33365, 33366)◀

▶(0259T has been deleted. To report, see 33365-33369)◀

0260T   Total body systemic hypothermia, per day, in the neonate 28 days of age or younger
Sunset January 2017
➔ *CPT Changes: An Insider's View* 2012

0261T   Selective head hypothermia, per day, in the neonate 28 days of age or younger
Sunset January 2017
➔ *CPT Changes: An Insider's View* 2012

0262T   Implantation of catheter-delivered prosthetic pulmonary valve, endovascular approach
Sunset January 2017
➔ *CPT Changes: An Insider's View* 2012

(0262T includes all congenital cardiac catheterization[s], intraprocedural contrast injection[s], fluoroscopic radiological supervision and interpretation, and imaging guidance performed to complete the pulmonary valve procedure. Do not report 0262T in conjunction with 76000, 76001, 93530, 93563, 93566-93568)

(0262T includes percutaneous balloon angioplasty/valvuloplasty of the pulmonary valve/conduit. Do not report 0262T in conjunction with 92990)

▶(0262T includes stent deployment within the pulmonary conduit. Do not report 37205, 37206, 75960 for stent placement within the pulmonary conduit. Report 37205, 37206, 92928-92944, 75960 separately when cardiovascular stent placement is performed at a site separate from the prosthetic valve delivery site. Report 92997, 92998 separately when pulmonary artery angioplasty is performed at a site separate from the prosthetic valve delivery site)◀

0263T   Intramuscular autologous bone marrow cell therapy, with preparation of harvested cells, multiple injections, one leg, including ultrasound guidance, if performed; complete procedure including unilateral or bilateral bone marrow harvest
Sunset January 2017
➔ *CPT Changes: An Insider's View* 2012

(Do not report 0263T in conjunction with 38204-38242, 76942, 93925, 93926)

0264T   complete procedure excluding bone marrow harvest
Sunset January 2017
➔ *CPT Changes: An Insider's View* 2012

(Do not report 0264T in conjunction with 38204-38242, 76942, 93925, 93926, 0265T)

0265T   unilateral or bilateral bone marrow harvest only for intramuscular autologous bone marrow cell therapy
Sunset January 2017
➔ *CPT Changes: An Insider's View* 2012

(Do not report 0265T in conjunction with 38204-38242, 0264T. For complete procedure, use 0263T)

0266T   Implantation or replacement of carotid sinus baroreflex activation device; total system (includes generator placement, unilateral or bilateral lead placement, intra-operative interrogation, programming, and repositioning, when performed)
Sunset January 2017
➔ *CPT Changes: An Insider's View* 2012

0267T   lead only, unilateral (includes intra-operative interrogation, programming, and repositioning, when performed)
Sunset January 2017
➔ *CPT Changes: An Insider's View* 2012

(For bilateral lead implantation or replacement, use 0267T with modifier 50)

Category III

0268T   pulse generator only (includes intra-operative interrogation, programming, and repositioning, when performed)
Sunset January 2017
➔ *CPT Changes: An Insider's View* 2012

(Do not report 0267T, 0268T in conjunction with 0266T, 0269T-0273T)

0269T   Revision or removal of carotid sinus baroreflex activation device; total system (includes generator placement, unilateral or bilateral lead placement, intra-operative interrogation, programming, and repositioning, when performed)
Sunset January 2017
➔ *CPT Changes: An Insider's View* 2012

(Do not report 0269T in conjunction with 0266T-0268T, 0270T-0273T)

0270T   lead only, unilateral (includes intra-operative interrogation, programming, and repositioning, when performed)
Sunset January 2017
➔ *CPT Changes: An Insider's View* 2012

(Do not report 0270T in conjunction with 0266T-0269T, 0271T-0273T)

(For bilateral lead removal, use 0270T with modifier 50)

(For removal of total carotid sinus baroreflex activation device, use 0269T)

0271T   pulse generator only (includes intra-operative interrogation, programming, and repositioning, when performed)
Sunset January 2017
➔ *CPT Changes: An Insider's View* 2012

(Do not report 0271T in conjunction with 0266T-0270T, 0272T, 0273T)

(For removal and replacement, see 0266T, 0267T, 0268T)

0272T   Interrogation device evaluation (in person), carotid sinus baroreflex activation system, including telemetric iterative communication with the implantable device to monitor device diagnostics and programmed therapy values, with interpretation and report (eg, battery status, lead impedance, pulse amplitude, pulse width, therapy frequency, pathway mode, burst mode, therapy start/stop times each day);
Sunset January 2017
➔ *CPT Changes: An Insider's View* 2012

(Do not report 0272T in conjunction with 0266T-0271T, 0273T)

0273T   with programming
Sunset January 2017
➔ *CPT Changes: An Insider's View* 2012

(Do not report 0273T in conjunction with 0266T-0272T)

0274T   Percutaneous laminotomy/laminectomy (interlaminar approach) for decompression of neural elements, (with or without ligamentous resection, discectomy, facetectomy and/or foraminotomy), any method, under indirect image guidance (eg, fluoroscopic, CT), with or without the use of an endoscope, single or multiple levels, unilateral or bilateral; cervical or thoracic
Sunset January 2017
➔ *CPT Assistant* Jan 12:14, Jul 12:3, 4; *CPT Changes: An Insider's View* 2012

0275T   lumbar
Sunset January 2017
➔ *CPT Assistant* Jan 12:14, Jul 12:3, 4; *CPT Changes: An Insider's View* 2012

(For laminotomy/hemilaminectomy performed using an open and endoscopically-assisted approach, see 63020-63035)

(For percutaneous decompression of the nucleus pulposus of intervertebral disc utilizing needle based technique, use 62287)

▶(0276T, 0277T have been deleted. To report, see 31660, 31661)◀

0278T   Transcutaneous electrical modulation pain reprocessing (eg, scrambler therapy), each treatment session (includes placement of electrodes)
Sunset January 2017
➔ *CPT Changes: An Insider's View* 2012

▶(0279T, 0280T have been deleted. To report, see 86152, 86153)◀

0281T   Percutaneous transcatheter closure of the left atrial appendage with implant, including fluoroscopy, transseptal puncture, catheter placement(s), left atrial angiography, left atrial appendage angiography, radiological supervision and interpretation
Sunset January 2017
➔ *CPT Changes: An Insider's View* 2012

(Do not report 0281T in conjunction with 93462 [left heart catheterization by transseptal puncture])

(Report cardiac catheterization procedures [93451-93461, 93530-93533] separately for indications distinct from the left atrial appendage closure procedure)

(For left ventriculography performed by transseptal approach for indications distinct from the left atrial appendage closure procedure, use 93565)

(Do not report 0281T in conjunction with 93452, 93453, 93458-93461, 93531-93533 unless catheterization of the left ventricle is performed by a non-transseptal approach for indications distinct from the left atrial appendage closure procedure)

(Do not report 0281T in conjunction with 93451, 93453, 93456, 93460, 93461, 93530-93533 unless complete right heart catheterization is performed for indications distinct from the left atrial appendage closure procedure)

⊙ **0282T**   Percutaneous or open implantation of neurostimulator electrode array(s), subcutaneous (peripheral subcutaneous field stimulation), including imaging guidance, when performed, cervical, thoracic or lumbar; for trial, including removal at the conclusion of trial period

Sunset January 2017

➔ *CPT Changes: An Insider's View* 2012

⊙ **0283T**   permanent, with implantation of a pulse generator

Sunset January 2017

➔ *CPT Changes: An Insider's View* 2012

⊙ **0284T**   Revision or removal of pulse generator or electrodes, including imaging guidance, when performed, including addition of new electrodes, when performed

Sunset January 2017

➔ *CPT Changes: An Insider's View* 2012

0285T   Electronic analysis of implanted peripheral subcutaneous field stimulation pulse generator, with reprogramming when performed

Sunset January 2017

➔ *CPT Changes: An Insider's View* 2012

(Do not report 0282T-0285T in conjunction with 64550-64595, 77002, 77003, 95970-95973)

0286T   Near-infrared spectroscopy studies of lower extremity wounds (eg, for oxyhemoglobin measurement)

Sunset January 2017

➔ *CPT Assistant* Jun 12:16; *CPT Changes: An Insider's View* 2012

0287T   Near-infrared guidance for vascular access requiring real-time digital visualization of subcutaneous vasculature for evaluation of potential access sites and vessel patency

Sunset January 2017

➔ *CPT Changes: An Insider's View* 2012

0288T   Anoscopy, with delivery of thermal energy to the muscle of the anal canal (eg, for fecal incontinence)

Sunset January 2017

➔ *CPT Changes: An Insider's View* 2012

(Do not report 0288T in conjunction with 46600-46615)

+ 0289T   Corneal incisions in the donor cornea created using a laser, in preparation for penetrating or lamellar keratoplasty (List separately in addition to code for primary procedure)

Sunset January 2017

➔ *CPT Changes: An Insider's View* 2012

(Use 0289T in conjunction with 65710, 65730, 65750, 65755)

+ 0290T   Corneal incisions in the recipient cornea created using a laser, in preparation for penetrating or lamellar keratoplasty (List separately in addition to code for primary procedure)

Sunset January 2017

➔ *CPT Changes: An Insider's View* 2012

(Use 0290T in conjunction with 65710, 65730, 65750, 65755)

⊙+● **0291T**   Intravascular optical coherence tomography (coronary native vessel or graft) during diagnostic evaluation and/or therapeutic intervention, including imaging supervision, interpretation, and report; initial vessel (List separately in addition to primary procedure)

Sunset January 2018

➔ *CPT Changes: An Insider's View* 2013

▶(Use 0291T in conjunction with cardiac catheterization codes 92920, 92924, 92928, 92933, 92937, 92941, 92943, 92975, 93454-93461, 93563, 93564)◀

▶(Intravascular optical coherence tomography services include all transducer manipulations and repositioning within the specific vessel being examined, both before and after therapeutic intervention [eg, stent placement])◀

⊙+● **0292T**   each additional vessel (List separately in addition to primary procedure)

Sunset January 2018

➔ *CPT Changes: An Insider's View* 2013

▶(Use 0292T in conjunction with 0291T)◀

▶(For intravascular spectroscopy, use 0205T)◀

⊙● **0293T**   Insertion of left atrial hemodynamic monitor; complete system, includes implanted communication module and pressure sensor lead in left atrium including transseptal access, radiological supervision and interpretation, and associated injection procedures, when performed

Sunset January 2018

➔ *CPT Changes: An Insider's View* 2013

▶(Do not report 0293T in conjunction with 93462, 93662)◀

⊙+● **0294T**   pressure sensor lead at time of insertion of pacing cardioverter-defibrillator pulse generator including radiological supervision and interpretation and associated injection procedures, when performed (List separately in addition to code for primary procedure)

Sunset January 2018

➔ *CPT Changes: An Insider's View* 2013

▶(Use 0294T in conjunction with 33230, 33231, 33240, 33262-33264, 33249)◀

▶(Do not report 0294T in conjunction with 93462, 93662)◀

▶(Do not report 0293T or 0294T in conjunction with 33202-33249, 93451-93453 unless performed for separate and distinct clinical indication other than for placement or calibration of left atrial hemodynamic monitoring system)◀

● **0295T**   External electrocardiographic recording for more than 48 hours up to 21 days by continuous rhythm recording and storage; includes recording, scanning analysis with report, review and interpretation

Sunset January 2018

➔ *CPT Changes: An Insider's View* 2013

● **0296T**   recording (includes connection and initial recording)

Sunset January 2018

➔ *CPT Changes: An Insider's View* 2013

▲=Revised code   ●=New code   ▶ ◀=Contains new or revised text   ⊘=Modifier 51 exempt   American Medical Association   **591**

● **0297T**   scanning analysis with report
Sunset January 2018
➜ *CPT Changes: An Insider's View* 2013

● **0298T**   review and interpretation
Sunset January 2018
➜ *CPT Changes: An Insider's View* 2013

►(Do not report 0295T-0298T in conjunction with 93224-93272 for same monitoring period)◄

● **0299T**   Extracorporeal shock wave for integumentary wound healing, high energy, including topical application and dressing care; initial wound
Sunset January 2018
➜ *CPT Changes: An Insider's View* 2013

+● **0300T**   each additional wound (List separately in addition to code for primary procedure)
Sunset January 2018
➜ *CPT Changes: An Insider's View* 2013

►(Use 0300T in conjunction with 0299T)◄

►(Do not report 0300T in conjunction with 28890, 0101T, 0102T when treating same area)◄

⊙● **0301T**   Destruction/reduction of malignant breast tumor with externally applied focused microwave, including interstitial placement of disposable catheter with combined temperature monitoring probe and microwave focusing sensocatheter under ultrasound thermotherapy guidance
Sunset January 2018
➜ *CPT Changes: An Insider's View* 2013

►(Do not report 0301T in conjunction with 76645, 76942, 76998, 77600-77615)◄

⊙● **0302T**   Insertion or removal and replacement of intracardiac ischemia monitoring system including imaging supervision and interpretation when performed and intra-operative interrogation and programming when performed; complete system (includes device and electrode)
Sunset January 2018
➜ *CPT Changes: An Insider's View* 2013

⊙● **0303T**   electrode only
Sunset January 2018
➜ *CPT Changes: An Insider's View* 2013

⊙● **0304T**   device only
Sunset January 2018
➜ *CPT Changes: An Insider's View* 2013

►(Do not report 0302T-0304T in conjunction with 93000-93010)◄

● **0305T**   Programming device evaluation (in person) of intracardiac ischemia monitoring system with iterative adjustment of programmed values, with analysis, review, and report
Sunset January 2018
➜ *CPT Changes: An Insider's View* 2013

►(Do not report 0305T in conjunction with 93000-93010, 0302T-0304T, 0306T)◄

● **0306T**   Interrogation device evaluation (in person) of intracardiac ischemia monitoring system with analysis, review, and report
Sunset January 2018
➜ *CPT Changes: An Insider's View* 2013

►(Do not report 0306T in conjunction with 93000-93010, 0302T-0305T)◄

⊙● **0307T**   Removal of intracardiac ischemia monitoring device
Sunset January 2018
➜ *CPT Changes: An Insider's View* 2013

⊙⊘● **0308T**   Insertion of ocular telescope prosthesis including removal of crystalline lens
Sunset January 2018
➜ *CPT Changes: An Insider's View* 2013

►(Do not report 0308T in conjunction with 65800-65815, 66020, 66030, 66600-66635, 66761, 66825, 66982-66986, 69990)◄

+● **0309T**   Arthrodesis, pre-sacral interbody technique, including disc space preparation, discectomy, with posterior instrumentation, with image guidance, includes bone graft, when performed, lumbar, L4-L5 interspace (List separately in addition to code for primary procedure)
Sunset January 2018
➜ *CPT Changes: An Insider's View* 2013

►(Use 0309T in conjunction with 22586)◄

►(Do not report 0309T in conjunction with 20930-20938, 22840, 22848, 72275, 77002, 77003, 77011, 77012)◄

● **0310T**   Motor function mapping using non-invasive navigated transcranial magnetic stimulation (nTMS) for therapeutic treatment planning, upper and lower extremity
Sunset January 2018
➜ *CPT Changes: An Insider's View* 2013

►(Do not report 0310T in conjunction with 95860-95870, 95928, 95929, 95939)◄

● **0311T**   Non-invasive calculation and analysis of central arterial pressure waveforms with interpretation and report
Sunset January 2018
➜ *CPT Changes: An Insider's View* 2013

● **0312T**   Vagus nerve blocking therapy (morbid obesity); laparoscopic implantation of neurostimulator electrode array, anterior and posterior vagal trunks adjacent to esophagogastric junction (EGJ), with implantation of pulse generator, includes programming
Sunset January 2018
➜ *CPT Changes: An Insider's View* 2013

● **0313T**   laparoscopic revision or replacement of vagal trunk neurostimulator electrode array, including connection to existing pulse generator
Sunset January 2018
➜ *CPT Changes: An Insider's View* 2013

● **0314T**   laparoscopic removal of vagal trunk neurostimulator
             electrode array and pulse generator
             Sunset January 2018
             ➔ *CPT Changes: An Insider's View* 2013

● **0315T**   removal of pulse generator
             Sunset January 2018
             ➔ *CPT Changes: An Insider's View* 2013

● **0316T**   replacement of pulse generator
             Sunset January 2018
             ➔ *CPT Changes: An Insider's View* 2013

             ►(Do not report 0315T in conjunction with 0316T)◄

● **0317T**   neurostimulator pulse generator electronic analysis,
             includes reprogramming when performed
             Sunset January 2018
             ➔ *CPT Changes: An Insider's View* 2013

             ► (For implantation, revision, replacement, and/or
             removal of vagus [cranial] nerve neurostimulator
             electrode array and/or pulse generator for vagus nerve
             stimulation performed other than at the EGJ [eg,
             epilepsy], see 64568-64570)◄

             ► (For analysis and/or [re]programming for vagus nerve
             stimulator, see 95970, 95974, 95975) ◄

● **0318T**   Implantation of catheter-delivered prosthetic aortic heart
             valve, open thoracic approach, (eg, transapical, other
             than transaortic)
             Sunset January 2018
             ➔ *CPT Changes: An Insider's View* 2013

             ►(For percutaneous femoral artery, open femoral artery,
             open axillary artery, open iliac artery, or transaortic
             approach, see 33361-33365)◄

             ►(To report cardiopulmonary bypass in conjunction with
             0318T, see 33367, 33368, or 33369)◄

Notes

Appendix A

Modifiers

This list includes all of the modifiers applicable to CPT 2013 codes.

A modifier provides the means to report or indicate that a service or procedure that has been performed has been altered by some specific circumstance but not changed in its definition or code. Modifiers also enable health care professionals to effectively respond to payment policy requirements established by other entities.

22 Increased Procedural Services: When the work required to provide a service is substantially greater than typically required, it may be identified by adding modifier 22 to the usual procedure code. Documentation must support the substantial additional work and the reason for the additional work (ie, increased intensity, time, technical difficulty of procedure, severity of patient's condition, physical and mental effort required). **Note:** This modifier should not be appended to an E/M service.

➔ *CPT Assistant* Jan 09:8, Apr 09:8, Jun 09:8,10 *CPT Changes: An Insider's View* 2008

23 Unusual Anesthesia: Occasionally, a procedure, which usually requires either no anesthesia or local anesthesia, because of unusual circumstances must be done under general anesthesia. This circumstance may be reported by adding modifier 23 to the procedure code of the basic service.

24 ▶Unrelated Evaluation and Management Service by the Same Physician or Other Qualified Health Care Professional During a Postoperative Period: The physician or other qualified health care professional may need to indicate that an evaluation and management service was performed during a postoperative period for a reason(s) unrelated to the original procedure. This circumstance may be reported by adding modifier 24 to the appropriate level of E/M service.◀

➔ *CPT Changes: An Insider's View* 2013

25 ▶Significant, Separately Identifiable Evaluation and Management Service by the Same Physician or Other Qualified Health Care Professional on the Same Day of the Procedure or Other Service: It may be necessary to indicate that on the day a procedure or service identified by a CPT code was performed, the patient's condition required a significant, separately identifiable E/M service above and beyond the other service provided or beyond the usual preoperative and postoperative care associated with the procedure that was performed. A significant, separately identifiable E/M service is defined or substantiated by documentation that satisfies the relevant criteria for the respective E/M service to be reported (see **Evaluation and Management Services Guidelines** for instructions on determining level of E/M service). The E/M service may be prompted by the symptom or condition for which the procedure and/or service was provided. As such, different

diagnoses are not required for reporting of the E/M services on the same date. This circumstance may be reported by adding modifier 25 to the appropriate level of E/M service. **Note:** This modifier is not used to report an E/M service that resulted in a decision to perform surgery. See modifier 57. For significant, separately identifiable non-E/M services, see modifier 59.◀

➔ *CPT Assistant* Feb 09:22, Mar 09:3, Apr 09:4; Jun 09:11 *CPT Changes: An Insider's View* 2008, 2013

26 ▶Professional Component: Certain procedures are a combination of a physician or other qualified health care professional component and a technical component. When the physician or other qualified health care professional component is reported separately, the service may be identified by adding modifier 26 to the usual procedure number.◀

➔ *CPT Assistant* Jan 09:7, Apr 09:4, May 09:7; *CPT Changes: An Insider's View* 2013

32 Mandated Services: Services related to *mandated* consultation and/or related services (eg, third party payer, governmental, legislative or regulatory requirement) may be identified by adding modifier 32 to the basic procedure.

33 Preventive Services: When the primary purpose of the service is the delivery of an evidence based service in accordance with a US Preventive Services Task Force A or B rating in effect and other preventive services identified in preventive services mandates (legislative or regulatory), the service may be identified by adding 33 to the procedure. For separately reported services specifically identified as preventive, the modifier should not be used.

➔ *CPT Changes: An Insider's View* 2012

47 Anesthesia by Surgeon: Regional or general anesthesia provided by the surgeon may be reported by adding modifier 47 to the basic service. (This does not include local anesthesia.) **Note:** Modifier 47 would not be used as a modifier for the anesthesia procedures.

50 Bilateral Procedure: Unless otherwise identified in the listings, bilateral procedures that are performed at the same session, should be identified by adding modifier 50 to the appropriate 5 digit code.

➔ *CPT Assistant* Apr 09:9, *CPT Changes: An Insider's View* 2011

51 ▶Multiple Procedures: When multiple procedures, other than E/M services, Physical Medicine and Rehabilitation services or provision of supplies (eg, vaccines), are performed at the same session by the same individual, the primary procedure or service may be reported as listed. The additional procedure(s) or service(s) may be identified by appending modifier 51 to the additional procedure or service code(s). **Note:** This modifier should not be appended to designated "add-on" codes (see Appendix D).◀

➔ *CPT Assistant* Feb 09:6, Mar 09:10, Apr 09:8 *CPT Changes: An Insider's View* 2008, 2013

52 ▶Reduced Services: Under certain circumstances a service or procedure is partially reduced or eliminated at the

Appendixes A–E

discretion of the physician or other qualified health care professional. Under these circumstances the service provided can be identified by its usual procedure number and the addition of modifier 52, signifying that the service is reduced. This provides a means of reporting reduced services without disturbing the identification of the basic service. **Note:** For hospital outpatient reporting of a previously scheduled procedure/service that is partially reduced or cancelled as a result of extenuating circumstances or those that threaten the well-being of the patient prior to or after administration of anesthesia, see modifiers 73 and 74 (see modifiers approved for ASC hospital outpatient use).◄

➔ *CPT Assistant* Mar 09:11, Apr 09:5, May 09:8, Jun 09:10; *CPT Changes: An Insider's View* 2013

53 ▶**Discontinued Procedure:** Under certain circumstances, the physician or other qualified health care professional may elect to terminate a surgical or diagnostic procedure. Due to extenuating circumstances or those that threaten the well being of the patient, it may be necessary to indicate that a surgical or diagnostic procedure was started but discontinued. This circumstance may be reported by adding modifier 53 to the code reported by the individual for the discontinued procedure. **Note:** This modifier is not used to report the elective cancellation of a procedure prior to the patient's anesthesia induction and/or surgical preparation in the operating suite. For outpatient hospital/ambulatory surgery center (ASC) reporting of a previously scheduled procedure/service that is partially reduced or cancelled as a result of extenuating circumstances or those that threaten the well being of the patient prior to or after administration of anesthesia, see modifiers 73 and 74 (see modifiers approved for ASC hospital outpatient use).◄

➔ *CPT Changes: An Insider's View* 2013

54 ▶**Surgical Care Only:** When 1 physician or other qualified health care professional performs a surgical procedure and another provides preoperative and/or postoperative management, surgical services may be identified by adding modifier 54 to the usual procedure number.◄

➔ *CPT Changes: An Insider's View* 2013

55 ▶**Postoperative Management Only:** When 1 physician or other qualified health care professional performed the postoperative management and another performed the surgical procedure, the postoperative component may be identified by adding modifier 55 to the usual procedure number.◄

➔ *CPT Changes: An Insider's View* 2013

56 ▶**Preoperative Management Only:** When 1 physician or other qualified health care professional performed the preoperative care and evaluation and another performed the surgical procedure, the preoperative component may be identified by adding modifier 56 to the usual procedure number.◄

➔ *CPT Changes: An Insider's View* 2013

57 **Decision for Surgery:** An evaluation and management service that resulted in the initial decision to perform the surgery may be identified by adding modifier 57 to the appropriate level of E/M service.

➔ *CPT Assistant* May 09:9

58 ▶**Staged or Related Procedure or Service by the Same Physician or Other Qualified Health Care Professional During the Postoperative Period :** It may be necessary to indicate that the performance of a procedure or service during the postoperative period was: (a) planned or anticipated (staged); (b) more extensive than the original procedure; or (c) for therapy following a surgical procedure. This circumstance may be reported by adding modifier 58 to the staged or related procedure. **Note:** For treatment of a problem that requires a return to the operating/procedure room (eg, unanticipated clinical condition), see modifier 78.◄

➔ *CPT Changes: An Insider's View* 2008, 2013

59 **Distinct Procedural Service:** Under certain circumstances, it may be necessary to indicate that a procedure or service was distinct or independent from other non-E/M services performed on the same day. Modifier 59 is used to identify procedures/services, other than E/M services, that are not normally reported together, but are appropriate under the circumstances. Documentation must support a different session, different procedure or surgery, different site or organ system, separate incision/excision, separate lesion, or separate injury (or area of injury in extensive injuries) not ordinarily encountered or performed on the same day by the same individual. However, when another already established modifier is appropriate it should be used rather than modifier 59. Only if no more descriptive modifier is available, and the use of modifier 59 best explains the circumstances, should modifier 59 be used. **Note:** Modifier 59 should not be appended to an E/M service. To report a separate and distinct E/M service with a non-E/M service performed on the same date, see modifier 25.

➔ *CPT Assistant* Feb 09:17, Apr 09:4,8, May 09:6, Jun 09:8 *CPT Changes: An Insider's View* 2008

62 ▶**Two Surgeons:** When 2 surgeons work together as primary surgeons performing distinct part(s) of a procedure, each surgeon should report his/her distinct operative work by adding modifier 62 to the procedure code and any associated add-on code(s) for that procedure as long as both surgeons continue to work together as primary surgeons. Each surgeon should report the co-surgery once using the same procedure code. If additional procedure(s) (including add-on procedure(s) are performed during the same surgical session, separate code(s) may also be reported with modifier 62 added. **Note:** If a co-surgeon acts as an assistant in the performance of additional procedure(s), other than those reported with the modifier 62, during the same surgical session, those services may be reported using separate procedure code(s) with modifier 80 or modifier 82 added, as appropriate.◄

➔ *CPT Changes: An Insider's View* 2013

63 ▶**Procedure Performed on Infants less than 4 kg:** Procedures performed on neonates and infants up to a present body weight of 4 kg may involve significantly increased complexity and physician or other qualified health care professional work commonly associated with these patients. This circumstance may be reported by adding modifier 63 to the procedure number. **Note:** Unless otherwise designated, this modifier may only be appended to procedures/services listed in the 20005-69990 code series. Modifier 63 should not be appended to any CPT

codes listed in the **Evaluation and Management Services, Anesthesia, Radiology, Pathology/Laboratory, or Medicine** sections.◀

➔ *CPT Changes: An Insider's View* 2013

66 ▶**Surgical Team:** Under some circumstances, highly complex procedures (requiring the concomitant services of several physicians or other qualified health care professionals, often of different specialties, plus other highly skilled, specially trained personnel, various types of complex equipment) are carried out under the "surgical team" concept. Such circumstances may be identified by each participating individual with the addition of modifier 66 to the basic procedure number used for reporting services.◀

➔ *CPT Changes: An Insider's View* 2013

76 ▶**Repeat Procedure or Service by Same Physician or Other Qualified Health Care Professional:** It may be necessary to indicate that a procedure or service was repeated by the same physician or other qualified health care professional subsequent to the original procedure or service. This circumstance may be reported by adding modifier 76 to the repeated procedure or service. **Note:** This modifier should not be appended to an E/M service.◀

➔ *CPT Assistant* Feb 09:6 *CPT Changes: An Insider's View* 2008, 2011, 2013

77 ▶**Repeat Procedure by Another Physician or Other Qualified Health Care Professional:** It may be necessary to indicate that a basic procedure or service was repeated by another physician or other qualified health care professional subsequent to the original procedure or service. This circumstance may be reported by adding modifier 77 to the repeated procedure or service. **Note:** This modifier should not be appended to an E/M service.◀

➔ *CPT Changes: An Insider's View* 2008, 2011, 2013

78 ▶**Unplanned Return to the Operating/Procedure Room by the Same Physician or Other Qualified Health Care Professional Following Initial Procedure for a Related Procedure During the Postoperative Period :** It may be necessary to indicate that another procedure was performed during the postoperative period of the initial procedure (unplanned procedure following initial procedure). When this procedure is related to the first, and requires the use of an operating/procedure room, it may be reported by adding modifier 78 to the related procedure. (For repeat procedures, see modifier 76.)◀

➔ *CPT Changes: An Insider's View* 2008, 2011, 2013

79 ▶**Unrelated Procedure or Service by the Same Physician or Other Qualified Health Care Professional During the Postoperative Period :** The individual may need to indicate that the performance of a procedure or service during the postoperative period was unrelated to the original procedure. This circumstance may be reported by using modifier 79. (For repeat procedures on the same day, see modifier 76.)◀

➔ *CPT Changes: An Insider's View* 2013

80 **Assistant Surgeon:** Surgical assistant services may be identified by adding modifier 80 to the usual procedure number(s).

81 **Minimum Assistant Surgeon:** Minimum surgical assistant services are identified by adding modifier 81 to the usual procedure number.

82 **Assistant Surgeon (when qualified resident surgeon not available):** The unavailability of a qualified resident surgeon is a prerequisite for use of modifier 82 appended to the usual procedure code number(s).

90 ▶**Reference (Outside) Laboratory:** When laboratory procedures are performed by a party other than the treating or reporting physician or other qualified health care professional, the procedure may be identified by adding modifier 90 to the usual procedure number.◀

➔ *CPT Changes: An Insider's View* 2013

91 **Repeat Clinical Diagnostic Laboratory Test:** In the course of treatment of the patient, it may be necessary to repeat the same laboratory test on the same day to obtain subsequent (multiple) test results. Under these circumstances, the laboratory test performed can be identified by its usual procedure number and the addition of modifier 91. **Note:** This modifier may not be used when tests are rerun to confirm initial results; due to testing problems with specimens or equipment; or for any other reason when a normal, one-time, reportable result is all that is required. This modifier may not be used when other code(s) describe a series of test results (eg, glucose tolerance tests, evocative/suppression testing). This modifier may only be used for laboratory test(s) performed more than once on the same day on the same patient.

➔ *CPT Assistant* May 09:6

92 **Alternative Laboratory Platform Testing:** When laboratory testing is being performed using a kit or transportable instrument that wholly or in part consists of a single use, disposable analytical chamber, the service may be identified by adding modifier 92 to the usual laboratory procedure code (HIV testing 86701-86703, and 87389). The test does not require permanent dedicated space, hence by its design may be hand carried or transported to the vicinity of the patient for immediate testing at that site, although location of the testing is not in itself determinative of the use of this modifier.

➔ *CPT Changes: An Insider's View* 2008, 2012

99 **Multiple Modifiers:** Under certain circumstances 2 or more modifiers may be necessary to completely delineate a service. In such situations modifier 99 should be added to the basic procedure, and other applicable modifiers may be listed as part of the description of the service.

Anesthesia Physical Status Modifiers

The Physical Status modifiers are consistent with the American Society of Anesthesiologists ranking of patient physical status, and distinguishing various levels of complexity of the anesthesia service provided. All anesthesia services are reported by use of the anesthesia five-digit procedure code (00100-01999) with the appropriate physical status modifier appended.

Example: 00100-P1

Under certain circumstances, when another established modifier(s) is appropriate, it should be used in addition to the physical status modifier.

Example: 00100-P4-53

Physical Status Modifier P1: A normal healthy patient

Physical Status Modifier P2: A patient with mild systemic disease

Physical Status Modifier P3: A patient with severe systemic disease

Physical Status Modifier P4: A patient with severe systemic disease that is a constant threat to life

Physical Status Modifier P5: A moribund patient who is not expected to survive without the operation

Physical Status Modifier P6: A declared brain-dead patient whose organs are being removed for donor purposes

Modifiers Approved for Ambulatory Surgery Center (ASC) Hospital Outpatient Use

CPT Level I Modifiers

25 ►**Significant, Separately Identifiable Evaluation and Management Service by the Same Physician or Other Qualified Health Care Professional on the Same Day of the Procedure or Other Service :** It may be necessary to indicate that on the day a procedure or service identified by a CPT code was performed, the patient's condition required a significant, separately identifiable E/M service above and beyond the other service provided or beyond the usual preoperative and postoperative care associated with the procedure that was performed. A significant, separately identifiable E/M service is defined or substantiated by documentation that satisfies the relevant criteria for the respective E/M service to be reported (see **Evaluation and Management Services Guidelines** for instructions on determining level of E/M service). The E/M service may be prompted by the symptom or condition for which the procedure and/or service was provided. As such, different diagnoses are not required for reporting of the E/M services on the same date. This circumstance may be reported by adding modifier 25 to the appropriate level of E/M service. **Note:** This modifier is not used to report an E/M service that resulted in a decision to perform surgery. See modifier 57. For significant, separately identifiable non-E/M services, see modifier 59.◄

➔ *CPT Changes: An Insider's View* 2013

27 **Multiple Outpatient Hospital E/M Encounters on the Same Date:** For hospital outpatient reporting purposes, utilization of hospital resources related to separate and distinct E/M encounters performed in multiple outpatient hospital settings on the same date may be reported by adding modifier 27 to each appropriate level outpatient and/or emergency

department E/M code(s). This modifier provides a means of reporting circumstances involving evaluation and management services provided by physician(s) in more than one (multiple) outpatient hospital setting(s) (eg, hospital emergency department, clinic). **Note:** This modifier is not to be used for physician reporting of multiple E/M services performed by the same physician on the same date. For physician reporting of all outpatient evaluation and management services provided by the same physician on the same date and performed in multiple outpatient setting(s) (eg, hospital emergency department, clinic), see **Evaluation and Management, Emergency Department, or Preventive Medicine Services** codes.

50 **Bilateral Procedure:** Unless otherwise identified in the listings, bilateral procedures that are performed at the same session, should be identified by adding modifier 50 to the appropriate 5 digit code.

52 ►**Reduced Services:** Under certain circumstances a service or procedure is partially reduced or eliminated at the discretion of the physician or other qualified health care professional. Under these circumstances the service provided can be identified by its usual procedure number and the addition of modifier 52, signifying that the service is reduced. This provides a means of reporting reduced services without disturbing the identification of the basic service. **Note:** For hospital outpatient reporting of a previously scheduled procedure/service that is partially reduced or cancelled as a result of extenuating circumstances or those that threaten the well-being of the patient prior to or after administration of anesthesia, see modifiers 73 and 74 (see modifiers approved for ASC hospital outpatient use).◄

➔ *CPT Changes: An Insider's View* 2013

58 ►**Staged or Related Procedure or Service by the Same Physician or Other Qualified Health Care Professional During the Postoperative Period :** It may be necessary to indicate that the performance of a procedure or service during the postoperative period was: (a) planned or anticipated (staged); (b) more extensive than the original procedure; or (c) for therapy following a surgical procedure. This circumstance may be reported by adding modifier 58 to the staged or related procedure. **Note:** For treatment of a problem that requires a return to the operating/procedure room (eg, unanticipated clinical condition), see modifier 78.◄

➔ *CPT Changes: An Insider's View* 2013

59 **Distinct Procedural Service:** Under certain circumstances, it may be necessary to indicate that a procedure or service was distinct or independent from other non-E/M services performed on the same day. Modifier 59 is used to identify procedures/services, other than E/M services, that are not normally reported together, but are appropriate under the circumstances. Documentation must support a different session, different procedure or surgery, different site or organ system, separate incision/excision, separate lesion, or separate injury (or area of injury in extensive injuries) not ordinarily encountered or performed on the same day by the same individual. However, when another already established modifier is appropriate it should be used rather than modifier 59. Only if no more descriptive modifier is available, and the use of modifier 59 best explains the circumstances, should modifier 59 be used. **Note:** Modifier 59 should not be appended to an E/M service. To report a separate and distinct E/M service with a non-E/M service performed on the same date, see modifier 25.

73 Discontinued Out-Patient Hospital/Ambulatory Surgery Center (ASC) Procedure Prior to the Administration of Anesthesia: Due to extenuating circumstances or those that threaten the well being of the patient, the physician may cancel a surgical or diagnostic procedure subsequent to the patient's surgical preparation (including sedation when provided, and being taken to the room where the procedure is to be performed), but prior to the administration of anesthesia (local, regional block(s) or general). Under these circumstances, the intended service that is prepared for but cancelled can be reported by its usual procedure number and the addition of modifier 73. **Note:** The elective cancellation of a service prior to the administration of anesthesia and/or surgical preparation of the patient should not be reported. For physician reporting of a discontinued procedure, see modifier 53.

74 Discontinued Out-Patient Hospital/Ambulatory Surgery Center (ASC) Procedure After Administration of Anesthesia: Due to extenuating circumstances or those that threaten the well being of the patient, the physician may terminate a surgical or diagnostic procedure after the administration of anesthesia (local, regional block(s), general) or after the procedure was started (incision made, intubation started, scope inserted, etc). Under these circumstances, the procedure started but terminated can be reported by its usual procedure number and the addition of modifier 74. **Note:** The elective cancellation of a service prior to the administration of anesthesia and/or surgical preparation of the patient should not be reported. For physician reporting of a discontinued procedure, see modifier 53.

76 ▶Repeat Procedure or Service by Same Physician or Other Qualified Health Care Professional: It may be necessary to indicate that a procedure or service was repeated by the same physician or other qualified health care professional subsequent to the original procedure or service. This circumstance may be reported by adding modifier 76 to the repeated procedure or service. **Note:** This modifier should not be appended to an E/M service.◀
→ *CPT Changes: An Insider's View* 2013

77 ▶Repeat Procedure by Another Physician or Other Qualified Health Care Professional: It may be necessary to indicate that a basic procedure or service was repeated by another physician or other qualified health care professional subsequent to the original procedure or service. This circumstance may be reported by adding modifier 77 to the repeated procedure or service. **Note:** This modifier should not be appended to an E/M service.◀
→ *CPT Changes: An Insider's View* 2013

78 ▶Unplanned Return to the Operating/Procedure Room by the Same Physician or Other Qualified Health Care Professional Following Initial Procedure for a Related Procedure During the Postoperative Period : It may be necessary to indicate that another procedure was performed during the postoperative period of the initial procedure (unplanned procedure following initial procedure). When this procedure is related to the first, and requires the use of an operating/procedure room, it may be reported by adding modifier 78 to the related procedure. (For repeat procedures, see modifier 76.)◀
→ *CPT Changes: An Insider's View* 2013

79 ▶Unrelated Procedure or Service by the Same Physician or Other Qualified Health Care Professional During the Postoperative Period : The individual may need to indicate that the performance of a procedure or service during the postoperative period was unrelated to the original procedure. This circumstance may be reported by using modifier 79. (For repeat procedures on the same day, see modifier 76.)◀
→ *CPT Changes: An Insider's View* 2008, 2011

91 Repeat Clinical Diagnostic Laboratory Test: In the course of treatment of the patient, it may be necessary to repeat the same laboratory test on the same day to obtain subsequent (multiple) test results. Under these circumstances, the laboratory test performed can be identified by its usual procedure number and the addition of modifier 91. **Note:** This modifier may not be used when tests are rerun to confirm initial results; due to testing problems with specimens or equipment; or for any other reason when a normal, one-time, reportable result is all that is required. This modifier may not be used when other code(s) describe a series of test results (eg, glucose tolerance tests, evocative/suppression testing). This modifier may only be used for laboratory test(s) performed more than once on the same day on the same patient.

Level II (HCPCS/National) Modifiers

E1 Upper left, eyelid

E2 Lower left, eyelid

E3 Upper right, eyelid

E4 Lower right, eyelid

F1 Left hand, second digit

F2 Left hand, third digit

F3 Left hand, fourth digit

F4 Left hand, fifth digit

F5 Right hand, thumb

F6 Right hand, second digit

F7 Right hand, third digit

F8 Right hand, fourth digit

F9 Right hand, fifth digit

FA Left hand, thumb

GG Performance and payment of a screening mammogram and diagnostic mammogram on the same patient, same day

GH Diagnostic mammogram converted from screening mammogram on same day

LC Left circumflex coronary artery

LD Left anterior descending coronary artery

LT Left side (used to identify procedures performed on the left side of the body)

QM Ambulance service provided under arrangement by a provider of services

QN Ambulance service furnished directly by a provider of services

RC Right coronary artery

RT Right side (used to identify procedures performed on the right side of the body)

T1 Left foot, second digit

T2 Left foot, third digit

T3 Left foot, fourth digit

T4 Left foot, fifth digit

T5 Right foot, great toe

T6 Right foot, second digit

T7 Right foot, third digit

T8 Right foot, fourth digit

T9 Right foot, fifth digit

TA Left foot, great toe

Appendixes A–E

Appendix B

Summary of Additions, Deletions, and Revisions

Appendix B shows the actual changes that were made to the code descriptors. New codes appear with a bullet (●) and are indicated as "Code Added." Revised codes are preceded with a triangle (▲). Within revised codes, the deleted language appears with a ~~strikethrough~~, while new text is underlined. Codes with which moderate sedation would not be separately reported when performed at the same session by the same individual are denoted with the bullseye (⊙). The symbol ∕ is used to identify codes for vaccines that are pending FDA approval (see **Appendix K**). The symbol # is used to identify codes that have been resequenced (see **Appendix N**). CPT add-on codes are annotated by the symbol ✚ (see **Appendix D**). The symbol ⊘ is used to identify codes that are exempt from the use of modifier 51 (see **Appendix E**).

Evaluation and Management

▲ 99201   **Office or other outpatient visit** for the evaluation and management of a new patient, which requires these 3 key components:

- **A problem focused history;**
- **A problem focused examination;**
- **Straightforward medical decision making.**

Counseling and/or coordination of care with <u>other physicians,</u> other ~~providers~~<u>qualified health care professionals,</u> or agencies are provided consistent with the nature of the problem(s) and the patient's and/or family's needs.

Usually, the presenting problem(s) are self-limited or minor. ~~Physicians typically spend~~<u>Typically,</u> 10 minutes <u>are spent</u> face-to-face with the patient and/or family.

▲ 99202   **Office or other outpatient visit** for the evaluation and management of a new patient, which requires these 3 key components:

- **An expanded problem focused history;**
- **An expanded problem focused examination;**
- **Straightforward medical decision making.**

Counseling and/or coordination of care with <u>other physicians,</u> other ~~providers~~<u>qualified health care professionals,</u> or agencies are provided consistent with the nature of the problem(s) and the patient's and/or family's needs.

Usually, the presenting problem(s) are of low to moderate severity. ~~Physicians typically spend~~<u>Typically,</u> 20 minutes <u>are spent</u> face-to-face with the patient and/or family.

▲ 99203   **Office or other outpatient visit** for the evaluation and management of a new patient, which requires these 3 key components:

- **A detailed history;**
- **A detailed examination;**
- **Medical decision making of low complexity.**

Counseling and/or coordination of care with <u>other physicians,</u> other ~~providers~~<u>qualified health care professionals,</u> or agencies are provided consistent with the nature of the problem(s) and the patient's and/or family's needs.

Usually, the presenting problem(s) are of moderate severity. ~~Physicians typically spend~~<u>Typically,</u> 30 minutes <u>are spent</u> face-to-face with the patient and/or family.

▲ 99204   **Office or other outpatient visit** for the evaluation and management of a new patient, which requires these 3 key components:

- **A comprehensive history;**
- **A comprehensive examination;**
- **Medical decision making of moderate complexity.**

Counseling and/or coordination of care with <u>other physicians,</u> other ~~providers~~<u>qualified health care professionals,</u> or agencies are provided consistent with the nature of the problem(s) and the patient's and/or family's needs.

Usually, the presenting problem(s) are of moderate to high severity. ~~Physicians typically spend~~<u>Typically,</u> 45 minutes <u>are spent</u> face-to-face with the patient and/or family.

▲ 99205   **Office or other outpatient visit** for the evaluation and management of a new patient, which requires these 3 key components:

- **A comprehensive history;**
- **A comprehensive examination;**
- **Medical decision making of high complexity.**

Counseling and/or coordination of care with <u>other physicians,</u> other ~~providers~~<u>qualified health care professionals,</u> or agencies are provided consistent with the nature of the problem(s) and the patient's and/or family's needs.

Usually, the presenting problem(s) are of moderate to high severity. ~~Physicians typically spend~~<u>Typically,</u> 60 minutes <u>are spent</u> face-to-face with the patient and/or family.

▲ 99211   **Office or other outpatient visit** for the evaluation and management of an established patient, that may not require the presence of a physician <u>or other qualified health care professional</u>. Usually, the presenting problem(s) are minimal. Typically, 5 minutes are spent performing or supervising these services.

▲ 99212   **Office or other outpatient visit** for the evaluation and management of an established patient, which requires at least 2 of these 3 key components:

- **A problem focused history;**
- **A problem focused examination;**
- **Straightforward medical decision making.**

Counseling and/or coordination of care with <u>other physicians,</u> other ~~providers~~<u>qualified health care professionals,</u> or agencies are provided consistent with the nature of the problem(s) and the patient's and/or family's needs.

Usually, the presenting problem(s) are self-limited or minor. ~~Physicians typically spend~~<u>Typically,</u> 10 minutes <u>are spent</u> face-to-face with the patient and/or family.

▲ 99213 **Office or other outpatient visit** for the evaluation and management of an established patient, which requires at least 2 of these 3 key components:

■ **An expanded problem focused history;**

■ **An expanded problem focused examination;**

■ **Medical decision making of low complexity.**

Counseling and coordination of care with other physicians, other ~~providers~~qualified health care professionals, or agencies are provided consistent with the nature of the problem(s) and the patient's and/or family's needs.

Usually, the presenting problem(s) are of low to moderate severity. ~~Physicians typically spend~~Typically, 15 minutes are spent face-to-face with the patient and/or family.

▲ 99214 **Office or other outpatient visit** for the evaluation and management of an established patient, which requires at least 2 of these 3 key components:

■ **A detailed history;**

■ **A detailed examination;**

■ **Medical decision making of moderate complexity.**

Counseling and/or coordination of care with other physicians, other ~~providers~~qualified health care professionals, or agencies are provided consistent with the nature of the problem(s) and the patient's and/or family's needs.

Usually, the presenting problem(s) are of moderate to high severity. ~~Physicians typically spend~~Typically, 25 minutes are spent face-to-face with the patient and/or family.

▲ 99215 **Office or other outpatient visit** for the evaluation and management of an established patient, which requires at least 2 of these 3 key components:

■ **A comprehensive history;**

■ **A comprehensive examination;**

■ **Medical decision making of high complexity.**

Counseling and/or coordination of care with other physicians, other ~~providers~~qualified health care professionals, or agencies are provided consistent with the nature of the problem(s) and the patient's and/or family's needs.

Usually, the presenting problem(s) are of moderate to high severity. ~~Physicians typically spend~~Typically, 40 minutes are spent face-to-face with the patient and/or family.

▲ 99217 **Observation care discharge** day management (This code is to be utilized ~~by the physician~~ to report all services provided to a patient on discharge from "observation status" if the discharge is on other than the initial date of "observation status." To report services to a patient designated as "observation status" or "inpatient status" and discharged on the same date, use the codes for Observation or Inpatient Care Services [including Admission and Discharge Services, 99234-99236 as appropriate.])

▲ 99218 **Initial observation care,** per day, for the evaluation and management of a patient which requires these 3 key components:

■ **A detailed or comprehensive history;**

■ **A detailed or comprehensive examination; and**

■ **Medical decision making that is straightforward or of low complexity.**

Counseling and/or coordination of care with other physicians, other ~~providers~~qualified health care professionals, or agencies are provided consistent with the nature of the problem(s) and the patient's and/or family's needs.

Usually, the problem(s) requiring admission to "observation status" are of low severity. ~~Physicians typically spend~~Typically, 30 minutes are spent at the bedside and on the patient's hospital floor or unit.

▲ 99219 **Initial observation care,** per day, for the evaluation and management of a patient, which requires these 3 key components:

■ **A comprehensive history;**

■ **A comprehensive examination; and**

■ **Medical decision making of moderate complexity.**

Counseling and/or coordination of care with other physicians, other ~~providers~~qualified health care professionals, or agencies are provided consistent with the nature of the problem(s) and the patient's and/or family's needs.

Usually, the problem(s) requiring admission to "observation status" are of moderate severity. ~~Physicians typically spend~~Typically, 50 minutes are spent at the bedside and on the patient's hospital floor or unit.

▲ 99220 **Initial observation care,** per day, for the evaluation and management of a patient, which requires these 3 key components:

■ **A comprehensive history;**

■ **A comprehensive examination; and**

■ **Medical decision making of high complexity.**

Counseling and/or coordination of care with other physicians, other ~~providers~~qualified health care professionals, or agencies are provided consistent with the nature of the problem(s) and the patient's and/or family's needs.

Usually, the problem(s) requiring admission to "observation status" are of high severity. ~~Physicians typically spend~~Typically, 70 minutes are spent at the bedside and on the patient's hospital floor or unit.

#▲ 99224 **Subsequent observation care,**~~per day, for the evaluation and management of a patient, which requires at least 2 of these 3 key components:

■ **Problem focused interval history;**

■ **Problem focused examination;**

■ **Medical decision making that is straightforward or of low complexity.**

Counseling and/or coordination of care with other physicians, other ~~providers~~qualified health care professionals, or agencies are provided consistent with the nature of the problem(s) and the patient's and/or family's needs.

Usually, the patient is stable, recovering, or improving. ~~Physicians typically spend~~Typically, 15 minutes are spent at the bedside and on the patient's hospital floor or unit.

#▲ 99225 **Subsequent observation care,** per day, for the evaluation and management of a patient, which requires at least 2 of these 3 key components:

■ **An expanded problem focused interval history;**

■ **An expanded problem focused examination;**

■ **Medical decision making of moderate complexity.**

Counseling and/or coordination of care with other physicians, other ~~providers~~qualified health care professionals, or agencies are provided consistent with the nature of the problem(s) and the patient's and/or family's needs.

Appendixes A–E

Usually, the patient is responding inadequately to therapy or has developed a minor complication. ~~Physicians typically spend~~Typically, 25 minutes are spent at the bedside and on the patient's hospital floor or unit.

#▲ 99226 **Subsequent observation care,** per day, for the evaluation and management of a patient, which requires at least 2 of these 3 key components:

■ **A detailed interval history;**

■ **A detailed examination;**

■ **Medical decision making of high complexity.**

Counseling and/or coordination of care with other physicians, other ~~providers~~qualified health care professionals, or agencies are provided consistent with the nature of the problem(s) and the patient's and/or family's needs.

Usually, the patient is unstable or has developed a significant complication or a significant new problem. ~~Physicians typically spend~~Typically, 35 minutes are spent at the bedside and on the patient's hospital floor or unit.

▲ 99221 **Initial hospital care,** per day, for the evaluation and management of a patient, which requires these 3 key components:

■ **A detailed or comprehensive history;**

■ **A detailed or comprehensive examination; and**

■ **Medical decision making that is straightforward or of low complexity.**

Counseling and/or coordination of care with other physicians, other ~~providers~~qualified health care professionals, or agencies are provided consistent with the nature of the problem(s) and the patient's and/or family's needs.

Usually, the problem(s) requiring admission are of low severity. ~~Physicians typically spend~~Typically, 30 minutes are spent at the bedside and on the patient's hospital floor or unit.

▲ 99222 **Initial hospital care,** per day, for the evaluation and management of a patient, which requires these 3 key components:

■ **A comprehensive history;**

■ **A comprehensive examination; and**

■ **Medical decision making of moderate complexity.**

Counseling and/or coordination of care with other physicians, other ~~providers~~qualified health care professionals, or agencies are provided consistent with the nature of the problem(s) and the patient's and/or family's needs.

Usually, the problem(s) requiring admission are of moderate severity. ~~Physicians typically spend~~Typically, 50 minutes are spent at the bedside and on the patient's hospital floor or unit.

▲ 99223 **Initial hospital care,** per day, for the evaluation and management of a patient, which requires these 3 key components:

■ **A comprehensive history;**

■ **A comprehensive examination; and**

■ **Medical decision making of high complexity.**

Counseling and/or coordination of care with other physicians, other ~~providers~~qualified health care professionals, or agencies are provided consistent with the nature of the problem(s) and the patient's and/or family's needs.

Usually, the problem(s) requiring admission are of high severity. ~~Physicians typically spend~~Typically, 70 minutes are spent at the bedside and on the patient's hospital floor or unit.

▲ 99231 **Subsequent hospital care,** per day, for the evaluation and management of a patient, which requires at least 2 of these 3 key components:

■ **A problem focused interval history;**

■ **A problem focused examination;**

■ **Medical decision making that is straightforward or of low complexity.**

Counseling and/or coordination of care with other physicians, other ~~providers~~qualified health care professionals, or agencies are provided consistent with the nature of the problem(s) and the patient's and/or family's needs.

Usually, the patient is stable, recovering or improving. ~~Physicians typically spend~~Typically, 15 minutes are spent at the bedside and on the patient's hospital floor or unit.

▲ 99232 **Subsequent hospital care,** per day, for the evaluation and management of a patient, which requires at least 2 of these 3 key components:

■ **An expanded problem focused interval history;**

■ **An expanded problem focused examination;**

■ **Medical decision making of moderate complexity.**

Counseling and/or coordination of care with other physicians, other ~~providers~~qualified health care professionals, or agencies are provided consistent with the nature of the problem(s) and the patient's and/or family's needs.

Usually, the patient is responding inadequately to therapy or has developed a minor complication. ~~Physicians typically spend~~Typically, 25 minutes are spent at the bedside and on the patient's hospital floor or unit.

▲ 99233 **Subsequent hospital care,** per day, for the evaluation and management of a patient, which requires at least 2 of these 3 key components:

■ **A detailed interval history;**

■ **A detailed examination;**

■ **Medical decision making of high complexity.**

Counseling and/or coordination of care with other physicians, other ~~providers~~qualified health care professionals, or agencies are provided consistent with the nature of the problem(s) and the patient's and/or family's needs.

Usually, the patient is unstable or has developed a significant complication or a significant new problem. ~~Physicians typically spend~~Typically, 35 minutes are spent at the bedside and on the patient's hospital floor or unit.

▲ 99234 **Observation or inpatient hospital care,** for the evaluation and management of a patient including admission and discharge on the same date, which requires these 3 key components:

■ **A detailed or comprehensive history;**

■ **A detailed or comprehensive examination; and**

■ **Medical decision making that is straightforward or of low complexity.**

Counseling and/or coordination of care with other physicians, other ~~providers~~qualified health care professionals, or agencies are provided consistent with the nature of the problem(s) and the patient's and/or family's needs.

Usually the presenting problem(s) requiring admission are of low severity. Typically, 40 minutes are spent at the bedside and on the patient's hospital floor or unit.

▲ 99235 **Observation or inpatient hospital care,** for the evaluation and management of a patient including admission and discharge on the same date, which requires these 3 key components:

■ **A comprehensive history;**

■ **A comprehensive examination; and**

■ **Medical decision making of moderate complexity.**

Counseling and/or coordination of care with other physicians, other ~~providers~~qualified health care professionals, or agencies are provided consistent with the nature of the problem(s) and the patient's and/or family's needs.

Usually the presenting problem(s) requiring admission are of moderate severity. Typically, 50 minutes are spent at the bedside and on the patient's hospital floor or unit.

▲ 99236 **Observation or inpatient hospital care,** for the evaluation and management of a patient including admission and discharge on the same date, which requires these 3 key components:

■ **A comprehensive history;**

■ **A comprehensive examination; and**

■ **Medical decision making of high complexity.**

Counseling and/or coordination of care with other physicians, other ~~providers~~qualified health care professionals, or agencies are provided consistent with the nature of the problem(s) and the patient's and/or family's needs.

Usually the presenting problem(s) requiring admission are of high severity. Typically, 55 minutes are spent at the bedside and on the patient's hospital floor or unit.

▲ 99241 **Office consultation** for a new or established patient, which requires these 3 key components:

■ **A problem focused history;**

■ **A problem focused examination; and**

■ **Straightforward medical decision making.**

Counseling and/or coordination of care with other physicians, other ~~providers~~qualified health care professionals, or agencies are provided consistent with the nature of the problem(s) and the patient's and/or family's needs.

Usually, the presenting problem(s) are self limited or minor. ~~Physicians typically spend~~Typically, 15 minutes are spent face-to-face with the patient and/or family.

▲ 99242 **Office consultation** for a new or established patient, which requires these 3 key components:

■ **An expanded problem focused history;**

■ **An expanded problem focused examination; and**

■ **Straightforward medical decision making.**

Counseling and/or coordination of care with other physicians, other ~~providers~~qualified health care professionals, or agencies are provided consistent with the nature of the problem(s) and the patient's and/or family's needs.

Usually, the presenting problem(s) are of low severity. ~~Physicians typically spend~~Typically, 30 minutes are spent face-to-face with the patient and/or family.

▲ 99243 **Office consultation** for a new or established patient, which requires these 3 key components:

■ **A detailed history;**

■ **A detailed examination; and**

■ **Medical decision making of low complexity.**

Counseling and/or coordination of care with other physicians, other ~~providers~~qualified health care professionals, or agencies are provided consistent with the nature of the problem(s) and the patient's and/or family's needs.

Usually, the presenting problem(s) are of moderate severity. ~~Physicians typically spend~~Typically, 40 minutes are spent face-to-face with the patient and/or family.

▲ 99244 **Office consultation** for a new or established patient, which requires these 3 key components:

■ **A comprehensive history;**

■ **A comprehensive examination; and**

■ **Medical decision making of moderate complexity.**

Counseling and/or coordination of care with other physicians, other ~~providers~~qualified health care professionals, or agencies are provided consistent with the nature of the problem(s) and the patient's and/or family's needs.

Usually, the presenting problem(s) are of moderate to high severity. ~~Physicians typically spend~~Typically, 60 minutes are spent face-to-face with the patient and/or family.

▲ 99245 **Office consultation** for a new or established patient, which requires these 3 key components:

■ **A comprehensive history;**

■ **A comprehensive examination; and**

■ **Medical decision making of high complexity.**

Counseling and/or coordination of care with other physicians, other ~~providers~~qualified health care professionals, or agencies are provided consistent with the nature of the problem(s) and the patient's and/or family's needs.

Usually, the presenting problem(s) are of moderate to high severity. ~~Physicians typically spend~~Typically, 80 minutes are spent face-to-face with the patient and/or family.

▲ 99251 **Inpatient consultation** for a new or established patient, which requires these 3 key components:

■ **A problem focused history;**

■ **A problem focused examination; and**

■ **Straightforward medical decision making.**

Counseling and/or coordination of care with other physicians, other ~~providers~~qualified health care professionals, or agencies are provided consistent with the nature of the problem(s) and the patient's and/or family's needs.

Usually, the presenting problem(s) are self limited or minor. ~~Physicians typically spend~~Typically, 20 minutes are spent at the bedside and on the patient's hospital floor or unit.

▲ 99252 **Inpatient consultation** for a new or established patient, which requires these 3 key components:

■ **An expanded problem focused history;**

■ **An expanded problem focused examination; and**

■ **Straightforward medical decision making.**

Counseling and/or coordination of care with other physicians, other ~~providers~~qualified health care professionals, or agencies are provided consistent with the nature of the problem(s) and the patient's and/or family's needs.

Appendixes A–E

Usually, the presenting problem(s) are of low severity. ~~Physicians typically spend~~Typically, 40 minutes are spent at the bedside and on the patient's hospital floor or unit.

▲ 99253   **Inpatient consultation** for a new or established patient, which requires these 3 key components:

- **A detailed history;**
- **A detailed examination; and**
- **Medical decision making of low complexity.**

Counseling and/or coordination of care with <u>other physicians,</u> other ~~providers~~<u>qualified health care professionals,</u> or agencies are provided consistent with the nature of the problem(s) and the patient's and/or family's needs.

Usually, the presenting problem(s) are of moderate severity. ~~Physicians typically spend~~Typically, 55 minutes <u>are spent</u> at the bedside and on the patient's hospital floor or unit.

▲ 99254   **Inpatient consultation** for a new or established patient, which requires these 3 key components:

- **A comprehensive history;**
- **A comprehensive examination; and**
- **Medical decision making of moderate complexity.**

Counseling and/or coordination of care with <u>other physicians,</u> other ~~providers~~<u>qualified health care professionals,</u> or agencies are provided consistent with the nature of the problem(s) and the patient's and/or family's needs.

Usually, the presenting problem(s) are of moderate to high severity. ~~Physicians typically spend~~Typically, 80 minutes <u>are spent</u> at the bedside and on the patient's hospital floor or unit.

▲ 99255   **Inpatient consultation** for a new or established patient, which requires these 3 key components:

- **A comprehensive history;**
- **A comprehensive examination; and**
- **Medical decision making of high complexity.**

Counseling and/or coordination of care with <u>other physicians,</u> other ~~providers~~<u>qualified health care professionals,</u> or agencies are provided consistent with the nature of the problem(s) and the patient's and/or family's needs.

Usually, the presenting problem(s) are of moderate to high severity. ~~Physicians typically spend~~Typically, 110 minutes <u>are spent</u> at the bedside and on the patient's hospital floor or unit.

▲ 99281   **Emergency department visit** for the evaluation and management of a patient, which requires these 3 key components:

- **A problem focused history;**
- **A problem focused examination; and**
- **Straightforward medical decision making.**

Counseling and/or coordination of care with <u>other physicians,</u> other ~~providers~~<u>qualified health care professionals,</u> or agencies are provided consistent with the nature of the problem(s) and the patient's and/or family's needs.

Usually, the presenting problem(s) are self limited or minor.

▲ 99282   **Emergency department visit** for the evaluation and management of a patient, which requires these 3 key components:

- **An expanded problem focused history;**
- **An expanded problem focused examination; and**
- **Medical decision making of low complexity.**

Counseling and/or coordination of care with <u>other physicians,</u> other ~~providers~~<u>qualified health care professionals,</u> or agencies are provided consistent with the nature of the problem(s) and the patient's and/or family's needs.

Usually, the presenting problem(s) are of low to moderate severity.

▲ 99283   **Emergency department visit** for the evaluation and management of a patient, which requires these 3 key components:

- **An expanded problem focused history;**
- **An expanded problem focused examination; and**
- **Medical decision making of moderate complexity.**

Counseling and/or coordination of care with <u>other physicians,</u> other ~~providers~~<u>qualified health care professionals,</u> or agencies are provided consistent with the nature of the problem(s) and the patient's and/or family's needs.

Usually, the presenting problem(s) are of moderate severity.

▲ 99284   **Emergency department visit** for the evaluation and management of a patient, which requires these 3 key components:

- **A detailed history;**
- **A detailed examination; and**
- **Medical decision making of moderate complexity.**

Counseling and/or coordination of care with <u>other physicians,</u> other ~~providers~~<u>qualified health care professionals,</u> or agencies are provided consistent with the nature of the problem(s) and the patient's and/or family's needs.

Usually, the presenting problem(s) are of high severity, and require urgent evaluation by the physician <u>physicians, or other health care professionals</u> but do not pose an immediate significant threat to life or physiologic function.

▲ 99285   **Emergency department visit** for the evaluation and management of a patient, which requires these 3 key components within the constraints imposed by the urgency of the patient's clinical condition and/or mental status:

- **A comprehensive history;**
- **A comprehensive examination; and**
- **Medical decision making of high complexity.**

Counseling and/or coordination of care with <u>other physicians,</u> other ~~providers~~<u>qualified health care professionals,</u> or agencies are provided consistent with the nature of the problem(s) and the patient's and/or family's needs.

Usually, the presenting problem(s) are of high severity and pose an immediate significant threat to life or physiologic function.

▲ 99288   **Physician** ~~direction of~~<u>or other qualified health care professional direction of</u> emergency medical systems (EMS) emergency care, advanced life support;

▲ 99304   Initial nursing facility care, per day, for the evaluation and management of a patient, which requires these 3 key components:

- **A detailed or comprehensive history;**
- **A detailed or comprehensive examination; and**
- **Medical decision making that is straightforward or of low complexity.**

Counseling and/or coordination of care with ~~other physicians,~~ other ~~providers~~qualified health care professionals, or agencies are provided consistent with the nature of the problem(s) and the patient's and/or family's needs.

Usually, the problem(s) requiring admission are of low severity. ~~Physicians typically spend~~Typically, 25 minutes are spent at the bedside and on the patient's facility floor or unit.

▲ 99305   Initial nursing facility care, per day, for the evaluation and management of a patient, which requires these 3 key components:

- A comprehensive history;
- A comprehensive examination; and
- Medical decision making of moderate complexity.

Counseling and/or coordination of care with other physicians, other ~~providers~~qualified health care professionals, or agencies are provided consistent with the nature of the problem(s) and the patient's and/or family's needs.

Usually, the problem(s) requiring admission are of moderate severity. ~~Physicians typically spend~~Typically, 35 minutes are spent at the bedside and on the patient's facility floor or unit.

▲ 99306   Initial nursing facility care, per day, for the evaluation and management of a patient, which requires these 3 key components:

- A comprehensive history;
- A comprehensive examination; and
- Medical decision making of high complexity.

Counseling and/or coordination of care with other physicians, other ~~providers~~qualified health care professionals, or agencies are provided consistent with the nature of the problem(s) and the patient's and/or family's needs.

Usually, the problem(s) requiring admission are of high severity. ~~Physicians typically spend~~Typically, 45 minutes are spent at the bedside and on the patient's facility floor or unit.

▲ 99307   Subsequent nursing facility care, per day, for the evaluation and management of a patient, which requires at least 2 of these 3 key components:

- A problem focused interval history;
- A problem focused examination;
- Straightforward medical decision making.

Counseling and/or coordination of care with other physicians, other ~~providers~~qualified health care professionals, or agencies are provided consistent with the nature of the problem(s) and the patient's and/or family's needs.

Usually, the patient is stable, recovering, or improving. ~~Physicians typically spend~~Typically, 10 minutes are spent at the bedside and on the patient's facility floor or unit.

▲ 99308   Subsequent nursing facility care, per day, for the evaluation and management of a patient, which requires at least 2 of these 3 key components:

- An expanded problem focused interval history;
- An expanded problem focused examination;
- Medical decision making of low complexity.

Counseling and/or coordination of care with other physicians, other ~~providers~~qualified health care professionals, or agencies are provided consistent with the nature of the problem(s) and the patient's and/or family's needs.

Usually, the patient is responding inadequately to therapy or has developed a minor complication. ~~Physicians typically spend~~Typically, 15 minutes are spent at the bedside and on the patient's facility floor or unit.

▲ 99309   Subsequent nursing facility care, per day, for the evaluation and management of a patient, which requires at least 2 of these 3 key components:

- A detailed interval history;
- A detailed examination;
- Medical decision making of moderate complexity.

Counseling and/or coordination of care with other physicians, other ~~providers~~qualified health care professionals, or agencies are provided consistent with the nature of the problem(s) and the patient's and/or family's needs.

Usually, the patient has developed a significant complication or a significant new problem. ~~Physicians typically spend~~Typically, 25 minutes are spent at the bedside and on the patient's facility floor or unit.

▲ 99310   Subsequent nursing facility care, per day, for the evaluation and management of a patient, which requires at least 2 of these 3 key components:

- A comprehensive interval history;
- A comprehensive examination;
- Medical decision making of high complexity.

Counseling and/or coordination of care with other physicians, other ~~providers~~qualified health care professionals, or agencies are provided consistent with the nature of the problem(s) and the patient's and/or family's needs.

The patient may be unstable or may have developed a significant new problem requiring immediate physician attention. ~~Physicians typically spend~~Typically, 35 minutes are spent at the bedside and on the patient's facility floor or unit.

▲ 99318   Evaluation and management of a patient involving an annual nursing facility assessment, which requires these 3 key components:

- A detailed interval history;
- A comprehensive examination; and
- Medical decision making that is of low to moderate complexity.

Counseling and/or coordination of care with other physicians, other ~~providers~~qualified health care professionals, or agencies are provided consistent with the nature of the problem(s) and the patient's and/or family's needs.

Usually, the patient is stable, recovering, or improving. ~~Physicians typically spend~~Typically, 30 minutes are spent at the bedside and on the patient's facility floor or unit.

▲ 99324   Domiciliary or rest home visit for the evaluation and management of a new patient, which requires these 3 key components:

- A problem focused history;
- A problem focused examination; and
- Straightforward medical decision making.

Counseling and/or coordination of care with other physicians, other ~~providers~~qualified health care professionals, or agencies are provided consistent with the nature of the problem(s) and the patient's and/or family's needs.

Usually, the presenting problem(s) are of low severity. ~~Physicians typically spend~~Typically, 20 minutes ~~are spent~~ with the patient and/or family or caregiver

▲ 99325   Domiciliary or rest home visit for the evaluation and management of a new patient, which requires these 3 key components:

- **An expanded problem focused history;**

- **An expanded problem focused examination; and**

- **Medical decision making of low complexity.**

Counseling and/or coordination of care with other physicians, other ~~providers~~qualified health care professionals, or agencies are provided consistent with the nature of the problem(s) and the patient's and/or family's needs.

Usually, the presenting problem(s) are of moderate severity. ~~Physicians typically spend~~Typically, 30 minutes ~~are spent~~ with the patient and/or family or caregiver

▲ 99326   Domiciliary or rest home visit for the evaluation and management of a new patient, which requires these 3 key components:

- **A detailed history;**

- **A detailed examination; and**

- **Medical decision making of moderate complexity.**

Counseling and/or coordination of care with other physicians, other ~~providers~~qualified health care professionals, or agencies are provided consistent with the nature of the problem(s) and the patient's and/or family's needs.

Usually, the presenting problem(s) are of moderate to high severity. ~~Physicians typically spend~~Typically, 45 minutes ~~are spent~~ with the patient and/or family or caregiver

▲ 99327   Domiciliary or rest home visit for the evaluation and management of a new patient, which requires these 3 key components:

- **A comprehensive history;**

- **A comprehensive examination; and**

- **Medical decision making of moderate complexity.**

Counseling and/or coordination of care with other physicians, other ~~providers~~qualified health care professionals, or agencies are provided consistent with the nature of the problem(s) and the patient's and/or family's needs.

Usually, the presenting problem(s) are of high severity. ~~Physicians typically spend~~Typically, 60 minutes ~~are spent~~ with the patient and/or family or caregiver

▲ 99328   Domiciliary or rest home visit for the evaluation and management of a new patient, which requires these 3 key components:

- **A comprehensive history;**

- **A comprehensive examination; and**

- **Medical decision making of high complexity.**

Counseling and/or coordination of care with other physicians, other ~~providers~~qualified health care professionals, or agencies are provided consistent with the nature of the problem(s) and the patient's and/or family's needs.

Usually, the patient is unstable or has developed a significant new problem requiring immediate physician attention. ~~Physicians typically spend~~Typically, 75 minutes ~~are spent~~ with the patient and/or family or caregiver

▲ 99334   Domiciliary or rest home visit for the evaluation and management of an established patient, which requires at least 2 of these 3 key components:

- **A problem focused interval history;**

- **A problem focused examination;**

- **Straightforward medical decision making.**

Counseling and/or coordination of care with other physicians, other ~~providers~~qualified health care professionals, or agencies are provided consistent with the nature of the problem(s) and the patient's and/or family's needs.

Usually, the presenting problem(s) are self-limited or minor. ~~Physicians typically spend~~Typically, 15 minutes ~~are spent~~ with the patient and/or family or caregiver

▲ 99335   Domiciliary or rest home visit for the evaluation and management of an established patient, which requires at least 2 of these 3 key components:

- **An expanded problem focused interval history;**

- **An expanded problem focused examination;**

- **Medical decision making of low complexity.**

Counseling and/or coordination of care with other physicians, other ~~providers~~qualified health care professionals, or agencies are provided consistent with the nature of the problem(s) and the patient's and/or family's needs.

Usually, the presenting problem(s) are of low to moderate severity. ~~Physicians typically spend~~Typically, 25 minutes ~~are spent~~ with the patient and/or family or caregiver

▲ 99336   Domiciliary or rest home visit for the evaluation and management of an established patient, which requires at least 2 of these 3 key components:

- **A detailed interval history;**

- **A detailed examination;**

- **Medical decision making of moderate complexity.**

Counseling and/or coordination of care with other physicians, other ~~providers~~qualified health care professionals, or agencies are provided consistent with the nature of the problem(s) and the patient's and/or family's needs.

Usually, the presenting problem(s) are of moderate to high severity. ~~Physicians typically spend~~Typically, 40 minutes ~~are spent~~ with the patient and/or family or caregiver

▲ 99337   Domiciliary or rest home visit for the evaluation and management of an established patient, which requires at least 2 of these 3 key components:

- **A comprehensive interval history;**

- **A comprehensive examination;**

- **Medical decision making of moderate to high complexity.**

Counseling and/or coordination of care with other physicians, other ~~providers~~qualified health care professionals, or agencies are provided consistent with the nature of the problem(s) and the patient's and/or family's needs.

Usually, the presenting problem(s) are of moderate to high severity. The patient may be unstable or may have developed a significant new problem requiring immediate physician attention. ~~Physicians typically spend~~Typically, 60 minutes ~~are spent~~ with the patient and/or family or caregiver

▲ 99341   **Home visit** for the evaluation and management of a new patient, which requires these 3 key components:

- **A problem focused history;**

- **A problem focused examination; and**

- **Straightforward medical decision making.**

Counseling and/or coordination of care with other physicians, other providersqualified health care professionals, or agencies are provided consistent with the nature of the problem(s) and the patient's and/or family's needs.

Usually, the presenting problem(s) are of low severity. Physicians typically spendTypically, 20 minutes are spent face-to-face with the patient and/or family

▲ 99342 **Home visit** for the evaluation and management of a new patient, which requires these 3 key components:

- **An expanded problem focused history;**

- **An expanded problem focused examination; and**

- **Medical decision making of low complexity.**

Counseling and/or coordination of care with other physicians, other providersqualified health care professionals, or agencies are provided consistent with the nature of the problem(s) and the patient's and/or family's needs.

Usually, the presenting problem(s) are of moderate severity. Physicians typically spendTypically, 30 minutes are spent face-to-face with the patient and/or family

▲ 99343 **Home visit** for the evaluation and management of a new patient, which requires these 3 key components:

- **A detailed history;**

- **A detailed examination; and**

- **Medical decision making of moderate complexity.**

Counseling and/or coordination of care with other physicians, other providersqualified health care professionals, or agencies are provided consistent with the nature of the problem(s) and the patient's and/or family's needs.

Usually, the presenting problem(s) are of moderate to high severity. Physicians typically spendTypically, 45 minutes are spent face-to-face with the patient and/or family

▲ 99344 **Home visit** for the evaluation and management of a new patient, which requires these 3 key components:

- **A comprehensive history;**

- **A comprehensive examination; and**

- **Medical decision making of moderate complexity.**

Counseling and/or coordination of care with other physicians, other providersqualified health care professionals, or agencies are provided consistent with the nature of the problem(s) and the patient's and/or family's needs.

Usually, the presenting problem(s) are of high severity. Physicians typically spendTypically, 60 minutes are spent face-to-face with the patient and/or family

▲ 99345 **Home visit** for the evaluation and management of a new patient, which requires these 3 key components:

- **A comprehensive history;**

- **A comprehensive examination; and**

- **Medical decision making of high complexity.**

Counseling and/or coordination of care with other physicians, other providersqualified health care professionals, or agencies are provided consistent with the nature of the problem(s) and the patient's and/or family's needs.

Usually, the patient is unstable or has developed a significant new problem requiring immediate physician attention. Physicians typically spendTypically, 75 minutes are spent face-to-face with the patient and/or family

▲ 99347 **Home visit** for the evaluation and management of an established patient, which requires at least 2 of these 3 key components:

- **A problem focused interval history;**

- **A problem focused examination;**

- **Straightforward medical decision making.**

Counseling and/or coordination of care with other physicians, other providersqualified health care professionals, or agencies are provided consistent with the nature of the problem(s) and the patient's and/or family's needs.

Usually, the presenting problem(s) are self limited or minor. Physicians typically spendTypically, 15 minutes are spent face-to-face with the patient and/or family

▲ 99348 **Home visit** for the evaluation and management of an established patient, which requires at least 2 of these 3 key components:

- **An expanded problem focused interval history;**

- **An expanded problem focused examination;**

- **Medical decision making of low complexity.**

Counseling and/or coordination of care with other physicians, other providersqualified health care professionals, or agencies are provided consistent with the nature of the problem(s) and the patient's and/or family's needs.

Usually, the presenting problem(s) are of low to moderate severity. Physicians typically spendTypically, 25 minutes are spent face-to-face with the patient and/or family

▲ 99349 **Home visit** for the evaluation and management of an established patient, which requires at least 2 of these 3 key components:

- **A detailed interval history;**

- **A detailed examination;**

- **Medical decision making of moderate complexity.**

Counseling and/or coordination of care with other physicians, other providersqualified health care professionals, or agencies are provided consistent with the nature of the problem(s) and the patient's and/or family's needs.

Usually, the presenting problem(s) are moderate to high severity. Physicians typically spendTypically, 40 minutes are spent face-to-face with the patient and/or family

▲ 99350 **Home visit** for the evaluation and management of an established patient, which requires at least 2 of these 3 key components:

- **A comprehensive interval history;**

- **A comprehensive examination;**

- **Medical decision making of moderate to high complexity.**

Counseling and/or coordination of care with other physicians, other providersqualified health care professionals, or agencies are provided consistent with the nature of the problem(s) and the patient's and/or family's needs.

Usually, the presenting problem(s) are of moderate to high severity. The patient may be unstable or may have developed a significant new problem requiring immediate physician attention. Physicians typically spendTypically, 60 minutes are spent face-to-face with the patient and/or family.

▲ 99360 **Physician standbyStandby service,** requiring prolonged physician attendance, each 30 minutes (eg, operative standby, standby for frozen section, for cesarean/high risk delivery, for monitoring EEG)

▲ 99374   ~~Physician supervision~~<u>Supervision</u> of a patient under care of home health agency (patient not present) in home, domiciliary or equivalent environment (eg, Alzheimer's facility) requiring complex and multidisciplinary care modalities involving regular ~~physician~~ development and/or revision of care plans <u>by that individual</u>, review of subsequent reports of patient status, review of related laboratory and other studies, communication (including telephone calls) for purposes of assessment or care decisions with health care professional(s), family member(s), surrogate decision maker(s) (eg, legal guardian) and/or key caregiver(s) involved in patient's care, integration of new information into the medical treatment plan and/or adjustment of medical therapy, within a calendar month; 15-29 minutes

▲ 99375   30 minutes or more

▲ 99377   ~~Physician supervision~~<u>Supervision</u> of a hospice patient (patient not present) requiring complex and multidisciplinary care modalities involving regular ~~physician~~ development and/or revision of care plans <u>by that individual</u>, review of subsequent reports of patient status, review of related laboratory and other studies, communication (including telephone calls) for purposes of assessment or care decisions with health care professional(s), family member(s), surrogate decision maker(s) (eg, legal guardian) and/or key caregiver(s) involved in patient's care, integration of new information into the medical treatment plan and/or adjustment of medical therapy, within a calendar month; 15-29 minutes

▲ 99378   30 minutes or more

▲ 99379   ~~Physician supervision~~<u>Supervision</u> of a nursing facility patient (patient not present) requiring complex and multidisciplinary care modalities involving regular ~~physician~~ development and/or revision of care plans <u>by that individual</u>, review of subsequent reports of patient status, review of related laboratory and other studies, communication (including telephone calls) for purposes of assessment or care decisions with health care professional(s), family member(s), surrogate decision maker(s) (eg, legal guardian) and/or key caregiver(s) involved in patient's care, integration of new information into the medical treatment plan and/or adjustment of medical therapy, within a calendar month; 15-29 minutes

▲ 99380   30 minutes or more

▲ 99441   Telephone evaluation and management service ~~provided~~ by a physician <u>or other qualified health care professional who may report evaluation and management services provided</u> to an established patient, parent, or guardian not originating from a related E/M service provided within the previous 7 days nor leading to an E/M service or procedure within the next 24 hours or soonest available appointment; 5-10 minutes of medical discussion

▲ 99442   11-20 minutes of medical discussion

▲ 99443   21-30 minutes of medical discussion

▲ 99444   Online evaluation and management service provided by a physician <u>or other qualified health care professional who may report an evaluation and management services provided</u> to an established patient~~;~~ <u>or</u> guardian, ~~or health care provider~~ not originating from a related E/M service provided within the previous 7 days, using the Internet or similar electronic communications network

▲ 99464   Attendance at delivery (when requested by the delivering physician<u> or other qualified health care professional</u>) and initial stabilization of newborn

▲ 99466   **Critical care** ~~services delivered by a physician,~~ face-to-face <u>services</u>, during an interfacility transport of critically ill or critically injured pediatric patient, 24 months of age or younger; first 30-74 minutes of hands-on care during transport

+▲ 99467   each additional 30 minutes (List separately in addition to code for primary service)

#● 99485   Code added

+#● 99486   Code added

● 99487   Code added

● 99488   Code added

+● 99489   Code added

● 99495   Code added

● 99496   Code added

Anesthesia

▲ 01991   Anesthesia for diagnostic or therapeutic nerve blocks and injections (when block or injection is performed by a different ~~provider~~<u>physician or other qualified health care professional</u>); other than the prone position

▲ 01992   prone position

Surgery

▲ 15740   Flap; island pedicle<u> requiring identification and dissection of an anatomically named axial vessel</u>

▲ 20665   Removal of tongs or halo applied by another ~~physician~~<u>individual</u>

+⊙▲ 22522   each additional thoracic or lumbar vertebral body (List separately in addition to code for primary procedure)

● 22586   Code added

● 23473   Code added

● 23474   Code added

● 24370   Code added

● 24371   Code added

▲ 28890   Extracorporeal shock wave, high energy, performed by a physician<u> or other qualified health care professional</u>, requiring anesthesia other than local, including ultrasound guidance, involving the plantar fascia

29590   ~~Denis-Browne splint strapping~~

⊙● 31647   Code added

⊙● 31648   Code added

+⊙● 31649   Code added

+⊙● 31651   Code added

31656   ~~with injection of contrast material for segmental bronchography (fiberscope only)~~

⊙● 31660   Code added

⊙● 31661   Code added

31715   ~~Transtracheal injection for bronchography~~

32420   ~~Pneumocentesis, puncture of lung for aspiration~~

32421   ~~Thoracentesis, puncture of pleural cavity for aspiration, initial or subsequent~~

32422   ~~Thoracentesis with insertion of tube, includes water seal (eg, for pneumothorax), when performed (separate procedure)~~

⊙▲ **32551** Tube thoracostomy, includes ~~water seal~~connection to drainage system (eg, ~~for abscess, hemothorax, empyema~~water seal), when performed, open (separate procedure)

● **32554** Code added

● **32555** Code added

● **32556** Code added

● **32557** Code added

● **32701** Code added

+▲ **33225** Insertion of pacing electrode, cardiac venous system, for left ventricular pacing, at time of insertion of pacing cardioverter-defibrillator or pacemaker pulse generator (~~including~~eg, for upgrade to dual chamber system ~~and pocket revision~~) (List separately in addition to code for primary procedure)

● **33361** Code added

● **33362** Code added

● **33363** Code added

● **33364** Code added

● **33365** Code added

+● **33367** Code added

+● **33368** Code added

+● **33369** Code added

⊙● **33990** Code added

⊙● **33991** Code added

⊙● **33992** Code added

⊙● **33993** Code added

⊙▲ **36010** Introduction of catheter, superior or inferior vena cava

⊙▲ **36140** extremity artery

⊙● **36221** Code added

⊙● **36222** Code added

⊙● **36223** Code added

⊙● **36224** Code added

⊙● **36225** Code added

⊙● **36226** Code added

+⊙● **36227** Code added

+⊙● **36228** Code added

▲ **36400** Venipuncture, younger than age 3 years, necessitating ~~physician's~~the skill of a physician or other qualified health care professional, not to be used for routine venipuncture; femoral or jugular vein

▲ **36405** scalp vein

▲ **36406** other vein

▲ **36410** Venipuncture, age 3 years or older, necessitating ~~physician's~~the skill of a physician or other qualified health care professional (separate procedure), for diagnostic or therapeutic purposes (not to be used for routine venipuncture)

⊙● **37197** Code added

37201 ~~Transcatheter therapy, infusion for thrombolysis other than coronary;~~

⊙#● **37211** Code added

⊙#● **37212** Code added

⊙#● **37213** Code added

⊙#● **37214** Code added

37203 ~~Transcatheter retrieval, percutaneous, of intravascular foreign body (eg, fractured venous or arterial catheter)~~

37209 ~~Exchange of a previously placed intravascular catheter during thrombolytic therapy~~

▲ **38240** ~~Bone marrow or blood-derived peripheral stem~~Hematopoietic progenitor cell transplantation(HPC); allogeneic transplantation per donor

▲ **38241** autologous transplantation

#● **38243** Code added

▲ **38242** ~~allogenic~~Allogeneic ~~donor~~lymphocyte infusions

⊙● **43206** Code added

43234 ~~Upper gastrointestinal endoscopy, simple primary examination (eg, with small diameter flexible endoscope) (separate procedure)~~

⊙● **43252** Code added

● **44705** Code added

● **52287** Code added

▲ **59300** Episiotomy or vaginal repair, by other than attending ~~physician~~;

▲ **62370** with reprogramming and refill (requiring skill~~physician's~~ of a physician or other qualified health care professional)

▲ **64561** sacral nerve (transforaminal placement) including image guidance, if performed

▲ **64612** Chemodenervation of muscle(s); muscle(s) innervated by facial nerve, unilateral (eg, for blepharospasm, hemifacial spasm)

▲ **64614** extremity~~(s)~~ and/or trunk muscle(s) (eg, for dystonia, cerebral palsy, multiple sclerosis)

● **64615** Code added

▲ **65800** Paracentesis of anterior chamber of eye (separate procedure); with ~~diagnostic aspiration~~removal of aqueous

65805 ~~with therapeutic release of aqueous~~

#▲ **67810** ~~Biopsy~~Incisional biopsy of eyelid skin including lid margin

Radiology

71040 ~~Bronchography, unilateral, radiological supervision and interpretation~~

71060 ~~Bronchography, bilateral, radiological supervision and interpretation~~

▲ **72040** Radiologic examination, spine, cervical; ~~23 views~~ or ~~3 views~~less

▲ **72050** ~~4~~minimum of or 5 views

▲ **72052** ~~complete, including oblique and flexion and/~~6 or ~~extension studies~~more views

75650 ~~Angiography, cervicocerebral, catheter, including vessel origin, radiological supervision and interpretation~~

75660 ~~Angiography, external carotid, unilateral, selective, radiological supervision and interpretation~~

75662 ~~Angiography, external carotid, bilateral, selective, radiological supervision and interpretation~~

75665 ~~Angiography, carotid, cerebral, unilateral, radiological supervision and interpretation~~

75671 ~~Angiography, carotid, cerebral, bilateral, radiological supervision and interpretation~~

75676 ~~Angiography, carotid, cervical, unilateral, radiological supervision and interpretation~~

75680 ~~Angiography, carotid, cervical, bilateral, radiological supervision and interpretation~~

75685 ~~Angiography, vertebral, cervical, and/or intracranial, radiological supervision and interpretation~~

▲ 75896 Transcatheter therapy, infusion~~, any method (eg, thrombolysis other than ~~coronary~~)~~for thrombolysis, radiological supervision and interpretation

▲ 75898 Angiography through existing catheter for follow-up study for transcatheter therapy, embolization or infusion, other than for thrombolysis

75900 ~~Exchange of a previously placed intravascular catheter during thrombolytic therapy with contrast monitoring, radiological supervision and interpretation;~~

75961 ~~Transcatheter retrieval, percutaneous, of intravascular foreign body (eg, fractured venous or arterial catheter), radiological supervision and interpretation;~~

▲ 76000 Fluoroscopy (separate procedure), up to 1 hour physician or other qualified health care professional time, other than 71023 or 71034 (eg, cardiac fluoroscopy)

▲ 76001 Fluoroscopy, physician or other qualified health care professional time more than 1 hour, assisting a nonradiologic physician or other qualified health care professional (eg, nephrostolithotomy, ERCP, bronchoscopy, transbronchial biopsy)

▲ 76376 3D rendering with interpretation and reporting of computed tomography, magnetic resonance imaging, ultrasound, or other tomographic modality with image postprocessing under concurrent supervision; not requiring image postprocessing on an independent workstation

▲ 76377 requiring image postprocessing on an independent workstation

▲ 76885 Ultrasound, infant hips, real time with imaging documentation; dynamic (requiring physician or other qualified health care professional manipulation)

▲ 76886 limited, static (not requiring physician or other qualified health care professional manipulation)

+▲ 77051 Computer-aided detection (computer algorithm analysis of digital image data for lesion detection) with further ~~physician~~ review for interpretation, with or without digitization of film radiographic images; diagnostic mammography (List separately in addition to code for primary procedure)

+▲ 77052 screening mammography (List separately in addition to code for primary procedure)

▲ 77071 Manual application of stress performed by physician or other qualified health care professional for joint radiography, including contralateral joint if indicated

78000 ~~Thyroid uptake; single determination~~

78001 ~~multiple determinations~~

78003 ~~stimulation, suppression or discharge (not including initial uptake studies)~~

78006 ~~Thyroid imaging, with uptake; single determination~~

78007 ~~multiple determinations~~

78010 ~~Thyroid imaging; only~~

78011 ~~with vascular flow~~

● 78012 Code added

● 78013 Code added

● 78014 Code added

▲ 78070 Parathyroid planar imaging (including subtraction, when performed)

● 78071 Code added

● 78072 Code added

Pathology and Laboratory

● 81201 Code added

● 81202 Code added

● 81203 Code added

● 81235 Code added

● 81252 Code added

● 81253 Code added

● 81254 Code added

● 81321 Code added

● 81322 Code added

● 81323 Code added

● 81324 Code added

● 81325 Code added

● 81326 Code added

▲ 81400 Molecular pathology procedure, Level 1 ~~(eg, identification of single germline variant [eg, SNP] by techniques such as restriction enzyme digestion or melt curve analysis)~~(eg, identification of single germline variant [eg, SNP] by techniques such as restriction enzyme digestion or melt curve analysis)

ABCC8 (ATP-binding cassette, sub-family C [CFTR/MRP], member 8) (eg, familial hyperinsulinism), F1388del variant

~~ACADM (acyl-CoA dehydrogenase, C-4 to C-12 straight chain, MCAD) (eg, medium chain acyl dehydrogenase deficiency), K304E variant~~ACADM (acyl-CoA dehydrogenase, C-4 to C-12 straight chain, MCAD) (eg, medium chain acyl dehydrogenase deficiency), K304E variant

~~ACE (angiotensin converting enzyme) (eg, hereditary blood pressure regulation), insertion/deletion variant~~ACE (angiotensin converting enzyme) (eg, hereditary blood pressure regulation), insertion/deletion variant

~~AGTR1 (angiotensin II receptor, type 1) (eg, essential hypertension), 1166A>C variant~~AGTR1 (angiotensin II receptor, type 1) (eg, essential hypertension), 1166A>C variant

~~CCR5 (chemokine C-C motif receptor 5) (eg, HIV resistance), 32-bp deletion mutation/794 825del32 deletion~~CCR5 (chemokine C-C motif receptor 5) (eg, HIV resistance), 32-bp deletion mutation/794 825del32 deletion

CLRN1 (clarin 1) (eg, Usher syndrome, type 3), N48K variant

~~DPYD (dihydropyrimidine dehydrogenase) (eg, 5-fluorouracil/5-FU and capecitabine drug metabolism), IVS14+1G>A variant~~DPYD (dihydropyrimidine dehydrogenase) (eg, 5-fluorouracil/5-FU and capecitabine drug metabolism), IVS14+1G>A variant

~~F2 (coagulation factor 2) (eg, hereditary hypercoagulability), 1199G>A variant~~F2 (coagulation factor 2) (eg, hereditary hypercoagulability), 1199G>A variant

~~F5 (coagulation factor V) (eg, hereditary hypercoagulability), HR2 variant~~F5 (coagulation factor V) (eg, hereditary hypercoagulability), HR2 variant

F7 (coagulation factor VII [serum prothrombin conversion accelerator]) (eg, hereditary hypercoagulability), R353Q variant*F7 (coagulation factor VII [serum prothrombin conversion accelerator]) (eg, hereditary hypercoagulability), R353Q variant*

F13B (coagulation factor XIII, B polypeptide) (eg, hereditary hypercoagulability), V34L variant*F13B (coagulation factor XIII, B polypeptide) (eg, hereditary hypercoagulability), V34L variant*

FGB (fibrinogen beta chain) (eg, hereditary ischemic heart disease), -455G>A variant*FGB (fibrinogen beta chain) (eg, hereditary ischemic heart disease), -455G>A variant*

FGFR3 (fibroblast growth factor receptor 3) (eg, Muenke syndrome), P250R variant

Human Platelet Antigen 1 genotyping (HPA-1), ITGB3 (integrin, beta 3 [platelet glycoprotein IIIa], antigen CD61 [GPIIIa]) (eg, neonatal alloimmune thrombocytopenia [NAIT], post-transfusion purpura), HPA-1a/b (L33P)*Human Platelet Antigen 1 genotyping (HPA-1), ITGB3 (integrin, beta 3 [platelet glycoprotein IIIa], antigen CD61 [GPIIIa]) (eg, neonatal alloimmune thrombocytopenia [NAIT], post-transfusion purpura), HPA-1a/b (L33P)*

Human Platelet Antigen 2 genotyping (HPA-2), GP1BA (glycoprotein Ib [platelet], alpha polypeptide [GPIbα]) (eg, neonatal alloimmune thrombocytopenia [NAIT], post-transfusion purpura), HPA-2a/b (T145M)*Human Platelet Antigen 2 genotyping (HPA-2), GP1BA (glycoprotein Ib [platelet], alpha polypeptide [GPIbα]) (eg, neonatal alloimmune thrombocytopenia [NAIT], post-transfusion purpura), HPA-2a/b (T145M)*

Human Platelet Antigen 3 genotyping (HPA-3), ITGA2B (integrin, alpha 2b [platelet glycoprotein IIb of IIb/IIIa complex], antigen CD41 [GPIIb]) (eg, neonatal alloimmune thrombocytopenia [NAIT], post-transfusion purpura), HPA-3a/b (I843S)*Human Platelet Antigen 3 genotyping (HPA-3), ITGA2B (integrin, alpha 2b [platelet glycoprotein IIb of IIb/IIIa complex], antigen CD41 [GPIIb]) (eg, neonatal alloimmune thrombocytopenia [NAIT], post-transfusion purpura), HPA-3a/b (I843S)*

Human Platelet Antigen 4 genotyping (HPA-4), ITGB3 (integrin, beta 3 [platelet glycoprotein IIIa], antigen CD61 [GPIIIa]) (eg, neonatal alloimmune thrombocytopenia [NAIT], post-transfusion purpura), HPA-4a/b (R143Q)*Human Platelet Antigen 4 genotyping (HPA-4), ITGB3 (integrin, beta 3 [platelet glycoprotein IIIa], antigen CD61 [GPIIIa]) (eg, neonatal alloimmune thrombocytopenia [NAIT], post-transfusion purpura), HPA-4a/b (R143Q)*

Human Platelet Antigen 5 genotyping (HPA-5), ITGA2 (integrin, alpha 2 [CD49B, alpha 2 subunit of VLA-2 receptor] [GPIa]) (eg, neonatal alloimmune thrombocytopenia [NAIT], post-transfusion purpura), HPA-5a/b (K505E)*Human Platelet Antigen 5 genotyping (HPA-5), ITGA2 (integrin, alpha 2 [CD49B, alpha 2 subunit of VLA-2 receptor] [GPIa]) (eg, neonatal alloimmune thrombocytopenia [NAIT], post-transfusion purpura), HPA-5a/b (K505E)*

Human Platelet Antigen 6 genotyping (HPA-6w), ITGB3 (integrin, beta 3 [platelet glycoprotein IIIa, antigen CD61] [GPIIIa]) (eg, neonatal alloimmune thrombocytopenia [NAIT], post-transfusion purpura), HPA-6a/b (R489Q)*Human Platelet Antigen 6 genotyping (HPA-6w), ITGB3 (integrin, beta 3 [platelet glycoprotein IIIa, antigen CD61] [GPIIIa]) (eg, neonatal alloimmune thrombocytopenia [NAIT], post-transfusion purpura), HPA-6a/b (R489Q)*

Human Platelet Antigen 9 genotyping (HPA-9w), ITGA2B (integrin, alpha 2b [platelet glycoprotein IIb of IIb/IIIa complex, antigen CD41] [GPIIb]) (eg, neonatal alloimmune thrombocytopenia [NAIT], post-transfusion purpura), HPA-9a/b (V837M)*Human Platelet Antigen 9 genotyping (HPA-9w), ITGA2B (integrin, alpha 2b [platelet glycoprotein IIb of IIb/IIIa complex, antigen CD41] [GPIIb]) (eg, neonatal alloimmune thrombocytopenia [NAIT], post-transfusion purpura), HPA-9a/b (V837M)*

Human Platelet Antigen 15 genotyping (HPA-15), CD109 (CD109 molecule) (eg, neonatal alloimmune thrombocytopenia [NAIT], post-transfusion purpura), HPA-15a/b(S682Y)*Human Platelet Antigen 15 genotyping (HPA-15), CD109 (CD109 molecule) (eg, neonatal alloimmune thrombocytopenia [NAIT], post-transfusion purpura), HPA-15a/b (S682Y)*

IVD (isovaleryl-CoA dehydrogenase) (eg, isovaleric acidemia), A282V variant

SERPINE1 (serpine peptidase inhibitor clade E, member 1, plasminogen activator inhibitor -1, PAI-1) (eg, thrombophilia), 4G variant*SERPINE1 (serpine peptidase inhibitor clade E, member 1, plasminogen activator inhibitor -1, PAI-1) (eg, thrombophilia), 4G variant*

SHOC2 (soc-2 suppressor of clear homolog) (eg, Noonan-like syndrome with loose anagen hair), S2G variant

MN1 (survival of motor neuron 1, telomeric) (eg, spinal muscular atrophy), exon 7 deletion

SRY (sex determining region Y) (eg, 46,XX testicular disorder of sex development, gonadal dysgenesis), gene analysis

TOR1A (torsin family 1, member A [torsin A])(eg, early-onset primary dystonia [DYT1]), 907_909delGAG (904_906delGAG) variant

▲ 81401   Molecular pathology procedure, Level 2 (eg, 2-10 SNPs, 1 methylated variant, or 1 somatic variant [typically using nonsequencing target variant analysis], or detection of a dynamic mutation disorder/triplet repeat)

ABL (c-abl oncogene 1, receptor tyrosine kinase) (eg, acquired imatinib resistance), T315I variant

ACADM (acyl-CoA dehydrogenase, C-4 to C-12 straight chain, MCAD) (eg, medium chain acyl dehydrogenase deficiency), commons variants (eg, K304E, Y42H)

ADRB2 (adrenergic beta-2 receptor surface) (eg, drug metabolism), common variants (eg, G16R, Q27E) *APOB (apolipoprotein B)* (eg, familial hypercholesterolemia type B), common variants (eg, R3500Q, R3500W)

APOE (apolipoprotein E) (eg, hyperlipoproteinemia type III, cardiovascular disease, Alzheimer disease), common variants (eg, *2, *3, *4)

AR (androgen receptor) (eg, spinal and bulbar muscular atrophy, Kennedy disease, X chromosome inactivation), characterization of alleles (eg, expanded size or methylation status)

ATN1 (atrophin 1) (eg, dentatorubral-pallidoluysian atrophy), evaluation to detect abnormal (eg, expanded) alleles

CBFB/MYH11 (inv(16)) (eg, acute myeloid leukemia), qualitative, and quantitative, if performed

CBS (cystathionine-beta-synthase) (eg, homocystinuria, cystathionine beta-synthase deficiency), common variants (eg, I278T, G307S)

CCND1/IGH (BCL1/IgH, t(11;14)) (eg, mantle cell lymphoma) translocation analysis, major breakpoint, qualitative, and quantitative, if performed

CFH/ARMS2 (complement factor H/age-related maculopathy susceptibility 2)(eg, macular degeneration), common variants (eg, Y402H [CFH], A69S [ARMS2])

CYP3A4 (cytochrome P450, family 3, subfamily A, polypeptide 4) (eg, drug metabolism), common variants (eg, *2, *3, *4, *5, *6)

CYP3A5 (cytochrome P450, family 3, subfamily A, polypeptide 5) (eg, drug metabolism), common variants (eg, *2, *3, *4, *5, *6)

DMPK (dystrophia myotonica-protein kinase) (eg, myotonic dystrophy, type 1), evaluation to detect abnormal (eg, expanded) alleles

<u>*E2A/PBX1 (t(1;19))* (eg, acute lymphocytic leukemia), translocation analysis, qualitative, and quantitative, if performed</u>

<u>*EML4/ALK (inv(2))* (eg, non-small cell lung cancer), translocation or inversion analysis</u>

<u>*ETV6/RUNX1 (t(12;21))* (eg, acute lymphocytic leukemia), translocation analysis, qualitative, and quantitative, if performed</u>

<u>*EWSR1/ERG (t(21;22))* (eg, Ewing sarcoma/peripheral neuroectodermal tumor), translocation analysis, qualitative, and quantitative, if performed</u>

<u>*EWSR1/FLI1 (t(11;22))* (eg, Ewing sarcoma/peripheral neuroectodermal tumor), translocation analysis, qualitative, and quantitative, if performed</u>

F11 (coagulation factor XI) (eg, coagulation disorder), common variants (eg, E117X [Type II], F283L [Type III], IVS14del14, and IVS14+1G>A [Type I])

FGFR3 (fibroblast growth factor receptor 3) (eg, achondroplasia, hypochondroplasia), common variants (eg, 1138G>A, 1138G>C, 1620C>A, 1620C>G)

FIP1L1/PDGFRA (del[4q12]) (eg, imatinib-sensitive chronic eosinophilic leukemia), qualitative, and quantitative, if performed

<u>*FOXO1/PAX3 (t(1;13))* (eg, Ewing sarcoma/peripheral neuroectodermal tumor), translocation analysis, qualitative, and quantitative, if performed</u>

<u>*FOXO1/PAX7 (t(2;13))* (eg, Ewing sarcoma/peripheral neuroectodermal tumor), translocation analysis, qualitative, and quantitative, if performed</u>

<u>*FXN (frataxin)* (eg, Friedreich ataxia), evaluation to detect abnormal (expanded) alleles</u>

GALT (galactose-1-phosphate uridylyltransferase) (eg, galactosemia), common variants (eg, Q188R, S135L, K285N, T138M, L195P, Y209C, IVS2-2A>G, P171S, del5kb, N314D, L218L/N314D)

<u>*H19 (imprinted maternally expressed transcript [non-protein coding])* (eg, Beckwith-Wiedemann syndrome), methylation analysis</u>

HBB (hemoglobin, beta) (eg, sickle cell anemia, hemoglobin C, hemoglobin E), common variants (eg, HbS, HbC, HbE)

HTT (huntingtin) <u>*(eg, Huntington disease), evaluation to detect abnormal*</u> (eg, ~~Huntington disease), evaluation to detect abnormal~~ expanded alleles)expanded

<u>*KCNQ1OT1 (KCNQ1 overlapping transcript 1 [non-protein coding])* (eg, Beckwith-Wiedemann syndrome), methylation analysis</u>

<u>*MEG3/DLK1 (maternally expressed 3 [non-protein coding]/delta-like 1 homolog [Drosophila])* (eg, intrauterine growth retardation), methylation analysis</u>

<u>*MLL/AFF1 (t(4;11))* (eg, acute lymphoblastic leukemia), translocation analysis, qualitative, and quantitative, if performed</u>

<u>*MLL/MLLT3 (t(9;11))* (eg, acute myeloid leukemia), translocation analysis, qualitative, and quantitative, if performed</u>

<u>*MT-RNR1 (mitochondrially encoded 12S RNA)* (eg, nonsyndromic hearing loss), common variants (eg, m.1555A>G, m.1494C>T)</u>

<u>*MUTYH (mutY homolog [E. coli])* (eg, MYH-associated polyposis), common variants (eg, Y165C, G382D)</u>

<u>*MT-ATP6 (mitochondrially encoded ATP synthase 6)* (eg, neuropathy with ataxia and retinitis pigmentosa [NARP], Leigh syndrome), common variants (eg, m.8993T>G, m.8993T>C)</u>

<u>*MT-ND4, MT-ND6 (mitochondrially encoded NADH dehydrogenase 4, mitochondrially encoded NADH dehydrogenase 6)* (eg, Leber hereditary optic neuropathy [LHON]), common variants (eg, m.11778G>A, m.3460G>A, m.14484T>C)</u>

<u>*MT-TK (mitochondrially encoded tRNA lysine)* (eg, myoclonic epilepsy with ragged-red fibers [MERRF]), common variants (eg, m.8344A>G, m.8356T>C)</u>

<u>*MT-TL1 (mitochondrially encoded tRNA leucine 1 [UUA/G])* (eg, diabetes and hearing loss), common variants (eg, m.3243A>G, m.14709 T>C) MT-TL1</u>

<u>*MT-ND5 (mitochondrially encoded tRNA leucine 1 [UUA/G], mitochondrially encoded NADH dehydrogenase 5)* (eg, mitochondrial encephalopathy with lactic acidosis and stroke-like episodes [MELAS]), common variants (eg, m.3243A>G, m.3271T>C, m.3252A>G, m.13513G>A)</u>

<u>*MT-TS1, MT-RNR1 (mitochondrially encoded tRNA serine 1 [UCN], mitochondrially encoded 12S RNA)* (eg, nonsyndromic sensorineural deafness [including aminoglycoside-induced nonsyndromic deafness]), common variants (eg, m.7445A>G, m.1555A>G)</u>

<u>*NPM1/ALK (t(2;5))* (eg, anaplastic large cell lymphoma), translocation analysis</u>

<u>*PAX8/PPARG (t(2;3) (q13;p25))* (eg, follicular thyroid carcinoma), translocation analysis</u>

<u>*PRSS1 (protease, serine, 1 [trypsin 1])* (eg, hereditary pancreatitis), common variants (eg, N29I, A16V, R122H)</u>

<u>*PYGM (phosphorylase, glycogen, muscle)* (eg, glycogen storage disease type V, McArdle disease), common variants (eg, R50X, G205S)</u>

RUNX1/RUNX1T1 (t(8;21)) (eg, acute myeloid leukemia) translocation analysis, qualitative, and quantitative, if performed

SEPT9 (Septin 9) (eg, colon cancer), methylation analysis

<u>*SMN1/SMN2 (survival of motor neuron 1, telomeric/survival of motor neuron 2, centromeric)* (eg, spinal muscular atrophy), dosage analysis (eg, carrier testing)</u>

TPMT (thiopurine S-methyltransferase) (eg, drug metabolism), common variants (eg, *2, *3)

<u>*TYMS (thymidylate synthetase)* (eg, 5-fluorouracil/5-FU drug metabolism), tandem repeat variant</u>

VWF (von Willebrand factor) (eg, von Willebrand disease type 2N), common variants (eg, T791M, R816W, R854Q)

▲ 81402   Molecular pathology procedure, Level 3 (eg, >10 SNPs, 2-10 methylated variants, or 2-10 somatic variants [typically using non-sequencing target variant analysis], immunoglobulin and T-cell receptor gene rearrangements, duplication/deletion variants of 1 exon, loss of heterozygosity [LOH], uniparental disomy [UPD])

<u>Chromosome 18q- (eg, D18S55, D18S58, D18S61, D18S64, and D18S69) (eg, colon cancer), allelic imbalance assessment (ie, loss of heterozygosity)</u>

Appendixes A–E

CYP21A2 (cytochrome P450, family 21, subfamily A, polypeptide 2) (eg, congenital adrenal hyperplasia, 21-hydroxylase deficiency), common variants (eg, IVS2-13G, P30L, I172N, exon 6 mutation cluster [I235N, V236E, M238K], V281L, L307FfsX6, Q318X, R356W, P453S, G110VfsX21, 30-kb deletion variant)

ESR1/PGR (receptor 1/progesterone receptor) ratio (eg, breast cancer)

KIT (v-kit Hardy-Zuckerman 4 feline sarcoma viral oncogene homolog) (eg, mastocytosis), common variants (eg, D816V, D816Y, D816F)

MEFV (Mediterranean fever) (eg, familial Mediterranean fever), common variants (eg, E148Q, P369S, F479L, M680I, I692del, M694V, M694I, K695R, V726A, A744S, R761H)

MPL (myeloproliferative leukemia virus oncogene, thrombopoietin receptor, TPOR) (eg, myeloproliferative disorder), common variants (eg, W515A, W515K, W515L, W515R)

TCD@ (T cell antigen receptor, delta) (eg, leukemia and lymphoma), gene rearrangement analysis, evaluation to detect abnormal clonal population

<u>Uniparental disomy (UPD) (eg, Russell-Silver syndrome, Prader-Willi/Angelman syndrome), short tandem repeat (STR) analysis</u>

▲ **81403** Molecular pathology procedure, Level 4 (eg, analysis of single exon by DNA sequence analysis, analysis of >10 amplicons using multiplex PCR in 2 or more independent reactions, mutation scanning or duplication/deletion variants of 2-5 exons)

ABL1 (c-abl oncogene 1, receptor tyrosine kinase) (eg, acquired imatinib tyrosine kinase inhibitor resistance), variants in the kinase domain

<u>*ANG (angiogenin, ribonuclease, RNase A family, 5)* (eg, amyotrophic lateral sclerosis), full gene sequence</u>

<u>*CEBPA (CCAAT/enhancer binding protein [C/EBP], alpha)* (eg, acute myeloid leukemia), full gene sequence</u>

<u>*CEL (carboxyl ester lipase [bile salt-stimulated lipase])* (eg, maturity-onset diabetes of the young [MODY]), targeted sequence analysis of exon 11 (eg, c.1785delC, c.1686delT)</u>

DAZ/SRY (deleted in azoospermia and sex determining region Y) (eg, male infertility), common deletions (eg, AZFa, AZFb, AZFc, AZFd)

<u>*F8 (coagulation factor VIII)* (eg, hemophilia A), inversion analysis, intron 1 and intron 22A</u>

<u>*FGFR3 (fibroblast growth factor receptor 3)* (eg, isolated craniosynostosis), targeted sequence analysis (eg, exon 7)</u>

<u>(For targeted sequence analysis of multiple FGFR3 exons, use 81404)</u>

<u>*GJB1 (gap junction protein, beta 1)* (eg, Charcot-Marie-Tooth X-linked), full gene sequence</u>

<u>*HBB (hemoglobin, beta, beta-globin)* (eg, beta thalassemia), duplication/deletion analysis</u>

<u>*HRAS (v-Ha-ras Harvey rat sarcoma viral oncogene homolog)* (eg, Costello syndrome), exon 2 sequence</u>

<u>*IDH1 (isocitrate dehydrogenase 1 [NADP+], soluble)* (eg, glioma), common exon 4 variants (eg, R132H, R132C)</u>

<u>*IDH2 (isocitrate dehydrogenase 2 [NADP+], mitochondrial)* (eg, glioma), common exon 4 variants (eg, R140W, R172M)</u>

JAK2 (Janus kinase 2) (eg, myeloproliferative disorder), exon 12 sequence and exon 13 sequence, if performed

<u>Known familial variant not otherwise specified, for gene listed in Tier 1 or Tier 2, DNA sequence analysis, each variant exon</u>

<u>(For a known familial variant that is considered a common variant, use specific common variant Tier 1 or Tier 2 code)</u>

KRAS (v-Ki-ras2 Kirsten rat sarcoma viral oncogene) (eg, carcinoma), gene analysis, variant(s) in exon ~~2~~3 (eg, codon 61)

MPL (myeloproliferative leukemia virus oncogene, thrombopoietin receptor, TPOR) (eg, myeloproliferative disorder), exon 10 sequence

<u>*MT-RNR1 (mitochondrially encoded 12S RNA)* (eg, nonsyndromic hearing loss), full gene sequence</u>

<u>*MT-TS1 (mitochondrially encoded tRNA serine 1)* (eg, nonsyndromic hearing loss), full gene sequence</u>

<u>*SMN1 (survival of motor neuron 1, telomeric)* (eg, spinal muscular atrophy), known familial sequence variant(s)</u>

VHL (von Hippel-Lindau tumor suppressor) (eg, von Hippel-Lindau familial cancer syndrome), deletion/duplication analysis

VWF (von Willebrand factor) (eg, von Willebrand disease types 2A, 2B, 2M), targeted sequence analysis (eg, exon 28)

▲ **81404** Molecular pathology procedure, Level 5 (eg, analysis of 2-5 exons by DNA sequence analysis, mutation scanning or duplication/deletion variants of 6-10 exons, or characterization of a dynamic mutation disorder/triplet repeat by Southern blot analysis)

<u>*ACADS (acyl-CoA dehydrogenase, C-2 to C-3 short chain)* (eg, short chain acyl-CoA dehydrogenase deficiency), targeted sequence analysis (eg, exons 5 and 6)</u>

<u>*AQP2 (aquaporin 2 [collecting duct])* (eg, nephrogenic diabetes insipidus), full gene sequence</u>

<u>*ARX (aristaless related homeobox)* (eg, X-linked lissencephaly with ambiguous genitalia, X-linked mental retardation), full gene sequence</u>

BTD (biotinidase) (eg, biotinidase deficiencysequence gene full ,)

<u>*CAV3 (caveolin 3)* (eg, CAV3-related distal myopathy, limb-girdle muscular dystrophy type 1C), full gene sequence</u>

<u>*CDKN2A (cyclin-dependent kinase inhibitor 2A)* (eg, CDKN2A-related cutaneous malignant melanoma, familial atypical mole-malignant melanoma syndrome), full gene sequence</u>

<u>*CLRN1 (clarin 1)* (eg, Usher syndrome, type 3), full gene sequence</u>

<u>*CPT2 (carnitine palmitoyltransferase 2)* (eg, carnitine palmitoyltransferase II deficiency), full gene sequence</u>

CYP1B1 (cytochrome P450, family 1, subfamily B, polypeptide 1) (eg, primary congenital glaucoma), full gene sequence

DMPK (dystrophia myotonica-protein kinase) (eg, myotonic dystrophy type 1), characterization of abnormal (eg, expanded) alleles

EGR2 (early growth response 2) (eg, Charcot-Marie-Tooth), full gene sequence

<u>*FGFR2 (fibroblast growth factor receptor 2)* (eg, craniosynostosis, Apert syndrome, Crouzon syndrome), targeted sequence analysis (eg, exons 8, 10)</u>

<u>*FGFR3 (fibroblast growth factor receptor 3)* (eg, achondroplasia, hypochondroplasia), targeted sequence analysis (eg, exons 8, 11, 12, 13)</u>

FKRP (Fukutin related protein) (eg, congenital muscular dystrophy type 1C [MDC1C], limb-girdle muscular dystrophy [LGMD] type 2I), full gene sequence

FOXG1 (forkhead box G1) (eg, Rett syndrome), full gene sequence

FSHMD1A (facioscapulohumeral muscular dystrophy 1A) (eg, facioscapulohumeral muscular dystrophy), evaluation to detect abnormal (eg, deleted) alleles

FSHMD1A (facioscapulohumeral muscular dystrophy 1A) (eg, facioscapulohumeral muscular dystrophy), characterization of haplotype(s) (ie, chromosome 4A and 4B haplotypes)

FXN (frataxin) (eg, Friedreich ataxia), full gene sequence

HBA1/HBA2 (alpha globin 1 and alpha globin 2) (eg, alpha thalassemia), duplication/deletion analysis

(For common deletion variants of alpha globin 1 and alpha globin 2 genes, use 81257)

HBB (hemoglobin, beta, Beta-Globin) (eg, thalassemia), full gene sequence

HNF1B (HNF1 homeobox B) (eg, maturity-onset diabetes of the young [MODY]), duplication/deletion analysis

HRAS (v-Ha-ras Harvey rat sarcoma viral oncogene homolog) (eg, Costello syndrome), full gene sequence

KCNJ10 (potassium inwardly-rectifying channel, subfamily J, member 10) (eg, SeSAME syndrome, EAST syndrome, sensorineural hearing loss), full gene sequence

KIT (C-kit) (v-kit Hardy-Zuckerman 4 feline sarcoma viral oncogene homolog) (eg, GIST, acute myeloid leukemia, melanoma), targeted gene analysis (eg, exons 8, 11, 13, 17, 18)

LITAF (lipopolysaccharide-induced TNF factor) (eg, Charcot-Marie-Tooth), full gene sequence

MEFV (Mediterranean fever) (eg, familial Mediterranean fever), full gene sequence

MEN1 (multiple endocrine neoplasia I) (eg, multiple endocrine neoplasia type 1, Wermer syndrome), duplication/deletion analysis

NRAS (neuroblastoma RAS viral oncogene homolog) (eg, colorectal carcinoma), exon 1 and exon 2 sequences

PDGFRA (platelet-derived growth factor receptor alpha polypeptide) (eg, gastrointestinal stromal tumor), targeted sequence analysis (eg, exons 12, 18)

PDX1 (pancreatic and duodenal homeobox 1) (eg, maturity-onset diabetes of the young [MODY]), full gene sequence

PRNP (prion protein) (eg, genetic prion disease), full gene sequence

PRSS1 (protease, serine, 1 [trypsin 1]) (eg, hereditary pancreatitis), full gene sequence

RAF1 (v-raf-1 murine leukemia viral oncogene homolog 1) (eg, LEOPARD syndrome), targeted sequence analysis (eg, exons 7, 12, 14, 17)

RET (ret proto-oncogene) (eg, multiple endocrine neoplasia, type 2B and familial medullary thyroid carcinoma), common variants (eg, M918T, 2647_2648delinsTT, A883F)

SDHD (succinate dehydrogenase complex, subunit D, integral membrane protein) (eg, hereditary paraganglioma), full gene sequence

SLC25A4 (solute carrier family 25 [mitochondrial carrier; adenine nucleotide translocator], member 4) (eg, progressive external ophthalmoplegia), full gene sequence

TP53 (tumor protein 53) (eg, tumor samples), targeted sequence analysis of 2-5 exons

TTR (transthyretin) (eg, familial transthyretin amyloidosis), full gene sequence

TYR (tyrosinase [oculocutaneous albinism IA]) (eg, oculocutaneous albinism IA), full gene sequence

USH1G (Usher syndrome 1G [autosomal recessive]) (eg, Usher syndrome, type 1), full gene sequence

VHL (von Hippel-Lindau tumor suppressor) (eg, von Hippel-Lindau familial cancer syndrome), full gene sequence

VWF (von Willebrand factor) (eg, von Willebrand disease type 1C), targeted sequence analysis (eg, exons 26, 27, 37)

▲ 81405 ~~Molecular pathology procedure, Level 6~~*Molecular pathology procedure, Level 6* (eg, analysis of 6-10 exons by DNA sequence analysis, mutation scanning or duplication/deletion variants of 11-25 exons)

ABCD1 (ATP-binding cassette, sub-family D [ALD], member 1) (eg, adrenoleukodystrophy), full gene sequence

ACADS (acyl-CoA dehydrogenase, C-2 to C-3 short chain) (eg, short chain acyl-CoA dehydrogenase deficiency), full gene sequence

ACTC1 (actin, alpha, cardiac muscle 1) (eg, familial hypertrophic cardiomyopathy), full gene sequence

APTX (aprataxin) (eg, ataxia with oculomotor apraxia 1), full gene sequence

AR (androgen receptor) (eg, androgen insensitivity syndrome), full gene sequence

CHRNA4 (cholinergic receptor, nicotinic, alpha 4) (eg, nocturnal frontal lobe epilepsy), full gene sequence

CHRNB2 (cholinergic receptor, nicotinic, beta 2 [neuronal]) (eg, nocturnal frontal lobe epilepsy), full gene sequence

CYP21A2 (cytochrome P450, family 21, subfamily A, polypeptide2) (eg, steroid 21-hydroxylase isoform, congenital adrenal hyperplasia), full gene sequence

DFNB59 (deafness, autosomal recessive 59) (eg, autosomal recessive nonsyndromic hearing impairment), full gene sequence

DHCR7 (7-dehydrocholesterol reductase) (eg, Smith-Lemli-Opitz syndrome), full gene sequence

EYA1 (eyes absent homolog 1 [Drosophila]) (eg, branchio-oto-renal [BOR] spectrum disorders), duplication/deletion analysis

F9 (coagulation factor IX) (eg, hemophilia B), full gene sequence

FH (fumarate hydratase) (eg, fumarate hydratase deficiency, hereditary leiomyomatosis with renal cell cancer), full gene sequence

FKTN (fukutin) (eg, limb-girdle muscular dystrophy [LGMD] type 2M or 2L), full gene sequence

GFAP (glial fibrillary acidic protein) (eg, Alexander disease), full gene sequence

GLA (galactosidase, alpha) (eg, Fabry disease), full gene sequence

HBA1/HBA2 (alpha globin 1 and alpha globin 2) (eg, thalassemia), full gene sequence

HNF1A (HNF1 homeobox A) (eg, maturity-onset diabetes of the young [MODY]), full gene sequence

HNF1B (HNF1 homeobox B) (eg, maturity-onset diabetes of the young [MODY]), full gene sequence

KRAS (v-Ki-ras2 Kirsten rat sarcoma viral oncogene homolog) (eg, Noonan syndrome), full gene sequence

LAMP2 (lysosomal-associated membrane protein 2) (eg, Danon disease), full gene sequence

MEN1 (multiple endocrine neoplasia I) (eg, multiple endocrine neoplasia type 1, Wermer syndrome), full gene sequence

MPZ (myelin protein zero) (eg, Charcot-Marie-Tooth), full gene sequence

MYL2 (myosin, light chain 2, regulatory, cardiac, slow) (eg, familial hypertrophic cardiomyopathy), full gene sequence

MYL3 (myosin, light chain 3, alkali, ventricular, skeletal, slow) (eg, familial hypertrophic cardiomyopathy), full gene sequence

MYOT (myotilin) (eg, limb-girdle muscular dystrophy), full gene sequence

NEFL (neurofilament, light polypeptide) (eg, Charcot-Marie-Tooth), full gene sequence

NF-2 (neurofibromin 2 [merlin]) (eg, neurofibromatosis, type 2), duplication/deletion analysis

NSD1 (nuclear receptor binding SET domain protein 1) (eg, Sotos syndrome), duplication/deletion analysis

OTC (ornithine carbamoyltransferase) (eg, ornithine transcarbamylase deficiency), full gene sequence

PDHB (pyruvate dehydrogenase [lipoamide] beta) (eg, lactic acidosis), full gene sequence

PSEN1 (presenilin 1) (eg, Alzheimer disease), full gene sequence

RET (ret proto-oncogene) (eg, multiple endocrine neoplasia, type 2A and familial medullary thyroid carcinoma), targeted sequence analysis (eg, exons 10, 11, 13-16)

SDHB (succinate dehydrogenase complex, subunit B, iron sulfur) (eg, hereditary paraganglioma), full gene sequence

SDHC (succinate dehydrogenase complex, subunit C, integral membrane protein, 15kDa) (eg, hereditary paraganglioma-pheochromocytoma syndrome), full gene sequence

SGCA (sarcoglycan, alpha [50kDa dystrophin-associated glycoprotein]) (eg, limb-girdle muscular dystrophy), full gene sequence

SGCB (sarcoglycan, beta [43kDa dystrophin-associated glycoprotein]) (eg, limb-girdle muscular dystrophy), full gene sequence

SGCD (sarcoglycan, delta [35kDa dystrophin-associated glycoprotein]) (eg, limb-girdle muscular dystrophy), full gene sequence

SGCG (sarcoglycan, gamma [35kDa dystrophin-associated glycoprotein]) (eg, limb-girdle muscular dystrophy), full gene sequence

SHOC2 (soc-2 suppressor of clear homolog) (eg, Noonan-like syndrome with loose anagen hair), full gene sequence

SMN1 (survival of motor neuron 1, telomeric) (eg, spinal muscular atrophy), full gene sequence

SPRED1 (sprouty-related, EVH1 domain containing 1) (eg, Legius syndrome), full gene sequence

TGFBR1 (transforming growth factor, beta receptor 1) (eg, Marfan syndrome), full gene sequence

TGFBR2 (transforming growth factor, beta receptor 2) (eg, Marfan syndrome), full gene sequence

THRB (thyroid hormone receptor, beta) (eg, thyroid hormone resistance, thyroid hormone beta receptor deficiency), full gene sequence or targeted sequence analysis of >5 exons

TNNI3 (troponin I, type 3 [cardiac]) (eg, familial hypertrophic cardiomyopathy), full gene sequence

TP53 (tumor protein 53) (eg, Li-Fraumeni syndrome, tumor samples), full gene sequence or targeted sequence analysis of >5 exons

TPM1 (tropomyosin 1 [alpha]) (eg, familial hypertrophic cardiomyopathy), full gene sequence

TSC1 (tuberous sclerosis 1) (eg, tuberous sclerosis), duplication/deletion analysis

VWF (von Willebrand factor) (eg, von Willebrand disease type 2N), targeted sequence analysis (eg, exons 18-20, 23-25)

▲ 81406 Molecular pathology procedure, Level 7 (eg, analysis of 11-25 exons by DNA sequence analysis, mutation scanning or duplication/deletion variants of 26-50 exons, cytogenomic array analysis for neoplasia)

ACADVL (acyl-CoA dehydrogenase, very long chain) (eg, very long chain acyl-coenzyme A dehydrogenase deficiency), full gene sequence

ACTN4 (actinin, alpha 4) (eg, focal segmental glomerulosclerosis), full gene sequence

ANO5 (anoctamin 5) (eg, limb-girdle muscular dystrophy), full gene sequence

APP (amyloid beta [A4] precursor protein) (eg, Alzheimer disease), full gene sequence

ATP7B (ATPase, Cu++ transporting, beta polypeptide) (eg, Wilson disease), full gene sequence

BRAF (v-raf murine sarcoma viral oncogene homolog B1) (eg, Noonan syndrome), full gene sequence

CAPN3 (Calpain 3) (eg, limb-girdle muscular dystrophy [LGMD] type 2A, calpainopathy), full gene sequence

CBS (cystathionine-beta-synthase) (eg, homocystinuria, cystathionine beta-synthase deficiency), full gene sequence

CDH1 (cadherin 1, type 1, E-cadherin [epithelial]) (eg, hereditary diffuse gastric cancer), full gene sequence

CDKL5 (cyclin-dependent kinase-like 5) (eg, early infantile epileptic encephalopathy), full gene sequence

Cytogenomic microarray analysis, neoplasia (eg, interrogation of copy number, and loss-of-heterozygosity via single nucleotide polymorphism [SNP]-based comparative genomic hybridization [CGH] microarray analysis)

DLAT (dihydrolipoamide S-acetyltransferase) (eg, pyruvate dehydrogenase E2 deficiency), full gene sequence

DLD (dihydrolipoamide dehydrogenase) (eg, maple syrup urine disease, type III), full gene sequence

EYA1 (eyes absent homolog 1 [Drosophila]) (eg, branchio-oto-renal [BOR] spectrum disorders), full gene sequence

F8 (coagulation factor VIII) (eg, hemophilia A), duplication/deletion analysis

GAA (glucosidase, alpha; acid) (eg, glycogen storage disease type II [Pompe disease]), full gene sequence

GALT (galactose-1-phosphate uridylyltransferase) (eg, galactosemia), full gene sequence

GCDH (glutaryl-CoA dehydrogenase) (eg, glutaricacidemia type 1), full gene sequence

GCK (glucokinase [hexokinase 4]) (eg, maturity-onset diabetes of the young [MODY]), full gene sequence

Appendixes A–E

HADHA (hydroxyacyl-CoA dehydrogenase/3-ketoacyl-CoA thiolase/enoyl-CoA hydratase [trifunctional protein] alpha subunit) (eg, long chain acyl-coenzyme A dehydrogenase deficiency), full gene sequence

HEXA (hexosaminidase A, alpha polypeptide) (eg, Tay-Sachs disease), full gene sequence

HNF4A (hepatocyte nuclear factor 4, alpha) (eg, maturity-onset diabetes of the young [MODY]), full gene sequence

IVD (isovaleryl-CoA dehydrogenase) (eg, isovaleric acidemia), full gene sequence

JAG1 (jagged 1) (eg, Alagille syndrome), duplication/deletion analysis

LDB3 (LIM domain binding 3) (eg, familial dilated cardiomyopathy, myofibrillar myopathy), full gene sequence

LMNA (lamin A/C) (eg, Emery-Dreifuss muscular dystrophy [EDMD1, 2 and 3] limb-girdle muscular dystrophy [LGMD] type 1B, dilated cardiomyopathy [CMD1A], familial partial lipodystrophy [FPLD2]), full gene sequence

MAP2K1 (mitogen-activated protein kinase 1) (eg, cardiofaciocutaneous syndrome), full gene sequence

MAP2K2 (mitogen-activated protein kinase 2) (eg, cardiofaciocutaneous syndrome), full gene sequence

MCCC2 (methylcrotonoyl-CoA carboxylase 2 [beta]) (eg, 3-methylcrotonyl carboxylase deficiency), full gene sequence

MUTYH (mutY homolog [E. coli]) (eg, MYH-associated polyposis), full gene sequence

NF2 (neurofibromin 2 [merlin]) (eg, neurofibromatosis, type 2), full gene sequence

NOTCH3 (notch 3) (eg, cerebral autosomal dominant arteriopathy with subcortical infarcts and leukoencephalopathy [CADASIL]), targeted sequence analysis (eg, exons 1-23)

NSD1 (nuclear receptor binding SET domain protein 1) (eg, Sotos syndrome), full gene sequence

OPA1 (optic atrophy 1) (eg, optic atrophy), duplication/deletion analysis

PAH (phenylalanine hydroxylase) (eg, phenylketonuria), full gene sequence

PALB2 (partner and localizer of BRCA2) (eg, breast and pancreatic cancer), full gene sequence

PAX2 (paired box 2) (eg, renal coloboma syndrome), full gene sequence

PC (pyruvate carboxylase) (eg, pyruvate carboxylase deficiency), full gene sequence

PCCB (propionyl CoA carboxylase, beta polypeptide) (eg, propionic acidemia), full gene sequence

PDHA1 (pyruvate dehydrogenase [lipoamide] alpha 1) (eg, lactic acidosis), full gene sequence

PDHX (pyruvate dehydrogenase complex, component X) (eg, lactic acidosis), full gene sequence

POLG (polymerase [DNA directed], gamma) (eg, Alpers-Huttenlocher syndrome, autosomal dominant progressive external ophthalmoplegia), full gene sequence

POMGNT1 (protein O-linked mannose beta1,2-N acetylglucosaminyltransferase) (eg, muscle-eye-brain disease, Walker-Warburg syndrome), full gene sequence

POMT1 (protein-O-mannosyltransferase 1) (eg, limb-girdle muscular dystrophy [LGMD] type 2K, Walker-Warburg syndrome), full gene sequence

POMT2 (protein-O-mannosyltransferase 2) (eg, limb-girdle muscular dystrophy [LGMD] type 2N, Walker-Warburg syndromesequence gene full)

PRKAG2 (protein kinase, AMP-activated, gamma 2 non-catalytic subunit) (eg, familial hypertrophic cardiomyopathy with Wolff-Parkinson-White syndrome, lethal congenital glycogen storage disease of heart), full gene sequence

PSEN2 (presenilin 2 [Alzheimer disease 4]) (eg, Alzheimer disease), full gene sequence

PTPN11 (protein tyrosine phosphatase, non-receptor type 11) (eg, Noonan syndrome, LEOPARD syndrome), full gene sequence

PYGM (phosphorylase, glycogen, muscle) (eg, glycogen storage disease type V, McArdle disease), full gene sequence

RAF1 (v-raf-1 murine leukemia viral oncogene homolog 1) (eg, LEOPARD syndrome), full gene sequence

RET (ret proto-oncogene) (eg, Hirschsprung disease), full gene sequence

RYR1 (ryanodine receptor 1, skeletal) (eg, malignant hyperthermia), targeted sequence analysis of exons with functionally-confirmed mutations

SLC9A6 (solute carrier family 9 [sodium/hydrogen exchanger], member 6) (eg, Christianson syndrome), full gene sequence

SLC26A4 (solute carrier family 26, member 4) (eg, Pendred syndrome), full gene sequence

SOS1 (son of sevenless homolog 1) (eg, Noonan syndrome, gingival fibromatosis), full gene sequence

TAZ (tafazzin) (eg, methylglutaconic aciduria type 2, Barth syndrome), full gene sequence

TNNT2 (troponin T, type 2 [cardiac]) (eg, familial hypertrophic cardiomyopathy), full gene sequence

TSC1 (tuberous sclerosis 1) (eg, tuberous sclerosis), full gene sequence

TSC2 (tuberous sclerosis 2) (eg, tuberous sclerosis), duplication/deletion analysis

UBE3A (ubiquitin protein ligase E3A) (eg, Angelman syndrome), full gene sequence

VWF (von Willebrand factor) (von Willebrand disease type 2A), extended targeted sequence analysis (eg, exons 11-16, 24-26, 51, 52)

▲ 81407 Molecular pathology procedure, Level 8 (eg, analysis of 26-50 exons by DNA sequence analysis, mutation scanning or duplication/deletion variants of >50 exons, sequence analysis of multiple genes on one platform)

ABCC8 (ATP-binding cassette, sub-family C [CFTR/MRP], member 8) (eg, familial hyperinsulinism), full gene sequence

CHD7 (chromodomain helicase DNA binding protein 7) (eg, CHARGE syndrome), full gene sequence

F8 (coagulation factor VIII) (eg, hemophilia A), full gene sequence

JAG1 (jagged 1) (eg, Alagille syndrome), full gene sequence

MYBPC3 (myosin binding protein C, cardiac) (eg, familial hypertrophic cardiomyopathy), full gene sequence

MYH6 (myosin, heavy chain 6, cardiac muscle, alpha) (eg, familial dilated cardiomyopathy), full gene sequence

MYH7 (myosin, heavy chain 7, cardiac muscle, beta) (eg, familial hypertrophic cardiomyopathy, Liang distal myopathy), full gene sequence

MYO7A (myosin VIIA) (eg, Usher syndrome, type 1), full gene sequence

NOTCH1 (notch 1) (eg, aortic valve disease), full gene sequence

OPA1 (optic atrophy 1) (eg, optic atrophy), full gene sequence

PCDH15 (protocadherin-related 15) (eg, Usher syndrome, type 1), full gene sequence

SCN1A (sodium channel, voltage-gated, type 1, alpha subunit) (eg, generalized epilepsy with febrile seizures), full gene sequence

SCN5A (sodium channel, voltage-gated, type V, alpha subunit) (eg, familial dilated cardiomyopathy), full gene sequence

TSC2 (tuberous sclerosis 2) (eg, tuberous sclerosis), full gene sequence

USH1C (Usher syndrome 1C [autosomal recessive, severe]) (eg, Usher syndrome, type 1), full gene sequence

▲ **81408** Molecular pathology procedure, Level 9 (eg, analysis of > 50 exons in a single gene by DNA sequence analysis)

ATM (ataxia telangiectasia mutated) (eg, ataxia telangiectasia), full gene sequence

CDH23 (cadherin-related 23) (eg, Usher syndrome, type 1), full gene sequence

COL1A1 (collagen, type I, alpha 1) (eg, osteogenesis imperfecta, type I), full gene sequence

COL1A2 (collagen, type I, alpha 2) (eg, osteogenesis imperfecta, type I), full gene sequence

DYSF (dysferlin, limb girdle muscular dystrophy 2B [autosomal recessive]) (eg, limb-girdle muscular dystrophy), full gene sequence

FBN1 (fibrillin 1) (eg, Marfan syndrome), full gene sequence

NF1 (neurofibromin 1) (eg, neurofibromatosis, type 1), full gene sequence

RYR1 (ryanodine receptor 1, skeletal) (eg, malignant hyperthermia), full gene sequence

USH2A (Usher syndrome 2A [autosomal recessive, mild]) (eg, Usher syndrome, type 2), full gene sequence

VWF (von Willebrand factor) (eg, von Willebrand disease types 1 and 3), full gene sequence;

● **81479** Code added

● **81500** Code added

● **81503** Code added

● **81506** Code added

● **81508** Code added

● **81509** Code added

● **81510** Code added

● **81511** Code added

● **81512** Code added

● **81599** Code added

▲ **82009** ~~Acetone or other ketone bodies~~Ketone body(s) (eg, acetone, acetoacetic acid, ~~serum~~beta-hydroxybutyrate); qualitative

▲ **82010** quantitative

● **82777** Code added

83890 ~~Molecular diagnostics; molecular isolation or extraction, each nucleic acid type (ie, DNA or RNA)~~

83891 ~~isolation or extraction of highly purified nucleic acid, each nucleic acid type (ie, DNA or RNA)~~

83892 ~~enzymatic digestion, each enzyme treatment~~

83893 ~~dot/slot blot production, each nucleic acid preparation~~

83894 ~~separation by gel electrophoresis (eg, agarose, polyacrylamide), each nucleic acid preparation~~

83896 ~~nucleic acid probe, each~~

83897 ~~nucleic acid transfer (eg, Southern, Northern), each nucleic acid preparation~~

83898 ~~amplification, target, each nucleic acid sequence~~

83900 ~~amplification, target, multiplex, first 2 nucleic acid sequences~~

83901 ~~amplification, target, multiplex, each additional nucleic acid sequence beyond 2 (List separately in addition to code for primary procedure)~~

83902 ~~reverse transcription~~

83903 ~~mutation scanning, by physical properties (eg, single strand conformational polymorphisms [SSCP], heteroduplex, denaturing gradient gel electrophoresis [DGGE], RNA'ase A), single segment, each~~

83904 ~~mutation identification by sequencing, single segment, each segment~~

83905 ~~mutation identification by allele specific transcription, single segment, each segment~~

83906 ~~mutation identification by allele specific translation, single segment, each segment~~

83907 ~~lysis of cells prior to nucleic acid extraction (eg, stool specimens, paraffin embedded tissue), each specimen~~

83908 ~~amplification, signal, each nucleic acid sequence~~

83909 ~~separation and identification by high resolution technique (eg, capillary electrophoresis), each nucleic acid preparation~~

83912 ~~interpretation and report~~

83913 ~~RNA stabilization~~

83914 ~~Mutation identification by enzymatic ligation or primer extension, single segment, each segment (eg, oligonucleotide ligation assay [OLA], single base chain extension [SBCE], or allele-specific primer extension [ASPE]);~~

#● **86152** Code added

#● **86153** Code added

● **86711** Code added

● **86828** Code added

● **86829** Code added

● **86830** Code added

● **86831** Code added

● **86832** Code added

● **86833** Code added

● **86834** Code added

● **86835** Code added

▲ **87498** enterovirus, reverse transcription and amplified probe technique

▲ **87521** hepatitis C, reverse transcription and amplified probe technique

▲ 87522   hepatitis C, <u>reverse transcription and</u> quantification

▲ 87535   HIV-1, <u>reverse transcription and</u> amplified probe technique

▲ 87536   HIV-1, <u>reverse transcription and</u> quantification

▲ 87538   HIV-2, <u>reverse transcription and</u> amplified probe technique

▲ 87539   HIV-2, <u>reverse transcription and</u> quantification

● 87631   Code added

● 87632   Code added

● 87633   Code added

#● 87910   Code added

▲ 87901   HIV-1, reverse transcriptase and protease regions

#● 87912   Code added

● 88375   Code added

88384   ~~Array-based evaluation of multiple molecular probes; 11 through 50 probes~~

88385   ~~51 through 250 probes~~

88386   ~~251 through 500 probes~~

Medicine

✎● 90653   Code added

▲ 90655   Influenza virus vaccine<u>, trivalent</u>, split virus, preservative free, when administered to children 6-35 months of age, for intramuscular use

▲ 90656   Influenza virus vaccine<u>, trivalent</u>, split virus, preservative free, when administered to individuals 3 years and older, for intramuscular use

▲ 90657   Influenza virus vaccine<u>, trivalent</u>, split virus, when administered to children 6-35 months of age, for intramuscular use

▲ 90658   Influenza virus vaccine<u>, trivalent</u>, split virus, when administered to individuals 3 years of age and older, for intramuscular use

▲ 90660   Influenza virus vaccine<u>, trivalent</u>, live, for intranasal use

#● 90672   Code added

90665   ~~Lyme disease vaccine, adult dosage, for intramuscular use~~

90701   ~~Diphtheria, tetanus toxoids, and whole cell pertussis vaccine (DTP), for intramuscular use~~

90718   ~~Tetanus and diphtheria toxoids (Td) adsorbed when administered to individuals 7 years or older, for intramuscular use;~~

✎● 90739   Code added

▲ 90746   Hepatitis B vaccine, adult dosage <u>(3 dose schedule)</u>, for intramuscular use

+● 90785   Code added

● 90791   Code added

● 90792   Code added

90801   ~~Psychiatric diagnostic interview examination;~~

90802   ~~Interactive psychiatric diagnostic interview examination using play equipment, physical devices, language interpreter, or other mechanisms of communication~~

90804   ~~Individual psychotherapy, insight oriented, behavior modifying and/or supportive, in an office or outpatient facility, approximately 20 to 30 minutes face-to-face with the patient~~

90805   ~~with medical evaluation and management services~~

90806   ~~Individual psychotherapy, insight oriented, behavior modifying and/or supportive, in an office or outpatient facility, approximately 45 to 50 minutes face-to-face with the patient;~~

90807   ~~with medical evaluation and management services~~

90808   ~~Individual psychotherapy, insight oriented, behavior modifying and/or supportive, in an office or outpatient facility, approximately 75 to 80 minutes face-to-face with the patient;~~

90809   ~~with medical evaluation and management services~~

90810   ~~Individual psychotherapy, interactive, using play equipment, physical devices, language interpreter, or other mechanisms of non-verbal communication, in an office or outpatient facility, approximately 20 to 30 minutes face-to-face with the patient;~~

90811   ~~with medical evaluation and management services~~

90812   ~~Individual psychotherapy, interactive, using play equipment, physical devices, language interpreter, or other mechanisms of non-verbal communication, in an office or outpatient facility, approximately 45 to 50 minutes face-to-face with the patient;~~

90813   ~~with medical evaluation and management services~~

90814   ~~Individual psychotherapy, interactive, using play equipment, physical devices, language interpreter, or other mechanisms of non-verbal communication, in an office or outpatient facility, approximately 75 to 80 minutes face-to-face with the patient;~~

90815   ~~with medical evaluation and management services~~

90816   ~~Individual psychotherapy, insight oriented, behavior modifying and/or supportive, in an inpatient hospital, partial hospital or residential care setting, approximately 20 to 30 minutes face-to-face with the patient;~~

90817   ~~with medical evaluation and management services~~

90818   ~~Individual psychotherapy, insight oriented, behavior modifying and/or supportive, in an inpatient hospital, partial hospital or residential care setting, approximately 45 to 50 minutes face-to-face with the patient;~~

90819   ~~with medical evaluation and management services~~

90821   ~~Individual psychotherapy, insight oriented, behavior modifying and/or supportive, in an inpatient hospital, partial hospital or residential care setting, approximately 75 to 80 minutes face-to-face with the patient;~~

90822   ~~with medical evaluation and management services~~

90823   ~~Individual psychotherapy, interactive, using play equipment, physical devices, language interpreter, or other mechanisms of non-verbal communication, in an inpatient hospital, partial hospital or residential care setting, approximately 20 to 30 minutes face-to-face with the patient;~~

90824   ~~with medical evaluation and management services~~

90826   ~~Individual psychotherapy, interactive, using play equipment, physical devices, language interpreter, or other mechanisms of non-verbal communication, in an inpatient hospital, partial hospital or residential care setting, approximately 45 to 50 minutes face-to-face with the patient;~~

90827   ~~with medical evaluation and management services~~

90828   ~~Individual psychotherapy, interactive, using play equipment, physical devices, language interpreter, or other mechanisms of non-verbal communication, in an inpatient hospital, partial hospital or residential care setting, approximately 75 to 80 minutes face-to-face with the patient;~~

90829   ~~with medical evaluation and management services~~

Appendixes A–E

● 90832   Code added

✚● 90833   Code added

● 90834   Code added

✚● 90836   Code added

● 90837   Code added

✚● 90838   Code added

● 90839   Code added

✚● 90840   Code added

90857   ~~Interactive group psychotherapy~~

90862   ~~Pharmacologic management, including prescription, use, and review of medication with no more than minimal medical psychotherapy~~

✚● 90863   Code added

▲ 90875   Individual psychophysiological therapy incorporating biofeedback training by any modality (face-to-face with the patient), with psychotherapy (eg, insight oriented, behavior modifying or supportive psychotherapy); ~~approximately 20-~~30 minutes

▲ 90876   ~~approximately 45-50~~ minutes

▲ 90889   Preparation of report of patient's psychiatric status, history, treatment, or progress (other than for legal or consultative purposes) for other ~~physicians~~individuals, agencies, or insurance carriers

▲ 90935   Hemodialysis procedure with single evaluation by a physician ~~evaluation~~or other qualified health care professional

▲ 90945   Dialysis procedure other than hemodialysis (eg, peritoneal dialysis, hemofiltration, or other continuous renal replacement therapies), with single evaluation by a physician ~~evaluation~~or other qualified health care professional

▲ 90947   Dialysis procedure other than hemodialysis (eg, peritoneal dialysis, hemofiltration, or other continuous renal replacement therapies) requiring repeated evaluation by a physician ~~evaluations~~or other qualified health care professional, with or without substantial revision of dialysis prescription

▲ 90951   End-stage renal disease (ESRD) related services monthly, for patients younger than 2 years of age to include monitoring for the adequacy of nutrition, assessment of growth and development, and counseling of parents; with 4 or more face-to-face visits by a physician ~~visits~~or other qualified health care professional per month

▲ 90952   with 2-3 face-to-face visits by a physician ~~visits~~or other qualified health care professional per month

▲ 90953   with 1 face-to-face visit by a physician ~~visit~~or other qualified health care professional per month

▲ 90954   End-stage renal disease (ESRD) related services monthly, for patients 2-11 years of age to include monitoring for the adequacy of nutrition, assessment of growth and development, and counseling of parents; with 4 or more face-to-face visits by a physician ~~visits~~or other qualified health care professional per month

▲ 90955   with 2-3 face-to-face visits by a physician ~~visits~~or other qualified health care professional per month

▲ 90956   with 1 face-to-face visit by a physician ~~visit~~or other qualified health care professional per month

▲ 90957   End-stage renal disease (ESRD) related services monthly, for patients 12-19 years of age to include monitoring for the adequacy of nutrition, assessment of growth and development, and counseling of parents; with 4 or more face-to-face visits by a physician ~~visits~~or other qualified health care professional per month

▲ 90958   with 2-3 face-to-face visits by a physician ~~visits~~or other qualified health care professional per month

▲ 90959   with 1 face-to-face visit by a physician ~~visit~~or other qualified health care professional per month

▲ 90960   End-stage renal disease (ESRD) related services monthly, for patients 20 years of age and older; with 4 or more face-to-face visits by a physician ~~visits~~or other qualified health care professional per month

▲ 90961   with 2-3 face-to-face visits by a physician ~~visits~~or other qualified health care professional per month

▲ 90962   with 1 face-to-face visit by a physician ~~visit~~or other qualified health care professional per month

▲ 91110   Gastrointestinal tract imaging, intraluminal (eg, capsule endoscopy), esophagus through ileum, with ~~physician~~ interpretation and report

▲ 91111   Gastrointestinal tract imaging, intraluminal (eg, capsule endoscopy), esophagus with ~~physician~~interpretation and report

● 91112   Code added

▲ 92286   ~~Special anterior~~Anterior segment ~~photography~~imaging with interpretation and report; with specular ~~endothelial~~microscopy and endothelial cell ~~count~~analysis

▲ 92287   with fluorescein angiography

▲ 92613   ~~physician~~interpretation and report only

▲ 92615   ~~physician~~interpretation and report only

▲ 92617   ~~physician~~interpretation and report only

92980   ~~Transcatheter placement of an intracoronary stent(s), percutaneous, with or without other therapeutic intervention, any method; single vessel~~

92981   ~~each additional vessel (List separately in addition to code for primary procedure)~~

92982   ~~Percutaneous transluminal coronary balloon angioplasty; single vessel~~

92984   ~~each additional vessel (List separately in addition to code for primary procedure)~~

92995   ~~Percutaneous transluminal coronary atherectomy, by mechanical or other method, with or without balloon angioplasty; single vessel~~

92996   ~~each additional vessel (List separately in addition to code for primary procedure)~~

⊙#● 92920   Code added

✚⊙#● 92921   Code added

⊙#● 92924   Code added

✚⊙#● 92925   Code added

⊙#● 92928   Code added

✚⊙#● 92929   Code added

⊙#● 92933   Code added

✚⊙#● 92934   Code added

⊙#● 92937   Code added

+⊙#● **92938**   Code added

⊙#● **92941**   Code added

⊙#● **92943**   Code added

+⊙#● **92944**   Code added

+⊙#▲ **92973**   Percutaneous transluminal coronary thrombectomy mechanical (List separately in addition to code for primary procedure)

▲ **93015**   Cardiovascular stress test using maximal or submaximal treadmill or bicycle exercise, continuous electrocardiographic monitoring, and/or pharmacological stress; with ~~physician~~ supervision, ~~with~~ interpretation and report

▲ **93016**   ~~physician~~ supervision only, without interpretation and report

▲ **93224**   External electrocardiographic recording up to 48 hours by continuous rhythm recording and storage; includes recording, scanning analysis with report, ~~physician~~ review and interpretation by a physician or other qualified health care professional

▲ **93227**   ~~physician~~ review and interpretation by a physician or other qualified health care professional

▲ **93228**   External mobile cardiovascular telemetry with electrocardiographic recording, concurrent computerized real time data analysis and greater than 24 hours of accessible ECG data storage (retrievable with query) with ECG triggered and patient selected events transmitted to a remote attended surveillance center for up to 30 days; ~~physician~~ review and interpretation with report by a physician or other qualified health care professional

▲ **93229**   technical support for connection and patient instructions for use, attended surveillance, analysis and ~~physician prescribed~~ transmission of daily and emergent data reports as prescribed by a physician or other qualified health care professional

▲ **93268**   External patient and, when performed, auto activated electrocardiographic rhythm derived event recording with symptom-related memory loop with remote download capability up to 30 days, 24-hour attended monitoring; includes transmission, ~~physician~~ review and interpretation by a physician or other qualified health care professional

▲ **93272**   ~~physician~~ review and interpretation by a physician or other qualified health care professional

▲ **93279**   Programming device evaluation (in person) with iterative adjustment of the implantable device to test the function of the device and select optimal permanent programmed values with ~~physician~~ analysis, review and report by a physician or other qualified health care professional; single lead pacemaker system

▲ **93280**   dual lead pacemaker system

▲ **93281**   multiple lead pacemaker system

▲ **93282**   single lead implantable cardioverter-defibrillator system

▲ **93283**   dual lead implantable cardioverter-defibrillator system

▲ **93284**   multiple lead implantable cardioverter-defibrillator system

▲ **93285**   implantable loop recorder system

▲ **93286**   Peri-procedural device evaluation (in person) and programming of device system parameters before or after a surgery, procedure, or test with ~~physician~~ analysis, review and report by a physician or other qualified health care professional; single, dual, or multiple lead pacemaker system

▲ **93287**   single, dual, or multiple lead implantable cardioverter-defibrillator system

▲ **93288**   Interrogation device evaluation (in person) with ~~physician~~ analysis, review and report by a physician or other qualified health care professional, includes connection, recording and disconnection per patient encounter; single, dual, or multiple lead pacemaker system

▲ **93289**   single, dual, or multiple lead implantable cardioverter-defibrillator system, including analysis of heart rhythm derived data elements

▲ **93290**   implantable cardiovascular monitor system, including analysis of 1 or more recorded physiologic cardiovascular data elements from all internal and external sensors

▲ **93291**   implantable loop recorder system, including heart rhythm derived data analysis

▲ **93292**   wearable defibrillator system

▲ **93293**   Transtelephonic rhythm strip pacemaker evaluation(s) single, dual, or multiple lead pacemaker system, includes recording with and without magnet application with ~~physician~~ analysis, review and report(s) by a physician or other qualified health care professional, up to 90 days

▲ **93294**   Interrogation device evaluation(s) (remote), up to 90 days; single, dual, or multiple lead pacemaker system with interim ~~physician~~ analysis, review(s) and report(s) by a physician or other qualified health care professional

▲ **93295**   single, dual, or multiple lead implantable cardioverter-defibrillator system with interim ~~physician~~ analysis, review(s) and report(s) by a physician or other qualified health care professional

▲ **93297**   Interrogation device evaluation(s), (remote) up to 30 days; implantable cardiovascular monitor system, including analysis of 1 or more recorded physiologic cardiovascular data elements from all internal and external sensors, ~~physician~~ analysis, review(s) and report(s) by a physician or other qualified health care professional

▲ **93298**   implantable loop recorder system, including analysis of recorded heart rhythm data, ~~physician~~ analysis, review(s) and report(s) by a physician or other qualified health care professional

▲ **93351**   including performance of continuous electrocardiographic monitoring, with supervision by a physician ~~supervision~~ or other qualified health care professional

93651   ~~Intracardiac catheter ablation of arrhythmogenic focus; for treatment of supraventricular tachycardia by ablation of fast or slow atrioventricular pathways, accessory atrioventricular connections or other atrial foci, singly or in combination~~

93652   ~~for treatment of ventricular tachycardia~~

⊙● **93653**   Code added

⊙● **93654**   Code added

+⊙● **93655**   Code added

⊙● **93656**   Code added

+⊙● **93657**   Code added

▲ **93745**   Initial set-up and programming by a physician or other qualified health care professional of wearable cardioverter-defibrillator includes initial programming of system, establishing baseline electronic ECG, transmission of data to data repository, patient instruction in wearing system and patient reporting of problems or events

▲ **93750**   Interrogation of ventricular assist device (VAD), in person, with physician or other qualified health care professional analysis of device parameters (eg, drivelines, alarms, power surges), review of device function (eg, flow and volume status, septum status, recovery), with programming, if performed, and report

▲ 93790 ~~physician~~ review with interpretation and report

▲ 93797 Physician <u>or other qualified health care professional</u> services for outpatient cardiac rehabilitation; without continuous ECG monitoring (per session)

▲ 93798 with continuous ECG monitoring (per session)

▲ 94014 Patient-initiated spirometric recording per 30-day period of time; includes reinforced education, transmission of spirometric tracing, data capture, analysis of transmitted data, periodic recalibration and ~~physician~~ review and interpretation <u>by a physician or other qualified health care professional</u>

▲ 94016 ~~physician~~ review and interpretation only <u>by a physician or other qualified health care professional</u>

▲ 94452 High altitude simulation test (HAST), with ~~physician~~ interpretation and report <u>by a physician or other qualified health care professional</u>

▲ 94453 with supplemental oxygen titration

⊘▲ 94610 Intrapulmonary surfactant administration by a physician <u>or other qualified health care professional</u> through endotracheal tube

▲ 94774 Pediatric home apnea monitoring event recording including respiratory rate, pattern and heart rate per 30-day period of time; includes monitor attachment, download of data, ~~physician~~ review, interpretation, and preparation of a report <u>by a physician or other qualified health care professional</u>

▲ 94777 ~~physician~~ review, interpretation and preparation of report only <u>by a physician or other qualified health care professional</u>

▲ 95004 Percutaneous tests (scratch, puncture, prick) with allergenic extracts, immediate type reaction, including test interpretation and report ~~by a physician~~, specify number of tests

95010 ~~Percutaneous tests (scratch, puncture, prick) sequential and incremental, with drugs, biologicals or venoms, immediate type reaction, including test interpretation and report by a physician, specify number of tests~~

95015 ~~Intracutaneous (intradermal) tests, sequential and incremental, with drugs, biologicals, or venoms, immediate type reaction, including test interpretation and report by a physician, specify number of tests~~

● 95017 Code added

● 95018 Code added

▲ 95024 Intracutaneous (intradermal) tests with allergenic extracts, immediate type reaction, including test interpretation and report ~~by a physician~~, specify number of tests

▲ 95027 Intracutaneous (intradermal) tests, sequential and incremental, with allergenic extracts for airborne allergens, immediate type reaction, including test interpretation and report ~~by a physician~~, specify number of tests

95075 ~~Ingestion challenge test (sequential and incremental ingestion of test items, eg, food, drug or other substance such as metabisulfite~~

● 95076 Code added

+● 95079 Code added

▲ 95120 Professional services for allergen immunotherapy in ~~prescribing physicians~~<u>the</u> office or institution <u>of the prescribing physician or other qualified health care professional</u>, including provision of allergenic extract; single injection

▲ 95125 2 or more injections

▲ 95130 single stinging insect venom

▲ 95131 2 stinging insect venoms

▲ 95132 3 stinging insect venoms

▲ 95133 4 stinging insect venoms

▲ 95134 5 stinging insect venoms

▲ 95808 Polysomnography; <u>any age,</u> sleep staging with 1-3 additional parameters of sleep, attended by a technologist

▲ 95810 <u>age 6 years or older,</u> sleep staging with 4 or more additional parameters of sleep, attended by a technologist

▲ 95811 <u>age 6 years or older,</u> sleep staging with 4 or more additional parameters of sleep, with initiation of continuous positive airway pressure therapy or bilevel ventilation, attended by a technologist

#● 95782 Code added

#● 95783 Code added

▲ 95830 Insertion by physician <u>or other qualified health care professional</u> of sphenoidal electrodes for electroencephalographic (EEG) recording;

95900 ~~Nerve conduction, amplitude and latency/velocity study, each nerve; motor, without F-wave study~~

95903 ~~motor, with F-wave study~~

95904 ~~sensory~~

● 95907 Code added

● 95908 Code added

● 95909 Code added

● 95910 Code added

● 95911 Code added

● 95912 Code added

● 95913 Code added

95920 ~~Intraoperative neurophysiology testing, per hour (List separately in addition to code for primary procedure)~~

+#● 95940 Code added

+#● 95941 Code added

● 95924 Code added

#● 95943 Code added

95934 ~~H-reflex, amplitude and latency study; record gastrocnemius/soleus muscle~~

95936 ~~record muscle other than gastrocnemius/soleus muscle~~

▲ 95954 Pharmacological or physical activation requiring physician <u>or other qualified health care professional</u> attendance during EEG recording of activation phase (eg, thiopental activation test)

▲ 95961 Functional cortical and subcortical mapping by stimulation and/or recording of electrodes on brain surface, or of depth electrodes, to provoke seizures or identify vital brain structures; initial hour of <u>attendance by a</u> physician ~~attendance~~<u>or other qualified health care professional</u>

+▲ 95962 each additional hour of <u>attendance by a</u> physician ~~attendance~~<u>or other qualified health care professional</u> (List separately in addition to code for primary procedure)

▲ 95991 requiring <u>skill of a</u> physician~~'s skill~~ <u>or other qualified health care professional</u>

▲ 96004 ~~Physician review~~Review and interpretation by physician or other qualified health care professional of comprehensive computer-based motion analysis, dynamic plantar pressure measurements, dynamic surface electromyography during walking or other functional activities, and dynamic fine wire electromyography, with written report

▲ 96020 Neurofunctional testing selection and administration during noninvasive imaging functional brain mapping, with test administered entirely by a physician or other qualified health care professional (ie, psychologist), with review of test results and report

▲ 97530 Therapeutic activities, direct (one-on-one) patient contact ~~by the provider~~ (use of dynamic activities to improve functional performance), each 15 minutes

▲ 97532 Development of cognitive skills to improve attention, memory, problem solving (includes compensatory training), direct (one-on-one) patient contact ~~by the provider~~, each 15 minutes

▲ 97533 Sensory integrative techniques to enhance sensory processing and promote adaptive responses to environmental demands, direct (one-on-one) patient contact ~~by the provider~~, each 15 minutes

▲ 97535 Self-care/home management training (eg, activities of daily living (ADL) and compensatory training, meal preparation, safety procedures, and instructions in use of assistive technology devices/adaptive equipment) direct one-on-one contact ~~by provider~~, each 15 minutes

▲ 97537 Community/work reintegration training (eg, shopping, transportation, money management, avocational activities and/or work environment/modification analysis, work task analysis, use of assistive technology device/adaptive equipment), direct one-on-one contact ~~by provider~~, each 15 minutes

▲ 97755 Assistive technology assessment (eg, to restore, augment or compensate for existing function, optimize functional tasks and/or maximize environmental accessibility), direct one-on-one contact ~~by provider~~, with written report, each 15 minutes

▲ 98969 Online assessment and management service provided by a qualified nonphysician health care professional to an established patient~~,~~ or guardian, ~~or health care provider~~ not originating from a related assessment and management service provided within the previous 7 days, using the Internet or similar electronic communications network

▲ 99000 Handling and/or conveyance of specimen for transfer from the ~~physician's~~ office to a laboratory

▲ 99001 Handling and/or conveyance of specimen for transfer from the patient in other than ~~a physician's~~an office to a laboratory (distance may be indicated)

▲ 99002 Handling, conveyance, and/or any other service in connection with the implementation of an order involving devices (eg, designing, fitting, packaging, handling, delivery or mailing) when devices such as orthotics, protectives, prosthetics are fabricated by an outside laboratory or shop but which items have been designed, and are to be fitted and adjusted by the attending physician or other qualified health care professional

▲ 99070 Supplies and materials (except spectacles), provided by the physician or other qualified health care professional over and above those usually included with the office visit or other services rendered (list drugs, trays, supplies, or materials provided)

▲ 99071 Educational supplies, such as books, tapes, and pamphlets, ~~provided by the physician~~ for the patient's education at cost to physician or other qualified health care professional

▲ 99078 Physician or other qualified health care professional qualified by education, training, licensure/regulation (when applicable) educational services rendered to patients in a group setting (eg, prenatal, obesity, or diabetic instructions)

▲ 99091 Collection and interpretation of physiologic data (eg, ECG, blood pressure, glucose monitoring) digitally stored and/or transmitted by the patient and/or caregiver to the physician or other qualified health care professional, qualified by education, training, licensure/regulation (when applicable) requiring a minimum of 30 minutes of time

⊘▲ 99143 Moderate sedation services (other than those services described by codes 00100-01999) provided by the same physician or other qualified health care professional performing the diagnostic or therapeutic service that the sedation supports, requiring the presence of an independent trained observer to assist in the monitoring of the patient's level of consciousness and physiological status; younger than 5 years of age, first 30 minutes intra-service time

⊘▲ 99144 age 5 years or older, first 30 minutes intra-service time

+▲ 99145 each additional 15 minutes intra-service time (List separately in addition to code for primary service)

▲ 99148 Moderate sedation services (other than those services described by codes 00100-01999), provided by a physician or other qualified health care professional other than the health care professional performing the diagnostic or therapeutic service that the sedation supports; younger than 5 years of age, first 30 minutes intra-service time

▲ 99149 age 5 years or older, first 30 minutes intra-service time

+▲ 99150 each additional 15 minutes intra-service time (List separately in addition to code for primary service)

▲ 99174 ~~Ocular photoscreening with interpretation and report~~Instrument-based ocular screening (eg, photoscreening, automated-refraction), bilateral

▲ 99183 Physician or other qualified health care professional attendance and supervision of hyperbaric oxygen therapy, per session

Category II Codes

▲ 1005F Asthma symptoms evaluated (includes ~~physician~~ documentation of numeric frequency of symptoms or patient completion of an asthma assessment tool/survey/questionnaire) (NMA –No Measure Associated)

● 1052F Code added

▲ 2060F Patient interviewed directly ~~by evaluating clinician~~ on or before date of diagnosis of major depressive disorder (MDD ADOL)[1];

● 3517F Code added

● 3520F Code added

● 3750F Code added

4009F ~~Angiotensin converting enzyme (ACE) inhibitor or angiotensin-receptor blocker (ARB) therapy prescribed (HF, CAD, CKD)PCPI, (DM)NCQA-HEDIS~~

● 4069F Code added

● 4142F Code added

▲ 4240F Instruction in therapeutic exercise with follow-up ~~by the physician~~ provided to patients during episode of back pain lasting longer than 12 weeks (BkP)[2];

▲ 5010F Findings of dilated macular or fundus exam communicated to the physician or other qualified health care professional managing the diabetes care (EC)[5];

Appendixes A–E

▲ **5020F** Treatment summary report communicated to physician(s) or other qualified health care professional(s) managing continuing care and to the patient within 1 month of completing treatment (ONC)[1];

▲ **5100F** Potential risk for fracture communicated to the referring physician or other qualified health care professional within 24 hours of completion of the imaging study (NUC_MED)[1];

● **6150F** Code added

Category III Codes

~~0030T~~ ~~Antiprothrombin (phospholipid cofactor) antibody, each Ig class;~~

~~0048T~~ ~~Implantation of a ventricular assist device, extracorporeal, percutaneous transseptal access, single or dual cannulation;~~

~~0050T~~ ~~Removal of a ventricular assist device, extracorporeal, percutaneous transseptal access, single or dual cannulation;~~

~~0173T~~ ~~Monitoring of intraocular pressure during vitrectomy surgery (List separately in addition to code for primary procedure)~~

▲ **0195T** Arthrodesis, pre-sacral interbody technique, disc space preparation, discectomy, ~~including~~without instrumentation, imaging (when performed)with image guidance, ~~and discectomy to prepare interspace, lumbar~~includes bone graft when performed; ~~single~~L5-S1 interspace

+▲ **0196T** ~~each additional~~L4-L5 interspace (List separately in addition to code for primary procedure)

▲ **0206T** ~~Algorithmic~~Computerized database analysis of multiple cycles of digitized cardiac electrical data from two or more ECG leads, including transmission to a remote center, application of ~~electrocardiographic-derived data~~multiple nonlinear mathematical transformations, with ~~computer probability assessment, including report~~coronary artery obstruction severity assessment

~~0242T~~ ~~Gastrointestinal tract transit and pressure measurement, stomach through colon, wireless capsule, with interpretation and report~~

~~0250T~~ ~~Airway sizing and insertion of bronchial valve(s), each lobe (List separately in addition to code for primary procedure)~~

~~0251T~~ ~~Bronchoscopy, rigid or flexible, including fluoroscopic guidance, when performed; with removal of bronchial valve(s), initial lobe~~

~~0252T~~ ~~with removal of bronchial valve(s), each additional lobe (List separately in addition to code for primary procedure)~~

~~0256T~~ ~~Implantation of catheter-delivered prosthetic aortic heart valve; endovascular approach~~

~~0257T~~ ~~open thoracic approach (eg, transapical, transventricular)~~

~~0258T~~ ~~Transthoracic cardiac exposure (eg, sternotomy, thoracotomy, subxiphoid) for catheter-delivered aortic valve replacement; without cardiopulmonary bypass~~

~~0259T~~ ~~with cardiopulmonary bypass~~

~~0276T~~ ~~Bronchoscopy, rigid or flexible, including fluoroscopic guidance, when performed; with bronchial thermoplasty, 1 lobe~~

~~0277T~~ ~~with bronchial thermoplasty, 2 or more lobes~~

~~0279T~~ ~~Cell enumeration using immunologic selection and identification in fluid specimen (eg, circulating tumor cells in blood)~~

~~0280T~~ ~~interpretation and report~~

+⊙● **0291T** Code added

+⊙● **0292T** Code added

⊙● **0293T** Code added

+⊙● **0294T** Code added

● **0295T** Code added

● **0296T** Code added

● **0297T** Code added

● **0298T** Code added

● **0299T** Code added

+● **0300T** Code added

⊙● **0301T** Code added

⊙● **0302T** Code added

⊙● **0303T** Code added

⊙● **0304T** Code added

● **0305T** Code added

● **0306T** Code added

⊙● **0307T** Code added

⊘⊙● **0308T** Code added

+● **0309T** Code added

● **0310T** Code added

● **0311T** Code added

● **0312T** Code added

● **0313T** Code added

● **0314T** Code added

● **0315T** Code added

● **0316T** Code added

● **0317T** Code added

● **0318T** Code added

Appendixes A–E

Appendix C

Clinical Examples

►As described in *CPT 2013*, clinical examples of the CPT codes for Evaluation and Management (E/M) services are intended to be an important element of the coding system. The clinical examples, when used with the E/M descriptors contained in the full text of the CPT code set, provide a comprehensive and powerful tool for individuals to report the services provided to their patients.◄

The American Medical Association is pleased to provide you with these clinical examples for CPT 2013. The clinical examples that are provided in this supplement are limited to Office or Other Outpatient Services, Hospital Inpatient Services, Consultations, Critical Care, Prolonged Services and Care Plan Oversight.

These clinical examples do not encompass the entire scope of medical practice. Inclusion or exclusion of any particular specialty group does not infer any judgment of importance or lack thereof; nor does it limit the applicability of the example to any particular specialty.

►Of utmost importance is that these clinical examples are just that: examples. A particular patient encounter, depending on the specific circumstances, must be judged by the services provided by the physician or other qualified health care professional for that particular patient. Simply because the patient's complaints, symptoms, or diagnoses match those of a particular clinical example, does not automatically assign that patient encounter to that particular level of service. The three components (history, examination, and medical decision making) must be met and documented in the medical record to report a particular level of service.◄

Office or Other Outpatient Service

New Patient

99201   Initial office visit for a 50-year-old male from out-of-town who needs a prescription refill for a nonsteroidal anti-inflammatory drug. (Anesthesiology)

Initial office visit for a 40-year-old female, new patient, requesting information about local pain clinics. (Anesthesiology/Pain Medicine)

Initial office visit for a 10-year-old girl for determination of visual acuity as part of a summer camp physical (does not include determination of refractive error). (Ophthalmology)

Initial office visit for an out-of-town patient requiring topical refill. (Dermatology)

Initial office visit for a 65-year-old male for reassurance about an isolated seborrheic keratosis on upper back. (Plastic Surgery)

Initial office visit for an out-of-state visitor who needs refill of topical steroid to treat lichen planus. (Dermatology)

Initial office visit for an 86-year-old male, out-of-town visitor, who needs prescription refilled for an anal skin preparation that he forgot. (General Surgery/Colon & Rectal Surgery)

Initial office visit for a patient with alveolar osteitis for repacking. (Oral & Maxillofacial Surgery)

Initial office visit for a patient with a pedunculated lesion of the neck which is unsightly. (Dermatology)

Initial office visit for a 10-year-old male, for limited subungual hematoma not requiring drainage. (Internal Medicine)

Initial office visit with an out-of-town visitor who needs a prescription refilled because she forgot her hay fever medication. (Allergy & Immunology/Internal Medicine)

Initial office visit with a 9-month-old female with diaper rash. (Pediatrics)

Initial office visit with a 10-year-old male with severe rash and itching for the past 24 hours, positive history for contact with poison oak 48 hours prior to the visit. (Family Medicine)

Initial office visit with a 5-year-old female to remove sutures from simple wound placed by another physician. (Plastic Surgery)

Initial office visit for a 22-year-old male with a small area of sunburn requiring first aid. (Dermatology/Family Medicine/Internal Medicine)

Initial office visit for the evaluation and management of a contusion of a finger. (Orthopaedic Surgery)

99202   Initial office visit for a 13-year-old patient with comedopapular acne of the face unresponsive to over-the-counter medications. (Family Medicine)

Initial office visit for a patient with a clinically benign lesion or nodule of the lower leg that has been present for many years. (Dermatology)

Initial office visit for a patient with a circumscribed patch of dermatitis of the leg. (Dermatology)

Initial office visit for a patient with papulosquamous eruption of elbows. (Dermatology)

Initial office visit for a 9-year-old patient with erythematous grouped, vesicular eruption of the lip of three days duration. (Pediatrics)

Initial office visit for an 18-year-old male referred by an orthodontist for advice regarding removal of four wisdom teeth. (Oral & Maxillofacial Surgery)

Initial office visit for a 14-year-old male, who was referred by his orthodontist, for advice on the exposure of impacted maxillary cuspids. (Oral & Maxillofacial Surgery)

Initial office visit for a patient presenting with itching patches on the wrists and ankles. (Dermatology)

Initial office visit for a 30-year-old male for evaluation and discussion of treatment of rhinophyma. (Plastic Surgery)

Initial office visit for a 16-year-old male with severe cystic acne, new patient. (Dermatology)

Initial office evaluation for gradual hearing loss, 58-year-old male, history and physical examination, with interpretation of complete audiogram, air bone, etc. (Otolaryngology)

Initial evaluation and management of recurrent urinary infection in female. (Internal Medicine)

Initial office visit with a 10-year-old girl with history of chronic otitis media and a draining ear. (Pediatrics)

Initial office visit for a 10-year-old female with acute maxillary sinusitis. (Family Medicine)

Initial office visit for a patient with recurring episodes of herpes simplex who has developed a clustering of vesicles on the upper lip. (Internal Medicine)

Initial office visit for a 25-year-old patient with a single season allergic rhinitis. (Allergy & Immunology)

99203 Initial office visit of a 76-year-old male with a stasis ulcer of three months' duration. (Dermatology)

Initial office visit for a 30-year-old female with pain in the lateral aspect of the forearm. (Physical Medicine & Rehabilitation)

Initial office visit for a 15-year-old patient with a four-year history of moderate comedopapular acne of the face, chest, and back with early scarring. Discussion of use of systemic medication. (Dermatology)

Initial office visit for a patient with papulosquamous eruption of the elbow with pitting of nails and itchy scalp. (Dermatology)

Initial office visit for a 57-year-old female who complains of painful parotid swelling of one week's duration. (Oral & Maxillofacial Surgery)

Initial office visit for a patient with an ulcerated non-healing lesion or nodule on the tip of the nose. (Dermatology)

Initial office visit for a patient with dermatitis of the antecubital and popliteal fossae. (Dermatology)

Initial office visit for a 22-year-old female with irregular menses. (Family Medicine)

Initial office visit for a 50-year-old female with dyspepsia and nausea. (Family Medicine)

Initial office visit for a 53-year-old laborer with degenerative joint disease of the knee with no prior treatment. (Orthopaedic Surgery)

Initial office visit for a 60-year-old male with Dupuytren's contracture of one hand with multiple digit involvement. (Orthopaedic Surgery)

Initial office visit for a 33-year-old male with painless gross hematuria without cystoscopy. (Internal Medicine)

Initial office visit for a 55-year-old female with chronic blepharitis. There is a history of use of many medications. (Ophthalmology)

Initial office visit for an 18-year-old female with a two-day history of acute conjunctivitis. Extensive history of possible exposures, prior normal ocular history, and medication use is obtained. (Ophthalmology)

Initial office visit for a 14-year-old male with unilateral anterior knee pain. (Physical Medicine & Rehabilitation)

Initial office visit of an adult who presents with symtoms of an upper-respiratory infection that has progressed to unilateral purulent nasal discharge and discomfort in the right maxillary teeth. (Otolaryngology/Head & Neck Surgery)

Initial office visit of a 40-year-old female with symptoms of atopic allergies including eye and sinus congestion, often associated with infections. She would like to be tested for allergies. (Otolaryngology/Head & Neck Surgery)

Initial office visit of a 65-year-old with nasal stuffiness. (Otolaryngology/Head & Neck Surgery)

Initial office visit for initial evaluation of a 48-year-old man with recurrent low back pain radiating to the leg. (General Surgery)

Initial office visit for evaluation, diagnosis, and management of painless gross hematuria in a new patient, without cystoscopy. (Internal Medicine)

Initial office visit with couple for counseling concerning voluntary vasectomy for sterility. Spent 30 minutes discussing procedure, risks and benefits, and answering questions. (Urology)

Initial office visit of a 49-year-old male with nasal obstruction. Detailed exam with topical anesthesia. (Plastic Surgery)

Initial office visit for evaluation of a 13-year-old female with progressive scoliosis. (Physical Medicine & Rehabilitation)

Initial office visit for a 21-year-old female desiring counseling and evaluation of initiation of contraception. (Family Practice/Internal Medicine/Obstetrics & Gynecology)

Initial office visit for a 49-year-old male presenting with painless blood per rectum associated with bowel movement. (Colon & Rectal Surgery)

Initial office visit for a 19-year-old football player with three-day-old acute knee injury; now with swelling and pain. (Orthopaedic Surgery)

99204 Initial office visit for a 13-year-old female with progressive scoliosis. (Orthopaedic Surgery)

Initial office visit for a 34-year-old female with primary infertility for evaluation and counseling. (Obstetrics & Gynecology)

Initial office visit for a 6-year-old male with multiple upper respiratory infections. (Allergy & Immunology)

Initial office visit for a patient with generalized dermatitis of 80 percent of the body surface area. (Dermatology)

Initial office visit for an adolescent who was referred by school counselor because of repeated skipping school. (Psychiatry)

Initial office visit for a 50-year-old machinist with a generalized eruption. (Dermatology)

Initial office visit for a 45-year-old female who has been abstinent from alcohol and benzodiazepines for three months but complains of headaches, insomnia, and anxiety. (Psychiatry)

Initial office visit for a 60-year-old male with recent change in bowel habits, weight loss, and abdominal pain. (Abdominal Surgery/General Surgery)

Initial office visit for a 50-year-old male with an aortic aneurysm who is considering surgery. (General Surgery)

Initial office visit for a 17-year-old female with depression. (Internal Medicine)

Initial office visit of a 40-year-old with chronic draining ear, imbalance, and probable cholesteatoma. (Otolaryngology/Head & Neck Surgery)

Initial office visit for initial evaluation of a 63-year-old male with chest pain on exertion. (Cardiology/Internal Medicine)

Initial office visit for evaluation of a 70-year-old patient with recent onset of episodic confusion. (Internal Medicine)

Initial office visit for a 7-year-old female with juvenile diabetes mellitus, new to area, past history of hospitalization times three. (Pediatrics)

Initial office visit of a 50-year-old female with progressive solid food dysphagia. (Gastroenterology)

Initial office visit for a 34-year-old patient with primary infertility, including counseling. (Obstetrics & Gynecology)

Initial office visit for evaluation of a 70-year-old female with polyarthralgia. (Rheumatology)

Initial office visit for a patient with papulosquamous eruption involving 60 percent of the cutaneous surface with joint pain. Combinations of topical and systemic treatments discussed. (Dermatology)

99205 Initial office visit for a patient with disseminated lupus erythematosus with kidney disease, edema, purpura, and scarring lesions on the extremities plus cardiac symptoms. (Dermatology/General Surgery/Internal Medicine)

Initial office visit for a 25-year-old female with systemic lupus erythematosus, fever, seizures, and profound thrombocytopenia. (Rheumatology/Allergy & Immunology)

Initial office visit for an adult with multiple cutaneous blisters, denuded secondarily infected ulcerations, oral lesions, weight loss, and increasing weakness refractory to high dose corticosteroid. Initiation of new immunosuppressive therapy. (Dermatology)

Initial office visit for a 28-year-old male with systemic vasculitis and compromised circulation to the limbs. (Rheumatology)

Initial office visit for a 41-year-old female new to the area requesting rheumatologic care, on disability due to scleroderma and recent hospitalization for malignant hypertension. (Rheumatology)

Initial office visit for a 52-year-old female with acute four extremity weakness and shortness of breath one week post-flu vaccination. (Physical Medicine & Rehabilitation)

Initial office visit for a 60-year-old male with previous back surgery; now presents with back and pelvic pain, two-month history of bilateral progressive calf and thigh tightness and weakness when walking, causing several falls. (Orthopaedic Surgery)

Initial office visit for an adolescent referred from emergency room after making suicide gesture. (Psychiatry)

Initial office visit for a 49-year-old female with a history of headaches and dependence on opioids. She reports weight loss, progressive headache, and depression. (Psychiatry)

Initial office visit for a 50-year-old female with symptoms of rash, swellings, recurrent arthritic complaints, and diarrhea and lymphadenopathy. Patient has had a 25 lb weight loss and was recently camping in the Amazon. (Allergy & Immunology)

Initial office visit for a 34-year-old uremic Type I diabetic patient referred for ESRD modality assessment and planning. (Nephrology)

Initial office visit for a 75-year-old female with neck and bilateral shoulder pain, brisk deep tendon reflexes, and stress incontinence. (Physical Medicine & Rehabilitation)

Initial office visit for an 8-year-old male with cerebral palsy and spastic quadriparesis. (Physical Medicine & Rehabilitation)

Initial office visit for a 73-year-old male with known prostate malignancy, who presents with severe back pain and a recent onset of lower extremity weakness. (Physical Medicine & Rehabilitation)

Initial office visit for a 38-year-old male with paranoid delusions and a history of alcohol abuse. (Psychiatry)

Initial office visit for a 12-week-old with bilateral hip dislocations and bilateral club feet. (Orthopaedic Surgery)

Initial office visit for a 29-year-old female with acute orbital congestion, eyelid retraction, and bilateral visual loss from optic neuropathy. (Ophthalmology)

Initial office visit for a 70-year-old diabetic patient with progressive visual field loss, advanced optic disc cupping, and neovascularization of retina. (Ophthalmology)

Initial office visit for a newly diagnosed Type I diabetic patient. (Endocrinology)

Initial office evaluation of a 65-year-old female with exertional chest pain, intermittent claudication, syncope, and a murmur of aortic stenosis. (Cardiology)

Initial office visit for a 73-year-old male with an unexplained 20 lb weight loss. (Hematology/Oncology)

Initial office evaluation, patient with systemic lupus erythematosus, fever, seizures, and profound thrombodytopenia. (Allergy & Immunology/Internal Medicine/Rheumatology)

Initial office evaluaton and management of patient with systemic vasculitis and compromised circulation to the limbs. (Rheumatology)

Initial office visit for a 24-year-old homosexual male who has a fever, a cough, and shortness of breath. (Infectious Disease)

Initial outpatient evaluation of a 69-year-old male with severe chronic obstructive pulmonary disease, congestive heart failure, and hypertension. (Family Medicine)

Initial office visit for a 17-year-old female, who is having school problems and has told a friend that she is considering suicide. The patient and her family are consulted in regard to treatment options. (Psychiatry)

Initial office visit for a female with severe hirsutism, amenorrhea, weight loss, and a desire to have children. (Endocrinology/Obstetrics & Gynecology)

Initial office visit for a 42-year-old male on hypertensive medication, newly arrived to the area, with diastolic blood pressure of 110, history of recurrent calculi, episodic headaches, intermittent chest pain, and orthopnea. (Internal Medicine)

Established Patient

99211 Office visit for an 82-year-old female, established patient, for a monthly B12 injection with documented Vitamin B12 deficiency. (Geriatrics/Internal Medicine/Family Medicine)

Office visit for a 50-year-old male, established patient, for removal of uncomplicated facial sutures. (Plastic Surgery)

Office visit for an established patient who lost prescription for lichen planus. Returned for new copy. (Dermatology)

Office visit for an established patient undergoing orthodontics who complains of a wire that is irritating his/her cheek and asks you to check it. (Oral & Maxillofacial Surgery)

Office visit for a 50-year-old female, established patient, seen for her gold injection by the nurse. (Rheumatology)

Office visit for a 73-year-old female, established patient, with pernicious anemia for weekly B12 injection. (Gastroenterology)

Office visit for an established patient for dressing change on a skin biopsy. (Dermatology)

Office visit for a 19-year-old, established patient, for removal of sutures from a 2 cm laceration of forehead, which you placed four days ago in ER. (Plastic Surgery)

Office visit of a 20-year-old female, established patient, who receives an allergy vaccine injection and is observed for a reaction by the nurse. (Otolaryngology/Head & Neck Surgery)

Office visit for a 45-year-old male, established patient, with chronic renal failure for the administration of erythropoietin. (Nephrology)

Office visit for an established patient, a Peace Corps enlistee, who requests documentation that third molars have been removed. (Oral & Maxillofacial Surgery)

Office visit for a 69-year-old female, established patient, for partial removal of antibiotic gauze from an infected wound site. (Plastic Surgery)

Office visit for a 9-year-old, established patient, successfully treated for impetigo, requiring release to return to school. (Dermatology/Pediatrics)

Office visit for an established patient requesting a return-to-work certificate for resolving contact dermatitis. (Dermatology)

Office visit for an established patient who is performing glucose monitoring and wants to check accuracy of machine with lab blood glucose by technician who checks accuracy and function of patient machine. (Endocrinology)

Follow-up office visit for a 65-year-old female with a chronic indwelling percutaneous nephrostomy catheter seen for routine pericatheter skin care and dressing change. (Interventional Radiology)

Outpatient visit with 19-year-old male, established patient, for supervised drug screen. (Addiction Medicine)

Office visit with 12-year-old male, established patient, for cursory check of hematoma one day after venipuncture. (Internal Medicine)

Office visit with 31-year-old female, established patient, for return to work certificate. (Anesthesiology)

Office visit for a 42-year-old, established patient, to read tuberculin test results. (Allergy & Immunology)

Office visit for 14-year-old, established patient, to re-dress an abrasion. (Orthopaedic Surgery)

Office visit for a 45-year-old female, established patient, for a blood pressure check. (Obstetrics & Gynecology)

Office visit for a 23-year-old, established patient, for instruction in use of peak flow meter. (Allergy & Immunology)

Office visit for prescription refill for a 35-year-old female, established patient, with schizophrenia who is stable but has run out of neuroleptic and is scheduled to be seen in a week. (Psychiatry)

99212 Office visit for an 11-year-old, established patient, seen in follow-up for mild comedonal acne of the cheeks on topical desquamating agents. (Dermatology/Family Medicine/Pediatrics)

Office visit for a 10-year-old female, established patient, who has been swimming in a lake, now presents with a one-day history of left ear pain with purulent drainage. (Family Medicine)

Office visit for a child, established patient, with chronic secretory otitis media. (Otolaryngology/Head & Neck Surgery)

Office visit for an established patient seen in follow-up of clearing patch of localized contact dermatitis. (Family Medicine/Dermatology)

Office visit for an established patient returning for evaluation of response to treatment of lichen planus on wrists and ankles. (Dermatology)

Office visit for an established patient with tinea pedis being treated with topical therapy. (Dermatology)

Office visit for an established patient with localized erythematous plaque of psoriasis with topical hydration. (Dermatology)

Office visit for a 50-year-old male, established patient, recently seen for acute neck pain, diagnosis of spondylosis, responding to physical therapy and intermittent cervical traction. Returns for evaluation for return to work. (Neurology)

Office visit for an established patient with recurring episodes of herpes simplex who has developed a clustering of vesicles on the upper lip. (Oral & Maxillofacial Surgery)

Evaluation of a 50-year-old male, established patient, who has experienced a recurrence of knee pain after he discontinued NSAID. (Anesthesiology/Pain Medicine)

Office visit for an established patient with an irritated skin tag for reassurance. (Dermatology)

Office visit for a 40-year-old, established patient, who has experienced a systemic allergic reaction following administration of immunotherapy. The dose must be readjusted. (Allergy & Immunology)

Office visit for a 33-year-old, established patient, for contusion and abrasion of lower extremity. (Orthopaedic Surgery)

Office visit for a 22-year-old male, established patient, one month after I & D of "wrestler's ear." (Plastic Surgery)

Office visit for a 21-year-old, established patient, who is seen in follow-up after antibiotic therapy for acute bacterial tonsillitis. (Otolaryngology/Head & Neck Surgery)

Office visit for a 4-year-old, established patient, with tympanostomy tubes, check-up. (Otolaryngology/Head & Neck Surgery)

Office visit for an established patient who has had needle aspiration of a peritonsillar abscess. (Otolaryngology/Head & Neck Surgery)

Follow-up office examination for evaluation and treatment of acute draining ear in a 5-year-old with tympanotomy tubes. (Otolaryngology/Head & Neck Surgery)

Office visit, established patient, 6-year-old with sore throat and headache. (Family Medicine/Pediatrics)

Office evaluation for possible purulent bacterial conjunctivitis with one- to two-day history of redness and discharge, 16-year-old female, established patient. (Pediatrics/Internal Medicine/Family Medicine)

Office visit for a 65-year-old female, established patient, returns for three-week follow-up for resolving severe ankle sprain. (Orthopaedic Surgery)

Office visit, sore throat, fever, and fatigue in a 19-year-old college student, established patient. (Internal Medicine)

Office visit with a 33-year-old female, established patient, recently started on treatment for hemorrhoidal complaints, for re-evaluation. (Colon & Rectal Surgery)

Office visit with a 36-year-old male, established patient, for follow-up on effectiveness of medicine management of oral candidiasis. (Oral & Maxillofacial Surgery)

Office visit for a 27-year-old female, established patient, with complaints of vaginal itching. (Obstetrics & Gynecology)

Office visit for a 65-year-old, established patient, with eruptions on both arms from poison oak exposure. (Allergy & Immunology/Internal Medicine)

99213 Office visit for an established patient with new lesions of lichen planus in spite of topical therapies. (Dermatology)

Office visit for the quarterly follow-up of a 45-year-old male with stable chronic asthma requiring regular drug therapy. (Allergy & Immunology)

Office visit for a 13-year-old, established patient, with comedopapular acne of the face that has shown poor response to topical medication. Discussion of use of systemic medication. (Dermatology)

Office visit for a 62-year-old female, established patient, for follow-up for stable cirrhosis of the liver. (Internal Medicine/Family Medicine)

Office visit for a 3-year-old, established patient, with atopic dermatitis and food hypersensitivity for quarterly follow-up evaluation. The patient is on topical lotions and steroid creams as well as oral antihistamines. (Allergy & Immunology)

Office visit for an 80-year-old female, established patient, to evaluate medical management of osteoarthritis of the temporomandibular joint. (Rheumatology)

Office visit for a 70-year-old female, established patient, one year post excision of basal cell carcinoma of nose with nasolabial flap. Now presents with new suspicious recurrent lesion and suspicious lesion of the back. (Plastic Surgery)

Office visit for a 68-year-old female, established patient, with polymyalgia rheumatic, maintained on chronic low-dose corticosteroid, with no new complaints. (Rheumatology)

Office visit for a 3-year-old female, established patient, for earache and dyshidrosis of feet. (Pediatrics/Family Medicine)

Office visit for an established patient for 18-months post-operative follow-up of TMJ repair. (Oral & Maxillofacial Surgery)

Office visit for a 45-year-old male, established patient, being re-evaluated for recurrent acute prostatitis. (Urology)

Office visit for a 43-year-old male, established patient, with known reflex sympathetic dystrophy. (Anesthesiology)

Office visit for an established patient with an evenly pigmented superficial nodule of leg that is symptomatic. (Dermatology)

Office visit for an established patient with psoriasis involvement of the elbows, pitting of the nails, and itchy scalp. (Dermatology)

Office visit for a 27-year-old male, established patient, with deep follicular and perifollicular inflammation unable to tolerate systemic antibiotics due to GI upset, requires change of systemic medication. (Dermatology)

Office visit for a 16-year-old male, established patient, who is on medication for exercise-induced bronchospasm. (Allergy & Immunology)

Office visit for a 60-year-old, established patient, with chronic essential hypertension on multiple drug regimen, for blood pressure check. (Family Medicine)

Office visit for a 20-year-old male, established patient, for removal of sutures in hand. (Family Medicine)

Office visit for a 58-year-old female, established patient, with unilateral painful bunion. (Orthopaedic Surgery)

Office visit for a 45-year-old female, established patient, with known osteoarthritis and painful swollen knees. (Rheumatology)

Office visit for a 25-year-old female, established patient, complaining of bleeding and heavy menses. (Obstetrics & Gynecology)

Office visit for a 55-year-old male, established patient, with hypertension managed by a beta blocker/thiazide regime; now experiencing mild fatigue. (Nephrology)

Office visit for a 65-year-old female, established patient, with primary glaucoma for interval determination of intraocular pressure and possible adjustment of medication. (Ophthalmology)

Office visit for a 56-year-old man, established patient, with stable exertional angina who complains of new onset of calf pain while walking. (Cardiology)

Office visit for a 63-year-old female, established patient, with rheumatoid arthritis on auranofin and ibuprofen, seen for routine follow-up visit. (Rheumatology)

Office visit for an established patient with Graves' disease, three months post I-131 therapy, who presents with lassitude and malaise. (Endocrinology)

Office visit for the quarterly follow-up of a 63-year-old male, established patient, with chronic myofascial pain syndrome, effectively managed by doxepin, who presents with new onset urinary hesitancy. (Pain Medicine)

Office visit for the biannual follow-up of an established patient with migraine variant having infrequent, intermittent, moderate to severe headaches with nausea and vomiting, which are sometimes effectively managed by ergotamine tartrate and an antiemetic, but occasionally requiring visits to an emergency department. (Pain Medicine)

Office visit for an established patient after discharge from a pain rehabilitation program to review and adjust medication dosage. (Pain Medicine)

Office visit with 55-year-old male, established patient, for management of hypertension, mild fatigue, on beta blocker/thiazide regimen. (Family Medicine/Internal Medicine)

Outpatient visit with 37-year-old male, established patient, who is three years post total colectomy for chronic ulcerative colitis, presents for increased irritation at his stoma. (General Surgery)

Office visit for a 70-year-old diabetic hypertensive established patient with recent change in insulin requirement. (Internal Medicine/Nephrology)

Office visit with 80-year-old female, established patient, for follow-up osteoporosis, status-post compression fractures. (Rheumatology)

Office visit for an established patient with stable cirrhosis of the liver. (Gastroenterology)

Routine, follow-up office evaluation at a three-month interval for a 77-year-old female, established patient, with nodular small cleaved-cell lymphoma. (Hematology/Oncology)

Quarterly follow-up office visit for a 45-year-old male, established patient, with stable chronic asthma, on steroid and bronchodilator therapy. (Pulmonary Medicine)

Office visit for a 50-year-old female, established patient, with insulin-dependent diabetes mellitus and stable coronary artery disease, for monitoring. (Family Medicine/Internal Medicine)

99214 Office visit for an established patient now presenting with generalized dermatitis of 80% of the body surface area. (Dermatology)

Office visit for a 32-year-old female, established patient, with new onset right lower quadrant pain. (Family Medicine)

Office visit for reassessment and reassurance/counseling of a 40-year-old female, established patient, who is experiencing increased symptoms while on a pain management treatment program. (Pain Medicine)

Office visit for a 30-year-old, established patient, under management for intractable low back pain, who now presents with new onset right posterior thigh pain. (Pain Medicine)

Office visit for an established patient with frequent intermittent, moderate to severe headaches requiring beta blocker or tricyclic antidepressant prophylaxis, as well as four symptomatic treatments, but who is still experiencing headaches at a frequency of several times a month that are unresponsive to treatment. (Pain Medicine)

Office visit for an established patient with psoriasis with extensive involvement of scalp, trunk, palms, and soles with joint pain. Combinations of topical and systemic treatments discussed and instituted. (Dermatology)

Office visit for a 55-year-old male, established patient, with increasing night pain, limp, and progressive varus of both knees. (Orthopaedic Surgery)

Follow-up visit for a 15-year-old withdrawn patient with four-year history of papulocystic acne of the face, chest, and back with early scarring and poor response to past treatment. Discussion of use of systemic medication. (Dermatology)

Office visit for a 28-year-old male, established patient, with regional enteritis, diarrhea, and low-grade fever. (Internal Medicine)

Office visit for a 25-year-old female, established patient, following recent arthrogram and MR imaging for TMJ pain. (Oral & Maxillofacial Surgery)

Office visit for a 32-year-old female, established patient, with large obstructing stone in left mid-ureter, to discuss management options including urethroscopy with extraction or ESWL. (Urology)

Evaluation for a 28-year-old male, established patient, with new onset of low back pain. (Anesthesiology/Pain Medicine)

Office visit for a 28-year-old female, established patient, with right lower quadrant abdominal pain, fever, and anorexia. (Internal Medicine/Family Medicine)

Office visit for a 45-year-old male, established patient, four months follow-up of L4-5 diskectomy, with persistent incapacitating low back and leg pain. (Orthopaedic Surgery)

Outpatient visit for a 77-year-old male, established patient, with hypertension, presenting with a three-month history of episodic substernal chest pain on exertion. (Cardiology)

Office visit for a 25-year-old female, established patient, for evaluation of progressive saddle nose deformity of unknown etiology. (Plastic Surgery)

Office visit for a 65-year-old male, established patient, with BPH and severe bladder outlet obstruction, to discuss management options such as TURP. (Urology)

Office visit for an adult diabetic established patient with a past history of recurrent sinusitis who presents with a one-week history of double vision. (Otolaryngology/Head & Neck Surgery)

Office visit for an established patient with lichen planus and 60% of the cutaneous surface involved, not responsive to systemic steroids, as well as developing symptoms of progressive heartburn and paranoid ideation. (Dermatology)

Office visit for a 52-year-old male, established patient, with a 12-year history of bipolar disorder responding to lithium carbonate and brief psychotherapy. Psychotherapy and prescription provided. (Psychiatry)

Office visit for a 63-year-old female, established patient, with a history of familial polyposis, status post-colectomy with sphincter sparing procedure, who now presents with rectal bleeding and increase in stooling frequency. (General Surgery)

Office visit for a 68-year-old male, established patient, with the sudden onset of multiple flashes and floaters in the right eye due to a posterior vitreous detachment. (Ophthalmology)

Office visit for a 55-year-old female, established patient, on cyclosporin for treatment of resistant, small vessel vasculitis. (Rheumatology)

Follow-up office visit for a 55-year-old male, two months after iliac angioplasty with new onset of contralateral extremity claudication. (Interventional Radiology)

Office visit for a 68-year-old male, established patient, with stable angina, two months post myocardial infarction, who is not tolerating one of his medications. (Cardiology)

Weekly office visit for 5FU therapy for an ambulatory established patient with metastatic colon cancer and increasing shortness of breath. (Hematology/Oncology)

Follow-up office visit for a 60-year-old male, established patient, whose post-traumatic seizures have disappeared on medication and who now raises the question of stopping the medication (Neurology)

Office evaluation on new onset RLQ pain in a 32-year-old female, established patient. (Urology/General Surgery/ Internal Medicine/Family Medicine)

Office evaluation of 28-year-old, established patient, with regional enteritis, diarrhea, and low-grade fever. (Family Medicine/Internal Medicine)

Office visit with 50-year-old female, established patient, diabetic, blood sugar controlled by diet. She now complains of frequency of urination and weight loss, blood sugar of 320 and negative ketones on dipstick. (Internal Medicine)

Follow-up office visit for a 45-year-old, established patient, with rheumatoid arthritis on gold, methotrexate, or immunosuppressive therapy. (Rheumatology)

Office visit for a 60-year-old male, established patient, two years post-removal of intracranial meningioma, now with new headaches and visual disturbance. (Neurosurgery)

Office visit for a 68-year-old female, established patient, for routine review and follow-up of non-insulin dependent diabetes, obesity, hypertension, and congestive heart failure. Complains of vision difficulties and admits dietary noncompliance. Patient is counseled concerning diet and current medications adjusted. (Family Medicine)

99215 Office visit for an established patient who developed persistent cough, rectal bleeding, weakness, and diarrhea plus pustular infection on skin. Patient on immunosuppressive therapy. (Dermatology)

Office visit for an established patient with disseminated lupus erythematosus, extensive edema of extremities kidney disease, and weakness requiring monitored course on azathioprene, corticosteroid and complicated by acute depression. (Dermatology/Internal Medicine/ Rheumatology)

Office visit for an established patient with progressive dermatomyositis and recent onset of fever, nasal speech, and regurgitation of fluids through the nose. (Dermatology)

Office visit for a 28-year-old female, established patient, who is abstinent from previous cocaine dependence but reports progressive panic attacks and chest pains. (Psychiatry)

Office visit for an established adolescent patient with history of bipolar disorder treated with lithium; seen on urgent basis at family's request because of severe depressive symptoms. (Psychiatry)

Office visit for an established patient having acute migraine with new onset neurological symptoms and whose headaches are unresponsive to previous attempts at management with a combination of preventive and abortive medication. (Pain Medicine)

Office visit for an established patient with exfoliative lichen planus with daily fever spikes, disorientation, and shortness of breath. (Dermatology)

Office visit for a 25-year-old, established patient, two years post-burn with bilateral ectropion, hypertrophic facial burn scars, near absence of left breast, and burn syndactyly of both hands. Discussion of treatment options following examination. (Plastic Surgery)

Office visit for a 6-year-old, established patient, to review newly diagnosed immune deficiency with recommendations for therapy including IV immunoglobulin and chronic antibiotics. (Allergy & Immunology)

Office visit for a 36-year-old, established patient, three-month status post-transplant, with new onset of peripheral edema, increased blood pressure, and progressive fatigue. (Nephrology)

Office visit for an established patient with Kaposi's sarcoma who presents with fever and widespread vesicles. (Dermatology)

Office visit for a 27-year-old female, established patient, with bipolar disorder who was stable on lithium carbonate and monthly supportive psychotherapy but now has developed symptoms of hypomania. (Psychiatry)

Office visit for a 25-year-old male, established patient with a history of schizophrenia who has been seen bi-monthly but is complaining of auditory hallucinations. (Psychiatry)

Office visit for a 62-year-old male, established patient, three years postoperative abdominal perineal resection, now with a rising carcinoembryonic antigen, weight loss, and pelvic pain. (Abdominal Surgery)

Office visit for a 42-year-old male, established patient, nine months postoperative emergency vena cava shunt for variceal bleeding, now presents with complaints of one episode of "dark" bowel movement, weight gain, tightness in abdomen, whites of eyes seem yellow, and occasional drowsiness after eating hamburgers. (Abdominal Surgery)

Office visit for a 68-year-old male, established patient, with biopsy-proven rectal carcinoma, for evaluation and discussion of treatment options. (General Surgery)

Office visit for a 60-year-old, established patient, with diabetic nephropathy with increasing edema and dyspnea. (Endocrinology)

Office visit with 30-year-old male, established patient for three-month history of fatigue, weight loss, intermittent fever, and presenting with diffuse adenopathy and splenomegaly. (Family Medicine)

Office visit for restaging of an established patient with new lymphadenopathy one year post-therapy for lymphoma. (Hematology/Oncology)

Office visit for evaluation of recent onset syncopal attacks in a 70-year-old female, established patient. (Internal Medicine)

Follow-up visit, 40-year-old mother of three, established patient, with acute rheumatoid arthritis, anatomical Stage 3, ARA function Class 3 rheumatoid arthritis, and deteriorating function. (Rheumatology)

Follow-up office visit for a 65-year-old male, established patient, with a fever of recent onset while on outpatient antibiotic therapy for endocarditis. (Infectious Disease)

Office visit for a 75-year-old, established patient, with ALS (amyotrophic lateral sclerosis), who is no longer able to swallow. (Neurology)

Office visit for a 70-year-old female, established patient, with diabetes mellitus and hypertension, presenting with a two-month history of increasing confusion, agitation, and short-term memory loss. (Family Medicine/Internal Medicine)

Hospital Inpatient Services

Initial Hospital Care

New or Established Patient

99221   Initial hospital visit following admission for a 42-year-old male for observation following an uncomplicated mandible fracture. (Plastic Surgery/Oral & Maxillofacial Surgery)

Initial hospital visit for a 40-year-old patient with a thrombosed synthetic arteriovenous conduit. (Nephrology)

Initial hospital visit for a healthy 24-year-old male with an acute onset of low back pain following a lifting injury. (Internal Medicine/Anesthesiology/Pain Medicine)

Initial hospital visit for a 69-year-old female with controlled hypertension, scheduled for surgery. (Internal Medicine/Cardiology)

Initial hospital visit for a 24-year-old healthy female with benign tumor of palate. (Oral & Maxillofacial Surgery)

Initial hospital visit for a 14-year-old female with infectious mononucleosis and dehydration. (Internal Medicine)

Initial hospital visit for a 62-year-old female with stable rheumatoid arthritis, admitted for total joint replacement. (Rheumatology)

Initial hospital visit for a 12-year-old patient with a laceration of the upper eyelid, involving the lid margin and superior canaliculus, admitted prior to surgery for IV antibiotic therapy. (Plastic Surgery)

Initial hospital visit for a 69-year-old female with controlled hypertension, scheduled for surgery. (Cardiology)

Hospital admission, examination, and initiation of treatment program for a 67-year-old male with uncomplicated pneumonia who requires IV antibiotic therapy. (Internal Medicine)

Hospital admission for an 18-month-old with 10% dehydration. (Pediatrics)

Hospital admission for a 12-year-old with a laceration of the upper eyelid involving the lid margin and superior canaliculus, admitted prior to surgery for IV antibiotic therapy. (Ophthalmology)

Hospital admission for a 32-year-old female with severe flank pain, hematuria, and presumed diagnosis of ureteral calculus as determined by Emergency Department physician. (Urology)

Initial hospital visit for a patient with several large venous stasis ulcers not responding to outpatient therapy. (Dermatology)

Initial hospital visit for 21-year-old pregnant patient (nine-weeks gestation) with hyperemesis gravidarum. (Obstetrics & Gynecology)

Initial hospital visit for a 73-year-old female with acute pyelonephritis who is otherwise generally healthy. (Geriatrics)

Initial hospital visit for 62-year-old patient with cellulitis of the foot requiring bedrest and intravenous antibiotics. (Orthopaedic Surgery)

99222   Initial hospital visit for a 50-year-old patient with lower quadrant abdominal pain and increased temperature, but without septic picture. (General Surgery/Abdominal Surgery/Colon & Rectal Surgery)

Initial hospital visit for airway management, due to a benign laryngeal mass. (Otolaryngology/Head & Neck Surgery)

Initial hospital visit for a 66-year-old female with an L-2 vertebral compression fracture with acute onset of paralytic ileus; seen in the office two days previously. (Orthopaedic Surgery)

Initial hospital visit and evaluation of a 15-year-old male admitted with peritonsillar abscess or cellulitis requiring intravenous antibiotic therapy. (Otolaryngology/Head & Neck Surgery)

Initial hospital visit for a 42-year-old male with vertebral compression fracture following a motor vehicle accident. (Orthopaedic Surgery)

Initial hospital visit for a patient with generalized atopic dermatitis and secondary infection. (Dermatology)

Initial hospital visit for a 3-year-old patient with high temperature, limp, and painful hip motion of 18 hours' duration. (Pediatrics/Orthopaedic Surgery)

Initial hospital visit for a young adult, presenting with an acute asthma attack unresponsive to outpatient therapy. (Allergy & Immunology)

Initial hospital visit for an 18-year-old male who has suppurative sialoadenitis and dehydration. (Oral & Maxillofacial Surgery)

Initial hospital visit for a 65-year-old female for acute onset of thrombotic cerebrovascular accident with contralateral paralysis and aphasia. (Neurology)

Initial hospital visit for a 50-year-old male chronic paraplegic patient with pain and spasm below the lesion. (Anesthesiology)

Partial hospital admission for an adolescent patient from chaotic blended family, transferred from inpatient setting, for continued treatment to control symptomatic expressions of hostility and depression. (Psychiatry)

Initial hospital visit for a 15-year-old male with acute status asthmaticus, unresponsive to outpatient therapy. (Internal Medicine)

Initial hospital visit for a 61-year-old male with history of previous myocardial infarction, who now complains of chest pain. (Internal Medicine)

Initial hospital visit of a 15-year-old on medications for a sore throat over the last two weeks. The sore throat has worsened and patient now has dysphagia. The exam shows large necrotic tonsils with an adequate airway and small palpable nodes. The initial mono test was negative. (Otolaryngology/Head & Neck Surgery)

Initial hospital evaluation of a 23-year-old allergy patient admitted with eyelid edema and pain on fifth day of oral antibiotic therapy. (Otolaryngology/Head & Neck Surgery)

Hospital admission, young adult patient, failed previous therapy and now presents in acute asthmatic attack. (Family Medicine/Allergy & Immunology)

Hospital admission of a 62-year-old smoker, established patient, with bronchitis in acute respiratory distress. (Internal Medicine/Pulmonary Medicine)

Hospital admission, examination, and initiation of a treatment program for a 65-year-old female with new onset of right-sided paralysis and aphasia. (Neurology)

Hospital admission, examination, and initiation of treatment program for a 66-year-old chronic hemodialysis patient with fever and a new pulmonary infiltrate. (Nephrology)

Hospital admission for an 8-year-old febrile patient with chronic sinusitis and severe headache, unresponsive to oral antibiotics. (Allergy & Immunology)

Hospital admission for a 40-year-old male with submaxillary cellulitis and trismus from infected lower molar. (Oral & Maxillofacial Surgery)

99223 Initial hospital visit for a 45-year-old female, who has a history of rheumatic fever as a child and now has anemia, fever, and congestive heart failure. (Cardiology)

Initial hospital visit for a 50-year-old male with acute chest pain and diagnostic electrocardiographic changes of an acute anterior myocardial infarction. (Cardiology/Family Medicine/Internal Medicine)

Initial hospital visit of a 75-year-old with progressive stridor and dysphagia with history of cancer of the larynx treated by radiation therapy in the past. Exam shows a large recurrent tumor of the glottis with a mass in the neck. (Otolaryngology/Head & Neck Surgery)

Initial hospital visit for a 70-year-old male admitted with chest pain, complete heart block, and congestive heart failure. (Cardiology)

Initial hospital visit for an 82-year-old male who presents with syncope, chest pain, and ventricular arrhythmias. (Cardiology)

Initial hospital visit for a 75-year-old male with history of arteriosclerotic coronary vascular disease, who is severely dehydrated, disoriented, and experiencing auditory hallucinations. (Psychiatry)

Initial hospital visit for a 70-year-old male with alcohol and sedative-hypnotic dependence, admitted by family for severe withdrawal, hypertension, and diabetes mellitus. (Psychiatry)

Initial hospital visit for a persistently suicidal latency-aged child whose parents have requested admission to provide safety during evaluation but are anxious about separation from her. (Psychiatry)

Initial psychiatric visit for an adolescent patient without previous psychiatric history, who was transferred from the medical ICU after a significant overdose. (Psychiatry)

Initial hospital visit for a 35-year-old female with severe systemic lupus erythematosus on corticosteroid and cyclophosphamide, with new onset of fever, chills, rash, and chest pain. (Rheumatology)

Initial hospital visit for a 52-year-old male with known rheumatic heart disease who presents with anasarca, hypertension, and history of alcohol abuse. (Cardiology)

Initial hospital visit for a 55-year-old female with a history of congenital heart disease; now presents with cyanosis. (Cardiology)

Initial hospital visit for a psychotic, hostile, violently combative adolescent, involuntarily committed, for seclusion and restraint in order to provide for safety on unit. (Psychiatry)

Initial hospital visit for a now subdued and sullen teenage male with six-month history of declining school performance, increasing self-endangerment, and resistance of parental expectations, including running away past weekend after physical fight with father. (Psychiatry)

Initial partial hospital admission for a 17-year-old female with history of borderline mental retardation who has developed auditory hallucinations. Parents are known to abuse alcohol, and Child Protective Services is investigating allegations of sexual abuse of a younger sibling. (Psychiatry)

Initial hospital visit of a 67-year-old male admitted with a large neck mass, dysphagia, and history of myocardial infarction three months before. (Otolaryngology/Head & Neck Surgery)

Initial hospital visit for a patient with suspected cerebrospinal fluid rhinorrhea that developed two weeks after head injury. (Otolaryngology/Head & Neck Surgery)

Initial hospital visit for a 25-year-old female with history of poly-substance abuse and psychiatric disorder. The patient appears to be psychotic with markedly elevated vital signs. (Psychiatry)

Initial hospital visit for a 70-year-old male with cutaneous T-cell lymphoma who has developed fever and lymphadenopathy. (Internal Medicine)

Initial hospital visit for a 62-year-old female with known coronary artery disease, for evaluation of increasing edema, dyspnea on exertion, confusion, and sudden onset of fever with productive cough. (Internal Medicine)

Initial hospital visit for a 3-year-old female with 36-hour history of sore throat and high fever; now with sudden onset of lethargy, irritability, photophobia, and nuchal rigidity. (Pediatrics)

Initial hospital visit for a 26-year-old female for evaluation of severe facial fractures (LeFort's II/III). (Plastic Surgery)

Initial hospital visit for a 55-year-old female for bilateral mandibular fractures resulting in flail mandible and airway obstruction. (Plastic Surgery)

Initial hospital visit for a 71-year-old patient with a red painful eye four days following uncomplicated cataract surgery due to endophthalmitis. (Ophthalmology)

Initial hospital visit for a 45-year-old patient involved in a motor vehicle accident who suffered a perforating corneoscleral laceration with loss of vision. (Ophthalmology)

Initial hospital visit for a 58-year-old male who has Ludwig's angina and progressive airway compromise. (Oral & Maxillofacial Surgery)

Initial hospital visit for a patient with generalized systemic sclerosis, receiving immunosuppressive therapy because of recent onset of cough, fever, and inability to swallow. (Dermatology)

Initial hospital visit for an 82-year-old male who presents with syncope, chest pain, and ventricular arrhythmias. (Cardiology)

Initial hospital visit for a 62-year-old male with history of previous myocardial infarction, comes in with recurrent, sustained ventricular tachycardia. (Cardiology)

Initial hospital visit for a chronic dialysis patient with infected PTFE fistula, septicemia, and shock. (Nephrology)

Initial hospital visit for a 1-year-old male, victim of child abuse, with central nervous system depression, skull fracture, and retinal hemorrhage. (Family Medicine/Neurology)

Initial hospital visit for a 25-year-old female with recent C4-C5 quadriplegia, admitted for rehabilitation. (Physical Medicine & Rehabilitation)

Initial hospital visit for an 18-year-old male, post-traumatic brain injury with multiple impairment. (Physical Medicine & Rehabilitation)

Initial partial hospital admission for 16-year-old male, sullen and subdued, with six-month history of declining school performance, increasing self-endangerment, and resistance to parental expectations. (Psychiatry)

Initial hospital visit for a 16-year-old primigravida at 32-weeks gestation with severe hypertension (200/110), thrombocytopenia, and headache. (Obstetrics & Gynecology)

Initial hospital visit for a 49-year-old male with cirrhosis of liver with hematemesis, hepatic encephalopathy, and fever. (Gastroenterology)

Initial hospital visit for a 55-year-old female in chronic pain who has attempted suicide. (Psychiatry)

Initial hospital visit for a 70-year-old male, with multiple organ system disease, admitted with history of being aneuric and septic for 24 hours prior to admission. (Urology)

Initial hospital visit for a 3-year-old female with 36-hour history of sore throat and high fever, now with sudden onset of lethargy, irritability, photophobia, and nuchal rigidity. (Internal Medicine)

Initial hospital visit for a 78-year-old male, transfers from nursing home with dysuria and pyuria, increasing confusion, and high fever. (Internal Medicine)

Initial hospital visit for a 1-day-old male with cyanosis, respiratory distress, and tachypnea. (Cardiology)

Initial hospital visit for a 3-year-old female with recurrent tachycardia and syncope. (Cardiology)

Initial hospital visit for a thyrotoxic patient who presents with fever, atrial fibrillation, and delirium. (Endocrinology)

Initial hospital visit for a 50-year-old Type I diabetic who presents with diabetic ketoacidosis with fever and obtundation. (Endocrinology)

Initial hospital visit for a 40-year-old female with anatomical stage 3, ARA functional class 3 rheumatoid arthritis on methotrexate, corticosteroid, and nonsteroidal anti-inflammatory drugs. Patient presents with severe arthritis flare, new oral ulcers, abdominal pain, and leukopenia. (Rheumatology)

Initial hospital exam of a pediatric patient with high fever and proptosis. (Otolaryngology/Head & Neck Surgery)

Initial hospital visit for a 25-year-old patient admitted for the first time to the rehab unit, with recent C4-C5 quadriplegia. (Physical Medicine & Rehabilitation)

Hospital admission, examination, and initiation of treatment program for a previously unknown 58-year-old male who presents with acute chest pain. (Cardiology)

Hospital admission, examination, and initiation of induction chemotherapy for a 42-year-old patient with newly diagnosed acute myelogenous leukemia. (Hematology/Oncology)

Hospital admission following a motor vehicle accident of a 24-year-old male with fracture dislocation of C5-C6; neurologically intact. (Neurosurgery)

Hospital admission for a 78-year-old female with left lower lobe pneumonia and a history of coronary artery disease, congestive heart failure, osteoarthritis, and gout. (Family Medicine)

Hospital admission, examination, and initiation of treatment program for a 65-year-old immunosuppressed male with confusion, fever, and a headache. (Infectious Disease)

Hospital admission for a 9-year-old with vomiting, dehydration, fever, tachypnea, and an admitting diagnosis of diabetic ketoacidosis. (Pediatrics)

Initial hospital visit for a 65-year-old male who presents with acute myocardial infarction, oliguria, hypotension, and altered state of consciousness. (Cardiology)

Initial hospital visit for a hostile/resistant adolescent patient who is severely depressed and involved in poly-substance abuse. Patient is experiencing significant conflict in his chaotic family situation and was suspended from school following an attack on a teacher with a baseball bat. (Psychiatry)

Initial hospital visit for 89-year-old female with fulminant hepatic failure and encephalopathy. (Gastroenterology)

Initial hospital visit for a 42-year-old female with rapidly progressing scleroderma, malignant hypertension, digital infarcts, and oligurea. (Rheumatology)

Subsequent Hospital Care

99231 Subsequent hospital visit for a 65-year-old female, post-open reduction and internal fixation of a fracture. (Physical Medicine & Rehabilitation)

Subsequent hospital visit for a 33-year-old patient with pelvic pain who is responding to pain medication and observation. (Obstetrics & Gynecology)

Subsequent hospital visit for a 21-year-old female with hyperemesis who has responded well to intravenous fluids. (Obstetrics & Gynecology)

Subsequent hospital visit to re-evaluate postoperative pain and titrate patient-controlled analgesia for a 27-year-old female. (Anesthesiology)

Follow-up hospital visit for a 35-year-old female, status post-epidural analgesia. (Anesthesiology/Pain Medicine)

Subsequent hospital visit for a 56-year-old male, post-gastrectomy, for maintenance of analgesia using an intravenous dilaudid infusion. (Anesthesiology)

Subsequent hospital visit for a 4-year-old on day three receiving medication for uncomplicated pneumonia. (Allergy & Immunology)

Subsequent hospital visit for a 30-year-old female with urticaria that has stabilized with medication. (Allergy & Immunology)

Subsequent hospital visit for a 76-year-old male with venous stasis ulcers. (Dermatology)

Subsequent hospital visit for a 24-year-old female with otitis externa, seen two days before in consultation, now to have otic wick removal. (Otolaryngology/Head & Neck Surgery)

Subsequent hospital visit for a 27-year-old with acute labyrinthitis. (Otolaryngology/Head & Neck Surgery)

Subsequent hospital visit for a 10-year-old male admitted for lobar pneumonia with vomiting and dehydration; is becoming afebrile and tolerating oral fluids. (Family Medicine/Pediatrics)

Subsequent hospital visit for a 62-year-old patient with resolving cellulitis of the foot. (Orthopaedic Surgery)

Subsequent hospital visit for a 25-year-old male admitted for supra-ventricular tachycardia and converted on medical therapy. (Cardiology)

Subsequent hospital visit for a 27-year-old male two days after open reduction and internal fixation for malar complex fracture. (Plastic Surgery)

Subsequent hospital visit for a 76-year-old male with venous stasis ulcers. (Geriatrics)

Subsequent hospital visit for a 67-year-old female admitted three days ago with bleeding gastric ulcer; now stable. (Gastroenterology)

Subsequent hospital visit for stable 33-year-old male, status post-lower gastrointestinal bleeding. (General Surgery/Gastroenterology)

Subsequent hospital visit for a 29-year-old auto mechanic with effort thrombosis of left upper extremity. (General Surgery)

Subsequent hospital visit for a 14-year-old female in middle phase of inpatient treatment, who is now behaviorally stable and making satisfactory progress in treatment. (Psychiatry)

Subsequent hospital visit for an 18-year-old male with uncomplicated asthma who is clinically stable. (Allergy & Immunology)

Subsequent hospital visit for a 55-year-old male with rheumatoid arthritis, two days following an uncomplicated total joint replacement. (Rheumatology)

Subsequent hospital visit for a 60-year-old dialysis patient with an access infection, now afebrile on antibiotic. (Nephrology)

Subsequent hospital visit for a 36-year-old female with stable post-rhinoplasty epistaxis. (Plastic Surgery)

Subsequent hospital visit for a 66-year-old female with L-2 vertebral compression fracture with resolving ileus. (Orthopaedic Surgery)

Subsequent hospital visit for a patient with peritonsillar abscess. (Otolaryngology/Head & Neck Surgery)

Subsequent hospital visit for an 18-year-old female responding to intravenous antibiotic therapy for ear or sinus infection. (Otolaryngology/Head & Neck Surgery)

Subsequent hospital visit for a 70-year-old male admitted with congestive heart failure who has responded to therapy. (Cardiology)

Follow-up hospital visit for a 32-year-old female with left ureteral calculus; being followed in anticipation of spontaneous passage. (Urology)

Subsequent hospital visit for a 4-year-old female, admitted for acute gastroenteritis and dehydration, requiring IV hydration; now stable. (Family Medicine)

Subsequent hospital visit for a 50-year-old Type II diabetic who is clinically stable and without complications requiring regulation of a single dose of insulin daily. (Endocrinology)

Subsequent hospital visit to reassesses the status of a 65-year-old patient post-open reduction and internal fixation of hip fracture, on the rehab unit. (Physical Medicine & Rehabilitation)

Subsequent hospital visit for a 78-year-old male with cholangiocarcinoma managed by biliary drainage. (Interventional Radiology)

Subsequent hospital visit for a 50-year-old male with uncomplicated myocardial infarction who is clinically stable and without chest pain. (Family Medicine/Cardiology/Internal Medicine)

Subsequent hospital visit for a stable 72-year-old lung cancer patient undergoing a five-day course of infusion chemotherapy. (Hematology/Oncology)

Subsequent hospital visit, two days post admission for a 65-year-old male with a CVA (cerebral vascular accident) and left hemiparesis, who is clinically stable. (Neurology/Physical Medicine & Rehabilitation)

Subsequent hospital visit for now stable, 33-year-old male, status post lower gastrointestinal bleeding. (General Surgery)

Subsequent visit on third day of hospitalization for a 60-year-old female recovering from an uncomplicated pneumonia. (Infectious Disease/Internal Medicine/Pulmonary Medicine)

Subsequent hospital visit for a 3-year-old patient in traction for a congenital dislocation of the hip. (Orthopaedic Surgery)

Subsequent hospital visit for a 4-year-old female, admitted for acute gastroenteritis and dehydration, requiring IV hydration; now stable. (Family Medicine/Internal Medicine)

Subsequent hospital visit for 50-year-old female with resolving uncomplicated acute pancreatitis. (Gastroenterology)

99232 Subsequent hospital visit for a patient with venous stasis ulcers who developed fever and red streaks adjacent to the ulcer. (Dermatology/Internal Medicine/Family Medicine)

Subsequent hospital visit for a 66-year-old male for dressing changes and observation. Patient has had a myocutaneous flap to close a pharyngeal fistula and now has a low-grade fever. (Plastic Surgery)

Subsequent hospital visit for a 54-year-old female admitted for myocardial infarction, but who is now having frequent premature ventricular contractions. (Internal Medicine)

Subsequent hospital visit for an 80-year-old patient with a pelvic rim fracture, inability to walk, and severe pain; now 36 hours post-injury, experiencing urinary retention. (Orthopaedic Surgery)

Subsequent hospital visit for a 17-year-old female with fever, pharyngitis, and airway obstruction, who after 48 hours develops a maculopapular rash. (Pediatrics/Family Medicine)

Follow-up hospital visit for a 32-year-old patient admitted the previous day for corneal ulcer. (Dermatology)

Follow-up visit for a 67-year-old male with congestive heart failure who has responded to antibiotics and diuretics and has now developed a monoarthropathy. (Internal Medicine)

Follow-up hospital visit for a 58-year-old male receiving continuous opioids who is experiencing severe nausea and vomiting. (Pain Medicine)

Subsequent hospital visit for a patient after an auto accident who is slow to respond to ambulation training. (Physical Medicine & Rehabilitation)

Subsequent hospital visit for a 14-year-old with unstable bronchial asthma complicated by pneumonia. (Allergy & Immunology)

Subsequent hospital visit for a 50-year-old diabetic, hypertensive male with back pain not responding to conservative inpatient management with continued radiation of pain to the lower left extremity. (Orthopaedic Surgery)

Subsequent hospital visit for a 37-year-old female on day five of antibiotics for bacterial endocarditis, who still has low-grade fever. (Cardiology)

Subsequent hospital visit for a 54-year-old patient, post MI (myocardial infarction), who is out of the CCU (coronary care unit) but is now having frequent premature ventricular contractions on telemetry. (Cardiology/Internal Medicine)

Subsequent hospital visit for a patient with neutropenia, a fever responding to antibiotics, and continued slow gastrointestinal bleeding on platelet support. (Hematology/Oncology)

Subsequent hospital visit for a 50-year-old male admitted two days ago for sub-acute renal allograft rejection. (Nephrology)

Subsequent hospital visit for a 35-year-old drug addict, not responding to initial antibiotic therapy for pyelonephritis. (Urology)

Subsequent hospital visit of an 81-year-old male with abdominal distention, nausea, and vomiting. (General Surgery)

Subsequent hospital care for a 62-year-old female with congestive heart failure, who remains dyspneic and febrile. (Internal Medicine)

Subsequent hospital visit for a 73-year-old female with recently diagnosed lung cancer, who complains of unsteady gait. (Pulmonary Medicine)

Subsequent hospital visit for a 20-month-old male with bacterial meningitis treated one week with antibiotic therapy; has now developed a temperature of 101 degrees. (Pediatrics)

Subsequent hospital visit for 13-year-old male admitted with left lower quadrant abdominal pain and fever, not responding to therapy. (General Surgery)

Subsequent hospital visit for a 65-year-old male with hemiplegia and painful paretic shoulder. (Physical Medicine & Rehabilitation)

99233 Subsequent hospital visit for a 38-year-old male, quadriplegic with acute autonomic hyperreflexia, who is not responsive to initial care. (Physical Medicine & Rehabilitation)

Follow-up hospital visit for a teenage female who continues to experience severely disruptive, violent, and life-threatening symptoms in a complicated multi-system illness. Family/social circumstances also a contributing factor. (Psychiatry)

Subsequent hospital visit for a 42-year-old female with progressive systemic sclerosis (scleroderma), renal failure on dialysis, congestive heart failure, cardiac arrhythmias, and digital ulcers. (Allergy & Immunology)

Subsequent hospital visit for a 50-year-old diabetic, hypertensive male with nonresponding back pain and radiating pain to the lower left extremity, who develops chest pain, cough, and bloody sputum. (Orthopaedic Surgery)

Subsequent hospital visit for a 64-year-old female, status post-abdominal aortic aneurysm resection, with non-responsive coagulopathy, who has now developed lower GI bleeding. (Abdominal Surgery/Colon & Rectal Surgery/General Surgery)

Follow-up hospital care of a patient with pansinusitis infection complicated by a brain abscess and asthma; no response to current treatment. (Otolaryngology/Head & Neck Surgery)

Subsequent hospital visit for a patient with a laryngeal neoplasm who develops airway compromise, suspected metastasis. (Otolaryngology/Head & Neck Surgery)

Subsequent hospital visit for a 49-year-old male with significant rectal bleeding, etiology undetermined, not responding to treatment. (Abdominal Surgery/General Surgery/Colon & Rectal Surgery)

Subsequent hospital visit for a 50-year-old male, post-aortocoronary bypass surgery; now develops hypotension and oliguria. (Cardiology)

Subsequent hospital visit for an adolescent patient who is violent, unsafe, and noncompliant, with multiple expectations for participation in treatment plan and behavior on the treatment unit. (Psychiatry)

Subsequent hospital visit for an 18-year-old male being treated for presumed PCP psychosis. Patient is still moderately symptomatic with auditory hallucinations and is insisting on signing out against medical advice. (Psychiatry)

Subsequent hospital visit for an 8-year-old female with caustic ingestion, who now has fever, dyspnea, and dropping hemoglobin. (Gastroenterology)

Follow-up hospital visit for a chronic renal failure patient on dialysis who develops chest pain and shortness of breath and a new onset pericardial friction rub. (Nephrology)

Subsequent hospital visit for a 44-year-old patient with electrical burns to the left arm with ascending infection. (Orthopaedic Surgery)

Subsequent hospital visit for a patient with systemic sclerosis who has aspirated and is short of breath. (Dermatology)

Subsequent hospital visit for a 65-year-old female, status postoperative resection of abdominal aortic aneurysm, with suspected ischemic bowel. (General Surgery)

Subsequent hospital visit for a 50-year-old male, post-aortocoronary bypass surgery, now develops hypotension and oliguria. (Cardiology)

Subsequent hospital visit for a 65-year-old male, following an acute myocardial infarction, who complains of shortness of breath and new chest pain. (Cardiology)

Subsequent hospital visit for a 65-year-old female with rheumatoid arthritis (stage 3, class 3) admitted for urosepsis. On the third hospital day, chest pain, dyspnea, and fever develop. (Rheumatology)

Follow-up hospital care of a pediatric case with stridor, laryngomalacia, established tracheostomy, complicated by multiple medical problems in PICU. (Otolaryngology/Head & Neck Surgery)

Subsequent hospital visit for a 60-year-old female, four days post uncomplicated inferior myocardial infarction who has developed severe chest pain, dyspnea, diaphoresis, and nausea. (Family Medicine)

Subsequent hospital visit for a patient with AML (acute myelogenous leukemia), fever, elevated white count and uric acid undergoing induction chemotherapy. (Hematology/Oncology)

Subsequent hospital visit for a 38-year-old quadriplegic male with acute autonomic hyperreflexia, who is not responsive to initial care. (Physical Medicine & Rehabilitation)

Subsequent hospital visit for a 65-year-old female postoperative resection of abdominal aortic aneurysm, with suspected ischemic bowel. (General Surgery)

Subsequent hospital visit for a 60-year-old female with persistent leukocytosis and a fever seven days after a sigmoid colon resection for carcinoma. (Infectious Disease)

Subsequent hospital visit for a chronic renal failure patient on dialysis, who develops chest pain, shortness of breath, and new onset of pericardial friction rub. (Nephrology)

Subsequent hospital visit for a 65-year-old male with acute myocardial infarction who now demonstrates complete heart block and congestive heart failure. (Cardiology)

Subsequent hospital visit for a 25-year-old female with hypertension and systemic lupus erythematosus, admitted for fever and respiratory distress. On the third hospital day, the patient presented with purpuric skin lesions and acute renal failure. (Allergy & Immunology)

Subsequent hospital visit for a 55-year-old male with severe chronic obstructive pulmonary disease and bronchospasm; initially admitted for acute respiratory distress requiring ventilatory support in the ICU. The patient was stabilized, extubated, and transferred to the floor but has now developed acute fever, dyspnea, left lower lobe rhonchi, and laboratory evidence of carbon dioxide retention and hypoxemia. (Family Medicine/ Internal Medicine)

Subsequent hospital visit for 46-year-old female, known liver cirrhosis patient, with recent upper gastrointestinal hemorrhage from varices; now with worsening ascites and encephalopathy. (Gastroenterology)

Subsequent hospital visit for 62-year-old female admitted with acute subarachnoid hemorrhage, negative cerebral arteriogram, increased lethargy, and hemiparesis with fever. (Neurosurgery)

Consultations

Office or Other Outpatient Consultations

New or Established Patient

99241 Initial office consultation for a 40-year-old female in pain from blister on lip following a cold. (Oral & Maxillofacial Surgery)

Initial office consultation for a 62-year-old construction worker with olecranon bursitis. (Orthopaedic Surgery)

Office consultation with 25-year-old postpartum female with severe symptomatic hemorrhoids. (Colon & Rectal Surgery)

Office consultation with 58-year-old male, referred for follow-up of creatinine level and evaluation of obstructive uropathy, relieved two months ago. (Nephrology)

Office consultation for 30-year-old female tennis player with sprain or contusion of the forearm. (Orthopaedic Surgery)

Office consultation for a 45-year-old male, requested by his internist, with asymptomatic torus palatinus requiring no further treatment. (Oral & Maxillofacial Surgery)

99242 Initial office consultation for a 20-year-old male with acute upper respiratory tract symptoms. (Allergy & Immunology)

Initial office consultation for a 29-year-old soccer player with painful proximal thigh/groin injury. (Orthopaedic Surgery)

Initial office consultation for a 66-year-old female with wrist and hand pain, numbness of finger tips, suspected median nerve compression by carpal tunnel syndrome. (Plastic Surgery)

Initial office consultation for a patient with a solitary lesion of discoid lupus erythematosus on left cheek to rule out malignancy or self-induced lesion. (Dermatology)

Office consultation for management of systolic hypertension in a 70-year-old male scheduled for elective prostate resection. (Geriatrics)

Office consultation with 27-year-old female, with old amputation, for evaluation of existing above-knee prosthesis. (Physical Medicine & Rehabilitation)

Office consultation with 66-year-old female with wrist and hand pain, and finger numbness, secondary to suspected carpal tunnel syndrome. (Orthopaedic Surgery)

Office consultation for 61-year-old female, recently on antibiotic therapy, now with diarrhea and leukocytosis. (Abdominal Surgery)

Office consultation for a patient with papulosquamous eruption of elbow with pitting of nails and itchy scalp. (Dermatology)

Office consultation for a 30-year-old female with single season allergic rhinitis. (Allergy & Immunology)

99243 Initial office consultation for a 60-year-old male with avascular necrosis of the left femoral head with increasing pain. (Orthopaedic Surgery)

Office consultation for a 31-year-old woman complaining of palpitations and chest pains. Her internist had described a mild systolic click. (Cardiology)

Office consultation for a 65-year-old female with persistent bronchitis. (Infectious Disease)

Office consultation for a 65-year-old man with chronic low-back pain radiating to the leg. (Neurosurgery)

Office consultation for 23-year-old female with Crohn's disease not responding to therapy. (Abdominal Surgery/Colon & Rectal Surgery)

Office consultation for 25-year-old patient with symptomatic knee pain and swelling, with torn anterior cruciate ligament and/or torn meniscus. (Orthopaedic Surgery)

Office consultation for a 67-year-old patient with osteoporosis and mandibular atrophy with regard to reconstructive alternatives. (Oral & Maxillofacial Surgery)

Office consultation for 39-year-old patient referred at a perimenopausal age for irregular menses and menopausal symptoms. (Obstetrics & Gynecology)

99244 Initial office consultation for a 28-year-old male, HIV+, with a recent change in visual acuity. (Ophthalmology)

Initial office consultation for a 15-year-old male with failing grades, suspected drug abuse. (Pediatrics)

Initial office consultation for a 36-year-old factory worker, status four months post-occupational low back injury and requires management of intractable low back pain. (Pain Medicine)

Initial office consultation for a 45-year-old female with a history of chronic arthralgia of TMJ and associated myalgia and sudden progressive symptomatology over last two to three months. (Oral & Maxillofacial Surgery)

Initial office consultation for evaluation of a 70-year-old male with appetite loss and diminished energy. (Psychiatry)

Initial office consultation for an elementary school-aged patient, referred by pediatrician, with multiple systematic complaints and recent onset of behavioral discontrol. (Psychiatry)

Initial office consultation for a 23-year-old female with developmental facial skeletal anomaly and subsequent abnormal relationship of jaw(s) to cranial base. (Oral & Maxillofacial Surgery)

Initial office consultation for a 45-year-old myopic patient with a one-week history of floaters and a partial retinal detachment. (Ophthalmology)

Initial office consultation for a 65-year-old female with moderate dementia, mild unsteadiness, back pain fatigue on ambulation, intermittent urinary incontinence. (Neurosurgery)

Initial office consultation for a 33-year-old female referred by endocrinologist with amenorrhea and galactorrhea, for evaluation of pituitary tumor. (Neurosurgery)

Initial office consultation for a 34-year-old male with new onset nephrotic syndrome. (Nephrology)

Initial office consultation for a 39-year-old female with intractable chest wall pain secondary to metastatic breast cancer. (Anesthesiology/Pain Medicine)

Initial office consultation for a patient with multiple giant tumors of jaws. (Oral & Maxillofacial Surgery)

Initial office consultation for a patient with a failed total hip replacement with loosening and pain upon walking. (Orthopaedic Surgery)

Initial office consultation for a 60-year-old female with three-year history of intermittent tic-like unilateral facial pain; now constant pain for six weeks without relief by adequate carbamazepine dosage. (Neurosurgery)

Initial office consultation for a 45-year-old male heavy construction worker with prior lumbar disk surgery two years earlier; now gradually recurring low back and unilateral leg pain for three months, unable to work for two weeks. (Neurosurgery)

Initial office consultation of a patient who presents with a 30-year history of smoking and right neck mass. (Otolaryngology/Head & Neck Surgery)

Office consultation with 38-year-old female, with inflammatory bowel disease, who now presents with right lower quadrant pain and suspected intra-abdominal abscess. (General Surgery/Colon & Rectal Surgery)

Office consultation with 72-year-old male with esophageal carcinoma, symptoms of dysphagia and reflux. (Thoracic Surgery)

Office consultation for discussion of treatment options for a 40-year-old female with a 2 cm adenocarcinoma of the breast. (Radiation Oncology)

Office consultation for young patient referred by pediatrician because of patient's short attention span, easy distractibility, and hyperactivity. (Psychiatry)

Office consultation for 66-year-old female, history of colon resection for adenocarcinoma six years earlier, now with severe mid-back pain; X-rays showing osteoporosis and multiple vertebral compression fractures. (Neurosurgery)

Office consultation for a patient with chronic pelvic inflammatory disease who now has left lower quadrant pain with a palpable pelvic mass. (Obstetrics & Gynecology)

Office consultation for a patient with long-standing psoriasis with acute onset of erythroderma, pustular lesions, chills, and fever. Combinations of topical and systemic treatments discussed and instituted. (Dermatology)

99245 Initial office consultation for a 35-year-old multiple-trauma male patient with complex pelvic fractures, for evaluation and formulation of management plan. (Orthopaedic Surgery)

Initial emergency room consultation for 10-year-old male in status epilepticus, recent closed head injury, information about medication not available. (Neurosurgery)

Initial emergency room consultation for a 23-year-old patient with severe abdominal pain, guarding, febrile, and unstable vital signs. (Obstetrics & Gynecology)

Office consultation for a 67-year-old female longstanding uncontrolled diabetic who presents with retinopathy, nephropathy, and a foot ulcer. (Endocrinology)

Office consultation for a 37-year-old male for initial evaluation and management of Cushing's disease. (Endocrinology)

Office consultation for a 60-year-old male who presents with thyrotoxicosis, exophthalmos, frequent premature ventricular contractions, and congestive heart failure. (Endocrinology)

Initial office consultation for a 36-year-old patient, one year status post occupational herniated cervical disk treated by laminectomy, requiring management of multiple sites of intractable pain, depression, and narcotic dependence. (Pain Medicine)

Office consultation for a 58-year-old man with a history of MI and CHF who complains of the recent onset of rest angina and shortness of breath. The patient has a systolic blood pressure of 90 mmHG and is in Class IV heart failure. (Cardiology)

Emergency room consultation for a 1-year-old with a three-day history of fever with increasing respiratory distress who is thought to have cardiac tamponade by the ER physician. (Cardiology)

Office consultation in the emergency room for a 25-year-old male with severe, acute, closed head injury. (Neurosurgery)

Office consultation for a 23-year-old female with Stage II A Hodgkins disease with positive supraclavicular and mediastinal nodes. (Radiation Oncology)

Office consultation for a 27-year-old juvenile diabetic patient with severe diabetic retinopathy, gastric atony, nephrotic syndrome, and progressive renal failure, now with a serum creatinine of 2.7, and a blood pressure of 170/114. (Nephrology)

Office consultation for independent medical evaluation of a patient with a history of complicated low back and neck problems with previous multiple failed back surgeries. (Orthopaedic Surgery)

Office consultation for an adolescent referred by pediatrician for recent onset of violent and self-injurious behavior. (Psychiatry)

Office consultation for a 6-year-old male for evaluation of severe muscle and joint pain and a diffuse rash. Patient well until 4-6 weeks earlier, when he developed arthralgia, myalgias, and a fever of 102 degrees for one week. (Rheumatology)

Inpatient Consultations

New or Established Patient

99251 Initial hospital consultation for a 27-year-old female with fractured incisor post-intubation. (Oral & Maxillofacial Surgery)

Initial hospital consultation for an orthopaedic patient on IV antibiotics who has developed an apparent candida infection of the oral cavity. (Oral & Maxillofacial Surgery)

Initial inpatient consultation for a 30-year-old female complaining of vaginal itching, post orthopaedic surgery. (Obstetrics & Gynecology)

Initial inpatient consultation for a 36-year-old male on orthopaedic service with complaint of localized dental pain. (Oral & Maxillofacial Surgery)

99252 Initial hospital consultation for a 45-year-old male, previously abstinent alcoholic, who relapsed and was admitted for management of gastritis. The patient readily accepts the need for further treatment. (Addiction Medicine)

Initial hospital consultation for a 35-year-old dialysis patient with episodic oral ulcerations. (Oral & Maxillofacial Surgery)

Initial inpatient preoperative consultation for a 43-year-old woman with cholecystitis and well-controlled hypertension. (Cardiology)

Initial inpatient consultation for recommendation of antibiotic prophylaxis for a patient with a synthetic heart valve who will undergo urologic surgery. (Internal Medicine)

Initial inpatient consultation for possible drug induced skin eruption in 50-year-old male. (Dermatology)

Preoperative inpatient consultation for evaluation of hypertension in a 60-year-old male who will undergo a cholecystectomy. Patient had a normal annual check-up in your office four months ago. (Internal Medicine)

Initial inpatient consultation for 66-year-old patient with wrist and hand pain and finger numbness, secondary to carpal tunnel syndrome. (Orthopaedic Surgery/Plastic Surgery)

Initial inpatient consultation for a 66-year-old male smoker referred for pain management immediately status post-biliary tract surgery done via sub-costal incision. (Anesthesiology/Pain Medicine)

99253 Initial hospital consultation for a 50-year-old female with incapacitating knee pain due to generalized rheumatoid arthritis. (Orthopaedic Surgery)

Initial hospital consultation for a 60-year-old male with avascular necrosis of the left femoral heel with increasing pain. (Orthopaedic Surgery)

Initial hospital consultation for a 45-year-old female with compound mandibular fracture and concurrent head, abdominal, and/or orthopaedic injuries. (Oral & Maxillofacial Surgery)

Initial hospital consultation for a 22-year-old female, paraplegic, to evaluate wrist and hand pain. (Orthopaedic Surgery)

Initial hospital consultation for a 40-year-old male with 10-day history of incapacitating unilateral sciatica, unable to walk now, not improved by bed rest. (Neurosurgery)

Initial hospital consultation, requested by pediatrician, for treatment recommendations for a patient admitted with persistent inability to walk following soft tissue injury to ankle. (Physiatry)

Initial hospital consultation for a 27-year-old previously healthy male who vomited during IV sedation and may have aspirated gastric contents. (Anesthesiology)

Initial hospital consultation for a 33-year-old female, post-abdominal surgery, who now has a fever. (Internal Medicine)

Initial inpatient consultation for a 57-year-old male, post lower endoscopy, for evaluation of abdominal pain and fever. (General Surgery)

Initial inpatient consultation for rehabilitation of a 73-year-old female one week after surgical management of a hip fracture. (Physical Medicine & Rehabilitation)

Initial inpatient consultation for diagnosis/management of fever following abdominal surgery. (Internal Medicine)

Initial inpatient consultation for a 35-year-old female with a fever and pulmonary infiltrate following cesarean section. (Pulmonary Medicine)

Initial inpatient consultation for a 42-year-old non-diabetic patient, postoperative cholecystectomy, now with an acute urinary tract infection. (Nephrology)

Initial inpatient consultation for 53-year-old female with moderate uncomplicated pancreatitis. (Gastroenterology)

Initial inpatient consultation for 45-year-old patient with chronic neck pain with radicular pain of the left arm. (Orthopaedic Surgery)

Initial inpatient consultation for 8-year-old patient with new onset of seizures who has a normal examination and previous history. (Neurology)

99254 Initial hospital consultation for a 15-year-old patient with painless swelling of proximal humerus with lytic lesion by X-ray. (Orthopaedic Surgery)

Initial hospital consultation for evaluation of a 29-year-old female with a diffusely positive medical review of systems and history of multiple surgeries. (Psychiatry)

Initial hospital consultation for a 70-year-old diabetic female with gangrene of the foot. (Orthopaedic Surgery)

Initial inpatient consultation for a 47-year-old female with progressive pulmonary infiltrate, hypoxemia, and diminished urine output. (Anesthesiology)

Initial hospital consultation for a 13-month-old with spasmodic cough, respiratory distress, and fever. (Allergy & Immunology)

Initial hospital consultation for a patient with failed total hip replacement with loosening and pain upon walking. (Orthopaedic Surgery)

Initial hospital consultation for a 62-year-old female with metastatic breast cancer to the femoral neck and thoracic vertebra. (Orthopaedic Surgery)

Initial hospital consultation for a 39-year-old female with nephrolithiasis requiring extensive opioid analgesics, whose vital signs are now elevated. She initially denied any drug use but today gives history of multiple substance abuse, including opioids and prior treatment for a personality disorder. (Psychiatry)

Initial hospital consultation for a 70-year-old female without previous psychiatric history, who is now experiencing nocturnal confusion and visual hallucinations following hip replacement surgery. (Psychiatry)

Initial inpatient consultation for evaluation of a 63-year-old in the ICU with diabetes and chronic renal failure who develops acute respiratory distress syndrome 36 hours after a mitral valve replacement. (Anesthesiology)

Initial inpatient consultation for a 66-year-old female with enlarged supraclavicular lymph nodes, found on biopsy to be malignant. (Hematology/Oncology)

Initial inpatient consultation for a 43-year-old female for evaluation of sudden painful visual loss, optic neuritis, and episodic paresthesia. (Ophthalmology)

Initial inpatient consultation for evaluation of a 71-year-old male with hyponatremia (serum sodium 114) who was admitted to the hospital with pneumonia. (Nephrology)

Initial inpatient consultation for a 72-year-old male with emergency admission for possible bowel obstruction. (Internal Medicine/General Surgery)

Initial inpatient consultation for a 35-year-old female with fever, swollen joints, and rash of one-week duration. (Rheumatology)

99255 Initial inpatient consultation for a 76-year-old female with massive, life-threatening gastrointestinal hemorrhage and chest pain. (Gastroenterology)

Initial inpatient consultation for a 75-year-old female, admitted to intensive care with acute respiratory distress syndrome, who is hypersensitive, and has a moderate metabolic acidosis, and a rising serum creatinine. (Nephrology)

Initial hospital consultation for patient with a history of complicated low back pain and neck problems with previous multiple failed back surgeries. (Orthopaedic Surgery/Neurosurgery)

Initial hospital consultation for a 66-year-old female, two days post-abdominal aneurysm repair, with oliguria and hypertension of one-day duration. (Nephrology/Internal Medicine)

Initial hospital consultation for a patient with shotgun wound to face with massive facial trauma and airway obstruction. (Oral & Maxillofacial Surgery)

Initial hospital consultation for patient with severe pancreatitis complicated by respiratory insufficiency, acute renal failure, and abscess formation. (General Surgery/Colon & Rectal Surgery)

Initial hospital consultation for a 35-year-old multiple-trauma male patient with complex pelvic fractures to evaluate and formulate management plan. (Orthopaedic Surgery)

Initial inpatient consultation for adolescent patient with fractured femur and pelvis who pulled out IVs and disconnected traction in attempt to elope from hospital. (Psychiatry)

Initial hospital consultation for a 16-year-old primigravida at 32-weeks gestation requested by a family practitioner for evaluation of severe hypertension, thrombocytopenia, and headache. (Obstetrics & Gynecology)

Initial hospital consultation for a 58-year-old insulin-dependent diabetic with multiple antibiotic allergies, now with multiple fascial plane abscesses and airway obstruction. (Oral & Maxillofacial Surgery)

Initial inpatient consultation for a 55-year-old male with known cirrhosis and ascites, now with jaundice, encephalopathy, and massive hematemesis. (Gastroenterology)

Initial hospital consultation for a 25-year-old male, seen in emergency room with severe, closed head injury. (Neurosurgery)

Initial hospital consultation for a 2-day-old male with single ventricle physiology and subaortic obstruction. Family counseling following evaluation for multiple, staged surgical procedures. (Thoracic Surgery)

Initial hospital consultation for a 45-year-old male admitted with subarachnoid hemorrhage and intracranial aneurysm on angiogram. (Neurosurgery)

Initial inpatient consultation for myxedematous patient who is hypoventilating and obtunded. (Endocrinology)

Initial hospital consultation for a 45-year-old patient with widely metastatic lung carcinoma, intractable back pain, and a history that includes substance dependence, NSAID allergy, and two prior laminectomies with fusion for low back pain. (Pain Medicine)

Initial hospital consultation for evaluation of treatment options in a 50-year-old patient with cirrhosis, known peptic ulcer disease, hypotension, encephalopathy, and massive acute upper gastrointestinal bleeding that cannot be localized by endoscopy. (Interventional Radiology)

Initial inpatient consultation in the ICU for a 70-year-old male who experienced a cardiac arrest during surgery and was resuscitated. (Cardiology)

Initial inpatient consultation for a patient with severe pancreatitis complicated by respiratory insufficiency, acute renal failure, and abscess formation. (Gastroenterology)

Initial inpatient consultation for a 70-year-old cirrhotic male admitted with ascites, jaundice, encephalopathy, and massive hematemesis. (Gastroenterology)

Initial inpatient consultation in the ICU for a 51-year-old patient who is on a ventilator and has a fever two weeks after a renal transplantation. (Infectious Disease)

Initial inpatient consultation for evaluation and formulation of plan for management of multiple-trauma patient with complex pelvic fracture, 35-year-old male. (General Surgery/Orthopaedic Surgery)

Initial inpatient consultation for a 50-year-old male with a history of previous myocardial infarction, now with acute pulmonary edema and hypotension. (Cardiology)

Initial inpatient consultation for 45-year-old male with recent, acute subarachnoid hemorrhage, hesitant speech, mildly confused, drowsy. High risk group for HIV+ status. (Neurosurgery)

Initial inpatient consultation for 36-year-old female referred by her internist to evaluate a patient being followed for abdominal pain and fever. The patient has developed diffuse abdominal pain, guarding, rigidity, and increased fever. (Obstetrics & Gynecology)

Emergency Department Services

New or Established Patient

99281 Emergency department visit for a patient for removal of sutures from a well-healed, uncomplicated laceration. (Emergency Medicine)

Emergency department visit for a patient for tetanus toxoid immunization. (Emergency Medicine)

Emergency department visit for a patient with several uncomplicated insect bites. (Emergency Medicine)

99282
Emergency department visit for a 20-year-old student who presents with a painful sunburn with blister formation on the back. (Emergency Medicine)

Emergency department visit for a child presenting with impetigo localized to the face. (Emergency Medicine)

Emergency department visit for a patient with a minor traumatic injury of an extremity with localized pain, swelling, and bruising. (Emergency Medicine)

Emergency department visit for an otherwise healthy patient whose chief complaint is a red, swollen cystic lesion on his/her back. (Emergency Medicine)

Emergency department visit for a patient presenting with a rash on both legs after exposure to poison ivy. (Emergency Medicine)

Emergency department visit for a young adult patient with infected sclera and purulent discharge from both eyes without pain, visual disturbance, or history of foreign body in either eye. (Emergency Medicine)

99283
Emergency department visit for a sexually active female complaining of vaginal discharge who is afebrile and denies experiencing abdominal or back pain. (Emergency Medicine)

Emergency department visit for a well-appearing 8-year-old who has a fever, diarrhea, and abdominal cramps; is tolerating oral fluids and is not vomiting. (Emergency Medicine)

Emergency department visit for a patient with an inversion ankle injury, who is unable to bear weight on the injured foot and ankle. (Emergency Medicine)

Emergency department visit for a patient who has a complaint of acute pain associated with a suspected foreign body in the painful eye. (Emergency Medicine)

Emergency department visit for a healthy, young adult patient who sustained a blunt head injury with local swelling and bruising without subsequent confusion, loss of consciousness, or memory deficit. (Emergency Medicine)

99284
Emergency department visit for a 4-year-old who fell off a bike sustaining a head injury with brief loss of consciousness. (Emergency Medicine)

Emergency department visit for an elderly female who has fallen and is now complaining of pain in her right hip and is unable to walk. (Emergency Medicine)

Emergency department visit for a patient with flank pain and hematuria. (Emergency Medicine)

Emergency department visit for a female presenting with lower abdominal pain and a vaginal discharge. (Emergency Medicine)

99285
Emergency department visit for a patient with a complicated overdose requiring aggressive management to prevent side effects from the ingested materials. (Emergency Medicine)

Emergency department visit for a patient with a new onset of rapid heart rate requiring IV drugs. (Emergency Medicine)

Emergency department visit for a patient exhibiting active, upper gastrointestinal bleeding. (Emergency Medicine)

Emergency department visit for a previously healthy young adult patient who is injured in an automobile accident and is brought to the emergency department immobilized and has symptoms compatible with intra-abdominal injuries or multiple extremity injuries. (Emergency Medicine)

Emergency department visit for a patient with an acute onset of chest pain compatible with symptoms of cardiac ischemia and/or pulmonary embolus. (Emergency Medicine)

Emergency department visit for a patient who presents with a sudden onset of "the worst headache of her life," and complains of a stiff neck, nausea, and inability to concentrate. (Emergency Medicine)

Emergency department visit for a patient with a new onset of a cerebral vascular accident. (Emergency Medicine)

Emergency department visit for acute febrile illness in an adult, associated with shortness of breath and an altered level of alertness. (Emergency Medicine)

Critical Care Services

99291
First hour of critical care of a 65-year-old man with septic shock following relief of ureteral obstruction caused by a stone.

First hour of critical care of a 15-year-old with acute respiratory failure from asthma.

First hour of critical care of a 45-year-old who sustained a liver laceration, cerebral hematoma, flailed chest, and pulmonary contusion after being struck by an automobile.

First hour of critical care of a 65-year-old woman who, following a hysterectomy, suffered a cardiac arrest associated with a pulmonary embolus.

First hour of critical care of a 6-month-old with hypovolemic shock secondary to diarrhea and dehydration.

First hour of critical care of a 3-year-old with respiratory failure secondary to pneumocystis carinii pneumonia.

Prolonged Services

Prolonged Service With Direct Patient Contact

Office or Other Outpatient

99354 A 20-year-old female with history of asthma presents with acute bronchospasm and moderate respiratory distress. Initial evaluation shows respiratory rate 30, labored breathing and wheezing heard in all lung fields. Office treatment is initiated which includes intermittent bronchial dilation and subcutaneous epinephrine. Requires intermittent time with patient over a period of 2-3 hours. (Family Medicine/Internal Medicine)

99355 A 20-year-old female with history of asthma presents with acute bronchospasm and moderate respiratory distress. Initial evaluation shows respiratory rate 30, labored breathing and wheezing heard in all lung fields. Office treatment is initiated which includes intermittent bronchial dilation and subcutaneous epinephrine. Requires intermittent time with patient over a period of 2-3 hours. (Family Medicine/Internal Medicine)

Inpatient

99356 A 34-year-old primigravida presents to hospital in early labor. Admission history and physical reveals severe preeclampsia. Physician supervises management of preeclampsia, IV magnesium initiation and maintenance, labor augmentation with pitocin, and close maternal-fetal monitoring. Involvement includes 40 minutes of continuous bedside care until the patient is stable, then is intermittent over several hours until the delivery. (Family Medicine/Internal Medicine/Obstetrics & Gynecology)

Prolonged Service Without Direct Patient Contact

99358 An 85-year-old new patient with multiple complicated medical problems has moved to the area to live closer to her daughter. She is brought to the primary care office by her daughter and has been seen and examined by the physician. The physician indicated that past medical records would be obtained from the patient's prior physicians' and that he will communicate further with the daughter upon review of them.

99359 An 85-year-old new patient with multiple complicated medical problems has moved to the area to live closer to her daughter. She is brought to the primary care office by her daughter and has been seen and examined by the physician. The physician indicated that past medical records would be obtained from the patient's prior physicians' and that he will communicate further with the daughter upon review of them.

Physician Standby Services

99360 A 24-year-old patient is admitted to OB unit attempting VBAC. Fetal monitoring shows increasing fetal distress. Patient's blood pressure is rising and labor progressing slowly. A primary care physician is requested by the OB/GYN to standby in the unit for possible cesarean delivery and neonatal resuscitation. (Family Medicine/Internal Medicine)

Care Plan Oversight Services

99375 First month of care plan oversight for terminal care of a 58-year-old female with advanced intraabdominal ovarian cancer. Care plan includes home oxygen, diuretics IV for edema and ascites control and pain control management involving IV morphine infusion when progressive ileus occurred. Physician phone contacts with nurse, family, and MSW. Discussion with MSW concerning plans to withdraw supportive measures per patient wishes. Documentation includes review and modification of care plan and certifications from nursing, MSW, pharmacy, and DME. (Family Medicine/Internal Medicine)

Appendix D

Summary of CPT Add-on Codes

This listing is a summary of CPT add-on codes for CPT 2013. The codes listed below are identified in CPT 2013 with a **+** symbol.

01953	15272	22552	32674
01968	15274	22585	33141
01969	15276	22614	33225
11001	15278	22632	33257
11008	15777	22634	33258
11045	15787	22840	33259
11046	15847	22841	33367
11047	16036	22842	33368
11101	17003	22843	33369
11201	17312	22844	33508
11732	17314	22845	33517
11922	17315	22846	33518
13102	19001	22847	33519
13122	19126	22848	33521
13133	19291	22851	33522
13153	19295	26125	33523
14302	19297	26861	33530
15003	20930	26863	33572
15005	20931	27358	33768
15101	20936	27692	33884
15111	20937	29826	33924
15116	20938	31620	34806
15121	20985	31627	34808
15131	22103	31632	34813
15136	22116	31633	34826
15151	22208	31637	35306
15152	22216	31649	35390
15156	22226	31651	35400
15157	22328	32501	35500
15201	22522	32506	35572
15221	22525	32507	35600
15241	22527	32667	35681
15261	22534	32668	35682

35683	48400	63088
35685	49326	63091
35686	49327	63103
35697	49412	63295
35700	49435	63308
36148	49568	63621
36218	49905	64480
36227	51797	64484
36228	56606	64491
36248	57267	64492
36476	58110	64494
36479	58611	64495
37185	59525	64634
37186	60512	64636
37206	61316	64727
37208	61517	64778
37222	61609	64783
37223	61610	64787
37232	61611	64832
37233	61612	64837
37234	61641	64859
37235	61642	64872
37250	61781	64874
37251	61782	64876
38102	61783	64901
38746	61797	64902
38747	61799	65757
38900	61800	66990
43273	61864	67225
43283	61868	67320
43338	62148	67331
43635	62160	67332
44015	63035	67334
44121	63043	67335
44128	63044	67340
44139	63048	69990
44203	63057	74301
44213	63066	75565
44701	63076	75774
44955	63078	75946
47001	63082	75964
47550	63086	75968

76125	92925	95915	99602
76802	92929	95916	99607
76810	92934	95940	0054T
76812	92938	95941	0055T
76814	92944	95962	0076T
76937	92973	95967	0079T
77001	92974	95973	0081T
77051	92978	95975	0092T
77052	92979	95979	0095T
78020	92998	96361	0098T
78496	93320	96366	0159T
78730	93321	96367	0163T
81266	93325	96368	0164T
82952	93352	96370	0165T
86826	93462	96371	0172T
87187	93463	96375	0174T
87503	93464	96376	0189T
87904	93563	96411	0190T
88155	93564	96415	0196T
88177	93565	96417	0205T
88185	93566	96423	0214T
88311	93567	96570	0215T
88314	93568	96571	0217T
88332	93571	97546	0218T
88334	93572	97598	0222T
88388	93609	97811	0229T
90461	93613	97814	0231T
90472	93621	99100	0241T
90474	93622	99116	0289T
90785	93623	99135	0290T
90833	93655	99140	0291T
90836	93657	99145	0292T
90838	93662	99150	0294T
90840	94645	99292	0300T
90863	94729	99354	0309T
91013	94781	99355	
92547	95079	99356	
92608	95873	99357	
92618	95874	99359	
92621	95885	99467	
92627	95886	99486	
92921	95887	99489	

Appendix E

Summary of CPT Codes Exempt from Modifier 51

This listing is a summary of CPT codes that are exempt from the use of modifier 51. Procedures on this list are typically performed with another procedure but may be a stand alone procedure and not always be performed with other specified procedures. For add-on codes see Appendix D. This is not an exhaustive list of procedures that are typically exempt from multiple procedure reductions. The codes listed below are identified in CPT 2013 with a ⊘ symbol.

17004	93451	93616
20697	93456	93618
20974	93503	93631
20975	93600	94610
31500	93602	95905
33961	93603	95992
36620	93610	99143
44500	93612	99144
61107	93615	0308T

Appendices A–E

Appendix F

Summary of CPT Codes Exempt from Modifier 63

The listing is a summary of CPT codes that are exempt from the use of modifier 63. The codes listed below are additionally identified in *CPT 2013* with the parenthetical instruction "(Do not report modifier 63 in conjunction with…)"

30540	36415	49496
30545	36420	49600
31520	36450	49605
33401	36460	49606
33403	36510	49610
33470	36660	49611
33472	39503	53025
33502	43313	54000
33503	43314	54150
33505	43520	54160
33506	43831	63700
33610	44055	63702
33611	44126	63704
33619	44127	63706
33647	44128	65820
33670	46070	99337
33690	46705	
33694	46715	
33730	46716	
33732	46730	
33735	46735	
33736	46740	
33750	46742	
33755	46744	
33762	47700	
33778	47701	
33786	49215	
33922	49491	
33960	49492	
33961	49495	

Appendixes F–J

Appendix G

Summary of CPT Codes That Include Moderate (Conscious) Sedation

The following list of procedures includes conscious sedation as an inherent part of providing the procedure. These codes are identified in the CPT codebook with a ⊙ symbol.

►Since these services include moderate sedation, it is not appropriate for the same physician or other qualified health care professional to report both the service and the sedation codes 99143-99145. It is expected that if conscious sedation is provided to the patient as part of one of these services, it is provided by the same physician or other qualified health care professional who is providing the service.

In the unusual event when a second physician or other qualified health care professional other than the health care professional performing the diagnostic or therapeutic services provides moderate sedation in the facility setting (eg, hospital, outpatient hospital/ambulatory surgery center, skilled nursing facility) for the procedures listed in Appendix G, the second individual can report 99148-99150. However, for the circumstance in which these services are performed by the second individual in the nonfacility setting (eg, office, freestanding imaging center), codes 99148-99150 would not be reported. Moderate sedation does not include minimal sedation (anxiolysis), deep sedation, or monitored anesthesia care (00100-01999).

The inclusion of a procedure on this list does not prevent separate reporting of an associated anesthesia procedure/service (CPT codes 00100-01999) when performed by a physician or other qualified health care professional other than the health care professional performing the diagnostic or therapeutic procedure. In such cases, the person providing anesthesia services shall be present for the purpose of continuously monitoring the patient and shall not act as a surgical assistant. When clinical conditions of the patient require such anesthesia services or in the circumstances when the patient does not require sedation, the operating physician or other qualified health care professional is not required to report the procedure as a reduced service using modifier 52.◄

19298	22522	31620	31625
20982	22526	31622	31626
22520	22527	31623	31627
22521	31615	31624	31628

31629	33235	36560
31634	33240	36561
31635	33241	36563
31645	33244	36565
31646	33249	36566
31647	33262	36568
31648	33263	36570
31649	33264	36571
31651	33990	36576
31660	33991	36578
31661	33992	36581
31725	33993	36582
32201	35471	36583
32405	35472	36585
32550	35475	36590
32551	35476	36870
32553	36010	37183
33010	36140	37184
33011	36147	37185
33206	36148	37186
33207	36200	37187
33208	36221	37188
33210	36222	37191
33211	36223	37192
33212	36224	37193
33213	36225	37197
33214	36226	37210
33216	36227	37211
33217	36228	37212
33218	36245	37213
33220	36246	37214
33221	36247	37215
33222	36248	37216
33223	36251	37220
33227	36252	37221
33228	36253	37222
33229	36254	37223
33230	36481	37224
33231	36555	37225
33233	36557	37226
33234	36558	37227

Appendixes F–J

37228	43251	44386	45385	92925	93464	0291T
37229	43252	44388	45386	92928	93505	0292T
37230	43255	44389	45387	92929	93530	0293T
37231	43256	44390	45391	92933	93561	0294T
37232	43257	44391	45392	92934	93562	0301T
37233	43258	44392	47000	92937	93563	0302T
37234	43259	44393	47011	92938	93564	0303T
37235	43260	44394	47382	92941	93565	0304T
43200	43261	44397	47525	92943	93566	0307T
43201	43262	44500	48511	92944	93567	0308T
43202	43263	44901	49021	92953	93568	
43204	43264	45303	49041	92960	93571	
43205	43265	45305	49061	92961	93572	
43206	43267	45307	49411	92973	93609	
43215	43268	45308	49418	92974	93613	
43216	43269	45309	49440	92975	93615	
43217	43271	45315	49441	92978	93616	
43219	43272	45317	49442	92979	93618	
43220	43273	45320	49446	92986	93619	
43226	43453	45321	50021	92987	93620	
43227	43456	45327	50200	93312	93621	
43228	43458	45332	50382	93313	93622	
43231	44360	45333	50384	93314	93624	
43232	44361	45334	50385	93315	93640	
43235	44363	45335	50386	93316	93641	
43236	44364	45337	50387	93317	93642	
43237	44365	45338	50592	93318	93650	
43238	44366	45339	50593	93451	93653	
43239	44369	45340	57155	93452	93654	
43240	44370	45341	58823	93453	93655	
43241	44372	45342	66720	93454	93656	
43242	44373	45345	69300	93455	93657	
43243	44376	45355	77371	93456	94011	
43244	44377	45378	77600	93457	94012	
43245	44378	45379	77605	93458	94013	
43246	44379	45380	77610	93459	0200T	
43247	44380	45381	77615	93460	0201T	
43248	44382	45382	92920	93461	0282T	
43249	44383	45383	92921	93462	0283T	
43250	44385	45384	92924	93463	0284T	

Appendix H

Alphabetical Clinical Topics Listing (AKA – Alphabetical Listing)

The Alphabetical Clinical Topics Listing (formerly Appendix H) has been removed from the CPT codebook. Since this document is a dynamic and rapidly expanding source of information to link CPT Category II codes, clinical conditions, and measure abstracts, the Alphabetical Listing is now solely accessed on the AMA Web site at www.ama-assn.org/go/cpt.

In addition, new codes for the publication cycle (ie, **the Update to the List of Category II Codes**) will continue to be located on the AMA Web site prior to publication in the next edition of the CPT codebook (subsequent to its listing to the Web).

Appendix I

Genetic Testing Code Modifiers

The Genetic Testing Code Modifiers (formerly Appendix I) has been removed from the CPT codebook.

The addition of more than 100 molecular pathology codes to the 2012 code set and still more codes to the 2013 CPT code set resulted in the deletion of the stacking codes (83890–83914). The genetic testing code modifiers formerly described in Appendix I applied to those stacking codes, and therefore, the Appendix and modifiers have been removed from the 2013 code set.

The rapidly evolving science of molecular pathology genetic testing will be an important part of the physician's tools for diagnosis and management of patients. To help explain the new codes that will be reported for these molecular pathology services, an article titled "Molecular Pathology" has been added to the Front Matter on page xix of the codebook. This article is an update to the article in the May 2012 *CPT Assistant*, the official AMA document of record for the CPT code set.

For the most up-to-date information on future updates for molecular pathology coding in the CPT code set, see www.ama-assn.org/ama/pub/physician-resources/solutions-managing-your-practice/coding-billing-insurance/cpt/about-cpt/mopath-codes.page.

Appendixes F–J

Appendix J

Electrodiagnostic Medicine Listing of Sensory, Motor, and Mixed Nerves

This summary assigns each sensory, motor, and mixed nerve with its appropriate nerve conduction study code in order to enhance accurate reporting of codes 95907-95913. Each nerve constitutes one unit of service.

Motor Nerves Assigned to Codes 95900 and 95907-95913

I. Upper extremity, cervical plexus, and brachial plexus motor nerves
   A. Axillary motor nerve to the deltoid
   B. Long thoracic motor nerve to the serratus anterior
   C. Median nerve
      1. Median motor nerve to the abductor pollicis brevis
      2. Median motor nerve, anterior interosseous branch, to the flexor pollicis longus
      3. Median motor nerve, anterior interosseous branch, to the pronator quadratus
      4. Median motor nerve to the first lumbrical
      5. Median motor nerve to the second lumbrical
   D. Musculocutaneous motor nerve to the biceps brachii
   E. Radial nerve
      1. Radial motor nerve to the extensor carpi ulnaris
      2. Radial motor nerve to the extensor digitorum communis
      3. Radial motor nerve to the extensor indicis proprius
      4. Radial motor nerve to the brachioradialis
   F. Suprascapular nerve
      1. Suprascapular motor nerve to the supraspinatus
      2. Suprascapular motor nerve to the infraspinatus
   G. Thoracodorsal motor nerve to the latissimus dorsi

H. Ulnar nerve
   1. Ulnar motor nerve to the abductor digiti minimi
   2. Ulnar motor nerve to the palmar interosseous
   3. Ulnar motor nerve to the first dorsal interosseous
   4. Ulnar motor nerve to the flexor carpi ulnaris
I. Other

II. Lower extremity motor nerves
   A. Femoral motor nerve to the quadriceps
      1. Femoral motor nerve to vastus medialis
      2. Femoral motor nerve to vastus lateralis
      3. Femoral motor nerve to vastus intermedialis
      4. Femoral motor nerve to rectus femoris
   B. Ilioinguinal motor nerve
   C. Peroneal (fibular) nerve
      1. Peroneal motor nerve to the extensor digitorum brevis
      2. Peroneal motor nerve to the peroneus brevis
      3. Peroneal motor nerve to the peroneus longus
      4. Peroneal motor nerve to the tibialis anterior
   D. Plantar motor nerve
   E. Sciatic nerve
   F. Tibial nerve
      1. Tibial motor nerve, inferior calcaneal branch, to the abductor digiti minimi
      2. Tibial motor nerve, medial plantar branch, to the abductor hallucis
      3. Tibial motor nerve, lateral plantar branch, to the flexor digiti minimi brevis
   G. Other

III. Cranial nerves and trunk
   A. Cranial nerve VII (facial motor nerve)
      1. Facial nerve to the frontalis
      2. Facial nerve to the nasalis
      3. Facial nerve to the orbicularis oculi
      4. Facial nerve to the orbicularis oris
   B. Cranial nerve XI (spinal accessory motor nerve)
   C. Cranial nerve XII (hypoglossal motor nerve)
   D. Intercostal motor nerve
   E. Phrenic motor nerve to the diaphragm
   F. Recurrent laryngeal nerve
   G. Other

IV. Nerve Roots
   A. Cervical nerve root stimulation
      1. Cervical level 5 (CT)
      2. Cervical level 6 (C6)
      3. Cervical level 7 (C7)
      4. Cervical level 8 (C8)

B. Thoracic nerve root stimulation
   1. Thoracic level 1 (T1)
   2. Thoracic level 2 (T2)
   3. Thoracic level 3 (T3)
   4. Thoracic level 4 (T4)
   5. Thoracic level 5 (T5)
   6. Thoracic level 6 (T6)
   7. Thoracic level 7 (T7)
   8. Thoracic level 8 (T8)
   9. Thoracic level 9 (T9)
   10. Thoracic level 10 (T10)
   11. Thoracic level 11 (T11)
   12. Thoracic level 12 (T12)
C. Lumbar nerve root stimulation
   1. Lumbar level 1 (L1)
   2. Lumbar level 2 (L2)
   3. Lumbar level 3 (L3)
   4. Lumbar level 4 (L4)
   5. Lumbar level 5 (L5)
D. Sacral nerve root stimulation
   1. Sacral level 1 (S1)
   2. Sacral level 2 (S2)
   3. Sacral level 3 (S3)
   4. Sacral level 4 (S4)

Sensory and Mixed Nerves Assigned to Codes 95907-95913

I. Upper extremity sensory and mixed nerves
   A. Lateral antebrachial cutaneous sensory nerve
   B. Medial antebrachial cutaneous sensory nerve
   C. Medial brachial cutaneous sensory nerve
   D. Median nerve
      1. Median sensory nerve to the first digit
      2. Median sensory nerve to the second digit
      3. Median sensory nerve to the third digit
      4. Median sensory nerve to the fourth digit
      5. Median palmar cutaneous sensory nerve
      6. Median palmar mixed nerve
   E. Posterior antebrachial cutaneous sensory nerve
   F. Radial sensory nerve
      1. Radial sensory nerve to the base of the thumb
      2. Radial sensory nerve to digit 1
   G. Ulnar nerve
      1. Ulnar dorsal cutaneous sensory nerve
      2. Ulnar sensory nerve to the fourth digit
      3. Ulnar sensory nerve to the fifth digit
      4. Ulnar palmar mixed nerve
   H. Intercostal sensory nerve
   I. Other

II. Lower extremity sensory and mixed nerves
   A. Lateral femoral cutaneous sensory nerve
   B. Medial calcaneal sensory nerve
   C. Medial femoral cutaneous sensory nerve
   D. Peroneal nerve
      1. Deep peroneal sensory nerve
      2. Superficial peroneal sensory nerve, medial dorsal cutaneous branch
      3. Superficial peroneal sensory nerve, intermediate dorsal cutaneous branch
   E. Posterior femoral cutaneous sensory nerve
   F. Saphenous nerve
      1. Saphenous sensory nerve (distal technique)
      2. Saphenous sensory nerve (proximal technique)
   G. Sural nerve
      1. Sural sensory nerve, lateral dorsal cutaneous branch
      2. Sural sensory nerve
   H. Tibial sensory nerve (digital nerve to toe 1)
   I. Tibial sensory nerve (medial plantar nerve)
   J. Tibial sensory nerve (lateral plantar nerve)
   K. Other
III. Head and trunk sensory nerves
   A. Dorsal nerve of the penis
   B. Greater auricular nerve
   C. Ophthalmic branch of the trigeminal nerve
   D. Pudendal sensory nerve
   E. Suprascapular sensory nerves
   F. Other

Appendixes F–J

The following table provides a reasonable maximum number of studies performed per diagnostic category necessary for a physician to arrive at a diagnosis in 90% of patients with that final diagnosis. The numbers in each column represent the number of studies recommended. The appropriate number of studies to be performed is based upon the physician's discretion.

	Type of Study/Maximum Number of Studies		
Indication	**Limbs Studied by Needle EMG (95860-95864, 95867-95870, 95885-95887)**	**Nerve Conduction Studies (Total nerves studied, 95907-95913)**	**Neuromuscular Junction Testing (Repetitive Stimulation, 95937)**
Carpal Tunnel (Unilateral)	1	7	—
Carpal Tunnel (Bilateral)	2	10	—
Radiculopathy	2	7	—
Mononeuropathy	1	8	—
Polyneuropathy/Mononeuropathy Multiplex	3	10	—
Myopathy	2	4	2
Motor Neuronopathy (eg, ALS)	4	6	2
Plexopathy	2	12	—
Neuromuscular Junction	2	4	3
Tarsal Tunnel Syndrome (Unilateral)	1	8	—
Tarsal Tunnel Syndrome (Bilateral)	2	11	—
Weakness, Fatigue, Cramps, or Twitching (Focal)	2	7	2
Weakness, Fatigue, Cramps, or Twitching (General)	4	8	2
Pain, Numbness, or Tingling (Unilateral)	1	9	—
Pain, Numbness, or Tingling (Bilateral)	2	12	—

Appendix K

Product Pending FDA Approval

Some vaccine products have been assigned a CPT Category I code in anticipation of future approval from the Food and Drug Administration (FDA). Following is a list of the vaccine product codes pending FDA approval status that are identified in the CPT codebook with the (✔) symbol. Upon revision of the approval status by the FDA, notation of this revision will be provided via the AMA CPT "Category I Vaccine Codes" Internet listing (www.ama-assn.org/ama/pub/category/10902.html) and in subsequent publications of the CPT codebook.

90653
90661
90666
90667
90668
90739

Appendix L

Vascular Families

Assignment of branches to first, second, and third order in this table makes the assumption that the starting point is catheterization of the aorta. This categorization would not be accurate, for instance, if a femoral or carotid artery were catheterized directly in an antegrade direction. Arteries highlighted in bold are those more commonly reported during arteriographic procedures.

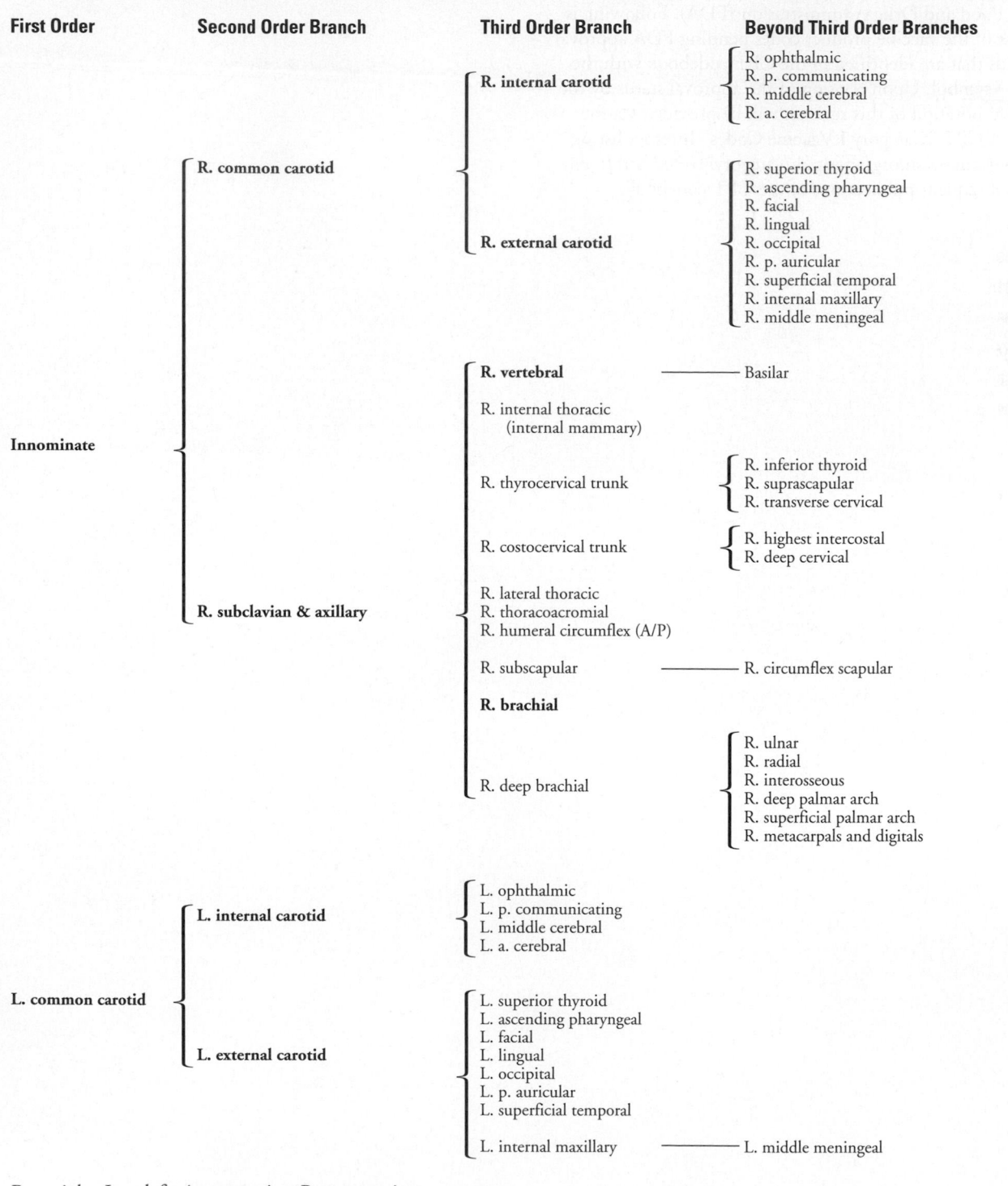

First Order	Second Order Branch	Third Order Branch	Beyond Third Order Branches
	R. common carotid	**R. internal carotid**	R. ophthalmic R. p. communicating R. middle cerebral R. a. cerebral
		R. external carotid	R. superior thyroid R. ascending pharyngeal R. facial R. lingual R. occipital R. p. auricular R. superficial temporal R. internal maxillary R. middle meningeal
Innominate		**R. vertebral**	Basilar
		R. internal thoracic (internal mammary)	
		R. thyrocervical trunk	R. inferior thyroid R. suprascapular R. transverse cervical
		R. costocervical trunk	R. highest intercostal R. deep cervical
	R. subclavian & axillary	R. lateral thoracic R. thoracoacromial R. humeral circumflex (A/P)	
		R. subscapular	R. circumflex scapular
		R. brachial	
		R. deep brachial	R. ulnar R. radial R. interosseous R. deep palmar arch R. superficial palmar arch R. metacarpals and digitals
L. common carotid	**L. internal carotid**	L. ophthalmic L. p. communicating L. middle cerebral L. a. cerebral	
	L. external carotid	L. superior thyroid L. ascending pharyngeal L. facial L. lingual L. occipital L. p. auricular L. superficial temporal	
		L. internal maxillary	L. middle meningeal

R = right, L = left, A = anterior, P = posterior

First Order	Second Order Branch	Third Order Branch	Beyond Third Order Branches

L. subclavian & axillary

- **L. vertebral**
- L. internal thoracic (internal mammary)
- L. thyrocervical trunk
  - L. inferior thyroid
  - L. suprascapular
  - L. transverse cervical
- L. costocervical trunk
  - L. highest intercostal
  - L. deep cervical
- L. lateral thoracic
- L. thoracoacromial
- L. humeral circumflex (A/P)
- L. subscapular —— L. circumflex scapular
- **L. brachial**
- L. deep brachial
  - L. ulnar
  - L. radial
  - L. interosseous
    - L. deep palmar arch
    - L. superficial palmar arch
    - L. metacarpals and digitals

Intercostals

Bronchials

Recurrent esophageal

Inferior phrenic —— Superior suprarenal

Celiac trunk

- L. gastric —— Esophageal branch
- Splenic
  - Dorsal pancreatic —— Inferior transverse pancreatic
  - Great pancreatic
  - Caudal pancreatic
  - Gastroepiploic
  - Short gastrics
- Common hepatic
  - Gastroduodenal
    - P. superior pancreaticoduodenal
    - A. superior pancreaticoduodenal
  - Proper Hepatic
    - L. hepatic
    - R. hepatic
    - Cystic
    - Gastroepiploic
    - Supraduodenal
    - Intermediate hepatic

Middle suprarenal

Superior mesenteric

- Middle colic
- Inferior pancreaticoduodenal
  - P. inferior pancreaticoduodenal
  - A. inferior pancreaticoduodenal
- Jejunal
- Ileocolic
- Appendicular
- P. cecal
- A. cecal
- Marginal
- R. colic

R = right, L = left, A = anterior, P = posterior

First Order	Second Order Branch	Third Order Branch	Beyond Third Order Branches

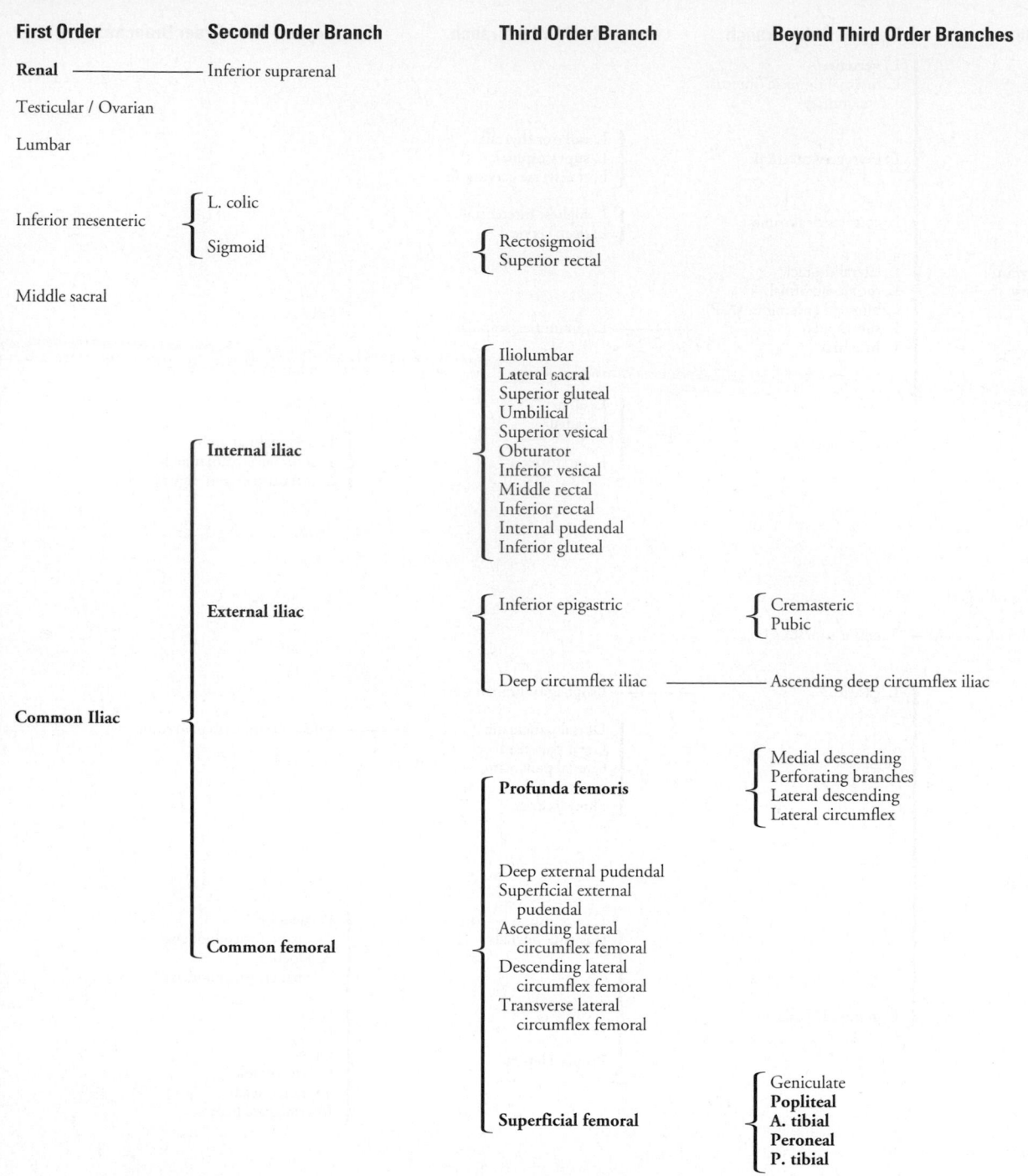

Renal ——————— Inferior suprarenal

Testicular / Ovarian

Lumbar

Inferior mesenteric
- L. colic
- Sigmoid
  - Rectosigmoid
  - Superior rectal

Middle sacral

Common Iliac

Internal iliac
- Iliolumbar
- Lateral sacral
- Superior gluteal
- Umbilical
- Superior vesical
- Obturator
- Inferior vesical
- Middle rectal
- Inferior rectal
- Internal pudendal
- Inferior gluteal

External iliac
- Inferior epigastric
  - Cremasteric
  - Pubic
- Deep circumflex iliac ——————— Ascending deep circumflex iliac

Common femoral
- **Profunda femoris**
  - Medial descending
  - Perforating branches
  - Lateral descending
  - Lateral circumflex
- Deep external pudendal
- Superficial external pudendal
- Ascending lateral circumflex femoral
- Descending lateral circumflex femoral
- Transverse lateral circumflex femoral
- **Superficial femoral**
  - Geniculate
  - **Popliteal**
  - **A. tibial**
  - **Peroneal**
  - **P. tibial**

R. & L. main pulmonary arteries (venous selective)

Reference: Kadir S. *Atlas of Normal and Variant Angiographic Anatomy.* Philadephia, Pa: WB Saunders Co; 1991.
R = right, L = left, A = anterior, P = posterior

Appendix M

Deleted CPT Codes

This listing is a summary of crosswalked deleted and renumbered codes and descriptors with the associated *CPT Assistant* references for the deleted codes. This listing includes codes deleted and renumbered from 2007 to 2009. Additional codes will not be added, since the principle of deleting and renumbering is no longer being utilized in the CPT code set.

Current Code(s)	Deleted/Former Code	Year Code Deleted	Citations Referencing Former Code— Applicable to Current Code(s)
89240	0058T	2009	Jun 04:8 CPT Changes: An Insider's View 2004
89240	0059T	2009	CPT Changes: An Insider's View 2004
41530	0088T	2009	May 05:7, Sep 05:9 CPT Changes: An Insider's View 2005
95803	0089T	2009	Jun 05:6, Feb 06:1 CPT Changes: An Insider's View 2006
22856	0090T	2009	Jun 05:6, Feb 06:1 CPT Changes: An Insider's View 2006, 2007
22864	0093T	2009	Jun 05:6, Feb 06:1 CPT Changes: An Insider's View 2006, 2007
22861	0096T	2009	Jun 05:6, Feb 06:1 CPT Changes: An Insider's View 2006, 2007
55706	0137T	2009	CPT Changes: An Insider's View 2006
95980-95982	0162T	2009	CPT Changes: An Insider's View 2007
1123F, 1124F	1080F	2009	CPT Changes: An Insider's View 2008
0054T, 0055T	20986	2009	CPT Changes: An Insider's View 2008
0054T, 0055T	20987	2009	CPT Changes: An Insider's View 2008
4177F	4007F	2009	CPT Changes: An Insider's View 2008
52214	52606	2009	Apr 01:4
52601	52612	2009	Apr 01:4
52601	52614	2009	Apr 01:4
52630	52620	2009	Apr 01:4
61796-61800, 63020, 63621	61793	2009	Nov 97:23, May 03:19, Apr 04:15, Jan 06:46
77785, 77786	77781	2009	Winter 90:10, Winter 91:23, Mar 99:3, Feb 02:7, Mar 02:2, Sep 05:1, Nov 05:15
77785-77787	77782	2009	Winter 90:10, Winter 91:23, Mar 99:3, Feb 02:7, Mar 02:2, Sep 05:1, Nov 05:15
77785-77787	77783	2009	Winter 90:10, Winter 91:23, Mar 99:3, Feb 02:7, Mar 02:2, Sep 05:1, Nov 05:15
77785-77787	77784	2009	Winter 90:10, Winter 91:23, Mar 99:3, Feb 02:7, Mar 02:2, Sep 05:1, Nov 05:15
88720	88400	2009	Aug 05:9
96360	90760	2009	Nov 05:1, Jul 06:4, Sep 06:14, Dec 06:14 CPT Changes: An Insider's View 2006, 2008
96361	90761	2009	Nov 05:1, Jul 06:4, Sep 06:14, Dec 06:14, Mar 07:10 CPT Changes: An Insider's View 2006, 2007
96365	90765	2009	Nov 05:1, Sep 06:14, Nov 06:22, Dec 06:14 CPT Changes: An Insider's View 2006
96366	90766	2009	Nov 05:1, Sep 06:14, Dec 06:14, Mar 07:10 CPT Changes: An Insider's View 2006, 2007
96367	90767	2009	Nov 05:1, Sep 06:14, Nov 06:22, Dec 06:14 CPT Changes: An Insider's View 2006
96368	90768	2009	Nov 05:1, Aug 06:11, Sep 06:14, Nov 06:22, Dec 06:14 CPT Changes: An Insider's View 2006
96369	90769	2009	CPT Changes: An Insider's View 2008
96370	90770	2009	CPT Changes: An Insider's View 2008
96371	90771	2009	CPT Changes: An Insider's View 2008
96372	90772	2009	Nov 05:1, Sep 06:14, Dec 06:14 CPT Changes: An Insider's View 2006
96373	90773	2009	Nov 05:1, Sep 06:14, Dec 06:14 CPT Changes: An Insider's View 2006

Current Code(s)	Deleted/Former Code	Year Code Deleted	Citations Referencing Former Code— Applicable to Current Code(s)
96374	90774	2009	Nov 05:1, Sep 06:14, Dec 06:14 CPT Changes: An Insider's View 2006
96375	90775	2009	Nov 05:1, Sep 06:14, Dec 06:14 CPT Changes: An Insider's View 2006
96376	90776	2009	CPT Changes: An Insider's View 2008
96379	90779	2009	Nov 05:1, Sep 06:14, Dec 06:14 CPT Changes: An Insider's View 2006
90951-90953, 90963, 90967	90918	2009	Fall 93:5, May 96:4, May 02:17, Jan 03:22
90954-90956, 90964, 90968	90919	2009	Fall 93:5, May 96:5, May 02:17, Jan 03:22
90957-90959, 90965, 90969	90920	2009	Fall 93:5, May 96:5, May 02:17, Jan 03:22
90960-90962, 90966, 90970	90921	2009	Fall 93:5, May 96:5, May 02:17, Jan 03:22
90951-90953, 90963, 90967	90922	2009	Fall 93:5, May 96:5, May 02:17, Jan 03:22
90954-90956, 90964, 90968	90923	2009	May 96:5, May 02:17, Jan 03:22
90957-90959, 90965, 90969	90924	2009	May 96:5, May 02:17, Jan 03:22
90960-90962, 90966, 90970	90925	2009	May 96:5, May 02:17, Jan 03:22
93285, 93291, 93298	93727	2009	Nov 99:50, Jul 00:5, CPT Changes: An Insider's View 2000
93280, 93288, 93294	93731	2009	Summer 94:23, Feb 98:11
93280, 93288, 93294	93732	2009	Summer 94:23, Feb 98:11, Mar 00:10
93293	93733	2009	Summer 94:23
93279, 93288, 93294	93734	2009	Summer 94:23, Feb 98:11
93279, 93288, 93294	93735	2009	Summer 94:23, Feb 98:11
93293	93736	2009	Summer 94:23
93282, 93289, 93292, 93295	93741	2009	Nov 99:50-51, Jul 00:5, Nov 00:9, Sep 05:8 CPT Changes: An Insider's View 2000, 2005
93282, 93289, 93292, 93295	93742	2009	Nov 99:50-51, Jul 00:5, Nov 00:9 CPT Changes: An Insider's View 2000, 2005
93283, 93289, 93295	93743	2009	Nov 99:50-51, Jul 00:5, Nov 00:9, Sep 05:8 CPT Changes: An Insider's View 2000
93283, 93289, 93295	93744	2009	Nov 99:50-51, Jul 00:5, Nov 00:9 CPT Changes: An Insider's View 2000
99466	99289	2009	May 05:1, Jul 06:4 CPT Changes: An Insider's View 2002, 2003
99467	99290	2009	CPT Changes: An Insider's View 2002
99471	99293	2009	Feb 03:15, Oct 03:2, Aug 04:7, 10, May 05:1, Nov 05:10, Jul 06:4, Apr 07:3 CPT Changes: An Insider's View 2003, 2004, 2005
99472	99294	2009	Feb 03:15, Oct 03:2, Aug 04:7, Nov 05:10, Jul 06:4, Apr 07:3 CPT Changes: An Insider's View 2003, 2004, 2005
99468	99295	2009	Summer 93:1, Nov 97:4-5, Mar 98:11, Nov 99:5-6, Dec 00:14, Feb 03:15, Oct 03:1, May 05:1, Nov 05:10, CPT Changes: An Insider's View 2000, 2003, 2004, 2005
99469	99296	2009	Summer 93:1, Nov 97:4-5, Mar 98:11, Nov 99:5-6, Dec 00:14, Feb 03:15, Oct 03:1, Nov 05:10, CPT Changes: An Insider's View 2000, 2003, 2004, 2005, 2008

Current Code(s)	Deleted/Former Code	Year Code Deleted	Citations Referencing Former Code— Applicable to Current Code(s)
99478	99298	2009	Nov 98:2-3, Nov 99: 5-6, Aug 00:4, Dec 00:15, Oct 03:2, May 05:1, Nov 05:10; CPT Changes: An Insider's View 2000, 2003
99479	99299	2009	Oct 03:2, Nov 05:10; CPT Changes: An Insider's View 2003
99480	99300	2009	CPT Changes: An Insider's View 2006
99460	99431	2009	Apr 97:10, Nov 97:9, Sep 98:5, Apr 04:14, May 05:1
99461	99432	2009	Sep 98:5, May 99:11, Apr 04:14
99462	99433	2009	Sep 98:5, Apr 03:27
99463	99435	2009	Sep 98:5, Apr 04:14
99464	99436	2009	Nov 97:9-10, Sep 98:5, Nov 99:5-6, Aug 00:3, Aug 04:9, Nov 05:15
99465	99440	2009	Summer 93:3, Mar 96:10, Nov 97:9, Sep 98:5, Nov 99:5-6, Aug 00:3, Oct 03:3, Aug 04:9, Apr 07:3
20985-20987	0054T	2008	May 04:14, Jun 04:8 CPT Changes: An Insider's View 2004
20985-20987	0055T	2008	May 04:14, Jun 04:8 CPT Changes: An Insider's View 2004, 2005
20985-20987	0056T	2008	May 04:14, Jun 04:8 CPT Changes: An Insider's View 2004
99174	0065T	2008	Mar 05:1, 3-4 CPT Changes: An Insider's View 2005
99444	0074T	2008	May 05:7, Sep 05:6 CPT Changes: An Insider's View 2005
99605-99607	0115T	2008	CPT Changes: An Insider's View 2006
99605-99607	0116T	2008	CPT Changes: An Insider's View 2006
99605-99607	0117T	2008	CPT Changes: An Insider's View 2006
50593	0135T	2008	CPT Changes: An Insider's View 2006, Clinical Examples in Radiology Winter 06:18
34806	0153T	2008	CPT Changes: An Insider's View 2007, Clinical Examples in Radiology Winter 06:19
93982	0154T	2008	CPT Changes: An Insider's View 2007, Clinical Examples in Radiology Winter 06:19
01935, 01936	01905	2008	Mar 06:15 CPT Changes: An Insider's View 2002
24357-24359	24350	2008	
24357-24359	24351	2008	
24357-24359	24352	2008	
24357-24359	24354	2008	
24357-24359	24356	2008	
3044F-3045F	3047F	2008	CPT Changes: An Insider's View 2007
3074F-3075F	3076F	2008	CPT Changes: An Insider's View 2007
32421	32000	2008	Spring 91:4, Winter 92:20
32422	32002	2008	Nov 03:14
32560	32005	2008	
32550	32019	2008	CPT Changes: An Insider's View 2005
32551	32020	2008	Fall 92:13, Nov 03:14
36591	36540	2008	Jan 02:11, Nov 02:3, Apr 03:26, Nov 05:1 CPT Changes: An Insider's View 2001, 2003
36593	36550	2008	Nov 99:20, Nov 05:1 CPT Changes: An Insider's View 2000
49203-49205, 58957, 58958	49200	2008	CPT Changes: An Insider's View 2003
49203-49205, 58957, 58958	49201	2008	
51100	51000	2008	Nov 99:32-33, Aug 00:3, Oct 03:2
51101	51005	2008	
51102	51010	2008	
60300	60001	2008	
67041, 67042, 67043	67038	2008	Aug 03:15, Sep 05:12

Current Code(s)	Deleted/Former Code	Year Code Deleted	Citations Referencing Former Code— Applicable to Current Code(s)
75557-75564	75552	2008	Fall 95:2
75557-75564	75553	2008	Fall 95:2
75557-75564	75554	2008	Fall 95:2
75557-75564	75555	2008	Fall 95:2
75557-75564	75556	2008	Fall 95:2
78610	78615	2008	CPT Changes: An Insider's View 2002
86356, 86486	86586	2008	Jul 98:11
99366-99368	99361	2008	May 05:1
99366-99368	99362	2008	
99441-99443	99371	2008	Spring 94:34, May 00:11, May 05:1, Nov 05:10
99441-99443	99372	2008	Spring 94:34, May 00:11, Nov 05:10
99441-99443	99373	2008	Spring 94:34, May 00:11, Nov 05:10
0160T, 0161T	0018T	2007	CPT Changes: An Insider's View 2002
96904	0044T	2007	CPT Changes: An Insider's View 2003, 2004
96904	0045T	2007	Jul 04:7 CPT Changes: An Insider's View 2004
77371-77373	0082T	2007	CPT Changes: An Insider's View 2005
77371-77373	0083T	2007	CPT Changes: An Insider's View 2005
22857	0091T	2007	CPT Changes: An Insider's View 2006
22865	0094T	2007	CPT Changes: An Insider's View 2006
22862	0097T	2007	CPT Changes: An Insider's View 2006
19105	0120T	2007	CPT Changes: An Insider's View 2006
15002, 15004	15000	2007	Fall 93:7, Apr 97:4, Aug 97:6, Sep 97:2, Nov 98:5, Jan 99:4, Apr 99:10, May 99:10, Nov 02:7, Aug 03:14 CPT Changes: An Insider's View 2001, 2006
15003, 15005	15001	2007	Nov 98:5-6, Jan 99:4, May 99:10, Aug 03:14
15830, 15847, 17999	15831	2007	May 01:11 CPT Changes: An Insider's View 2007
17311	17304	2007	Winter 94:19, Mar 99:11, Jun 99:10, Nov 02:7, Nov 03:15, Feb 04:11, Jul 04:2 CPT Changes: An Insider's View 2003
17312, 17314	17305	2007	Winter 94:19, Mar 99:11, Jun 99:10, Nov 02:7, Feb 04:11, Jul 04:3
17312, 17314	17306	2007	Winter 94:19, Mar 99:11, Jun 99:10, Nov 02:7, Feb 04:11, Jul 04:4
17312, 17314	17307	2007	Winter 94:19, Mar 99:11, Jun 99:10, Nov 02:7, Nov 03:15, Feb 04:11, Jul 04:4
17315	17310	2007	Winter 94:19, Mar 99:11, Jun 99:10, Nov 02:7, Feb 04:11, May 04:14, Jul 04:4 CPT Changes: An Insider's View 2003
19300	19140	2007	Feb 96:9, Apr 05:13
19301	19160	2007	Apr 05:7 CPT Changes: An Insider's View 2005
19302	19162	2007	Jun 00:11, Apr 05:7
19303	19180	2007	Apr 05:7
19304	19182	2007	Apr 05:7
19305	19200	2007	Apr 05:7
19306	19220	2007	Apr 05:7
19307	19240	2007	Apr 05:7
25606	25611	2007	Fall 93:23, Oct 99:5
25607-25609	25620	2007	
26390	26504	2007	
27325	27315	2007	
27326	27320	2007	

Current Code(s)	Deleted/Former Code	Year Code Deleted	Citations Referencing Former Code—Applicable to Current Code(s)
28055	28030	2007	
33254-33256	33253	2007	
35302-35306	35381	2007	
35506	35507	2007	
35537, 35538	35541	2007	
35539, 35540	35546	2007	
35637, 35638	35641	2007	Dec 01:7
44799	44152	2007	
44799	44153	2007	
47719	47716	2007	
48105	48005	2007	
48548	48180	2007	
49402	49085	2007	
54150	54152	2007	Sep 96:11, Dec 96:10, May 98:11, Apr 03:27 CPT Changes: An Insider's View 2007
54865	54820	2007	Oct 01:8
55875	55859	2007	Apr 04:6
56442	56720	2007	
57558	57820	2007	
67346	67350	2007	
77001	75998	2007	Dec 04:12-13 CPT Changes: An Insider's View 2004 Clinical Examples in Radiology Inaugural 04:1-2, Winter 05:9
77002	76003	2007	Fall 93:14, Jul 01:7 CPT Changes: An Insider's View 2001 Clinical Examples in Radiology Spring 05:5-6
77003	76005	2007	Nov 99:32, 34, 41, Jan 00:2, Feb 00:6, Aug 00:8, Sep 02:11, Sep 04:5 CPT Changes: An Insider's View 2000
77071	76006	2007	Nov 98:21 CPT Changes: An Insider's View 2003
72291	76012	2007	Mar 01:2 CPT Changes: An Insider's View 2001, 2006
72292	76013	2007	Mar 01:2 CPT Changes: An Insider's View 2001
77072	76020	2007	
77073	76040	2007	
77074	76061	2007	
77075	76062	2007	
77076	76065	2007	
77077	76066	2007	CPT Changes: An Insider's View 2002
77078	76070	2007	Nov 97:24 CPT Changes: An Insider's View 2002, 2003
77079	76071	2007	CPT Changes: An Insider's View 2003
77080	76075	2007	Nov 97:24, Jun 03:11 CPT Changes: An Insider's View 2005
77081	76076	2007	Nov 97:24
77082	76077	2007	CPT Changes: An Insider's View 2005
77083	76078	2007	Nov 97:24 CPT Changes: An Insider's View 2002
77051	76082	2007	CPT Changes: An Insider's View 2004
77052	76083	2007	CPT Changes: An Insider's View 2004
77053	76086	2007	
77054	76088	2007	
77055	76090	2007	Jul 96:6, Jun 99:10 CPT Changes: An Insider's View 2004
77056	76091	2007	Jul 96:6 CPT Changes: An Insider's View 2004

Appendixes K–O

Current Code(s)	Deleted/Former Code	Year Code Deleted	Citations Referencing Former Code—Applicable to Current Code(s)
77057	76092	2007	Jul 96:6, Jun 99:10 CPT Changes: An Insider's View 2004
77058	76093	2007	
77059	76094	2007	
77031	76095	2007	Apr 96:9, Nov 97:24, Jan 01:9 CPT Changes: An Insider's View 2001
77032	76096	2007	Jan 01:10 CPT Changes: An Insider's View 2001
77011	76355	2007	CPT Changes: An Insider's View 2002, 2003
77012	76360	2007	Fall 93:12, Fall 94:2, Jan 01:9-10, Mar 05:2 CPT Changes: An Insider's View 2001, 2002, 2003
77013	76362	2007	Oct 02:4 CPT Changes: An Insider's View 2002, 2004
77014	76370	2007	Fall 91:12 CPT Changes: An Insider's View 2002, 2003
77021	76393	2007	Jan 01:10, Mar 05:2 CPT Changes: An Insider's View 2001, 2002
77022	76394	2007	Oct 02:4, Mar 05:5 CPT Changes: An Insider's View 2002, 2004
77084	76400	2007	
76775, 76776	76778	2007	CPT Changes: An Insider's View 2002
76998	76986	2007	CPT Changes: An Insider's View 2001
78707-78709	78704	2007	
78701-78709	78715	2007	
78761	78760	2007	
92700	92573	2007	
94002, 94004	94656	2007	Fall 92:30, Spring 95:4, Summer 95:4, Feb 96:9, Aug 00:2, Oct 03:2
94003, 94004	94657	2007	Fall 92:30, Spring 95:4, Summer 95:4, Feb 96:9, Aug 00:2, Oct 03:2

Appendix N

Summary of Resequenced CPT Codes

This is a summary of CPT codes that do not apear in numeric sequence in the listing of CPT codes. Rather than deleting and renumbering, resequencing allows existing codes to be relocated to an appropriate location for the code concept, regardless of the numeric sequence. The codes listed below are identified in CPT 2013 with a # symbol for location of the resequenced number within the family of related concepts. Numerically placed references (eg, **Code is out of numerical sequence. See...**) are used as navigational alerts to direct the user to the location of out-of-sequence code.

11045	33227	80104	92975
11046	33228	82652	92977
21552	33229	86152	92978
21554	33230	86153	92979
23071	33231	87906	95782
23073	33262	87910	95783
24071	33263	87912	95800
24073	33264	88177	95801
25071	37211	90672	95885
25073	37212	92558	95886
26111	37213	92618	95887
26113	37214	92920	95938
27043	38243	92921	95939
27045	46220	92924	95940
27059	46320	92925	95941
27329	46945	92928	95943
27337	46946	92929	99224
27339	46947	92933	99225
27632	51797	92934	99226
27634	64633	92937	99485
28039	64634	92938	99486
28041	64635	92941	0253T
29914	64636	92943	
29915	67810	92944	
29916	77424	92973	
33221	77425	92974	

Appendix O

Multianalyte Assays with Algorithmic Analyses

The following list includes a set of administrative codes for Multianalyte Assays with Algorithmic Analyses (MAAA) procedures that by their nature are typically unique to a single clinical laboratory or manufacturer.

Multianalyte Assays with Algorithmic Analyses (MAAAs) are procedures that utilize multiple results derived from assays of various types, including molecular pathology assays, fluorescent in situ hybridization assays and non-nucleic acid based assays (eg, proteins, polypeptides, lipids, carbohydrates). Algorithmic analysis using the results of these assays as well as other patient information (if used) is then performed and reported typically as a numeric score(s) or as a probability. MAAAs are typically unique to a single clinical laboratory or manufacturer. The results of individual component procedure(s) that are inputs to the MAAAs may be provided on the associated laboratory report, however these assays are not reported separately using additional codes.

The list includes a proprietary name and clinical laboratory or manufacturer in the first column, an alpha-numeric code in the second column and code descriptor in the third column. The format for the code descriptor usually includes (in order):

- Disease type (eg, oncology, autoimmune, tissue rejection),
- Chemical(s) analyzed (eg, DNA, RNA, protein, antibody),
- Number of markers (eg, number of genes, number of proteins),
- Methodology(s) (eg, microarray, real-time [RT]-PCR, in situ hybridization [ISH], enzyme linked immunosorbent assays [ELISA]),
- Number of functional domains (if indicated),
- Specimen type (eg, blood, fresh tissue, formalin-fixed paraffin embedded),
- Algorithm result type (eg, prognostic, diagnostic),
- Report (eg, probability index, risk score).

MAAA procedures that have been assigned a Category I code are noted in the list below and additionally listed in the Category I MAAA section (81500-81599). The Category I MAAA section introductory language and associated parenthetical instruction(s) should be used to govern the appropriate use for Category I MAAA codes. If a specific MAAA procedure has not been assigned a Category I code, it is indicated as a four-digit number followed by the letter M.

When a specific MAAA procedure is not included in either the list below or in the Category I MAAA section, report the analysis using the Category I MAAA unlisted code (81599). The codes below are specific to the assays identified in Appendix O by proprietary name. When an analysis is performed that may potentially fall within a specific descriptor, however the proprietary name is not included in the list below, the MAAA unlisted code (81599) should be used.

Additions in this section may be released tri-annually via the AMA/CPT Internet site to expedite dissemination for reporting. The list will be published annually in the CPT codebook. Go to www.ama-assn.org/go/cpt for the most current listing.

These administrative codes encompass all analytical services required for the algorithmic analysis (eg, cell lysis, nucleic acid stabilization, extraction, digestion, amplification, hybridization and detection) in addition to the algorithmic analysis itself. Procedures that are required prior to cell lysis (eg, microdissection, codes 88380 and 88381) should be reported separately.

The codes in this list are provided as an administrative coding set to facilitate accurate reporting of MAAA services. The minimum standard for inclusion in this list is that an analysis is generally available for patient care. The AMA has not reviewed procedures in the administrative coding set for clinical utility. The list is not a complete list of all MAAA procedures.

Appendixes K–0

Proprietary Name and Clinical Laboratory or Manufacturer	Alpha-Numeric Code	Code Descriptor
Administrative Codes for Multianalyte Assays with Algorithmic Analyses (MAAA)		
HCV FibroSURE™, LabCorp	● 0001M	Infectious disease, HCV, six biochemical assays (ALT, A2-macroglobulin, apolipoprotein A-1, total bilirubin, GGT, and haptoglobin) utilizing serum, prognostic algorithm reported as scores for fibrosis and necroinflammatory activity in liver
ASH FibroSURE™, LabCorp	● 0002M	Liver disease, ten biochemical assays (ALT, A2-macroglobulin, apolipoprotein A-1, total bilirubin, GGT, haptoglobin, AST, glucose, total cholesterol and triglycerides) utilizing serum, prognostic algorithm reported as quantitative scores for fibrosis, steatosis and alcoholic steatohepatitis (ASH)
NASH FibroSURE™, LabCorp	● 0003M	Liver disease, ten biochemical assays (ALT, A2-macroglobulin, apolipoprotein A-1, total bilirubin, GGT, haptoglobin, AST, glucose, total cholesterol and triglycerides) utilizing serum, prognostic algorithm reported as quantitative scores for fibrosis, steatosis and nonalcoholic steatohepatitis (NASH)
Category I Codes for Multianalyte Assays with Algorithmic Analyses (MAAA)		
Risk of Ovarian Malignacy Algorithm (ROMA)™, Fujirebio Diagnostics	● 81500	Oncology (ovarian), biochemical assays of two proteins (CA-125 and HE4), utilizing serum, with menopausal status, algorithm reported as a risk score
OVA1™, Vermillion, Inc.	● 81503	Oncology (ovarian), biochemical assays of five proteins (CA-125, apoliprotein A1, beta-2 microglobulin, transferrin, and pre-albumin), utilizing serum, algorithm reported as a risk score
PreDx Diabetes Risk Score™, Tethys Clinical Laboratory	● 81506	Endocrinology (type 2 diabetes), biochemical assays of seven analytes (glucose, HbA1c, insulin, hs-CRP, adoponectin, ferritin, interleukin 2-receptor alpha), utilizing serum or plasma, algorithm reporting a risk score
Maternal serum screening procedures are well established procedures and are performed by many labs throughout the country. The concept of prenatal screens has existed and evolved for over ten years and is not exclusive to any one facility.	● 81509	Fetal congenital abnormalities, biochemical assays of three proteins (PAPP-A, hCG [any form], DIA), utilizing maternal serum, algorithm reported as a risk score
	● 81510	Fetal congenital abnormalities, biochemical assays of three analytes (AFP, uE3, hCG (any form)), utilizing maternal serum, algorithm reported as a risk score
	● 81511	Fetal congenital abnormalities, biochemical assays of four analytes (AFP, uE3, hCG (any form), DIA) utilizing maternal serum, algorithm reported as a risk score (may include additional results from previous biochemical testing)
	● 81512	Fetal congenital abnormalities, biochemical assays of five analytes (AFP, uE3, total hCG, hyperglycosylated hCG, DIA) utilizing maternal serum, algorithm reported as a risk score

Notes

Index

Instructions for the Use of the CPT Index

The alphabetical index is not a substitute for the main text of the CPT codebook, and therefore, should not be used to code. Even if only one code is listed in the index, the user must refer to the main text to ensure that the code selected accurately identifies the service or procedure performed.

Main Terms

The index is organized by main terms. Each main term can stand alone, or be followed by up to three modifying terms. There are four primary classes of main entries:

1. Procedure or service.
   For example: Endoscopy; Anastomosis; Splint

2. Organ or other anatomic site.
   For example: Tibia; Colon; Salivary Gland

3. Condition.
   For example: Abscess; Entropion; Tetralogy of Fallot

4. Synonyms, Eponyms, and Abbreviations.
   For example: EEG; Bricker Operation; Clagett Procedure

Anesthesia-section codes are indexed under the Anesthesia main entry and are not double-entered under the anatomical sites. Only specific codes within the Surgery, Medicine, Category II, and Category III sections that reference the service of anesthesia are indexed under the anatomical sites.

Modifying Terms

A main term may be followed by up to three indented terms that modify the terms they follow. For example, the main term Endoscopy is subdivided by the anatomical sites in which it is used, and within these anatomical sites, the specific purpose of the procedure is identified. In the following example, the code for an endoscopic removal of calculus from the urethra could be located:

Urethra
  Removal
    Calculus 52352

Note that in this entry, the inclusion of a subentry under "Removal" implies the reading "Removal [of]" the term that follows it. If no subheads followed "Removal," the procedure would relate to the subhead that preceded it, as in this entry for the endoscopic removal of the spleen:

Spleen
  Removal 38120

When modifying terms appear, one should review the list, as these subterms further qualify the selection of the appropriate code for the procedure.

Code Ranges

Whenever more than one code applies to a given index entry, a code range is listed. If several nonsequential codes apply, they will be separated by a comma. In the following example, three nonsequential codes apply:

Esophagus
  Reconstruction 43300, 43310, 43313

If two or more sequential codes apply, they will be separated by a hyphen. If more than one code range applies, the code ranges will be separated by a comma as in the following example:

Monitoring
  Electroencephalogram 95812-95813, 95950-95953

Conventions

As a space-saving convention, certain terms carry meaning inferred from the context. This convention is primarily used when a procedure or service is listed as a subterm. For example:

Knee
  Incision (of)

In this example, the bracketed qualifier "[of]" does not appear in the index; "of" is understood in the context of the term "Exploration." As another example:

Lung
  Aspiration[puncture of lung for] 32420

In this example, as there is no such entity as "lung aspiration," the bracketed words are inferred.

Pathology and Laboratory

The Pathology and Laboratory listing in the index presents the headings, subheadings, procedures, and analytes appearing in the Pathology and Laboratory section of the CPT codebook. Analytes are either listed alphabetically (eg, the Chemistry analytes) or cross-referenced to the index main heads in which they are alphabetically listed (eg, to reference infectious agent analytes, the entry will indicate "See Infectious Agents").

A

A Vitamin
See Vitamin, A

A-II
See Angiotensin II

Abbe-Estlander Procedure
Lip Reconstruction 40527, 40761
See Reconstruction; Repair, Cleft Lip

Abdomen
Ahdominal Aorta
    Angiography. 75635
Abdominal Wall
    Debridement
      Infected. 11005-11006
    Removal
      Mesh. 11008
      Prosthesis. 11008
    Repair
      Hernia. 49491-49496, 49501,
                     49507, 49521, 49590
    Tumor
      Excision. 22900-22903
      Radical Resection. 22904-22905
Abscess
    Incision and Drainage
      Open 49020, 49040
      Percutaneous 49021, 49041
Anesthesia
    See Anesthesia, Abdomen
Angiography. 74174-74175, 74185, 75635
Aorta
    See Abdomen, Abdominal Aorta; Aorta,
    Abdominal
Aortic Aneurysm
    See Aorta, Abdominal, Aneurysm
Artery
    Ligation 37617
Biopsy. 49000
Bypass Graft
    Excision 35907
Catheter
    Removal. 49422
Celiotomy
    See Laparotomy
    for Staging 49220
CT Scan. 74150, 74160, 74170,
                  74174-74178, 75635
Cyst
    Destruction/Excision 49203-49205
Deliveries
    See Caesarean Delivery
Drainage
    Fluid 49082-49083
Ectopic Pregnancy 59130
Endometrioma
    Destruction/Excision 49203-49205
Exploration 49000, 49010
    Blood Vessel. 35840
    Staging. 58960
Hysterectomy
    See Hysterectomy, Abdominal
Incision 49000-49084
    Staging. 58960
Incision and Drainage
    Pancreatitis 48000
Infraumbilical Panniculectomy 15830

Injection
    Air. 49400
    Contrast Material. 49400
Insertion
    Catheter 49324, 49418-49419, 49421
    Venous Shunt. 49425
Intraperitoneal
    Catheter Exit Site. 49436
    Catheter Insertion 49418-49421, 49435
    Catheter Removal 49422
    Catheter Revision. 49325
    Shunt
      Insertion 49425
      Ligation. 49428
      Removal 49429
      Revision 49426
Laparoscopy 49320-49327, 49329
Laparotomy
    Reopening 49002
    Staging. 49220, 58960
Lymphangiogram
    See Lymphangiography, Abdomen
Magnetic Resonance Imaging
(MRI). 74181-74183
Needle Biopsy (Mass) 49180
Paracentesis. 49082-49083
Radical Resection 51597
Radiation Therapy
    Placement of Guidance
    Devices. 49411-49412
Radiographies
    See Abdomen, X-ray
Removal
    Node(s). 49220
Repair
    Blood Vessel. 35221
      with Other Graft 35281
      with Vein Graft 35251
    Hernia. 49491-49525,
               49560-49587, 49590
    Suture. 49900
Revision
    Venous Shunt. 49426
Suture. 49900
Tumor
    Destruction/Excision 49203-49205
Ultrasound 76700-76705
Unlisted Services and Procedures 49999
Wall
    See Abdomen, Abdominal Wall
Wound Exploration
    Penetrating. 20102
X-ray 74000, 74010, 74020, 74022

Abdominal
See Abdomen
Aorta
    See Abdomen, Abdominal Aorta; Aorta,
    Abdominal
Aortic Aneurysm
    See Aorta, Abdominal, Aneurysm
Deliveries
    See Caesarean Delivery
Hysterectomy
    See Hysterectomy, Abdominal
Lymphangiogram
    See Lymphangiography, Abdomen
Paracentesis
    See Abdomen, Drainage
Radiographies
    See Abdomen, X-ray
Wall
    See Abdomen, Abdominal Wall

Abdominohysterectomy
See Hysterectomy, Abdominal

Abdominopelvic Amputation
See Amputation, Interpelviabdominal

Abdominoplasty
See Panniculectomy
Excision, Skin and Tissue 15830, 15847
Unlisted Procedure. 17999

Ablation
Anus
    Polyp. 46615
    Tumor 46615
Bone
    Tumor 20982
Colon
    Polyp. 44393
    Tumor 44393, 45339
Cryosurgical
    Fibroadenoma 19105
    Liver Tumor. 47381
    Renal Mass 50250
    Renal Tumor
      Percutaneous 50593
CT Scan Guidance 77013
Endometrial 58353, 58356, 58563
    with Ultrasound Guidance. 58356
Heart
    Arrhythmogenic Focus . . 33250-33251, 33261,
               93653, 93654, 93655
    Atrioventricular 93650, 93653, 93654
Liver (Tumor)
    Cryosurgical 47381
    Laparoscopic 47370-47371
    Radiofrequency 47380-47382
Lung
    Tumor
      Radiofrequency. 32998
Parenchymal Tissue
    CT Scan Guidance 77013
    Magnetic Resonance Guidance. 77022
    Ultrasound Guidance 76940
Prostate 55873
Pulmonary Tumor 32998
Radiofrequency
    Liver Tumor. 47382
    Lung Tumor. 32998
    Renal Tumor 50592
    Tongue Base. 41530
Rectum
    Polyp. 45339
    Tumor 45339
Renal Cyst. 50541
Renal Mass 50542
Renal Tumor
    Cryotherapy
      Percutaneous 50593
      Radiofrequency 50592
Tongue Base
    Radiofrequency 41530
Turbinate Mucosa 30801-30802
Uterine Tumor
    Ultrasound, Focused 0071T-0072T
Vein
    Endovenous 36475-36479

Abortion
See Obstetrical Care
Incomplete 59812
Induced
    by Dilation and Curettage 59840
    by Dilation and Evacuation 59841

by Saline 59850-59851
by Vaginal Suppositories 59855-59856
with Hysterotomy 59100, 59852, 59857
Missed
First Trimester 59820
Second Trimester 59821
Septic 59830
Spontaneous
Complete
See Hospital Services
Incomplete 59812
Therapeutic
by Saline 59850
with Dilation and Curettage 59851
with Hysterotomy 59852

Abrasion (Skin)
Chemical Peel 15788-15789, 15792-15793
Dermabrasion 15780-15783
Lesion 15786-15787

Abscess
Bone
Ankle
Incision 27607
Clavicle
Sequestrectomy 23170
Elbow
Incision 23930, 23935
Facial
Excision 21026
Femur
Incision 27303
Finger
Incision 26034
Foot
Incision 28005
Forearm
Incision 25035
Sequestrectomy 25145
Humeral Head
Incision 23174
Humerus
Excision 24134
Incision and Drainage 23935
Knee
Incision 27303
Leg, Lower
Incision 27607
Olecranon Process 24138
Sequestrectomy 24136
Pelvis
Incision 26992
Radius
Incision, Deep 25035
Sequestrectomy 24136
Scapula
Sequestrectomy 23172
Shoulder
Incision 23035
Thorax
Incision 21510
Wrist
Incision 25035
Sequestrectomy 25145
Drainage
with X-ray 75989
Localization
Nuclear Medicine 78806-78807
Tissue
Abdomen 49040-49041
Incision and Drainage 49021, 49040
Anus
Incision and Drainage 46045-46060

Ankle
Incision and Drainage 27603
Appendix
Incision and Drainage 44900-44901
Arm, Lower
Incision and Drainage 25028
Auditory Canal, External
Incision and Drainage 69020
Bartholin's Gland
Incision and Drainage 56420
Bladder
Incision and Drainage 51080
Brain
Drainage via Burr Hole 61150-61151
Drainage via Craniotomy 61320-61321
Excision 61514, 61522
Breast
Incision and Drainage 19020
Ear, External
Incision and Drainage 69000, 69005
Elbow
Incision and Drainage 23930-23931
Epididymis
Incision and Drainage 54700
Eyelid
Incision and Drainage 67700
Finger
Incision and Drainage 26010-26011
Forearm
Incision and Drainage 25028
Gums
Incision and Drainage 41800
Hand
Incision and Drainage 26034
Hip
Incision and Drainage 26990-26992
Kidney
Incision and Drainage
Open 50020
Percutaneous 50021
Knee
Incision and Drainage 27301
Leg, Lower
Incision and Drainage 27603
Liver
sub21 . . . . Drainage
Open 47010
Percutaneous 47011
Injection 47015
Marsupialization 47300
Lung
Percutaneous Drainage 32200-32201
Lymph Node
Incision and Drainage 38300, 38305
Lymphocele Drainage 49062
Mandible
Excision 21025
Mouth 41015-41018
Incision and Drainage
Dentoalveolar 41800
Lingual 41000
Masticator Space 41009, 41018
Sublingual 41005-41006, 41015
Submandibular 41008, 41017
Submental 41007, 41016
Vestibular 40800-40801
Musculoskeletal
Incision and Drainage 20005
Nasal
Incision and Drainage 30000, 30020
Neck
Incision and Drainage 21501-21502

Olecranon Process
Excision 24138
Ovary
Incision and Drainage 58820, 58822
Percutaneous Drainage 58823
Abdominal Approach 58822
Vaginal Approach 58820
Palate
Incision and Drainage 42000
Paraurethral Gland
Incision and Drainage 53060
Parotid Gland
Drainage 42300, 42305
Pelvis
Incision and Drainage . . . 26990-26991, 45000
Percutaneous 58823
Pericolic
Percutaneous Drainage 58823
Perineum
Incision and Drainage 56405
Perirenal or Renal
Incision and Drainage 50020-50021
Peritoneum
Incision and Drainage 49020-49021
Pharynx
Incision and Drainage 42720, 42725
Prostate
Incision and Drainage 55720, 55725
Transurethral Drainage 52700
Rectum
Incision and Drainage . 45005, 45020, 46040,
　　　　　　　　　　　　　　　　　　46060
Renal
Incision and Drainage 50020-50021
Retroperitoneal
Incision and Drainage 49060-49061
Salivary Gland
Drainage 42300-42320
Scrotum
Incision and Drainage 54700, 55100
Shoulder
Incision and Drainage 23030
Skene's Gland
Incision and Drainage 53060
Skin/Superficial
Incision and Drainage 10060-10061
Puncture Aspiration 10160
Spine
Incision and Drainage 22010, 22015
Subdiaphragmatic
Drainage 49040-49041
Sublingual Gland
Drainage 42310-42320
Submaxillary Gland
Drainage 42310, 42320
Subphrenic
Drainage 49040-49041
Testis
Incision and Drainage 54700
Thigh
Incision and Drainage 27301
Thorax
Incision and Drainage 21501-21502
Throat
Incision and Drainage 42700-42725
Tongue
Incision and Drainage 41000-41006
Tonsil
Incision and Drainage 42700
Urethra
Incision and Drainage 53040
Uvula
Incision and Drainage 42000

Index

Acupuncture
with Electrical Stimulation 97813-97814
without Electrical Stimulation 97810-97811

Acute Poliomyelitis
See Polio

Acylcarnitines 82016-82017

Adamantinoma, Pituitary
See Craniopharyngioma

Addam Operation
See Dupuytren's Contracture

Adductor Tenotomy of Hip
See Tenotomy, Hip, Adductor

Adenoidectomy
See Adenoids, Excision

Adenoids
Excision 42830-42836
    with Tonsils 42820-42821
Unlisted Services and Procedures 42999

Adenoma
Pancreas
    Excision 48120
Parathyroid
    Localization
        Injection Procedure 78808
Thyroid Gland Excision 60200

Adenosine 3'5' Monophosphate
See Cyclic AMP

Adenosine Diphosphate
Blood 82030

Adenosine Monophosphate (AMP)
Blood 82030

Adenovirus
Antibody Detection 86603
Antigen Detection
    Enzyme Immunoassay 87301
    Immunofluorescence 87260

Adenovirus Vaccine
See Vaccines

Adenylic Acid
See Adenosine Monophosphate (AMP)

ADH
See Antidiuretic Hormone

Adhesions
Epidural 62263-62264
Eye
    Corneovitreal 65880
    Incision
        Anterior Segment . . . . 65860, -65870
        Posterior Segment 65875
    Construction 67880
        Transposition of Tarsal Plate 67882
Intestinal
    Enterolysis 44005
    Laparoscopic 44180
Intracranial
    Dissection 62161
Intrauterine
    Lysis 58559
Labial
    Lysis 56441
Liver
    Lysis 58660

Lungs
    Pneumonolysis 32124, 32940
Nose
    Lysis 30560
Pelvic
    Lysis 58660, 58740
Penile
    Lysis
        Post-circumcision 54162
Preputial
    Lysis 54450
Urethral
    Lysis 53500

Adipectomy
See Lipectomy

ADL
See Activities of Daily Living

Administration
Immunization
    Each Additional
        Vaccine/Toxoid 90472, 90474
            with Counseling 90461
        One Vaccine/Toxoid 90471, 90473
            with Counseling 90460
Occlusive Substance 31634
Pharmacologic Agent 93463

ADP
See Adenosine Diphosphate

ADP Phosphocreatine Phosphotransferase
See CPK

Adrenal Cortex Hormone
See Corticosteroids

Adrenal Gland
Biopsy 60540-60545
Excision 60540
    Laparoscopy 60650
    Retroperitoneal Tumor 60545
Exploration 60540, 60545
Nuclear Medicine
    Imaging 78075

Adrenal Medulla
See Medulla

Adrenalectomy
Partial 60540, 60545, 60650
Complete 60540, 60545, 60650
Anesthesia 00866
Laparoscopic 50545

Adrenalin
See Catecholamines
Blood 82383
Urine 82382, 82384

Adrenaline-Noradrenaline
Testing 82382-82384

Adrenocorticotropic Hormone (ACTH) 80400-80406, 80412, 80418, 82024
Blood or Urine 82024
Stimulation Panel 80400-80406

Adrenogenital Syndrome 56805, 57335

Adult T Cell Leukemia Lymphoma Virus I
See HTLV-I (Human T-cell Lymphotrophic Virus Type I)

Advanced Life Support
See Emergency Department Services
Physician/Health Care
Professional Direction 99288

Advancement
Genioglossus 21199
Tendon
    Tibia 28238

Advancement Flap
See Skin, Adjacent Tissue Transfer

Aerosol Inhalation
See Pulmonology, Therapeutic
Pentamidine 94642

AFB
See Acid-Fast Bacilli (AFB)

Afferent Nerve
See Sensory Nerve

AFP
See Alpha-Fetoprotein (AFP)

After Hours Medical Services 99050

Agents, Anticoagulant
See Clotting Inhibitors

Agglutinin
Cold 86156-86157
Febrile 86000

Aggregation
Platelet 85576

AHG
See Clotting Factor

AICD (Automated Implantable Cardioverter-Defibrillator)
See Cardioverter-Defibrillator

Aid, Hearing
See Hearing Aid

AIDS Antibodies
See Antibody, HIV

AIDS Virus
See HIV-1

Airway
Leak
See Bronchoscopy

Akin Operation
See Bunion Repair

ALA
See Aminolevulinic Acid (ALA)

Alanine 2 Oxoglutarate Aminotransferase
See Transaminase, Glutamic Pyruvic

Alanine Amino Transferase (ALT) 84460

Alanine Transaminase
See Transaminase, Glutamic Pyruvic

Albumin
Ischemia modified 82045
Serum, Plasma or Whole Blood 82040
Urine 82042-82044

Alcohol
Breath 82075
Ethanol
   Blood 82055
   Urine 82055
   Ethylene Glycol 82693

Alcohol Dehydrogenase
See Antidiuretic Hormone

Alcohol, Isopropyl
See Isopropyl Alcohol

Alcohol, Methyl
See Methanol

Aldolase
Blood 82085

Aldosterone
Blood 82088
Suppression Evaluation 80408
Urine 82088

Alimentary Canal
See Gastrointestinal Tract

Alkaline Phosphatase 84075, 84078,
84080
Leukocyte 85540
WBC 85540

Alkaloids
See Specific Drug
Urine 82101

Allergen Bronchial Provocation Tests
See Allergy Tests; Bronchial Challenge Test

Allergen Challenge, Endobronchial
See Bronchial Challenge Test

Allergen Immunotherapy
Allergen
   IgE 86003, 86005
   IgG 86001
   Multiallergen Screen 86005
Allergenic Extracts
   Injection 95115, 95117
   Injection and Provision 95120-95134
      Insect Venom 95130-95134
Antigens
   Preparation and Provision 95144-95165
      Insect Venom 95145-94149
Insect, Whole Body Extract 95170
Rapid Desensitization 95180

Allergy Services/Procedures
See Allergen Immunotherapy;Office and/or Other Outpatient Services
Education and Counseling 99201-99215
Unlisted Services and Procedures 95199

Allergy Tests
Challenge Test
   Bronchial 95070-95071
   Ingestion 95076, 95079
Eye Allergy 95060
Food Allergy 95076, 95079
Intradermal
   Allergen Extract 95024-95028
   Biologicals 95018
   Drugs 95018
   Incremental 95027
   Venoms 95017

Nasal Mucous Membrane Test 95065
Nose Allergy 95065
Patch
   Application Tests 95044
   Photo Patch 95052
Photosensitivity 95056
Skin Tests
   Allergen Extract 95004, 95024, 95027
   Biologicals 95018
   Drugs 95018
   Venoms 95017

Allogeneic Donor
Lymphocyte Infusion 38242

Allogeneic Transplantation
See Homograft
Hematopoietic progenitor cells 38420

Allograft
Aortic Valve 33406, 33413
Bone
   Elbow Joint 24370, 24371
   Shoulder Joint 23473-23474
   Spine Surgery
      Morselized 20930
      Structural 20931
Cartilage
   Knee 27415
Lung Transplant 32850

Allograft Preparation
Cornea 65757
Heart 33933, 33944
Intestines 44715-44721
Kidney 50323-50329
Liver 47143-47147
Lung 32855-32856, 33933
Pancreas 48551-48552
Renal 50323-50329

Allotransplantation
Intestines 44135-44136
   Removal 44137
Renal 50360-50365
   Removal 50370

Almen Test
See Blood, Feces

Alpha-1-Antitrypsin 82103-82104

Alpha-2 Antiplasmin 85410

Alpha-Fetoprotein (AFP)
Amniotic Fluid 82106
Serum 82105, 82107

Alpha-tocopherol 84446

ALT
See Transaminase, Glutamic-Pyruvic

Altemeier Procedure
See Procidentia, Rectum; Rectum, Prolapse, Excision

Aluminum
Blood 82108

Alveola
Fracture
   Closed Treatment 21421
   Open Treatment 21422-21423

Alveolar Cleft
Ungrafted Bilateral 21147
Ungrafted Unilateral 21146

Alveolar Nerve
Avulsion 64738
Incision 64738
Transection 64738

Alveolar Ridge
Fracture
   Closed Treatment 21440
   Open Treatment 21445

Alveolectomy 41830

Alveoloplasty 41874

Alveolus
Excision 41830

Amide, Procaine
See Procainamide

Amikacin
Assay 80150

Amine
Vaginal Fluid 82120

Amino Acids 82127-82139

Aminolevulinic Acid (ALA)
Blood or Urine 82135

Aminotransferase
See Transaminase

Aminotransferase, Alanine
See Transaminase, Glutamic-Pyruvic

Aminotransferase, Aspartate
See Transaminase, Glutamic-Oxaloacetic

Amitriptyline
Assay 80152

Ammonia
Blood 82140

Amniocenteses
See Amniocentesis

Amniocentesis
See Chromosome Analysis
Diagnostic 59000
Induced Abortion 59850
   with Dilation and Curettage 59851
   with Dilation and Evacuation 59851
   with Hysterotomy 59852
Therapeutic
   Amniotic Fluid Reduction 59001

Amnioinfusion
Transabdominal 59070

Amnion
Amniocentesis 59000
   with Amniotic Fluid Reduction 59001
Amnioinfusion
   Transabdominal 59070
Membrane Placement
   Eye 65778-65779

Amniotic Fluid
Alpha-Fetoprotein 82106
Scan 82143
Testing 83661, 83663-83664

Amniotic Membrane
See Amnion

Amobarbital 82205

AMP
See Adenosine Monophosphate (AMP)

AMP, Cyclic
See Cyclic AMP

Amphetamine
Blood or Urine 82145

Amputation
See Radical Resection; Replantation
Ankle. 27888
Arm, Lower. 25900-25905, 25915
   Revision 25907, 25909
Arm, Upper. 24900-24920
   and Shoulder 23900-23921
   Cineplasty 24940
   Revision 24925-24930
   with Implant. 24931-24935
Cervix
   Total 57530
Ear
   Partial. 69110
   Total 69120
Finger 26910-26952
Foot. 28800-28805
Hand at Metacarpal. 25927
   at Wrist 25920
     Revision 25922
   Revision 25924, 25929, 25931
Interpelviabdominal. 27290
Interthoracoscapular 23900
Leg, Lower 27598, 27880-27882
   Revision 27884, 27886
Leg, Upper 27590-27592
   at Hip 27290, 27295
   Revision 27594, 27596
Metacarpal. 26910
Metatarsal 28810
Penis
   Partial. 54120
   Radical 54130, 54135
   Total 54125
Thumb. 26910, 26951-26952
Toe 28810, 28820, 28825
Tuft of Distal Phalanx. 11752
Upper Extremity 24900-24940
   Revision 24925, 24930, 24935
   with Implant. 24931-24935
   Cineplasty 24940

Amputation through Hand
See Hand, Amputation

Amputation, Nose
See Resection, Nose

Amylase
Blood. 82150
Urine 82150

ANA
See Antinuclear Antibodies (ANA)

Anabolic Steroid
See Androstenedione

Anal Abscess
See Abscess, Anal

Anal Bleeding
See Anus, Hemorrhage

Anal Fistula
See Fistula, Anal

Anal Fistulectomy
See Excision, Fistula, Anal

Anal Fistulotomy
See Fistulotomy, Anal

Anal Sphincter
Dilation. 45905
Incision. 46080

Anal Ulceration
See Anus, Fissure

Analgesia
See Anesthesia; Sedation

Analgesic Cutaneous Electrostimulation
See Application, Neurostimulation

Analysis
Biochemical Assay Algorithm
   Risk Score 81500, 81503, 81506,
                      81508-81512
   Unlisted Assay. 81599
Computer Data. 99090
   Cardiovascular Monitoring 93290, 93297,
                          93299
   Device Evaluation and Programming
     Cardioverter-Defibrillator . . . 93282-93299,
     Loop Recorder. 93285, 93291,
                      93298-93299
     Pacemaker. 93279-93281,
                      93293-93294
   Electrocardiograph
     Data Analysis 0206T
   Multivariate Probability Assessment . . . 0185T
   Pacemaker 93288, 93293-93294
   Electroencephalogram
     Digital. 95957
   Electronic
     Drug Infusion Pump 62367-62370
     Pacing Cardioverter-Defibrillator
       Data Analysis 93289, 93295-93296
       Initial Evaluation. 93640, 93641
        See Pacemaker, Heart
     Pulse Generator
       Neurostimulator 95970-95982
Physiologic Data, Remote 99091
Protein
   Tissue
     Western Blot 88372
Semen. 89320-89322
   Sperm Isolation 89260-89261

Analysis, Spectrum
See Spectrophotometry

Anaspadias
See Epispadias

Anastomosis
Arteriovenous Fistula
   Direct 36821
   with Bypass Graft 35686
   with Graft. 36825, 36830, 36832
Artery
   to Aorta 33606
   to Artery
     Cranial 61711
Bile Duct
   to Bile Duct 47800
   to Intestines. 47760, 47780
Bile Duct
   to Gastrointestinal Tract. 47780, 47785

Broncho-Bronchial 32486
Caval to Mesenteric 37160
Cavopulmonary. 33622, 33768
Colorectal 44626
Epididymis
   to Vas Deferens
     Bilateral 54901
     Unilateral 54900
Excision
   Trachea. 31780-31781
Fallopian Tube 58750
Gallbladder to Intestines 47720-47740
Hepatic Duct to Intestines. 47765, 47802
Ileum to Anus. 45113
Intestine to Intestine 44130
Intestines
   Colon to Anus. 45119
   Cystectomy. 51590
   Enterocystoplasty. 51960
   Ileoanal 44157-44158
   Resection
     Laparoscopic. 44202-44205
Intrahepatic Portosystemic 37182-37183
Jejunum 43820-43825
Microvascular
   Free Transfer
     Jejunum 43496
Nerve
   Facial to Hypoglossal 64868
   Facial to Phrenic. 64870
Oviduct 58750
Pancreas to Intestines 48520, 48540, 48548
Portocaval. 37140
Pulmonary. 33606
Renoportal 37145
Splenorenal 37180-37181
Stomach
   to Duodenum 43810, 43855
     Revision 43850
   to Jejunum 43820-43825, 43860-43865
Tubotubal 58750
Ureter
   to Bladder. 50780-50785
   to Colon 50810-50815
     Removal 50830
   to Intestine. 50800, 50820, 50825
     Removal 50830
   to Kidney 50727-50750
   to Ureter. 50725-50727, 50760, 50770
Vein
   Saphenopopliteal. 34530
Vein to Vein 37140-37160, 37182-37183

Anastomosis of Lacrimal Sac to Conjunctival Sac
See Conjunctivorhinostomy

Anastomosis of Pancreas
See Pancreas, Anastomosis

Anastomosis, Aorta-Pulmonary Artery
See Aorta, Anastomosis, to Pulmonary Artery

Anastomosis, Bladder, to Intestine
See Enterocystoplasty

Anastomosis, Hepatic Duct
See Hepatic Duct, Anastomosis

Anderson Tibial Lengthening. 27715
See Ankle; Tibia, Osteoplasty, Lengthening

Index

Index

Index

Index

Antibody Identification

Antibody Neutralization Test
See Neutralization Test

Antibody Receptor
See FcReceptor

Antibody Screening

Anticoagulant
See Clotting Inhibitors

Anticoagulant Management

Antidiabetic Hormone
See Glucagon

Antidiuretic Hormone

AntiDNA Autoantibody
See Antinuclear Antibodies (ANA)

Antigen
See Antigen Detection

Antigen Bronchial Provocation Tests
See Bronchial Challenge Test

Antigen Detection

Antigen, Australia
See Hepatitis Antigen, B Surface

Antigen, CD4
See CD4

Antigen, CD8
See CD8

Antigens, CD142
See Thromboplastin

Antigens, CD143
See Angiotensin Converting Enzyme (ACE)

Antigens, E
See Hepatitis Antigen, Be

Antigens, Hepatitis
See Hepatitis Antigen

Antigens, Hepatitis B
See Hepatitis Antigen, B

Antihemophilic Factor B
See Christmas Factor

Antihemophilic Factor C
See Plasma Thromboplastin, Antecedent

Antihemophilic Globulin (AHG) 85240

Antihuman Globulin 86880-86886

Antimony 83015

Antinuclear Antibodies (ANA) 86038-86039

Antiplasmin, Alpha-2 85410

Antiplatelet Therapy
See Performance Measures, Interventions

Antiprotease, Alpha-1
See Alpha-1 Antitrypsin

Antistreptococcal Antibody 86215

Antistreptokinase Titer 86590

Antistreptolysin O 86060-86063

Antithrombin III 85300-85301

Antithrombin VI
See Fibrin Degradation Products

Antitoxin Assay 87230

Antiviral Antibody
See Viral Antibodies

Antrostomy

Antrotomy

Antrum of Highmore
See Sinus, Maxillary

Antrum Puncture

Index

Index

Index

Index

Index

Index

Biopsy, Skin
See Skin, Biopsy

Biopsy, Vein
See Vein, Biopsy

Biostatistics
See Biometry

Biosterol
See Vitamin, A

Birthing Room

Bischof Procedure
See Laminectomy, Surgical

Bizzozero's Corpuscle/Cell
See Blood, Platelet

Bladder

Index

Blood Banking
Frozen Blood Preparation. . . . 86930-86932, 88240
Frozen Plasma Preparation 86927
Physician Services 86077-86079

Blood Cell
CD4 and CD8
   Including Ratio. 86360
Enzyme Activity 82657
Exchange 36511-36513
Sedimentation Rate
   Automated 85652
   Manual. 85651

Blood Cell Count
Automated 85049
BCells 86355
Blood Smear. 85007-85008
Complete (CBC) 85025-85027
Differential WBC Count. 85004-85007, 85009
Hematocrit 85014
Hemoglobin 85018
Hemogram
   Added Indices 85025-85027
   Automated 85025-85027
   Manual. 85032
Microhematocrit 85013
Natural Killer (NK) Cells 86357
Red Blood Cells 85032-85041
Reticulocyte 85044-85046
Stem Cells 86367
TCells 86359-86361
White Blood Cells 85032, 85048, 89055

Blood Cell Count, Red
See Red Blood Cell (RBC), Count

Blood Cell Count, White
See White Blood Cell (WBC), Count

Blood Cell, Red
See Red Blood Cell (RBC)

Blood Cell, White
See Leukocyte

Blood Coagulation
See Clotting
Clot
   See Clot
Defect
   See Coagulopathy
Disorders
   See Clot
Factor
   See Clotting Factor
Test
   See Coagulation

Blood Component Removal
See Apheresis

Blood Count, Complete
See Complete Blood Count (CBC)

Blood Flow Check, Graft. 15860, 90940

Blood Gases
CO2. 82803
HCO3. 82803
O2 Saturation. 82805, 82810
pCO2 82803
pH 82800, 82803, 82930
pO2 . . . . 82803, 82820

Blood Letting

See Phlebotomy

Blood Lipoprotein
See Lipoprotein

Blood Pool Imaging
Cardiac 78472-78473,
             78481-78483, 78494-78496

Blood Pressure
See Performance Measures, Diagnostic/Screening
Processes or Results
Baroreflex
   Activation Device. 0266T-0273T
Central Arterial
   Calculation/Analysis 0311T
Diastolic. 3078F-3080F
Monitoring, 24-Hour 93784, 93786,
                   93788, 93790
Ocular
   Measurement. 0198T
Systolic. 3074F-3075F, 3077F
Venous 93770

Blood Products
Irradiation. 86945
Pooling 86965
Splitting 86985
Volume Reduction 86960

Blood Sample
Fetal 59030

Blood Serum
See Serum

Blood Smear
Microorganism Identification 87205-87207
Microscopic Examination 85007-85008
Peripheral 85060
Sex Chromatin 88140
Surgical Pathology. 88312-88313, 88319

Blood Syndrome
Chromosome Analysis. 88245, 88248-88249

Blood Tests
Coagulation
   See Blood Coagulation, Tests
Cell Count
   See Blood Cell Count
Culture, Bacteria
   See Bacteria Culture
Gas Analysis
   See Blood Gases
Iron Stores 3160F
Kt/V. 3082F-3084F
Nuclear Medicine
   Plasma Volume. 78110-78111
   Platelet Survival. 78190-78191
   Red Cell Survival 78130, 78135
   Red Cell Volume. 78120-78121
   Whole Blood Volume. 78122
Panels
   Electrolyte 80051
   General Health. 80050
   Hepatic Function 80076
   Hepatitis, Acute. 80074
   Lipid 80061
   Metabolic
      Basic 80047-80048
      Comprehensive. 80053
   Obstetric. 80055
   Renal Function 80069
Typing

See Blood Typing
Urea Nitrogen. 84520-84525
Volume Determination. 78122

Blood Transfusion, Autologous
See Autotransfusion

Blood Typing
ABO Only 86900
Antigen Screen. 86904
Antigen Testing, Donor Blood 86902
Compatibility 86920-86923
Other RBC Antigens 86905
Paternity Testing 86910-86911
Rh (D) 86901
Rh Phenotype 86906

Blood Urea Nitrogen 84520-84525

Blood Vessels
See Artery, specific site; Vascular Procedures; Vein, specific site
Angioscopy. 35400
Endoscopy. 37500-37501
Excision
   See Arteriovenous Malformation; Bypass Graft
Exploration
   Abdomen 35840
   Carotid Artery. 35701
   Chest 35820
   Extremity 35860
   Femoral Artery 35721
   Neck. 35800
   Popliteal Artery 35741
   Vessel, Other 35761
Harvest
   See Bypass Graft, Harvest
Repair
   Aneurysm
      See Aneurysm Repair
   Aorta 33320-33322
   Fistula
      See Fistula, Repair
   Direct 35201-35226
      Finger 35207
      Hand 35207
      Intra-abdominal 35221, 35281
      Intrathoracic . . . 35211, 35216, 35271, 35276
      Lower Extremity 35226, 35286
      Neck 35201, 35231, 35261
   Great Vessel. 33320-33322
   Kidney 50100
   Upper Extremity 35236, 35266
   Malformation
      See Arteriovenous Malformation
Shunt Creation
   Direct 36818, 36821
   ECMO. 36822
   Thomas Shunt 36835
   with Bypass Graft 35686
   with Graft. 36825-36830
   with Transposition 36818-36820
Shunt Revision
   with Graft. 36832

Blood, Occult
See Occult Blood

Bloom Syndrome
Chromosome Analysis. 88245
Gene Analysis 81209

Blot Test, Ink
See Inkblot Test

Borreliosis, Lyme
See Lyme Disease

Bost Fusion
See Arthrodesis, Wrist

Bosworth Operation
See Acromioclavicular Joint, Dislocation;
Arthrodesis, Vertebrae; Fasciotomy

Bottle Procedure
Repair of Tunica Vaginalis Hydrocele 55060

Botulinum Toxin
See Chemodenervation

Boutonniere Deformity 26426-26428

Bowel
See Intestine

Bowleg Repair 27455-27457

Boyd Hip Disarticulation
See Amputation, Leg, Upper; Radical Resection;
Replantation

Brace
See Cast
for Leg Cast 29358
Vertebral Fracture 22310, 22315

Brachial Arteries
See Artery, Brachial

Brachial Plexus
Anesthetic Injection 64415-64416
Decompression 64713
Neuroplasty 64708, 64713
Release 64713
Repair/Suture 64861

Brachiocephalic Artery
See Artery, Brachiocephalic

Brachycephaly
Reconstruction 21175

Brachytherapy
High Dose Electronic 0182T
Intracavitary Application 77761-77763
Interstitial Radioelement
Application 77776-77779
  Device Placement
    Breast 19296-19298
    Genitalia 55920
    Head 41019
    Intraocular 0190T
    Neck 41019
    Pelvis 55920
    Uterus 57155
    Vagina 57155-57156
    Heyman Capsule Insertion 58346
  Planning
    Isodose Plan 77326-77328
    Prostate Volume Study 76873
  Radioelement Solution
    Infusion 77750
    Instillation 77750
  Remote Afterloading 77785-77787
  Surface Application 77789-77790
  Unlisted Clinical Procedures 77799

Bradykinin
Blood or Urine 82286

Brain
See Brainstem; Mesencephalon; Skull Base
Surgery
Abscess
  Drainage 61150-61151
  Excision 61514, 61522
  Incision and Drainage 61320-61321
Adhesions 62161
Angiography 36100, 70444, 70496
Biopsy 61140
  Stereotactic 61750-61751
Catheter
  Insertion 61210
  Irrigation 62194, 62225
  Replacement 62160, 62194, 62225
Catheter Placement
  for Chemotherapy 0169T
  for Radiation Source 61770
Cingulotomy 61490
Computer Assisted
  Procedure 61781-61782
Cortex
  Magnetic Stimulation 0310T, 90867-90869
  Mapping 90867, 96020
    Motor Function 0310T
Cyst
  Drainage 61150-61151, 62161-62162
  Excision 61516, 61524, 62162
Debridement 62010
Diagnostic Radiology
  CT Scan 0042T, 70450,
                 70460, 70470, 70496
  Imaging 70010-70015, 78600-78601,
                       78605-78610
    Cerebrospinal Fluid 78630-78650
    Cisternography 70015
    Vascular Flow 78601, 78606, 78610
    Ventriculography 78635
  Doppler Study 93886, 93888, 93890,
                      93892-93893
  Magnetic Resonance Imaging . . . 70551-70555,
                       70557-70559
  Perfusion Analysis 0042T
  Positron Emission
  Tomography (PET) 78608-78609
Electrocorticography 61536, 61538
Electroencephalography
  Cerebral Death Evaluation 95824
  Monitored 95812-95813
  Recorded 95816, 95819, 95822, 95827
Epileptogenic Focus
  Excision 61534, 61536
  Monitoring 61531, 61533, 61535, 61760
Excision
  Amygdala 61566
  Choroid Plexus 61544
  Craniopharyngioma 61545
  Hemisphere 61542-61543
  Hippocampus 61566
  Meningioma 61512, 61519
  Other Lobe 61323, 61539-61540
  Temporal Lobe 61537-61538
  Tumor 61510, 61518, 61520-61521,
                61526-61530, 61545, 62164
Exploration
  Infratentorial 61305
  Supratentorial 61304
Hematoma
  Drainage 61154
  Incision and Drainage 61312-61315
Implantation
  Chemotherapy Agent 61517

Electrode 61210, 61850,
             61860, 61863-61864, 61875
Pulse Generator 61885-61886
Reservoir 61210, 61215
Incision
  Frontal Lobe 61490
  Mesencephalic Tract 61480
Infusion 0169T, 95990-95991
Lesion
  Aspiration, Stereotactic 61750-61751
  Excision 61600-61601, 61605-61608,
                       61615-61616
Lobectomy 61537-61540
Lobotomy 61490
Magnetoencephalography 95965-95967
Mapping 90867-90869, 95961-95962, 96020
Meningioma
  Excision 61512, 61519
Neurostimulation
  Analysis 95970, 95978-95982
  Electrode
    Implantation 61210, 61850, 61860,
                61863-61864, 61875
    Removal 61880
    Revision 61880
  Pulse Generator
    Insertion 61885-61886
    Removal 61880
    Revision 61880
Radiosurgery
  for Lesion 61796-61800
  Radiation Treatment Delivery . . . 77371-77373
Removal
  Electrode 61535, 61880
  Foreign Body 61570, 62163
  Pulse Generator 61888
  Shunt 62256-62258
Repair
  Dura 61618
  Wound 61571
Shunt
  Creation 62190, 62192, 62200, 62223
  Removal 62256-62258
  Replacement 62160, 62194, 62225,
                62230, 62256, 62258
  Reprogramming 62252
Skull Surgery
  See Skull Base Surgery
Stereotaxis-aided Procedures
  Aspiration 61750-61751
  Biopsy 61750-61751
  Catheter Placement 0169T, 61770
  Navigation 61781-61782
  Create Lesion 61720, 61735, 61790-61791
  Procedure 61781-61782
  Radiation Treatment 77432
  Radiosurgery 61796-61800, 77371-77373
  Trigeminal Tract 61791
Transcranial Magnetic
Stimulation (TMS) 90867-90869
Transection
  Corpus Callosum 61541
  Subpial 61567
Tumor
  Excision
    Supratentorial 61510
    Infratentorial 61518
    Cerebellopontine Angle 61520, 61526
Ventriculocisternostomy 62200-62201
  Torkildsen Type 62180

Brain Coverings
See Meninges

Index (side tab)

Index

Graft Repair 31770
Stenosis 31775
Removal 32501
Foreign Body 31635
Repair 32501
Fistula 32815, 32906
Stenosis 31641, 96570-96571
Stent
Placement 31636-31637
Revision 31638
Tests
See Bronchial Challenge Test
Air Leak Assessment 31647, 31651
Airway Sizing 31647, 31651
Bronchospasm Evaluation 94070, 94620
Wheeze Rate 0243T
Thermoplasty 31660-31661
Tumor
Destruction 31641
Excision 31640
Ultrasound 31620
Unlisted Services and Procedures 31899

Bronchial Allergen Challenge
See Bronchial Challenge Test

Bronchial Alveolar Lavage 31624

Bronchial Brush Biopsy
with Catheterization 31717

Bronchial Brushings/Protected Brushing 31623

Bronchial Challenge Test
See Allergy Tests
Bronchospasm Evaluation 94070, 94620
for Wheeze Rate 0243T
with Antigens 95071
with Gases 95071
with Histamine 95070
with Methacholine 95070
with Chemicals 95070

Bronchial Provocation Tests
See Bronchial Challenge Test

Bronchioalveolar Lavage
See Lung, Lavage

Bronchial Thermoplasty . . . 31660, 31661

Broncho-Bronchial Anastomosis 32486

Bronchoalveolar Lavage
See Lung, Lavage

Bronchoplasty 32501
See Reconstruction, Bronchi
Excision Stenosis and Anastomosis 31775
Graft Repair 31770

Bronchopneumonia, Hiberno-Vernal
See Q Fever

Bronchopulmonary Lavage
See Lung, Lavage

Bronchoscopy
Ablation
Photodynamic Therapy 96570-96571
Alveolar Lavage 31624
Aspiration 31629, 31633, 31645-31646
Balloon Occlusion 31634, 31647, 31651

Biopsy 31625-31629, 31632-31633
with Bronchial Thermoplasty 31660-31661
with airway resizing 31647, 31648, 31649
with assessment airway
leak 31647, 31648, 31649
with balloon occlusion 31647, 31648, 31649
with insertion bronchial
valves 31647, 31648, 31649
Brushing/Protected Brushing 31623
Catheter Placement
Aspiration 31725
Intracavitary Radioelement 31643
Computer-assisted Navigation 31627
Dilation 31630-31631, 31636-31638
Exploration 31622, 31634, 31647, 31651
Fiducial Marker Placement 31626
Fracture Reduction 31630
Insertion of Bronchial Valve(s) 31647, 31651
Needle Biopsy 31629, 31633
Removal
Bronchial Valve 31648-31649
Foreign Body 31635
Tumor 31640-31641
Stenosis 31641
Stent Placement 31631, 31636-31637
Stent Revision 31638
Ultrasound 31620

Bronchospasm Evaluation
See Pulmonology, Diagnostic, Spirometry

Bronkodyl
See Theophylline

Brow Ptosis
Repair 67900, 67909

Brucella
Antibody 86622
Antigen 86000

Bruise
See Hematoma

Brunschwig Operation
Pelvic Exenteration 58240

Brush Biopsy
See Biopsy; Needle Biopsy
Bronchi 31717

Brush Border Ab
See Antibody, Heterophile

Bucca
See Cheek

Buccal Mucosa
See Mouth, Mucosa

Bulbourethral Gland
Excision 53250

Bulla
Incision and Drainage
Puncture Aspiration 10160
Lung
Resection-plication 32141, 32655

BUN
See Blood Urea Nitrogen; Urea Nitrogen

Bunion Repair
by Phalanx Osteotomy 28298-28299
Chevron Procedure 28296
Concentric Procedure 28296

Joplin Procedure 28294
Keller Procedure 28292
Lapidus Procedure 28297
Mayo Procedure 28292
McBride Procedure 28292
Mitchell Procedure 28296
Silver Procedure 28290
Simple Exostectomy 29290
with Implant 28293
with Metatarsal Osteotomy 28296
with Tendon Transplants 28294

Burgess Amputation
See Disarticulation, Ankle

Burkitt Herpesvirus
See Epstein-Barr Virus

Burns
Debridement 15002-15005,
16020, 16025, 16030
Dressings 16020, 16025, 16030
Escharotomy 15002-15005, 16035-16036
First Degree, Initial Treatment 16000
Tissue Cultured Skin Grafts 15150-15152,
15155-15157
Total Body Surface Area (TBSA)
Calculation 16000

Burr Hole
for Aspiration
Cyst 61156
Hematoma 61156
for Biopsy
Brain 61140
Lesion 61140, 61750-61751
for Catheterization 61210
for Drainage
Abscess 61150-61151
Cyst 61150-61151
Hematoma 61154-61156
for Exploration
Infratentorial 61253
Supratentorial 61250
for Implantation
Catheter 61210
Cerebral Monitoring Device 61210
EEG Electrode 61210
Neurostimulator Array 61850,
61863-61864, 61867-61868
Pressure Recording Device 61210
Reservoir 61210
Strip Electrodes 61531
for Insertion
Pump 61210
Reservoir 61210
for Lesion Creation 61720-61721
for Stereotactic Localization 61770
for Ventricular Puncture 61020
with Injection, Contrast Media 61120
with Injection, Diagnostic or Therapeutic
Substance 61026

Burrow's Operation
See Skin, Adjacent Tissue Transfer

Bursa
Ankle
Aspiration 20605
Incision and Drainage 27604
Injection 20605
Arm, Lower
Aspiration 20605
Incision and Drainage 25031

Index

Index

Index

Index

Index

Index

Conisation
See Cervix, Conization

Conization
Cervix 57461, 57520, 57522

Conjoint Psychotherapy
See Psychiatric Treatment, Family

Conjunctiva
Biopsy 68100
Cyst
   Incision and Drainage 68020
Fistulization for Drainage 68745, 68750
Follicle Expression 68040
Graft 65150, 65782
   Harvesting, Living Donor 68371
Injection 68200
Insertion Stent 68750
Lesion
   Destruction 68135
   Excision 68110, 68115
     with Adjacent Sclera 68130
Reconstruction 68320, 68325-68326, 68328
   with Flap 67971, 68360, 68362
Removal
   Foreign Body 65205, 65210
Repair
   Eyelid Wound 67961, 67966
     Direct Closure 65270, 67930, 67935
     Mobilization and Rearrangement . . . .
                      65272-65273
   Symblepharon
     Division 68340
     with Graft 68335
     without Graft 68330
Unlisted Services and Procedures 68399

Conjunctivo-Tarso-Muller Resection
. . . . 67908

Conjunctivocystorhinostomy
See Conjunctivorhinostomy

Conjunctivodacryocystostomy
See Conjunctivorhinostomy

Conjunctivoplasty 68320-68330
Reconstruction Cul de Sac
   with Extensive Rearrangement 68326
   with Graft 68326
     Buccal Mucous Membrane 68328
Repair of Symblepharon 68330, 68335, 68340

Conjunctivorhinostomy
with Tube 68750
without Tube 68745

Conscious Sedation
See Sedation

Construction
Arterial
   Conduit 33920, 33608
   Tunnel 33505
Bladder from Sigmoid Colon 50810
Eye Adhesions 67880
Finger
   Toe to Hand Transfer 26551-26556
Gastric Tube 43832
Neobladder 51596
Tracheoesophageal Fistula 31611
Vagina
   with Graft 57292
   without Graft 57291
Valve
   Apical-Aortic Conduit 33404

Consultation
Clinical Pathology 80500, 80502
Inpatient 99251-99255
   New or Established Patient 99251-99255
Office and/or Other Outpatient 99241-99245
   New or Established Patient 99241-99245
Psychiatric, with Family 90887
Radiation Therapy
   Radiation Physics 77336, 77370
Surgical Pathology 88321, 88323, 88325
   Intraoperative 88329, 88331-88334
X-ray 76140

Consumption Test, Antiglobulin
See Coombs Test

Contact Lens Services
Fittings and Prescription 92071-92072,
                           92310-92317
Modification 92325
Prescription 92314-92317
Replacement 92326

Continuous Negative Pressure Breathing (CNPB) 94662

Continuous Positive Airway Pressure (CPAP) 94660
See Pulmonology, Therapeutic

Contouring
Cranial
   Bones 21181
   Sutures 61559
Forehead 21137-21138
Frontal Sinus Wall 21139
Septoplasty 30520
Subcutaneous Injections 11950-11952, 11954
Tumor
   Facial Bone 21029

Contraception
Cervical Cap
   Fitting 57170
Diaphragm
   Fitting 57170
Intrauterine Device (IUD)
   Insertion 58300
   Removal 58301

Contraceptive Capsules, Implantable
Removal 11976

Contraceptive Device, Intrauterine
See Intrauterine Device (IUD)

Contracture
Bladder Neck
   Resection 52640
Elbow
   Release
     with Radical Resection of Capsule . . . 24149
Finger Cast 29086
Palm
   Release 26121-26125
Scar
Shoulder
   Capsular Release 23020
Thumb
   Thenar Muscle Release 26508
Volkmann 25315
Wrist
   Capsulotomy 25085

Contracture of Palmar Fascia
See Dupuytren's Contracture

Contralateral Ligament
Repair
   Knee 27405

Contrast Aortogram
See Aortography

Contrast Bath Therapy
See Physical Medicine/Therapy/Occupational Therapy
Application of Modality 97034

Contrast Material
Injection
   Arteriovenous Dialysis Shunt 36147
   Central Venous Access Device 36598
   Colonic Tube
     for Insertion 49440-49442
     for Radiological Evaluation 49465
     for Removal of Obstruction 49460
     for Replacement 49446, 49450-49452
   Cranial
     for Ventricular Puncture 61120
   Dacryocystography 68850
   Peritoneal
     for Assessment of Abscess or Cyst . . . 49424
     for Evaluation of Venous Shunt 49427
     for Insertion of Tunneled Catheter 49418
   Peritoneal Cavity 49400
   Renal Angiography 36251-36254
   Saline Infusion Sonohysterography
   (SIS) 58340
   Spine
     for Localization . 62310-62311, 62318-62319,
                          62263
   Urethrocystography 51605

Contrast Phlebogram
See Venography

Contusion
See Hematoma

Converting Enzyme, Angiotensin
See Angiotensin Converting Enzyme (ACE)

Coombs Test
   Antihuman Globulin
     Direct 86880
     Indirect 86885-86886
RBC Antibody Screen 86850, 86860

Copper 82525

Coprobilinogen
Feces Test 84577

Coproporphyrin 84119-84120

Coracoacromial Ligament
Release 23415, 29826

Coracoid Process Transfer 23462

Cord, Spermatic
See Spermatic Cord

Cord, Spinal
See Spinal Cord

Cord, Vocal
See Vocal Cords

Cordectomy 31300

Index

Cortisol 80400, 80402, 80406,
80418, 80420, 80436, 82530
Stimulation............................ 80412
Total 82533

Cortisol Binding Globulin 84449

Costectomy
See Resection, Ribs

Costen Syndrome
See Temporomandibular Joint (TMJ)

Costotransversectomy 21610

Cothromboplastin
See Proconvertin

Cotte Operation
Uterine Suspension 58400, 58410

Cotton Procedure
Bohler Procedure 28405

Counseling
See Preventive Medicine
Smoking and Tobacco Use Cessation 99406-99407

Counseling and/or Risk Factor Reduction Intervention, Preventive Medicine, Individual Counseling
See Preventive Medicine, Counseling and/or Risk Factor Reduction Intervention, Individual Counseling

Count
Blood Cell
   See Blood Cell Count
Blood Platelet
   See Blood, Platelet, Count
Cell
   See Cell Count
Complete Blood
   See Complete Blood Count (CBC)
Erythrocyte
   See Red Blood Cell (RBC), Count
Leukocyte
   See White Blood Cell, Count
Reticulocyte
   See Reticulocyte, Count

Counterimmuno-electrophoresis 86185

Counters, Cell
See Cell Count

Countershock, Electric
See Cardioversion

Coventry Tibial Wedge Osteotomy
See Osteotomy, Tibia

Cowper's Gland
Excision. 53250

Coxa
See Hip

Coxiella Burnetii
Antibody........................... 86638

Coxsackie
Antibody........................... 86658

CPAP
See Continuous Positive Airway Pressure

CPK
Blood....................... 82550-82552

CPR (Cardiopulmonary Resuscitation)
Cardiac Arrest 92950

Cranial Bone
See Craniectomy; Craniotomy
Bone Graft
   See Bone Graft
Burr Hole
   See Burr Hole
Frontal Bone Flap............... 61556-61557
Halo Application
   Thin Skull Osteology 20664
Parietal Bone Flap 61556
Reconstruction
   Extracranial 21181-21184
Temporal Bone
   Implantation
      Cochlear Device 69930
      Hearing Device........... 69710-69711
      Osseointegrated Implant ... 69714-69715
   Removal of Tumor 69970
   Resection 69535
   Unlisted Procedure................. 69979
Tumor
   Excision 61563-61564

Cranial Halo.................... 20661

Cranial Nerve
Avulsion 64732-64760, 64771
Cranial Nerve II
   See Optic Nerve
Cranial Nerve V
   See Trigeminal Nerve
Cranial Nerve VII
   See Facial Nerve
Cranial Nerve X
   See Vagus Nerve
Cranial Nerve XI
   See Accessory Nerve
Cranial Nerve XII
   See Hypoglossal Nerve
Decompression............ 61458, 61460, 64716
Injection
   Anesthetic
      Trigeminal Nerve 64400
      Vagus Nerve.............. 64408, 64412
   Neurolytic.......... 64600, 64605, 64610
Neuroplasty 64716
Neurostimulator
   See Neurostimulators
Release 64716
Repair
   Suture, with or without Graft ... 64864-64865
Transection.............. 64732-64760, 64771
Transposition 64716

Cranial Tongs
Application/Removal 20660
Removal 20665

Craniectomy................... 61501
See Craniotomy
Abscess Drainage 61320-61321
Anesthesia 00211
Compression........................ 61450
Craniosynostosis
   Single Suture 61550
   Multiple Sutures 61552, 61558-61559
Decompression...... 61322-61323, 61340, 61343
   Cranial Nerves 61458
   Sensory Root of Gasserian Ganglion. ... 61450
Exploratory 61304-61305, 61458

for Electrode
   Cortical.................... 61860, 61870
   Subcortical 61863-61864,
      61867-61868, 61875
Release Stenosis 61550-61552
Section 61450, 61460
Tractotomy 61470, 61480
with Craniotomy...................... 61530
Wound Treatment 61571
Surgical......... 61312-61315, 61320-61323,
   61440-61480, 61500-61516, 61518-61522

Craniofacial Procedures
Unlisted Services and Procedures 21299

Craniofacial Separation
Bone Graft 21436
Closed Treatment..................... 21431
External Fixation 21435
Open Treatment 21432-21433, 21435-21436
Wire Fixation 21431-21432

Craniomegalic Skull
Reduction 62115-62117

Craniopharyngioma
Excision.............................61545

Cranioplasty
Autograft 62146-62147
Bone Graft 61316, 62146-62147
Bone Graft Retrieval 62148
Encephalocele Repair 62120
Skull Defect 62140-62141, 62145

Craniostenosis
See Craniosynostosis

Craniosynostosis
Bifrontal Craniotomy 61557
Extensive Craniectomy 61558-61559
Front or Parietal 61556
Multiple Sutures 61552
Single Suture 61550

Craniotomy
See Burr Hole; Craniectomy; Drill Hole
Anesthesia.......................... 00211
Bifrontal 61557
Decompression................. 61322-61323
Exploratory 61304-61305
for Craniosynostosis 61556-61557
for Encephalocele 62121
for Implant of Neurostimulators 61850-61875
Frontal.............................. 61556
Parietal............................. 61556
Surgery 61312-61315, 61320-61323,
   61440, 61490, 61546, 61570-61571,
   61582-61583, 61590, 61592, 61760, 62120
with Bone Flap...... 61510-61516, 61526-61530,
   61533-61545, 61566-61567

Cranium
See Skull

Craterization
Calcaneus.......................... 28120
Clavicle............................ 23180
Femur 27070-27071, 27360
Fibula 27360, 27641
Hip................................ 27070
Humerus....................... 23184, 24140
Ileum 27070
Metacarpal......................... 26230
Metatarsal 28122
Olecranon Process 24147

Index

Index

Index

Index

Index

Toe
  Closed Treatment............ 26770, 26775,
                                    28630-28635
  Open Treatment...................... 28645
  Percutaneous Fixation 26776, 28636
Trans-Scaphoperilunar
  Closed Treatment................... 25680
  Open Treatment 25685
Vertebra
  Additional Segment
    Open Treatment 22328
  Cervical
    Open Treatment 22318-22319, 22326
  Closed Treatment
    with Manipulation, Casting and/or
    Bracing 22315
  Lumbar
    Open Treatment 22325
  Thoracic
    Open Treatment 22327
Wrist
  Closed Treatment....... 25660, 25675, 25680
  Intercarpal 25660
    Open Treatment 25670
  Open Treatment 25670, 25685
  Percutaneous Fixation 25671
  Radiocarpal 25660
    Open Treatment 25670
  Radioulnar
    Closed Treatment 25675
    Open Treatment 25676
    Percutaneous Fixation 25671
  with Fracture
    Closed Treatment 25680
    Open Treatment 25685
  with Manipulation 25660, 25675, 25680

Dislocation, Radiocarpal Joint
See Radiocarpal Joint, Dislocation

Disorder
Blood Coagulation
  See Coagulopathy
Penis
  See Penis
Retinal
  See Retina

Displacement Therapy
Nose 30210

Dissection
Axial Vessel
  for Island Pedicle 15740
Cavernous Sinus 61613
Cranial Adhesions 62161
Donor Organ
  Heart 33944
  Heart/Lung........................ 33933
  Kidney 50323, 50325
  Liver 47143
  Lung 32855
  Pancreas.......................... 48551
Facial Nerve 42420
for Debulking 58952-58953
Hygroma, Cystic
  Axillary/Cervical.............. 38550, 38555
Infrarenal Aneurysm 34825-34826, 34800,
                              34802, 34830-34832
Lymph Nodes 38542
Mediastinal 60521-60522
Neck
  See Radical Neck Dissection
Neurovascular 32503

Sclera 67107
Urethra 54328, 54332, 54336, 54348, 54352

Dissection, Neck, Radical
See Radical Neck Dissection

Distention
See Dilation

Diverticula, Meckel's
See Diverticulum, Meckel's

Diverticulectomy 44800
Esophagus 43130, 43135

Diverticulectomy, Meckel's
See Meckel's Diverticulum, Excision

Diverticulum
Bladder
  See Bladder, Diverticulum
Large Intestine 44604-44605
Meckel's
  Excision 44800
  Unlisted Procedure................. 44899
Small Intestine 44602-44603
Urethra
  Excision 53230, 53235
  Marsupialization 53240
  Urethroplasty 53400, 53405

Division
Anal Sphincter 46080
Flap.............. 15600, 15610, 15620, 15630
Intrauterine Septum................... 58560
Muscle
  Foot 28250
  Neck
    Scalenus Anticus 21700, 21705
    Sternocleidomastoid 21720, 21725
Plantar Fascia
  Foot 28250
Rectal Stricture 45150
Saphenous Vein 37700, 37722, 37735
Symblepharon 68340

Division, Isthmus, Horseshoe Kidney
See Symphysiotomy, Horseshoe Kidney

Division, Scalenus Anticus Muscle
See Division, Scalenus Anticus

Dl-Amphetamine
See Amphetamine

DMO
See Dimethadione

DNA
See Deoxyribonucleic Acid (DNA)

DNA Endonuclease
See DNAse

DNA Probe
See Cytogenetics Studies; DNA Probe

DNAse
Antibody............................ 86215

Domiciliary Services
See Nursing Facility Services
Care Plan Oversight............. 99339-99340
Discharge Services 99315-99316
Established Patient 99334-99337
New Patient 99324-99328
Supervision................... 99374-99375

Donor Procedures
See Harvesting
Bone Harvesting.............. 20900-20902
Bone Marrow Harvesting 38230, 38232
Conjunctival Graft 68371
Heart Excision 33940
Heart/Lung Excision................ 33930
Intestine Excision........... 44132, 44133
Kidney Excision 50300, 50320
Liver Excision 47133
  Segment.................. 47140-47142
Lung Excision 32850
Mucosa of Vestibule of Mouth Excision... 40818
Pancreas Excision 48550
Preparation of Fecal Microbiota 44705
Stem Cells 38204
  Donor Search 38204
  Harvesting 38205-38206

Dopamine
See Catecholamines

Doppler Echocardiography 76827-76828,
                          93306-93308, 93320-93350
Intracardiac 93662
Transesophageal 93318
Transthoracic 93303-93317

Doppler Scan
Arterial Studies
  Coronary Flow Reserve 93571-93572
  Extremities.................. 93922-93924
  Fetal
    Middle Cerebral Artery............ 76821
    Umbilical Artery 76820
Duplex
  Transplanted Kidney 76776
Extremity Veins 93965
Intracranial Arteries
  Complete Study 93886
  Emboli Detection 93892-93893
  Limited Study..................... 93888
  Vasoreactivity Study 93890
Saline Infusion Sonohysterography (SIS)... 76831
Transplanted Kidney 76776

Dorsal Vertebra
See Vertebra, Thoracic

Dose Plan
See Dosimetry

Dosimetry
Radiation Therapy
  Basic Calculation................. 77300
    Oncology....................... 0520F
  Brachytherapy 77326-77328
  Intensity Modulation 77301, 77338
  Special....................... 77331
  Teletherapy 77305, 77310, 77315, 77321
Unlisted Radiation Dosimetry Procedure ... 77399

Double-Stranded DNA
See Deoxyribonucleic Acid (DNA)

Doxepin
Assay 80166

DPH
See Phenytoin

Drainage
See Incision and Drainage; Paracentesis; Puncture Aspiration
Abscess
  Anal 46045, 46050, 46060

Index

Drainage Implant, Glaucoma
See Aqueous Shunt

Dressings

DREZ Procedure
See Incision, Spinal Cord; Incision and Drainage

DRIL
See Revascularization, Distal

Drill Hole

Drinking Test for Glaucoma
See Glaucoma, Provocative Test

Drug
See Specific Drug
Administration
　　Allergenic Extracts
　　See Allergen Immunotherapy
　　　for Cancer
　　　See Chemotherapy
　　　for Cardiac Assessments............ 93463
　　　for Helicobacter Pylori Breath Test..... 83014
　　Infusion
　　　Epidural................... 62360-62362
　　　Home.................... 99601-99602
　　　Intravenous......... 4100F, 96365-96368
　　Injection.................... 96372-96376
　　Instillation
　　　See Instillation, Drugs
　　Unlisted Injection or Infusion......... 96379
Aspirin........................... 4084F
Metabolism
　See Gene Analysis
Resistance Analysis
　HIV 1................... 87903-87904
Susceptibility Prediction
　Infectious Agent.................. 87900
Testing
　Confirmation.................... 80102
　Qualitative
　　Multiple............. 80100, 80104
　　Single..................... 80101
　　Tissue Preparation.............. 80103
　Quantitative
　　See Drug Assay

Drug Assay
Amikacin......................... 80150
Amitriptyline...................... 80152
Benzodiazepine.................... 80154
Carbamazepine.............. 80156-80157
Cyclosporine...................... 80158
Desipramine...................... 80160
Digoxin.......................... 80162
Dipropylacetic Acid................. 80164
Doxepin......................... 80166
Ethosuximide..................... 80168
Gentamicin....................... 80170
Gold............................ 80172
Haloperidol....................... 80173
Imipramine....................... 80174
Lidocaine........................ 80176
Lithium.......................... 80178
Nortriptyline...................... 80182
Phenobarbital..................... 80184
Phenytoin.................. 80185-80186
Primidone........................ 80188
Procainamide............... 80190-80192
Quantitative
　Other.......................... 80299
Quinidine........................ 80194
Salicylate........................ 80196
Sirolimus......................... 80195
Tacrolimus....................... 80197
Theophylline...................... 80198
Tobramycin....................... 80200
Topiramate....................... 80201
Vancomycin...................... 80202

Drug Delivery Implant
See Infusion Pump
Insertion......................... 11981
Irrigation......................... 96523
Maintenance and Refill

Brain........................ 95990-95991
Epidural..................... 95990-95991
Intra-arterial...................... 96522
Intrathecal................... 95990-95991
Intravenous...................... 96522
Intraventricular............... 95990-95991
Removal..................... 11982-11983
　with Reinsertion................. 11983

Drug Instillation
See Instillation, Drugs

Drug Management
by Pharmacist.................. 99605-99607
Psychiatric.......................... 90863

Drug Screen.... 80100-80101, 80104, 82486,
99408-99409

Drugs, Anticoagulant
See Anticoagulant Management; Clotting Inhibitors

DST
See Dexamethasone, Suppression Test

DT Shots......................... 90702

DTaP Immunization............. 90721

DTaP-HepB-IPV
Immunization................... 90723

DTP Immunization............. 90720

Dual Photon Absorptiometry
See Absorptiometry, Dual Photon

Dual X-ray Absorptiometry (DXA)
Appendicular....................... 77081
Axial Skeleton...................... 77080
Vertebral Fracture................... 77082

Duct, Bile
See Bile Duct

Duct, Hepatic
See Hepatic Duct

Duct, Nasolacrimal
See Nasolacrimal Duct

Duct, Omphalomesenteric
See Omphalomesenteric Duct

Duct, Pancreatic
See Pancreatic Duct

Duct, Salivary
See Salivary Duct

Duct, Stensen
See Parotid Duct

Duct, Thoracic
See Thoracic Duct

Ductogram, Mammary
See Galactogram

Ductus Arteriosus
Repair....................... 33820, 33824

Ductus Deferens
See Vas Deferens

Duhamel Procedure
See Proctectomy, Total

Dunn Operation
See Arthrodesis, Foot Joint

Duodenectomy
Partial...................... 48153-48154
Total..................... 48150, 48152

Duodenostomy
Contrast Injection.................... 49465
Insertion......................... 49441
Obstructive Material Removal.......... 49460
Radiological Evaluation............... 49465
Replacement...................... 49451

Duodenotomy
Biopsy................... 43239, 44010
　Fine Needle Aspiration............. 43242
Exploration....................... 44010
Foreign Body Removal................ 44010

Duodenum
Bariatric Surgery
　See Bariatric Surgery
Biopsy................... 43239, 44010
　Fine Needle Aspiration............. 43242
Donor Transplant............... 48550-48551
Duodenostomy
　See Duodenostomy
Endoscopy......................... 43235
　Catheter Placement............... 43241
　Cholangiopancreatography.......... 43260
　Diagnostic..................... 43235
　Dilation....................... 43245
　Drainage, Pseudocyst............. 43240
　Examination.................... 43259
　Foreign Body Removal........ 43247, 43269
　with Control of Bleeding........... 43255
　with Injection
　　Sclerotic Varix................. 43243
　　Submucosal................... 43236
　with Ligation
　　Sclerotic Varix................. 43244
　with Lithotripsy.................. 43265
　with Stent Placement/Change... 43256, 43269
Excision............... 48150, 48152-48154
Exclusion........................ 48547
Exploration....................... 44010
Foreign Body Removal................ 44010
Incision......................... 44010
Intubation and Aspiration......... 43756-43757
Lysis........................... 44055
Motility Study...................... 91022
Naso- or Oro-gastric Feeding Tube
Repositioning...................... 43761
Removal
　Lesion......... 43250-43251, 43258, 43272
　Polyp.......... 43250-43251, 43258, 43272
　Tumor......... 43250-43251, 43258, 43272
X-ray............................ 74260
Contrast Injection.................... 49465

Duplex Scan
See Vascular Studies
Arterial Studies
　Aorta...................... 93978-93979
　Extracranial................ 93880-93882
　Lower Extremity............. 93925-93926
　Penile.................... 93980-93981
　Upper Extremity............. 93930-93931
　Visceral................... 93975-93979
Doppler
　See Doppler Scan, Duplex
Hemodialysis Access.................. 93990
Venous Studies
　Extremity.................. 93970-93971
　Penile.................... 93980-93981

Index

Congenital Cardiac Anomaly
  Fetal 76825-76826
    Doppler, Fetal 76827-76828
  Transesophageal 93315-93317
  Transthoracic 93303-93304
Intracardiac 93662
Transesophageal 93312-93318
Transthoracic 93306-93308, 93350-93352
  Congenital Cardiac Anomalies 93303-93304
    with Stress Test 93350-93352

Echoencephalography
Intracranial 76506

Echography
See Ultrasound

Echotomography
See Echography

ECMO
See Extracorporeal Membrane Oxygenation

ECS
See Emission Computerized Tomography

ECSF (Erythrocyte Colony Stimulating Factor)
See Erythropoietin

ECT
See Emission Computerized Tomography

Ectasia
See Dilation

Ectopic Pregnancy
See Obstetrical Care
Abdominal 59130
Cervix 59140
Laparoscopy 59150
  with Salpingectomy and/or
  Oophorectomy 59151
Ovarian 59121
  with Salpingectomy and/or
  Oophorectomy 59120
Tubal 59121
  with Salpingectomy and/or
  Oophorectomy 59120
Uterine
  with Hysterectomy 59135
  with Partial Uterine Resection 59136

Ectropion
Repair
  Excision Tarsal Wedge 67916
  Extensive 67917
  Suture 67914
  Thermocauterization 67915

Education Services
Group 98961-98962, 99078
Individual
  Pediatric Gastroenteritis Education 4058F

Education Supplies
Provided to Patient 99071

EEG
See Electroencephalography (EEG)

Egg
See Ova

Ehrlichia
Antibody 86666

EKG
See Electrocardiography

Elastase 82656
Elbow
See Humerus; Radius; Ulna
Abscess
  Incision and Drainage 23930, 23935
Anesthesia
  See Anesthesia, Elbow
Arthrectomy 24155
Arthrocentesis 20605
Arthrodesis 24800, 24802
Arthrography 73085
  Contrast Injection 24220
Arthroplasty 24360
  Total Replacement 24361-24363, 24365-24366
    Revision 24370-24371
    Implant Removal 24160, 24164
    with Implant 24361-24362
Arthroscopy
  Diagnostic 29830
  Surgical 29834-29838
Arthrotomy 24000
  Capsular Release 24006
  Drainage 24000
  Exploration 24000, 24101
  Removal of Foreign Body 24000
  Synovectomy 24102
  Synovial Biopsy 24100
Biopsy 24065-24066, 24101
  Synovial 24100, 29830
Bone Cortex Incision 23935
Capsule
  Excision 24006
  Radical Resection 24149
Contracture Release 24149
Dislocation
  Closed Treatment 24600, 24605, 24640
  Nursemaid Elbow 24640
  Open Treatment 24615
  Subluxate 24640
Epicondylitis 24357-24359
Excision
  Bursa 24105
  Synovium 24102, 29835-29836
  Tumor
  Soft Tissue 24077, 24079
    Subcutaneous 24071, 24075
    Subfascial 24076
Exploration 24000, 24101
Fracture
  Monteggia 24620, 24635
  Open Treatment 24586-24587
Hematoma
  Incision and Drainage 23930
Implant
  Removal 24164
Incision and Drainage
  Abscess, Deep 23930
  Bursa 23931
  Hematoma 23930
Injection
  Arthrography
    Radiologic 24220
  Magnetic Resonance Imaging (MRI) 73221
Manipulation 24300
Resection
  Capsule 24149
  Heterotropic Bone 24149
  Joint 24155
  Soft Tissue 24149
    with Contracture Release 24149
Removal

Foreign Body 24000, 24101, 24200-24201,
                                           29834
  Implant 24160
  Loose Body 24101, 29834
Repair
  Advancement 24330-24331
  Epicondylitis 24357-24359
  Flexorplasty 24330
  Graft 24320
  Hemiepiphyseal Arrest 24470
  Ligament 24343-24346
  Muscle 24341
  Muscle Transfer 24301, 24320
  Tendon 24340-24342, 24357-24359
    Lengthening 24305
    Repair 24341, 24359
    Tenodesis 24340
    Tenotomy 24310, 24357-24359
    Transfer 24301
  Tennis Elbow 24357-24359
Seddon-Brookes Procedure 24320
Steindler Advancement 24330
Strapping 29260
Tumor
  Excision 24071-24076
  Radical Resection 24077-24079
Ulnar Neuroplasty 64718
Unlisted Elbow Procedure 24999
X-ray 73070, 73080
  with Contrast 73085

Elbow, Golfer
See Elbow, Tendon; Tennis Elbow

Elbows, Tennis
See Elbow, Tendon; Tennis Elbow

Electric Countershock
See Cardioversion

Electric Stimulation
See Electrical Stimulation

Electric Stimulation, Transcutaneous
See Application, Neurostimulation

Electrical Modulation Pain Reprocessing, Transcutaneous 0278T

Electrical Stimulation
Acupuncture 97813-97814
Arrhythmia Induction 93618
Bone Healing
  Invasive 20975
  Noninvasive 20974
Brain Surface 95961-95962
Guidance
  for Chemodenervation 95873
Physical Therapy
  Attended, Manual 97032
  Unattended 97014
Spine 63650, 63655, 63661-63664,
                                    63685, 63688

Electro-Hydraulic Procedure . . . 52325

Electro-Oculography 92270

Electroanalgesia
See Application, Neurostimulation

Electrocardiography
12 Lead 3120F, 93000

Index

Index

Index

Index

Index

Index

Index

Skin
  Benign.. 11400-11404, 11406, 11420-11424,
    11426, 11440-11444, 11446, 11450-11451,
      11462-11464, 11470-11471
  Malignant.................11600-11604, 11606,
    11620-11624, 11626, 11640-11644, 11646
Skull.................61500, 61615-61616
  Anterior.................61600-61601
  Base.................61575-61576
  Middle.................61605-61608
  Posterior.................61615-61616
Spermatic Cord.................55520
Spinal Cord
  Intraspinal..... 63265-63268, 63270-63273,
    63300-63308
  Upper.................61575-61576
Tendon Sheath
  Ankle and/or Leg.................27630
  Forearm or Wrist.................25110
Testis.................54512
Toe.................28092
Tongue.............41110, 41112-41114
Urethra.................52224
Uterus
Uvula.................42104, 42106-42107
Vertebral Column.............22100-22103
  Without Decompression..... 22110, 22112,
    22114, 22116
Wrist Tendon Sheath.................25110
Lip.................40500, 40510, 40520, 40525
Liver
  See Hepatectomy
Lung
  Bronchus Resection.................32486
  Bullae
    Completion.................32488
    Lobe.................32480-32482
  Pleurectomy.................32310, 32320
  Pneumonectomy.............32440-32445
  Segment.................32484
  Tumor, Apical.............32503-32504
Lung/Heart, Donor.................33930
Lymphatic System
  Hygroma, Cystic.............38550, 38555
  Nodes... 38500, 38510 , 38520, 38525, 38530
  See Lymphadenectomy
Mandible
  Cyst.................21040, 21046-21047
  Tumor.................21040, 21044-21047
  Mandibular Torus
    Exostosis.................21031
Mass
  Mediastinum.................32662
  Pericardium.................32661
Mastoid Process
  See Mastoidectomy
Maxilla
  Cyst.................21030, 21048-21049
  Tumor.........21030, 21034, 21048-21049
Maxillary Torus Palatinus.................21032
Mediastinum
  Cyst.................32662, 39200
  Tumor.................32662
Meningioma
  Brain.................61512, 61519
Meniscus
  Temporomandibular Joint.................21060
Mesentary
  Lesion.................44820
  Meckle's Diverticulum.................44800
Metacarpal.................26230
  Cyst.................26200, 26205
  Tumor.................26200-26205

Metatarsal
  Cyst.................28104, 28106-28107
  Head..... 28110-28114, 28122, 28140, 28288
  Tumor.................28104, 28106-28107
Mouth
  Frenum.................40819, 41115
  Lesion.............40810-40816, 41116
  Mucosa.................40818
  Ranula.................42408
Mucosa
  Gums.................41828
  Vestibule of Mouth.................40818
Nail Fold.................11765
Nails.................11750-11752
Neck
  Tumor.................21552, 21554-21556
Neoplasm
  Spine.................63275-63290
Nerve
  Foot.................28055
  Hamstring Muscle.................27325
  Neurofibroma.................64788-64792
  Neurolemmoma.................64788-64792
  Neuroma.................64774-64786
  Popliteal.................27326
  Sympathetic
    See Sympathectomy
  Neurofibroma.................64788-64790
  Neurolemmoma.................64788-64792
  Neuroma.................64774-64786
Nose
  Cyst.................30124-30125
  Lesion.................30117-30118
  Polyp.................30110-30115
  Rhinectomy.................30150, 30160
  Skin.................30120
  Turbinate, Inferior.................30130, 30140
Odontoid Process.................22548
Olecranon Process.................24147
  Cyst.................24120, 24125-24126
  Tumor.................24120, 24125-24126
Omentum.................49255
Operculum.................41821
Orbit
  Lesion.................61333, 67412, 67420
Ovary
  Cystectomy.................58925
  Oophorectomy.........58940, 58943
  Salpingo-oophorectomy.................58720
  Wedge Resection/Bisection.........58920
Oviduct.................58700, 58720
Palate.................42120, 42145
  Lesion.............42104, 42106-42107
Pancreas
  See Pancreatectomy
  Ampulla of Vater.................48148
  Lesion.................48120
  Peripancreatic Tissue.................48105
Parathyroid Gland.........60500, 60502, 60505
  Tumor.... 42410, 42415, 42420, 42425-42426
Parotid Gland
  Partial.................42410-42415
  Total.................42420-42426
Patella.................27350
Pelvis
  Tumor.... 27043, 27045, 27047-27049, 27059
Penis
  Amputation..... 54120, 54125, 54130, 54135
  Circumcision..... 54150, 54160-54161, 54163
  Frenulotomy.................54164
  Lesion.................54060
  Plaque.................54110-54112
  Post-Circumcision Adhesion.........54162

Pericardium.................33030-33031
  Cyst.................32661
  Mass.................32661
  Tumor.................32661
Peritoneum
  Tumor.................49203-49205
Petrous Temporal Apex.................69530
Phalanges
  Cyst
    Finger.................26210, 26215
    Toe.................28108
  Finger.................26235-26236
  Toe.........28124, 28126, 28150, 28153
  Hemiphalangectomy.................28160
  Tumor... 26210, 26215, 26260, 26262, 28108,
    28175
Pharynx.........42145, 42890, 42892, 42894
  Cyst.................42810, 42815
  Lesion.................42808
  with Larynx.................31390, 31395
Pituitary Gland.................61546, 61548
  Tumor.........61546, 61548, 62165
Plaque
  Penis.................54110-54112
Pleura.................32310-32320
  Thoracoscopic.................32656
Polyp
  Nose.................30110, 30115
    Endoscopic.................31237
  Urethra.................53260
    Caruncle.................53265
Presacral
  Tumor.................49215
Prostate
  See Proctectomy
Pterygium.................65420, 65426
Pulmonary Artery.........33910, 33915-33916
Pubic Symphysis.................27070-27071
  Cyst.................27065-27067
  Tumor.................27065-27067
Radius.................24130, 24145, 25151
  Cyst.................24120, 24125-24126,
    25120, 25125-25126
  Styloid Process.................25230
  Tumor.... 24120, 24125, 25120, 25125-25126
Rectum
  See Proctectomy
  Lesion.................45108
  Prolapse.................45130, 45135
  Stricture.................45150
  Tumor.................45160, 45171-45172
Redundant Skin of Eyelid
  See Blepharoplasty
Retroperineal
  Tumor.................49203-49205
Ribs.............21600, 21610, 21615-21616
Sacrococcygeal
  Tumor.................49215
Salivary Gland Duct
  Cyst.................42408
Scalp
  Tumor.................21011-21014
Scapula.................23172, 23182, 23190
  Cyst.................23140, 23145, 23146
  Tumor.................23140, 23145, 23146
Sclera.................66150, 66155, 66160, 66165, 66170
  Lesion.................66130
Scrotum.................55150
Semilunar Cartilage of Knee
  See Knee, Meniscectomy
Seminal Vesicle.................55650
  Mullerian Duct Cyst.................55680

Index

Index

Index

Factor, Antinuclear
See Antinuclear Antibodies (ANA)

Factor, Blood Coagulation
See Clotting Factor

Factor, Fitzgerald
See Fitzgerald Factor

Factor, Fletcher
See Fletcher Factor

Factor, Hyperglycemic-Glycogenolytic
See Glucagon

Factor Inhibitor Tests
See Pathology and Laboratory, Factor Inhibitor Tests

Factor, Intrinsic
See Intrinsic Factor

Factor, Rheumatoid
See Rheumatoid Factor

Factor, Sulfation
See Somatomedin

Fallopian Tube
Anastomosis.........................58750
Biopsy.............................49321
Cannulation 58565
Catheterization.................58345, 74742
Destruction
    Endoscopic 58670
Ectopic Pregnancy 59121
    with Salpingectomy and/or
    Oophorectomy 59120, 59151
Excision.......... 58661, 58700, 58720, 58943,
                58950, 58953, 58956
Ligation..................58600, 58606, 58611
Lysis
    Adhesions 58740
Occlusion 58615
    Endoscopic......................58671
Placement
    Implant for Occlusion...............58565
Repair 58752
    Anastomosis 58750
    Create Stoma...............58673, 58770
Tumor
    Resection............58950, 58952-58954,
                  58956-58958
Unlisted Services and Procedures 58999
X-ray
Hysterosalpingography 74740

Fallopian Tube Pregnancy
See Ectopic Pregnancy, Tubal

Fallot, Tetralogy of
See Tetralogy of Fallot

Family Psychotherapy
See Psychotherapy, Family

Fanconi Anemia
Chromosome Analysis...........81242, 88248

Farnsworth-Munsell Color Test
See Color Vision Examination

Farr Test
See Gammaglobulin, Blood

Fasanella-Servat Procedure ... 67908

Fascia Graft 15840

Fascia Lata Graft
Harvesting 20920-20922

Fascial Defect
Leg 27656
Urostomy 50728

Fascial Graft
Cheek 15840
Fascia and Skin
    Flap...........15732, 15734, 15736, 15738
Free
    Microvascular Anastomosis 15758
Harvest...................... 20920, 20922
Reconstruction
    Collateral Ligament 26541
    Hamstring Muscle 27386
    Infrapatellar Tendon. 27381
    Quadriceps Muscle 27386
    Tendon Pulley. 26502
Sternoclavicular Dislocation 23532

Fasciectomy
Foot.......................... 28060-28062
Palm 26121-26125

Fasciocutaneous Flaps
Muscle 15732-15738
Pharyngeal Wall..................... 42894

Fasciotomy
Arm, Lower............... 24495, 25020-25025
Buttock
    Decompression 27027
    with Debridement. 27057
Foot.............................. 28008
Hand Decompression.................. 26037
Hip.............................. 27025
Knee 27305, 27496-27499
Leg, Lower 27600-27602, 27892-27894
Leg, Upper 27305, 27496-27499, 27892-27894
Palm 26040-26045
Pelvis
    Decompression 27027
    with Debridement. 27057
Plantar
    Endoscopic...................... 29893
Thigh............................. 27025
Toe.............................. 28008
Wrist......................... 25020-25025

FAST
See Allergen Immunotherapy

Fat
Feces.......................... 82705-82715
Removal
    Lipectomy.................. 15876-15879

Fat Stain
Feces............................. 89125
Respiratory Secretions 89125
Sputum........................... 89125
Urine............................. 89125

Fatty Acid
Blood............................ 82725
Long-Chain Omega-3
    Red Blood Cell (RBC) Membranes...... 0111T
Very Long Chain 82726

Favre-Durand Disease
See Lymphogranuloma Venereum

FcReceptor 86243

FDP
See Fibrin Degradation Products

Fecal Microbiota Transplant ... 44705

Feedback, Psychophysiologic
See Biofeedback; Training, Biofeedback

Female Castration
See Oophorectomy

Female Gonad
See Ovary

Femoral Arteries
See Artery, Femoral

Femoral Nerve
Injection
    Anesthetic 64447-64448

Femoral Stem Prosthesis
See Arthroplasty, Hip

Femoral Vein
See Vein, Femoral

Femur
See Hip; Knee; Leg, Upper
Abscess
    Incision......................... 27303
Amputation........................ 27590
Bone Graft 27170, 27177, 27470
Bursa
    Excision 27062
Craterization........... 27070-27071, 27360
Cyst
    Excision 27065-27067, 27355-27358
Diaphysectomy...................... 27360
Drainage........................... 27303
Excision. 27070-27071, 27360
Femoroplasty 29914
Fracture........................... 27244
    Closed Treatment...........27501-27503,
                   27267-27268
    Distal 27508, 27510, 27514
    Distal, Medial or Lateral Condyle 27509
      Open Treatment 27514
    Epiphysis 27516-27519
      Open Treatment 27519
    Intertrochanteric 27244
      Closed Treatment 27238
      Treatment with Implant 27244
      with Implant................... 27245
      with Manipulation 27240
    Neck
      Closed Treatment 27230-27232
      Open Treatment 27236, 27177-27179,
                      27181
      Percutaneous Fixation 27235
    Open Treatment 27245, 27269,
             27506-27507, 27511-27513
    Percutaneous Fixation 27509
    Peritrochanteric 27244
      Closed Treatment 27238
      Open Treatment 27236, 27269
      Treatment with Implant 27244
      with Implant................... 27245
      with Manipulation 27240
    Proximal End, Head
      Closed Treatment 27267-27268
    Shaft......... 27500, 27502, 27506-27507
    Subtrochanteric 27244
      Closed Treatment 27238
      Treatment with Implant 27244
      with Implant................... 27245

Index

Index

Index

Index

Fructose Intolerance Breath Test..................91065

Fruit Sugar
See Fructose

FSF............................85290-85291

FSH
See Follicle Stimulating Hormone (FSH)

FSP
See Fibrin Degradation Products

FT-4............................84439

Fulguration
Bladder..........................51020, 52285
Cervix........................57500, 57520
Cystourethroscopy with..........52214, 52400
    Lesion............................52224
    Tumor..........52234-52235, 52240, 52250
Kidney
    Endoscopic..................50557, 50576
Lesion
    Ovary.............................58662
    Pelvis.............................58662
    Peritoneal.........................58662
Oviducts.............................58670
Ureter................50957, 50976, 52354
Ureterocele
    Ectopic............................52301
    Orthotopic.........................52300
Urethra................52285, 53220, 53260

Fulguration, Endocavitary
See Electrocautery

Full Thickness Graft........15200-15261

Function Test, Lung
See Pulmonology, Diagnostic

Function Test, Vestibular
See Vestibular Function Tests

Function, Study, Nasal
See Nasal Function Study

Functional Ability
See Activities of Daily Living

Fundoplasty
Esophagogastric.........................43325
    Laparoscopic..........43279, 43280, 43283
    Laparotomy.........................43327
    Thoracotomy.........................43328
Esophagomyotomy
    Laparoscopic.......................43279
Paraesophageal Hiatal Hernia Repair
    Laparoscopic..................43281-43282
    with Fundoplication
        Laparotomy.................43332-43333
        Thoracoabdominal Incisional...43336-43337
        Thoracotomy..............43334-43335

Fundoplication
Paraesophageal Hiatal Hernia Repair
    via Laparotomy...............43332-43333
    via Thoracoabdominal Incision....43336-43337
    via Thoracotomy..............43334-43335

Fungus
Antibody............................86671
Culture
    Blood..........................87103
    Hair............................87101
    Identification...................87106

Nail................................87101
Other...............................87102
Skin................................87101
Tissue Exam.........................87220

Funnel Chest
See Pectus Excavatum

Furuncle
Incision and Drainage...........10060-10061

Furuncle, Vulva
See Abscess, Vulva

Fusion
Great Toe............................28760
Interphalangeal......................28285
Motatarsocuneiform...................28297
Pleural Cavity
    Instillation of Agent for Pleurodesis....32560
Thumb
    in Opposition.....................26820
Vertebrae
See Arthrodesis

Fusion, Epiphyseal-Diaphyseal
See Epiphyseal Arrest

Fusion, Joint
See Arthrodesis

Fusion, Joint, Ankle
See Ankle, Arthrodesis

Fusion, Joint, Interphalangeal, Finger
See Arthrodesis, Finger Joint, Interphalangeal

G

Gait Training.....................97116

Galactogram..............77053-77054
Injection............................19030

Galactokinase
Blood................................82759

Galactose
Blood................................82760
Urine................................82760

Galactose-1-Phosphate
Uridyl Transferase...............82775-82776

Galeazzi Fracture/Dislocation
Radial Shaft..............25520, 25525-25526

Gall Bladder
See Gallbladder

Gallbladder
See Bile Duct
Anastomosis
    with Intestines....47720-47721, 47740-47741
Biopsy...............................43261
Diagnostic Imaging
    Nuclear Medicine............78226-78227
    X-ray with Contrast..........74290-74291
Excision
    See Cholecystectomy
Exploration.........................47480

Endoscopic Retrograde
    Cholangiopancreatography (ERCP).....43260
Fistulization.....................47480, 47490
Incision............................47480
Incision and Drainage................47480
Pharmacologic Intervention...........78227
Removal
    Calculi (Stone)...................47480
Repair
    with Gastroenterostomy.............47741
    with Intestines....47720-47721, 47740-47741
Stimulation..........................43757
Unlisted Services and Procedures........47999

Galvanocautery
See Electrocautery

Galvanoionization
See Iontophoresis

Gamete Intrafallopian Transfer (GIFT)............................58976

Gamete Transfer
In Vitro Fertilization.................58976

Gamma Camera Imaging
See Nuclear Medicine

Gamma Glutamyl Transferase......................82977

Gamma Seminoprotein
See Antigen, Prostate Specific

Gammacorten
See Dexamethasone

Gammaglobulin
Blood...................82784-82785, 82787

Gamulin Rh
See Immune Globulins, Rho(D)

Ganglia, Trigeminal
See Gasserian Ganglion

Ganglion
Cyst
    Aspiration/Injection...............20612
    Drainage..........................20612
    Wrist
        Excision..................25111-25112
Gasserian
    See Gasserian Ganglion
Geniculate
    Facial Nerve
        Decompression...........69720, 69725
        Suture...................69740, 69745
Injection
    Anesthetic
        Sphenopalatine.................64505
        Stellate........................64510
Stellate
    See Stellate Ganglion

Ganglion Cervicothoracicum
See Stellate Ganglion

Ganglion Pterygopalatinum
See Sphenopalatine Ganglion

Ganglion, Gasser's
See Gasserian Ganglion

Gardner Operation
See Meningocele Repair

Index

Gene Product
See Protein

Genioplasty

Genitourinary Sphincter, Artificial
See Prosthesis, Urethral Sphincter

Genotype Analysis

Gentamicin

Gentamycin Level
See Gentamicin

Gentiobiase
See Beta Glucosidase

Genus: Human Cytomegalovirus Group
See Cytomegalovirus

GERD
See Gastroesophageal Reflux Test

German Measles
See Rubella

Gestational Trophoblastic Tumor
See Hydatidiform Mole

GGT
See Gamma Glutamyl Transferase

GI Tract
See Gastrointestinal Tract

Giardia

Giardia Lamblia

Gibbons Stent

GIF
See Somatostatin

GIFT
See Gamete Intrafallopian Transfer

Gill Operation

Gillies Approach

Gingiva
See Gums

Gingiva, Abscess

Gingivectomy

Gingivoplasty

Girdlestone Laminectomy
See Laminectomy

Girdlestone Procedure
See Acetabulum, Reconstruction

Gla Protein (Bone)
See Osteocalcin

Gland
See Specific Gland

Gland, Adrenal
See Adrenal Gland

Gland, Bartholin's
See Bartholin's Gland

Gland, Bulbourethral
See Bulbourethral Gland

Gland, Lacrimal
See Lacrimal Gland

GMP, Cyclic
See Cyclic GMP

Goeckerman Treatment
Photochemotherapy........ 96910, 96912-96913

Gol-Vernet Operation
See Pyelotomy, Exploration

Gold
Assay 80172

Goldwaite Procedure
Knee 27422

Golfer's Elbow
See Tennis Elbow

Gonadectomy, Female
See Oophorectomy

Gonadectomy, Male
See Excision, Testis

Gonadotropin
Chorionic....................... 84702-84704
   Stimulation Panel.................. 80414
FSH 83001
ICSH 83002
LH 83002
Stimulation Panel..................... 80426

Gonadotropin Panel
Stimulation............................ 80426

Gonioscopy
Ophthalmic........................... 92020

Goniotomy
Congenital Glaucoma 65820

Gonococcus
See Neisseria Gonorrhoeae

Goodenough Harris Drawing Test
Psychological Testing............. 96101-96103

GOTT
See Transaminase, Glutamic Oxaloacetic

GPUT
See Galactose-1-Phosphate, Uridyl Transferase

Graft
Anal...................................... 46753
Aorta...............33840-33851, 33860-33877
Artery
   Bypass Graft
      See Bypass Graft, Arterial/Arterial-Venous
   Coronary........................... 33503
Bone
 See Bone Graft
Bone Marrow
   See Bone Marrow, Transplantation
Bone and Skin 20969-20970, 20972-20973
Cartilage
   See Cartilage Graft
Conjunctiva........................... 65782
   Harvesting 68371
Cornea
   with Lesion Excision 65426
Cornea Transplant
   See Cornea, Transplantation
Dura
   Cranial

Craniectomy 61343
   Anterior Cranial Fossa 61601
   Middle Cranial Fossa 61606, 61608
   Posterior Cranial Fossa............ 61616
Spinal Cord............................ 63710
   Laminectomy 63180, 63182
Eye
   Amniotic Membrane 65778-65780
   Conjunctiva 65782
   Stem Cell 65781
for Facial Nerve Paralysis
   Fascia 15840
   Muscle 15841-15842, 15845
Fascia
   See Fascial Grafts
Fascia Lata
   Harvesting 20920, 20922
Gum Mucosa 41870
Intestine 43116, 46748
Muscle
   See Muscle Flaps; Muscle Grafts
Nail Bed
   Reconstruction................... 11762
Nerve
   See Nerve Graft
Oral Mucosa.......................... 40818
Organ
   See Transplantation
Pancreas
   See Pancreas, Transplantation
Patency
   Blood Flow Check.................. 15860
   Vascular Flow Check 15860
Skin
   See Skin Graft and Flap
Skin Substitute
   See Skin Substitute Graft
Tendon
   Finger 26392, 26416, 26420, 26428, 26434
   Hand.............. 26392, 26412, 26416
   Harvesting 20924
Tissue
   Harvesting 20926
Vein
   Bypass Graft
      See Bypass Graft, Venous
   Cross-Over 34520

Grain Alcohol
See Alcohol, Ethyl

Granulation Tissue
Cauterization, Chemical................ 17250

Gravis, Myasthenia
See Myasthenia Gravis

Gravities, Specific
See Specific Gravity

Great Toe
Arthrodesis
   Interphalangeal Joint............... 28755
      with Tendon Transfer 28760
   Metatarsophalangeal Joint........... 28750
Fracture
   Skeletal Fixation 28496
   Closed Treatment.................. 28490
   Open Treatment 28505
Osteocutaneous Flap................... 20973
Toe-to-Hand Transfer.................. 20973
   Wrap-around with Bone Graft........ 26551

Great Vessels
Graft Insertion 33330, 33332, 33335
Shunt
   Aorta to Pulmonary Artery
      Ascending.....................33755
      Descending.....................33762
   Central 33764
   Subclavian to Pulmonary Artery 33750
   Vena Cava to Pulmonary
      Artery.................. 33766-33767
Suture Repair..................... 33320-33322
Translocation
   Aortic Root.................. 33782-33783
Transposition Repair
   Aortic Pulmonary Artery
      Reconstruction.............. 33778-33781
   Atrial Baffle Procedure 33774-33777
   with Subpulmonary Stenosis.... 33770-33771
   with Ventricular Septal
      Defect.................... 33770-33771
Unlisted Services and Procedures 33999

Great Vessels Transposition
See Transposition, Great Arteries

Greater Tuberosity Fracture
Humeral
   Closed Treatment....... 23620, 23625, 23665
   Open Treatment 23630, 23670
with Shoulder Dislocation
   Closed Treatment.................. 23665
   Open Treatment 23670

Greater Vestibular Gland
See Bartholin's Gland

Green Operation
See Scapulopexy

Grippe, Balkan
See Q Fever

Gritti Operation
See Amputation, Leg, Upper; Radical Resection;
Replantation

Groin Area
Incision
   Femoral Artery Exposure 34812
Repair
   Hernia...................... 49550-49557
Revision
   Femoral Arterial Bypass Graft........ 35883

Group Health Education
   Genetic.............. 98961-98962, 99078
   Physical 99078
   Preventive Medicine 99411
   Self-Management, Condition or
      Treatment.................. 98961-98962

Grouping, Blood
See Blood Typing

Growth Factors, Insulin-Like
See Somatomedin

Growth Hormone 83003
Human
   Measurement...................... 83003
   Antibody.......................... 86277
Growth Hormone Stimulation Panel...... 80428
Growth Hormone Suppression Panel 80430
Insulin Tolerance Panel 80435
Pituitary Evaluation Panel 80418

Growth Hormone Release Inhibiting Factor
See Somatostatin

GTT
See Hydatidiform Mole

Guaiac Test
See Blood, Feces

Guanosine Monophosphate
Measurement 83008

Guanosine Monophosphate, Cyclic
See Cyclic GMP

Guanylic Acids
See Guanosine Monophosphate

Guard Stain
Special Stain, Group II 88313

Gullet
See Esophagus

Gums
Abscess
   Incision and Drainage 41800
Alveolus
   Excision 41830
Cyst
   Incision and Drainage 41800
Excision
   Gingiva 41820
   Operculum 41821
Graft
   Mucosa 41870
Hematoma
   Incision and Drainage 41800
Lesion
   Destruction 41850
   Excision 41825-41827
Mucosa
   Excision 41828
   Graft 41870
Reconstruction
   Alveolus 41874
   Gingiva 41872
Removal
   Bone 41806
   Foreign Body 41805
Tuberosities
   Excision 41822-41823
Tumor
   Excision 41825-41827
Unlisted Services and Procedures 41899

Gunning-Lieben Test
See Acetone, Blood or Urine

Guthrie Test
Phenylalanine (PKU) 84030

H

H Flu
See Hemophilus Influenza

H1N1
Immunization
  See Vaccines

HAA (Hepatitis Associated Antigen)
See Hepatitis Antigen, B Surface

HAAb
See Antibody, Hepatitis

Haemoglobin F
See Fetal Hemoglobin

Haemorrhage
See Hemorrhage

Haemorrhage Rectum
See Hemorrhage, Rectum

Hageman Factor
Clotting Factor XII 85280

HAI Test
See Hemagglutination Inhibition Test

Hair
Cell
   Ear, Function Analysis 92588
Electrolysis 17380
Fungi Isolation 87101
KOH Examination 87220
Microscopic Evaluation 96902
Transplant
   Punch Graft 15775-15776
   Strip Graft 15220-15221

Hair Removal
See Removal, Hair

Hallux
See Great Toe

Halo
Body Cast 29000
Cranial 20661
   for Thin Skull Osteology 20664
Femur 20663
Maxillofacial 21100
Pelvic 20662
Removal 20665

Haloperidol
Assay 80173

Halstead-Reitan Neuropsychological Battery
Neuropsychological Testing 96118-96119

Halsted Mastectomy
See Mastectomy, Radical

Halsted Repair
See Hernia, Repair, Inguinal

Ham Test
See Hemolysins

Hammertoe Repair
Correction 28285-28286

Hamster Penetration Test
Sperm Evaluation 89329

Hand
Amputation
   at Metacarpal 25927, 26910
   at Wrist 25920
     Revision 25922
   Ray Amputation 26910
     Revision 25924, 25929, 25931

Bone
  Cyst
   Curettage 26210, 26215
   Excision 26210, 26215
   Osteotomy, Metacarpal 26565
  Incision and Drainage 26034
Casts, Splints, and Strapping 29065, 29085
  Compression System 29584
  Gauntlet Cast 29085
  Long Arm Cast 29065
  Long Arm Splint 29105
  Short Arm Cast 29075
  Short Arm Splint 29125-29126
  Strapping 29280
Decompression 26035
Diagnostic Imaging
  Magnetic Resonance Imaging
  (MRI) 73218-73220
   Angiography 73225
  X-ray 73120, 73130
Fasciectomy 26121, 26123, 26125
Fasciotomy
  Decompressive 26037
  Injection, Enzyme 20527, 26341
  Open 36045
  Percutaneous 26040
Drainage
  Bursa 26025, 26030
Fracture
  Carpometacarpal 26645, 26650
  Interphalangeal
   See Phalanx, Finger
  Metacarpal
   Closed Treatment 26600, 26605, 26607
   Open Treatment 26615
   Skeletal Fixation 26608
  Metacarpophalangeal 26740-26746
  Phalangeal 26720-26735, 26750-26765
Insertion
  Tendon Graft 26392
Joint
  See Carpometacarpal Joint; Intercarpal Joint
Manipulation
  Carpometacarpal Fracture 26645, 26650
  Dupuytren's Cord 26341
  Joint Dislocation
   See Carpometacarpal Joint; Intercarpal
   Joint
  Metacarpal Fracture 26605, 26607
  Palmar Fascial Cord 26341
Nerve
  Graft 64890-64891, 64895-64896
  Neuroma, Excision 64782-64783
  Neuroplasty 64704
  Suture
   Additional Nerve 64837
   Common Sensory 64834
   Digital 64831
Reconstruction
  Tendon Pulley 26500-26502
Removal
  Implantation 26320
  Tube/Rod 26390-26392, 26416
Repair
  Blood Vessel 35207
  Cleft Hand 26580
  Muscle 26591-26593
   Release, Thenar 26508
   Transfer, Hypothenar 26494
  Non-Union, Metacarpal 26546
Tendon
  Extensor
   Delayed Tendon Graft 26416

Index

Index

Index

Index

Muscle
Incision and Suspension 21685

Hyperbaric Oxygen Pressurization 99183

Hypercycloidal X-ray 76101-76102

Hyperdactylies
See Supernumerary Digit

Hyperglycemic Glycogenolytic Factor
See Glucagon

Hyperhidrosis 64650-64653

Hypertelorism of Orbit
See Orbital Hypertelorism

Hyperthermia Therapy
See Thermotherapy

Hyperthermia Treatment 77600-77620

Hypnotherapy 90880

Hypodermis
See Subcutaneous Tissue

Hypogastric Plexus
Destruction 64681
Injection
Anesthetic 64517
Neurolytic 64680-64681

Hypoglossal Nerve
Anastomosis
Facial-Hypoglossal 64868
Facial-Phrenic 64870
Facial-Spinal 64866

Hypoglossal-Facial Anastomosis
See Hypoglossal Nerve, Anastomosis, Facial-Hypoglossal

Hypopharynges
See Hypopharynx

Hypopharynx
Biopsy 42802

Hypophysectomy 61546-61548, 62165

Hypophysis
See Pituitary Gland

Hypopyrexia
See Hypothermia

Hypospadias
Repair 54300, 54352
Complications 54340-54348
First Stage 54304
Proximal Penile or Penoscrotal 54332
One Stage
Meatal Advancement 54322
Perineal 54336
Urethroplasty
Local Skin Flaps 54324
Local Skin Flaps and Mobilization of Urethra 54326
Local Skin Flaps, Skin Graft Patch and/or Island Flap 54328
Urethroplasty for Second Stage 54308, 54312, 54316
Free Skin Graft 54316
Urethroplasty for Third Stage 54318

Hypothermia
Treatment
Neonatal
Selective 0261T
Systemic 0260T

Hypoxia
Breathing Response 94450
High Altitude Simulation Test 94452-94453

Hysterectomy
Abdominal
Radical 58210
Resection of Ovarian Malignancy 58951, 58953-58954, 58956
Supracervical 58180
Total 50150, 58200, 58956
with Colpo-Urethrocystopexy 58152
with Omentectomy 58956
with Partial Vaginectomy 58200
Cesarean
after Cesarean Delivery 59525
with Closure of Vesicouterine Fistula . . . 51925
Laparoscopic 58541-58544
Radical 58548
Total 58570-58573
Removal
Lesion 59100
Supracervical
Laparoscopic 58541-58544
Vaginal 58260-58270, 58290-58294, 58550-58554
Laparoscopic 58550, 58570-58573
Radical 58285
Removal Tubes/Ovaries 58262-58263, 58291-58292, 58552, 58554
Repair of Enterocele . . . 58263, 58292, 58294
with Colpectomy 58275-58280
with Colpo-Urethrocystopexy . . . 58267, 58293

Hysterolysis
See Lysis, Adhesions, Uterus

Hysteroplasty 58540

Hysterorrhaphy 58520, 59350

Hysterosalpingography 74740
Catheterization 58345
Injection Procedure 58340

Hysterosalpingostomy
See Implantation, Tubouterine

Hysteroscopy
Ablation
Endometrial 58563
Diagnostic 58555
Lysis
Adhesions 58559
Placement
Fallopian Tube Implants 58565
Removal
Impacted Foreign Body 58562
Leiomyomata 58561
Resection
of Intrauterine Septum 58560
Surgical with Biopsy 58558
Unlisted Services and Procedures 58578-58579

Hysterosonography
See Ultrasound; Sonohysterography

Hysterotomy
See Cesarean Delivery

Abdominal 59100
with FailedAbortion 59852, 59857
with Tubal Ligation 58611

Hysterotrachelectomy
See Amputation, Cervix

I

I Antibodies, HTLV
See Antibody, HTLV-I

I, Angiotensin
See Angiotensin I

I, Coagulation Factor
See Fibrinogen

I, Heparin Co-Factor
See Antithrombin III

ICCE
See Extraction, Lens, Intracapsular

Ichthyosis, Sex Linked
See Syphilis Test

ICSH
See Luteinizing Hormone (LH)

Identification
Antibody
See Antibody Identification
Antigen
See Antigen Detection
Axial Vessel
for Island Pedicle 15740
Crystal, Light Microscopy 89060
Microbe
See Infectious Agent; Bacteria Culture; Ova; Parasites
Oocyte
from Follicular Fluid 89254
Sex Chromatin 88130, 88140
Sperm
Medicolegal 88125
from Aspiration 89257
from Tissue 89264
Urate Crystal 89060

IDH
See Isocitric Dehydrogenase, Blood

IG
See Immune Globulins

IgA 82784

IgD 82784

IgE 82785, 86003-86005

IgG 82784, 82787, 86001

IgM 82784

II, Coagulation Factor
See Prothrombin
See Gene Analysis

II, Cranial Nerve
See Optic Nerve

Index

Biological Implant
  Soft Tissue Reinforcement. 15777
Bone
  for External Speech Processor/
  Cochlear Stimulator. 69714-69718
Brain
  Chemotherapy 61517
Cardiac Event Recorder 33282
Cochlear Device. 69930
Drug Delivery Device 11981, 11983, 61517
Electrode
  Brain. 61850-61875
  Gastric 43647-43648
  Spinal Cord. 63650-63655
Electrode Array. 0282T-0283T
  Nerve 0312T, 64553-64581
Embryo 58974
Eye
  Anterior Segment. 65920
  Aqueous Shunt to Extraocular Placement or
  Replacement of Pegs 65125
  Corneal Ring Segments 0099T
  Posterior Segment
    Extraocular 67120
    Intraocular 67121
  Reservoir 66180
  Vitreous
    Drug Delivery System. 67027
Fallopian Tube 58565
Hearing Aid Hormone Pellet(s)
  Bone Conduction 69710
Hip Prosthesis
  See Arthroplasty, Hip
Hormone Pellet. 11980
Intraocular Lens
  See Insertion, Intraocular Lens
Joint
  See Arthroplasty
Left Atrial Appendage 0281T
Load
  Upper Eyelid. 67912
Mesh. 49568
  Hernia Repair. . . 43333, 43335, 43337, 49568,
                  49652-49657
  Vaginal Repair 57267
Nerve
  into Bone 64787
  into Muscle 64787
Neurostimulators
  Gastric 95980-95982
  Pulse Generator 61885
  Receiver 61886
Ovum. 58976
Pulmonary Valve Prosthesis 0262T
Pulse Generator
  Brain. 61885-61886
  Spinal Cord Electrode Array. 63685
Receiver
  Brain. 61885-61886
  Spinal Cord. 63685
Removal 20670-20680
  Ankle 27704
  Breast. 19328-19330
  Contraceptive Capsules. 11976
  Disc 22865
  Elbow 24164
  Eye 67120-67121
  Finger 26320
  Hand. 26320
  Radius 24164
  Wrist 25449
Reservoir Vascular Access Device
  Declotting. 36593

Retinal Electrode Array 0100T
Total Replacement Heart System
  Intracorporeal. 0051T
Tubouterine. 58752
Ventricular Assist Device
  See Ventricular Assist Device (VAD)

Impression, Maxillofacial
Auricular Prosthesis. 21086
Definitive Obturator Prosthesis. 21080
Facial Prosthesis 21088
Interim Obturator 21079
Mandibular Resection Prosthesis. 21081
Nasal Prosthesis 21087
Oral Surgical Splint 21085
Orbital Prosthesis. 21077
Palatal Augmentation Prosthesis 21082
Palatal Lift Prosthesis 21083
Speech Aid Prosthesis. 21084
Surgical Obturator 21076

IMT
See Intima-Media Thickness Study

In Situ Hybridization
See Nucleic Acid Probe, Cytogenetic Studies,
Morphometric Analysis

In Vitro Fertilization 58321-58322

In Vivo Laboratory Procedures
Unlisted Service. 88749

In Vivo NMR Spectroscopy
See Magnetic Resonance Spectroscopy

Incision
See Incision and Drainage
Abdomen 49000
  Exploration. 58960
Abscess
  Soft Tissue
    Subfascial. 20005
Accessory Nerve 63191
Anal
  Fistula. 46270, 46280
  Septum. 46070
  Sphincter 46080
Ankle. 27607
  Tendon 27605-27606
Anus
  See Anus, Incision
Aortic Valve
  for Stenosis 33415
Artery
  Nose. 30915-30920
Atrial Septum. 33735-33737
Bile Duct
  Sphincter 43262, 47460
Bladder
  Catheterization. 51045
  with Destruction 51020-51030
  with Radiotracer 51020
Bladder Diverticulum. 52305
Brachial Artery
  Exposure. 34834
Brain
  Amygdalohippocampectomy 61566
  Subpial. 61567
Breast
  Capsules. 19370
Burn Scab 16035-16036
Buttock 27027, 27057

Cataract
  Secondary
    Laser Surgery 66821
    Stab Incision Technique 66820
Chest
  Biopsy. 32096-32098
  with Therapeutic Wedge
  Resection 32505-32506
Colon
  Exploration. 44025
  Stoma
    Creation 44320-44322
    Revision 44340-44346
Cornea
  for Astigmatism 65772
  Laser
    for Keratoplasty 0209T-0290T
Corpus Callosum 61541
Cricothyroid Membrane. 31605
Dentate Ligament 63180-63182
Duodenum 44010
Ear, Inner
  Labyrinth
    Transcanal 69801
Elbow 24000
Esophagus 43020, 43045
  Muscle. 43030
Exploration
  Heart 33310-33315
  Kidney 50010
Eye
  Adhesions 65880
    Anterior Segment. 65860-65865
    Anterior Synechiae. 65870
    Corneovitreal 65880
    Posterior 65875
  Anterior Chamber. 65820
  Conjunctiva 0124T
  Trabeculae 65850
Eyelid
  Canthus 67715
  Margin
    for Biopsy 67810
    Sutures. 67710
Femoral Artery
  Exposure. 34812-34813
Fibula 27607
Finger
  Decompression 26035
  Tendon 26060, 26455-26460
  Tendon Sheath. 26055
Foot. 28005
  Capsule 28260-28264
  Fasciotomy 28008
  for Infection 28002-28003
  Tendon 28230, 28234
Frontal Lobe 61490
Gallbladder. 47490
Hand Decompression. 26035-26037
  Tendon 26450, 26460
Heart
  Exploration. 33310-33315
Hemorrhoids
  External 46083
Hepatic Ducts
  See Hepaticostomy
Hip
  Denervation 27035
  Exploration. 27033
  Fasciotomy. 27025
  Joint Capsule
    for Flexor Release. 27036

Incisional Hernia Repair
See Hernia Repair, Incisional

Inclusion Bodies

Incomplete Abortion
See Abortion, Incomplete

Indicator Dilution Studies

Induced Abortion
See Abortion

Induced Hyperthermia
See Thermotherapy

Induced Hypothermia
See Hypothermia

Induratio Penis Plastica
See Peyronie Disease

Indwelling Catheter
Percutaneous, lung
　See Pleural Drainage

Index

Inspiratory Positive Pressure Breathing

Instillation

Instillation, Bladder

Instrumentation

Insufflation, Eustachian Tube

Insulin

Insulin C-Peptide Measurement

Insulin-Like Growth Factors

Insurance

Integumentary System

Integumentum Commune

Intelligence Test

Intensive Care

Interbody

Injection
Chemonucleolysis Agent............62292
X-ray........................62290-62291
Removal
Artificial Disc.....0095T, 0164T, 22864-22865
by Needle.......................62287
Revision
Artificial Disc Arthroplasty.....0098T, 0165T,
22861-22862

Intestinal Anastomosis
See Anastomosis, Intestines

Intestinal Invagination
See Intussusception

Intestinal Peptide, Vasoactive
See Vasoactive Intestinal Peptide

Intestines
Alimentation.........................44015
Allotransplantation...............44135-44136
Removal.......................44137
Anastomosis............44130, 44625-44626
Camey Enterocystoplasty............50825
Closure........................44227
Koch Pouch.......................50825
with Cystectomy...................51590
with Intestinal Replacement of Ureter..50840
Laparoscopic....................44227
Biopsy.........................44100
Closure
Enterostomy..........44620, 44625-44626
Large or Small......44227, 44625-44626
Fistula.........44640, 44650, 44660
with Resection....................44661
Stoma..................44620-44625
Construction
Neobladder.....................51596
Ureter........................50840
Enteroenterostomy....................44130
Enterolysis.......................44005
Laparoscopic....................44180
Enterostomy
Closure..............44620, 44625-44626
Laparoscopic........44227, 44625-44626
Excision
Donor.....................44132-44133
Fecal Microbiota Transplantation
Preparation of Specimen............44705
Graft.......................43116, 46748
Ladd Procedure.......................44055
Laparoscopic Resection
with Anastomosis
See Small Intestine, Anastomosis
Exteriorization..................44602-44605
Lesion
Excision....................44110-44111
Lysis
Laparoscopic....................44180
of Adhesions....................44005
of Duodenal Bands................44050
Malrotation
Correction......................44055
Mobilization...........43108, 43113, 43118,
43123, 43361
Nuclear Medicine
Imaging.......................78290
Obstruction
Stricturoplasty...................44615
Plication.......................44680
Reconstruction
Bladder.......................50820
Colonic Reservoir................45119

for Obstruction...................44615
Pouch................43622, 43634
Resection...........................44661
Laparoscopic....................44227
Transplantation
Allograft Preparation.........44715-44721
Donor Enterectomy..........44132-44133
Removal of Allograft...............44137
Unlisted Services and Procedures........44799
Laparoscopic....................44238
Ureteroenterostomy...................50800
Volvulus
Reduction......................44050

Intestines, Large
See Anus; Colon; Rectum

Intestines, Small
Anastomosis..................43845, 44130
Closure.....................44227
Laparoscopic Resection..........44202-44203
Biopsy.........................44020
Endoscopy....................44361
Catheterization
Jejunum......................44015
Decompression....................44021
Destruction
Lesion......................44369
Tumor.......................44369
Endoscopy........................44364
Ablation
Lesion......................44369
Polyp.......................44369
Tumor.......................44369
Biopsy.........44361, 44377, 44382, 44386
Collection of Specimen.......44360, 44376,
44380, 44385
Control of Bleeding...........44366, 44378
via Stoma....................44382
Destruction
Lesion......................44369
Tumor.......................44369
Diagnostic..........44360, 44376, 44380
Evaluation
Pouch.......................44305
Exploration....................44360
Hemorrhage..............44366, 44378
Insertion
Stent...................44370, 44379
Tube.......................44372
Pelvic Pouch..............44385-44386
Removal
Foreign Body..................44363
Lesion....................44364-44365
Polyp....................44364-44365
Tumor....................44364-44365
Repair
Fistula.......................46707
Tube Placement.................44372
Tube Revision..................44373
via Stoma
Biopsy......................44382
Diagnostic....................44380
Stent Placement................44383
Enterostomy
Placement.....................44300
Excision.........44120-44121, 44125-44128
Partial with Anastomosis..........44140
Exclusion........................44700
Exploration......................44020
Gastrostomy Tube.................44373
Hemorrhage......................44378
Hemorrhage Control...............44366
Ileostomy..............44310-44314, 45136

Continent......................44316
Incision.........................44020
Creation
Pouch.......................44316
Stoma.........44300-44310, 44314
Decompression..................44021
Exploration....................44020
Revision
Stoma.......................44312
Stoma Closure............44620-44626
Insertion
Catheter......................44015
Duodenostomy Tube.............49441
Jejunostomy Tube.........44372, 49441
Jejunostomy......................44310
Lysis
Adhesions....................44005
Removal
Foreign Body...........44020, 44363
Repair
Diverticula.............44602-44603
Enterocele
Abdominal Approach...........57270
Vaginal Approach.............57268
Fistula.................44640-44661
Hernia.................44050
Malrotation...................44055
Obstruction....................44050
Ulcer..................44602-44603
Volvulus....................44050
Wound.................44602-44603
Revision
Jejunostomy Tube......44373, 49451-49452
Specimen Collection............43756-43757
Suture
Diverticula...............44602-44603
Fistula..................44640-44661
Plication....................44680
Ulcer...................44602-44603
Wound.................44602-44603
X-ray....................74245, 74249-74251
Guide Intubation..................74355

Intestinovesical Fistula
See Fistula, Enterovesical

Intima-Media Thickness (IMT) Study
Artery
Carotid, Common...................0126T

Intimectomy
See Endarterectomy

Intra Arterial Injections
See Injection, Intra-Arterial

Intra-Abdominal Voiding Pressure Studies
Gastric.........................51797
Intraperitoneal....................51797
Rectal........................51797

Intra-Osseous Infusion
See Infusion, Intraosseous

Intracapsular Extraction of Lens
See Extraction, Lens, Intracapsular

Intracardiac Echocardiography
See Echocardiography, Cardiac

Intracranial
Biopsy.........................61140
Extracranial......................61623
Microdissection....................69990

Index

Reimplantation Kidney 50380
Removal Transplant Renal Autograft 50370
Tumor
   Ablation
      Cryotherapy 50593
Ultrasound 76770, 76775-76776
X-ray with Contrast
   Guide Catheter 74475

Kidney Stone
See Calculus, Removal, Kidney

Killian Operation
See Sinusotomy, Frontal

Kinase, Creatine
See CPK

Kineplasty
See Cineplasty

Kinetic Therapy 97530
See Physical Medicine/Therapy/Occupational Therapy

Kininase A
See Angiotensin Converting Enzyme (ACE)

Kininogen 85293

Kininogen, High Molecular Weight
See Fitzgerald Factor

Kleihauer-Betke Test 85460

Kloramfenikol
See Chloramphenicol

Knee
See Femur; Fibula; Patella; Tibia
Abscess 27301
Arthrocentesis 20610
Arthrodesis 27580
Arthroplasty 27440-27445, 27447
   Revision 27486-27487
Arthroscopy
   Diagnostic 29870
   Surgical 20006-29008, 29871,
                 29873-29877, 29879-29889
Arthrotomy 27310, 27330-27335, 27403
Autograft, Osteochondral, Open 27416
Biopsy 27323-27324, 27330-27331
   Synovium 27330
Bone
   Drainage 27303
   Graft 29885
Bone Graft 29885
Bursa 27301
   Excision 27340
Cyst
   Excision 27345-27347
Disarticulation 27598
Dislocation 27550-27552, 27556-27558,
               27560-27562, 27566
   Open Treatment 27556-27558, 27566
Drainage 27310
Excision
   Cartilage 27332-27333
   Ganglion 27347
   Lesion 27347
   Patella 27350, 27424
   Synovium 27334-27335
Exploration 27310, 27331
Fasciotomy 27305, 27496-27499
Fracture 27520-27524, 27538, 27540
   Arthroscopic Treatment 29850-29851
Fusion 27580

Hematoma 27301
Incision
   Capsule 27435
Injection
   X-ray 27370
Magnetic Resonance Imaging
  (MRI) 73721-73723
Manipulation 27570
Meniscectomy 27332-27333
Patella
   See Patella
Reconstruction 27437-27438
   Ligament 27427-27429
   with Prosthesis 27445
Removal
   Foreign Body 27310, 27331, 27372
   Loose Body 27331
   Prosthesis 27488
Repair
   Ligament 27405-27409
      Collateral 27405
      Collateral and Cruciate 27409
      Cruciate 27407-27409
   Meniscus 27403
   Tendon 27380-27381
Replacement 27447
Retinacular
   Release 27425
Strapping 29530
Suture
   Tendon 27380-27381
Transplantation
   Chondrocytes 27412
   Meniscus 29868
   Osteochondral
      Allograft 27415, 29867
      Autograft 27412, 29866
Tumor
   Excision 27327-27328, 27337-27339
   Radical Resection 27329, 27364-27365
Unlisted Services and Procedures 27599
X-ray 73560-73564
   Arthrography 73580
   Bilateral 73505
X-ray with Contrast
   Arthrography 73580
   Injection, Contrast 27370

Knee Joint
Arthroplasty 27437-27438, 27440-27443,
                  27445-27447
   Revision 27486
Biopsy 27331
Debridement 27441
Disarticulation 27598
Drainage 27310
Exploration 27310, 27331
Excision
   Semilunar Cartilage 27332-27333
   Synovium 27334-27335
Fusion 27580
Manipulation 27570
Removal
   Foreign Body 27310, 27331
Repair
   Condyle 27446-27447
   Debridement 27441
   Dislocation
      Patella 27420, 27424-27425
   Plateau 27446-27447
   Resurfacing 27447

Synovectomy
   Partial 27443
   with Prosthesis
      See Prosthesis, Knee

Knee Prosthesis
See Prosthesis, Knee

Kneecap
Excision 27350, 27424
Repair
   Instability 27420-27424
   Arthroplasty 27437-27438
      with Prosthesis 27438

Knock-Knee Repair 27455-27457

Kocher Operation 23650-23680
See Clavicle; Scapula; Shoulder, Dislocation, Closed Treatment

Kocher Pylorectomy
See Gastrectomy, Partial

Kock Pouch 44316
Formation 50825

Kock Procedure 44316

KOH
See Hair, Nails, Tissue, Examination for Fungi

Kraske Procedure 45116

Kroenlein Procedure 67420

Krukenberg Procedure 25915

Kuhlmann Test 96101-96103

Kyphectomy
More than Two Segments 22819
Up to Two Segments 22818

Kyphoplasty 22523-22525

L

L Ascorbic Acid
See Ascorbic Acid

L Aspartate 2 Oxoglutarate Aminotransferase
See Transaminase, Glutamic Oxaloacetic

L Glutamine
See Glutamine

L-Alanine
See Aminolevulinic Acid (ALA)

L-Leucylnaphthylamidase
See Leucine Aminopeptidase

L/S Ratio
Amniotic Fluid 83661

Labial Adhesions
Lysis 56441

Labyrinth
See Ear, Inner

Labyrinthectomy 69905
with Mastoidectomy 69910
with Skull Base Surgery 61596

Labyrinthotomy
Transcanal 69801

Laceration Repair
See Specific Site

Lacrimal Duct
Balloon 68816
Canaliculi
   Repair 68700
Dilation 68816
Exploration 68810
   Canaliculi 68840
   Stent 68815
   with Anesthesia 68811
Insertion
   Stent 68815
Nasolacrimal Duct Probing 68816
Removal
   Dacryolith 68530
   Foreign Body 68530
X-ray with Contrast 70170

Lacrimal Gland
Biopsy 68510
Close Fistula 68770
Excision
   Partial 68505
   Total 68500
Fistulization 68720
Incision and Drainage 68400
Injection
   X-ray 68850
Tear Flow Diagnostic Procedure
   Microfluidic Analysis 83861
   Nuclear Medicine 78660
Removal
   Dacryolith 68530
   Foreign Body 68530
Repair
   Fistula 68770
Tumor
   Excision
      Frontal Approach 68540
      with Osteotomy 68550
X-ray 70170

Lacrimal Punctum
Closure
   by Plug 68761
   by Thermocauterization, Ligation or Laser
   Surgery 68760
Dilation 68801
Incision 68440
Repair 68705

Lacrimal Sac
Biopsy 68525
Excision 68520
Incision and Drainage 68420

Lacrimal System
Unlisted Services and Procedures 68899

Lactase Deficiency Breath Test 91065

Lactate 83605

Lactate Dehydrogenase . . . 83615-83625

Lactic Acid 83605

Lactic Cytochrome Reductase
See Lactate Dehydrogenase

Lactic Dehydrogenase
See Lactate Dehydrogenase

Lactiferous Duct
See Mammary Duct; Mammary Ductogram
Excision 19112
Exploration 19110

Lactoferrin
Fecal 83630-83631

Lactogen, Human Placental 83632

Lactogenic Hormone
See Prolactin

Lactose
Urine 83633-83634

Ladd Procedure 44055

Lagophthalmos
Correction 67912

Laki-Lorand Factor
See Fibrin Stabilizing Factor

Lamblia Intestinalis
See Giardia Lamblia

Lambrinudi Operation
See Arthrodesis, Foot Joint

Lamellar Keratoplasties
See Keratoplasty, Lamellar

Laminaria
Insertion
   for Cervical Dilation 59200
   for Abortion 59855

Laminectomy
Arthrodesis 22630, 22632-22634
for Decompression
   Cervical 0274T, 61343, 63001, 63015,
                           63045, 63048
   Lumbar 0275T, 63005, 63012, 63017,
                           63047-63048
   Sacral 63011
   Thoracic 0274T, 63003, 63016,
                           63046, 63048
for Excision
   Arteriovenous Malformation 63250-63252
   Intraspinal Lesion 63300-63308
      Neoplasm 63275-63278, 63280-63283,
                      63285-63287, 63290
      Other than Neoplasm 63265-63268,
                      63270-63273
for Implantation of Electrodes 63655
Lumbar 0202T, 22630, 63012
with Discectomy 0274T-0275T, 63020
with Exploration
   Cervical 63001, 63015, 63045, 63048
   Lumbar 63005, 63017, 63047-63048
   Thoracic 63003, 63016, 63046, 63048
   Sacral 63011
with Cordotomy 63194-63199
with Creation of Shunt 63740
with Diagnostic/Therapeutic Injection 62351
with Drainage 63172-63173
with Dural/Cerebrospinal Fluid Leak
Repair 63709
with Facetectomy 0202T, 0274T-0275T,
                      63045-63048
with Foraminotomy 0202T, 0274T-0275T,
                      63045-63048

with Ligamentous Resection 0274T-0275T,
                      63180, 63182
with Myelotomy 63170
with Nerve Resection 63191
with Rhizotomy 63185, 63190
with Spinal Cord Release 63200

Laminoplasty
Cervical 63050-63051

Langerhans Islands
See Islet Cell

Language Evaluation
Otorhinolaryngologic 92506

Language Therapy
Individual 92507
Group 92508

LAP
See Leucine Aminopeptidase

Laparoscopic Appendectomy
See Appendectomy, Laparoscopic

Laparoscopic Biopsy of Ovary
See Biopsy, Ovary, Laparoscopic

Laparoscopy
Abdomen
   Aspiration
      Cavity 49322
      Cyst 49322
   Biopsy 49321
   Collection of Specimen 49320
   Diagnostic 49320
   Drainage
      Lymphocele 49323
   Placement
      Interstitial Radiation Device 49327
   Unlisted Procedures 49329
Adrenal Gland
   Biopsy 60650
   Excision 60650
Appendix
   Appendectomy 44970
Aspiration 49322
Biopsy 47561, 49321
   Lymph Nodes 38570
Bladder
   Repair
      Sling Operation 51992
      Urethral Suspension 51990
   Unlisted 51999
   Laparoscopic 44188
Biliary Tract
   Cholangiography 47560-47561, 47563
   Cholecystectomy 47562-47564
   Cholecystenterostomy 47570
Colon
   Cecostomy 44188
   Colectomy
      Partial 44204-44208, 44213
      Total 44210-44212
Colostomy 44188
Destruction
   Lesion 58662
Ectopic Pregnancy 59150
   with Salpingectomy and/
   or Oophorectomy 59151
Esophagus
   Lengthening 43283
   Esophagogastric Fundoplasty 43280
   Esophagomyotomy Fundoplasty 43279
   Heller Type Esophagomyotomy 43279

Index

Index

Index

Direct Probe 87540
Quantification 87542

Leiomyomata
Embolization 37210
Removal 58140, 58145, 58545-58546, 58561

Leishmania
Antibody 86717

Lengthening, Tendon
See Tendon, Lengthening

Lens
Contact
　See Contact Lens Services
Extracapsular 66940
Incision 66821, 66825
Intracapsular 66920
　Dislocated 66930
Intraocular
　Exchange 66986
　Reposition 66825
Laser 66821
Prosthesis
　Insertion 66983
　　Manual or Mechanical Technique . . . 66982,
　　　　　　　　　　　　　　　　　　66984
　　Not Associated with Concurrent Cataract
　　Removal 66985
　　Ocular Telescope 0308T
　Removal
　　Crystalline 0308T
　Repositioning 66825
Removal 67108, 67113
Cataract
　See Cataract
Foreign Body 65235
Lens Material
　Aspiration Technique 66840
　Extracapsular 66940
　Intracapsular 66920-66930
　Pars Plana Approach 66852
　Phacofragmentation Technique 66850

Lens Material
Removal
　Aspiration Technique 66840
　Extracapsular 66940
　Intracapsular 66920-66930
　Pars Plana Approach 66852
　Phacofragmentation Technique 66850

Leptomeningioma
See Meningioma

Leptospira
Antibody 86720

Leriche Operation 64809
See Sympathectomy, Thoracolumbar

Lesion
See Tumor
Anal
　Destruction 46900-46917, 46924
　Excision 45108, 46922
Ankle
　Tendon Sheath
　　Excision 27630
Arm, Lower
　Tendon Sheath
　　Excision 25110
Auditory Canal, External
　Excision

Exostosis 69140
Radical with Neck Dissection 69155
Radical without Neck Dissection 69150
Soft Tissue 69145
Bladder
　Destruction 51030
　Fulguration 52224, 52234-52235, 52240
　Resection 52234-52235, 52240
　Treatment 52224
Brain
　Excision 61534, 61536, 61600-61608,
　　　　　　　　　　　　　　　　61615-61616
Brainstem
　Excision 61575-61576
Breast
　Detection
　　Mammography 77051-77052
　Excision 19120-19126
Chemotherapy 96405-96406
Choroid 67220-67221, 67225
Ciliary Body
　Destruction 66770
Colon
　Ablation 44393, 45383
　Excision 44110-44111
Conjunctiva
　Destruction 68135
　Excision 68110-68130
　　Over 1 cm 68115
　　with Adjacent Sclera 68130
Cornea
　Destruction 65450
　Excision 65400
　　of Pterygium 65420-65426
Cranium
　Radiosurgery 61796-61800
　Stereotactic Radiation Therapy 77432
Ear, Middle
　Excision 69540
Epididymis
　Excision 54830
Esophagus
　Ablation 43228
　Excision 43100-43101
　Removal 43216
Eyelid
　Destruction 67850
　Excision
　　Multiple, Different Lids 67805
　　Multiple, Same Lid 67801
　　Single 67800
　　Under Anesthesia 67808
　　without Closure 67840
Facial
　Destruction 17000-17004, 17280-17286
Finger
　Tendon Sheath
　　Excision 26160
Foot
　Excision 28080, 28090
Gums
　Destruction 41850
　Excision 41825-41828
Hand Tendon Sheath 26160
Intestines
　Excision 44110
Intestines, Small
　Ablation 44369
　Excision 44111
Iris
　Destruction 66770
Larynx
　Removal 31512, 31545-31546, 31578

Leg, Lower
　Tendon Sheath
　　Excision 27630
Mesentery
　Excision 44820
Mouth
　Destruction 40820
　Excision 40810-40816, 41116
Vestibule
　Destruction 40820
　Repair 40830
Nose
　Intranasal
　　Excision 30117, 30118
Orbit
　Excision 61333, 67412, 67420
Ovary
　Excision 58662
Palate
　Destruction 42160
　Excision 42104, 42106-42107
Pancreas
　Excision 48120
Pelvis
　Excision 58662
Penis
　Destruction
　　Cryosurgery 54056
　　Electrodesiccation 54055
　　Extensive 54065
　　Laser Surgery 54057
　　Simple 54050-54060
　　Surgical Excision 54060
　Excision 54060
　　Penile Plaque 54110-54112
Peritoneum
　Excision 58662
Pharynx
　Destruction 42808
　Excision 42808
Radiosurgery
　Cranial 61796-61800
Rectum
　Excision 45108
Renal Pelvis
　Biopsy 52354
　Fulguration 52354
Retina
　Destruction
　　Extensive 67227-67228
　　Localized 67208-67210
　Radiation by Implantation of Source 67218
Sclera
　Excision 66130
Skin
　Abrasion 15786-15787
　Biopsy 11100-11101
　Destruction
　　Benign 17110-17111, 17250
　　Malignant 17260-17286
　　Premalignant 17000-17004
　Excision
　　Benign 11400-11471
　　Malignant 11600-11646
　Injection 11900-11901
　Paring or Curettement 11055-11057
　Shaving 11300-11313
Skin Tags
　Removal 11200-11201
Skull
　Excision . . . 61500, 61600-61608, 61615-61616
Spermatic Cord
　Excision 55520

Index

Lymphadenopathy Associated Antibodies/Virus
See Antibody, HIV

Lymphangiogram
See Lymphangiography

Lymphangiography
Abdomen 75805-75807
Arm 75801-75803
Injection 38790
Leg 75801-75803
Pelvis 75805-75807

Lymphangioma, Cystic
See Hygroma; Lymph Nodes, Hygroma

Lymphangiotomy 38308

Lymphatic Channels
Incision 38308

Lymphatic Cyst
See Lymphocele

Lymphatic System
Unlisted Procedure 38999

Lymphatics
See Specific Procedure
Imaging
    Nuclear Medicine 78195

Lymphoblast Transformation
See Blastogenesis

Lymphocele
Drainage
    Laparoscopic 49323
    Open 49062

Lymphocoele
See Lymphocele

Lymphocyte
Culture 86821-86822
    Tissue 88230
Toxicity Assay 86805-86806
Transformation 86353

Lymphocyte, Thymus-Dependent
See TCells

Lymphocytes, CD4
See CD4

Lymphocytes, CD8
See CD8

Lymphocytic Choriomeningitis
Antibody 86727

Lymphocytotoxicity 86805-86806

Lymphogranuloma Venereum
Antibody 86729

Lymphoma Virus, Burkitt
See Epstein-Barr Virus

Lynch Procedure 31075

Lysergic Acid Diethylamide 80102-80103, 80299

Lysergide
See Lysergic Acid Diethylamide

Lysis
Adhesions
    Epidural 62263-62264
    Fallopian Tube 58660, 58740
    Foreskin 54450
    Intestinal 44005, 44180
    Labial 56441
    Liver 58860
    Lung 32124, 32940
    Nose 30560
    Ovary 58660, 58740
    Oviduct 58660, 58740
    Pelvic 58860
    Penile
        Post-Circumcision 54162
    Ureter 50715-50725
    Urethra 53500
    Uterus 58559
Clot
    Time 85175
Euglobulin 85360
Fibrosis
    Urethral 52285
Hemoglobin 85460-85461
Intranasal Synechia 30560

Lysozyme 85549

M

Macrodactylia
Repair 26590

Macroscopic Examination
Arthropod 87168
Parasite 87169
Tissue 88387-88388

Magnesium 83735

Magnet Operation
See Ciliary Body; Cornea; Eye, Removal, Foreign
Body; Iris; Lens; Retina; Sclera; Vitreous

Magnetic Resonance Angiography (MRA)
Abdomen 74185
Arm 73225
Chest 71555
Head 70544-70546
Leg 73725
Neck 70547-70549
Pelvis 72198
Spine 72159

Magnetic Resonance Imaging (MRI)
Diagnostic
    3-D Rendering 76376-76377
        not Requiring Independent
        Workstation 76376
        Requiring Independent Workstation . . . 76377
    Abdomen 74181-74183
    Ankle 73721-73723
    Arm 73218-73220
        Joint 73221-73223
    Bone Marrow Study 77084
    Brain 70551-70555
        Intraoperative 70557-70559

Chest 71550-71552
Elbow 73221
Face 70540-70543
Finger Joint 73221-73223
Foot 73718-73719
Foot Joints 73721-73723
Hand 73218-73220, 73223
Heart 75557-75565
Joint
    Lower Extremity 73721-73723
    Upper Extremity 73221-73223
Knee 73721-73723
Leg 73718-73720
    Joint 73721-73723
Neck 70540-70543
Orbit 70540-70543
Pelvis 72195-72197
Spectroscopy 76390
Spine
    Cervical 72141-72142, 72156
    Lumbar 72148-72149, 72158
    Thoracic 72146-72147, 72157
Temporomandibular Joint (TMJ) 70336
Toe 73721-73723
Wrist 73221
Guidance
    Arthrography, Enhanced
        Shoulder
            Injection 23350
    Brain
        Stereotactic Lesion Biopsy 61751
    Breast 77058-77059
        with Computer-aided Detection 0159T
    Needle Placement 77021
    Orthopedic Procedure
        Computer-assisted Navigation 0055T
    Parenchymal Tissue Ablation 77022
Unlisted Procedure 76498

Magnetic Resonance Spectroscopy 76390

Magnetic Stimulation
Transcranial 0310T, 90867-90869

Magnetoencephalography (MEG) 95965-95967

Magnuson Procedure 23450

MAGPI Operation 54322

MAGPI Procedure
See Hypospadias, Repair

Major Vestibular Gland
See Bartholin's Gland

Malar Area
Augmentation 21270
Bone Graft 21210
Fracture
    Open Treatment 21360-21366
    with Bone Graft 21366
    with Manipulation 21355
Reconstruction 21270

Malar Bone
See Cheek, Bone

Malaria Antibody 86750

Malaria Smear 87207

Malate Dehydrogenase 83775

Maldescent, Testis
See Testis, Undescended

Maternity Care
See Abortion; Cesarean Delivery; Ectopic
Pregnancy; Obstetrical Care

Maternity Care and
Delivery............ 59612-59622, 59898

Maxilla
See Facial Bones; Mandible
Bone Graft 21210, 21348
CT Scan....................... 70486-70488
Cyst
　Excision 21030, 21048-21049
Excision................. 21030, 21032-21034
　Cyst 21030, 21048-21049
　Torus Palatinus................... 21032
　Tumor 21030, 21034, 21048-21049
Fracture
　Closed Treatment............ 21345, 21421
　Open Treatment ...21346-21348, 21422-21423
　with Fixation 21345-21347, 21435, 21485
Osteotomy 21206
Reconstruction
　with Implant......21245-21246, 21248-21249
Tumor
　Excision 21030, 21048-21049

Maxillary Arteries
See Artery, Maxillary

Maxillary Sinus
See Sinus/Sinuses, Maxillary

Maxillary Torus Palatinus
Excision.............................21032

Maxillectomy 31225-31230
Partial 21049
with Craniofacial Procedures 61581

Maxillofacial Fixation
See Fixation (Device), Maxillofacial

Maxillofacial Impressions
Auricular Prosthesis...................21086
Facial Prosthesis 21088
Mandibular Resection Prosthesis........21081
Nasal Prosthesis 21087
Obturator Prosthesis
　Definitive 21080
　Interim 21079
　Surgical 21076
Oral Surgical Splint 21085
Orbital Prosthesis....................21077
Palatal Prosthesis
　Augmentation 21082
　Lift 21083
Speech Aid Prosthesis.................21084

Maxillofacial Procedures
Fixation
　See Fixation (Device), Maxillofacial
Reconstruction
　See Face, Reconstruction
Unlisted Services and Procedures 21299

Maxillofacial
Prosthetics 21076-21088
Impressions
　See Maxillofacial Impressions
Unlisted Services and Procedures 21089

Maydl Operation.......... 45563, 50810
See Colostomy

Mayo Hernia Repair............. 49582

Mayo Procedure................. 28292

Maze Procedure
Endoscopic................. 33265-33266
Open...................... 33254-33256

McBride Procedure 28292

McBurney Operation........... 49582

McCannel Procedure 66682

McKissock Surgery 19318

McVay Operation 49582

Measles Uncomplicated
See Rubeola

Measles Vaccine
See Vaccines

Measles, German
See Rubella

Meat Fibers
Feces................................89160

Meatoplasty
External Auditory Canal................. 69310
Urethra 53450, 53460

Meatotomy
Cystourethroscopy.....................52281
Infant...............................53025
Prostate
　Laser Coagulation 52647
　Laser Enucleation..................52649
　Laser Vaporization 52648
　with Prostatectomy 55801, 55821
　Transurethral Resection............52630
　　Electrosurgical 52601
Ureter 52290
Urethral..................... 52285, 53020
　Infant 53025

Meckel's Diverticulum
Excision.............................44800
Unlisted Services and Procedures 44899

Median Nerve
Decompression.......................64721
Neuroplasty 64721
Release............................64721
Repair/Suture
　Motor Thenar 64835
Transposition 64721

Median Nerve Compression
See Carpal Tunnel Syndrome

Mediastinal Cyst
See Cyst, Mediastinal; Mediastinum, Cyst

Mediastinoscopy 39400

Mediastinotomy
Cervical Approach 39000
Transthoracic Approach................39010

Mediastinum
See Chest; Thorax
Cyst
　Excision 32662
　Resection 39200
Endoscopy
　Biopsy.........................39400
　Exploration.....................39400

Excision
Cyst 32662
Mass 32662
Lymph Node..... 19272, 21632, 32674, 38746
Tumor 32662
Exploration 39000-39010, 60505
Incision and Drainage 39000-39010
Lymphadenectomy... 19272, 21632, 32674, 38746
Mass
　Excision 32662
Needle Biopsy 32405
Radical Dissection 60522
Removal
　Foreign Body 39000-39010
Resection
　Cyst 39200
　Tumor 39220
Thoracoscopy
　Biopsy........................ 32606
　Diagnostic 32601
　Excision
　　Cyst......................... 32662
　　Mass........................ 32662
　　Tumor 32662
Tumor
　Excision 32662
　Resection 39220
Unlisted Procedures................. 39499

Medical Disability Evaluation
Services 99455-99456

Medical Genetics 96040
Genetic Counseling 96040

Medical Team
Conference................. 99366-99368

Medical Testimony 99075

Medication Therapy Management
Pharmacist Provided 99605-99607
Psychiatric 90863

Medicine, Preventive
See Preventive Medicine

Medicine, Pulmonary
See Pulmonology

Medulla
Creation of Lesion
　Stereotactic..................... 61791
Decompression
　Craniectomy.................... 61343
Tractotomy 61470

Medullary Tract
Incision........................... 61470
Section 61470

Meibomian Cyst
See Chalazion

Membrane Oxygenation,
Extracorporeal
See Extracorporeal Membrane Oxygenation

Membrane, Mucous
See Mucosa

Membrane, Tympanic
See Ear, Drum

Meninges
Excision
　Tumor....................61512, 61519

Index

Index

Index

Index

Incision
　　Esophagus 32665, 43130, 43279,
　　　　　　　　　　　　　　　43330-43331
　　　　Hyoid 21685
　　　　Pharynx. 43030, 43130
　　　　Pylorus 43520
　　Injection 20552-20553
Masseter, Reduction
　　See Masseter Muscle/Bone
Interstitial Fluid Pressure
　　Monitoring 20950
Neck
　　See Neck Muscle
Neurectomy
　　Hamstring. 27325
Placement
　　Catheter
　　　　Interstitial Radioelement Application . 20555
Range of Motion
　　See Range of Motion Test
Redirection/Rerouting/Repositioning
　　Extraocular. 67320
　　Leg. Lower 27690-27691
　　Leg, Upper 27396-27397
　　Mouth. 40845
Release
　　Foot 28240
　　Hand. 26508, 26593
　　Hip 27036
　　Knee. 27422
Removal
　　Foreign Body 20520-20525
Repair
　　Arm, Upper. 24341
　　Blepharoptosis. 67901-67908
　　Elbow. 24341
　　Extraocular. 65290, 67311-67316,
　　　　　　　　　　　　　67334, 67340, 67346
　　Forearm 25260-25274
　　Frontalis Technique 67901-67902
　　Hand. 26591, 26593
　　Wrist 25260-25274
Revision
　　Arm, Upper. 24330-24331
Suspension
　　Hyoid 21685
Suture
　　Hamstring. 27385
　　Quadriceps. 27385
Testing
　　See Muscle Testing
Transfer
　　Arm, Upper. 24301, 24320
　　Elbow. 24301
　　Femur. 27110
　　Hand. 26494
　　Hip 27100-27105, 27111
　　Regional. 15845
　　Rotator Cuff 23410, 23412
　　Shoulder. 23395-23397, 24301,
　　　　　　　　　　　　　24320, 23410, 23412
　　Thigh 27400
Transplant
　　Anus. 46760
Unlisted Ocular Muscle Procedure 67399

Muscle Compartment Syndrome
Detection 20950

Muscle Denervation
See Denervation

Muscle Division
Plantar 28250

Scalenus Anticus 21700-21705
Sternocleidomastoid 21720-21725

Muscle Flaps. 15731-15738
Fasciocutaneous 15732, 15734, 15736, 15738
Muscle, Free. 15842
　　with Microvascular
　　Anastomosis 15756, 42894
Myocutaneous 15732, 15734, 15736,
　　　　　　　　　　　　　　　15738, 61619

Muscle Grafts
　　Free 15841, 25265, 25274

Muscle Testing
Dynamometry, Eye 92260
Electromyography
　　See Electromyography
Extraocular Multiple Muscles. 92265
Ischemic Limb. 95875
Manual 95831-95834
Range of Motion
　　See Range of Motion Test
Reflex
　　See Reflex Test

Muscle, Oculomotor
See Eye Muscles

Muscles
See Muscle

Musculo-Skeletal System
See Musculoskeletal System

Musculoplasty
See Muscle, Repair

Musculoskeletal System
Computer-Assisted Surgical
Navigation 0054T-0055T, 20985
Unlisted Services and Procedures 20999,
　　24999, 25999, 26989, 27299, 27599, 27899
Unlisted Services and Procedures, Head . . . 21499

Musculotendinous (Rotator) Cuff
Repair 23410-23412

Mustard Procedure
See Repair, Great Arteries; Revision

Myasthenia Gravis
Cholinesterase Inhibitor Challenge Test. . . . 95857

Myasthenic, Gravis
See Myasthenia Gravis

Mycobacteria
Culture 87116
　　Identification 87118
Detection 87550-87562
Sensitivity Studies. 87190

Mycoplasma
Antibody. 86738
Culture 07109
Detection 87580-87582

Mycota
See Fungus

Myectomy, Anorectal
See Myomectomy, Anorectal

Myelencephalon
See Medulla

Myelin Basic Protein

Cerebrospinal Fluid 83873

Myelography
Brain 70010
Injection Procedure 62284
Spine
　　Cervical 72240
　　Lumbosacral. 72265
　　Thoracic 72255
　　Total 72270

Myelomeningocele
Repair 63704-63706

Myeloperoxidase (MPO). 83876

Myelotomy 63170

Myocardial
Perfusion Imaging 78451-78454
　　See Nuclear Medicine
Positron Emission Tomography (PET) 78459
Resection 33542
Revascularization. 33140-33141

Myocardial Imaging
Infarct Avid. 78466-78469
Metabolic Evaluation
　　PET 78459
Perfusion Study
　　Nuclear Medicine
　　　Planar 78453-78454
　　　PET 78491-78492
　　　SPECT 78451-78452
Repair
　　Postinfarction. 33542

Myocutaneous
Flaps 15731-15738, 15756

Myofascial Pain Dysfunction Syndrome
See Temporomandibular Joint (TMJ)

Myofibroma
See Leiomyomata

Myoglobin. 83874

Myomectomy
Anorectal 45108
Uterus. 58140-58146
　　Laparoscopic 58545-58546

Myoplasty
See Muscle, Repair

Myotomy
Esophagus . . . 32665, 43130, 43279, 43330-43331
Hyoid. 21685
Pharynx. 43030, 43130
Pylorus 43520

Myringoplasty 69620

Myringostomy
See Myringotomy

Myringotomy. 69420-69421

Myxoid Cyst
See Ganglion

N

Regional 88036
Unlisted Services and Procedures 88099

Needle Biopsy
See Biopsy
Abdomen Mass 49180
Bone 20220-20225
Bone Marrow 38221
Breast 19100
Bronchi 31629, 31633
Colon
    Endoscopy 45392
Colon-Sigmoid
    Endoscopy 45342
CT Scan Guidance 77012
Epididymis 54800
Esophagus
    Endoscopy 43232
Fluoroscopic Guidance. 77002
Gastrointestinal, Upper
    Endoscopy 43238, 43242
Intervertebral Disc 62267
Kidney. 50200
Liver 47000-47001
Lung 32405
Lymph Nodes 38505
Mediastinum 32405
Muscle 20206
Nucleus Pulposus. 62267
Pancreas. 48102
Paravertebral Tissue 62267
Pleura 32400
Prostate 55700
    Transperineal 55706
Retroperitoneal Mass 49180
Salivary Gland 42400
Spinal Cord. 62269
Testis. 54500
Thyroid Gland 60100
Transbronchial 31629, 31633

Needle Localization
Breast
    Placement 19290-19291
        Mammographic Guidance 77032
        Stereotactic Guidance 77031
    with Lesion Excision 19125-19126
CT Guidance 77012
Fluoroscopic Guidance. 77002
    Spine 77003
Magnetic Resonance Guidance 77021
Ultrasonic Guidance 76942

Needle Manometer Technique 20950

Needle Wire
Introduction
    Trachea. 31730
Placement
    Breast. 19290-19291

Neer Procedure 23470

Neisseria Gonorrhoeae 87590-87592, 87850

Neisseria Meningitidis
Antibody 86741

Neobladder
Construction 51596

Neonatal Critical Care
See Newborn Care

Initial. 99468
Subsequent 99469

Neoplasm
Cancer Photoradiation Therapy
    See Photochemotherapy
Cardiac
    See Heart, Tumor
Colon
    See Colon, Tumor
Esophageal
    See Tumor, Esophagus
Spinal Cord
    See Spinal Cord, Neoplasm
Unspecified Nature of Brain
    See Brain, Tumor

Neoplastic Growth
See Tumor

Nephelometry 83883

Nephrectomy
Donor 50300-50320, 50547
Laparoscopic 50545-50548
Partial 50240
    Laparoscopic 50543
Recipient. 50340
with Ureters 50220-50236, 50546, 50548

Nephrolith
See Calculus, Removal, Kidney

Nephrolithotomy 50060-50075

Nephropexy 50400-50405

Nephroplasty
See Kidney, Repair

Nephropyeloplasty
See Pyeloplasty

Nephrorrhaphy 50500

Nephroscopy
See Endoscopy, Kidney

Nephrostogram 50394

Nephrostolithotomy
Percutaneous 50080-50081

Nephrostomy 50040, 50400
Change Tube. 50398
Endoscopic 50562-50570
Insertion
    Guide Wire. 50395, 52334
Percutaneous 52334
with Drainage. 50040
X-ray with Contrast
    Guide Dilation 74485

Nephrostomy Tract
Establishment 50395

Nephrotomogram
See Nephrotomography

Nephrotomography 74415

Nephrotomy 50040-50045
with Drainage. 50040
with Exploration 50045

Nerve
Axillary
    See Axillary Nerve
Biopsy 64795

Cranial
    See Cranial Nerve
Facial
    See Facial Nerve
Intercostal
    See Intercostal Nerve
Lingual
    See Lingual Nerve
Median
    See Median Nerve
Neuroma
    Excision
        Cutaneous. 64774
        Digital. 64776, 64778
        Foot, Other than Digital 64782, 64783
        Hand, Other than Digital 64782, 64783
        Peripheral 64784
        Sciatic. 64786
Obturator
    See Obturator Nerve
Peripheral
    See Peripheral Nerve
Phrenic
    See Phrenic Nerve
Sciatic
    See Sciatic Nerve
Spinal
    See Spinal Nerve
Tibial
    See Tibial Nerve
Ulnar
    See Ulnar Nerve
Vestibular
    See Vestibular Nerve

Nerve Conduction
Motor/Sensory Nerve 95905, 95907-95913
Preconfigured Electrode Array 0197T

Nerve Graft
Additional Nerve 64901-64902
Arm or Leg 64892-64893, 64897-64898
Foot or Hand. 64890-64891, 64895-64896
Head or Neck 64885-64886
Neurovascular Pedicle. 15750
Pedicle 64905, 64907

Nerve Root
See Cauda Equina; Spinal Cord
Decompression. 22856, 63020-63048,
                        63055-63103
Incision 63185-63190
Section 63185-63190

Nerve Stimulation, Transcutaneous
See Application, Neurostimulation

Nerve Teasing 88362

Nerve II, Cranial
See Optic Nerve

Nerve V, Cranial
See Trigeminal Nerve

Nerve VII, Cranial
See Facial Nerve

Nerve X, Cranial
See Vagus Nerve

Nerve XI, Cranial
See Accessory Nerve

Nerve XII, Cranial
See Hypoglossal Nerve

Index

Index

Oophorectomy 58262-58263,
58291-58292, 58552, 58554,
58661, 58940-58943
Ectopic Pregnancy
　　Laparoscopic Treatment. 59120
　　Surgical Treatment. 59120

Oophorectomy, Partial
See Excision, Ovary, Partial

Oophorocystectomy
See Cystectomy, Ovarian

Open Axillary Artery Approach, Transcatheter Aortic Valve Replacement
See Artery, Femoral, Approach, Transcatheter
Aortic Valve replacement

Open Biopsy, Adrenal Gland
See Adrenal Gland, Biopsy

Operating Microscope 69990

Open Femoral Artery Approach, Transcatheter Aortic Valve Replacement
See Artery, Femoral, Approach, Transcatheter
Aortic Valve replacement

Open Illiac Artery Approach
See Artery, Femoral, Approach, Transcatheter
Aortic Valve replacement

Operation/Procedure
Abbe-Estlander 00102, 40527, 40761
Akin 28298
Bankart 23455
Barker 28120, 28130
Batch-Spittler-McFadden 01404, 27598
Bischof 63170
Blalock-Hanlon 33735-33737
Blalock-Taussig 33750
Bohler 28405
Bristow 23460
Brunschwig operation 58240
Burrow's 14000-14350
Camey Enterocystoplasty 50825
Campbell 27422
Chambers 28300
Chevron 28296
Clagett 32810
Colles Fracture 25600
Conjunctivo-Tarso-Müller Resection 67908
Coombs Test 86880
Cotte Operation 58400-58410
Damus-Kaye-Stansel Procedure 33606
Dandy Operation 62180, 62200-62201
Darrach Procedure 25240
de Quervain's Disease Treatment 25000
Denver-Krupin Procedure 66180
Dunn
　　See Arthrodesis, Foot Joint
Dupuytren's Contracture 26040-26045
Duvries
　　See Tenoplasty
Dwyer-type Procedure 28300
Ebstein Anomaly Repair 33468
Estes
　　See Ovary, Transposition
Estlander Procedure 40525
Fasanella-Servat Procedure 67908
Foley Y-pyeloplasty 50400-50405
Fontan
　　See Repair, Heart, Anomaly

Fowler-Stephens Orchiopexy 54650
Fowler-Stephens Procedure 54650
Fredet-Ramstedt Procedure 43520
Frost Suture 67875
Gibbons Stent 52332
Gill Operation 63012
Glenn Procedure 33766-33767
Goeckerman Treatment 96910-96913
Goldwaite Procedure 27422
Green
　　See Scapulopexy
Halsted Operation 49491
Harii Procedure 25430
Harrington Rod Technique 00670
Hauser Procedure 27420
Haygroves Procedure 27120
Heller Operation 32665
Heller Procedure 32665, 43330-43331
Heyman Procedure 27179, 28264
Hibb Operation 22610, 22612, 22614
Hill Procedure 43324
Ilizarov Procedure, Monticelli type 20692
Jaboulay Operation
Gastroduodenostomy 43810
Jaboulay Operation 43810
Jannetta Procedure 61458
Jatene type 33770-33781
Johannsen Procedure 53400
Jones Procedure 28760
Joplin Procedure 28294, 28294
Kasai Procedure 47701
Kelikian Procedure 28280
Keller Procedure 28292
Kelly Urethral Plication 57220
Kocher Operation 23650-23680
Kocher pylorectomy 43631
Kock Pouch 44316
Kock Procedure 44316
Kraske Procedure 45116
Kroenlein Procedure 67420
Krukenberg Procedure 25915
Ladd Procedure 44055
Lapidus Procedure 28297, 28297
Leadbetter Procedure 53431
Leriche Operation 00622, 64809
Linton Procedure 37760
Lisfranc Operation 28600-28615
Lynch Procedure 31075
Magnuson Procedure 23450
Maquet Procedure 27418
Marcellation Operation 00944
Marshall-Marchetti-Krantz
Procedure 51840-51841, 58152, 58267, 58293
Maydl Operation 45563, 50810
Mayo Hernia Repair 49582
Mayo Procedure 28292
Maze Procedure 33254-33256, 33265-33266
McBride Procedure 28292
McBurney Operation 49582
McCannel Procedure 66682
McKissock Surgery 19318
McVay Operation 49582
Meckel's Diverticulum 44899
Meckel's Excision 44800
Miller Procedure 28737
Miller-Abbott Intubation 44500, 74340
Mitchell Procedure 28296, 28296
Mitrofanoff Operation 50845
Mohs Micrographic Surgery 17311-17315
Molteno Procedure 66180
Monteggia Fracture 24620-24635
Monticelli Procedure 20690
Mumford Procedure 29824

Nissen Procedure 43324
Norwood Procedure 33611-33612, 33619
Nuss Procedure 21742-21743
Ober-Yount Procedure 27025
Peans' Operation 27290-72795
Pemberton Osteotomy of Pelvis 27158
Pereyra Procedure . . . 51845, 57289, 58267, 58293
Pirogoff Procedure 27888
Polya Gastrectomy 43631-43635, 43845
Potts-Smith Procedure 33762
Puestow Procedure 48548
Putti-Platt Procedure 23450
Ramstedt
　　See Pyloromyotomy
Raskind Procedure 33735-33737
Raz Procedure 51845
Richardson Procedure 53460
Ripstein Operation 45540-45541
Ross Procedure 33413
Roux-En-Y Procedure 43621, 43633-43634,
43644, 43846, 47740-47741,
47780-47785, 48540
Sang-Park Procedure 33735-33737
Schanz
　　See Femur, Osteotomy
Schede Procedure 32905-32906
Scheie Procedure 00147, 66155
Schlatter OperationTotal
Gastrectomy 43620-43622
Schocket Procedure 66180
Scribner Cannulization 36810
Seddon-Brookes Procedure 24320
Sengstaaken Tamponade, Esophagus 43460
Senning Procedure 33774-33777
Senning Type 33774-33777
Silver Procedure 28290
Smith-Robinson Operation 22614
Soave Procedure 45120
Sofield Procedure 24410
Ssbanejew-Frank Operation 43830-43832
Stamey Procedure 51845
Steindler Stripping 28250
Stenger Test 92565, 92577
Stookey-Scarff Procedures 62200
Strassman Procedure 58540
Strayer Procedure 01474
Sturmdorf Procedure 57520
Swanson Procedure 28309
Swenson Procedure 45120
Syme Procedure 27888
Takeuchi Procedure 33505
Tenago Procedure 53431
Thal-Nissen Procedure 43325
Thiersch Operation 15050
Thiersch Procedure 46753
Thompson Procedure 27430
Tompkins metroplasty 58540
Torek Procedure 00930
Torkildsen Procedure 62180
Touroff Operation 37615
Tuffier Vaginal Hysterectomy 00944, 58260
Von Kraske Proctectomy 45111
Waldius Procedure 27445
Walsh Modified Radical 00865
Waterston Procedure 33755
Watson-Jones Procedure 27695-27698
Wertheim Operation 00846
Whipple Procedure 48150
Whitman Astragalectomy 28120, 28130
Whitman Procedure 27120
Winiwater Operation 47720- 47740
Winter Procedure 54435
Witzel Operation 43500, 43520, 43830-43832

Maxilla 21206
   Extra-Oral 21049
   Intra-Oral 21048
Metacarpal 26565
Metatarsal 28306-28309
Orbit Reconstruction 21256
Pelvis 27158
Periorbital
   Orbital Hypertelorism 21260-21263
   Osteotomy with Graft 21267-21268
Phalanges
   Finger 26567
   Toe 28299, 28310-28312
Radius
   and Ulna 25365, 25375
   Distal Third 25350
   Middle or Proximal Third 25355
   Multiple 25370
Skull Base 61582-61585, 61592
Spine
   Anterior 22220-22226
   Posterior
      Posterolateral 22210-22214
   Posterior or Posterolateral
      Three-Column 22206-22208
Talus 28302
Tarsal 28304-28305
Tibia 27455-27457, 27705, 27709-27712
Ulna 25360
   and Radius 25365, 25375
   Multiple 25370
Vertebra
   Additional Segment
      Anterior Approach 22226
      Posterior/Posterolateral Approach 22216
   Cervical
      Anterior Approach 22220
      Posterior/Posterolateral Approach 22210
   Lumbar
      Anterior Approach 22224
      Posterior/Posterolateral Approach . . . 22214
   Thoracic
      Anterior Approach 22222
      Posterior/Posterolateral Approach . . . 22212
with Graft
   Reconstruction
      Periorbital Region 21267-21268

Otolaryngology
Diagnostic
   Exam Under Anesthesia 92502

Otomy
See Incision

Otoplasty 69300

Otorhinolaryngology
Unlisted Services and Procedures 92700

Ouchterlony
Immunodiffusion 86331

Outer Ear
See Ear, Outer

Outpatient Visit
See History and Physical; Office and/or Other
Outpatient Services

Output, Cardiac
See Cardiac Output

Ova
Smear 87177

Oval Window
Repair Fistula 69666

Oval Window Fistula
See Fistula, Oval Window

Ovarian Cyst
See Cyst, Ovarian; Ovary, Cyst

Ovarian Vein Syndrome
Ureterolysis 50722

Ovariectomies
See Oophorectomy

Ovariolysis 58740

Ovary
Abscess
   Incision and Drainage 58820-58822
      Abdominal Approach 58822
Biopsy 49321, 58900
Cryopreservation 0058T
Cyst
   Excision 58925
   Incision and Drainage 58800-58805
Excision 58662, 58720
   Cyst 58925
   Partial
      Oophorectomy 58661, 58940,
                  58953-58954
      Ovarian Malignancy 58943
      Peritoneal Malignancy 58943
      Tubal Malignancy 58943
      Wedge Resection 58920
   Total 58940-58943
Laparoscopy 58660-58662, 58679
Lesion
   Excision 58662
   Fulguration 58662
Lysis
   Adhesions 58660, 58740
Malignancy
   Resection 58950-58952, 58957-58958
   Staging Laparotomy 58960
Oncology
   Biochemical Assay
      Apoliproprotein A1 81503
      Beta-2 Microglobulin 81503
      CA-125 . . . . 81500, 81503
      HE4 81500
      Menopausal Status 81500
      Pre-albumin 81503
      Transferrin 81503
Pregnancy
   Surgical Treatment 59120-59121
Radical Resection 58950-58952
Removal
   with Pelvic Exenteration 45126, 58240
   with Radical Trachelectomy 57531
   with Hysterectomy
      Abdominal 58150, 58152, 58180,
                  58200, 58210
      Laparoscopic . . . 58542, 58544, 58548, 58554,
             58552, 58571, 58573
      Vaginal 58262-58263, 58291-58292
Transposition 58825
Tumor
   Resection 58950-58958
Unlisted Services and Procedures 58679, 58999
Wedge Resection 58920

Oviduct
Anastomosis 58750
Chromotubation 58350

Ectopic Pregnancy 59120-59121
Excision 58700-58720
Fulguration
   Laparoscopic 58670
Hysterosalpingography 74740
Laparoscopy 58679
Ligation 58600-58611
Lysis
   Adhesions 58740
Occlusion 58615
   Laparoscopic 58671
Repair 58752
   Anastomosis 58750
   Create Stoma 58770
Unlisted Services and
Procedures 58679, 58999
X-ray with Contrast 74740

Ovocyte
See Oocyte

Ovulation Tests 84830

Ovum Implantation
See Implantation

Ovum Transfer Surgery
See Gamete Intrafallopian Transfer (GIFT)

Oxalate 83945

Oxidase, Ceruloplasmin
See Ceruloplasmin

Oxidoreductase, Alcohol-Nad+
See Antidiuretic Hormone

Oximetry (Noninvasive)
See Pulmonology, Diagnostic
Blood O2 Saturation Determination
   Ear or Pulse 94760-94762
   Pulse, Recording
      Car Seat/Bed Testing 94780-94781
   with Pulmonary Stress Testing 94620-94621

Oxoisomerase
See Phosphohexose Isomerase

Oxosteroids
See Ketosteroids

Oxycodinone 80102-80103, 83925

Oxygen Saturation 82805-82810

Oxygenation, Extracorporeal Membrane
See Extracorporeal Membrane Oxygenation

Oxyproline
See Hydroxyproline

Oxytocin Stress Test, Fetal 59020

P

P&P
See Proconvertin

P B Antibodies
See Antibody, Heterophile

P-Acetamidophenol
See Acetaminophen

Index

Pacemaker, Heart
See Cardiology; Defibrillator, Heart;
Electrocardiography
Conversion
    Single to Dual Chamber.............33214
Data Analysis............93288, 93293-93294
Electronic Analysis.........................93288
    Antitachycardia System................93724
Evaluation and Programming
    Dual Lead.............93280, 93286, 93288
    In Person.......93279-93281, 93286, 93288
    Multiple Lead.........93281, 93286, 93288
    Remote.............93293-93294, 93296
    Single Lead........93279, 93286, 93288
Insertion.....................33206-33208
    Electrode.......33202-33203, 33216-33217,
                    33224-33225
        Temporary................33210-33211
    Pulse Generator Only....33212-33213, 33221
Lead
    Placement..................33202-33203
Removal
    Pulse Generator Only.................33233
    Transvenous Electrodes........33234-33235
    via Thoracotomy..............33236-33237
Repair
    Electrode..................33218-33220
Replacement
    Catheter......................33210
    Electrode..................33210-33211
    Insertion...................33206-33208
    Pulse Generator.............33227-33229
Repositioning
    Electrode................33215, 33226
Revise Pocket
    Chest.......................33222
Telephonic Analysis......................93293
Upgrade.............................33214

Pachymetry
Eye.................................76514

Packing
Nasal Hemorrhage..............30901-30906

Pain Management
Electrical Reprocessing.............0278T
Epidural/Intrathecal...............62350-62351,
              62360-62362, 99601-99602
Intravenous Therapy..........96365-96368,
96374-96379

Palate
Abscess
    Incision and Drainage..............42000
Biopsy..............................42100
Bone Graft...........................42210
Excision
    Lesion.........................42120
Fracture
    Closed Treatment..................21421
    Open Treatment..............21422-21423
Lesion
    Destruction.....................42160
    Excision...................42104-42120
Prosthesis
    Augmentation....................21082
    Impression.....................42280
    Insertion......................42281
    Lift..........................21083
Reconstruction
    Lengthening................42226-42227
Repair
    Cleft Palate...............42200-42225

Laceration..................42180-42182
Vomer Flap......................42235
Unlisted Services and Procedures........42299

Palate, Cleft
See Cleft Palate

Palatoplasty.........42145, 42200-42225

Palatoschisis
See Cleft Palate

Palm
Arch
    Sympathectomy...................64823
Bursa
    Incision and Drainage........26025-26030
Dupuytren's Contracture
    Injection.......................20527
    Manipulation....................26341
Fascial Cord
    Enzyme Injection.................20527
    Manipulation....................26341
Fasciectomy................26121-26123
Fasciotomy.................26040-26045
Injection, Enzyme
    Fascial Cord....................20527
    Dupuytren's Contracture...........20527
Tendon
    Excision.......................26170
    Incision.......................26450
    Lysis....................26440, 26442
    Transfer.................26485, 26489
Tendon Sheath
    Excision.......................26145
    Incision and Drainage.............26020

Palsy, Seventh Nerve
See Facial Nerve Paralysis

Pancreas
Anastomosis
    with Intestines........48520-48540, 48548
Biopsy..............................48100
    Needle Biopsy...................48102
Cyst
    Anastomosis..........48520-48540
    Repair.........................48500
Debridement
    Peripancreatic Tissue.............48105
Endoscopy
    See Endoscopy, Pancreatic Duct
Excision
    Ampulla of Vater.................48148
    Duct...........................48148
    Partial....48140-48146, 48150, 48154, 48160
    Peripancreatic Tissue.............48105
    Total......................48155-48160
Lesion
    Ablation.......................43272
    Excision.......................48120
Needle Biopsy........................48102
Placement
    Drainage...................48000-48001
Polyp
    Ablation.......................43272
Pseudocyst
    Drainage
        Open.......................48510
        Percutaneous................48511
Removal
    Calculi (Stone)..............43264, 48020
Removal Transplanted Allograft.........48556
Repair
    Cyst...........................48500

Resection..........................48105
Suture.............................48545
Transplantation.....48160, 48550, 48554-48556
    Allograft Preparation..........48550-48552
Tumor
    Ablation.......................43272
Unlisted Services and Procedures........48999
X-ray with Contrast.............74300-74305
    Injection Procedure...............48400

Pancreas, Endocrine Only
See Islet Cell

Pancreatectomy
Donor..............................48550
Partial........48140-48146, 48150-48154, 48160
Total......................48155-48160
with Transplantation................48160

Pancreatic DNAse
See DNAse

Pancreatic Duct
Destruction
    Calculi (Stone)..................43265
Dilation
    Endoscopy......................43271
Endoscopy..........................43273
    Collection
        Specimen...................43260
    Destruction
        Calculi (Stone).............43265
        Tumor......................43272
    Dilation.......................43271
    Removal (Endoscopic)
        Calculi (Stone).............43264
        Foreign Body................43269
        Stent......................43269
    Sphincter Pressure................43263
    Sphincterotomy..................43262
    Tube Placement.............43267-43268
Incision
    Sphincter......................43262
Removal
    Calculi (Stone)..................43264
    Foreign Body....................43269
    Stent..........................43269
Tube Placement
    Nasopancreatic..................43267
    Stent..........................43268
Tumor
    Destruction.....................43272
X-ray with Contrast
    Guide Catheter..............74329-74330

Pancreatic Elastase 1 (PE1)....82656

Pancreatic Islet Cell AB
See Antibody, Islet Cell

Pancreaticojejunostomy.......48145,
             48150, 48153, 48548

Pancreatography
Injection Procedure..................48400
Intraoperative.................74300-74301
Postoperative........................74305

Pancreatorrhaphy..............48545

Pancreatotomy
See Incision, Pancreas

Pancreozymin-Secretin Test...82938

Panel
See Blood Tests; Organ or Disease-Oriented Panel

Index

Index

Index

Index

Index

Index

Index

Index

Index

Pneumoperitoneum
Injection of Air 49400

Pneumothorax
Pleurodesis. 32560
Pleural Scarification for Repeat 32215
Therapeutic
    Injection Intrapleural Air 32960

Polio
Antibody Detection 86658
Vaccine 90712-90713

Poliovirus Vaccine
See Vaccines

Pollicization
Digit 26550

Polya Gastrectomy
See Gastrectomy, Partial

Polydactylism
See Polydactyly; Supernumerary Digit

Polydactyly
Finger
    Reconstruction. 26587
    Repair. 26587
Toe 28344

Polyp
Ablation
  Endoscopic
    Anus 46615
    Colon. 44393, 45383
    Esophagus 43228
    Rectum 45320, 45339
    Small Intestine 44369
    Upper Gastrointestinal
    Tract 43258, 43272
Antrochoanal
  Removal. 31032
Anus
  Ablation
    Endoscopic 46615
  Removal
    Endoscopic 46610-46612
Colon
  Ablation 44393, 45383
  Removal 44392, 44394, 45384-45385
Esophagus
  Ablation 43228
  Removal 43216-43217
Excision
  Ear 69540
  Nose
    Endoscopic 31237-31240
    Extensive 30115
    Simple. 30110
  Urethra. 53260
  Uterus. 58558
Fulguration
  Urethra 53260
  Endoscopic
    Bladder. 52285
    Urethra 52285
Nose
  Excision
    Endoscopic 31237-31240
    Extensive 30115
    Simple. 30110
Rectum
  Ablation
    Endoscopic 45320, 45339

Removal
  Endoscopic 45308-45309, 45315, 45333
Removal
  Endoscopic
    Anus 46610-46612
    Colon. 44392, 44394, 45384-45385
    Esophagus 43216-43217
    Rectum 45308-45309, 45315, 45333
    Small Intestine 44364-44365
    Upper Gastrointestinal Tract 43250-43251
Small Intestine
  Ablation
    Endoscopic 44369
  Removal
    Endoscopic 44364-44365
Sphenoid Sinus
  Removal 31051
Urethra
  Excision 53260
  Fulguration 53260
Uterus
  Excision 58558

Polypectomy
Nose
  Endoscopic 31237-31240
  Extensive 30115
  Simple 30110
Urethra 53260
Uterus 58558

Polypeptide, Vasoactive Intestinal
See Vasoactive Intestinal Peptide

Polysomnography 95782-95783,
                   95808-95811

Pomeroy's Operation
See Tubal Ligation

Pooling
Blood Products 86965
Cardiac Blood Pool Imaging
  See Heart, Blood Pool Imaging

Popliteal Arteries
See Artery, Popliteal

Popliteal Synovial Cyst
See Baker's Cyst

Poradenitistras
See Lymphogranuloma Venereum

PORP (Partial Ossicular Replacement Prosthesis) 69633, 69637

Porphobilinogen
Urine 84106-84110

Porphyrin Precursors 82135

Porphyrins
Feces. 84126-84127
Urine 84119-84120

Port Film 77417

Portal Vein
See Vein, Hepatic Portal

Portoenterostomies, Hepatic
See Hepaticoenterostomy

Portoenterostomy 47701

Positional Nystagmus Test
See Nystagmus Tests, Positional

Positive End Expiratory Pressure
See Pressure Breathing, Positive

Positive-Pressure Breathing, Inspiratory
See Intermittent Positive Pressure Breathing (IPPB)

Positron Emission Tomography (PET)
Brain 78608-78609
Chest. 78811
Head/Neck 78811
Heart 78459
Myocardial Imaging
    Perfusion Study 78491-78492
Skull Base to Mid-thigh. 78812
Whole Body 78813
with Computed Tomography (CT) . . . 78814-78815

Post-Op Visit 99024

Postauricular Fistula
See Fistula, Postauricular

Postcaval Ureter
See Retrocaval Ureter

Postmortem
See Autopsy

Postop Vas Reconstruction
See Vasovasorrhaphy

Postoperative Wound Infection
Incision and Drainage 10180

Postpartum Care
Cesarean Delivery 59515
    after Attempted Vaginal Delivery 59622
    Previous 59610, 59614-59618, 59622
Vaginal Delivery 59430
    after Previous Cesarean Delivery 59614

Potassium 84132
Urine 84133

Potential, Auditory Evoked
See Auditory Evoked Potentials

Potential, Evoked
See Evoked Potential

Potts-Smith Procedure 33762

Pouch, Kock
See Kock Pouch

PPP
See Fibrin Degradation Products

PRA
See Cytotoxic Screen

Prealbumin 84134

Prebeta Lipoproteins
See Lipoprotein, Blood

Pregnancy
Abortion
  Induced. 59855-59857
    by Amniocentesis Injection . . 59850-59852
    by Dilation and Curettage 59840
    by Dilation and Evaluation 59841
  Septic. 59830

Index

Index

Index

Index

Index

Index

Index

Roentgen Rays
See X-ray

Roentgenographic
See X-ray

Roentgenography
See Radiology, Diagnostic

Ropes Test 83872

Rorschach Test 96101

**Ross Information Processing
Assessment** 96125

Ross Procedure 33413

Rotation Flap
See Skin, Adjacent Tissue Transfer

Rotator Cuff
Repair 23410-23420

Rotavirus
Antibody 86759
Antigen Detection
    Enzyme Immunoassay 87425

Rotavirus Vaccine
3 Dose 90680
2 Dose 90681

Round Window
Repair Fistula 69667

Round Window Fistula
See Fistula, Round Window

Roux-En-Y Procedure 43621,
    43633-43634, 43644, 43846, 47740-47741,
              47780-47785, 48540

RPR
See Syphilis Test

RSV
See Immune Globulins; Respiratory Syncytial Virus

RT3
See Triiodothyronine, Reverse

Rubbing Alcohol
See Isopropyl Alcohol

Rubella
Antibody 86762
Vaccine 90706-90710

Rubella HI Test
See Hemagglutination Inhibition Test

Rubella/Mumps
See Vaccines

Rubeola
Antibody 86765
Antigen Detection
    Immunofluorescence 87283

Rubeolla
See Rubeola

**Russell Viper Venom
Time** 85612-85613

S

Sac, Endolymphatic
See Endolymphatic Sac

Saccomanno Technique 88108

Sacral Nerve
Implantation
    Electrode Array 64561, 64581

Sacral, Pre
Arthrodesis
    See Arthrodesis, Vertebra, Lumbar

Sacroiliac Joint
Arthrodesis 27280
Arthrotomy 27050
Biopsy 27050
Dislocation
    Open Treatment 27218
Fusion 27280
Injection for Arthrography 27096
X-ray 72200-72202

Sacrum
Augmentation
    Percutaneous .... .0200T-0201T
    with CT Guidance 72292
    with Fluoroscopic Guidance 72291
Sacroplasty
    Percutaneous .... .0200T-0201T
Tumor
    Excision 49215
X-ray 72220

Sahli Test
See Gastroenterology, Diagnostic, Stomach

Salicylate
Assay 80196

Saline-Solution Abortion
See Abortion, Induced, by Saline

Salivary Duct
Catheterization 42660
Dilation 42650-42660
Diversion 42507-42510
Ligation 42665, 42510
Repair 42500-42505
    Fistula 42600

Salivary Gland Virus
See Cytomegalovirus

Salivary Glands
Abscess
    Incision and Drainage
        Parotid 42300-42305
        Sublingual 42310
        Submaxillary 42310-42320
Biopsy 42405
Calculi (Stone)
    Excision 42330-42340
Chemodenervation 64611
Cyst
    Marsupialization 42409
    Excision 42408
Duct
    See Salivary Duct
Excision
    Parotid Gland 42410, 42415, 42420,
                              42425-42426

Sublingual Gland 42450
    Submandibular Gland ... 42440, 42508-42509
Injection
    X-ray 42550
Needle Biopsy 42400
Nuclear Medicine
    Function Study 78232
    Imaging 78230-78231
Tumor
    Parotid
        Excision 42410, 42415, 42420,
                              42425-42426
Unlisted Services and Procedures 42699
X-ray 70380-70390
    with Contrast 70390

Salmonella
Antibody 86768

Salpingectomy
Complete or Partial 58700
    Laparoscopic 58661
for Ectopic Pregnancy 59120
    Laparoscopic 59151
with Vaginal Hysterectomy 58262-58263,
                              58291-58292
    Laparoscopic 58552, 58554
with Oophorectomy 58943

Salpingo-Oophorectomy 58720
Resection Ovarian Malignancy 58950-58958
Resection Peritoneal Malignancy ... 58950-58958
Resection Tubal Malignancy 58950-58958

Salpingohysterostomy
See Implantation, Tubouterine

Salpingolysis 58740
Laparoscopic 58660

Salpingoneostomy 58673, 58770

Salpingoplasty
See Fallopian Tube, Repair

Salpingostomy 58673, 58770
Laparoscopic 58673

Salter Osteotomy of the Pelvis
See Osteotomy, Pelvis

Sampling
See Biopsy; Brush Biopsy; Needle Biopsy

Sang-Park Procedure 33735-33737

Sao Paulo Typhus
See Rocky Mountain Spotted Fever

Saucerization
Calcaneus 28120
Clavicle 23180
Femur 27070, 27360
Fibula 27360, 27641
Hip 27070
Humerus 23184, 24140
Ileum 27070
Metacarpal 26230
Metatarsal 28122
Olecranon Process 24147
Phalanges
    Finger 26235-26236
    Toe 28124
Pubis 27070
Radius 24145, 25151
Scapula 23182
Symphysis Pubis 27070-27071

Index

Index

Analysis
Remote Physiologic Data............99091
Computer Data Analysis...............99090
  Electrocardiographic, Remote.........0206T
Device Handling........................99002
Emergency Care In Office...............99058
Emergency Care Out of Office............99060
Extended Hours Medical Services....99051-99053
Group Education.......................99078
  Self-Management............98961-98962
Hyperbaric Oxygen.....................99183
Individual Education
  Self-management...................98960
Medical Testimony.....................99075
Non-Office Medical Services............99056
On Call Services.................99026-99027
Phlebotomy............................99199
Post-Op Visit..........................99024
Pump Services..................99190-99192
Reports and Forms
  Medical, Extended.................99080
  Psychiatric.......................90889
Specimen Handling........99000-99001
Supply of Materials....................99070
  Educational.......................99071
Unlisted Services and Procedures........99199
Unusual Travel........................99082

Specific Gravity
Body Fluid............................84315

Specimen Collection
Aspirate
  See Aspiration
Brushings
  Abdomen........................49320
  Anus...................0226T, 46600
  Biliary Tract......................47552
  Colon.........44388, 45300, 45330, 45378
  Duodenum..........43235, 44360, 44376
  Esophagus..................43200, 43235
  Hepatobiliary System...............43260
  Ileum....................44376, 44380
  Jejunum..........................43235
  Omentum........................49320
  Peritoneum......................49320
  Rectum...................45300, 45330
  Small Intestine....................44385
  Stomach.........................43235
Radiologic Guidance..................75989
Specimen
  Capillary Blood....................36416
  Duodenum..............43756-43757
  for Dark Field Examination..........87164
  Ear.............................36416
  Hematoma.......................10140
  Sputum.........................89220
  Stomach.........................43754
  Sweat...........................89230
  Tears...........................83861
  Venous Access Device..............36591
  Venous Blood........36415, 36591-36592
  Venous Catheter...................36592
Washings
  Abdomen........................49320
  Anus...................0226T, 46600
  Biliary Tract......................47552
  Colon.........44388, 45300, 45330, 45378
  Duodenum..........43235, 44360, 44376
  Esophagus..................43200, 43235
  Hepatobiliary System...............43260
  Ileum....................44376, 44380
  Jejunum..........................43235

Omentum............................49320
Peritoneum.........................49320
Rectum.......................45300, 45330
Small Intestine......................44385
Stomach............................43235

Specimen Concentration.......87015

Specimen Handling.......99000-99001

SPECT
Bone/Joint Imaging....................78320
Brain Imaging.........................78607
Cerebrospinal Fluid Flow Imaging.........78647
Heart
  Blood Pool Imaging................78494
  Myocardial Imaging................78469
  Perfusion Imaging..........78451-78452
  Multiple..................78452, 78454
  Single...................78451, 78453
Kidney Imaging........................78710
Liver Imaging.........................78205
Localization
  Inflammatory Process..............78807
  Parathyroid Gland.................78072
  Tumor..........................78803
Parathyroid Gland..............78071-78072

Spectacle Services
Fitting
  Low Vision Aid.............92354-92355
  Spectacle Prosthesis.........92352-92353
  Spectacles.................92340-92342
Repair.......................92370-92371

Spectrometry
Mass
  Analyte
    Qualitative.....................83788
    Quantitative....................83789
  Column Chromatography
    Qualitative.....................82541
    Quantitative...............82552-82544

Spectrophotometry.............84311
Atomic Absorption
  See Atomic Absorption Spectroscopy

Spectroscopy
Atomic Absorption.....................82190
Bioimpedance Spectroscopy (BIS)........0239T
Fluorescent
  Advanced Glycation Endproducts
  (AGE)..........................0233T
Infrared.............................82365
  Intravascular....................0205T
  Lower Extremity Wound............0286T
Magnetic Resonance...................76390
  Lipoprotein.....................83704

Spectrum Analyses
See Spectrophotometry

Speech Evaluation.............92506
Cine.................................70371
for Prosthesis.........92597, 92607-92608
Video................................70371

Speech Prosthesis.......21084, 92609
Creation.............................31611
Evaluation.............92597, 92607-92608
Insertion.............................31611

Speech Therapy
Evaluation...........................92506
Group...............................92508
Individual............................92507

Sperm
Cryopreservation......................89259
  Preparation......................58323
  Storage.........................89343
  Thawing.........................89353
Evaluation.....................89329-89331

Sperm Analysis
Antibodies...........................89325
Cervical Mucus Penetration Test........89330
Evaluation from Semen
  Count............89310, 89320, 89322
  Motility........89300, 89310, 89320-89322
  Differential..............89320, 89322
  Presence..............89300, 89321
for Retrograde Ejaculation.............89331
Forensic.............................88125
Hamster Penetration Test..............89329
Huhner Test..........................89300
Identification
  Aspiration.......................89257
  from Testis Tissue................89264
Isolation......................89260-89261

Sperm Washing.................58323

Spermatic Cord
Hydrocele
  Excision........................55500
Laparoscopy
  Ligation, Vein...................55550
Lesion
  Excision........................55520
Repair
  Veins.....................55530-55540
    Abdominal Approach.............55535
    with Hernia Repair.............55540
Unlisted Procedure....................55559
Varicocele
  Excision..................55530-55540

Spermatic Veins
Excision.....................55530-55540
Ligation.............................55550

Spermatocele
Excision.............................54840

Spermatocystectomy
See Spermatocele, Excision

Sphenoid Sinus
See Sinus/Sinuses, Sphenoid

Sphenoidotomy
Excision
  with Nasal/Sinus Endoscopy....31287-31288

Sphenopalatine Ganglion
Injection
  Anesthetic.......................64505

Sphincter
See Specific Sphincter
Anal
  See Anal Sphincter
Artificial Genitourinary
  See Prosthesis, Urethral Sphincter
Common Bile Duct
  Incision........47420, 47425, 47460, 47620
Electromyography..............51784-51785
Esophageal
  Delivery, Thermal Energy............43257
  Excision.........................43262
Pyloric
  See Pyloric Sphincter

Index

Index

Index

Index

Index

Index

Index

Index

Index

Tunica Vaginalis
Hydrocele
   Aspiration 55000
   Excision 55040-55041
   Repair 55060

Turbinate
Excision 30130-30140
Fracture
   Therapeutic 30930
Injection 30200
Submucous Resection
   Nose Excision 30140

Turbinate Mucosa
Cauterization 30801-30802

Turcica, Sella
See Sella Turcica

Turnbuckle Jacket 29020-29025
Removal 29715

TURP
See Prostatectomy, Transurethral

Tylectomy
See Breast, Excision, Lesion

Tylenol
Urine 82003

Tympanic Membrane
Create Stoma 69433, 69436
   Myringoplasty 69620
   Myringotomy 69421
   Neurectomy 69676
   Repair 69610
   Tympanolysis 69450
   Tympanoplasty
     See Tympanoplasty
   Tympanostomy 69433, 69436
     Removal of Tube 69424

Tympanic Nerve
Excision 69676

Tympanolysis 69450

Tympanomastoidectomy
See Tympanoplasty

Tympanometry 92550, 92567, 92570
See Audiologic Function Tests

Tympanoplasty
See Myringoplasty
   with Ossicular Chain Reconstruction 69646
with Antrotomy or Mastoidotomy 69635
   with Ossicular Chain Reconstruction . . . 69636
   and Synthetic Prosthesis 69637
with Mastoidectomy 69641
   Radical or Complete 69645
   with Intact or Reconstructed Wall 69643
   and Ossicular Chain Reconstruction . . . 69644
   with Ossicular Chain Reconstruction . . . 69642
without Mastoidectomy 69631
   with Ossicular Chain Reconstruction . . . 69632
   and Synthetic Prosthesis 69633

Tympanostomy
Local Anesthetic 69433
General Anesthesia 69436
Removal of Tube 69424

Tympanotomy
See Myringotomy

Typhoid Vaccine 90690-90693
AKD 90693
H-P 90692
Oral 90690
Polysaccharide 90691

Typhus
Endemic
   See Murine Typhus
Mite-Borne
   See Scrub Typhus
Sao Paulo
   See Rocky Mountain Spotted Fever
Tropical
   See Scrub Typhus

Typing, Blood
See Blood Typing

Typing, HLA
See HLA Typing

Typing, Tissue
See Tissue, Typing

Tyrosine 84510

Tzank Smear 88160-88161

U

UDP Galactose Pyrophosphorylase
See Galactose-1-Phosphate, Uridyl Transferase

UFR
See Uroflowmetry

Ulcer
Anal
   See Anus, Fissure
Decubitus
   Excision
     Coccygeal 15920, 15922
     Ischial 15940-15941, 15944-15946
     Sacral 15931, 15933-15937
     Trochanteric . . . 15950-15953, 15956, 15958
     Unlisted Procedure 15999
Pinch Graft 15050
Pressure 15920-15999
Stomach
   Excision 43610

Ulcerative, Cystitis
See Cystitis, Interstitial

Ulna
See Arm, Lower; Elbow; Humerus; Radius
Arthrodesis
   Radioulnar Joint
     with Bone Graft 25830
     with Resection 25830
Arthroplasty
   with Implant 25442
Bone Graft 25830
Centralization or Wrist 25335
Craterization 24147, 25150-25151
Cyst
   Excision 24125-24126, 25120-25126
Diaphysectomy 24147, 25150-25151
Excision 24147
   Abscess 24138

Complete 25240
Epiphyseal Bar 20150
Partial 25145-25151, 25240
Fracture
   Closed Treatment 25530-25535
   Olecranon 24670-24675
   Open Treatment 24685, 25545
   Shaft 25530-25545
     Open Treatment 25574
   Styloid
     Closed Treatment 25650
     Open Treatment 25652
     Percutaneous Fixation 25651
   with Dislocation
     Closed Treatment 24620
     Open Treatment 24635
   with Manipulation 25535
   with Radius 25560-25565
     Open Treatment 25575
   without Manipulation 25530
Incision and Drainage 25035
Osteoplasty 25390-25393
Prophylactic Treatment 25491-25492
Realignment 25370, 25375
Reconstruction
   Radioulnar Joint 25337
Repair
   Collateral Ligament 29902
   Epiphyseal Arrest 25450-25455
   Malunion or Nonunion 25400, 25415,
                    25415, 25420
   Osteotomy 25360, 25370-25375
     and Radius 25365
   with Graft 25405, 25420-25426
Saucerization 24147, 25150-25151
Sequestrectomy 24138, 25145
Tumor
   Cyst 24120
   Excision . . . 24125-24126, 25120-25126, 25170

Ulnar Arteries
See Artery, Ulnar

Ulnar Nerve
Decompression 64718
Neuroplasty 64718-64719
Reconstruction 64718-64719
Release 64718-64719
Repair/Suture
   Motor 64836
Transposition 64718-64719

Ultrasonic
See Ultrasound

Ultrasonic Cardiography
See Echocardiography

Ultrasonic Procedure 52325

Ultrasonography
See Echography

Ultrasound
See Echocardiography; Echography
3-D Rendering 76376-76377
   not Requiring Independent
     Workstation 76376
     Requiring Independent Workstation 76377
Abdomen 76700-76705
Arm
   Complete 76881
   Limited 76882
Artery
   Intracranial 93886-93893

Index

Ultraviolet Light Therapy

Umbilectomy 49250

Umbilical

Umbilical Cord

Umbilicus

Undescended Testicle

Unfertilized Egg

Unguis

Unilateral Simple Mastectomy

Unlisted Services and Procedures 99499, 99600

Index

Index

Index

Index

Arterial Studies (Non-Invasive)
  Extracranial 93880-93882
  Extremities 93922-93924
  Intracranial 93886-93890
  Lower Extremity 93925-93926
  Middle Cerebral Artery, Fetal 76821
  Umbilical Artery, Fetal 76820
Artery Studies
  Upper Extremity 93930-93931
Bioimpedance Cardiovascular Analysis 93701
Blood Pressure Monitoring,
24 Hour 93784-93790
Cardiac Catheterization
  Imaging 93452-93461
Hemodialysis Access 93990
Kidney
  Multiple Study
    with Pharmacological Intervention ... 78709
  Single Study
    with Pharmacological Intervention ... 78708
Penile Vessels 93980-93981
Spectroscopy
  Catheter Based 0205T
Temperature Gradient 93740
Unlisted Services and Procedures ... 93799, 93998
Venous Studies
  Extremity 93965-93971
  Venous Pressure 93770
Visceral Studies 93975-93979

Vascular Surgery
Arm, Upper
  Anesthesia 01770-01782
Elbow
  Anesthesia 01770-01782
Endoscopy 37500
Unlisted Services and Procedures 37799

Vasectomy 55250
Laser Coagulation of Prostate 52647
Laser Vaporization 52648
Reversal
  See Vasovasorrhaphy
Transurethral
  Cystourethroscopic 52402
Transurethral Electrosurgical Resection of
Prostate 52601
Transurethral Resection of Prostate 52648

Vasoactive Drugs
Injection
  Penis 54231

Vasoactive Intestinal
Peptide 84586

Vasogram
See Vasography

Vasography 74440

Vasointestinal Peptide
See Vasoactive Intestinal Peptide

Vasopneumatic Device
Therapy 97016
See Physical Medicine/Therapy/Occupational
Therapy

Vasopressin 84588

Vasotomy 55200, 55300
Transurethral
  Cystourethroscopic 52402

Vasovasorrhaphy 55400

Vasovasostomy 55400

VATS
See Thoracoscopy

VDRL
See Syphilis Test

Vein
Ablation
  Endovenous 36475-36479
Adrenal
  Venography 75840-75842
Anastomosis
  Caval to Mesenteric 37160
  Intrahepatic Portosystemic 37182-37183
  Portocaval 37140
  Reniportal 37145
  Saphenopopliteal 34530
  Splenorenal 37180-37181
  to Vein 37140-37160, 37182-37183
Angioplasty 75978
  Transluminal 35460
Arm
  Harvest of Vein for Bypass Graft 35500
  Venography 75820-75822
Axillary
  Thrombectomy 34490
Biopsy 37200
  Transcatheter 75970
Cannulization
  to Artery 36810-36815
  to Vein 36800
Catheterization
  Central Insertion 36555-36558
  Organ Blood 36500
  Peripheral Insertion 36568-36569
  Removal 36589
  Repair 36575
  Replacement 36578-36581, 36584
  Umbilical 36510
Division
  Saphenous 37718-37722
Endoscopic Harvest
  for Bypass Graft 33508
External Cannula
  Declotting 36860-36861
Extremity
  Non-Invasive Studies 93965-93971
Femoral
  Repair 34501
Femoropopliteal
  Thrombectomy 34421-34451
Guidance
  Fluoroscopic 77001
  Ultrasound 76937
Hepatic Portal
  Splenoportography 75810
  Venography 75885-75887
Iliac
  Thrombectomy 34401-34451
Injection
  Sclerosing Agent 36468-36471
Interrupt
  Femoral 37650
  Iliac 37660
Jugular
  Venography 75860
Leg
  Harvest for Vascular Reconstruction 35572
  Venography 75820-75822
Ligation
  Clusters 37785
  Esophagus 43205

  Jugular 37565
  Perforation 37760-37761
  Saphenous 37700-37735, 37780
  Secondary 37785
Liver
  Venography 75889-75891
Neck
  Venography 75860
Nuclear Medicine
  Thrombosis Imaging 78456-78458
Orbit
  Venography 75880
Portal
  Catheterization 36481
Pulmonary
  Isolation 93656
  Repair 33730
Removal
  Clusters 37785
  Saphenous 37720, 37730-37735, 37780
  Varicose 37765-37766
Renal
  Venography 75831-75833
Repair
  Angioplasty 75978
  Graft 34520
Sampling
  Venography 75893
Sinus
  Venography 75870
Skull
  Venography 75870-75872
Spermatic
  Excision 55530-55540
  Ligation 55550
Splenic
  Splenoportography 75810
Stripping
  Saphenous 37718-37735
Subclavian
  Thrombectomy 34471-34490
Thrombectomy 37187-37188
  Other than Hemodialysis Graft or
  Fistula 35875-35876
Thrombolysis
  Transcatheter Infusion 37212-37214
Unlisted Services and Procedures 37799
Valve Transposition 34510
Varicose
  See Varicose Vein
Vena Cava
  Thrombectomy 34401-34451
  Venography 75825-75827

Velpeau Cast 29058

Vena Cava
Catheterization 36010
Filter
  Insertion 37191
  Repositioning 37192
  Retrieval 37193
Ligation 37619
Reconstruction 34502
Resection with Reconstruction 37799

Vena Caval
Thrombectomy 50230

Venereal Disease Research
Laboratory
See VDRL

Venesection
See Phlebotomy

Index

Index

XI, Coagulation Factor
See Plasma Thromboplastin, Antecedent

XI, Cranial Nerve
See Accessory Nerve

XII, Coagulation Factor
See Hageman Factor

XII, Cranial Nerve
See Hypoglossal Nerve

XIII, Coagulation Factor
See Fibrin Stabilizing Factor

Xylose Absorption Test
Blood................................. 84620
Urine................................. 84620

Y

Yacoub Procedure
See Ascending Aorta Graft

Yeast
Culture 87106

Yellow Fever Vaccine 90717

Yersinia
Antibody............................ 86793

YHrium-Aluminum-Garnet (YAG) Laser
See Eye, Incision

Z

Ziegler Procedure
Discission Secondary Membranous
Cataract 66820

Zinc 84630

Zinc Manganese Leucine Aminopeptidase
See Leucine Aminopeptidase

Zygoma
See Cheekbone

Zygomatic Arch
Fracture
    Open Treatment 21356-21366
    with Manipulation 21355
Reconstruction 21255

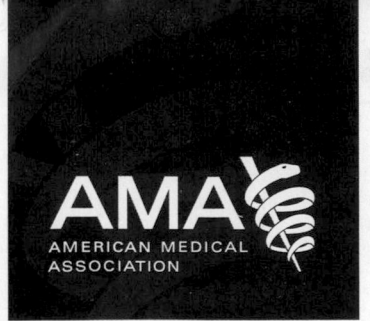

Interactive learning from the American Medical Association: Symposium and coding workshops

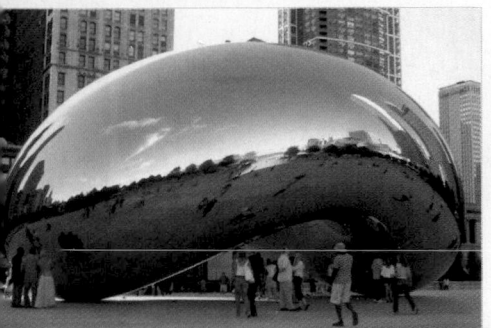

November 2012 Events

CPT® and RBRVS 2013 Annual Symposium
Nov. 14–16, 2012 • Marriott Chicago Magnificent Mile

Claim your seat at the coding industry's premier coding and reimbursement event. Meet and learn directly from the experts on CPT, the RBRVS, and Medicare. Ensure accurate and efficient claims submission in 2013.

ICD-10-CM Workshop
Nov. 13–14, 2012 • Marriott Chicago Magnificent Mile

Kick off your symposium experience with a workshop on one of the biggest changes to hit health care—the transition from ICD-9-CM to ICD-10-CM. Learn, implement, and code in a one-day ICD-10-CM workshop where subject experts will explain the details and how-to of ICD-10-CM coding.

To learn more and register, visit **ama-assn.org/go/symposia** or call **(800) 621-8335**.

December 2012 Events

CPT® Changes 2013 Workshops
A unique one-day, straight-from-the source CPT Changes Workshop educates you on the process, rationale, and application for numerous changes to the CPT code set. Expert instructors provide a hands-on, practical explanation of the changes to the 2013 code set along with some deeper insight into the subject and examples for better understanding.

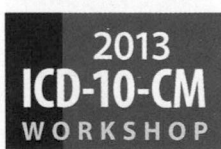

ICD-10-CM Workshops
Now is the time to increase your awareness of one of the biggest changes to hit health care—the transition from ICD-9-CM to ICD-10-CM. Learn, implement, and code in a one-day ICD-10-CM workshop where subject experts will explain the details and how-to of ICD-10-CM coding.

CPT Changes	ICD-10-CM	Location
Mon., Dec. 3	Tues., Dec. 4	Baltimore
Mon., Dec. 3	Tues., Dec. 4	New Brunswick, NJ
Wed., Dec. 5	Thurs, Dec. 6	Irving, TX
Mon., Dec. 10	Tues., Dec. 11	Las Vegas
Thurs., Dec. 13	Fri., Dec. 14	Atlanta

Sign up for both and make it a two-day learning retreat.

For more information on dates and locations and to register, visit **ama-assn.org/go/cptchangesworkshops** or **ama-assn.org/go/icd10workshops** or call **(800) 621-8335**.